KU-016-381

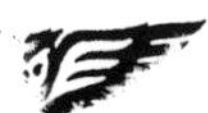

Leeds Metropolitan University
17 0062668 2

Nutritional Biochemistry and Metabolism

With Clinical Applications

SECOND EDITION

Nutritional Biochemistry and Metabolism

With Clinical Applications

SECOND EDITION

Edited by

Maria C. Linder, Ph.D.

Department of Chemistry and Biochemistry
California State University
Fullerton, California

With a Foreword by Hamish N. Munro

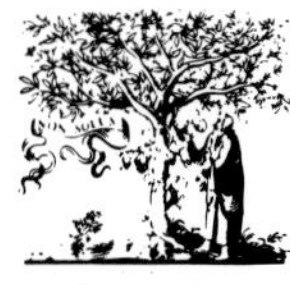

Elsevier

New York • Amsterdam • London • Tokyo

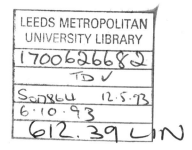

Elsevier Science Publishing Company, Inc.
655 Avenue of the Americas, New York, New York 10010

Sole distributors outside the United States and Canada:

Elsevier Science Publishers B.V.
P.O. Box 211, 1000 AE Amsterdam, The Netherlands

This book is printed on acid-free paper.

Library of Congress Cataloging in Publication Data

Nutritional biochemistry and metabolism : with clinical applications / edited by Maria C. Linder ; with a foreword by Hamish N. Munro.— 2nd ed.

p. cm.
Includes bibliographical references and index.
ISBN 0-444-01595-7 (hardcover : alk. paper)
1. Nutrition. 2. Metabolism. 3. Nutrition disorders. 4. Diet therapy. I. Linder, Maria C.
[DNLM: 1. Diet Therapy. 2. Metabolism. 3. Nutrition. 4. Nutrition Disorders. QU 145 N9763]
QP141.N86 1991
612'.3—dc20
DNLM/DLC
for Library of Congress 91-12807
CIP

Current printing (last digit):
10 9 8 7 6 5 4 3 2 1

Manufactured in the United States of America

This book is dedicated to the medical scientists—Sir Hans Krebs, Eric G. Ball, George F. Cahill Jr., Hamish N. Munro, and W. Eugene Knox among them—who have devoted themselves to arriving at an understanding of the physiology of human metabolism, and its relation to nutrition. It is also dedicated to the carbon dioxide physiologist, Karl E. Schaefer, who made the book possible, and to my father, Christoph U. Linder, who would have loved to see it.

Contents

Hamish N. Munro

Foreword

Gone are the days when instruction in nutritional science was adequately represented by a description of the chemistry of the major constituents of the diet, the diseases associated with gross insufficiency of each nutrient, and the amounts needed to prevent these deficiency diseases. Not only have florid deficiencies become rare events in Western medicine, but interest has been aroused in the much more subtle and pervasive relationships of long-term nutritional habits to chronic conditions such as atherosclerosis, hypertension, cancer, and osteoporosis, and in the role of nutrition as a therapeutic weapon in the treatment of patients postoperatively and in other clinical settings.

In order to capture the excitement of the new status of nutritional science as a component in health maintenance, a modern textbook not only should provide the basic information about nutrients, along with details of their functions in metabolism, but also must link this information to the role of nutrition in long-term health and in the prevention and treatment of disease. The present book meets this challenge with an imaginative selection of topics, some covered by Dr. Linder herself, some by other contributors. The popularity of the first edition fully justifies this revised edition.

For the second edition of this text, all chapters have undergone revision, some extensive. The first chapter, on human nutrition in context, now includes a description of biological variability and adaptation, the distribution of nutrients in plant and animal sources of our food, and contains an expanded section on factors affecting availability of nutrients. The next seven chapters, also authored by Dr. Linder, deal with individual classes of nutrients. Chapter 2, on carbohydrates, now identifies important food sources of these, and has been revised to include more details of biochemical mechanisms involved in carbohydrate metabolism in health and disease. The third chapter, on fats, includes new data on essential fatty acid metabolism and functions, as well as an extensive account of cholesterol and phospholipid metabolism and the current status of ω-3 fatty acids. The chapter on protein includes new or extensively revised sections dealing with tryptophan in sleep induction and in mental depression, special functions of glutathione in metabolism, and an account of food allergies. Chapter 5 provides an extensive account of the metabolism and functions of vitamins, with extended accounts of the role of vitamin B_6 and of vitamin B_{12}, and a new section on the functions of carotenoids independent of being precursors of vitamin A. The recently described essential nutrient pyrroloquinoline quinone also finds a place in this chapter. Chapter 6, on major minerals, deals with the role of potassium in hypertension and discusses the potentials of calcium and fluoride as well as estrogens and vitamin D in the treatment and prevention of osteoporosis. The description of the trace elements in Chapter 7 has undergone expansion to accommodate new information on most trace elements, and in particular on selenium, chromium, and the status of new elements such as boron, lithium, and aluminum.

These chapters on the metabolism and functions of individual nutrients are followed by three chapters that examine aspects of the diet not covered in the preceding descriptions. Dietary energy comes from several nutrients and is dealt with in Chapter 8, in which recent data on ideal body weight are included, as well as a new section on appetite and an extended account of diet-induced thermogenesis. Chapter 9 deals with non-nutrient constituents of the diet. It contains an updated section on food additives and food labeling and provides a new section on food irradiation. Chapter 10 describes the changes in food quality occurring from harvesting to the final stage of consumption, and includes a commentary on how quality is affected by agricultural practices, including genetic engineering.

The next four chapters are contributed by authors other than Dr. Linder and cover the nutrition of the neonate and that of the elderly, the procedures available for assessing nutritional status, and, finally, the metabolic consequences of parenteral administration of nutrients. Chapter 11 is a new presentation by Zlotkin of the nutrition of the neonate. It covers the topic of growth during the postnatal period and the need for specific nutrients, finally debating the provision of breast milk versus formula feeding. Chapter 12, by Ausman and Russell, also new, covers nutrition in relation to the elderly and begins with evidence provided by the studies on animal models of aging. Following a section on evaluation of the nutritional status of the elderly, it comments on the uses of supplements by the elderly. The remainder of this chapter is devoted to the needs of the elderly for individual nutrients and, finally, the interactions of drugs with nutrients. Chapter 13, on clinical assessment of the nutritional status of adults, by Morrow, Sahyoun, Jacob, and Russell, covers anthropometric evaluation, clinical evaluation, and biochemical evaluation, the last of these being extensively revised to reflect recent advances in this area. The inclusion of a lengthy table of appropriate tests for nutrient status will prove an attraction. Chapter 14, by Pichard and Jeejeebhoy, on metabolic consequences of total parenteral nutrition, has been updated since the last edition of this text. A new table covers strategies to be considered in parental nutrition.

The last five chapters relate to specific disease processes. In Chapter 15, Dr. Linder revises her account of nutrition and atherosclerosis, adding new or amended sections on prostaglandins, fish oils, and garlic. A new section evaluates the roles of coffee and ethanol in affecting blood cholesterol levels and the incidence of atherosclerosis. In addition, the status of fiber is also revised. The revised Chapter 16 on nutrition and cancer prevention by Dr. Linder contains many additional data. The sections on the roles of fat and fiber include much new information, and under vitamins there are expanded sections on carotenoids and on vitamin B_6 in relation to cancer. Four new tables and several new figures have been added to the text. Chapter 17, on nutrition and infection, by Beisel, has been revised to include new sections on hormonal cytokines and on host resistance factors, the latter covering the inflammatory reaction, phagocytic cell changes, and humoral and cell-mediated immunity. The text carries three new tables. Chapter 18, by Stanbury, on dietary treatment of inborn errors of metabolism, repeats the approach of illustrating this topic in a large table. Finally, Chapter 19, by Roe, on the interactions of drugs with food and nutrients, has particular relevance for the elderly. She discusses recent evidence on the effect of nutrient supplements on drug absorption. Two new tables have been added to the text.

For such a wide coverage, the text is relatively short, but is profusely illustrated by figures and tables, many of them created by Dr. Linder. In consequence, this book should continue to prove attractive to senior undergraduates, and graduate and medical students who need a survey of the current status of expertise in nutrition as it applies to health. Medical professionals will also find it an important reference. Its best recommendation will be if it attracts them to work in the field of nutrition.

Acknowledgments

I acknowledge with deep gratitude the advice and input of many colleagues, including Hamish N. Munro, George F. Cahill Jr., George Wolf, Luigi DeLuca, Hector DeLuca, Jean Pierre Flatt, Robert Rucker, Herbert Koepf, Walter Goldstein, and James Krochta, and the assistance of Joanne Wallick, Deborah Hawkins, and Carolyn Young with the preparation of the manuscript. I am also grateful for the support and encouragement of my husband, Gordon Nielson, which saw me through this often daunting task.

Contributors

Lynne M. Ausman, DSc, RD
USDA Human Nutrition Research Center on Aging
Boston, Massachusetts

William R. Beisel, MD, FAPC
Department of Immunology and Infectious Diseases
Johns Hopkins University
School of Hygiene and Public Health
Baltimore, Maryland

Robert A. Jacob, PhD
Department of Biochemistry
USDA Western Nutrition Research Center
San Francisco, California

Kursheed N. Jeejeebhoy, MBBS, PhD, FRCP(C)
Department of Medicine
University of Toronto
Toronto, Ontario, Canada

Maria C. Linder, PhD
Department of Chemistry and Biochemistry
California State University
Fullerton, California

Frank D. Morrow, PhD, FACN
USDA Human Nutrition Research Center on Aging
Boston, Massachusetts

Hamish N. Munro, MD
USDA Human Nutrition Research Center on Aging
Boston, Massachusetts

Claude Pichard, MD, PhD
Department of Medicine
University of Toronto
Toronto, Ontario, Canada

Daphne A. Roe, MD, FRCP
Division of Nutritional Sciences
Cornell University
Ithaca, New York

Robert M. Russell, MD
USDA Human Nutrition Research Center on Aging
Boston, Massachusetts

Nadine Sahyoun
USDA Human Nutrition Research Center on Aging
Boston, Massachusetts

John B. Stanbury, MD
Chestnut Hill, Massachusetts

Stanley Zlotkin, MD, PhD, FRCP(C)
Department of Pediatrics and Surgery
Division of Clinical Nutrition
Research Institute, The Hospital for Sick Children
University of Toronto
Toronto, Ontario, Canada

Maria C. Linder, Ph.D.*

1

Human Nutrition in Context

Introduction

This book describes the basic biochemical and physiologic processes through which the nourishment of the human organism is accomplished and how the interactions among nutrients, other aspects of the environment, and the body result in perturbations affecting human health. A basic knowledge of biochemistry, physiology, and biology (including molecular biology) is assumed, as is some basic medical knowledge in the clinical chapters.

The process of human nourishment proceeds within the context of an organism with an intricate structure, unique composition, and specific capacities for adaptive change. In this first chapter, basic information from many disciplines relating to body function and structure is summarized. The purpose is to set the stage for the detailed discussions that follow, which describe the nutritional biochemistry and metabolism of the body for the normal state and for states where nutrient availability is altered or disease is imposed. It is meant to serve as a background and reference, to help the reader organize details into a larger context.

* California State University, Fullerton, CA.

Growth, Structure, and Chemical Composition of the Human Organism

Growth and Structure of the Human Body

Body growth. Figure 1.1 delineates the body weight (or height) of Americans from birth to adulthood. The data plotted show the range from the 10th to the 90th percentile, by sex, for the U.S. population. (Upper and lower limits of ranges are indicated by pairs of solid or dashed lines.) If a 50th percentile line were drawn within each range, it would represent the median weight or height at each age.

The most rapid growth phase occurs in early infancy and childhood. There is also a second growth spurt at puberty, which is especially evident in the data for height and weight of male youths. There is little difference between the weight and height of boys and girls until puberty (in fact, girls may be larger than boys). At puberty, the height of the girls begins to stabilize, while that of the boys continues to grow. For both sexes, little or no change in height occurs after 17 years, but body weight continues to increase for some years thereafter, e.g., the bodies "fill out." With growth, the surface area of the body also changes. Surface area is often used in the calculation of normal parameters, such as rates of basal metabolism and glomerular filtration. A chart showing how surface area may be obtained from values for body weight and height is presented in Figure 1.2.

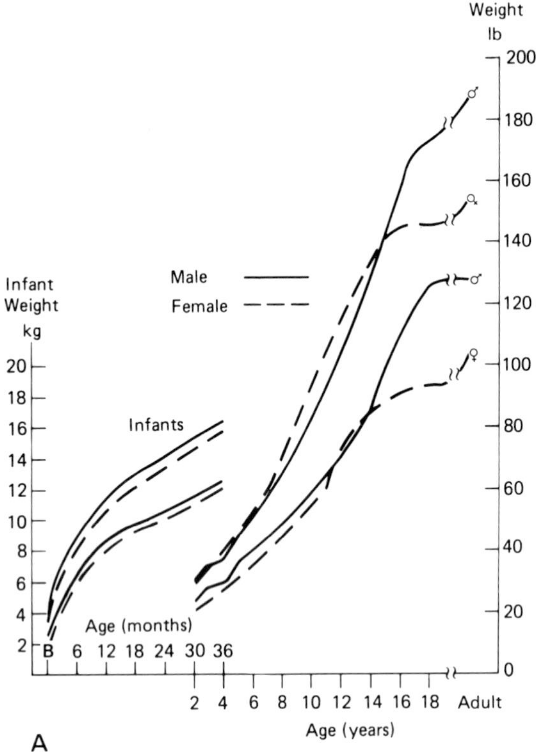

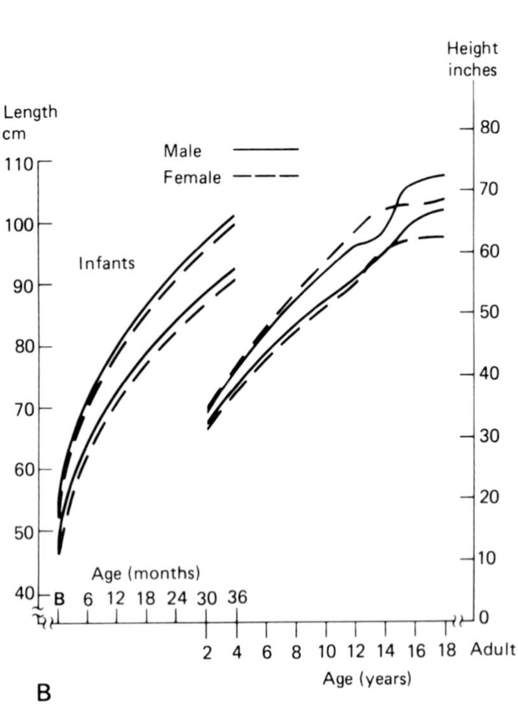

Figure 1.1. **(A)** Changes in body weight with age of U.S. infants, children, and youth. **(B)** Changes in height/length with age of U.S. infants, children, and youth. Upper and lower solid or dashed lines indicate limits of ranges from 10th–90th percentile.

Organ weights. The size of the individual organs in man is of interest when their various metabolic contributions and cooperative metabolism are considered (Table 1.1). Muscle comprises, by far, the largest single tissue. The value of 42% shown in Table 1.1 is an average that does not take into account sexual differences, as the percentage body weight of muscle in women is lower than in men. Fatty tissue is the most variable, but even in the lean person, it is quite abundant. It is followed by the skeleton and then the blood. Of the internal organs, per se, it is of interest that the brain is the largest, with the liver a close second. Kidneys and spleen represent a very small percentage of body weight, and it is noteworthy that the weight of both kidneys is considerably less than that of the heart.

Organ growth. The pattern of growth of the whole body is the same as that observed by a variety of body organs and has been termed the "general pattern" (Figure 1.3) first by Scammon

Table 1.1. Weight of Body Tissues and Organs[a]

Tissue or organ	Weight (kg)	Percent of body weight
Muscle	29.1	41.5
Fatty tissue	12.6	18
Skeleton	11.6	15.8
Blood	5.6	8.0
Skin	4.8	6.9
Brain	1.7	2.4
Liver	1.6	2.3
Stomach and intestines	1.27	1.8
Lungs	1.0	1.4
Heart	0.33	0.47
Kidneys	0.27	0.38
Spleen	0.13	0.18
Cerebrospinal fluid	0.13	0.18
Pancreas	0.10	0.14
Salivary glands	0.05	0.07
Testicles	0.03	0.04
Thyroid	0.03	0.04
Thymus	0.016	0.02
Adrenals	0.007	0.01
Parathyroids	0.0004	0.0006
Pituitary	0.0003	0.0004

Source: Data from Magnus-Levy (1910).

[a] 70-kg person.

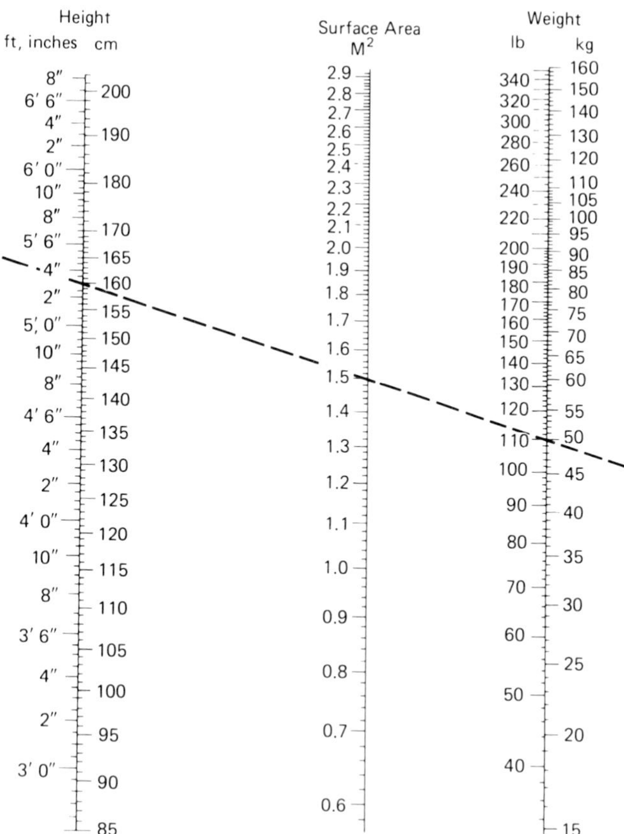

Figure 1.2. Chart for estimation of surface area from body weight and height for children, youths, and adults. When height and weight are aligned, the point at which the line intersects the center scale indicates surface area in square meters. [*Source:* Reprinted by permission from Boothby et al. (1936).]

(1930). In addition to this pattern, which is followed by the musculature, heart, liver, and many other tissues, three other patterns also exist (Figure 1.3). These are the "neural-type," where growth in volume is almost complete in early childhood; the "lymphoid pattern," where maximum volume and weight are attained prior to puberty and then decline; and the "genital-type," where the major growth spurt occurs after puberty. The pattern of brain growth is interesting in that most of it occurs prior to birth. There appear to be two spurts in brain growth: one at about 32 weeks of gestation (cellular) and the other at about 15 months of age (myelin) (Figure 1.4).

Cell growth. It should be noted that growth proceeds by two separate processes, each having different patterns of development: growth by cell proliferation (hyperplasia) and growth by cell expansion (hypertrophy). In general, and with the exception of the epithelial, blood-forming, and gonadal tissues, cell proliferation more or less ceases in midchildhood (before puberty). In the adult, there is very little evidence of cell proliferation in the major organs of the body, as evidenced by mitotic index or cell turnover studies (Table 1.2). In contrast, cells of the epithelia, glands, and blood-forming tissues do have a substantial mitotic index, and, even in the adult human (Table 1.2), some of these cells have quite a short lifespan, such as the cells of the intestinal mucosa, which are sloughed off after they migrate from the crypts to the tips of the villi. (In line with the higher basal metabolic rate and shorter lifespan of the rat, the mitotic indices are greater and cell lifespans shorter.)

Tissue regeneration and repair. Following injury, the regenerative capacity of the various human tissues and organs is related, in general, to the normal mitotic index and cell turnover. Thus, there is little or no regeneration of the central nervous system and skeletal and cardiac muscle, only a limited capacity for regeneration on the part of the kidney, and a moderate regeneration of the liver. At the same time, there is a good regen-

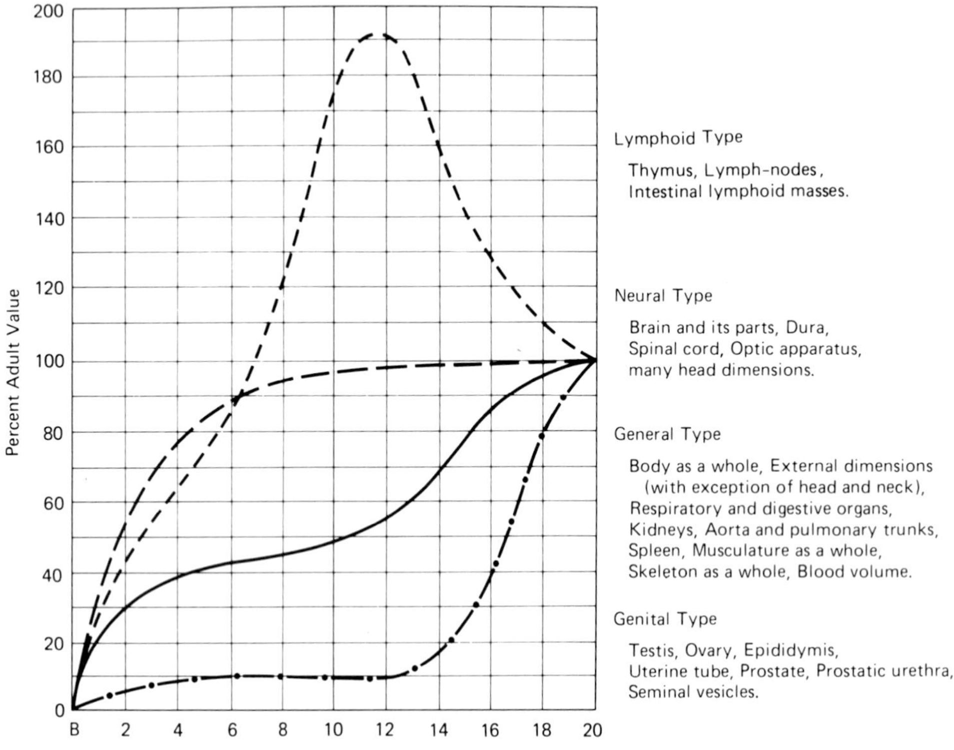

Figure 1.3. Major types of postnatal growth of various organs and parts of the body. The several curves are drawn to a common scale by computing their values at successive ages in terms of their total postnatal increments (to 20 years). [Based on Scammon (1930).]

erative capacity for the skin and various other epithelial tissues, blood-forming tissues, connective tissues, and so on.

Chemical Composition of the Body

Elemental and molecular composition. The approximate elementary composition of the human body, as a percentage of dry weight, is shown in Table 1.3. When water is excluded (as here), carbon is the most abundant element by far, followed by oxygen, hydrogen, and then nitrogen. The major minerals from calcium to magnesium follow, and starting with iron, the trace elements are listed. (Only three of the many present are shown.) If water were included in these calculations, oxygen would become the most abundant element, by far, at a ratio of about 3:1 for oxygen:carbon. Hydrogen would still be third, at about 10%.

The results of the direct elemental analysis of five whole human bodies are summarized in Table 1.4. These classic data (from the turn of the century) have since been verified by indirect methods: for example, lean body mass (and fat content) by body density, determined mainly by comparing weight to water displacement, and more recently by bioelectrical impedance analysis or total body electrical conductivity; cell mass (or potassium content) by counting ^{40}K (a constant proportion of the K in nature); extracellular water (and sodium content) by Na or Br isotope dilution; and some elements (such as N, Ca, and P) by activation analysis (Forbes, 1988). Alternatively, contents of some elements are determined on tissue aliquots and summed to approximate body content. Data in Table 1.4 have been extrapolated to 70 kg body weight. Here, water averaged 59% and fat 21% of body weight. Values vary from one individual to another; the variability in fat content in individual bodies determines the variability in water content, as one excludes the other. The concept of "lean body mass," which is the weight of the body after subtraction of the fat content, is useful in that the concentrations of various body substituents in the water-containing

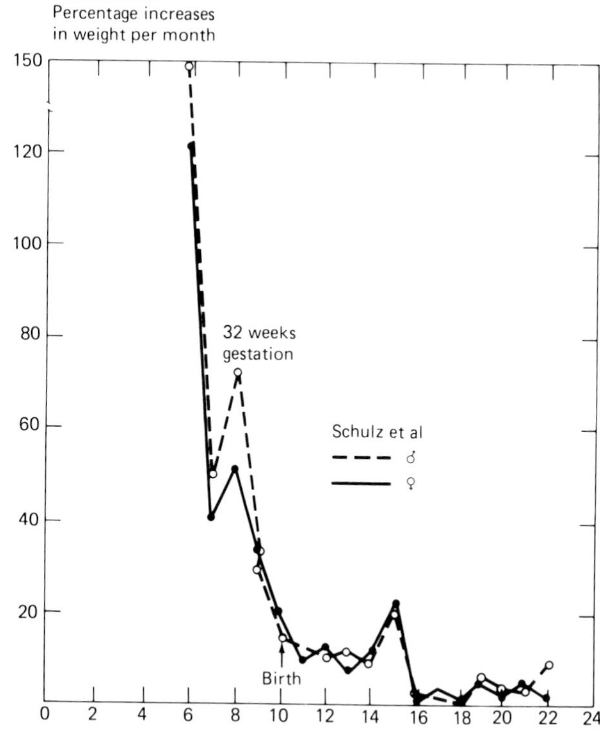

Figure 1.4. Human brain growth from conception (percent increase in weight per month). [*Source:* Reprinted by permission from the Pan American Health Organization (publication no. 251).]

Table 1.2. Tissue Cell Turnover and Regenerative Capacity in Man and Rats

	Mitotic index (divisions/1000 cells)		Cell lifespan (days)		Regenerative capacity[a]
	Rat	Man	Rat	Man	Man
Sebaceous glands	123.9	—	7.8	—	
Intestinal mucosa	13.7–92	29.2	1.35–1.57	2–8	+++
Cervix (epithelial)	—	—	5.5	5.7	
Bone marrow	11.5–22.6 (mouse)	9.0	—	120 (erythrocytes)	+++
Uterus (endometrial)	—	5.6	5.9–10.4	—	+++
Skin	5.7–52.4	0.37–0.90	19.1 (av.)	13–100	+++
Corneal epithelium	4–6.2	—	6.9	7	
Thymus	2.2	—	—	—	
Adrenal	1.2	—	—	—	+ (cortex)
Parathyroid	—	—	—	—	—
Lymph nodes	0.58–2.0	—	—	1 (lymphocytes)	
Ovary (epithelial)	—	low	32.8	—	+++
Lung (alveolar cells)	—	—	8–29	—	
(trachea-bronchioles)	—	—	47.6–200	—	
Pancreas	—	—	—	—	+
Salivary glands	0.006–0.01	0.05	—	—	(±)
Liver	0.005	—	400–450	—	+
Kidney	—	Rare	Life	Life	(±)
Brain	—	0	Life	Life	—
Heart	—	0	Life	Life	—
Muscle	—	0	Life	Life	(±)

Source: Data from FASEB Handbook, "Growth" (1962) and Cameron and Thrasher (1971).

[a] +++, good; +, some; (±), slight; −, negligible.

Table 1.3. Approximate Elementary Composition of the Body[a]

Element	Percent
Carbon	50.
Oxygen	20.
Hydrogen	10.
Nitrogen	8.5
Calcium	4.0
Phosphorus	2.5
Potassium	1.0
Sulfur	0.8
Sodium	0.4
Chlorine	0.4
Magnesium	0.1
Iron	0.01
Manganese	0.001
Iodine	0.00005

Source: Reprinted by permission from Williams (1942).

[a] Dry weight basis.

portions of the body are quite constant, as is the state of hydration of the lean body mass.

Next to carbon, hydrogen, and oxygen, nitrogen is the most abundant element, at 3.4% of lean body mass. Almost all of this is in the form of protein, much of it muscle protein. If the nitrogen content is multiplied by 6.25 (the average % N in amino acids is 1/6.25 or 16%) to obtain the body protein content, a figure of 21% is reached. A protein concentration of about 20% wet weight (or

Table 1.4. Body Composition of Hypothetical 70-kg Man[a]

Total weight	70 kg		
Water	41.3	59.0%[b]	
Fat (variable)	14.8	21.2	
Everything else	13.9		
Lean body mass[d]	55.2 kg		
Water	41.3	74.8%[c]	
Nitrogen	1877 g	3.4	
Calcium	1236	2.24	
Phosphorus	662	1.20	
Potassium	149	0.27	(69 meq/kg)
Sodium	99	0.18	(80 meq/kg)
Chlorine	99	0.18	(50 meq/kg)
Magnesium	26	0.047	
Iron	4.1	0.0074	
Zinc	1.5	0.0028	
Copper	0.094	0.00017	

Source: Reprinted by permission from Widdowson (1965).

[a] Based on data from five people.
[b] Percent of 70 kg.
[c] Percent of lean body mass.
[d] Fat-free man.

200 mg/g) is a typical figure, not only for the body as a whole, but also for most soft tissues.

Calcium and phosphorus are the next most abundant elements and are contained mostly in the skeletal structure. The potassium, sodium, and chlorine contents reflect the needs for intra- and extracellular electrolytes (see Chapter 6), which are important in the maintenance of osmotic pressure.

In addition to the minerals already mentioned, the body contains trace quantities of most elements found in nature. The concentrations of these elements in human tissues and fluids are partially known, and they include those that are essential for life, health, and procreation. The body probably also contains elements that have no essential function, based on our present knowledge, although this view may change as research continues. A list of most essential and nonessential trace elements found in the body is given in Chapter 7.

Age changes in body composition. Even though the water content of the lean body mass in adults is very constant at 75%, that of newborn infants and fetuses is somewhat greater. Indeed, there is a "drying out" of the body with age, as well as a change in the intra- and extracellular distribution of water. This is reflected in the values given in Table 1.5. The overall fat concentration of the body increases during gestation until birth, and the water content declines from birth to adulthood. If the infant is premature, there is an additional loss of water with age related to the change in fat content. Although the water content declines, the nitrogen content increases, reflecting a higher protein concentration in adult tissues as compared with that of the newborn infant or fetus. The changes from a greater to a lesser extracellular fluid volume with growth and development are reflected in the decreased sodium concentration of body tissues with age and the increase in potassium concentrations. The overall contributions of calcium, magnesium, and phosphorus, most of which are present in the bone, also increase dramatically from birth to adulthood, coinciding with the process of body "mineralization." The changes in trace elements can be explained on the basis of their function (see later chapters for specifics).

The relative changes in intracellular water, and the proportion of body water, in different organ systems from birth to adulthood are presented in a different way in Figure 1.5. While the proportion of body water in the central nervous

Table 1.5. Changes in Water and Elementary Composition of the Human Body from Gestation

	Fetus (20–25 weeks gestation)	Premature baby	Full-term baby	Adult man
Body weight (kg)	0.3	1.5	3.5	70
Fat (g/kg whole body)	5	35	160	160
Water (g/kg whole body)	880	830	690	600
Composition of lean *body mass*				
Water (g/kg)	880	850	820	720
Total N (g/kg)	15	19	23	34
Na (meq/kg)	100	100	82	80
K (meq/kg)	43	50	53	69
Cl (meq/kg)	76	—	55	44
Ca (g/kg)	4.2	7.0	9.6	22.4
Mg (g/kg)	0.18	0.24	0.26	0.50
P (g/kg)	3.0	3.8	5.6	12.0
Fe (mg/kg)	58	74	94	74
Cu (mg/kg)	3	4	5	2
Zn (mg/kg)	20	20	20	30

Source: Reprinted by permission from Widdowson (1965).

system, skin, and subcutaneous tissue declines, that of most other organs increases, especially in the muscles. Perhaps more importantly, most of the organ systems, including muscle and parenchymal tissues, increase their proportion of intracellular water, whereas the opposite is true of the skin and subcutaneous tissue.

Figure 1.5. Changes in intra- and extracellular water from birth to adulthood, in humans. ICW, intracellular H_2O; ECW, extracellular H_2O; BW, body weight. [*Source:* Redrawn from Friis-Hanson (1965).]

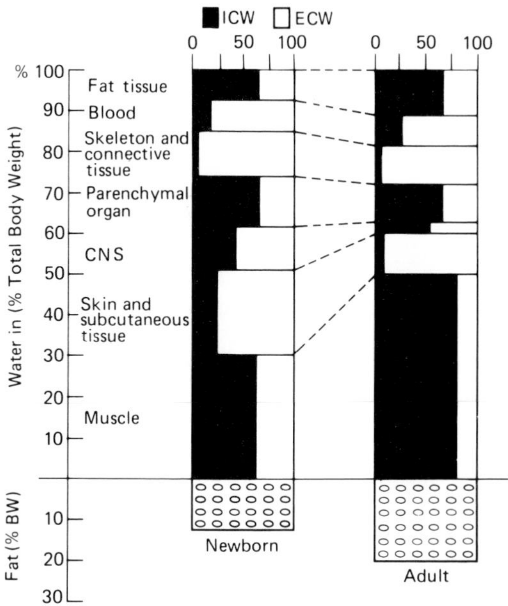

These trends continue during aging. Figure 1.6 shows that the average Western adult slowly loses lean body mass and accumulates more fat onward from early adulthood. The loss of lean body mass is more evident in men than women until after menopause, when it accelerates. This change is ascribable mainly to loss of cellular versus extracellular mass, reflected in losses of potassium and nitrogen that average 22.5% and 17.5%, respectively, from age 25 to 75 (for both sexes) (Cohn et al., 1984). Losses of skeletal calcium are also considerable (see Chapter 6).

Figure 1.6. Changes in average fat and lean body masses of men (—) and women (--) with age. [*Source:* Reprinted by permission from Forbes (1988).]

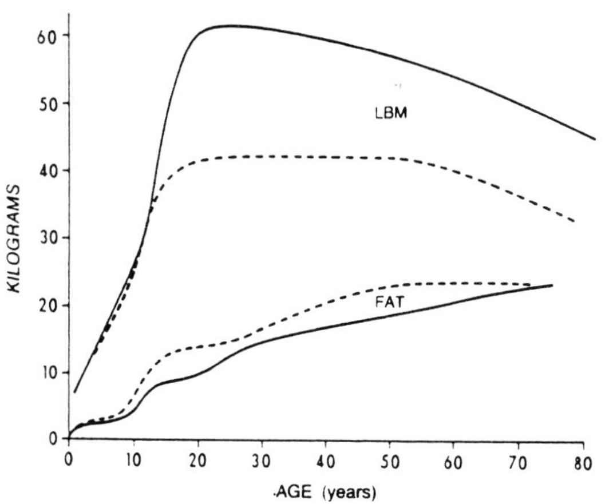

Metabolic and Adaptational Aspects of Body Function

Homeostasis Versus Chemical Individuality and Biological Variability

Biochemical and anatomical individuality and variation. Overall, there is a great deal of individual variability in the whole body and tissue content of individual chemical elements, as well as in the concentration of specific biochemical entities, from proteins, to sugars, to trace elements. Differences in chemical constitution may be ascribed to a great variety of normal and abnormal factors, including genetics, dietary habits, dietary history, immunological history, psychologic stresses (reflected in hormonal changes), disease, accidents and injuries, and so on. A classic example of individual variability is that of iron stores, which are altered by genetically determined variations in iron absorption, interactions of dietary factors, dietary abundance, sexual maturity, history of blood loss, number of pregnancies, etc. (see Chapter 7). Numerous examples of genetic variation leading to severe defects in metabolism are detailed throughout the book, notably in Chapter 18 (Dietary Treatment of the Inborn Errors of Metabolism), and include diabetes, phenylketonuria, homocystinuria, familial hypercholesterolemia, and pernicious anemia. It should also be stressed, however, that genetic makeup is an important variable underlying metabolic differences among normal individuals, and indeed that there is considerable "biological variation" among individuals within the "normal, healthy" population. As an example, numerous forms of hemoglobin have been described (with varying amino acid sequences) that are expressed by different subgroups of the normal human population. Each of these will vary to some extent in its ability to bind oxygen under a variety of different physiological conditions, but will still allow overall "normal" performance (not requiring medical intervention). The same is undoubtedly true for most enzymes in the body and for other proteins, such as those involved in nutrient transport. As molecular biological research continues, the extremes of "allowable" genetic differences for normal function will become ever clearer. For example, many variations in the genes for human apolipoproteins have already been described (Fisher et al., 1989), only some of which are known to be associated with a greatly increased risk of disease. In the case of receptors for low-density lipoproteins, many *nonallowable* mutations leading to diminished cell uptake of serum cholesterol are now being delineated (Odawara et al., 1989; Taira et al., 1989). Some of the "allowable" ones will eventually be determined also. At present, it is still hard to guess how much genetic variation will be tolerable, and whether any grand predictive generalizations will realistically be possible. [For example, there are currently at least a dozen known structural mutations in apolipoprotein A-I, but these are in only 0.1% of the population (Rall et al., 1986), whereas there are three structural alleles in apo E (Davignon et al., 1988) and at least six in apo(a) (Kraft et al., 1988) expressed differentially in human subpopulations.] Further examples of individual variation may be found in Linder (1979) and Williams (1956).

With regard to overall normal biological variability (not confined to differences in genes), the largest differences in biochemical and chemical constitution are usually intracellular. In general, the chemical changes catalyzed by enzymes and metabolic pathways occur *within* the different cells of the body. Relatively few enzymes are found extracellularly, except for traces that may leak out of cells during their normal functioning (and increasingly be lost if cells are damaged or diseased). The variations in trace levels of these enzymes among normal individuals may therefore reflect their normal intracellular differences. Examples of the normal ranges for two of these are given at the bottom of Table 1.6. Levels of intracellular enzymes in a given tissue will vary considerably depending on the metabolic state and habits of the individuals. Even greater variations may be found in storage substituents, such as liver or muscle glycogen (Chapter 2), or liver iron, due to dietary habits, sex, other environmental factors, etc.

The fact that there is so much variability in biochemical constitution, and also in the anatomic and physiologic makeup of men and women, has implications for therapy, whether it be dietary or medicinal. Specifically, it can be predicted that a given treatment for a given symptom will not have the same results in every individual. Thus, for example, iron supplementation in one case will prevent anemia, but in another, it may cause iron overload; treatment of glucose intolerance with chromium or vitamin B_6 may be useful in some individuals, but not in others (see later chapters).

Constancy of the extracellular fluid environment. The variability in biochemical and chemi-

Table 1.6. The Constancy and Variability of Plasma Substituents in Adults

Substituent	Concentration (normal range)			
	Conversion units		SI units	
Sodium	136–149	meq/L	136–149	mM
Chloride	118–132	meq/L	118–132	mM
Bicarbonate	18–23	meq/L	18–23	mM
Potassium	3.5–5.1	meq/L	3.5–5.1	mM
Protein (total)	6.4–8.3	g/dl	64–83	g/L
Albumin	3.5–5.0	g/dl	35–50	g/L
Transferrin	220–400	mg/dl	28–50	nM
Ceruloplasmin	18–45	mg/dl	1.4–3.4	nM
Glucose (fasting)	70–105	mg/dl	3.9–5.8	mM
Cholesterol (total)	150–260	mg/dl[a]	3.1–5.4	mM
Triglyceride[b]	56–298	mg/dl	0.63–3.4	mM
Calcium	8.4–10.2	mg/dl	21–2.6	mM
Glutamine	6–16	mg/dl	0.41–1.10	mM
Phenylalanine	0.8–1.8	mg/dl	0.05–0.11	mM
Iron	50–170	μg/dl	9.0–30	μM
Vitamin A	30–65	μg/dl	1.05–2.27	μM
Vitamin D (25-OH)[b]	14–42	ng/ml	35–105	nM
Alanine aminotransferase	8–20	U/L	8–20	U/L
Creatine kinase (30°)	10–105	U/L	10–105	U/L

[a] For 40-year-old men.
[b] Winter.

cal composition of individuals is largely confined to *intra*cellularly important substituents. In contrast, there is a great deal of adaptive action on the part of the body to maintain a constancy in the *extra*cellular fluid environment of cells. It is here that the term "homeostasis" most aptly applies. Homeostasis may be viewed as the result of cooperative attempts by various internal organs (especially the liver) to provide a constant nutritional, physical, and chemical milieu to the cells of the body. Thus, most major blood plasma substituents are maintained within a fairly narrow range, as illustrated by the data in the upper part of Table 1.6. The concentration of the major electrolytes, sodium and potassium, is quite rigidly controlled; concentrations of proteins, glucose, and other factors are also kept within a limited range. The maintenance of a constant level of any blood constituent requires a great deal of activity and a set of regulatory processes to deal with negative and positive trends. Very often, these involve hormones. The effect of a large amount of sucrose (or glucose) is a well known example (see Chapter 2), involving the secretions of insulin and later glucagon. Another is the effect of consuming a large amount of water (Figure 1.7). Within minutes, there is an increased production of urine to rid the body of the excess water that is beginning to dilute the extracellular fluid. After about 2 hr, sufficient additional water has been voided to return the system to its original balance. On the other hand, if isotonic saline solution is imbibed, the increase in urinary volume output occurs gradually over the ensuing hours because the osmotic balance of the extracellular fluid in the body has not been changed. Instead, another system involved on overall volume control comes

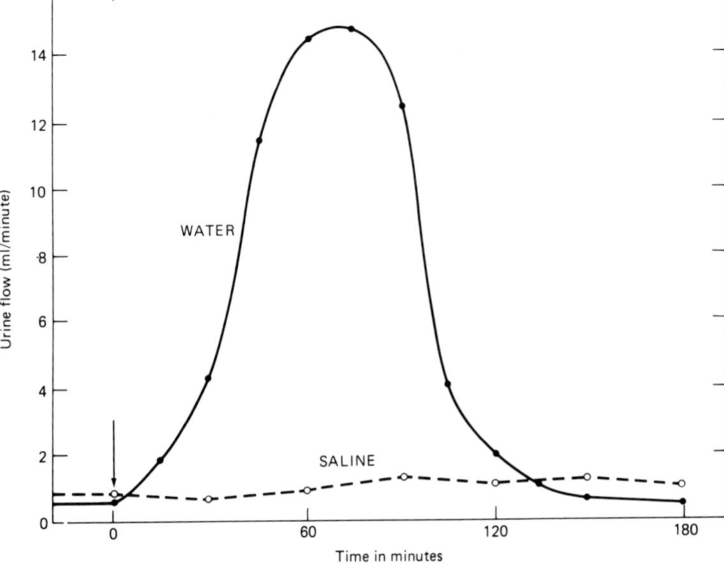

Figure 1.7. Rate of urine production as affected by intake of water or isotonic saline in humans. (Response after intake of 1 L of solution.) [*Source:* Reprinted by permission from Smith (1956).]

into play. Other examples of adaptive activities used to maintain homeostasis may be found throughout this book.

The Intracellular Localization of Metabolic Processes

Cell organelles. Mammalian (and eukaryotic) cells all contain various organelles, from nuclei and nucleoli to endoplasmic reticulum, myofibrils, mitochondria, and lysosomes (Figure 1.8A). Each organ contains more than one cell type, and each cell type is characterized by a particular abundance of one or more of these organelles (or cell parts). The characteristic architecture of a given cell type is the result of, and/or paralleled by, a characteristic set of metabolic capacities and characteristic amounts of specific substituents (from glycolysis and glycogenesis to steroid biosynthesis and urea production). The knowledgeable reader can predict many of the metabolic characteristics of a cell from its anatomy and vice versa. A summary of the localization of the major processes within various cells is given in Figure 1.8B.

Figure 1.8. **(A)** Cell structure and organelles. **(B)** Cellular location of the major metabolic pathways.

Overview of Nutrients and Nutritional Processes

Major Nutrients and Their Relation to Body Composition

Body composition and categories of nutrients. The average human body contains about 20% fat (Table 1.4), 15% protein, much smaller amounts of carbohydrate (perhaps 1%), and large amounts of water. It also contains substantial amounts of the "major minerals," from calcium and phosphorus down to sulfur and magnesium (Table 1.4), as well as trace quantities of most elements of the Periodic Table (Chapter 7). The human diet reflects this compositional need, and consists of large quantities of water-containing, proteinaceous, fatty, and carbohydrate foods, as well as others rich in the minerals. The trace elements are found in connection with these other nutrients, except where extensive processing and purification has occurred. In all, one may partition the nutrients into six categories: proteins, carbohydrates, lipids, vitamins, major minerals, and trace elements. This excludes a consideration of water and oxygen as nutrients, since no special efforts are required to produce and provide them. Individual chapters on these nutrients, their availability in foodstuffs, ingestion, absorption, distribution, storage, function, and excretion follow this chapter.

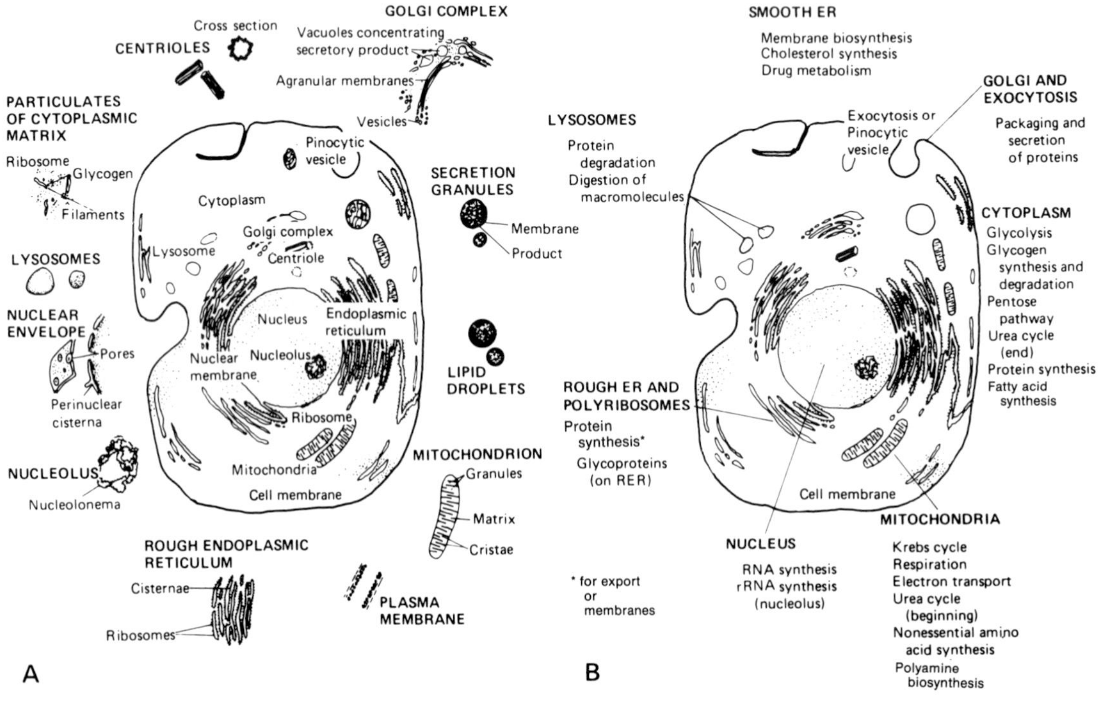

Location of "nutrients" in the body and in plant and animal foods. The general distribution of carbohydrates, fats, proteins, and other substituents within human cells and tissues, as well as in the plant and animal foods that are consumed, is summarized in Figure 1.9. In meats, fish, poultry, shellfish, etc., there is the same relative distribution as in human cells and tissues, but there are major differences in the plant. In general, lipids are found in two places, in lipid droplets (mostly triacylglycerol/triglyceride) or in cell membranes. Phospholipids (and sphingolipids) are used to form the membranes within and at the outside of cells. In humans and animals, the membranes also contain cholesterol (which is not the case for plants). Most of the phospholipid, sphingolipid, and/or cholesterol found in food or in the animal (or human) body is thus within cell membranes, an "exaggerated" form of which is the multilayered myelin sheath of the neurons of the central nervous system. Most of the triacylglycerol is in the form of lipid droplets, usually in specialized,

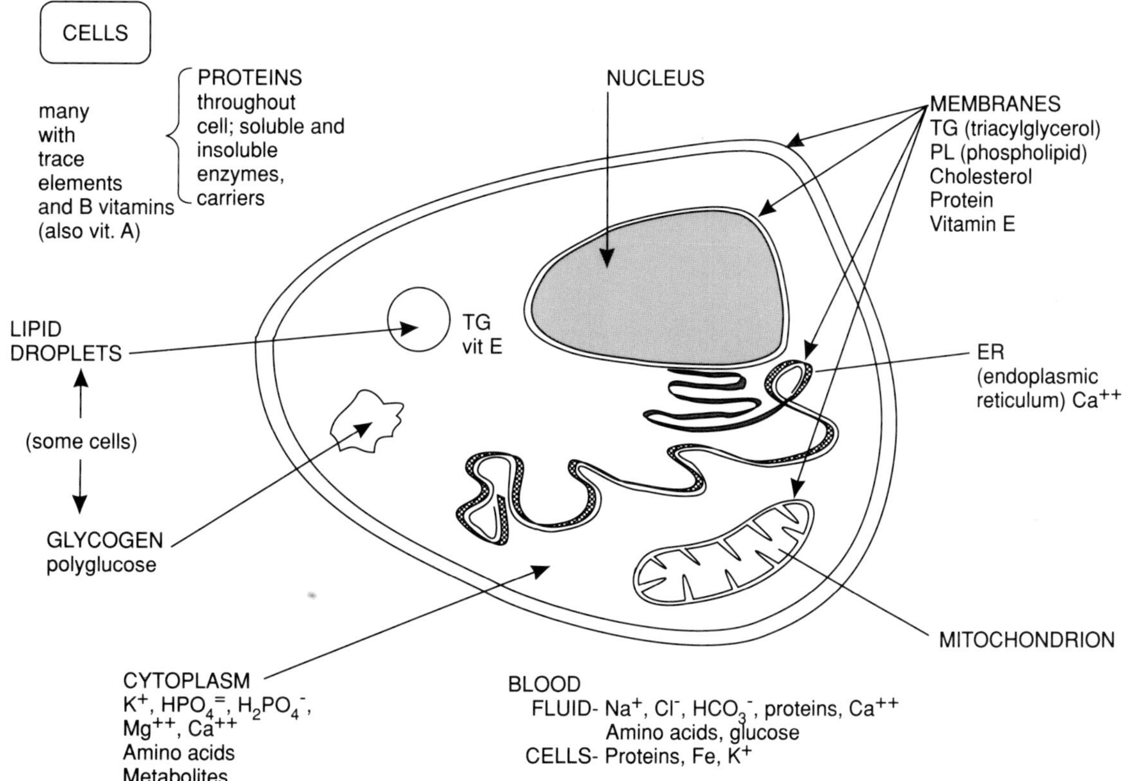

MEATS- MUSCLE rich in protein, fat, iron, Na^+, K^+, phosphate
LIVER rich in protein, iron, (fat) vitamins A, D, B12 folate, Na^+, K^+ etc.
FAT TISSUE rich in fat (triglyceride) (vit. E) (carotenes)
EGGS- rich in protein, vitamins, some trace elements, triglyceride, cholesterol
MILK- rich in protein, lactose, Ca^{++}, triglyceride

Figure 1.9. Locations of "nutrients" in cells and tissues of the human body **(A)** and of animal foods **(A)** and plant foods **(B)**.

B WHERE THE NUTRIENTS ARE IN PLANTS

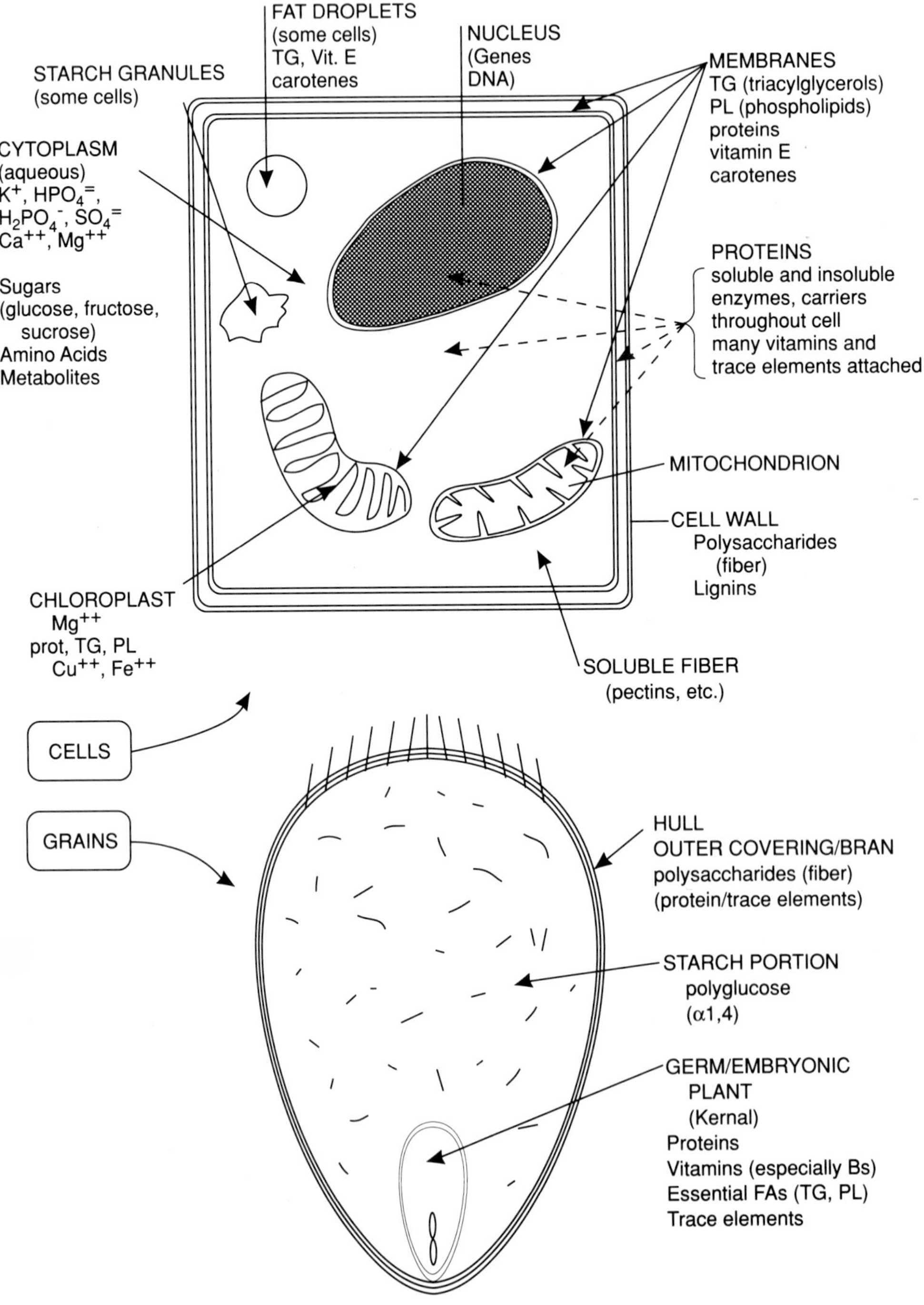
FAT DROPLETS
(some cells)
TG, Vit. E
carotenes
NUCLEUS
(Genes
DNA)
STARCH GRANULES
(some cells)
MEMBRANES
TG (triacylglycerols)
PL (phospholipids)
proteins
vitamin E
carotenes
CYTOPLASM
(aqueous)
K^+, $HPO_4^=$,
$H_2PO_4^-$, $SO_4^=$
Ca^{++}, Mg^{++}
Sugars
(glucose, fructose,
sucrose)
Amino Acids
Metabolites
PROTEINS
soluble and insoluble
enzymes, carriers
throughout cell
many vitamins and
trace elements attached
MITOCHONDRION
CELL WALL
Polysaccharides
(fiber)
Lignins
CHLOROPLAST
Mg^{++}
prot, TG, PL
Cu^{++}, Fe^{++}
SOLUBLE FIBER
(pectins, etc.)
CELLS
GRAINS
HULL
OUTER COVERING/BRAN
polysaccharides (fiber)
(protein/trace elements)
STARCH PORTION
polyglucose
(α1,4)
GERM/EMBRYONIC
PLANT
(Kernal)
Proteins
Vitamins (especially Bs)
Essential FAs (TG, PL)
Trace elements

fat storage cells (adipocytes). With regard to carbohydrates, animal foods (and the human body) have relatively little polysaccharide, whereas many plant foods are rich in starch and soluble "fiber," and plant cells also have a cell wall comprised mainly of nondigestible polysaccharide (also part of food "fiber"), not found in animals or humans. In plants, as well as humans and animals, proteins are found in all parts of the cell and in the extracellular fluids. Most vitamins and trace elements are associated with proteins, in all parts of cells. The plant has an additional intracellular organelle, the chloroplast, not found in humans or animal, that is rich in phospholipid, protein, and some minerals and trace elements (notably magnesium). Further details on these matters are presented in the chapters that follow.

Overview of Nutritional Processes, Their Localization, and Regulation

The gastrointestinal tract. The gastrointestinal (GI) tract is bordered by a layer of epithelial cells (with glands) sitting on a lamina propria (or basement membrane), comprising the mucosa and adjacent to the submucosa, which is penetrated by blood capillaries, lymphatics, and nerves. Beneath the mucosa and submucosa are two layers of smooth muscle, lying in longitudinal and transverse directions, to allow contractions and peristalsis. Within the stomach, but particularly in the small intestine, the surface area of the mucosa is greatly increased. The mucosal and submucosal layer is folded into microscopic villi on the surface of larger folds or ridges (Figure 1.10). At the bases of the villi are the "crypts," where new epithelial cells are formed that migrate upward to the villi. These cells are sloughed off at a fairly rapid rate; the lifespan of villus cells in the small intestine is as little as 2–3 days (in man), that of colonic cells 3–8 days (Wilson and Greene, 1988). Cells in the crypts include those with glandular and mucous-secreting functions, whereas those in the villi (of the small intestine and colon) are largely absorptive. Glandular cells are important in signaling the initiation and coordination of digestive processes, involving a large number of hormones, neurotransmitters, and paracrine factors (see below). Mucous provided by "goblet" cells promotes lubrication within the lumen of the GI tract. In the small intestine, crypt cells are also the source of some digestive juices.

The epithelial cells of the mucosa have an apical (lumen-oriented) surface that is often additionally invaginated to form microvilli (or a brush border) (Figure 1.10). In the small intestine the brush border contains transporters and some digestive enzymes. It is also more rigid than other parts of the cell membrane, a fact now attributable to high concentrations of sphingolipid in the outer half of the lipid bilayer (van Meer, 1988). Surface cells are held together by tight junctions near the apical (top) parts of the cells. At the opposite (serosal) end, the cell membrane has a different (less rigid) structure (high in phosphatidylcholine) and also serves different functions. Nutrients entering the blood or lymph for distribution to body tissues must first cross the brush border and ultimately the serosal surface of these cells to enter the interstitial fluid. Transport across either or both of these surfaces may be independently and/or differentially controlled, depending upon the nutrient. From there, capillaries and lymphatics take nutrients to the rest of the body. Nutrients not making it across the serosal membranes will remain with the mucosal cells until they are sloughed off, from whence they may be released by digestion and resorbed or lost with cell debris and bacteria in the feces.

Digestion and absorption of major nutrients. For the assimilation of nutrients by the body, the bulk of the foodstuffs must first undergo mastication and digestion. In this process, polymeric substances, such as starches, proteins, and triglycerides, are broken down into their "building blocks" of monomeric sugars, amino acids, fatty acids, etc. With the exception of most vitamins and inorganic substituents, this digestive breakdown process is necessary for absorption into the body. (It is also a factor in body defenses, preventing the potential absorption of "foreign" macromolecules.) During digestion/hydrolysis of the polymeric nutrients (especially the proteins), the vitamins and trace elements associated with them are released, allowing their more efficient absorption.

Gastrointestinal fluid secretions and digestion. The process of digestion begins in the mouth and ends in the small intestine. Breakdown of carbohydrate begins in the mouth, with salivary amylase, and ends in the brush border of the intestinal mucosa, where disaccharides are split. That of protein begins in the stomach, with acid denaturation and pepsin attack, then continues in the small intestine with pancreatic trypsin, chymotrypsin, and other proteases. Little fat breakdown occurs until it reaches the duodenum, where bile salts and lipases begin their action.

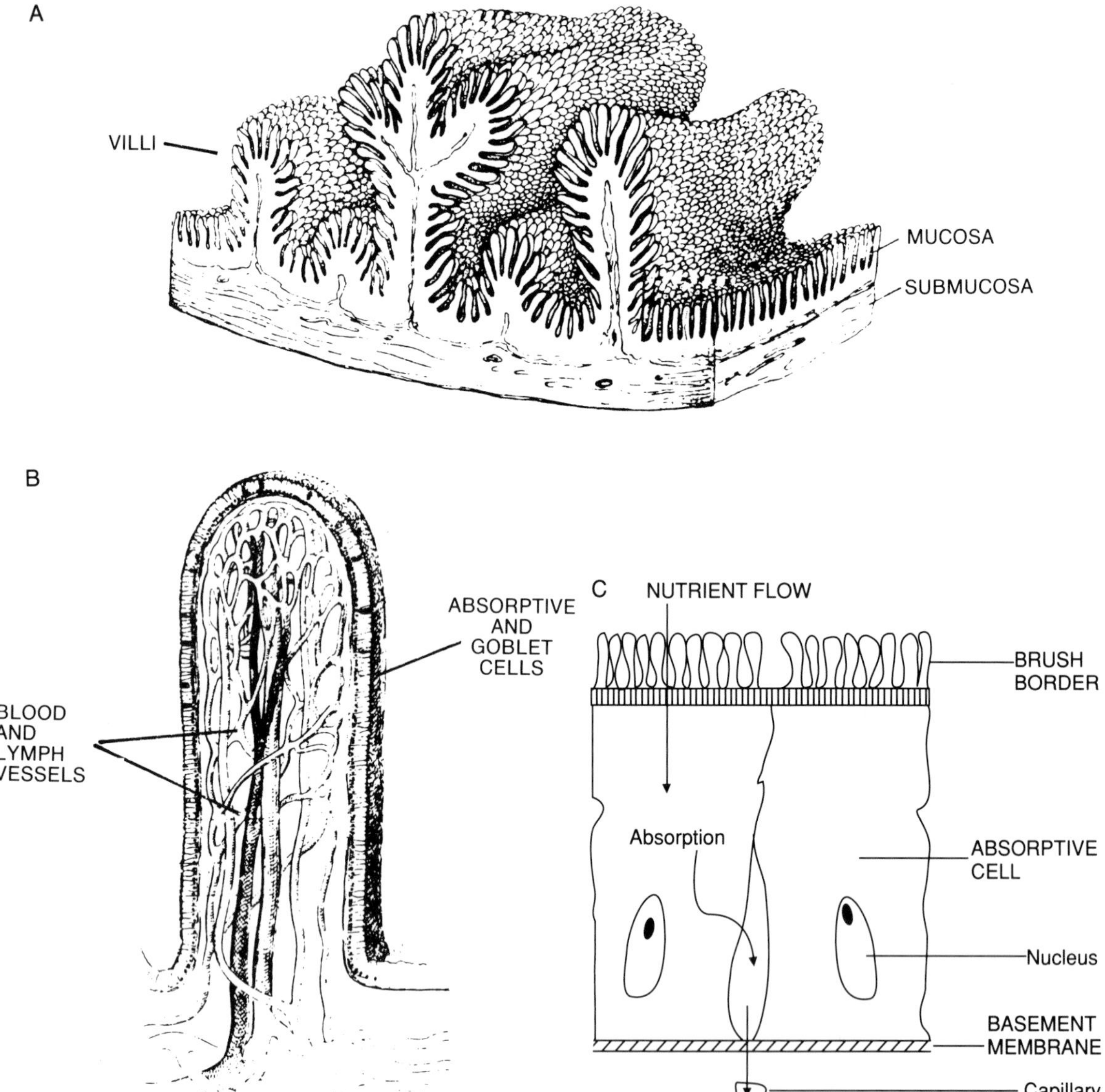

Figure 1.10. Histology of the intestine and mucosa. **(A)** Portion of the intestinal wall, showing the submucosa (which includes smooth muscle layers), and the mucosa, with its folds upon folds (villi). **(B)** A villus, showing the internal blood and lymph circulation, and the layer of absorptive (and goblet) cells. **(C)** Two absorptive cells, with their brush border microvilli, at the lumenal surface, and the basement membrane at the serosal end.

The hydrolysis of covalent bonds between sugars, amino acids, glycerides, etc. is catalyzed by enzymes secreted into the mouth, stomach, duodenum, and rest of the small intestine. Hydrolysis is promoted by other factors, such as acid (in the stomach) and detergents (in the bile). The whole process is beautifully coordinated, both mechanically and metabolically, through the autonomic nervous system (involving acetylcholine and norepinephrine), and by numerous hormones and neurotransmitters (Table 1.7) secreted locally into the lumen or into the blood by cells in various parts of the digestive tract, but especially in the stomach and upper small intestine. These factors promote or inhibit contractions of the smooth muscle sheaths around the GI tract, resulting in mixing and forward propulsion of the food. They also promote secretion of large quantities of the various fluids necessary for digestion, beginning

Table 1.7. Gastrointestinal Hormones: Their Locations and Effects

Gastrointestinal hormone	Location of secretory cells	Location and effect: Secretory (+ and −)[a]	Location and effect: Motor activity (+ and −)[a]	Location and effect: Growth (+ and −)[a]	Intestinal neurotransmitter and paracrine activities
Gastrin	Stomach and duodenum	Stomach (pyloric antrum) ++++ (HCl, pepsin) (pancreas and enzymes +)[b] (gallbladder bile +)[b]	Stomach + (gallbladder +)[b]	Gastric mucosa +	
Cholecystokinin[c]	Duodenum and jejunum	Pancreas ++++ (enzymes and HCO_3^-) (insulin +)[d] (intestine +)[b]	Gallbladder +++ Intestine ++/0 Stomach −−[e]	Pancreas + Upper small intestine + ?	
Secretin[c]	Duodenum and jejunum	Pancreas ++++ (HCO_3^- and enzymes) Biliary tract ++	Intestine −/0 Stomach −−[e]	Upper small intestine −	
Vasoactive intestinal peptide[c,f]	Intestine	Pancreas ++++ (enzymes) Bile ++ Intestine ++ (enzymes) Stomach −−	Stomach −−− Small intestine		Small intestine −−, vasodilation
Enteroglucagon	Intestine	Pancrease + (insulin released)	Intestine −−−		
Gastrointestinal inhibitory peptide	Intestine	Stomach −−− Intestine + (enzymes) Pancreas + (insulin released)		Upper small intestine + ?	
Motilin[c,f]	Intestine		Stomach ++++ Intestine ++++		
Pancreatic polypeptide		Pancreas − ?	?	?	
Somatostatin	Saliva/S	Throughout GI tract −− Throughout intestine	?	?	Inhibitory of paracrine effects
Bombesin[c]	Upper small intestine (from neurons)	Throughout GI tract + ? (release of gastrin)	?	?	
Neurotensin[c]	Lower small intestine	?	?	?	
Glucagon-like peptides[c]	Lower small intestine, colon	?	Stomach −−	?	(−−)
Neuromedin K/ Substance P[c]	Small intestine (neuronal and endocrine cells)	?	Intestine ++ (atropine resistant contractions)	?	
Enkephalins[c]	Throughout small intestine	?	?	?	− (acetylcholine release)
Endorphins[c]	Small intestine (endocrine cells)	GI tract −−	GI tract −−	?	(−−)

Source: Modified from Grossman (1976) and Wilson and Greene (1988).

[a] +, stimulatory; −, inhibitory; 0, no change.
[b] Perhaps at unphysiologic concentrations (?).
[c] Also found in brain.
[d] Potentiates blood amino acid effect (Liddle et al., 1988).
[e] Decreases stomach emptying (Green et al., 1988; Liddle et al., 1988; Moran and McHugh, 1982).
[f] Peptide neurotransmitters.

with the saliva in the mouth and ending with various enzyme-containing and mucous secretions of the small intestinal lining, totaling 6–12 L in the average adult per day. The types and quantities of secretions are given in Table 1.8.

Secretion of saliva is promoted by food anticipation and by nonconditioned (oral and GI) reflexes. It serves to begin digestion of starch with salivary amylase and also contains antibacterial thiocyanate (SCN^-), and somatostatin and growth factors (EGF, NGF) that will have effects further down. In the stomach, secretion of acid is promoted by vagal stimulation (food anticipation and stress) and/or by introduction of food, the latter resulting in localized release of histamine and gastrin (from specialized cells in the gastric mucosa) which act upon parietal cells, to release H^+. Similarly, pepsinogen is released from Chief cells and cleaved to begin digestion of proteins, which is promoted by their denaturation in the acid environment. The introduction of fat and protein into the stomach, and the beginning of its entry into the duodenum, also stimulates release of cholecystokinin (CCK) into the blood. This prepares for and coordinates (a) the final digestion of most foods in the duodenum and jejunum and (b) the distribution of their absorbed products that have entered the blood (Liddle et al., 1988). CCK immediately slows the rate of stomach emptying (Table 1.7) and stimulates the release of bile and pancreatic fluid into the duodenum, by causing gallbladder contraction and pancreatic enzyme release. It also promotes secretion of insulin into the blood (Liddle et al., 1988), as does food anticipation (Cahill, 1976). Other hormones also increase the rate of stomach emptying (Table 1.7). The response to food of cells secreting the various hormones (such as gastrin or CCK) follows the general pattern illustrated in Figure 1.11. Hormones released by sensor cells into the blood then interact with specific receptors in their target cells resulting in "second messenger" cascades leading to changes in cell function (such as fluid secretion). Some of the target cells (as in the pancreas and gallbladder) are at a distance from the GI tract; others are within the gastric or intestinal mucosa itself. Some of the factors affecting secretion, motility, and growth (Table 1.7) are released into the interstitial spaces to the mucosa to have much more local (paracrine) effects on neighboring cells.

Partially digested acidified food entering the duodenum through the pyloric sphincter is neutralized by pancreatic HCO_3^- and exposed to numerous pancreatic and intestinally derived digestive enzymes, mucous, and bile, which continue and complete hydrolysis of the macromolecular nutrients. The digestion of fats, mostly triacylglycerols (triglycerides), is accomplished with the help of bile and detergents that disperse it in the aqueous, lipase-containing medium of the duodenal lumen. Apart from CCK, several other hormones and paracrine factors (Table 1.7) stimulate the secretory activities of the pancreas and small intestine (the latter secretions coming from cells in the crypts).

The fluids and secretions that pour into the digestive tract serve not only the function of

Table 1.8. Secretions of the GI in the Adult Human

Secretion	Approximate normal daily volume (ml)	Average concentration of some electrolytes (meq/L)[a]				Other ingredients
		Na^+	K^+	Cl^-	HCO_3^-	
Saliva	1000–1500	10	26	10	8	Amylase, SCN^-, somatostatin, EGF, NGF
Gastric juice	1500	150	15	130	—	H^+, pepsin
Bile	1000	146	5	110	46	Bile acids, cholesterol, phospholipids Fe, Zn, Cu, Mn
Pancreatic juice and enzymes	1500	157	7	50	110	Digestive
Intestinal juices	4000	140	6	100	17	Digestive enzymes, IgA
Total	~9000 (all but 100–200 ml reabsorbed)					

Source: Modified from Wilson and Greene (1988).

[a] Concentrations may vary considerably (Shils and Randall, 1980).

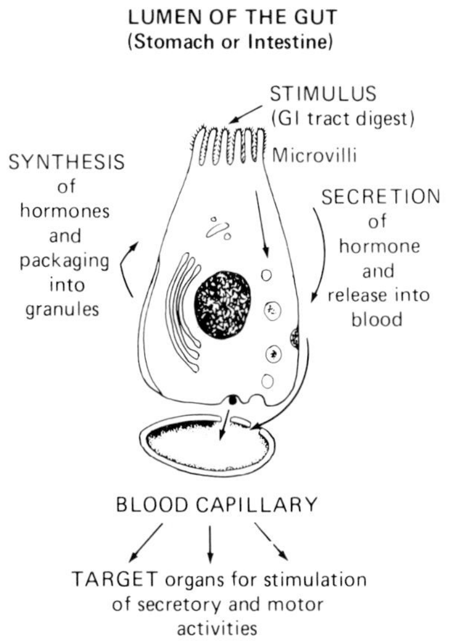

Figure 1.11. Regulation of hormone secretions in response to food intake. Endocrine cells of the intestinal tract are of many kinds and secrete a hormone and an amine (like serotonin) in response to digesting food, which is detected by the microvilli at the lumenal surface. This leads to release of hormone-containing granules into the interstitial space (by exocytosis). Hormone is then circulated to its target tissues (see Table 1.8). [*Source:* Redrawn from Iber (1980).]

breaking up polymeric nutrients for their absorption but also provide protection against invasion by foreign materials and organisms. Potentially antigenic substances, such as proteins, are broken apart; potentially transforming materials, such as nucleic acids and/or viruses, are also destroyed. Immunoglobulin A is secreted to bind bacterial toxins or to inactivate unusual invading organisms, such as parasites; the detergents (bile salts) secreted can also lyse such organisms. Nevertheless, a small percentage of the bacteria ingested with food do get through the pH 1 environment of the stomach, past the bile salts and pancreatic secretions, into the "safer" areas of the lower intestine and colon, where they play a somewhat symbiotic role (see later).

Most of the fluids and substituents secreted in response to food intake are reabsorbed. Most of the fluid is reabsorbed in the small intestine, but final resorption of excess water and electrolytes occurs in the colon. Secreted enzymes (or any other proteins) are first digested along with dietary proteins. Bile, which consists of phospholipid and bile acids (with smaller amounts of breakdown products of porphyrins from hemoglobin turnover) and some iron, manganese, zinc, and bile pigments (all in a supersaturated aqueous solution of cholesterol), is mostly recycled. Indeed, the average body content of bile salts is 5–6 g, and only about 1% of this (50 mg) on average is lost per day. Depending upon fat intake, the bile salts themselves may recycle through the enterohepatic circulation five to seven times a day (Iber, 1980). The degree of bile acid and cholesterol resorption is influenced by the fiber composition of the diet (see Chapters 2 and 3).

Bacterial composition of the gut. Most of the absorption of nutrients occurs in the duodenum and jejunum. The lower small intestine, and especially the colon, are populated by an immensely varied group of mostly anaerobic bacteria, including *Escherichia coli* and various strains of eubacteria, bacteroides, bifidobacteria, streptococci, clostridia, bacilli, peptococci, klebsiella, staphylococci, peptostreptococci, and lactobacilli (Finegold, 1975). More than 400 species comprised of more than 40 genera have been isolated from individual people. In general, the most abundant are bacteroides. Bifidobacteria (found especially in breast-fed infants) are also very numerous. People in developed countries probably have very few, if any, stable colonies of bacteria outside of the ileum, cecum, and colon (Savage, 1983). However, in less developed countries, in people with predominantly vegetarian and low-meat diets, small numbers of stable colonies may be found in the upper small intestine and even in the stomach (streptococci, lactobacilli) (Savage, 1983). Indeed, small numbers of bacteria (in transit) may be found in the stomach and duodenum of most people. Estimates show 10^1–10^2 and 10^2–10^4 bacteria/ml in the fluids of the stomach and duodenum, respectively, as compared with 10^6–10^8 and 10^{11}–10^{12} in the ileum and colon (Goldin et al., 1988). It is of some interest that the pattern of gut bacterial strains present, and their proportions, is quite individualized, and for a given person, does not vary appreciably with dietary pattern (at least over periods of days and weeks) (Moore and Holderman, 1975). In general, this has been borne out by more recent work, although some increases in the proportions of aerobes to anaerobes may occur in connection with a low-meat, higher complex carbohydrate diet in some people or populations (see Savage, 1986; Goldin et al., 1988).

Intestinal bacteria provide substantial portions of some vitamins to man (see Chapter 5) and also participate in ammonia and nitrate/nitrite balance (Tannenbaum et al., 1978), as well as in the modification of bile acids, bilirubin, and other degradation products of porphyrin metabolism (which color the urine and feces; Tietz, 1986). They also degrade dietary fiber and provide metabolites, such as butyrate, that may promote the health of the cells lining the colon (Roediger, 1980). Short-chain fatty and volatile acids (acetate through caproic) produced by colonic bacteria may indeed be a major energy source to the absorptive cells of the colon. (Further information on these aspects may be found in Chapters 2, 3, and 16.) Bacteria in the GI tract also degrade (and utilize) much of the mucin/mucoprotein secreted by goblet cells in the crypts (Hoskins and Zamchek, 1968), and they may enhance the loss of absorptive cells from the tips of intestinal villi (Savage et al., 1981). Thus, treatment with antibiotics does have some nutritional and clinically observable consequences.

The question arises as to whether medical antibiotic treatment can, or usually does, completely sterilize the intestinal tract, and further, whether ingestion of foods containing lactobacilli or streptococci (yogurt contains mainly *L. bulgaricus, L. acidophillus,* and *S. thermophillus*) is useful in repopulating the digestive tract after such treatment. The degree of sterilization of the intestine will depend on the breadth of "spectrum" of the antibiotic, as well as on the bacterial population present, and thus will vary. Clearly, some of the ingested bacteria will find their way past the stomach (where most are destroyed by acid), into the middle and lower intestinal tract, and into the colon, to proliferate.

Nutrient absorption and distribution. Absorption of nutrients occurs mainly in the upper half of the small intestine, although the lower half is perfectly capable of absorbing as well. Absorption of many nutrients occurs primarily by diffusion, or facilitated diffusion, but some, like glucose, are actively absorbed. With the exception of sugars, most molecules under 12,000 daltons diffuse into the intestinal mucosal cells without a great deal of difficulty if they are water soluble. It is noteworthy (see Chapter 4) that a small percentage of the proteins in the diet actually are absorbed as whole molecules and enter our blood circulation as such. Disaccharides, as well as very small peptides, are absorbed in the process of their digestion (splitting) in the brush border of the intestinal cells: sucrose, maltose, lactose, and tripeptides. An exception to upper intestinal absorption is the intake of vitamin B_{12}-intrinsic factor complexes and bile acids, which occurs in the lower half. (The lower portion of the small intestine is also a major site for excretion of uric acid.) The remnants of nutrients entering the colon ex-

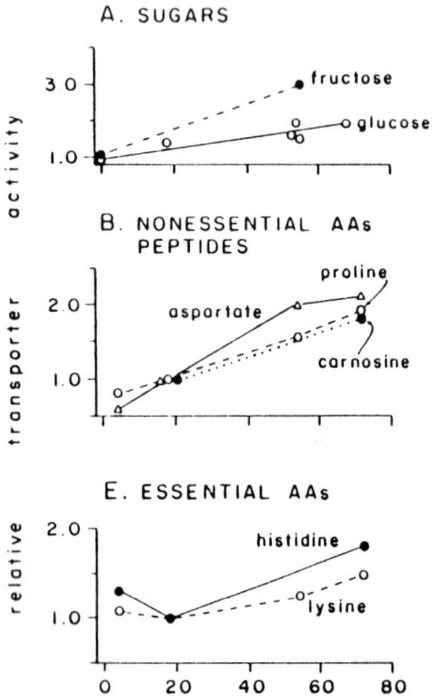

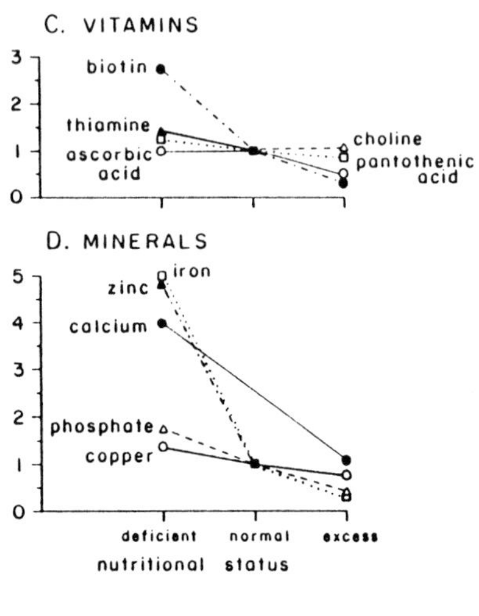

Figure 1.12. Effects of levels of intake of dietary substrates on levels of transporters in the intestinal mucosa. [*Source:* Reprinted by permission from Ferraris and Diamond (1989).]

perience their slowest transit in this portion of the GI tract. In the colon, most excess water is removed, and this is where the bulk of the bacteria proliferate. Indeed, the bulk of the feces of the average American on a Western diet (which is low in fiber) is comprised of bacteria.

During absorption, substances enter the body proper in two steps: first entering the mucosa and then the blood or the lymph. The second step, especially, may be controlled according to the body's needs. Overall, transport of many dietary nutrients into the blood adapts to dietary intake and/or body stores (Figure 1.12). Diets high in sugars and amino acids cause an adaptation of transporter activity to allow efficient absorption. In contrast, dietary status of some vitamins, major minerals, and trace elements is inversely related to ease of absorption via control of transport systems in the serosal and/or mucosal (brush border) membranes of endothelial cells. Cells lining the gastrointestinal tract migrate up the villi to be sloughed off and replaced generally within 3–5 days of their conception (Table 1.2). Substances caught in these cells and not transferred into the body *per se* are lost with them and partially or fully digested, with reabsorption of their substituents.

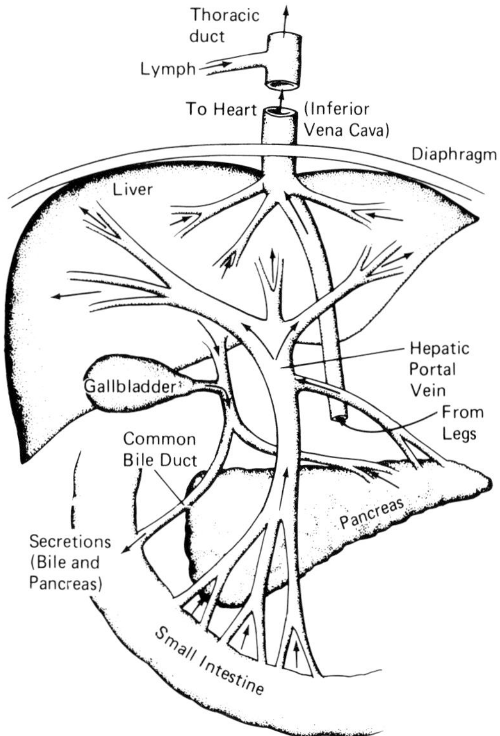

Figure 1.13. Enterohepatic/hepatic portal circulation. Blood flows from the small intestine (and pancreas) to the liver; bile produced by the liver travels to the gallbladder for storage and joins with pancreatic secretions to enter the small intestine via the common bile duct. (Blood in the liver leaves for the heart via the vena cava; lymph enters just prior to the heart.)

Nutrient distribution and the enterohepatic circulation. From the intestinal mucosa, most nutrients are distributed throughout the body via the blood, except for most fats, which first enter the lymph and then join the blood at the thoracic duct (Figure 1.13). Most of the entering nutrients are screened and acted upon by the liver, which is in the best position, vis-à-vis the circulation, to perform such a buffering function (Figure 1.13). Indeed, the liver and kidney are largely responsible for ensuring that the peripheral plasma and extracellular fluid do not undergo large fluctuations in composition.

Utilization and storage. The nutrients absorbed are either utilized immediately for synthetic or other bodily processes or stored after minor or major chemical transformation until further use. Of the major nutrients, carbohydrates are used in the form of hexoses or pentoses and are stored as polymeric glucose molecules (glycogen) or converted to triacylglycerols; fats are utilized or stored as triacylglycerols; proteins (as amino acids) are mainly utilized for protein synthesis or degraded for their carbon skeletons and converted to glucose or fat. Fat-soluble vitamins and smaller amounts of other vitamins are also stored, many in the liver, which is also a major site for storage of iron and perhaps other trace elements (Chapter 7). Bone represents a repository for the major minerals, other than Na^+, K^+, and Cl^-, as well as some trace elements.

Turnover of body substituents. The majority of complex substances within the body, including enzymes and structural proteins, are in a constant state of turnover, being degraded and resynthesized to maintain or change their concentrations as warranted. Exceptions are DNA and collagen fibers, especially in the adult. In the process of turnover, there is some loss of the amino acids and other "building blocks" required for formation of complex molecules; the energy needed for biosynthetic processes requires the complete catabolism of major nutrients (mainly carbohydrates and fats) to CO_2 and water (as well as to urea and ammonia, in the case of protein degradation). The bulk of the nutrients in our diet are needed to replace these daily losses.

Excretion. Excretion of nutrients and their metabolites from the body "proper" proceeds via the lungs (CO_2, acetone), the urine (urea, ammonia, most water-soluble metabolites of nonpeptide hormones and vitamins), the bile (cholesterol, bile acids, bile pigments, Fe, Mn, Cu), sweat (mainly electrolytes and some glycoproteins), and through the sloughing off of surface skin and cells lining the GI tract. Fecal excretion carries with it bile materials and sloughed cells, as well as dietary material undigested and/or unabsorbed. Overall, the metabolism of absorbed nutrients is extremely efficient, and with the possible exception of some water-soluble vitamins, bile acids, and cholesterol, there is little loss of substances that could be of use to the body.

References

Boothby WM, Berkson J, Dunn HL (1936): Am J Physiol 116:468.

Brozek J (1965): Human body composition. New York: Pergamon.

Cahill GF Jr (1976): Discussion. *In* Parsons JA, ed: Peptide hormones. Baltimore: University Park Press, p 101.

Cameron IL, Thrasher JD (1971): Cellular and molecular renewal in the mammalian body. New York: Academic.

Cheek DB (1975): Fetal and postnatal cellular growth. New York: Wiley.

Cohn SH, Vaswami AN, Yasumura S, Yeun MSf, Ellis KJ (1984): Am J Clin Nutr 40:255.

Davignon J, Gregg RE, Sing CF (1988): Arteriosclerosis 8:1.

Ferraris RP, Diamond JM (1989): Annu Rev Physiol 51:125.

Finegold SM, Flora DJ, Attebery HR, Sutter VL (1975): Cancer Res 35:3407.

Fisher EA, Coates PM, Cornter JA (1989): Annu Rev Nutr 9:139.

Forbes GB: *In* Shils ME, Young UR, eds: Modern nutrition in health and disease (7th ed). Philadelphia: Lea & Febiger, p 533.

Friis-Hanson B (1965): *In* Brozek J, ed: Human body composition. New York: Pergamon.

Goldin BR, Lichtenstein AH, Gorbach SL (1988): *In* Shils ME, Young VR, eds: Modern nutrition in health and disease. Philadelphia: Lea & Febiger, p 500.

Green T, Dimaline R, Peikin S, Dockray GJ (1988): Am J Physiol 255:G685.

Grossman MI (1976): *In* Parsons JA, ed: Peptide hormones. Baltimore: University Park Press, p 105.

Growth (1962): FASEB Handbook.

Hoskins LC, Zamchek N (1968): Gastroenterology 54:210.

Iber F (1980): *In* Goodhart RS, Shils MW, eds: Modern nutrition in health and disease. Philadelphia: Lea & Febiger, p 35.

Kraft H-G, Dieplinger H, Hoye E, Utermann G (1988): Arteriosclerosis 8:212.

Liddle RA, Rushakoff RJ, Morita ET, Becarria L, Carter JD, Goldfine ID (1988): J Clin Invest 81:1675.

Linder MC (1979): *In* Schaefer KE, Hildebrandt G, Macbeth W, eds: A new image of man in medicine, vol II. Mt Kisco, NY: Futura, p 109.

Magnus-Levy A (1910): Biochem Z 24:363.

Moore WEC, Holderman LV (1975): Cancer Res 35:3418.

Moran TH, McHugh PR (1982): Am J Physiol 242:R491.

Odawara M, Kadowski T, Yamamoto R, Shibasaki Y, Tobe K, Accilli D, Bevins C, Mikami Y, Matsuura N, Akanua Y, Takaku F, Taylor SI, Kasuga M (1989): Science 245:66.

Pan American Health Organization (publication no. 251).

Rall SC, Weisgraber KH, Mahley RW, Ehnholm C, Schamaun O (1986): J Lipid Res 27:436.

Roediger WEW (1980): Gut 21:793.

Savage DC (1983): *In* Henges DJ, ed: Human intestinal microflora in health and disease. New York: Academic, p 55.

Savage DC (1986): Annu Rev Nutr 6:155.

Savage DC, Siegel JE, Snellen JE, Whitt DD (1981): Appl Environm Microbiol 42:996.

Scammon RE (1930): The measurement of man. Minneapolis: University of Minnesota Press.

Shils ME, Randall HT (1980): *In* Goodhart RS, Shils ME, eds: Modern nutrition in health and disease. Philadelphia: Lea & Febiger, p 1082.

Smith HW (1956): Principles of renal physiology. New York: Oxford University Press, p 113.

Taira M, Taira M, Hashimoto N, Shimada F, Suzuki Y, Kanatsuka A, Nakamura F, Ebina Y, Tatibana M, Makino H, Yoshida S (1989): Science 245:63.

Tannenbaum SR, Fett D, Young VR, Land PD, Bruce WR (1978): Science 200:1487.

Tietz NW, ed (1986): Fundamentals of clinical chemistry. Philadelphia: WB Saunders.

van Meer G (1988): TIBS 13:242.

Widdowson E (1965): *In* Brozek J, ed: Human body composition. New York: Pergamon.

Williams RJ (1942): A textbook of biochemistry (2nd ed). New York: Van Nostrand.

Williams RJ (1956): Biochemical individuality. New York: Wiley.

Wilson PC, Greene HL (1988): *In* Shils ME, Young VR, eds: Modern nutrition in health and disease. Philadelphia: Lea & Febiger, p 481.

Maria C. Linder, Ph.D.*

2

Nutrition and Metabolism of Carbohydrates

Introduction to Carbohydrates

Consumption

Dietary carbohydrate presently comprises 40%–45% of the calories consumed by the average American, a decrease of 25%–30% since 1900 (Glinsmann et al., 1986; Gortner, 1975). About 60% of this absorbable carbohydrate is in the form of polysaccharides (mainly plant starches), the consumption of which has decreased from 75% in 1900 (Friend, 1976). The remainder is mostly sucrose and lactose (milk sugar), which are found in fruits, milk, table sugar, etc., although consumption of corn sweeteners (notably high fructose corn syrup) has increased dramatically. At present, there are about 65 lb of added sucrose and 40 lb of added high fructose corn-syrup solids available to the U.S. population per person annually (Glinsmann et al., 1986), and a total of about 126 lb of all added caloric sweeteners for each U.S. citizen. The added sweeteners are mainly in soda, candy, syrups, and breakfast cereals, but are also in other foods, from ice cream and catsup to salad dressing.

The proportion of absorbable carbohydrate represented by the disaccharides and monosaccharides has for some time now been much greater than it was at the turn of the century (about 40% versus 25%) (Friend, 1976); there has been a relatively high intake of refined sugar (20%–30% of carbohydrate intake) and a decreased ingestion of cereal grains, roots, and tubers (where plants accumulate their carbohydrate stores). The proportion of nonabsorbable carbohydrate, also called dietary fiber, has also been relatively low in proportion to the lower intake of complex carbohydrates (about 60% of the carbohydrate consumed). (Intake of complex carbohydrate and fiber is much higher in less developed countries.)

In 1977, a select committee of the U.S. Senate recommended a reversal in the dietary pattern of carbohydrate consumption to one closer to that of the early 1900s, with half as much sucrose and refined sugars (10% of calories), a greater amount of complex carbohydrate (totaling about 50% of calories), and more fiber. The reasons for these changes relate to (1) an effort to reduce consumption of fats that may be linked to cancer and atherosclerosis; (2) potential problems with large-scale sucrose and fructose consumption; and (3) the beneficial effects of dietary fiber. These recommendations were confirmed in the current (1989) report of the National Research Council of the National Academy, entitled "Diet and Health: Implications for Decreasing Chronic Disease Risk," in which it was emphasized that a reduced fat intake should be compensated by a higher intake of complex carbohydrates (and fiber) in the form of green and yellow vegetables, certain fruits, legumes, and especially whole grain cere-

* California State University, Fullerton, CA.

als and breads, as well as a reduction in added sugar.

Structure

Dietary carbohydrates come in complex (polymeric) or simple (monomeric and dimeric) forms. They also come in digestible and indigestible forms, the latter being the dietary fiber, of interest in relation to some disease states (see later). Figure 2.1 and Table 2.1 describe the structural characteristics and properties of these various classes of carbohydrate and their main dietary sources. Dietary fiber is discussed more fully at the end of the chapter. The principal sugars in all these carbohydrates are glucose, fructose, and galactose or their derivatives, whether available or unavailable for absorption by humans. With the exception of lactose, the linkages between units of digestible carbohydrates are mostly α1,4 or α1,6, whereas linkages in fiber tend to be β, often β1,4 (cellulose, pectins), for which we secrete no digestive enzymes.

Food Sources

As indicated in Tables 2.1 and 2.2, carbohydrates are mainly found in foods of plant origin and in processed foods. Very little carbohydrate is found in animal foods, such as meats, fish, or poultry, except for small amounts of glycogen in liver and muscle, and of course, milk, which contains 3%–6% lactose by weight (depending on its source). [This lactose is mostly (or completely) gone after milk has been fermented into yogurt or cheese.] In plant foods, starches are found especially in grains and seeds, but also in legumes, tubers, and in some vegetables and fruits. Branched starch (amylopectin) is about three times as abundant as the linear polyglucose, amylose. Sugars, notably sucrose, glucose, and fructose, are mainly found in fruits, sugar beets, and saps, such as those of the sugar cane or sugar maple. Honey (made by bees) is of course also a source. The distribution of fiber in foods generally follows that of starches, a major exception being the pectins, present mainly in fruits. Thus, whole grains (and seeds), legumes, and fruits/berries are the main sources of dietary fiber. Nevertheless, all vegetables also contain at least small amounts of fiber, as all plant cells have a rigid cell wall outside their lipid plasma membrane (see Chapter 1, Figure 1.9). Further details on fiber are given in other sections of this chapter.

Digestion

Digestion of complex carbohydrates begins in the mouth with salivary amylase, which begins the hydrolysis of starches (amylose, amylopectin, glycogen) to smaller units. From there, very little additional cleavage of complex carbohydrates (or disaccharides) occurs until the upper small intestine, where the bulk of carbohydrate digestion proceeds. Here, pancreatic and intestinal digestive enzymes, especially pancreatic amylase, reduce the complex carbohydrate to dimeric (and some oligomeric) units, primarily maltose (glucose–glucose), and to branched (α1,6) oligomers from digestion of amylopectin (MacDonald, 1988). [It should be noted that pancreatic synthesis of amylase is regulated by insulin (Owerbach et al., 1981); and this is depressed in the diabetic (Bunn et al., 1976).] The disaccharidases (enzymes) in the brush border of the intestinal mucosal cells then split maltose and dietary disaccharides (such as sucrose and lactose) into their constituent hexoses. Sucrose is split rapidly by sucrase, lactose more slowly by lactase. Maltose, maltotriose, and branched glucose oligomers (isomaltoses) are hydrolyzed rapidly to glucose, mainly by isomaltase but also by maltase (MacDonald, 1988). Sucrase also hydrolyzes some maltose and maltotriose. Sucrase (and maltase) activities may be positively influenced by the sucrose (or fructose) content of the diet. The resulting hexose units in the brush border are then all absorbed across the adjacent plasma membrane into the cells of the intestinal mucosa and are transported from there mainly to the liver via the portal circulation.

Absorption

Absorption of the monosaccharides, D-glucose and D-galactose, occurs by an energy-dependent process involving the Na^+ extracellular-to-intracellular chemical gradient across the brush border, and, thus, the Na^+ pump (or Na^+/K^+ ATPase) in the apical plasma membrane. Glucose and galactose compete for the same transport system, the carrier for which has not yet been identified. The capacity of the system for glucose uptake is so great it has been estimated an adult could theoretically absorb more than 20 lb over 24 hr (MacDonald, 1980). Glucose from the disaccharide, sucrose, is absorbed equally or even more rapidly as soon as it is split in the brush border. Absorption of fructose is not energy-dependent and is not quite as rapid, proceeding across the apical cell

MONOSACCHARIDES

D glucose (glu)

D-galactose (gal)

D-fructose (fru)

DISACCHARIDES

Sucrose — α1,4 linked glu and fru

Lactose — β1,4-linked gal and glu

Maltose — α1,4-linked glu and glu

POLYSACCHARIDES

α1,4(and α1,6)-linked glu Glycogen

β1,4-linked glu Cellulose

OTHERS (Mainly Components of Dietary Fiber Polymers)

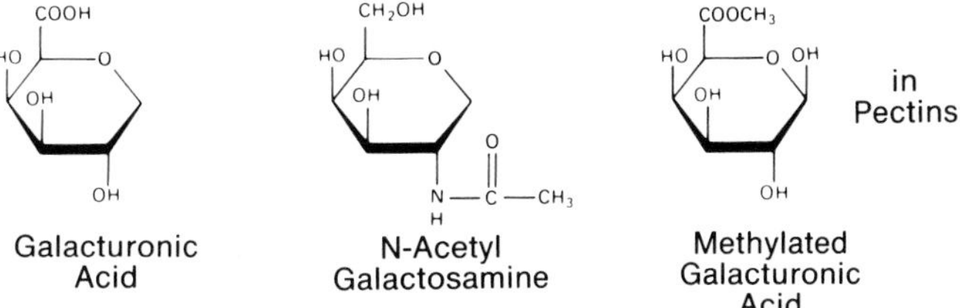

in Pectins

Galacturonic Acid

N-Acetyl Galactosamine

Methylated Galacturonic Acid

Ribose (Hemicellulose)

Gal-4-SO_4 (Carrageenan)

N-Acetyl Glucosamine (Chitin)

Phenyl Propane Derivatives (Lignin)

Figure 2.1. Components of dietary carbohydrates.

Table 2.1. Dietary Carbohydrates: Types, Sources, Structure, and Properties

Carbohydrate	Sources	Structure and properties
D-Glucose (dextrose)	Fruit; traces in most plant foods; honey; maple sugar	Water-soluble monosaccharide [molecular weight (MW) 180]
D-Fructose	Fruits; traces in most plant foods; honey; maple sugar	Water-soluble monosaccharide (MW 180)
D-Galactose	Component of lactose; produced during digestion	Water-soluble monosaccharide (MW 180)
Sucrose	Cane sugar; beet sugar; fruits; maple sugar	Water-soluble disaccharide (MW 360) (α1,4-linked glu-fru)
Lactose	Milk; dairy products (milk sugar)	Water-soluble disaccharide (MW 360) (β1,4-linked gal-glu)
Maltose	Sprouted grain; produced during digestion of starches	Water-soluble disaccharide (MW 360) (α1,4-linked glu-glu)
Amylose	Starchy plants; grains (starch)	Linear polymer of glucose (α1,4); water-soluble; MW 10^5–10^6
Amylopectin (starch)	Starchy plants; grains; used as thickener in processed foods	Branched polymer of glucose (α1,4 and α1,6); water-soluble; MW 10^7–10^8
Glycogen (animal starch)	Liver; muscle	Branched polymer of glucose (α1,4 and α1,6); water-soluble; MW 10^7–10^8
Cellulose[a]	Substituent of plant cell walls; major component of wheat bran	Linear polymer of glucose (β1,4); not water-soluble; MW 10^5–10^6
Hemicellulose[a]	Substituent of plant cell walls	Polymer of hexoses or pentoses, often branched; MW 10^4; not water-soluble
Pectins[a]	Fruits	Water-soluble linear polymers (β1,4) of galacturonic acids and/or modified galacturonic acid; gel forming; bile acid binding; MW 10^4–10^5
Carrageenan[a]	Red seaweed; used in candies and some processed foods	Linear polymer (β1,4) of disaccharide; units with gal-4-SO_4 and 3,6-anhydro-gal-2-SO_4 (linked β1,3); gel forming; water-soluble; MW 10^4
Inulin[a]	Jerusalem artichoke	Water-soluble fructose polymer; (β2,1)
Raffinose, stachyose, verbacose[a]	Pulses (plant "antifreeze")	Trimer of glucose, fructose, and galactose (β1,2; α1,6) plus/minus additional gal units (α1,6)
Dextrins	Used in processed foods	Short pieces of α1,4-glucose polymer
Invert sugar	Used in processed foods	Hydrolyzed sucrose (fru : glu = 1 : 1)
Corn syrup	Used in processed foods	Hydrolyzed starch (= glucose)
High fructose corn syrup	Used in processed foods	Starch hydrolyzed and partly isomerized (glu + fru)
Lignin[a]	Substituent of plant cell walls	Highly branched polymer of substituted phenylpropanes (not a carbohydrate); binds bile acids; not water-soluble; MW 1–5 × 10^3

Source: Anderson (1981); Gray and Fogel (1978); MacDonald (1988); Metzler (1977); White et al. (1973).

[a] Substituents of dietary fiber. See Figure 2.1 for actual structures.

Table 2.2. Carbohydrate Contents of Various Foods[a]

Food	Portion	Available carbohydrate[b] (g/portion)	Available carbohydrate[b] (g/100 g)	Fiber (g/100 g)
Apple (with peel, core)	1	32	18	3.0
Apricot (pitted)	3	12	11	2.1
Banana (peeled)	1	27	24	2.9
Dates (pitted, dried)	10	61	74	8.7
Orange (peeled, seeded)	1	15	12	2.3
Pear (cored)	1	25	15	3.0
(canned)				1.5
Strawberries	1 cup	11	7	2.2
Bread (whole wheat)	1 slice	13	45	11.4
(white)	1 slice	12	49	2.8
Macaroni	1 cup	39	30	1.1
Corn (cooked on cob)	1	19	25	4.7
Popcorn	1 cup	6	75	19.0
Rice (brown)	1 cup	50	26	2.0
(white)	1 cup	50	24	2.0
(wild)	1 cup	19	19	2.6
Almonds (raw)	1 cup	29	20	10.6
Cashews (roasted)	1 cup	45	33	5.8
Filberts (raw)	1 cup	18	16	6.8
Peanuts (roasted)	1 cup	27	19	8.3
Black beans (cooked)[c]	1 cup	41	24	8.8
Chick peas (cooked)	1 cup	45	28	5.3
Peas (cooked)	1 cup	11	14	9.6
Green beans (cooked)	1 cup	10	8	2.5
Beets (cooked)	2	7	7	2.3
Broccoli (cooked)	1 cup	9	6	4.1
Cabbage (raw)	1 cup	4	6	2.6
Carrots (raw)	1	7	10	2.8
Lettuce (raw)	Wedge	3	2	1.6
Potatoes (boiled, peeled)	1	27	20	2.4
(peeled, boiled)				1.6
Yams (baked, peeled)	1	28	24	2.6
Soda	12 oz	32–42	9–12	0
Milk (cow, whole)	1 cup	11	5	0
Cottage cheese	1 cup	6–8	3–4	0
Other cheeses	1 oz	0–1.1	0–4.8	0
Eggs	1	0.6	1.2	0
Meats (roasted, muscle)	3 oz	0	0	0
Fish	3 oz	0	0	0
Shellfish	3 oz	0	0	0

[a] *Source:* Whitney and Hamilton (1990).
[b] Available for absorption.
[c] From fresh.

membrane by facilitated diffusion at rates dependent upon its local concentration. (Uptake of free dietary fructose is less rapid than uptake of fructose from sucrose.) Most of the glucose, fructose, and galactose then diffuses rapidly through the cell and (crosses also by facilitated diffusion) the serosal border into the interstitial fluid and blood. As in the case of the hydrolyzing enzymes in the brush border, the activities of the serosal transport systems for glucose, galactose, and fructose appear to be influenced positively by diet, at least over days (see Chapter 1, Figure 1.12).

Due to the avidity of the intestinal mucosa for uptake of mono- and disaccharides, intake of these sugars and of many other carbohydrates results in rapid and substantial increases in plasma glucose, fructose, or galactose concentrations. These generate a series of adaptive activities to maintain plasma homeostasis (see below). The ingestion of some foods containing complex (polymeric) digestible carbohydrates does not change the blood glucose concentration as rapidly, partly perhaps because the slightly slower processes of starch digestion by salivary and pancreatic amylases is interposed. Consequently, less drastic adaptive actions (involving insulin secretion) may be required when carbohydrate is taken in the form of foods with starches versus sugars (see below, Carbohydrate Foods and Glucose Tolerance). In general, food starches in grains and legumes are only hydrolyzed efficiently when precooked (or baked), which releases the starch granules from their casings (MacDonald, 1988).

Figure 2.2. Absorption and distribution of carbohydrate: absorptive phase. Glucose, fructose, and galactose obtained from digestion of food products in the intestine are absorbed into the blood. Much of the glucose and almost all the fructose and galactose go to the liver; some glucose goes to the peripheral circulation increasing blood glucose concentrations. This releases insulin from the pancreas and lowers the secretion of glucagon. Insulin stimulates uptake of glucose from the blood by muscle and adipose cells. In the liver, glucose is trapped by phosphorylation to glucose-6-phosphate, which is then converted to glycogen and also used for energy in glycolysis and the tricarboxylic acid (Krebs) (TCA) cycle. Excess glucose is converted to fatty acids and incorporated into triglyceride. This glucose-derived fat is sent for storage to adipose tissue via VLDL. Abbreviations: CHO, carbohydrate; G6P, glucose-6-phosphate; G1P, glucose-1-phosphate; UDPG, uridine diphosphate glucose; VLDL, very low-density lipoprotein (see Chapter 3); FFA, free fatty acids; TG, triglyceride.

Carbohydrate Metabolism and Function

Glucose Metabolism

The influx of glucose into the blood raises blood glucose levels, causing increased diffusion of glucose into liver cells, secretion of pancreatic insulin, and reduced secretion of glucagon (Figure 2.2). The hormone changes result in increased uptake of glucose by muscle and adipose tissue cells. These changes also promote glycogen synthesis in liver and muscle by reducing the level of cyclic adenosine monophosphate (cAMP) production and the concomitant phosphorylation of otherwise active glycogen synthetase (see later). In the same process, glycogen phosphorylase activity is reduced. The synthesis and storage of glycogen are physically limited, since glycogen is a very bulky (hydrated) molecule, and it is esti-

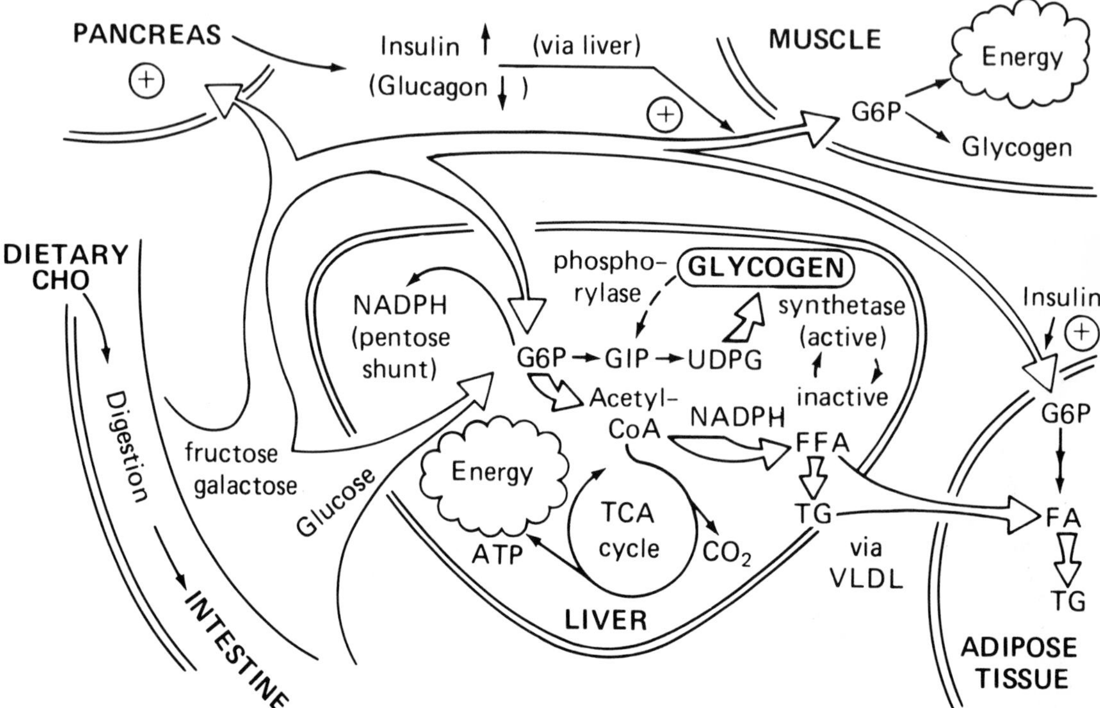

mated that not more than 10–15 hr worth of glucose energy can be stored as glycogen in the liver (approximately 100 g). It may be that an even larger amount of glycogen (about 0.5 kg), diluted in a much larger tissue mass, is stored in the total muscle under conditions of maximal glucose uptake. Traces of glycogen are also found in adipocytes (fat cells) (Vrana et al., 1988) and may also be deposited in the kidney.

Excess glucose is converted to fatty acids and triglyceride mainly by liver and adipose tissue (Figure 2.2). Enhanced glucose metabolism via the hexose monophosphate shunt (pentose shunt) produces the NADPH necessary for fatty acid synthesis. The triglyceride (triacylglycerol) formed in the liver is released into the plasma, as very low-density lipoprotein (VLDL), from where it is taken up by adipose tissue for storage (see Chapter 3). The main function of dietary carbohydrate is thus the initial and preferred source of energy after a meal, and as a continuing source of stored energy thereafter.

Upon cessation of glucose influx from the intestine (after the absorption of dietary carbohydrate has been mainly concluded), blood glucose levels begin to fall, which signals the reversal of the hormonal secretions by the pancreas (Figure 2.3). Now glucagon is released, and insulin secretion is greatly diminished. Glucagon mobilizes liver glycogen through the cAMP-protein kinase system (see later) and increases the synthesis of the enzymes necessary for reversal of glycolysis (gluconeogenesis from amino acids) (Table 2.3). Gluconeogenesis will be necessary if further carbohydrate is not soon available from the diet. [Glucagon may also release free fatty acids from the triglyceride stored in adipose tissue, but norepinephrine released from sympathetic nerve endings is probably more important (Figure 2.4) and so is simply a lack of insulin.] Glycogen phosphorylase in muscle (for glycogen breakdown) is also activated through the cAMP system, but by catecholamines (released by exercise and stress) rather than by glucagon. In stressful situations, catecholamines can cause glycogen mobilization and triglyceride hydrolysis, even in the absence of a direct need for the phenomenon. Muscle glucose stored as glycogen must be used in situ and can never be released into the circulation, because this tissue lacks glucose-6-phosphatase, an enzyme essentially unique to the liver and kidney (Table 2.3).

Table 2.3. Activities of Key Gluconeogenic Enzymes[a,b]

Tissue species	Pyruvate carboxylase	PEP carboxykinase	Fructose-diphosphatase	Glucose-6-phosphatase
Liver				
Rat	6.7	6.7	15	17
Other species[c]	8.3	13	20	12
Kidney				
Rat	5.8	6.7	17	13
Other species	—	—	14	—
Skeletal muscle				
Rat	0	<0.1	0.7	—
Other species	0	3	3.5	<0.1
Heart				
Rat	0	0.5	0.7	2
Other species	0	0	0.8	—
Brain				
Rat	0.5	0.3	2.3	0
Other species	0.3	—	—	—
Intestinal epithelium[d]				
Rat	1.0	0.7	1.7	0.5

Only the liver and kidney (and to a small extent the intestinal mucosa) have all the enzymes for formation of glucose from pyruvate (or oxaloacetate) and its net release into circulation. (The brain has traces of enzymes needed for "reversal" of glycolysis, but not net release.)

[a] μmol/min/g, 37°C.
[b] Data from Scrutton and Utter (1968).
[c] Man, guinea pig, miscellaneous [see Scrutton and Utter (1968)].
[d] Data from Anderson and Rosendall (1973).

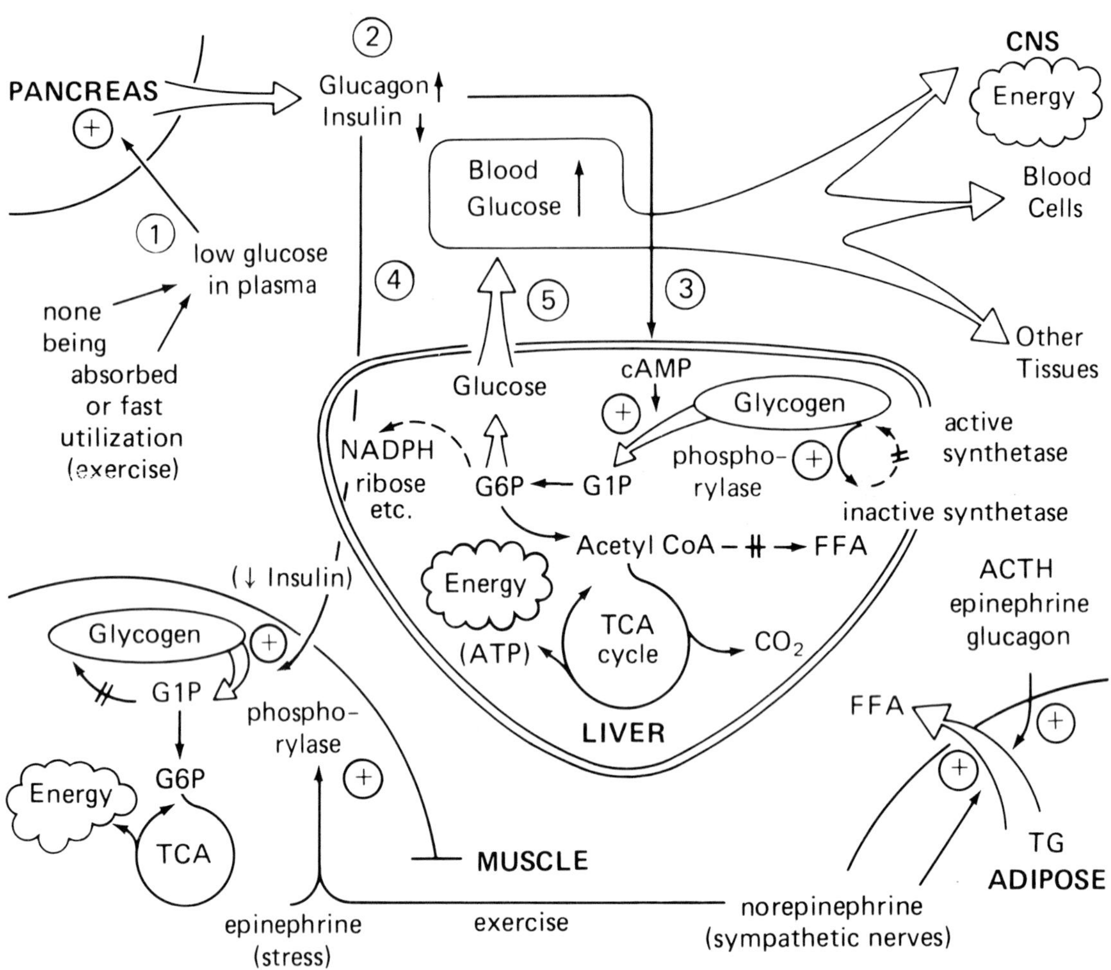

Figure 2.3. Carbohydrate metabolism in early fasting. (1) Decreased plasma glucose stimulates release of glucagon from the pancreas (and decreases secretion of insulin); (2, 3) glucagon goes to the liver and stimulates breakdown of glycogen via cAMP; (4) decreased insulin also enhances breakdown of muscle glycogen leading to its utilization for energy by muscle cells in glycolysis and the TCA cycle (exercise and catecholamines have the same effect, also beginning the release of free fatty acids from adipose cells; see Chapter 3); (5) breakdown of liver glycogen results in dephosphorylation of glucose-6-phosphate which allows release of glucose into the blood to maintain blood glucose concentrations. Blood glucose is needed especially by the central nervous system and by blood cells. Abbreviations: G6P, glucose-6-phosphate; G1P, glucose-1-phosphate; cAMP, cyclic AMP; TCA, tricarboxylic acid (Krebs) cycle; TG, triglyceride; FFA, free fatty acids; CNA, central nervous system.

Based on studies with perfused liver and isolated hepatocytes, there has been a recent interest in the possibility that liver glycogen is synthesized largely by an "indirect" pathway, from three-carbon metabolites, rather than directly from glucose (McGarry et al., 1987). Thus, after a carbohydrate-containing meal, the intestine (or other tissues) might produce substantial quantities of lactate that in the liver would be converted into glucose-6-phosphate (via a reversal of the glycolytic pathway) and then glycogen. Earlier and subsequent in vivo studies in animals and man do not support this concept (Landau and Wahren, 1988; Watford, 1988). Notably, neither the gut nor the muscle releases more than a small amount of any glucogenic precursors after an oral glucose load; the liver (even when isolated and perfused) *does* synthesize glycogen directly from glucose efficiently when blood oxygenation is normal. Indeed, it may release some lactate, indicating that glycolysis is in the "forward" mode. (This lactate can be utilized by muscle.) During the first 3–4 hr after a carbohydrate-containing meal, it appears that about equal thirds of the glucose are taken up by the liver, muscle, and the rest of the tissues (notably the central nervous system and adipocytes). As already indicated, the degree of conversion to fat will increase with the glucose load, because of the limitation on how much can be stored by the liver as glycogen. It is estimated that about 15 g/kg (or about 500 g) of glucose can be stored as glycogen (in liver and muscle) before lipid synthesis contributes to a net increase in body fat (Acheson et al., 1988).

Figure 2.4. Mechanisms of action of glucagon and insulin. **(A)** Glucagon binds to a cell membrane receptor (R) (1), activating a GTP-binding protein (G) (2) which in turn activates adenyl cyclase (AC) (3) and stimulates the production of cAMP. The latter combines with protein kinases (R2C2) (4) to free the catalytic subunits (C). These catalytic subunits activate (by phosphorylation) other protein kinases (5). The phosphorylated protein kinases produce phosphorylated proteins that promote transcription of specific genes in the nucleus (6) (or have other metabolic effects); or produce active enzymes such as glycogen phosphorylase (7). In the case of liver, this process results in increased synthesis of rate-limiting enzymes for the reversal of glycolysis and gluconeogenesis (8). The actions on gluconeogenesis and glycogen degradation only occur in the liver.

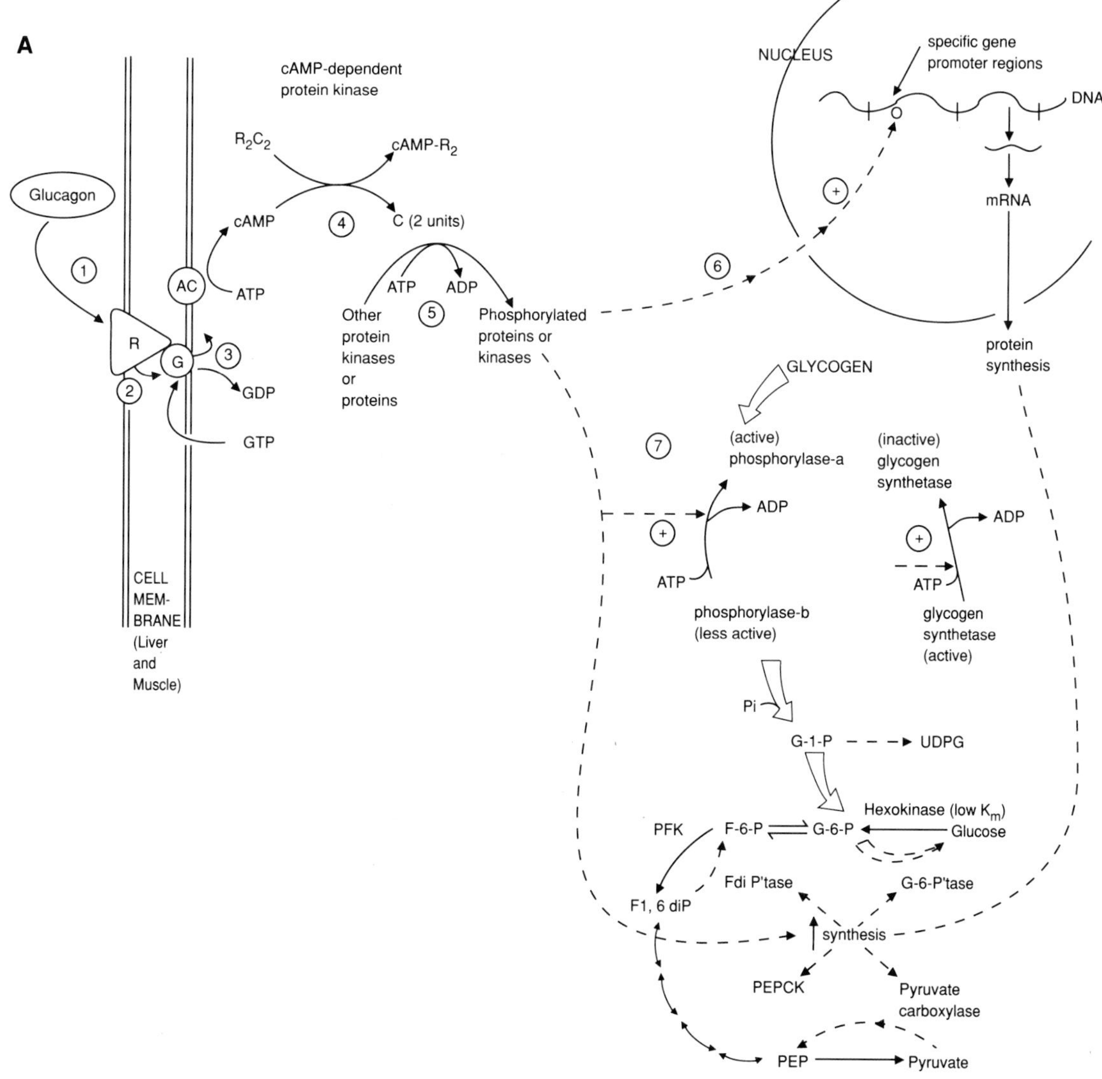

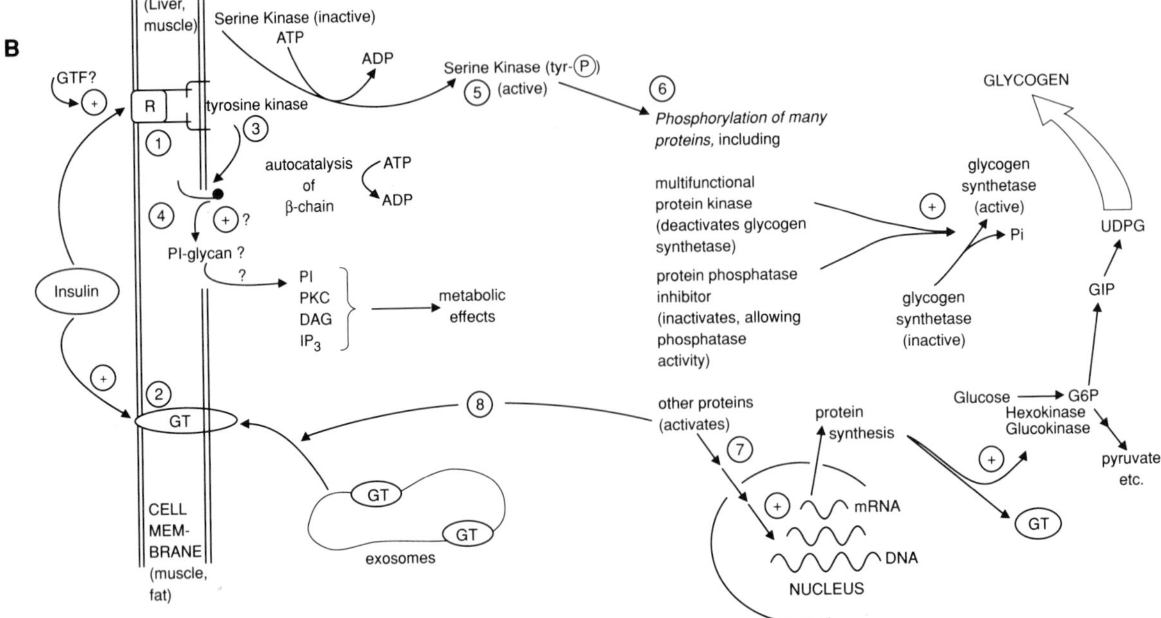

Figure 2.4. (*continued*) **(B)** Insulin (possibly with the help of a glucose tolerance factor; GTF) binds to cell surface membrane receptors (R) (1) and/or glucose transporters (GT) (2). Binding to receptors activates the tyrosine kinase activity of the receptor, which in turn autocatalyzes changes in the receptor that may lead to changes in the phosphoinositide metabolism (4) (described in Chapter 3). (5) It also results in activation of a serine kinase which causes the phosphorylation of many proteins, including a multifunctional protein kinase (MFPK). This increases transcription (7) of some proteins including the glucose transporter necessary for uptake of glucose by the cell membrane, and stimulates transfer (8) of existing glucose transporter from exosomes to the cell membrane. The net effect is also to activate glycogen synthetase (GS). [*Source:* Based on Czech et al. (1988); Garvey et al. (1989); Krebs (1989).] Other abbreviations: PEP, phosphoenolpyruvate; PEPCK, PEP carboxykinase; PFK, phosphofructokinase; PKC, protein kinase C; DAG, diacylglycerol; PI, phosphoinositide; IP3, inositol triphosphate. Effects (1) and (3–7) occur in liver, muscle, and fat cells; (2) in muscle and fat cells (not liver); glucokinase induction only in liver.

Mechanisms of action of hormones in glucose metabolism. Insulin and glucagon are peptide hormones secreted by beta and alpha cells of the pancreas, respectively, in response to changes in the glucose concentrations of the blood (and interstitial fluid). (The sensing mechanisms in these cells are not well understood.) Epinephrine and norepinephrine are catecholamines secreted by the adrenal medulla and sympathetic nervous system, respectively, in response to stress and exercise. The series of molecular events, leading to the actions of glucagon and norepinephrine/epinephrine on the carbohydrate metabolism of their target cells, is quite well understood. As summarized in Figure 2.4A, the hormone glucagon binds to a specific (high affinity) receptor on the cell surface. The resulting hormone–receptor complex interacts with a GTP-binding protein (G protein) that releases GDP and stimulates the adjacent enzyme, adenyl cyclase, to produce more cAMP from ATP. (These interactions are all thought to involve changes in protein conformation.) The resulting cAMP released into the cytoplasm binds to the regulatory subunits (R) of one or more protein kinases, releasing active catalytic subunits (C) (two from each R_2C_2 molecule) that now have protein kinase activity. These catalyze the phosphorylation of specific proteins, leading to at least two major kinds of effects: (1) direct activation and inactivation of specific (mostly rate limiting) enzymes, such as glycogen synthetase and glycogen phosphorylase in liver and muscle; (2) enhanced transcription of genes for specific proteins, including regulatory enzymes, such as pyruvate carboxylase, PEP carboxykinase, tyrosine aminotransferase (and some other enzymes concerned with amino acid catabolism and gluconeogenesis). Activations and inactivations occur either by direct phosphorylation (of some serine and threonine hydroxyl groups), via the activated cAMP-dependent protein kinase catalytic subunits or via specific kinases activated directly or indirectly by the cAMP-kinase (in a cascade). Such cascades are involved in the well-known activation/inactivation paths for glycogen phosphorylase and glycogen synthetase, respectively, by which glucagon (or catecholamines) enhances glycogen breakdown, simultaneously enhanced phosphorylase and inhibited synthetase activities. Various phosphatases (some of which are also regulated) serve to remove the added phosphate groups from these proteins; and a constant stream of new cAMP is needed to maintain the pattern of phosphorylation. [cAMP is rapidly degraded by inherent phosphodiesterases (sensitive to caffeine and theophylline inhibition).] Catecholamines use a mechanism similar to that of glucagon in carrying out their (very similar) effects on glycogen metabolism, although the pattern of phosphorylation of some target proteins is not entirely identical. The effects of glucagon on liver gluconeogenesis are not as fast and are accomplished by effects on the levels of mRNAs (and synthesis) of key enzymes, through increased (or decreased) rates of transcription and/or mRNA stabilization. The result is an accumulation and increased activity of enzymes, such as pyruvate carboxylase, necessary for the reversal of the three "irreversible" steps of glycolysis (Table 2.3), and concomitant decreases in other enzymes necessary for glucose oxidation or fatty acid synthesis (such as pyruvate kinase and malic enzyme) (see e.g., Goodridge, 1987).

Insulin secretion has (or is accompanied by) the opposite effect on these processes (Figure 2.2), including the phosphorylations, but the mechanism of action is still unclear. Some of the "effect" may simply be the indirect result of less glucagon. However, insulin also causes a host of changes, indicated by phosphorylation and dephosphorylation, leading to enzyme activation and inactivation, increased or decreased gene expression, and translocation of certain glucose transporter proteins that work in the plasma membrane (see Gould and Bell, 1990). Insulin also binds to specific cell surface receptors (Figure 2.4B). This binding may require glucose tolerance factors for optimal effectiveness (see Chapter 7, Chromium). The receptor complex has tyrosine kinase activity. This may result in the activation of some specific serine/threonine kinases that phosphorylate some important enzymes (including glycogen synthetase and pyruvate dehydrogenase) involved in glycogen synthesis and glucose oxidation, but at sites different from those phosphorylated through cAMP (Czech et al., 1988; E. Krebs, presentation of FASEB annual meeting, 1989). A key enzyme in this scheme may be casein kinase II, which appears to phosphorylate the same specific sites on those proteins as occurs with insulin. Insulin, however, also causes dephosphorylation, of other sites on the same and other proteins/enzymes, and this may be carried out by (1) deactivation of a protein phosphatase inhibitor (PPI), leading to activation of a phosphatase that hydrolyzes specific serine–phosphate residues on some enzymes (e.g., the cAMP-dependent sites on glycogen synthetase, causing synthetase activation); and (2) deactivation of a multifunctional protein kinase (MFPK) recently isolated (Ramakrishna and Benjamin, 1988) that phosphorylates some of these same sites. Some actions of insulin may also occur at the level of the cell membrane via phosphoinositides (Saltiel et al., 1986) (see Chapter 5, Inositol).

Apart from enzyme activation/inactivation, insulin has vital effects of glucose transport and also alters gene expression of some enzymes (notably glucokinase in the liver). (This enzyme aids in glucose phosphorylation when the hexokinase system is "overburdened.") It also releases lipoprotein lipase (LPL) from its inositide anchor to promote hydrolysis (and uptake) of incoming triacylglycerol (Chan et al., 1988) (see Chapter 3). Diffusion of glucose into cells is facilitated by a family of specific transporter proteins, expressed differentially in different cells (see Garvey et al., 1989). Only one of these (specific for adipocytes and cells of cardiac and skeletal muscle) is regulated by insulin. (Glucose uptake by liver is not regulated by insulin.) This regulation probably occurs at three levels: (1) activation of transporter activity, (2) translocation to the cell surface (both of which are rapid effects) (Calderhead and Lienhard, 1988), and (3) enhanced gene transcription and synthesis (Garvey et al., 1989). Regulation of this specific glucose transporter in muscle and fat provides the main mechanism for lowering blood glucose concentrations, and may be considered the most important action of insulin.

Glucose tolerance. The response of the body to the influx of glucose from the diet is monitored to determine "glucose tolerance." Glucose tolerance or intolerance is determined by the rate at which the inherent mechanisms for removing excess glucose from the blood perform their functions. Glucose tolerance is usually measured by following blood glucose concentrations 15 min to 2 or 3 hr after an oral load of 50–100 g glucose,

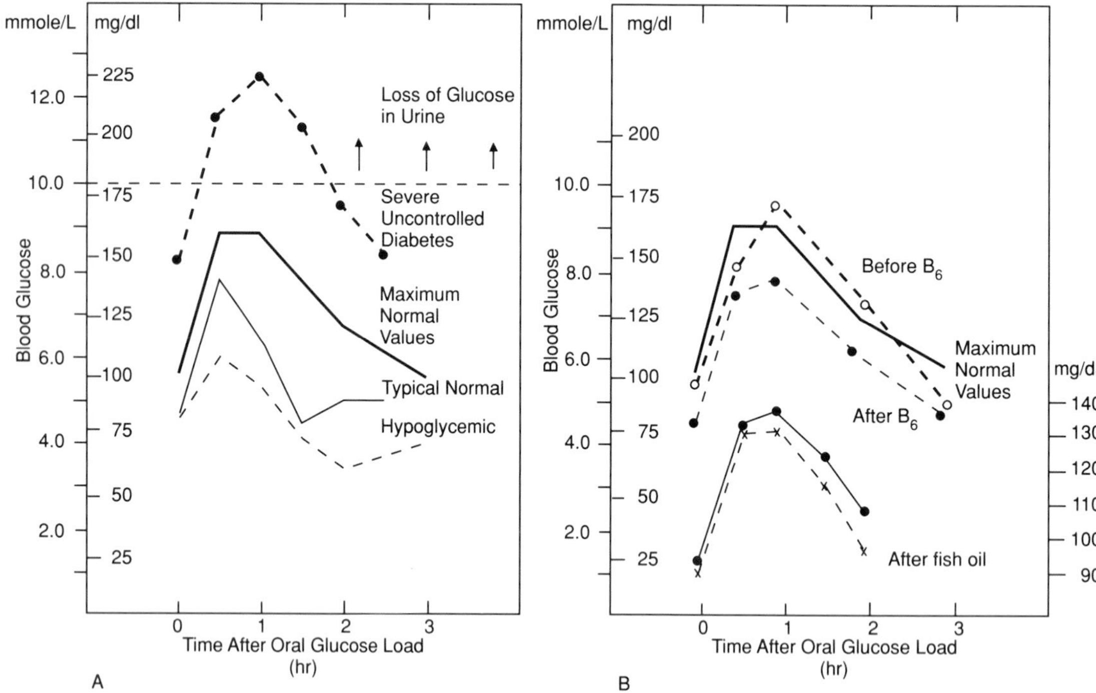

Figure 2.5. **(A)** Glucose tolerance in the normal state and in diabetes. [*Source:* Data for normal and diabetic subjects from Reed (1980). Data for maximum normal values from Coelingh-Benningk and Schreurs (1975).] **(B)** Glucose intolerance in pregnancy and effects of B_6 and fish oil treatments. Mean response of 14 women with gestational diabetes is presented, before and after treatment with vitamin B_6. [*Source:* Redrawn from Coelingh-Benningk and Schreurs (1975).] Mean response of 29 patients with various hyperlipoproteinemias (lower right-hand ordinate). [*Source:* Redrawn from Zak et al. (1989).]

given after fasting overnight (Figure 2.5A). The shape of the resulting curve is determined by (1) the capacity of the body to secrete adequate amounts of insulin; (2) the availability of other nutritional factors necessary for insulin binding and effectiveness (including glucose tolerance factors, chromium, fish oils, and fiber); (3) the rate of insulin catabolism; (4) the presence of insulin antagonists; and, finally, (5) the release of counterregulatory factors, like glucagon, to halt the continuing fall in blood glucose when the actions of insulin have been accomplished. Lesions in any aspect of the insulin pathway, from its synthesis to its binding and degradation, will alter glucose tolerance.

The degree of insulin release and its effectiveness determine how soon blood glucose reaches its peak and how high is the peak attained (normally not more than 160 mg/dl after 30–60 min) (Figure 2.5A). The same mechanisms determine how long it takes blood glucose to return to normal levels (70–105 mg/dl) (normally, 1.5–2 hr). A high "fasting glucose level" (at 0 time), a higher than normal and/or delayed peak, and delays in returning to normal are the hallmarks of glucose intolerance and diabetes. When blood glucose levels exceed 180 mg/dl, glucose is lost in the urine, because kidney tubules cannot reabsorb it fast enough. In the diabetic, repeated episodes of hyperglycemia are thought to be the primary cause of the neuropathy, microangiopathy, and other pathology associated with this disease (see more below). An overresponse to glucose intake, resulting in a lower peak, a more rapid return, and, in fact, an overshooting so that plasma glucose falls below normal, are the hallmarks of "hypoglycemia" (Figure 2.5A) and may precede the development of some forms of diabetes. (Nutritional factors that can influence glucose tolerance are discussed later in this chapter.)

Functions of glucose. The main function of glucose (and indeed of dietary carbohydrate) is to provide energy to cells for their numerous anabolic activities. (Energy is derived through glycolysis ± the Krebs cycle, which do not and do require oxygen, respectively.) Cells in certain tissues (notably the brain and blood) are limited in terms of the substrates they can absorb and use for energy. Blood cells can only burn glucose. (Red blood cells do not even have mitochondria and the Krebs cycle.) Brain cells are the same, except that many of them can switch to ketones when present in high concentrations (see Chapter 4 and Figures 4.9 and 4.10, for further discussion). It is thus essential that glucose always be available in the blood.

As already illustrated, the human and animal body is beautifully organized to maintain blood glucose concentrations within certain limits (Figure 2.5A; see also Table 1.6). Immediately after a carbohydrate meal, this is controlled by the actions of insulin; later on by the actions of glucagon on the liver. Indeed, the liver has a major role in the maintenance of blood glucose concentrations, through breakdown of glycogen and/or gluconeogenesis.

Additional functions of glucose are as a substrate for formation of other substances, including specific sugars (for glycoproteins, glycolipids, and nucleotides), nonessential amino acids, and specific fatty acids (see more below).

Galactose Metabolism

Depending on the diet, and certainly in the case of the infant, large amounts of galactose from milk lactose may also enter the blood from the small intestine. Galactose does not affect insulin secretion, and almost all of it enters the liver where it is converted to uridine diphosphate glucose (UDP-glucose) by the following pathway:

$$\text{gal} \xrightarrow{\text{ATP} \rightarrow \text{ADP}} \text{gal-1-phosphate} \xrightarrow[\text{(transferase)}]{\text{UDP-glu} \rightarrow \text{glu}} \text{UDP-gal} \xrightarrow[\text{(epimerase)}]{} \text{UDP-glu}$$

The resulting UDP-glucose is then ready for incorporation into glycogen (Figure 2.2) for later utilization in the maintenance of blood glucose concentrations. Since equal amounts of glucose are absorbed with the galactose when lactose is the source, the glucose will be used for immediate energy by most tissues and for glycogen production by the muscles and liver. Abnormally high levels of blood galactose (galactosemia) sometimes occur in newborn infants who have a genetic lack of the transferase enzyme. This can result in loss of galactose in the urine, and long-term cataract formation, neuropathy, and other pathologic symptoms that probably arise through formation of sugar alcohols (see below, Sugar Alcohol Production and Chapter 18). Traces of galactose will also be used to form the carbohydrate units added to membrane and serum/plasma glycoproteins and glycolipids (see below, Non-Energy-Related Functions of Carbohydrates).

Fructose Metabolism

The fate of fructose can be quite different. Again, the liver is the main site of its metabolism, and increased fructose levels in the blood do not evoke a release of insulin. Except in a situation where fructose is the only source of carbohydrate entering from the intestine and there are no appreciable glycogen stores, most of the fructose will be converted by the liver to intermediates of the glycolytic pathway. (See steps in Fig. 2.6.) Because the glycolytic pathway in the liver is working in the direction of pyruvate formation from glucose, after a meal containing glucose as well as fructose (as in the case of sucrose intake), the metabolites of fructose will also be converted to pyruvate and/or α-glycerophosphate (for triglyceride synthesis). Pyruvate will then be converted to acetyl-CoA; only small portions of this will be used for energy metabolism through the Krebs cycle, and the rest will be converted to fatty acid. Thus, when fructose enters the liver paired with glucose (which is the usual dietary situation), it becomes a direct source of carbons for fatty acid and triglyceride synthesis (Kupke and Lamprecht, 1967; MacDonald, 1980), rather than for glucose production. Indeed, it appears that fatty acid synthesis is a planned adaptation to fructose-containing diets, in that fructose itself increases the amounts and activities of key enzymes involved in fatty acid (FA) synthesis, including acetyl-CoA carboxylase (the first step in FA synthesis), FA synthetase itself, malic enzyme (which produces cytosolic NADPH needed for FA synthesis), and pyruvate kinase, the last step in glycolysis, producing pyruvate (Goodridge, 1987). The mechanism of the fructose effect is unknown, but it results in increased enzyme synthesis because of increased amounts of specific mRNAs. The increase in mRNAs is probably not due to increased transcription (Goodridge, 1987; Noguchi et al., 1982), indicating that enhanced stabilization of the message must be involved. Insulin and triiodothyronine also increase these enzymes, insulin by increasing transcription. (Glucagon has the opposite effect, suppressing transcription and probably accelerating degradation of the mRNAs.) But the fructose effect occurs even in the absence of insulin.

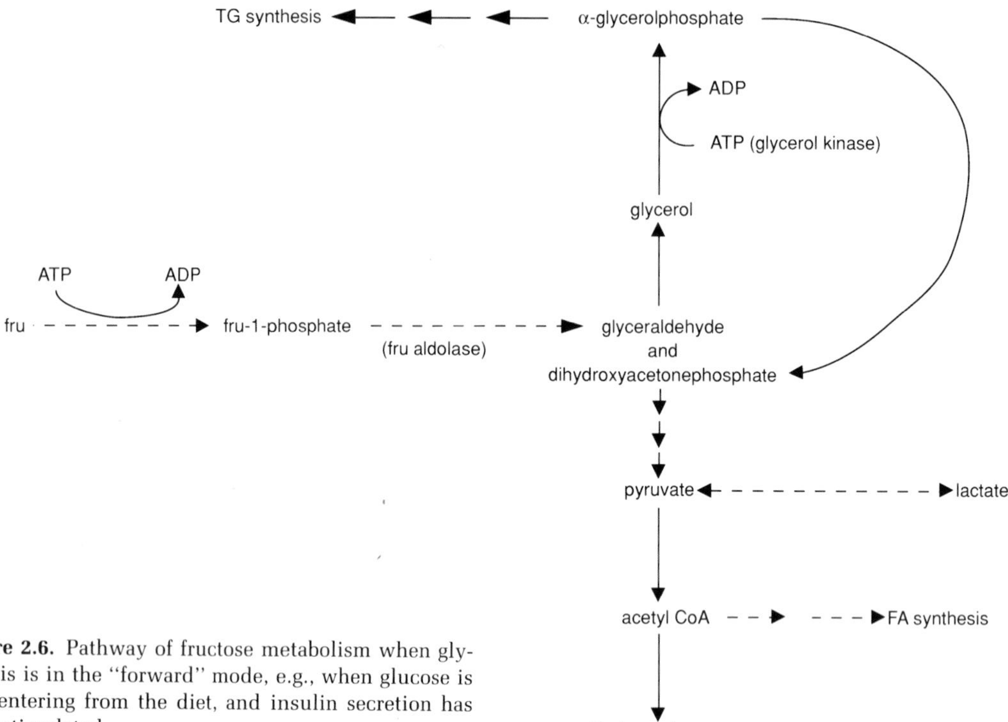

Figure 2.6. Pathway of fructose metabolism when glycolysis is in the "forward" mode, e.g., when glucose is also entering from the diet, and insulin secretion has been stimulated.

If fructose is the only carbohydrate in the ingested food, or dietary glucose concentrations are minimal, fructose metabolism is different. Fructose is again converted to dihydroxyacetone phosphate (DHAP) and glyceraldehyde (see above), but these are then used by the liver to form glucose or glucose-6-phosphate by a reversal of the first part of the glycolytic pathway, from aldolase back. (Glyceraldehyde is converted to glyceraldehyde-3-phosphate, via α-glycerol phosphate, and combines with DHAP.) The glucose-6-phosphate formed can then be used for glucose secretion into the blood or for storage as glycogen for later use.

One potential difficulty with ingestion of large amounts of fructose (or sucrose) is a reduction in the amount of liver cell adenosine triphosphate (ATP) through the rapid phosphorylation of fructose, leading to a reduction in the rate of biosynthetic processes, including protein synthesis (Maenpaa et al., 1968). It may also result in the formation of lactic acid and raise plasma uric acid concentrations (MacDonald, 1980), the former resulting mainly from a lag in the ability of the cells to regenerate NAD^+ from NADH produced through fructose glycolysis and the latter due to an increased breakdown of AMP to adenosine, inosine, and then uric acid, induced by the depression of ATP concentrations (MacDonald, 1980). At the same time, fructose does not require insulin for transport into cells (nor cause its secretion) and might thus theoretically be preferable as a sweetener for the diabetic. However, some studies on rats, where 15% fructose was substituted for some of the starch in the diet, showed that long-term, moderate fructose levels in the diet raised fasting levels of serum insulin and glucose and significantly enhanced the rate of insulin secretion in response to oral glucose (Blakley et al., 1981), suggesting some induction of glucose intolerance. Other evidence of pathology via high fructose/sucrose diets is accumulating and may involve the formation of sugar alcohols (see later in this chapter).

Non-Energy-Related Functions of Carbohydrate

Although carbohydrate (as glucose) may be regarded as the preferred energy source in the metabolism of man and animals, this is by far not the only function of carbohydrates in living systems and in man. Carbohydrates form polysaccharide chains attached to proteins or lipids, containing amino sugars (such as glucosamine and galactosamine), as well as more exotic sugars (such as fucose, mannose, and sialic acid) (Figure 2.7). As such, they are important constituents of tissue antigens (in the cell membrane) and secreted proteins. Ribose is, of course, also an important substituent of nucleotides and nucleic acids (formed in the pentose shunt from glucose-6-phosphate). Perhaps most importantly, large amounts of polysaccharides are found in the form of glycosaminoglycans, such as chondroitin sulfate, hyaluronic acid, and dermatan sulfate (Figure 2.7). These substances containing sugars with one or more oxidized carbons, such as glucuronic acid, are associated with protein (Figure 2.7), and as such, are part of the interstitial fluid matrix (gel) and the cartilage of connective tissue. The various sugars required are formed from glucose and not ingested as such. (Glucose itself need not even be eaten, since amino acids can also be converted to glucose.)

Carbohydrates in Health and Disease

Foods and Glucose Tolerance

Vitamins and trace elements necessary for the utilization and metabolism of digestible carbohydrates. Figure 2.8 presents the vitamins required for the activity of the various metabolic pathways directly involving glucose and other hexoses, as far as we understand them today. Obviously, a wide variety of B vitamins are utilized: most especially, nicotinamide (niacin) and pantothenic acid in the forms of NAD^+/NADH and coenzyme A, respectively, and thiamine.

What is not commonly known is that pyridoxine (vitamin B_6) may also play a role. Specifically, it was shown 30 years ago that pyridoxal phosphate is bound to glycogen phosphorylase (Krebs and Fischer, 1964; Tu et al., 1971). While this vitamin is not essential for the enzyme activity of phosphorylase, a deficiency of the vitamin can result in a 60%–70% reduction of total muscle phosphorylase in the liver (Krebs and Fischer, 1964). Evidence for another, more indirect, function of vitamin B_6 in carbohydrate metabolism comes from studies of the glucose intolerance of pregnancy (Figure 2.5B) and of some diabetics (see Chapter 5). Here, administration of 100 mg/day of pyridoxine was effective in improving glucose tolerance. The mechanism may involve a reduction (by B_6) of the accumulation of the tryptophan metabolite, xanthurenic acid, which may bind and reduce the biologic activity of insulin.

Among the other nutrients involved in carbohydrate metabolism, chromium is of interest. The essential nature of chromium intake for animals was first shown in 1959 by Schwartz and Mertz. (For a more detailed discussion of the functions and nutrition of chromium, see Chapter 7.) It has now been well established in animals that chromium is necessary for normal glucose tolerance, and it is thought this occurs through the need for a Cr^{3+}-dependent "glucose tolerance factor," which aids in the binding of insulin to its membrane receptors (see Chapter 7). The source of chromium used to counteract glucose intolerance is probably important: that present in Brewer's Yeast (but perhaps not in torula yeast) is effective. Using an appropriate source of chromium, the results of several studies in man have shown a reduction in glucose intolerance among more than half the persons so treated (see Chapter 7). Chromium deficiency may contribute to the prevalence of glucose intolerance in the American and Western European populations, as the trace amounts present may be depleted through the refining of whole grains and sugar cane in the production of flour, sugar, and other staples of the western diet (see Chapter 7).

Glucose tolerance with different foods. The generalization has been made that ingestion of complex carbohydrates (starches) requires a less drastic response on the part of the homeostatic mechanisms controlling blood glucose than does the ingestion of sugars, because of a slower release of glucose during digestion, but this is not always so. There is a considerable variation introduced by the food or diet in which the carbohydrate is incorporated. The structure of the various plant starches themselves (and their casings) also may not be identical, and this may contribute to the greater or lesser rise in blood glucose observed after eating them. Table 2.4 summarizes evidence on the response of blood glucose and insulin to ingestion of sucrose versus fructose, given in the form of cake or ice cream, and responses to ingestion of different forms of starch, in potatoes, grains, and beans. As is well known, sucrose (glu-fru) elicits more of an insulin (and blood glucose) response than fructose when given in comparable foods. [Indeed, that there is any insulin increase with fructose cake or ice cream is due to the presence of some glucose from lactose

A N-Acetyl glucosamine

CH_2OH
O OH
OH
HO
O
NH — C — CH_3

Galactose or Galactosamine (see Fig. 2-1)

D-Mannose

CH_2OH
O
OH HO
HO OH

L-Fucose

CH_3
O
OH HO
HO OH

Sialic Acid (N-acetyl neuraminic acid)

OH
HO
CH_2OH
O
OH
HN
COOH
C=O
CH_3

B

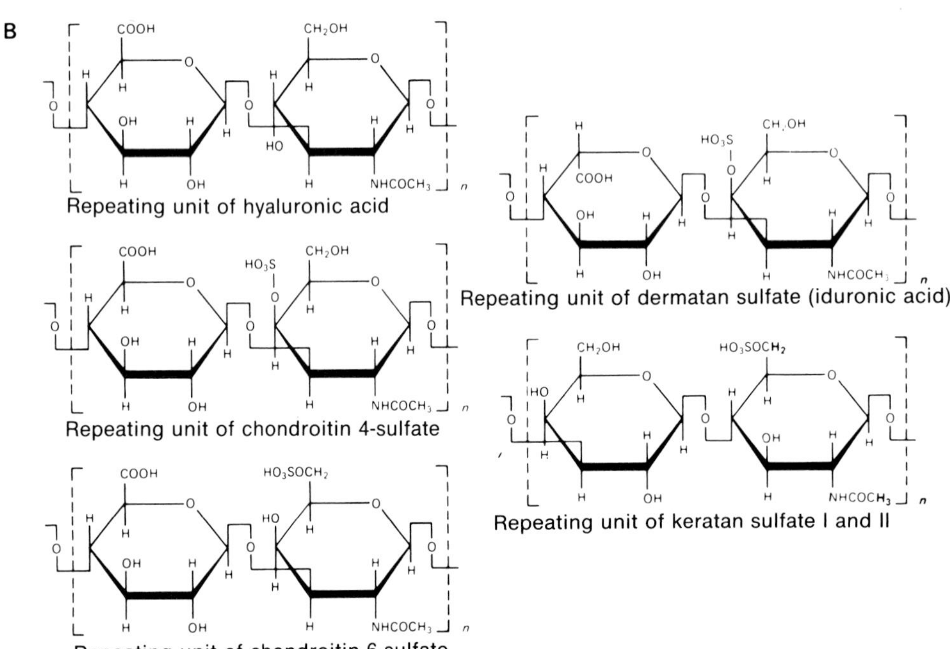

Figure 2.7. Other carbohydrates found in human and animal tissues. **(A)** On glycoproteins: polymeric units of hexoses and some other sugars (on plasma proteins, membrane proteins, etc.). **(B)** In connective tissue (glycosaminoglycans): cartilage, skin, tendon, ground substance; polymers of disaccharide units are attached to some proteins.

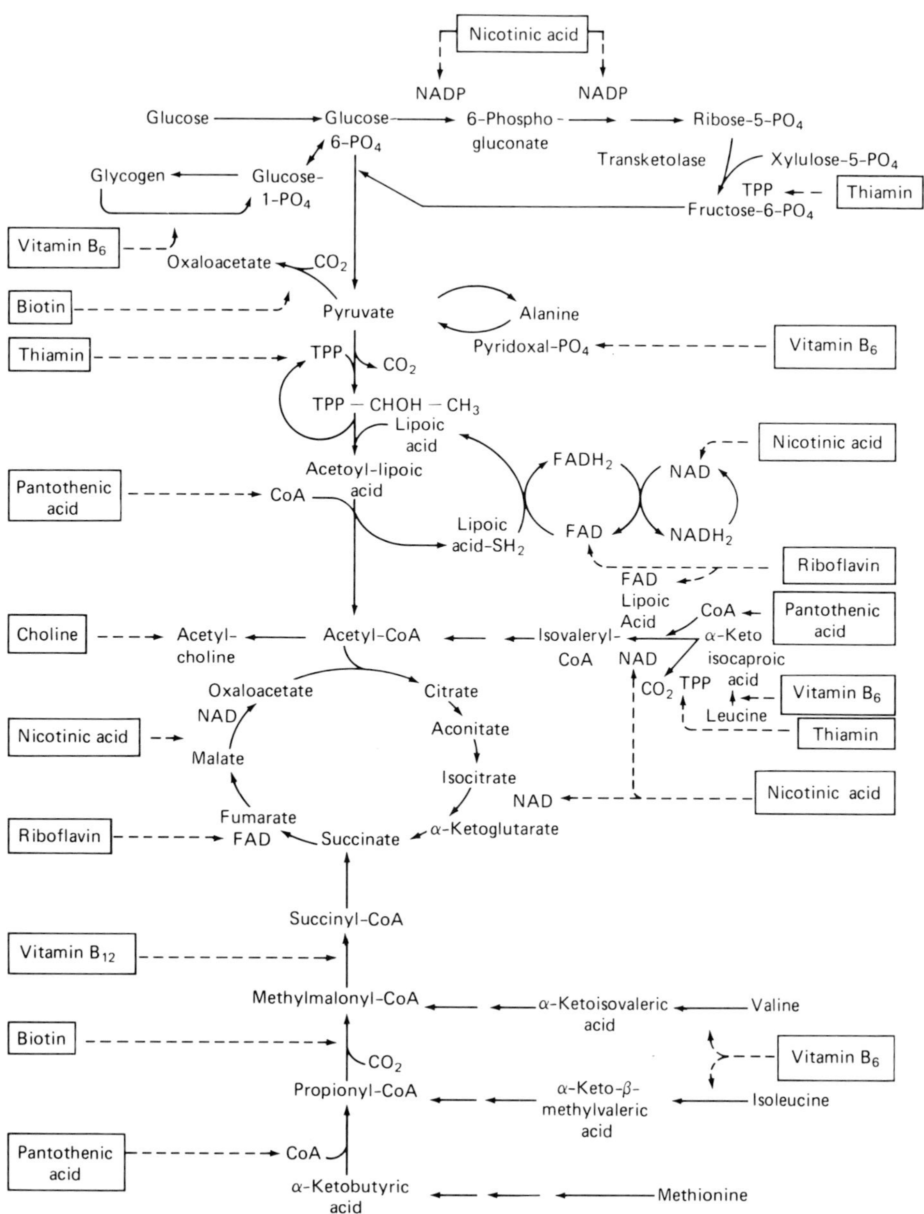

Figure 2.8. Involvement of vitamins in CHO metabolism. [*Source:* Reprinted with permission from Danforth and Munro (1980).]

and starches in the foods (see footnote *b*, Table 2.4).] What is more striking is that sucrose in ice cream puts much less of a demand on body mechanisms than sucrose in cake (despite a similar fat content). This appears to be so for both the normal individual and the diabetic. The varied responses of subjects to different starchy foods is also of great interest, notably the much more hyperglycemic effects of potatoes versus grains (Table 2.4-II) and the rather minimal effect of starches in legumes (Table 2.3). The bases for these differences are complex and poorly understood. They may involve changes in the rate of stomach emptying, differences in digestibility, and other factors determined by the protein, fat, fiber, and starch composition of the food. The rate of stomach emptying is decreased especially by fat (working via cholecystokinin; see Chapter 1) and is also diminished by dietary fibers (like pectin and guar gum) that reduce the viscosity of the contents of the stomach and duodenum (Meyer et al., 1988). With ice cream, the coldness of the

Table 2.4. Response of Serum Glucose and Insulin to Ingestion of Various Carbohydrates After Fasting Overnight

	Composition[a] (g)			Blood glucose		Insulin
Carbohydrate	Sugar or equivalent[b]	Fat	Protein	Maximum change (mg/dl)	Peak time (min)	Maximum change (IU/ml)
I. Normal subjects[c]						
Glucose only	70	—	—	67	45–60	75
Sucrose cake	63	21	7	53	30–45	75
Fructose cake	63	21	7	25	30	28
Sucrose ice cream	52	24	10	18	30–45	45
Fructose ice cream	52	24	10	—	—	10
II. Diabetics[c,d]						
Glucose only	50–70	—	—	110–140	45–60	36
Sucrose cake	63	21	7	101	60	140
Fructose cake	63	21	7	20	45	45
Sucrose ice cream	52	24	10	20	30–45	80
Fructose ice cream	52	24	10	15	45–60	40
Potato	50	(0)	(4)	125	60	44
White bread	50	(2)	(8)	87	60	25
Corn	50	(3)	(4)	73	45–60	23
Rice	50	(0)	(4)	69	45–60	14
III. Normal subjects[e]						
Glucose	50	—	—	62	30–45	—
Wheat	50	1	9	45	30	—
Rice	50	0	4	51	30	—
Chick peas	50	5	17	11	45	—
Red kidney beans	50	1	19	20	45	—

[a] Values in parentheses are from Food Tables.
[b] Glucose equivalent (mainly as starches) in the case of potato, bread, corn, rice, and legumes. Cakes contained an additional 28 g carbohydrate (mainly starch) and ice cream about 10 g lactose. These other carbohydrates account for the insulin release after eating the fructose foods.
[c] Data from Crapo et al. (1982).
[d] Data from Crapo et al. (1981).
[e] Data from Dilawari et al. (1981).

food might also play a role (Crapo et al., 1982). Diets with fish oil, rich in omega-3 (n-3) unsaturated fatty acids, also may have an ameliorating effect on glucose tolerance (Figure 2.5B). The mechanism of this effect is unknown, but may involve increased sensitivity to insulin at the cell level (Vrana et al., 1988), and changes in prostaglandins (see Chapter 3). The accumulating data will have a special significance for the diabetic.

Formation of Sugar Alcohols and Glycated Proteins

One of the potential consequences of elevations in blood hexose concentrations (whether glucose, fructose, or galactose) is the formation of sugar alcohols; another is the nonenzymatic glycosylation of proteins, also termed "glycation." Both of these processes are associated with long-term pathology of the nerves, blood vessels, kidney, lens (and pancreas), as occurs in diabetes and galactosemia (see below). Even in persons with a marginal or normal glucose tolerance (and perhaps also with a high fructose intake) some formation of sugar alcohols and/or "abnormal" glycoproteins may occur and contribute to the general deterioration of functions associated with the aging process.

Sugar alcohols. Formation from glucose and galactose is catalyzed by the enzyme, aldol reductase, producing sorbitol and dulcitol (or galactitol), respectively (Figure 2.9A). Sorbitol can be converted to fructose, but the opposite reaction also takes place, via polyol dehydrogenase, namely, the conversion of excess fructose to sorbitol. Indeed, this reaction is favored at physiological pH (Jedziniak et al., 1981), although the

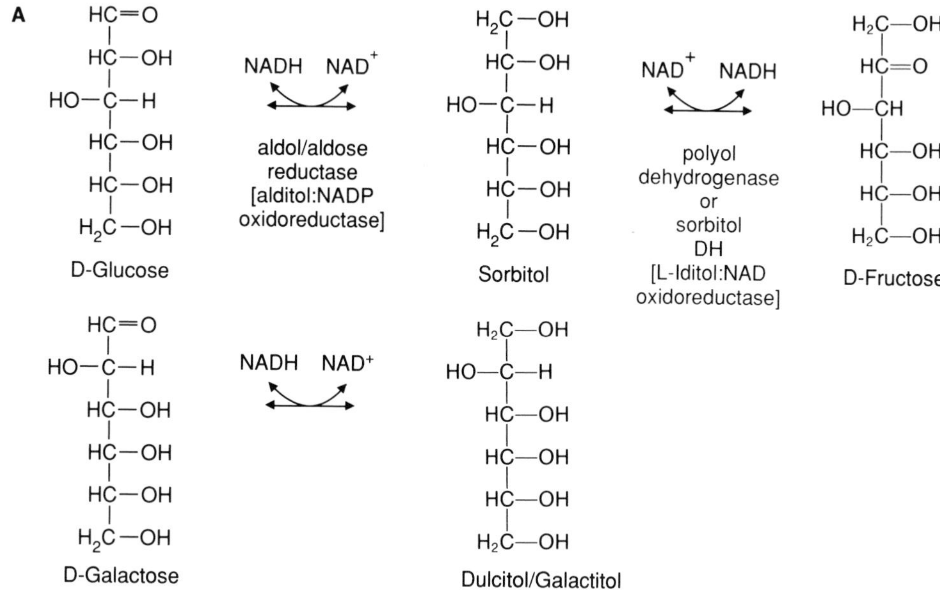

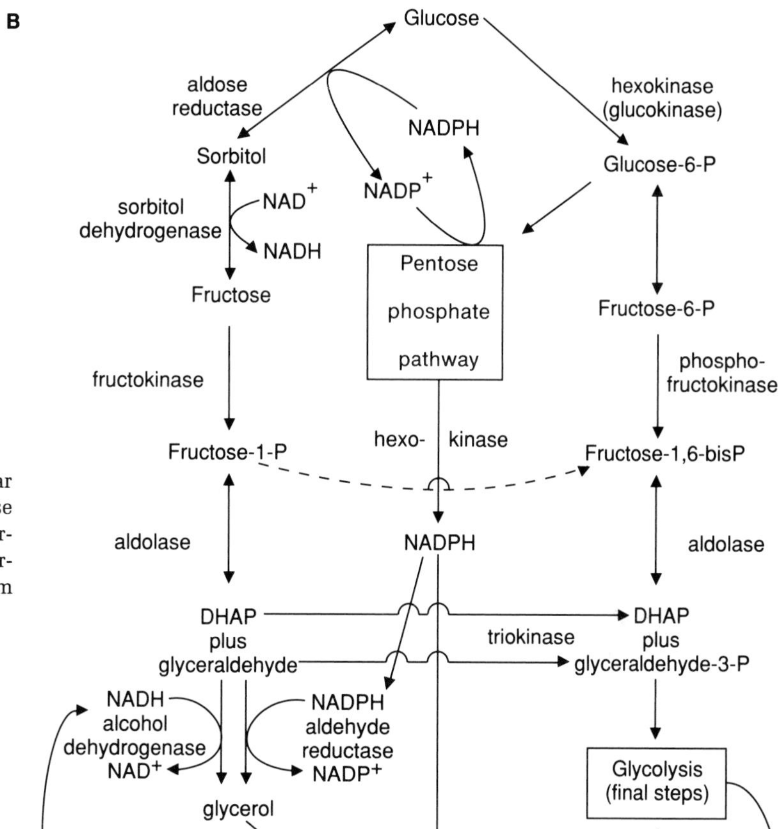

Figure 2.9. (A) Formation of sugar alcohols from glucose and galactose via aldol/aldose reductase. **(B)** Sorbitol metabolism in relation to intermediary metabolism, modified from Jeffery and Jornvall (1983).

overriding consideration for the direction of the reaction will be substrate (and cofactor) concentrations, pushing it one way or the other by "mass action." Excess fructose should also block the conversion of sorbitol (from glucose) to fructose, further promoting sorbitol accumulation (if the diet is high in sucrose). Isozymes of aldol reductase are present in most cells, including those of the liver (although the sorbitol pathway is not very active in this organ; Jeffery and Jornvall, 1983); but the aldol reductases are concentrated especially in the Schwann cells of peripheral nerves, in kidney papillae, and in the epithelium of the lens. They are also abundant in the pancreas (in cells of the insulin-forming islets of Langerhans), where sorbitol formation may be part of the signaling mechanism for insulin release (see Jeffery and Jornvall, 1983); and in male reproductive organs, where sorbitol (and fructose) are produced for seminal fluid. [Sperm utilize the fructose (and sorbitol) for energy after forming fructose-6-phosphate (rather than fructose-1-phosphate, as in the liver) to directly enter glycolysis.] Polyol dehydrogenase is present in all of these same tissues.

The polyol or sorbitol pathway fits into the rest of metabolism as generalized in Figure 2.9B, although cells will vary with regard to the relative activities of the enzymes involved, expression of isozymes, availabilities of NADPH/$NADP^+$, ATP/ADP, etc. (see Jeffery and Jornvall, 1983). It is noteworthy that there is considerable homology between aldol reductases and aldehyde reductases in terms of amino acid sequence, and similarly, between polyol/sorbitol dehydrogenases (iditol oxidoreductases) and alcohol dehydrogenases. Indeed, in the liver, the latter two may be the same enzyme (Jornvall et al., 1981). [The latter are also (in general) zinc-dependent (see Chapter 7, Zinc).] How and if total enzyme amounts are regulated is still unclear, although a high fructose diet will increase polyol dehydrogenase activity, at least in some tissues (Bellomo et al., 1987), and this may also be the case in diabetes.

Sorbitol accumulates in the tissues of animals and humans with diabetes (see next section on Diabetes, and Dyck et al., 1988). This can be explained on the basis that hyperglycemia increases concentrations of free glucose (over glucose-6-phosphate), in cells of sensitive tissues (like the central nervous system, pancreas, kidney, and lens) resulting in a greater production of sorbitol via aldol reductase. A high fructose diet has the same kind of effect (Bellomo et al., 1987; Lewis et al., 1990; Fields et al., 1989). On a theoretical basis, here the most likely mechanism of sorbitol accumulation would seem to be by mass action via polyol dehydrogenase (Figure 2.9). This still seems the most reasonable concept, although Bellomo et al. (1987) have reported that an inhibitor of *aldol reductase* blocked the increase in sorbitol in rat kidney that occurred with fructose feeding, suggesting that the sorbitol came from increased glucose rather than fructose. [However, in their studies, the activity of the sorbitol dehydrogenase also appeared to be lower in rats given the inhibitor (tolrestat).] It is noteworthy that the accumulation of sorbitol (and glucose) in rat tissues occurs whether the high fructose intake is in the form of sucrose or fructose per se (Fields et al., 1989). Moreover, the effect appears to be exacerbated by copper deficiency and occurs much more in men than in women.

Formation of excess galactitol (or dulcitol) occurs in the same sensitive nonhepatic tissues where sorbitol can be a problem, when blood (and thus cellular) galactose concentrations are increased, as in galactosemia (see later). Since the liver normally deals with most of the entering dietary fructose and galactose, and other tissues may have only low (or no) expression of the enzymes required for phosphorylation of these sugars, the excess galactose and fructose may, in general, only be metabolized by the enzymes of the polyol path (Figure 2.9A).

The presence of substantial sugar alcohol concentrations (e.g., >0.1 μmol sorbitol/g in sural nerves; Dyck et al., 1988) is associated with local pathologic changes. The mechanism by which sorbitol may produce these changes is not known, although cell swelling from osmosis may be a factor, as may the promotion of protein glycation (see more below). An indirect effect involving reductions in inositol ("myoinositol") concentrations does not appear to be involved (Dyck et al., 1988).

Protein glycation/glycosylation. Nonenzymatic addition of glucose, galactose, or fructose to proteins occurs upon their exposure to the free sugars over days and weeks. (For fructose glycation, see Monnier et al., 1986; McPherson et al., 1989; Oimomi et al., 1989; Suarez et al., 1989; for galactose glycation, see Hitz and Dain, 1988.) The major initial product appears to be the result of an interaction of the aldehyde (or keto) group of the sugar, with a lysine ε-amino group on the protein, to form a Schiff base that rearranges to a more stable "Amadori" product (Figure 2.10A) (Cerami, 1986; Cerami et al., 1987; Pongor et al., 1984). With time, there is further reaction and the

A

Aminoguanine inhibits

GLUCOSE

PROTEIN

SCHIFF BASE

AMADORI PRODUCT (more stable)

GLUCOSE-DERIVED CROSS-LINK (one kind of product)

B

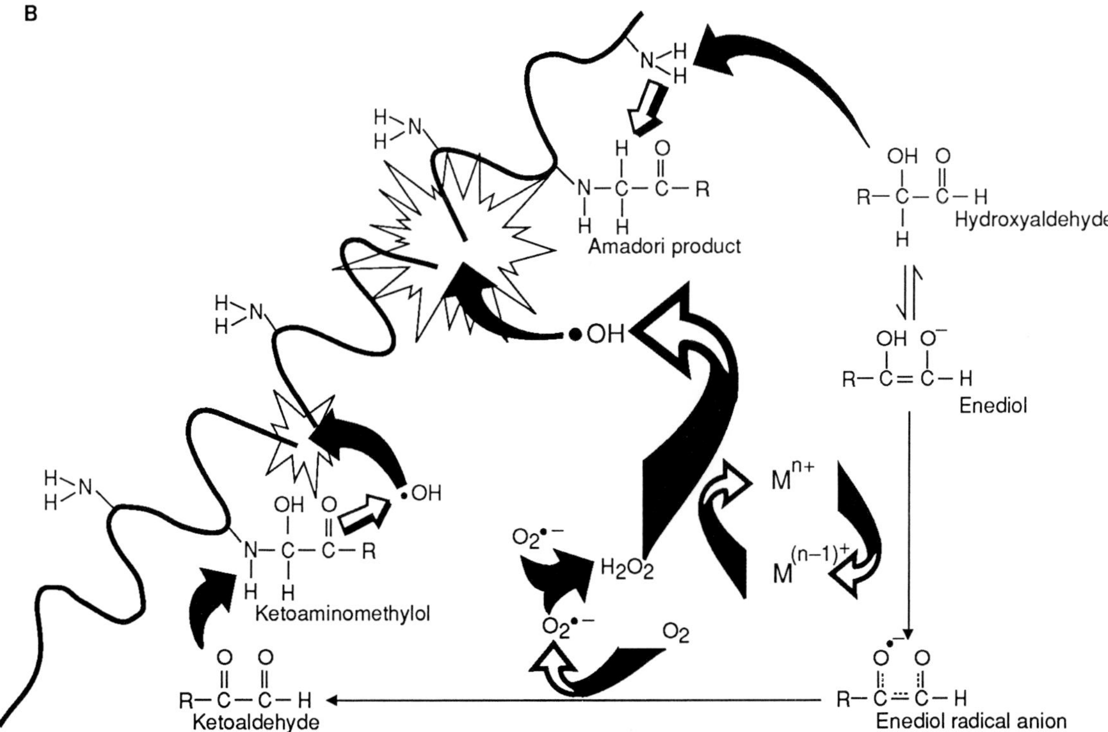

Figure 2.10. Glycation and fragmentation of proteins induced by hyperglycemia. **(A)** Glucose combines with lysine amino groups (or other amino groups) on proteins, forming a Schiff-base, which rearranges to an Amadori product. Later, two of these modified amino acid side chains can form a cross-linked derivative, the process of which is inhibited by aminoguanidine (interacting with the Amadori product). (Based on Cerami et al., 1987). **(B)** Interaction of Amadori product with hydroxyl radicals to produce fragmentation of the polypeptide chain. [*Source:* Reprinted by permission from Hunt et al. (1988).]

formation of fluorescent cross-links, one of which has been characterized (Figure 2.10A) and appears to result from interaction of two glucose–Amadori products. (The presence of free L-lysine appears to enhance the reaction.) The interaction of Amadori products is inhibited by aminoguanidine, which preferentially forms a Schiff base with the reactive hydroxyketone, thus preventing its further reaction and the formation of advanced glycosylation end products (or so-called AGE products). [Inhibition by aminoguanidine also occurs in vivo in diabetic and aging rats and is currently being tested in human diabetics (Cerami et al., 1987).]

An additional aspect of the reactions between hexoses and proteins may involve glucose autoxidation and ketoaldehyde formation, also leading to chromo- and fluorophoric products (Figure 2.10A) (Wolff and Dean, 1986, 1987, 1988). This process would be enhanced by some divalent metal ions (such as Cu^{2+}) or by other oxidation processes producing peroxide and hydroxyl radicals, as occurs in conjunction with inflammatory reactions (see Figure 5.33). It would be inhibited by antioxidants, deficiencies of which have been implicated in the formation of cataracts (Taylor, 1989) and in aging (see vitamin E, selenium). Another potential result is protein fragmentation (Figure 2.10B). Of special interest is the observation that sorbitol may *enhance* formation of ketoaldehydes produced experimentally by incubating bovine serum albumin with 25 m*M* glucose (Hunt et al., 1988). As both glucose and sorbitol are increased in certain dietary and disease conditions, this may explain some of the detrimental effects of sugar alcohols, as well. Finally, it should be noted that (as shown in bacteria) glycation of *DNA* probably also occurs and may result in changes in gene function. The potential damage to the human organism may thus not be confined to proteins.

High sugar diets. The question is then whether in normal individuals high sugar diets enhance the likelihood of sugar alcohol and macromolecular glycation reactions in the body, leading to some pathology. At least on a theoretical level, this is a reasonable supposition, although the body's tolerance (including its ability to degrade resulting products) may also be high. Certainly the final verdict is not in, but the following observations have been made.

Regarding sucrose and fructose, earlier (controversial) studies reported that high sucrose diets in rats resulted in glucose intolerance and insulin resistance (Cohen, 1975; Rosenmann et al., 1976). Recent work in rabbits indicates it also results in hypercholesterolemia and enhances atherogenesis (Sparks et al., 1986). The main factor in these studies may, however, be the fructose (in the sucrose), as suggested by numerous studies with sucrose-, starch-, and fructose-fed rats (see Lewis et al., 1990), also indicating the development of insulin resistance (decreased insulin effectiveness) (Blakley et al., 1981; Tobey et al., 1982) and retinopathy (Boot-Handford and Heath, 1980, 1981). Others have reported the development of impaired insulin binding and insulin resistance in humans on a high fructose intake (Beck-Nielson et al., 1980). Earlier human studies reported that a moderate fructose intake (72 g/day) for 2 years had no significant effects on fasting serum triglyceride or cholesterol concentrations (Huttanen et al., 1975) in normal subjects or in controlled juvenile diabetics (Akerblom et al., 1972). However, more sensitive parameters (such as tissue sorbitol and glycation) will need to be measured. This is especially so, as fructose intake has been increasing steadily through the rising use of high fructose corn sweetener ("HFCS") in processed foods. The latter is produced from glucose (released from corn starch) by isomerization, and the resulting preparations typically contain 42%–56% fructose solids (Glinsmann et al., 1986). Data for 1984 suggest that about half of the sugar (including sweetener) eaten daily by the average American is from fructose, amounting to 46 g/day. (Most is from processed foods.) This indicates that some individuals are taking in much larger amounts.

Lactose is less likely to produce a large rise in blood galactose because it is split much more slowly during its intestinal absorption than sucrose (see earlier). Fructose also tends to be absorbed more slowly than glucose (or fructose from sucrose), so only large intakes may be problematic.

Nutrition of the Diabetic

Diabetes is defined by an elevated fasting blood glucose concentration and an abnormally high glucose tolerance curve (see earlier discussion). Two forms are recognized: insulin-dependent diabetes mellitus (IDDM) (type I) and noninsulin-dependent diabetes mellitus (NIDDM) (type II). Type I, characterized by an insufficient endogenous production of insulin (or insulin autoimmunity; Johnson et al., 1990) and a tendency toward ketosis and ketoacidosis (see Chapter 3), is most commonly detected in childhood and is thus termed "juvenile onset." It tends to generate the most severe forms of the disease and requires insulin treatment. Type I diabetes is thought to arise from defects in the insulin gene or in genes for other aspects of pancreatic β-cell formation that lead to a decreased production or release of insulin. The second category is a catch-all for other forms of diabetes with ineffective or inadequate insulin. This usually develops in the adult ("adult onset"), is much more common, and can usually be managed by diet alone. Genetic alterations in the insulin receptor, leading to loss of its tyrosine kinase activity (Figure 2.4), and probably hypersecretion of "amylin," a newly discovered modulator of insulin action co-secreted from the β-cells (Leighton and Cooper, 1990), are some of the lesions responsible for this form of human diabetes and insulin resistance (Odawara et al., 1989; Taira et al., 1989). A majority of diabetics develop glucose intolerance as adults.

The diabetic not on insulin therapy must reduce his/her consumption of glucose, sucrose, and other simple sugars that are cleaved to glucose during absorption. If complex carbohydrate is consumed along with other nutrients, this may be better tolerated. It is generally thought that a carbohydrate intake of 40%–60% of calories is safe (Bantle et al., 1986; Friedman, 1980), and some studies suggest that, for mild diabetes, an even higher intake is beneficial (Brunzell et al., 1971). Recent studies suggest that replacing some of the carbohydrate calories with monounsaturated fat (to 33% of calories) (Garg et al., 1988), or supplementing with fish oil (see earlier, Glucose Tolerance and Figure 2.5B) may be beneficial. Additional considerations should be the intake of adequate fiber, pyridoxine, and chromium, for reasons already described above. It is still uncertain whether the long-term substitution of fructose would be useful (Wang and van Eys, 1981), although it may have some antiketogenic effects, and in short-term (controlled) studies on type I and II diabetics it lowered fasting blood glucose values (and albumin glycosylation) (Bantle et al., 1986). [In the latter studies, subjects were on diets with 55% of calories as carbohydrate (21% from fructose or sucrose, plus 20%–38% from starch.)]

The insulin-treated diabetic is faced with quite another situation and must, at all costs, consume carbohydrate in conjunction with insulin. Insulin comes in various forms, with rapid and slower release. The patient must match his or her schedule for insulin release with his or her schedule of carbohydrate consumption. Failure to coordinate the two could result in hypo- or hyperglycemia and glycosuria. With slow-release forms of insulin, a pattern of eating small meals is recommended. Above all, it is well established that obesity results in (and/or exacerbates) glucose intolerance. Thus, diabetics, who are usually obese, should be strongly encouraged to reduce their caloric intake and stay slim.

The point of dietary and drug therapy for diabetes is to prevent hyperglycemia, as this, in itself, is responsible for most of the long-term pathologic consequences of the disease. Chronic hyperglycemia results in the nonenzymatic (chemical) glycation of various proteins (see above section; Figure 2.10). This is expected to alter their functions. Thickening of basement membrane proteins in the vascular bed and in kidney glomeruli, observed in diabetes, may be some of the consequences, eventually leading to impaired blood capillary function and glomerular filtration, with proteinuria (loss of protein in the urine). Formation of fluorescent cross-linked collagen (AGE products; see earlier) also correlates with the degree of retinopathy, nephropathy, and angiopathy of diabetes (type I) (Monnier et al., 1986). Accumulation of sorbitol (Figure 2.10) in nerves, pancreas, kidney, and retinal tissue may also be related to this process and cause swelling, leading to a decrease in inositol and demyelination of the nerves (Friedman, 1980; Gabbay, 1975), and to cataract formation within the lens of the eye (Bunn and Higgins, 1981). Accumulation of sorbitol has been directly implicated in loss of nervous function, as shown by biopsy of the sural nerves of diabetics (Dyck et al., 1988). Long-term treatment with inhibitors of aldose reductase may reverse nerve degeneration in such patients (Sima et al., 1988), as may treatment with inositol ("myoinositol") per se (Greene et al., 1987), shown in rats.

With regard to control of hyperglycemia, the status of diabetic patients over the preceding 5–6 weeks is monitored by the degree of hemoglobin glycosylation (red cell hemoglobin has a lifespan of about 120 days); and for shorter (and more recent) periods by the degree of albumin glycosylation or level of fructosamine (Lloyd and Marples, 1988).

Galactosemia

This is a rare genetic disorder involving a deficiency or lack of the enzyme, UDP-galactose transferase which is involved in metabolism of galactose and its conversion to glucose (see the discussion of galactose metabolism, above, and in Chapter 18). In the absence of this enzyme, galactose accumulates in the circulation, and this can have deleterious effects, including the covalent (chemical) binding of galactose to proteins (Bunn and Higgins, 1981) and the development of cataracts and neurologic damage. As with diabetes, the latter may occur through osmotic effects from intracellular formation of sugar alcohol (dulcitol, from galactose) in the lens and nerves (Gabbay et al., 1966). Aldose reductase has been shown to be responsible for the thickening of basement membranes of the capillaries of the retina in galactosemia (Robison et al., 1983). If present, galactosemia will be noted in infancy upon exposure to large amounts of lactose (as in milk). Fermented milk products, such as cheeses and yogurt, and foods containing dextrose-maltose (glucose units) do not contain as much lactose and are thus better tolerated both by the galactosemic and the lactose-intolerant individual.

Sucrose Consumption and Intolerance

The average consumption of sucrose, as an additive, in the United States has been on the order of 100 lb/year (Friend, 1976). However, this value is quite misleading as far as individuals are concerned, in that it differs greatly with age and lifestyle. About one fifth of the sucrose is in the form of nonalcoholic beverages. Studies in both the United States (Page and Friend, 1974) and Canada (Department of National Health and Welfare) have shown that soft drink consumption varies enormously with age and sex, being highest in adolescent boys and young men, then decreasing with age. From the Canadian recall study, it was calculated that adolescent males consume an average of about 210 lb sucrose/year, with young men aged 20–39 consuming about 165 lb. Recently, sucrose consumption has been declining somewhat, in favor of high fructose corn syrup (HFCS) (see first part of chapter). HFCS has about the same proportions of glucose and fructose as sucrose, and total sugar consumption still appears to be increasing (Glinsmann et al., 1986).

The question arises as to whether consumption of average or larger than average amounts of sucrose and/or fructose/glucose combinations has unhealthful consequences. The least controversial negative aspects are that (a) it can tempt people to overeat (leading to obesity, which reduces glucose tolerance); (b) high sugar foods generally are of the "empty calorie" variety (leading to a possible reduction in the consumption of essential micronutrients, like Cr); and (c) that it promotes the formation of dental caries and plaque. Sucrose, glucose, and fructose, especially in chewy foods or treats, are utilized by bacteria in the mouth to form the dextran matrix of the plaque on the surfaces of the teeth, especially between the teeth and near the gums. They also provide a substrate for the production of lactic acid by the bacteria, an acid that slowly etches the tooth enamel; although starch digestion (releasing some glucose) begins in the mouth, in general the intake of carbohydrates mainly as starches in cereal grains (especially maize) is associated with a lower incidence of dental caries (Sreebny, 1983). Similarly, lactose is not so easily hydrolyzed by bacteria in the mouth.

More controversial is the supposition that high sucrose consumption will contribute directly to the development of diabetes in humans, as has been shown experimentally in rats (see above). Some epidemiologic evidence in humans is compatible with this concept, especially from the study of Cohen on Yemenites who emigrated to Israel and changed (from consuming little or no sugar) to the normal Western pattern of sucrose consumption. A large percentage of these Yemenites developed glucose intolerance; this did not happen among the population that remained in Yemen and consumed no sugar. However, the development of obesity (among the immigrants) as another contributing factor would need to be excluded, as obesity can cause glucose intolerance (by mechanisms that are as yet poorly understood).

The ingestion of sucrose and the subsequent rapid rise in blood glucose and fructose does require rapid and drastic responses on the part of the body in order to restore these concentrations to the normal range. It requires the release of more insulin and at a more rapid rate than if glucose is more slowly infused into the blood, as is the case when many polysaccharide foods are digested and absorbed (Swan et al., 1966) (see above).

The long-term "overrelease" of insulin due to above-average sucrose consumption would be consistent with one theory of the origin of adult-onset diabetes, namely, that it results from "exhaustion" of the β-cells of the pancreas. Another possibility is the formation of extra sorbitol (and enhanced protein glycation) in the pancreas, due to the periodic increase of fructose and glucose in the blood (see earlier section). The potential connections of a deficiency of Cr (and "glucose tolerance factor") to the degree of insulin release (and pancreas "exhaustion") is unknown but should also be investigated. [The sharp rise and fall in blood glucose concentrations may also have immediate effects on the release of growth hormones, which, through the liver, may enhance insulin degradation and insulin resistance (Vallance-Owen and Bajaj, 1975), although this is not well accepted.]

Finally, the response of certain individuals to carbohydrate (and especially sucrose) consumption is to increase blood triglyceride concentrations (familial hyperlipidemia, type IV; see Chapter 3). Elevated triglyceride concentrations (in the fasting state) are a secondary "risk factor" in the development of atherosclerosis, although this does not mean that there is a cause–effect relationship (see Chapter 15, Atherosclerosis).

Lactose Intolerance

Lactose intolerance results from the absence of lactase in the brush border of the small intestine. Consequently, lactose cannot be cleaved to its constituent hexoses and is not absorbed. It then becomes a nutrient for intestinal bacteria, which produce large amounts of methane, CO_2, and even H_2 "gas," causing flatulence and other intestinal discomforts. The lactose and its bacterially formed metabolites trapped there also osmotically draw water into the intestinal lumen, which can result in cramps and diarrhea. The condition of lactase deficiency is especially common in the American black population, where the incidence is estimated at 70% among adults and 35% in children under 11 years of age (Broitman and Zamchek, 1980). [It is equally high in Arabs and Ashkenazi Jews, and in American Indian groups (Saavedra and Perman, 1989).] In the white American, intolerance occurs in only about 10%.

Because of a correlation between patterns of low lactose intake and lactase deficiency, it seemed possible that, apart from genetic factors, a pattern of long-term low lactose intake, and low α-saccharide intake in general (Bustamante et al., 1981), might also contribute to lactase deficiency. This was also suggested by studies in rats (and other animals), where lactase activity was induced or stayed elevated with lactose feeding (Lebenthal et al., 1973; Saavedra and Perman, 1989). Repeated human studies do not support this idea (Saavedra and Perman, 1989). (Further information on lactose intolerance is found in Chapter 18.)

Dietary Fiber

Fiber has been defined as that portion of the diet that is not *enzymatically* digested by our digestive enzymes and thus does not directly serve as a source of nourishment. It includes cellulose and hemicellulose from plant walls (Figure 2.1, Table 2.5), pectins (part of the "ground" substance of fruits), mucillages, and gums, which are nonstructural components of plant cells (especially abundant in apples and the white portions of citrus) (Figure 2.11). Lignins are also part of food fiber but are not strictly carbohydrate in nature, being polymers of phenylpropane. The term, "fiber," is really a misnomer, in that the material is not fibrous nor long and stringy, and can even be a soluble material (see Tables 2.1 and 2.5). The most insoluble forms of fiber are the celluloses and lignins (Figure 2.11); the most soluble are the pectins and gums; the others lie in between. The digestibility also requires further definition, since the bacterial flora of the gut do attack and degrade much of the material, especially in the colon (our own digestive enzymes, however, do not). This is particularly true of the soluble forms (like pectins and gums), but not of the celluloses and lignins. Even neutral detergent fiber, however, is digested this way (Figure 2.11) (Brauer et al., 1981). Many forms of fiber are thus nutrients for gut bacteria. A considerable portion of the inherent energy is released by gut bacteria in the form of very short-chain FAs, principally acetate, propionate, and butyrate. The rest is used for energy and degraded aerobically to CO_2 and H_2O and anaerobically to H_2 and sometimes methane. The proportions of the various acids produced are fairly constant regardless of the form of fiber administered (Savage, 1986)—40%–50% being acetate, 20% propionate, and 20% butyrate. [These acids are also produced to some extent when there is little dietary fiber, and they may partly derive from digestion of mucins (and other materials) that come from (human) cells of the intestinal mucosa (Savage, 1986).] A portion of the short-chain acids is absorbed and used by the colonic epithelial cells. Some travel beyond the colon to the liver via the portal circulation. Acetate from colonic bacteria continues beyond the liver to peripheral tissues. It is estimated that in Americans about 10% of calories may derive from these products of colonic digestion (McNeil, 1984). The remaining acids are lost in the feces.

The dietary fiber content of the American diet is quite small (in the range of 10–20 g/day) relative to that of most less industrialized countries and some Western European countries, like Finland. This can be attributed to a lower consumption of whole grains, cereals, roots and tubers, and/or fruits. Foods high in fiber include brans, derived from whole grains (from wheat and oats to buckwheat and corn), unblanched nuts, legumes (from peas to limas, garbanza, pinto and

Table 2.5. Fiber Content of Common Foods

	Total fiber[a]	Soluble fiber[b]	Insoluble fiber			Percent glucose[d]	
			Polysaccharide[c]	Cellulose	Lignin	Soluble fiber[f]	Insoluble fiber
Cereals							
Wheat bran	46[e]	3.6	31	6	6	46	4
Oat bran	30	15.3	9	2	4	86	12
Rolled oats	15	8.5	5	1	1	80	29
Corn flakes	13	7.5	3	2	1	87	59
Grapenuts	14	6.0	6	1	1	63	16
Beans							
Pinto, raw	27	8.2	12	4	3	52	12
Pinto, canned	29	12.3	10	3	3	59	17
White, raw	27	11.6	11	3	2	58	14
Kidney, canned	29	13.2	10	3	3	51	13
Lentil, raw	21	4.5	10	4	3	72	13
Lima, canned/drained	25	8.6	11	4	2	69	8
Vegetables							
Corn, canned	17	9.5	6	1	1	83	4
Sweet potato	10	4.3	3	2	1	64	26
Kale, frozen	25	5.9	12	2	6	10	1
Green pepper, raw	19	7.1	6	2	4	1	1
Asparagus, raw	20	5.8	9	3	2	2	21
Cucumber, peeled/raw	11	4.4	4	2	1	2	1

Source: Data from Chen and Anderson (1981).

[a] Sum of various fiber forms shown.
[b] Extracted in boiling water (pectins, gums, and storage polysaccharides).
[c] The noncellulose, nonlignin portion of insoluble fiber released upon digestion with 1 *N* H_2SO_4 (2.5 hr) or 2 *N* trifluoroacetic acid (1 hr).
[d] Usually, uronic acid content was inversely related to glucose content. Increased glucose goes with decreased uronic acids, in general, and vice versa.
[e] g/100 g dry weight.
[f] High in arabinose and xylose.

other beans, to lentils), tubers (from potatoes to peanuts), and fruits (Tables 2.5 and 2.6). Populations consuming two to three times more fiber than Americans also have two or more bowel movements per day, and a smaller percentage of the excreted feces consists of bacterial cells.

The decreased consumption of fiber by our society since 1900 has been associated with an increased incidence of colon cancer (see Chapter 16). This potential link has been strengthened by epidemiologic studies comparing other populations around the world and is supported by animal experiments.

The potential connections between increased cancer and decreased fiber are discussed in Chapter 16, but may involve dilution and adsorption of "tumor promoting" bile acids and their decreased resorption, less formation of undesirable modified bile acids by gut bacteria, and enhanced health of the colonic epithelium.

Elevated cholesterol in the blood is a "risk factor" in atherosclerosis (see Chapter 15). Increased bile acid and cholesterol binding by certain dietary fiber components, especially pectins, gums, and carrageenans (from seaweed) has a lowering effect on levels of plasma cholesterol. [Bile acids are the major degradative products of cholesterol (see Chapters 3 and 15).] Brans, which contain mainly cellulose, do not have this action. Increased consumption of most kinds of fiber may also benefit the diabetic consuming carbohydrate, especially simple sugars, and in general will "flatten" the rise in blood glucose following a meal. Pectins, present in fruits, may slow the rate of transit of sugars from the stomach to the small intestine, thus working against a rapid increase in blood glucose concentrations following sugar ingestion. Other forms of fiber have the same result, slowing absorption by increasing the viscosity of the digesting food and inhibiting digestive en-

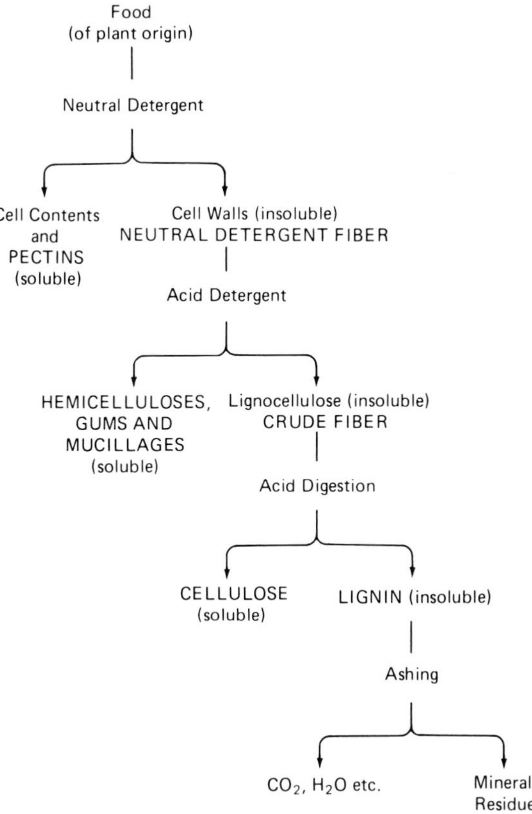

Figure 2.11. Separation of components/types of dietary fiber. Dietary fiber is material remaining after food is digested by enzymes secreted into the intestinal tract, in humans. Note positions of neutral detergent fiber and crude fiber. [*Source:* Modified from Ensminger et al. (1983).]

Table 2.6. Good Food Fiber Sources (Portions)

About 2 g of fiber	
Apple, 1 small	All Bran, 1 tbsp
Banana, 1 small	Cornflakes, 2/3 cup
Cherries, 10 large	Cracked wheat bread, 1 slice
Orange, 1 small	Grape-Nuts, 3 tbsp
Peach, 1 medium	Oatmeal, 3 tbsp (dry)
Pear, 1/2 small	Puffed wheat, 1-1/3 cup
Plums, 2 small	Rye bread, 1 slice
Strawberries, 1/3 cup	Wholewheat bread, 2 slices
Baked beans, canned, 2 tbsp	Corn-on-cob, 2 in
Broccoli, 1/2 stalk	Green beans, 1/2 cup
Brussel sprouts, 4	Lettuce, 2 cups
Carrots, 1/3 cup	Potato, 2-in diameter
Celery, 1 cup	Tomato, 1 medium
About 1 g of fiber	
Peanut butter, 2-1/2 tsp	Pickles, 1 large
Peanuts, 10	Strawberry jam, 5 tbsp

Source: From Nutrition and the MD, vol. VII, no. 7, based on Southgate and Bingham (1979).

zyme action (see Krichevsky, 1988). A beneficial effect is also seen in diverticular disease, where sacs or pouches may develop in the colon due to a weakening of the muscle and submucosal structure. Fiber is thought to "soften" the stool, thereby reducing pressure on the colonic wall and enhancing expulsion of the feces. The possibility that increased fiber consumption would lower the incidence of gallstones in gallbladder disease has only preliminary experimental support at this time (Thornton et al., 1983), although Burkitt points out that third world native populations (who are on high fiber diets) do not suffer from this disease (Burkitt, 1982).

Among the potential undesirable effects of a very high fiber diet are a reduction in the absorption of some trace elements, including iron (Monnier et al., 1980; Simpson et al., 1981), zinc, copper, calcium, and magnesium (Drews et al., 1979) (see Chapter 7), and bowel irritation in organic bowel disease. Diabetic patients should also be aware that changing to a high fiber diet may reduce their requirement for insulin.

The mechanisms by which dietary fiber has various long-term effects on health and disease are only partly understood, but may involve the following properties and effects. There is a direct correlation between the fiber content of the diet (especially the cellulose and hemicellulose portions) and the rate of transit of ingested nutrients through the gastrointestinal tract. Those diets high in cellulose fiber pass through much faster, a factor ascribed to the increased bulk of the stools. In contrast, the water-retaining, gel-forming pectins and gums delay gastric emptying, and by forming gels in the small intestine, they retard the rate of absorption of di- and monosaccharides (Anderson, 1981; Anderson and Chen, 1979), aiding the glucose-intolerant individual. [The latter is mainly a function of the increased viscosity of the contents of the digestive tract (see Krichevsky, 1988).] Many forms of fiber, but especially pectins and gums (in fruits and vegetables), and the lignin (in brans), adsorb bile acids, and some cholesterol and phospholipid (Story and Lord, 1987), from micelles such as those present in the upper small intestine. This may render the lipids less likely to be absorbed (or reabsorbed). As a consequence of one or more of these properties, fiber (except for cellulose) enhances fecal excretion of bile acids and even neutral sterols (cholesterol). Bile acid loss may also be enhanced by more conversion to less absorbable forms by colonic bacteria (Hillman et al., 1986). More indirect effects of fiber will be exerted by its bacterial metabolites, principally the CO_2, water, H_2, and acids that enter the colonic epithelium and blood. This may be an important aspect of the effects of fiber on blood cholesterol, as propionate can inhibit endogenous (liver) cholesterogenesis (Chen and Anderson, 1984; Shutler, 1987).

Additional plant substituents, not usually considered in connection with dietary fiber, may enhance the effects already described (Shutler, 1987). Plant sterols, especially β-sitosterol (Figure 2.12) (poorly absorbed themselves), may competitively inhibit cholesterol absorption (Mattson et al., 1982); and saponins may form nonabsorbable complexes with cholesterol $\pm$ bile acids, enhancing sterol excretion. Isoflavones (more easily absorbed) may also have minor effects, possibly mimicking actions of estrogens on hepatic low-density lipoprotein receptors (Shutler, 1987).

Dietary fiber also has effects on the morphology of intestinal villi (Krichevsky, 1988) and on the rate of turnover of mucosal cells (Savage, 1986). The villi of individuals who are vegetarians or are otherwise on high fiber diets (as in many developing nations) are not fingerlike, like those of most Westerners, but are broader, with additional convolutions or ridges. As fiber tends to enhance the rate of mucosal cell turnover by enhancing cell sloughing from off the villus tips, this may at least be partly responsible for the morphological differences. It also results in a smaller mass of endothelial (and thus absorptive) cells within the intestinal wall. How this may relate to decreased colonic (or other) diseases is not known.

Figure 2.12. Structure of the most common plant sterols in relation to cholesterol.

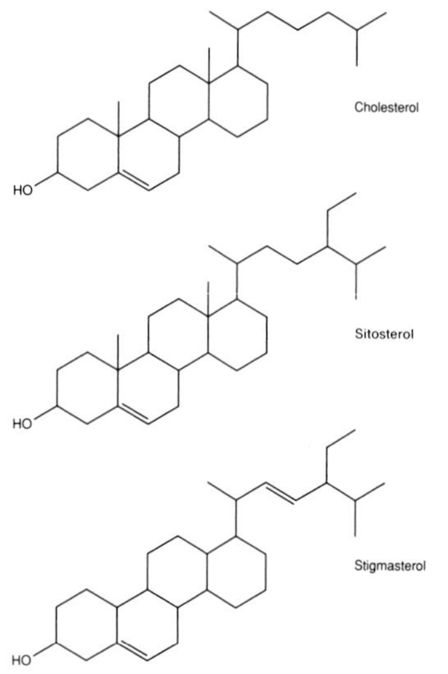

Starch Blockers for Dieting

Substances extracted from wheat, kidney beans, and other sources, capable of inhibiting the digestive (hydrolyzing) actions of amylases and maltase/glucoamylase in vitro, have appeared on the market as a product designed to aid in weight reduction. In theory, the "starch blockers," taken with starch in a meal, inhibit the full or partial depolymerization of these nutrients, thus preventing the absorption of the inherent glucose units. Several studies refute this theory and indicate that commercially available "blockers" have no effect on the efficiency of carbohydrate absorption from starches when taken in vivo (Bo-lin et al., 1982; Carlson et al., 1983; Hollenbeck et al., 1983). This suggests that the inhibitors are themselves destroyed or inactivated in vivo and/or are ineffective for other reasons.

References

Acheson KJ, Schutz Y, Bessard T, Anantharaman K, Flatt JP, Jequier E (1988): Am J Clin Nutr 48:240.

Akerblom HK, Siltanen, I, Kallio A-K (1972): Acta Med Scan (Suppl) 542:195.

Anderson JW (1981): *In* Garry PJ, ed: Human nutrition, clinical and biochemical aspects. Washington, DC: American Association for Clinical Chemistry, p 132.

Anderson JW, Chen WL (1979): Am J Clin Nutr 32:346.

Anderson JW, Rosendall AF (1973): Biochim Biophys Acta 304:384.

Anonymous (1983): Nutr Rev 41:174.

Bantle JP, Laine DC, Thomas JW (1986): JAMA 256:3241.

Basu SK, Goldstein JL, Brown MS (1983): Science 219:871.

Beck-Nielsen H, Peterson O, Lindskov HO (1980): Am J Clin Nutr 33:272.

Bellomo G, Comstock JP, Wen D, Hazelwood RL (1987): Proc Soc Exp Biol Med 186:348.

Blakley SR, Hallfrisch J, Reiser S, Prather ES (1981): J Nutr 111:307.

Bo-lin GW, Morawski SG, Fordtran JS (1982): N Engl J Med 307:1413.

Boot-Handford R, Heath H (1980): Metabolism 29:1247.

Boot-Handford R, Heath H (1981): Br J Exp Pathol 62:398.

Brauer PM, Slavin JL, Marlett JA (1981): Am J Clin Nutr 34:1061.

Broitman SA, Zamchek N (1980): *In* Goodhart RS, Shils ME, eds: Modern nutrition in health and disease. Philadelphia: Lea & Febiger, p 912.

Brunzell JD, Lerner RL, Hazzard WR, Porte D Jr, Bierman EL (1971): N Engl J Med 284:521.

Bunn HF, Haney DN, Kamin S, Gabbay KH, Gallop PM (1976): J Clin Invest 57:1652.

Bunn HF, Higgins PJ (1981): Science 213:222.

Burgoyne RD, Cheek TR, O'Sullivan AJ (1987): TIBS 12:332.

Burkitt DP (1982): *In* Rose J, ed: Nutrition and the killer diseases. Park Ridge, NJ: Noyes, p 1.

Bustamante S, Gasparo M, Kendall K, Coates P, Brown S, Somawaine B, Koldovsky O (1981): J Nutr 111:943.

Calderhead DM, Lienhard GE (1988): J Biol Chem 263:12171.

Carlson GL, Li BUK, Bass P, Olsen WA (1983): Science 219:393.

Cerami A (1986): Trends Biol Sci 11:311.

Cerami A, Vlassera M, Brownlee M (1987): Sci Am 72:90.

Chan BL, Lisanti MP, Rodriguez-Boulan E, Saltiel AR (1988): Science 241:1670.

Chen W-JL, Anderson JW (1981): Am J Clin Nutr 34:1077.

Chen W-JL, Anderson JW (1984): Proc Soc Exp Biol Med 175:215.

Coelingh-Benningk HJT, Schreurs WHP (1975): Br Med J 3:13.

Cohen AM (1975): High sucrose intake as a factor in the development of diabetes and its vascular complications. Washington, DC: Select Committee on Nutrition and Human Needs, p 167.

Crapo PA, Scarlett JA, Kolterman OG (1982): Am J Clin Nutr 36:256.

Crapo PA, Insel J, Sperling M, Kolterman OG (1981): Am J Clin Nutr 34:184.

Czech MP, Klarlund JK, Yagaloff KA, Bradford AP, Lewis RE (1988): J Biol Chem 263:11017.

Danford D, Munro HN (1980): *In:* Goodman LS, Gilman AG, eds: The pharmacological basis of therapeutics. New York: MacMillan, p 1560.

Department of National Health and Welfare: Food Consumption Patterns Report. Nutrition in Canada, from the Bureau of Nutritional Sciences, Health Protection Branch (1970–1972).

Dietary Goals for the United States (1977): Select Committee of the U.S. Senate.

Dilawari JB, Kamath PS, Batta RP, Mukewar S, Raghavan S (1981): Am J Clin Nutr 34:2450.

Drews LM, Kies C, Fox HM (1979): Am J Clin Nutr 32:1893.

Dyck PJ, Zimmerman BR, Vilen TH, Minnerath SR, Karnes JL, Yao JK, Poduslo JF (1988): N Engl J Med 319:542.

Ensminger AH, Ensminger ME, Konlands JE, Robson JRK (1983): Foods and nutrition encyclopedia, vol. 1. Clovis, CA: Pegus Press.

Fields M, Lewis CG, Beal T (1989): Metab Clin Exp 38:371.

Friedman GJ (1980): *In* Goodhart RS, Shils ME, eds: Modern nutrition in health and disease. Philadelphia: Lea & Febiger, p 977.

Friend B (1976): Am J Clin Nutr 20:8.

Gabbay KH (1975): Annu Rev Med 26:521.

Gabbay KH, Merola LO, Filed RA (1966): Science 151:209.

Garg A, Bonanome A, Grundy SM, Zhang Z-J, Unger RH (1988a): N Engl J Med 319:829.

Garg A, Sebokova E, Thomson ABR, Clandinin MT (1988b): Biochem J 249:351.

Garvey WT, Hueckstead TP, Birnbaum MJ (1989): Science 245:60.

Glinsmann WH, Irausquin H, Park YK (1986): J Nutr (Suppl) 116:S1.

Goodridge AG (1987): Annu Rev Nutr 7:157.

Gortner WA (1975): Cancer Res 35:3246.

Gould GW, Bell GI (1990): TIBS 15:18.

Gray GM, Fogel MR (1980): *In* Goodhart RS, Shils ME, eds: Modern nutrition in health and disease. Philadelphia: Lea & Febiger, p 99.

Greene DA, Lattimer SA, Sima AAF (1987): N Engl J Med 316:599.

Hillman LC, Peters SG, Fisher CA, Pomare EW (1986): Gut 27:29.

Hitz JB, Dain JA (1988): Biochem Arch 4:159.

Hollenbeck CB, Coulston AM, Quan R, Becker TR, Vreman HJ, Stevenson DK, Reaven GM (1983): Am J Clin Nutr 38:498.

Hunt JV, Dean RT, Wolff SP (1988): Biochem J 256:205.

Huttanen JK, Makinen KK, Schenin A (1975): Acta Odontol Scand 33(Suppl 70):239.

Jedziniak JA, Chylack LT, Cheng HM, Gillis MK, Kalustian AA, Tung WH (1981): Invest Ophthalmol 30:314.

Jeffery J, Jornvall H (1983): Proc Natl Acad Sci USA 80:901.

Johnson JH, Crider BP, McCorkle K, Alford M, Unger RH (1990): New Engl J Med 322:653.

Jornvall H, Persson M, Jeffery J (1981): Proc Natl Acad Sci USA 78:4226.

Krebs E (1989): FASEB presentation.

Krebs EG, Fischer EH (1964): Vitam Horm 22:399.

Krichevsky (1988): Annu Rev Nutr 8:301.

Kupke I, Lamprecht W (1967): Hoppe-Seylers Physiol Chem 348:17.

Landau BR, Wahren J (1988): FASEB J 2:2368.

Lebenthal E, Sunshine P, Krechmer N (1973): Gastroenterology 64:1136.

Lees AM, Mok HY, Lees RS, McCluskey MA, Grundy SM (1977): Atherosclerosis 28:325.

Leighton B, Cooper JS (1990): TIBS 15:295.

Lewis CG, Fields M, Beal T (1990): J Nutr Biochem 1:160.

Linscheer WG, Vergroesen AJ (1988): *In* Shils ME, Young V, eds: Modern nutrition in health and disease. Philadelphia: Lea & Febiger, p 72.

Lloyd DR, Marples J (1988): Ann Clin Biochem 25:432.

MacDonald I (1980): *In* Alfin-Slater RB, Krichevsky D, eds: Human nutrition, a comprehensive treatise. New York: Plenum, p 97.

MacDonald I (1988): *In* Shils ME, Young VY, eds: Modern nutrition in health and disease. Philadelphia: Lea & Febiger, p 38.

McPherson JD, Shilton BH, Walton DJ (1988): Biochem 27:1901.

Maenpaa PH, Raivio KO, Kekomaki MP (1968): Science 161:1253.

Mattson FH, Grundy SM, Crouse JR (1982): Am J Clin Nutr 35:697.

McGarry JD, Kuwajima M, Newgard CB, Foster DW (1987): Annu Rev Nutr 7:51.

Metzler DH (1977): Biochemistry. New York: Academic.

Meyer JH, Gu YG, Jehn D, Taylor IL (1988): Am J Clin Nutr 48:260.

Monnier L, Colette C, Aguirre L, Mirouze J (1980): Am J Clin Nutr 33:1225.

Monnier VM, Vishwanath V, Frank KE, Elmets CA, Dauchot P, Kohn RR (1986): N Engl J Med 314:403.

National Research Council (1989): Diet and health. Implications for reducing chronic disease risk. Washington, DC: National Academy Press.

Noguchi T, Inoue H, Tanaka T (1982): Eur J Biochem 128:583.

Odawara M, Kadowaki T, Yamamoto R, Shibasaki Y, Tobe K, Accili D, Bevins C, Mikami Y, Matsuura N, Akanua Y, Takaku F, Taylor SI, Kasuga M (1989): Science 245:66.

Oimomi M, Sakai M, Ohara T, Igaki N, Nakamichi T, Hata F, Baba S (1989) J Int Med Res 17:249.

Owerbach D, Quinto C, Rutter WJ (1981): Science 213:353.

Page L, Friend B (1974): *In* Sipple HL, McNutt KW, eds: Sugars in nutrition. New York: Academic.

Pongor S, Ulrich PC, Bencsath FA, Cerami A (1984): Proc Natl Acad Sci USA 81:2684.

Ramakrishna S, Benjamin WB (1988): J Biol Chem 263:12677.

Reed PB (1980): Nutrition, an applied science. Los Angeles: West.

Robison WG Jr, Kador PF, Kinoshita JH (1983): Science 221:1177.

Rosenmann E, Yanko L, Cohen AM (1976): Israel J Med Sci 11:753.

Saavedra JM, Perman JA (1989): Annu Rev Nutr 9:475.

Saltiel A, Fox JA, Sherline P, Cuatrecasas P (1986): Science 233:967.

Savage DC (1986): Annu Rev Nutr 6:155.

Schwarz K, Mertz W (1959): Arch Biochem Biophys 85:292.

Scrutton MC, Utter MF (1968): Annu Rev Biochem 37:249.

Shutler (1987): Human Nutr: Food Sci Nutr 41F:87.

Sima AAF, Bril V, Nathaniel V, McEwen TAJ, Brown MB, Lattimer SA, Greene DA (1988): N Engl J Med 319:548.

Simpson JM, Morris ER, Cook JD (1981): Am J Clin Nutr 34:1469.

Southgate DAT, Bingham SA (1979): Qual Plant Plant Foods Hum Nutr 29:49.

Sparks JD, Sparks CE, Kritchevsky D (1986): Atherosclerosis 60:183.

Sreebny LM (1983): Commun Dent Oral Epidemiol 11:148.

Stolz A, Takikawa H, Ookhtens M, Kaplowitz N (1989): Annu Rev Physiol 51:161.

Story JA, Lord SL (1987): Scand J Gastroenterol 22(Suppl):174.

Suarez G, Rajaram R, Oronsky AL, Gawinowicz MA (1989): J Biol Chem 264:3674.

Swan DC, Davidson P, Albrink MJ (1966): Lancet 1:60.

Taira M, Taira M, Hashimoto N, Shimada F, Suzuki Y, Kanatsuka A, Nakamura F, Ebina Y, Tatibana M, Makino H, Yoshida S (1989): Science 245:63.

Taylor A (1989): Nutr Rev 47:225.

Thornton JR, Emmett PM, Heaton KW (1983): Gut 24:2.

Tobey TA, Mondon CE, Zavaroni I, Reaven GM (1982): Metabolism 31:608.

Tu Ji-I, Jacobson GR, Graves DJ (1971): Biochemistry 10:1229.

Vallance-Owen J, Bajaj JS (1975): *In* Vallance-Owen J, ed: Diabetes, its physiological and biological basis. Baltimore: University Park Press, p 188.

Vrana A, Zak A, Kazdova L (1988): Nutr Rep Int 38:687.

Wang Y-M, van Eys J (1981): Annu Rev Nutr 1:437.

Watford M (1988): TIBS 13:329.

White W, Handler P, Smith E (1973): Principles of biochemistry (5th ed). New York: McGraw-Hill.

Whitney E, Hamilton EM (1990): Understanding nutrition. St. Paul: West Publishing.

Wolff SP, Dean RT (1986): Biochem J 243:399.

Wolff SP, Dean RT (1987): Biochem J 245:243.

Wolff SP, Dean RT (1988): Biochem J 249:617.

Zak A, Zemen M, Hrabak P, Vrana A, Svarcova H, Mares P (1989): Nutr Rep Int 39:235.

Maria C. Linder, Ph.D.*

3

Nutrition and Metabolism of Fats

Introduction to Fats

Consumption

It is estimated that the average American consumes about 38% of dietary calories as fat, down from a high of 40%–42% in the mid-1960s (National Research Council, 1989; Read et al., 1989). This is almost the same proportion of calories as that from carbohydrates. However, fat is much denser than carbohydrate in terms of potential energy content, containing 9.3 versus 4.1 kcal/g. In comparison with 1910, intake of fat is nearly 25% greater, while that of complex carbohydrate has declined. Not only has fat consumption increased, but there have been dramatic changes in the proportions of animal and vegetable fats ingested (Figure 3.1). Butter and lard, formerly 75% of fat intake, have been replaced by oils, margarine, and shortenings, all from vegetable sources. Consequently, the proportion of unsaturated to saturated fats (and especially linoleic acid) has greatly increased. Cholesterol in the food supply has not changed significantly, averaging 500 mg per person per day in 1909 and 480 in 1979 (after reaching a high of 570 in the late 1940s). [Actual per capita consumption, however, is somewhat lower (see below).] A new form of fat, containing trans fatty acids (see below), has also appeared, which is produced through the partial hydrogenation of polyunsaturated vegetable oils, especially in the production of margarines and shortenings. Of the fats currently consumed, about 6% are trans fatty acids (van den Reek et al., 1986).

Increased ingestion of fat (along with decreased fiber) has been linked to the increased incidence of certain forms of cancer (Chapter 16) and to atherosclerosis (Chapter 15). For these reasons, the National Research Council has recommended a reduction in the fat consumption of Americans to about 30% of calories. A reduction in cholesterol intake was also recommended, although the link between its *consumption* and atherogenesis is tenuous (see below).

Structure of Fats in the Diet

There are three main forms of fat found in the human diet and in the mammalian organism. These are glycerides, principally triacylglycerol (triglyceride), the form in which fat is stored for fuel and by far the most abundant form in foods and tissues (Figure 3.2A); the phospholipids; and the sterols, principally cholesterol. Triacylglycerols account for 95%–98% of the fat ingested in all forms of food (Table 3.1) and a similar percentage of the fat found in humans. The phospholipids and cholesterol are ingested in small amounts, being presented mainly as the constituents of cell membranes and myelin sheaths. Cholesterol is not found in food of plant origin (Table 3.1), as plant cell membranes do not contain cholesterol.

* California State University, Fullerton, CA.

A

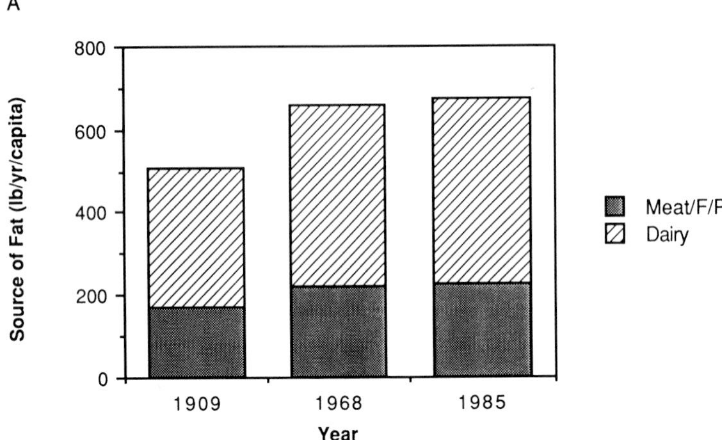

B

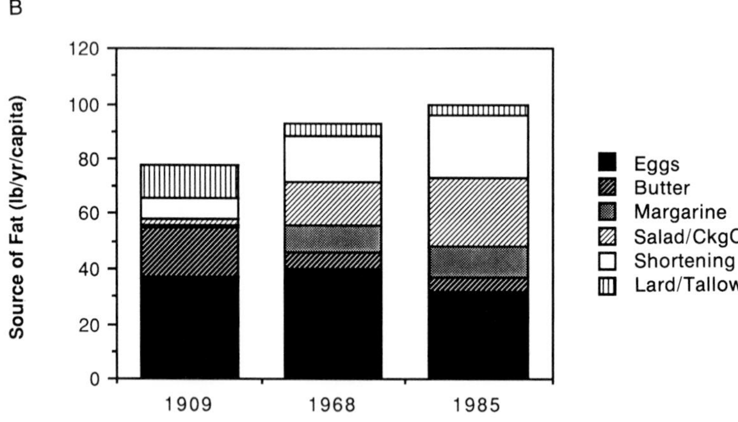

Figure 3.1. Trends in the consumption of fat and major dietary fat sources, from 1909 to the 1980s. **(A, B)** Data for average per capita utilization in the food supply. **(C)** Data for consumption of specific fatty acids. [*Source:* Unpublished data from RM Marston, given in NRC (1989).]

C

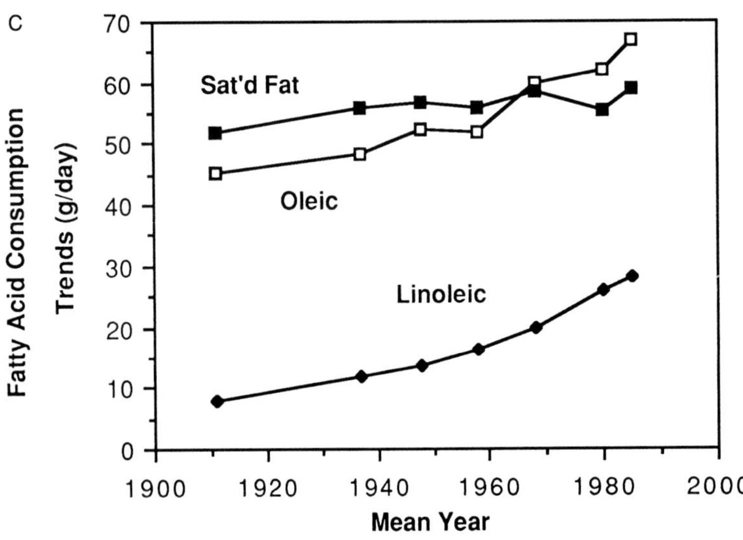

Source **Type**

95-98% of dietary fats and oils (storage fat)

Triglyceride

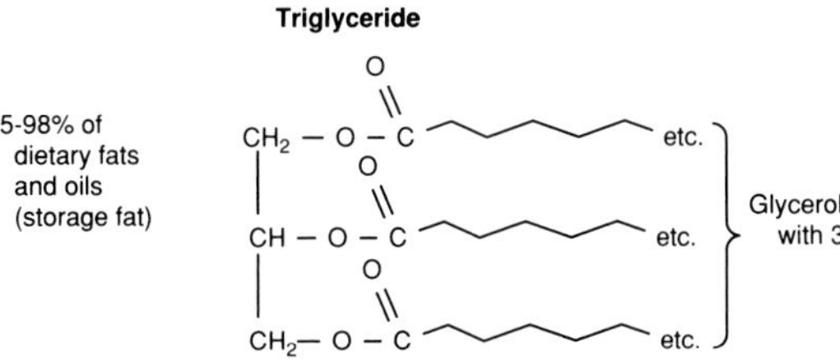

Glycerol esterified with 3 fatty acids

Cell membranes; especially high in brain

Phospholipids

O
CH2 – O – C etc.
O
CH – O – C etc.
O
CH2 – O – P – O – (base)
O–

Base is: choline HO – CH2 – CH2 – N – CH3 (+, CH3, CH3)

or

ethanol amine HO – CH2 – CH2 – NH3+

or

serine etc. HO – CH2 – CH (COO–, NH3+)

or inositol phosphate

OH OH HO O – P – OH (O, OH) HO OH

Cell membranes; cholesterol droplets in certain cells; not present in plant foods

Cholesterol

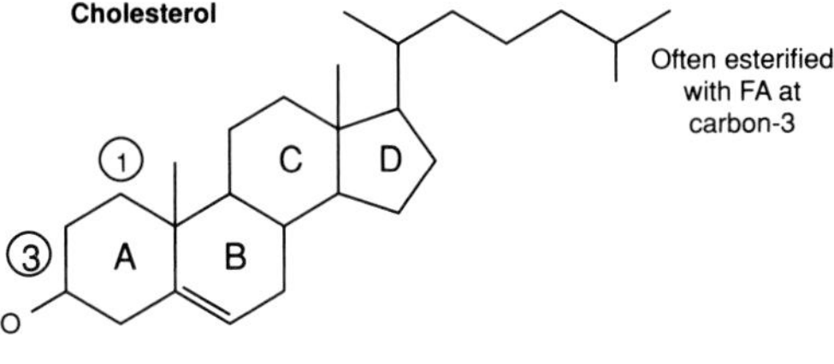

Often esterified with FA at carbon-3

COOH

Arachidonic acid (all *cis*)

COOH

Eicosapentaenoic acid (EPA)

COOH

Docosahexaenoic acid (DHA)

Linoleic Acid $C_{18} : \Delta^{9,12}$

O
HO – C
cis

O
HO – C
trans

Cardiolipin

O
CH2 – O – C etc.
O
CH – O – C etc.
O
CH2 – O – P – O – CH2
O–
CHOH
O
CH2 – O – P – O – CH2
O–
CH – O – C etc.
O
CH2 – O – C etc.
O

Sphingomyelin

O
R – C – N
O
(choline) or other base – O – P – O – H2C
O
OH

Figure 3.2. (A) *Dietary fats.* Forms of dietary fats and fatty acids found in the food supply and in human (and animal) tissues.

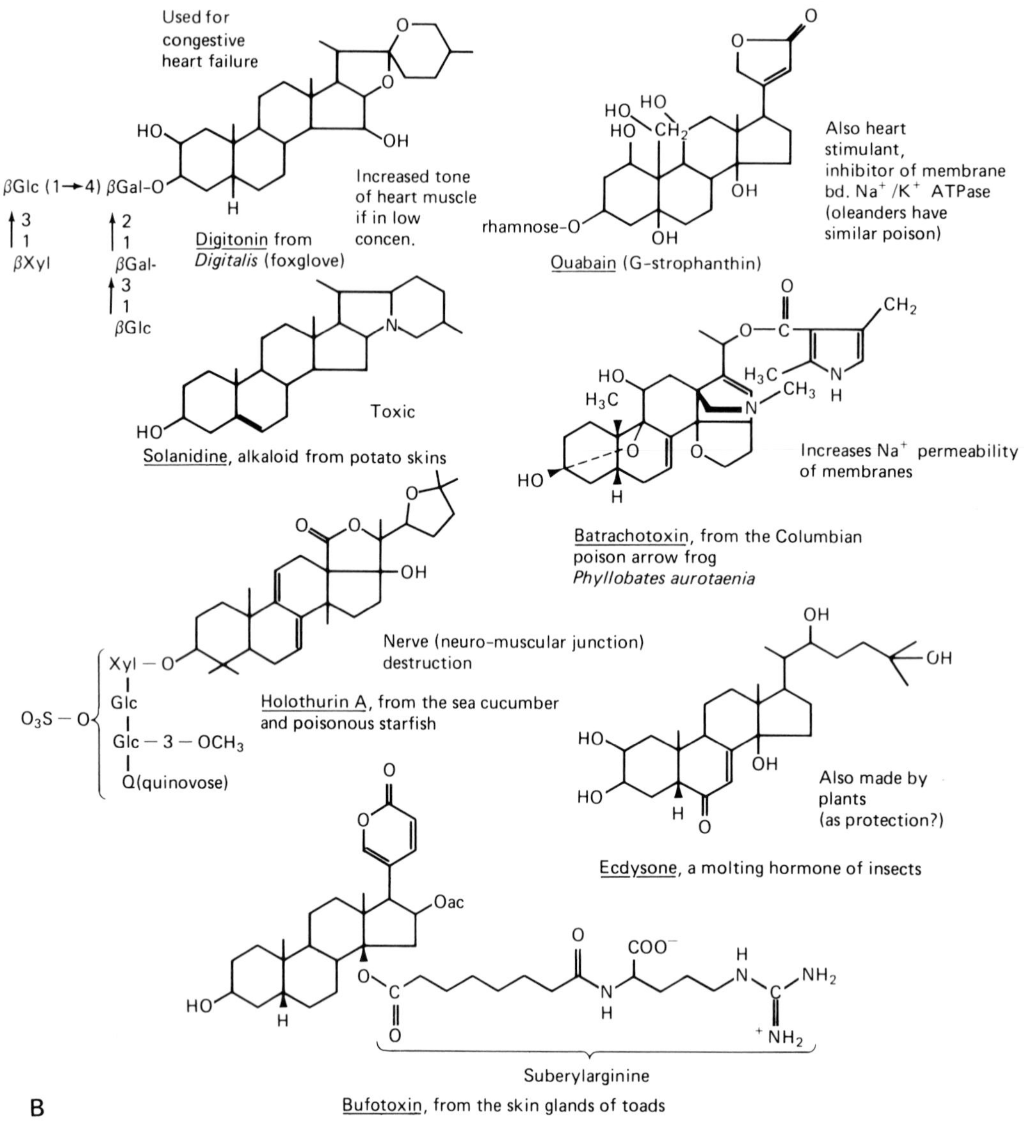

Used for congestive heart failure

Increased tone of heart muscle if in low concen.

Digitonin from *Digitalis* (foxglove)

Also heart stimulant, inhibitor of membrane bd. Na^+/K^+ ATPase (oleanders have similar poison)

Ouabain (G-strophanthin)

Toxic

Solanidine, alkaloid from potato skins

Increases Na^+ permeability of membranes

Batrachotoxin, from the Columbian poison arrow frog *Phyllobates aurotaenia*

Nerve (neuro-muscular junction) destruction

Holothurin A, from the sea cucumber and poisonous starfish

Also made by plants (as protection?)

Ecdysone, a molting hormone of insects

Suberylarginine

Bufotoxin, from the skin glands of toads

B

Figure 3.2. (*continued*) **(B)** Plant steroids generally found in trace quantities. The structures of more common plant sterols are given in the last chapter (Figure 2.11).

The structure of lipids is characterized by a relative lack of oxygen. Fats consist almost exclusively of carbon and hydrogen (Figure 3.2), a condition that renders them hydrophobic and mostly imiscible with water. (It also renders them richer in calories, as they have "further" to go in the oxidation process than do carbohydrates.) Oxygen is associated with one or more ester bonds in each of the categories of dietary lipids (Figure 3.2A). It is these ester bonds that are broken down during digestion and are reformed during the resynthesis of the fats after absorption of their substituent parts. The phospholipids are unique in containing a polar end, and thus having detergent properties, with negative and positive charges from phosphate and the additional substituents. It is the nature of the substituent on the phospholipid that determines its common name. Thus, phosphatidylcholine (lecithin) has choline as its substituent base, whereas phosphatidylserine and phosphatidylethanolamine have serine and ethanolamine, respectively. These three phospholipids are the most abundant in the body and foodstuffs. Smaller amounts of other phospholipids, such as sphingomyelin, cardiolipin, and

Table 3.1. Fat Content and Composition of Common Foods (Modified)

Food	Total lipid (g/100 g)[a]	Cholesterol (mg/100 g)	Percent fatty acid: Saturated	Oleic	Linoleic	Linolenic, EPA, DHA or arachidonic
Milk (whole)	3.5	12	59	25	3	1
Egg	11	548[b]	29	37	11	0.2
Beef, ground (lean only)	22	70	50	41	3	0.7
Pork (lean only)	14	85	37	42	9–14	1
Chicken leg (flesh only)	3.5	74	27	47	22	2
Salmon	14	35	18	16	2	20
Whole wheat	2.0	0	21	14	55	4
Corn (whole)	3.8	0	15	44	43	2
Soybeans (whole)	18	0	13	22	54	5
Peanuts (butter)	48	0	14	48	28	0.5
Coconut (fresh)	38	0	83	5	2	0
Avocado (fresh)	24	0	14	66	9	Tr

Source: Data from Souci et al. (1982).

[a] 95–98% triacylglycerols.
[b] Note: this is for more than one egg.

phosphotidylinositol phosphate, are also found (Figure 3.2A). The latter is of special recent interest as a mediator of cell regulatory processes (see below). Other lipids in animal tissues are the glycolipids, including ceramides found especially in the brain, and the steroids and bile acids that derive from cholesterol. Plants contain small amounts of phytosterols (Figure 2.11) (not in their cell membranes), which are very poorly absorbed and inhibit cholesterol absorption (see below). It is estimated that Americans may ingest 150–400 mg of these phytosterols per day (National Research Council, 1989). In some plants, there are also trace amounts of steroids, some of which have powerful pharmacologic effects (Figure 3.2B).

The properties of triacylglycerols (and phospholipids) vary a great deal, depending on their substituent fatty acids. Plant glycerides tend to be relatively liquid oils at room temperature due to a preponderance of mono- and polyunsaturated fatty acids, as well as shorter fatty acid chains than are usually found in animal glycerides. (Short chain length and especially unsaturated bonds lower the melting point of fatty acids.) Animal lard contains triglyceride with fewer unsaturated double bonds and with longer fatty acid chains (16 carbons or more). It is thus much more solid. (Human fat is more unsaturated than most animal fat.) Partial hydrogenation of vegetable oils, as in the production of margarine, raises the melting temperature by saturating double bonds. In nature, whether in plants or animals, the carbons on either side of the double bond are normally in the *cis* conformation, in effect, causing a bend (or bends) in the fatty acid chains. Commercial hydrogenation of plant fats, however, produces substantial quantities of *trans* fatty acids, with a more elongated structure (Figure 3.2A). The composition of the fat ingested influences the composition of the fat that accumulates (stored as triglyceride) in adipose tissue. Thus, diets high in unsaturated fats will tend to result in deposition of more unsaturated triglyceride, and vice versa, although considerable modification (saturation, desaturation, and chain elongation) of ingested fatty acids does occur. The composition of dietary fat also influences regulatory processes by altering the availability of fatty acids in cell membrane phospholipids, which are used to form prostaglandins, leukotrienes, and thromboxanes (see below).

Functions, Nutrition, and Metabolism

Functions of Fats in the Human Organism

Triacylglycerol (triglyceride). Triacylglycerol is the form of fat most efficient for storing the calories necessary for energy-requiring processes within the body. In contrast to glycogen, the principal carbohydrate storage compound, triacylglycerol is a space-saving (nonhydrated), less oxidized material, with about 9 kcal/g, as compared with 4 kcal/g for carbohydrate or protein. The bulk of triglyceride is found in adipose cells, where it comprises 99% of the cell volume (except in early infancy, where it is less). Adipocytes are found as discrete tissues in various parts of the body or are dispersed within the muscle and connective tissues. The total number of adipocytes is determined in childhood, where overfeeding increases the number [Table 3.2 (Knittle and Hirsch, 1968)]. Some triacylglycerol is also present in the form of small lipid droplets in nonadipose cells, like liver and muscle, where it may be of immediate use in energy metabolism. Aside from its use as fuel, triacylglycerol can be converted to cholesterol, phospholipid, and other lipids when required. As part of adipose tissue, triacylglycerol also serves the physical function of padding our skeleton and vital organs, thus protecting them from undue jarring or cracking. It is noteworthy that the heart, kidneys, epididymis, and mammary glands, for example, are enfolded by a layer of fatty tissue. Subcutaneous fat also serves as a means of heat or cold insulation.

Phospholipids and cholesterol. Phospholipids and cholesterol have as their principal function the formation of all interior and exterior cell membranes. In the present view of cell membrane structure, these lipids provide a semifluid matrix within which float various forms of membrane protein. The lipid matrix consists of a bilayer of interior cholesterol (mainly esterified) and two layers of phospholipid, with the polar groups facing the exterior and interior aqueous environment. The presence of specific polyunsaturated fatty acids on membrane phospholipids is important not only for cell membrane structure, but also as a source of substrate for the formation of prostaglandins, leukotrienes, and thromboxanes, which is essential for normal body function (see more below). The presence of specific phospholipids, notably phosphatidylinositides, is essential for cell regulatory signals via inositol phosphates and diacylglycerol (see below).

Table 3.2. Number and Size of Fat Cells in Normal and Obese Individuals

	Cell size (μg lipid/cell)	Total cell number (× 10⁹)
Normal weight	0.66 ± 0.06	26 ± 6.8
Juvenile-onset obese	0.90 ± 0.05	85 ± 6.9
Adult-onset obese	0.98 ± 0.14	62 ± 4.2
Reduced obese[a]	0.45 ± 0.05	62 ± 5.3

Source: Reproduced by permission from Grinker and Hirsch (1972). In Metabolic and Behavioural Correlates of Obesity, Ciba Foundation Symposium No 8, p 350.

[a] Each subject had lost 50 kg in weight.

Like phospholipid, cholesterol is also a substrate for the formation of other essential substances. Products include the bile acids made by the liver (Figure 3.3), which is the main route for cholesterol catabolism; the steroid hormones (from glucocorticoids and aldosterone in the adrenal cortex to progesterone, estrogens, and androgens in gonadal and some other tissue); and vitamin D_3, the only vitamin normally synthesized in sufficient quantities by the body not to be required in the diet. Synthesis of vitamin D in the skin requires the action of ultraviolet light to assist in the cleavage of "ring B" (Figure 3.3).

Essential fatty acids. For survival and optimal health, a portion of the triacylglycerol consumed must contain "essential fatty acids" (EFA), characterized by an unsaturated bond within the last seven carbons (and especially carbons 6 and 7) of the fatty acid chain, toward the methyl end (also called n-6 fatty acids). Fatty acids, such as linoleic acid (Figure 3.2A), that have this structure cannot be synthesized by the human organism. The category of EFA has now been broadened to also include polyunsaturated fatty acids with a double bond between carbons 3 and 4 from the methyl end, such as linolenic acid (Mead, 1980), eicosapentaenoic acid, and decosahexaenoic acid. These are also termed omega-3 (or n-3) fatty acids (the methyl end of a fatty acid being the "omega" end). They are especially abundant in brain phospholipid and are essential for the development and function of brain and retina (Neuringer et al., 1988), as well as sperm. It is estimated that adults require a minimum of 1%–2% of their calories as n-6 EFA per day, and probably 12%–14% of calories (40% of dietary fat) for optimal health (Mead, 1980). In this country, n-6 EFA deficiency is rare, as vegetable oils and their derivatives are ingested in large quantities. Deficiency of n-6 EFA is evidenced by reddish skin lesions, especially noticeable on the cheeks, and areas of abrasion. Neuringer et al. (1988) have recommended that the optimal ratio of n-6 to n-3 EFA ingested be 4 : 10, as high ratios will lead to a depletion of n-3 acids in the phospholipid of vital organs. Such a ratio is not that easy to achieve with present dietary patterns unless fish or fish oils are included in the diet (or more unusual vegetable sources high in linolenic acid) (see below, Fish Oils). Others agree that the ratio is im-

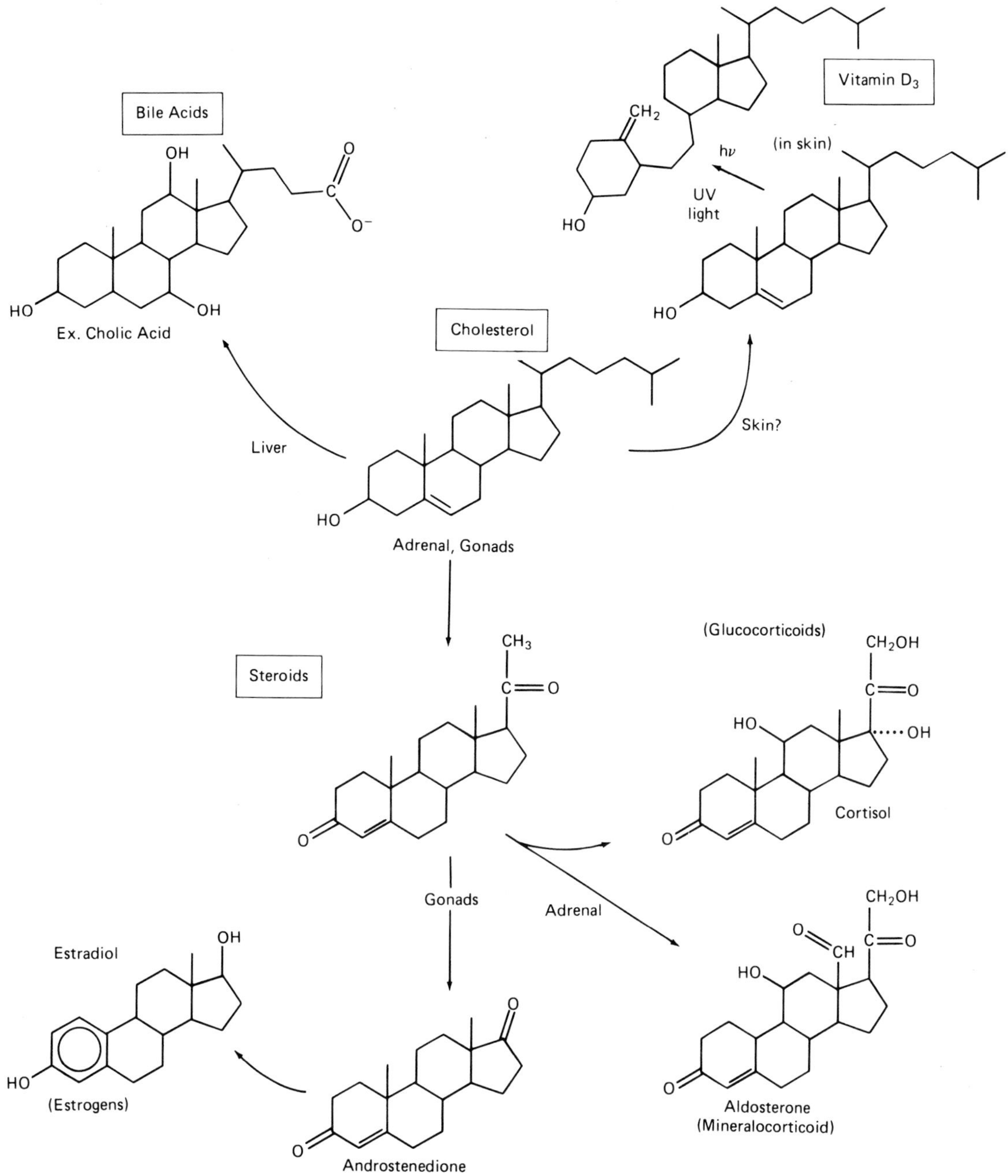

Figure 3.3. Cholesterol as a precursor for other important substances in the human organism.

portant, but are less sure what it should be (McCleod et al., 1985; *Nutr Rev*, 1987*a*, *b*). [The ratio in breast milk is 24 (*Nutr Rev*, 1987*a*).]

EFA, or their products (such as arachidonic acid) are needed for the formation of specific prostaglandins, leukotrienes, and thromboxanes (Figure 3.4), which are collectively termed eicosanoids, as they are formed from (unsaturated) 20-carbon fatty acids. These are hormonelike substances secreted for short-range action upon neighboring tissues. Prostaglandins are produced in all parts of the body and have been implicated

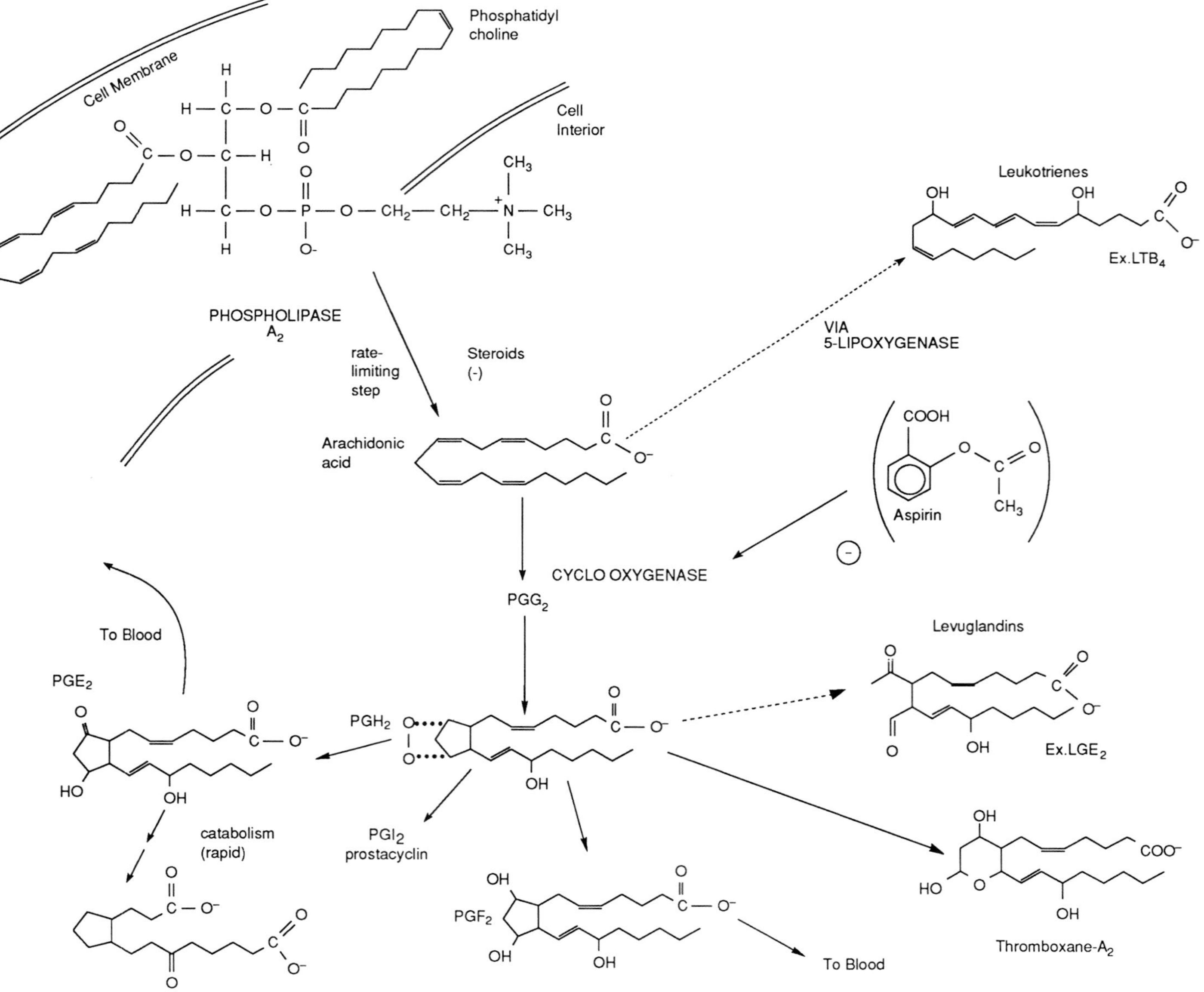

Figure 3.4. Synthesis of prostaglandins, thromboxanes, leukotrienes, and levuglandins, from fatty acids of membrane phospholipid.

in activities from the induction of labor, to inflammation, blood pressure maintenance, and headaches. Leukotrienes and thromboxanes are alternative products involved in platelet aggregation and the inflammatory response. They have been linked to the pathophysiology of some diseases, notably atherosclerosis. Thromboxane A_2 (TXA_2) stimulates formation of platelet-derived growth factor (PDGF) and stimulates blood clotting through enhanced platelet aggregation (see Chapter 15). Leukotrienes, especially those derived from arachidonic acid, are chemoattractants for phagocytes and polymorphonuclear leukocytes in inflammation and during plaque formation in arteries.

The forms of prostaglandins, thromboxanes, and leukotrienes produced depend upon the starting material (Figure 3.5), which is mostly arachidonic acid, but can also be eicosapentaenoic acid or (indirectly) decosahexaenoic acid, the major "omega-3" fatty acids in fish oils. As shown in Figure 3.6, the 20-carbon arachidonic and eicosapentaenoic acids (AA and EPA) are formed by elongation and desaturation of dietary 18-carbon linoleic and linolenic acids, respectively, a process that is initiated mainly in the liver and involves the so-called Δ^6-desaturase. Further elongation and desaturation occurs in peripheral tissues and includes the formation of DHA (docosahexaenoic acid). Alternatively, EPA and DHA can be provided by fish oils in the diet. Monounsaturated 18-carbon oleic acid (n-9) can undergo the same reactions, with less saturated products that cannot substitute for those of the EFA.

The prostanoid products of AA and EPA/DHA (Figure 3.5) have different and sometimes opposite effects. These are described in more detail below and in Chapter 15. Formation of prostaglandins and the other products occurs at the level of the cell plasma membrane (Figure 3.4)

Figure 3.5. Forms of prostaglandins, thromboxanes, and leukotrienes synthesized from n-3 and n-6 polyunsaturated fatty acids (in cell membrane phospholipid).

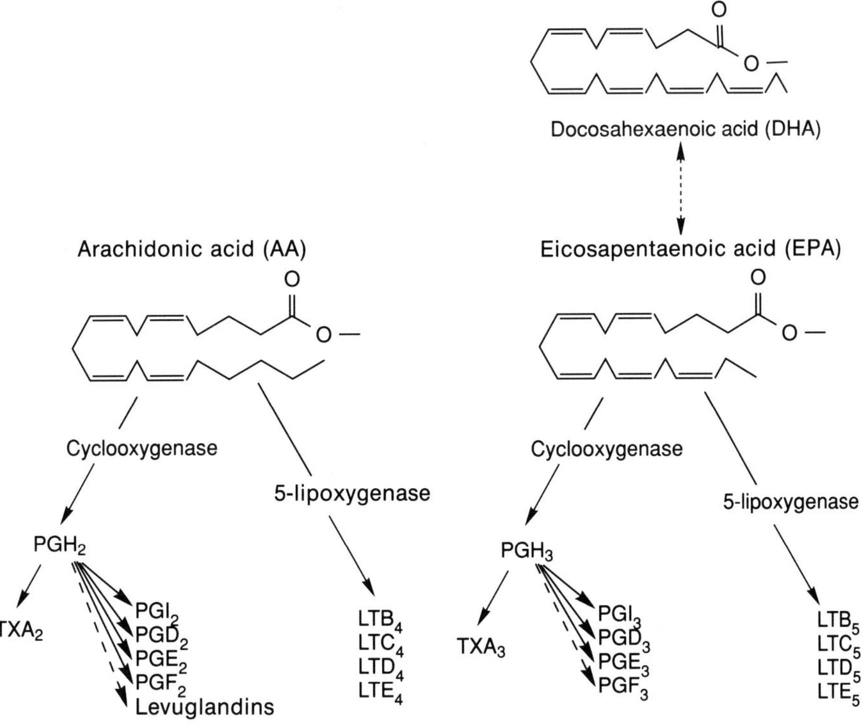

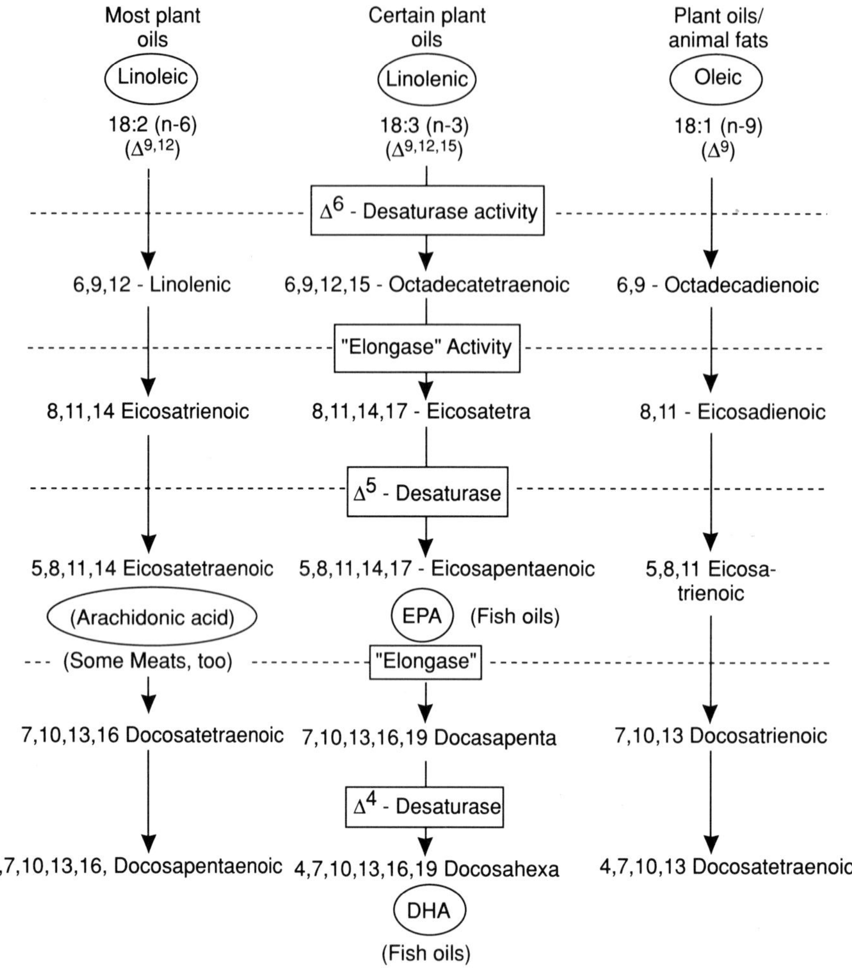

Figure 3.6. Formation of arachidonic acid, eicosapentaenoic acid (EPA), docosahexaenoic acid (DHA), and related fatty acids from 18 carbon n-6, n-3, and n-9 precursors. Based on Garg et al. (1988).

and is initiated by the release of a particular n-6 or n-3 fatty acid from the central glycerol carbon of membrane phospholipid (Figure 3.4) by a hormone/neurotransmitter-sensitive phospholipase A_2 (Levine and Moskowitz, 1979). [Alternatively, it may arise from the action of a diacylglycerol lipase on diacylglycerol, a product of the action of phospholipase C (Burgoyne et al., 1987).] This provides the substrate for prostaglandin synthetase/cyclooxygenase, the first enzyme on the pathway for production of the various prostaglandins and thromboxanes. The cyclooxygenase is inhibited by aspirin and other headache remedies. Leukotriene synthesis from the same fatty acids is initiated via a 5-lipoxygenase (Figure 3.4), and in gonadal tissues, leuglandins are also produced from the cyclooxygenase product, PGH_2 (Salomon et al., 1987).

An additional function of EFA has only recently emerged and helps to explain the classic skin symptomology of deficiency. A unique acyl acid composed of linoleic acid (Figure 3.6) ether bonded to a very long-chain monosaturated fatty acid has been identified free and bound to ceramides in the skin of man and animals (Figure 3.7). This form of interstitial lipid produced by stratum granulosum cells renders the skin impermeable to water (Hansen, 1986). Unsaturated n-3 fatty acids cannot substitute for n-6 linoleic acid in these compounds.

Arachidonic acid is found as 5%–15% of the fatty acid in most cell membrane phospholipids.

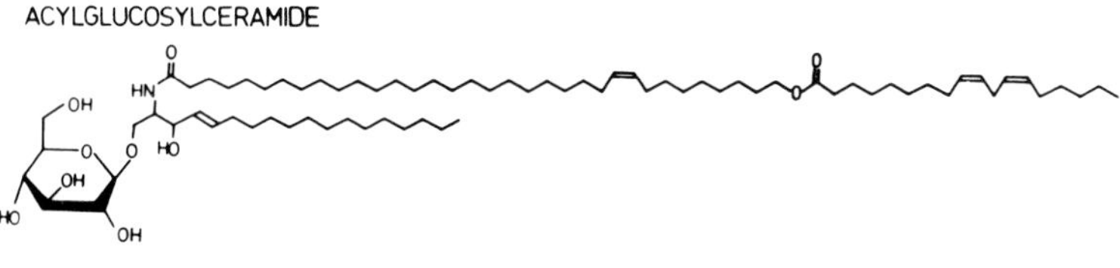

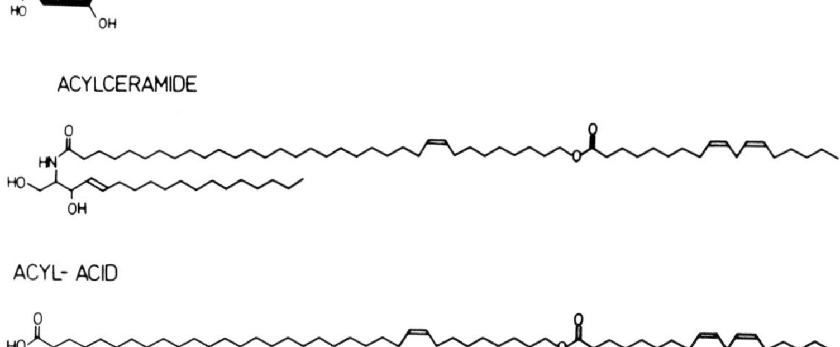

Figure 3.7. Forms of linoleic acid-derived lipid used to ensure the water impermeability of the skin. Reprinted, by permission, from Hansen (1986).

Normally, the n-3 fatty acids (EPA and DHA) are only a few percent of membrane fatty acids but achieve high concentrations in specific organs, notably DHA in retina, cerebral cortex, testes, and sperm (Neuringer et al., 1988). In cerebral gray matter, DHA is about 30% of the fatty acid in phosphatidylserine and ethanolamine and is not confined to the outer cell membranes.

Polyunsaturated fatty acids are also required in the esterification of plasma cholesterol (see below), necessary for its uptake as low density lipoprotein core material (LDL) and the normal excretion of sterols and bile acids (Mead, 1980). EFA or their derivatives may be more effective here.

EFA thus play numerous vital roles as substrates for regulatory signals and as structural elements in cell membranes and other barriers in the body. In the absence of these fatty acids or their dietary precursors, derivatives of monounsaturated oleic acid (18 : 1, n-9) (Figure 3.6) are substituted by the body, but are not able to fulfill the same roles.

Digestion

Breakdown of dietary fat to fatty acids, monoglycerides (monoacylglycerol), choline, etc., occurs almost exclusively in the duodenum and jejunum, through the combined actions of bile salts and pancreatic lipases, in the higher pH environment produced by secretion of bicarbonate. Some digestion (though probably minimal) by a lingual and a gastric lipase also occurs, especially in infancy (Lands, 1979). [These lipases are more efficient in the release of short-chain fatty acids (Linscheer and Vergroesen, 1988), as found in milk and coconuts.] In the duodenum, bile salts emulsify the fat, and with the help of peristaltic perturbation and inherent phospholipid, disperse it into small droplets with an estimated 10,000-fold increase in surface area. This allows the lipases access to the lipid. The partially digested lipid (still mainly water insoluble) forms stable micelles, consisting mainly of long-chain fatty acids, monoglycerides, and bile acids, which diffuse to the surface of mucosal cells and deliver the material for absorption. More polar products of digestion, such as short-chain fatty acids, phosphate, choline, etc., diffuse through the aqueous medium. In man, most of the triacylglycerol is broken down into monoacylglycerides (with the fatty acid retained on the central glycerol carbon), although some glycerol is also formed. Phospholipids are fully hydrolyzed or are left as lysophospholipids (the central fatty acid removed). Cholesterol is also deesterified, although this is a relatively slow process and thus reduces the absorption of dietary cholesterol. [Biliary nonesterified cholesterol is more readily reabsorbed (Linscheer and Vergroesen, 1988).]

Absorption

The fatty acids, monoacylglycerols, phosphate, free cholesterol, and other "building blocks" of fat formed by digestion are absorbed into the cells of the intestinal mucosa. Absorption occurs by passive diffusion, mainly in the upper half of the small intestine. The bile acids secreted to aid in digestion and absorption are mainly reabsorbed further down the intestinal tract (see Chapter 1). Phospholipids and free cholesterol in bile are pooled with, and have the same fate as, those in the diet. An overview of the process of digestion, absorption, and disposition of dietary fat after a meal is given in Figure 3.8.

Once within the intestinal mucosa, triacylglycerols, phospholipids, and some cholesterol esters are resynthesized, packaged with small amounts of protein, and then secreted as chylomicrons (Table 3.3) into the extracellular space, entering the lacteals of the lymphatic system. Chylomicrons are members of the class of lipoproteins eventually appearing in the plasma (Table 3.3) which have the common structural feature of a lipid core (containing triglyceride and cholesterol) and a surface of phospholipid and protein, the latter in contact with the aqueous phase. The proportions of various lipids and proteins (and the resultant densities) vary with the type of lipoprotein (Table 3.3). Short-chain free fatty acids (less than 14 carbons) in the intestinal mucosa enter the blood via the portal vein bound to albumin. These may be directly utilized by tissues as an energy source, or utilized for triacylglycerol synthesis by the liver. The intestinal mucosa also synthesizes some very low-density lipoprotein (VLDL) and high-density lipoprotein (HDL) (Figure 3.7). VLDL is primarily composed of triglycerides (but also contains some cholesterol and phospholipid) attached to several types of protein (Table 3.3). Most VLDL is synthesized by the liver. On entering the blood it is converted to LDL by removal of triglyceride and proteins. Triglyceride removal occurs mainly in adipose and/or muscle tissue, with the help of lipoprotein lipase (see below). VLDL produced by the intestine contains less cholesterol and a different form of apoprotein B than the more abundant VLDL produced by the liver (Hamosh et al., 1975; Linscheer and Vergroesen, 1988).

Distribution and Metabolism

The major portion of dietary fat (which has entered the lymphatic system) slowly enters into the bloodstream (as chylomicrons) through the thoracic duct, thus preventing large-scale changes in the lipid content of peripheral blood. Entry of chylomicrons into the blood from the lymph begins 1–2 hr after a meal and continues for many hours after consumption of meals heavy in fat. The chylomicrons and VLDL are mainly processed by adipose and muscle cells (Figure 3.8). One of the apoproteins on the surface of the chylomicron micelles (apo C II) activates lipoprotein lipase (LPL) attached to endothelial cells lining the small blood vessels and capillaries in these tissues. This causes the localized release of free fatty acids, which are quickly absorbed and utilized for energy or reincorporated into triglyceride for later use.

LPL is produced by most cell types, but is most abundant in fat and cardiac muscle tissues, as well as in the lactating mammary gland (Eckel, 1989). After secretion, it is bound to a polysaccharide structure protruding from the basement membrane underlying capillary endothelial cells, from which it can be released and stabilized directly by heparin. LPL is released into the circulation when insulin is secreted. This release is

Table 3.3. Structure, Composition, and Turnover of Plasma Lipoproteins in Man (Modified)

Parameter	VLDL[a]	LDL	HDL	Chylomicrons
Molecular weight (10^6)	5–10	2.5–2.8	0.18–0.36	400–30,000
Density (g/ml)	0.95–1.006	1.006–1.063[a]	1.063–1.25	<0.95
Lipid content (percent weight)				
Triacylglycerol	44–60 (15,700)[b]	8–11 (192)	4–9	84–95
Phospholipid	18–23 (4,400)	25–27 (743)	22–28 (94)	7–8
Cholesterol				
free	5–8 (1,600)	7–13 (538)	3–10 (6)	2
esterified	11–15 (3,700)	35–43 (1,390)	7–38 (32)	5
Protein content (percent weight)	4–11	23–28	21–48	2
Apoproteins present	C > B 100 > E (180 : 70 : 24)[c]	B 100 (63)	AI > AII > C > E [3–5 (AI + AII) : 1–2 : 0–1]	AI, AII, B 48, C
Turnover in plasma	1–3 hr	45%/day	~4 days	4–5 min

Source: Data mainly from Stein (1986) and Linscheer and Vergroesen (1988).

[a] Includes IDL.
[b] Average mol/mol.
[c] For intestinal VLDL, apoprotein B 48 is involved.

probably mediated by a phospholipase that attacks the phosphoinositide anchor of the enzyme (Chan et al., 1988).

During "digestion" of chylomicrons (and VLDL) by LPL, excess surface phospholipid and some proteins and cholesterol are transferred to HDL. Removal of apo C II (to HDL) allows the uptake of triglyceride-depleted "remnants" of chylomicrons, by the liver, via specific receptors and endocytosis, a process mediated by apoprotein E (Mahley, 1988). The half-life of chylomicrons in blood is normally only 4–5 min (Brown and Goldstein, 1979; Brown et al., 1981), but these particles are usually only fully cleared from the blood 8–10 hr after a meal, as they continue to dribble in from the (slower) lymph circulation. "Remnants" of intestinal VLDL are thought to enter the liver by the same pathway (Linscheer and Vergroesen, 1988), in contrast to liver VLDL, which goes on to form LDL (see below).

In the liver, any remaining triacylglycerol and phospholipid, and the cholesterol ester, are deesterified, and the fatty acids and cholesterol enter existing liver pools. Cholesterol is either excreted in the bile or incorporated into VLDL for further transport. If not required locally for energy or cell membranes, diet-derived fatty acids may be modified and pooled with fatty acids produced mainly from excess carbohydrate and reincorporated into triacylglycerol. Phospholipids, cholesterol, and protein are packaged and released in the form of liver VLDL. HDL (Figure 3.8 and Table 3.3) is also formed in the liver and small intestine. Liver VLDL enters the bloodstream and has the same initial fate as intestinal VLDL, losing its triglyceride to lipoprotein lipase (activated by apo C-II, which then transfers to HDL). It also has a much longer half-life in the plasma than chylomicrons (1–3 hr) (Brown et al., 1981).

Most of the fatty acids released from VLDL enter adipose tissue for storage as triglyceride (and/or muscle, for use as an energy source). The remaining lipoprotein (intermediate density lipoprotein, IDL) becomes LDL with the help of HDL and lecithin-cholesterol acyl transferase (LCAT), which esterifies the cholesterol with a polyunsaturated fatty acid from position 2 on lecithin. [LCAT is activated by apoprotein A-I.] LDL, which consists principally of a cholesterol-ester core, protein, and surface phospholipids (Table 3.3), is then taken up by most peripheral tissues, via receptor-mediated endocytosis involving apoprotein B recognition. [Some IDL is also removed by the same process (Mahley, 1988).] The turnover of LDL is much slower than that of VLDL, with a fractional removal rate of about 45% of the plasma pool per day in the normal adult (Brown et al., 1981). Especially at higher levels (but to some degree also normally; Stein, 1986), additional removal of LDL occurs with the help of reticuloendothelial macrophages (Brown et al., 1981), as well as by increased nonspecific uptake.

As in the liver (see later), the release of cholesterol from LDL represses endogenous cholesterol biosynthesis (feedback control). In contrast to LDL, HDL (also synthesized by the liver) is the main vehicle for transfer of cholesterol-ester between cells and back to the liver (Scanu, 1978) (see below). HDL has a higher protein-to-lipid ratio than LDL or VLDL and a phospholipid content exceeding that of cholesterol and triglyceride (Table 3.3). It is also involved in the delipidation of chylomicrons and VLDL, and the formation of LDL from VLDL, as already described. With apoprotein E, it may be viewed as a key mediator in the complex system of lipid transport and distribution. Further aspects of its function are described in the cholesterol section that follows. A schematized model of lipoprotein transport, for lipid derived from exogenous as well as endogenous sources, is shown in Figure 3.8 (see legend for details). A partial (simpler) version is in Figure 3.9.

During the early absorptive phase, especially after a carbohydrate-containing meal, the levels of key enzymes that promote storage of glucose carbon as fat are increased. These include acetyl-CoA carboxylase (ACC) and fatty acid synthetase, as well as malic enzyme and several enzymes of the pentose shunt which are necessary for fatty acid synthesis (the latter through formation of NADPH) in the liver and adipocytes. Also included is the extracellular lipoprotein lipase in adipose tissue, which would receive triacylglycerol coming from the liver on VLDL. Concomitantly, hormone-sensitive lipase (HSL) activity needed for release of fatty acids from adipocytes is reduced (Eckel, 1989). These events are promoted by insulin and thyroid hormone (triiodothyronine/T_3) via effects on transcription and translation (Eckel, 1989; Goodridge, 1987). [Effects of insulin on ACC and HSL also involve a 5′ AMP-dependent (not cAMP-dependent) kinase (Hardie et al., 1989).]

The distribution of fatty acid derived from the diet to various organs (on chylomicrons and intestinal VLDL) and their utilization will depend at least partly on their structure. For example, medium-chain length fatty acids tend to be used for energy, whereas saturated or monounsatu-

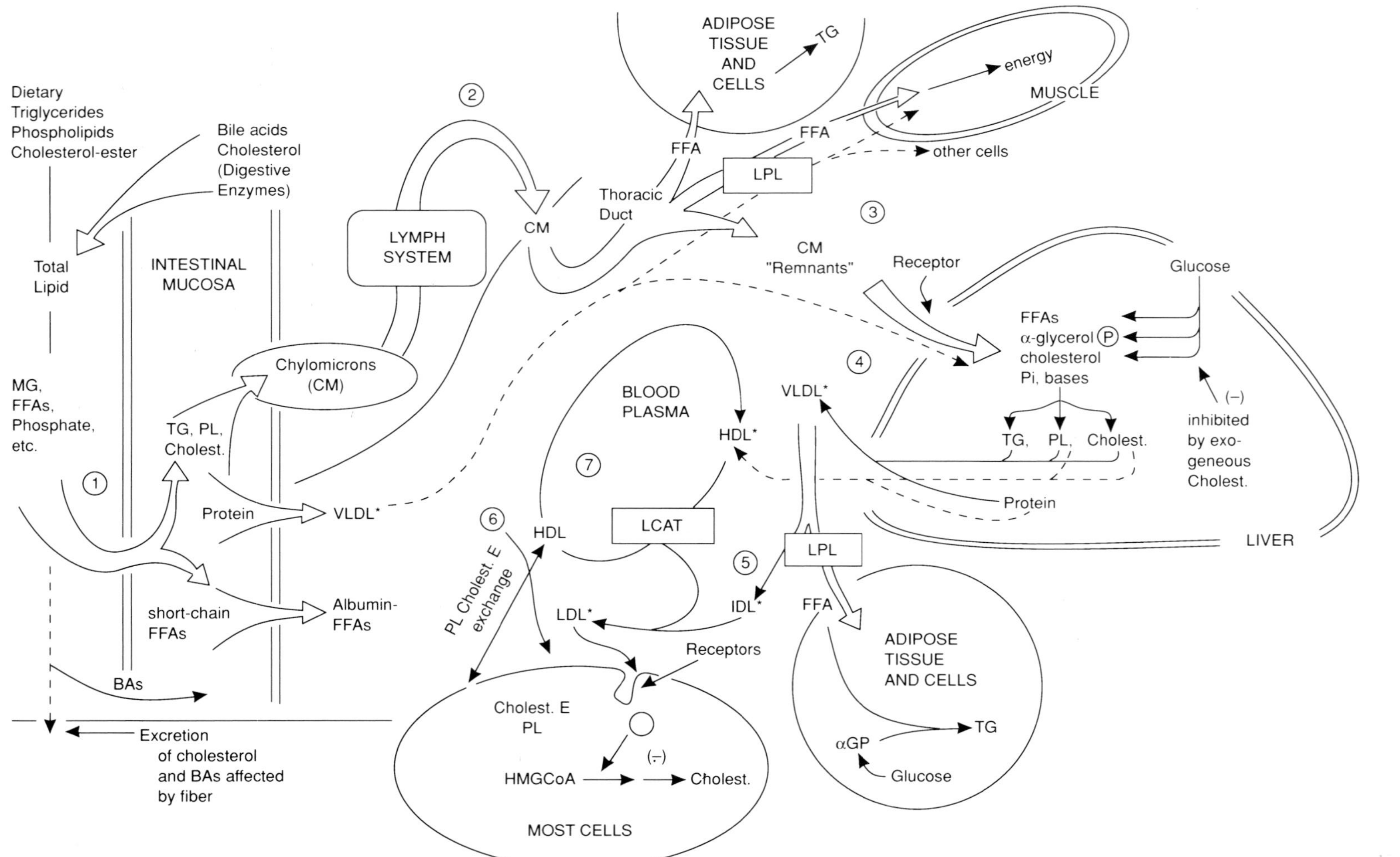

Figure 3.8. Disposal of dietary fat after a meal. Abbreviations: TG, triacylglycerol (triglyceride); PL, phospholipid; Cholest. E, cholesterol-ester; CM, chylomicrons; (square) plasma/capillary enzymes; LPL, lipoprotein lipase; LCAT, lecithin-cholesterol acyl transferase; BA, bile acids. Asterisk (*) means lipoproteins. Key: (1) Digestion of dietary fat and entry into the intestinal mucosa; (2) distribution via chylomicrons (removal of TG by LPL); (3) "remnants" enter liver (by receptor-mediated endocytosis); (4) output of VLDL by liver (and intestine); (5) conversion to LDL via IDL (after removal of TG by LPL and esterification of cholesterol by fatty acid from HDL); (6) cholesterol uptake (via LDL-receptor-mediated endocytosis); (7) synthesis and function of HDL, including return of cholesterol to the liver via HDL. (See Figure 3.12B.)

rated longer fatty acids tend to be used for storage, either directly or indirectly (via the liver) (Linscheer and Vergroesen, 1988). In the liver, especially, some desaturation may also occur. Polyunsaturated omega-3 (n-3) fatty acids, such as EPA and DHA (Figures 3.2A and 3.5), may be taken up directly by many cells for incorporation into their membrane phospholipid, and they may also be obtained indirectly from liver phospholipid distributed by HDL and other lipoproteins. Linoleic acid (n-6) from the diet is lengthened and used partly to form arachidonic acid for membrane phospholipid (Figure 3.6). Such fatty acids are important for the formation of prostaglandins, leukotrienes, and thromboxanes (Figures 3.4 and 3.5). Liver Δ^6-desaturase activity (which is rate-limiting for arachidonic acid synthesis) varies in relation to the fat composition of the diet (Garg et al., 1988) (at least in rats) and is reduced by dietary fish oil (n-3 fatty acids) or cholesterol.

As the body enters the postabsorptive period when glucose is no longer entering the blood from the intestine (so insulin is no longer released), the pattern of fat flow (and glucose) into storage is gradually reversed. As breakdown of glycogen begins in the liver to maintain blood glucose, the liver switches to fat as an energy source, and the same transition is increasingly made by other tissues. In support of this, fatty acids released from chylomicrons (and VLDL) are used increasingly for fuel; adipose tissue gradually slows its uptake of fatty acid (for storage) and eventually switches to triglyceride hydrolysis, releasing free fatty acids and glycerol into the blood (Figure 3.10).

Some of the same hormones that signal the liver and muscle to draw on their glycogen reserves signal activation of the hormone-sensitive lipase in adipose tissue (ACTH, glucagon) and reduce the activity of adipose tissue LPL. [LPL activity in muscle will increase or stay unchanged (Eckel, 1989).] The "fright–flight" mechanism that results in secretion of ACTH, glucocorticosteroids, and catecholamines also has this effect, as does sympathomimetic nerve stimulation. The action of all these hormones is via the cAMP–protein kinase system, which is also involved in glycogen breakdown (see Figure 2.4A, Chapter 2).

Free fatty acids released into the blood travel on albumin to most organs, where they diffuse across cell membranes and are carried into mitochondria for oxidation. [Transport across the mitochondrial membrane is accomplished with the help of carnitine (see Chapter 5 and Figure

Figure 3.9. Model for lipoprotein transport in humans, illustrating the division between the endogenous and exogenous cycles. Both cycles begin with the secretion of triglyceride-rich particles (chylomicrons and VLDL) that are converted to cholesterol-ester-rich particles (remnants, IDL, and LDL) through interaction with LPL. Abbreviations: LPL, lipoprotein lipase; VLDL, very low density lipoproteins; IDL, intermediate density lipoproteins; LDL, low density lipoproteins; HDL, high density lipoproteins; LCAT, lecithin-cholesterol acyl transferase. [*Source:* Reprinted by permission from Brown MS, Kovanen DT, Goldstein JL: (1981) Science 212:628. Copyright 1981 by the American Association for the Advancement of Science.]

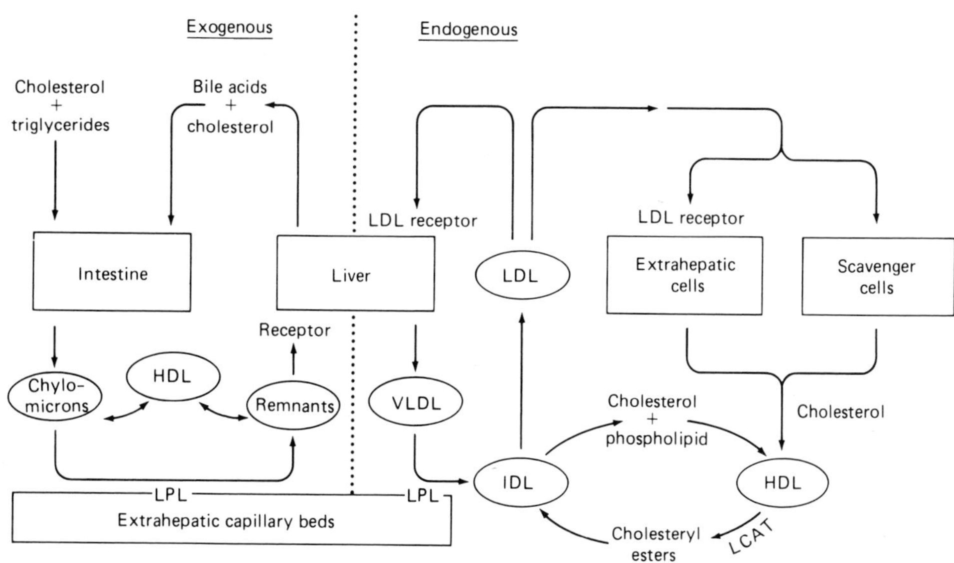

5.37).] Glycerol, on the other hand, travels mainly to the liver and, to a lesser degree, to the kidney, the only tissues where it can be utilized. The first step in utilization requires phosphorylation by α-glycerol kinase, which is not found in other tissues. The absence of the latter enzyme in adipose tissue probably helps to protect the body from futile cycles of triglyceride synthesis and breakdown, as the formation of α-glycerol phosphate in adipose tissue would allow resynthesis of triglyceride. Synthesis of triacylglycerol in adipocytes is dependent on α-glycerol phosphate generation from glucose, and under the conditions where fat is needed for fuel, glucose is not available for this process.

Because the signal for release of free fatty acid is similar to the signal that puts the liver into a gluconeogenic mode, the α-glycerol phosphate produced in the liver probably goes toward synthesis of glucose used to maintain blood glucose concentrations. Glycerol is only 5% of triglyceride carbon and is the only portion of fat that can be used for net production of glucose. Otherwise, no net production of glucose from lipid carbon can occur.

Increasingly, as fasting continues, larger proportions of the free fatty acid in the circulation are converted to ketone bodies, principally in the liver (Figure 3.10). Ketone bodies are a form of fuel much more water-soluble than fatty acids. The pathway for their synthesis is via acetyl-CoA (Figure 3.11). These ketones are used as fuel by

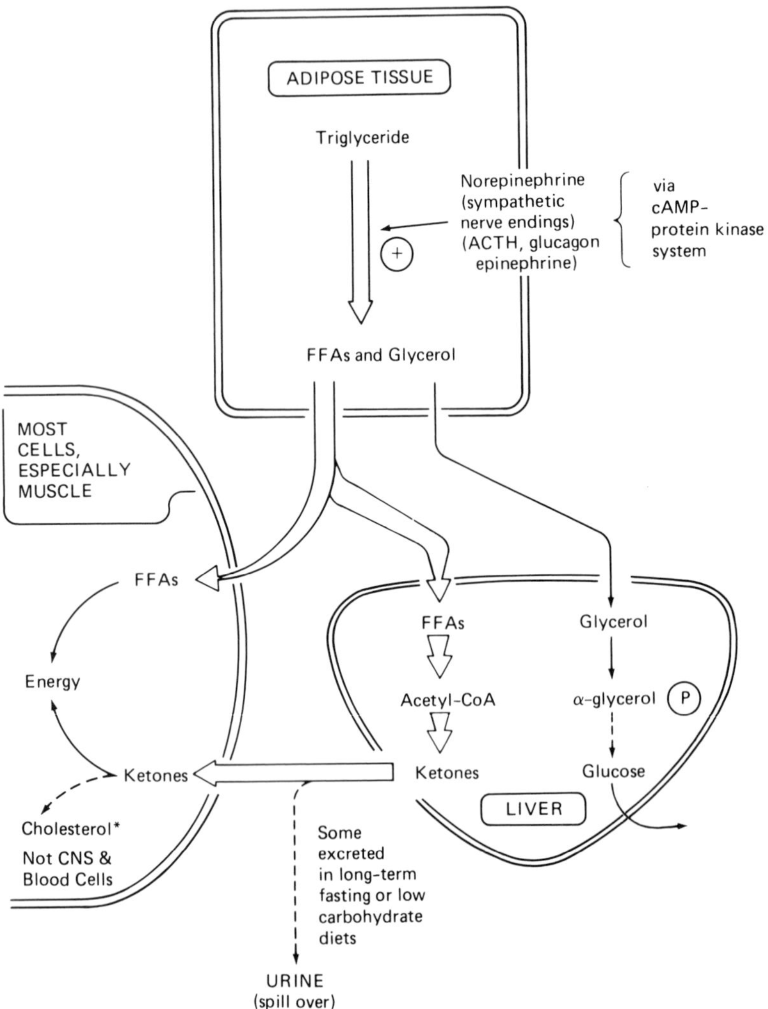

Figure 3.10. Utilization of stored triglyceride (triacylglycerol) between meals, in fasting, and on low carbohydrate diets. Asterisk (*) refers to findings of Bergstrom et al. (1981, 1982); ketone carbon also contributes to fatty acid synthesis in some cases.

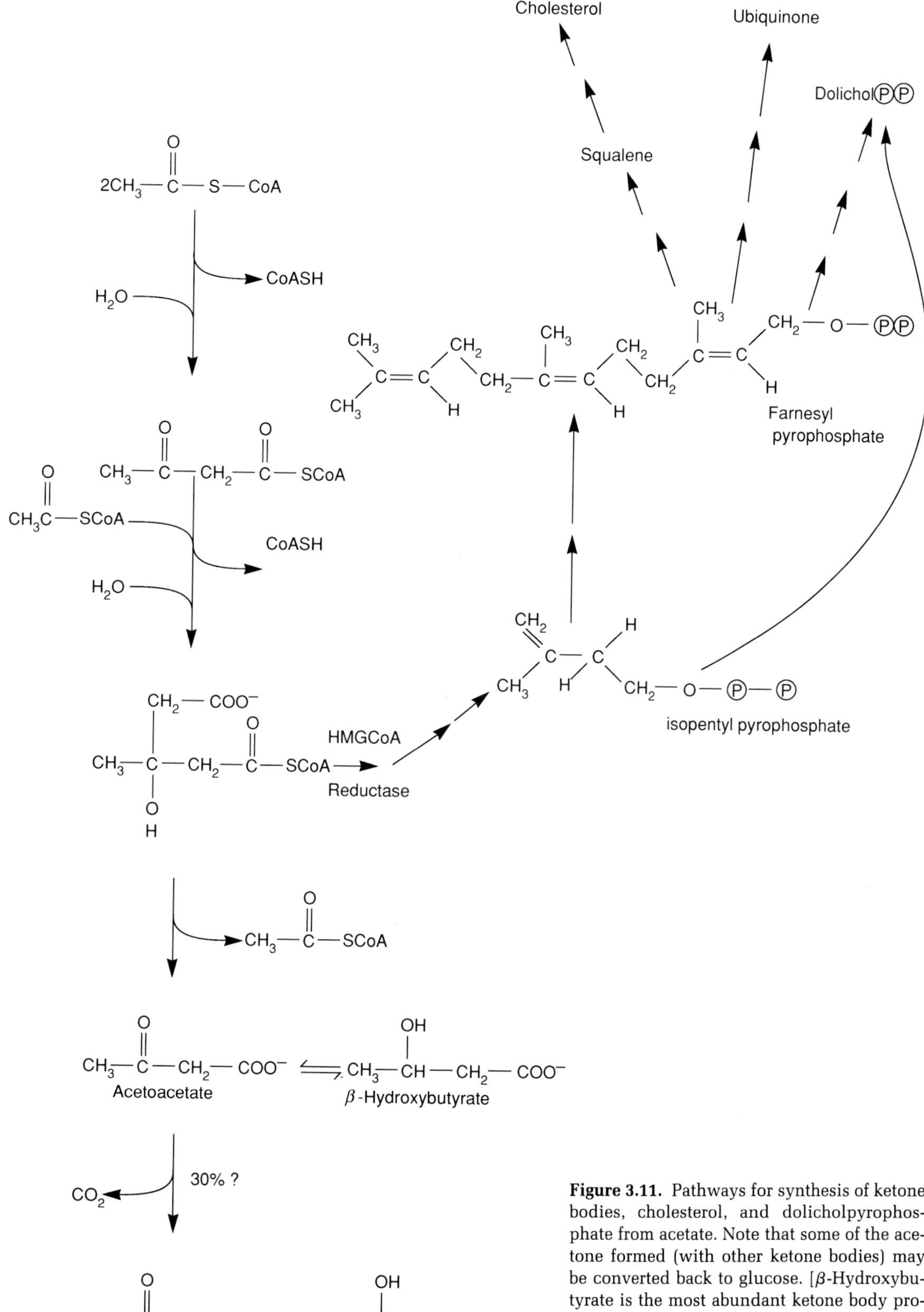

Figure 3.11. Pathways for synthesis of ketone bodies, cholesterol, and dolicholpyrophosphate from acetate. Note that some of the acetone formed (with other ketone bodies) may be converted back to glucose. [β-Hydroxybutyrate is the most abundant ketone body produced; acetone is only made in small amounts.]

the muscles and other tissues and, as fasting continues, eventually also by the central nervous system and brain, which does not utilize much fatty acid (Figure 3.10). Ketone production increases gradually during fasting, reaching its maximum by about 10 days (see Figure 4.10, Chapter 4). The same occurs in individuals consuming little or no carbohydrate. As calculated by Cahill and colleagues (1973), ketones become as important as glucose (from gluconeogenesis) as a source of energy, accounting for about 17% of total calories (see Figure 4.9, Chapter 4). When maximum amounts of ketones are produced, a proportion (about 18%) spills over into the urine. Long-term fasting is also characterized by "acetone breath," since small amounts of the latter, formed from the ketones, are exhaled. The formation of α-ketobutyric and acetoacetic acids, which travel in the bloodstream, requires an adjustment in acid/base balance. In the normal individual, increasing ammonia formation occurs in parallel with increased ketone production (see Figure 4.8, Chapter 4). The enzyme involved is the phosphate-dependent kidney glutaminase, which uses the most abundant plasma amino acid, glutamine, as a substrate. Consequently, a much smaller proportion of nitrogen is lost in the form of urea (Cahill et al., 1973).

Cholesterol and Phospholipid Metabolism

The pathway taken by cholesterol from the diet to tissues has already partly been described, beginning with its incorporation into chylomicrons (and intestinal VLDL) and delivery to the liver in the form of "remnants" absorbed via receptor-mediated endocytosis (Figure 3.8). Liver remnant receptors recognize apoprotein E (Mahley, 1988) associated with these particles (Table 3.3). Figure 3.12 further details the progression with regard to cholesterol.

After uptake into the hepatocytes, diet-derived cholesterol is released during "digestion" of remnants in the endocytic vesicles (Figure 3.12A). Attached to carrier proteins in the cytosol, it then has three effects on endogenous metabolism: (1) direct inhibition of the rate-limiting enzyme for cholesterol biosynthesis, hydroxymethylglutaryl (HMG)-CoA reductase; (2) decreased transcription of the gene for this enzyme, and thus a reduction in its rate of synthesis; (3) decreased transcription of the gene for liver LDL receptors (that depend on recognition of apoproteins B and E) (Mahley, 1988); this results in fewer receptors on hepatocyte plasma membranes. The extent of these effects will depend upon the amount of dietary cholesterol. Thus, endogenous cholesterol production, which occurs primarily in the liver (and to some extent in the intestine) will be decreased in relation to dietary intake. The more comes in, the less is produced, and vice versa. This "feedback" control is designed to prevent fluctuations in blood VLDL and LDL cholesterol concentrations and to maintain a consistent supply of the substance for use by peripheral cells (see below, Special Topics). Cholesterol synthesis by peripheral cells is similarly controlled by cholesterol released from LDL after endocytic uptake (Figure 3.12A). [Some membrane cholesterol is also replaced by HDL (see below).] Thus, peripheral cells control their cholesterol supplies by encouraging uptake (via more LDL receptors) and endogenous biosynthesis, or the reverse, depending on their needs.

Ultimately, all cholesterol must be returned to the liver for excretion, except that being used to form steroid hormones and vitamin D (Figure 3.3). HDL is the lipoprotein mainly responsible for this return (Figure 3.12A and B), where cholesterol is ultimately released into the bile as free cholesterol and bile acids. [Bile consists largely of bile acids and phospholipid in a supersaturated solution of cholesterol. It also carries bile pigments (from porphyrin degradation) and several trace elements (see Chapter 7).] Formation of bile acids occurs in hepatocytes, and bile is temporarily stored in the gallbladder. Biliary substituents put into the duodenum to aid in fat digestion are at least partly recycled. This "enterohepatic" recycling (between intestine and liver) is particularly efficient for the bile acids, which hepatocytes extract from portal blood (Stoltz et al., 1989). Phospholipid recycling is also efficient, and it is noteworthy that much more phospholipid enters the digestive tract in the bile than is present in the diet (12 versus 2 g on average, respectively) (Linscheer and Vergroesen, 1988). Biliary *cholesterol* is not as readily recycled, although it is absorbed more easily than dietary cholesterol-ester. [The efficiency of cholesterol absorption is simply not that great, which is as it should be if it is to be excreted.] Thus, in contrast to other types of fats, which are lost from the body as CO_2 and H_2O, cholesterol is not catabolized, but is lost largely unchanged or as its derivative bile acids. Dietary fiber enhances these losses by binding and dilution (which reduce the efficiency of resorption/absorption), and by enhancing the rate of transit of cholesterol and bile acids through the intestine and colon (see Chapter 2).

The manner in which cholesterol (and phospholipid) is returned to the liver and/or redistributed among cells after its delivery on LDL is of recent interest and summarized in Figure 3.12B. The key players in these processes are HDL and apoprotein E. [Lipid transfer protein (LTP) is important in that it mediates the extracellular lipid exchanges involved (Morton, 1988).] Apoprotein E is made by the liver for VLDL and released from IDL during LDL formation (Figures 3.8 and 3.12A). Apoprotein E is also produced independently of VLDL by the brain and most other tissues (except intestinal mucosa), where an important source is probably the macrophage (Mahley, 1988). This apoprotein E is released as discs formed with phospholipid (density, ~1.08) (Basu et al., 1983; Mahley, 1988). HDL devoid of apoprotein E picks up cholesterol-ester from the membranes of cells with too much cholesterol (including macrophages that may be metabolizing necrotic cells) (Figure 3.12B). In the process, it enlarges (fills) and then takes on apoprotein E (and phospholipid, in discs) present in the circulation and interstitial fluid. The apoprotein conveys the capacity for receptor-mediated uptake, via the LDL receptors, so that HDL and its cholesterol are absorbed. (LDL receptors recognize both apoprotein E and B.) Absorption is either by other peripheral cells needing cholesterol, or by liver hepatocytes for disposal and/or conversion to bile acids. A reduction in the reabsorption of bile acids from the intestine, and thus a drop in the bile acid concentration of the portal blood, will enhance formation and disposition of hepatocyte membrane LDL receptors, so that removal of LDL, IDL, and HDL cholesterol from the blood is enhanced. HDL (with apoprotein E) may also use hepatocyte chylomicron remnant receptors, as these appear to depend on recognition of apoprotein E as well (Mahley, 1988). Apoprotein E thus becomes pivotal in allowing redistribution and accelerated disposal of cholesterol in cells throughout the body, peripheral to the liver. Nevertheless, some individuals have just been discovered with a genetic incapacity to produce apoprotein E, and these individuals do not appear to be suffering from any gross defects in lipid metabolism (ref). Therefore, the apoprotein B-containing lipoproteins may be able to take up the task of cholesterol (and phospholipid) redistribution, when apoprotein E is lacking.

Special Topics

Cholesterol Nutrition and the Control of Serum Cholesterol Concentrations

The average American consumes about 0.3–0.5 g of cholesterol/day. The main food sources contributing exogenous cholesterol are meat, eggs, and dairy products (Table 3.1).

The average adult requires about 1.1 g cholesterol/day for maintenance of cell membranes and other functions. Of this, 10%–20% (100–200 mg) normally comes from the diet and the rest from endogenous biosynthesis, mainly by the liver and secondarily by the small intestine (Figure 3.8). As already indicated, there is no feedback regulation of cholesterol biosynthesis in the small intestine, but in the liver (on the microsomes) the rate-limiting enzyme for cholesterol biosynthesis (HMG-CoA reductase) is directly inhibited by dietary cholesterol entering on chylomicron remnants or LDL (Figure 3.12A). Consequently, if less cholesterol is eaten and absorbed, more is synthesized by the liver, and vice versa. As a result, a drastic reduction in cholesterol intake generally results in a small decrease in total plasma cholesterol concentrations (usually about 10%–15%). Similarly, there are no significant changes in serum cholesterol in most persons switching from one or more eggs per day to fewer or no eggs, or vice versa (Buzzard et al., 1983; Porter et al., 1977), except in a fraction of the population that is "cholesterol-sensitive" (Flynn et al., 1986; Katan and Beynen, 1987; Katan et al., 1986). [The extent of cholesterol sensitivity in the United States and other countries is still unclear, but the sensitivity appears not to be predicted by cholesterol intake, body weight, or levels of plasma HDL (Katan and Beynen, 1987).]

The small amount of cholesterol biosynthesis occurring in peripheral tissues other than the intestine is also feedback controlled. In this case, cholesterol enters on LDL, which originates mainly in the liver. This inhibits endogenous cholesterol production (Figure 3.12A). Entry of this cholesterol into peripheral (and liver) cells occurs by receptor-mediated endocytosis. The hereditary absence of receptors, or presence of altered receptors, prevents normal removal of cholesterol from the blood. The reduction in the rate of plasma cholesterol uptake mediated by these receptors thus causes an abnormal elevation of plasma/serum cholesterol, as in the case of homozygous familial hypercholesterolemia, where pe-

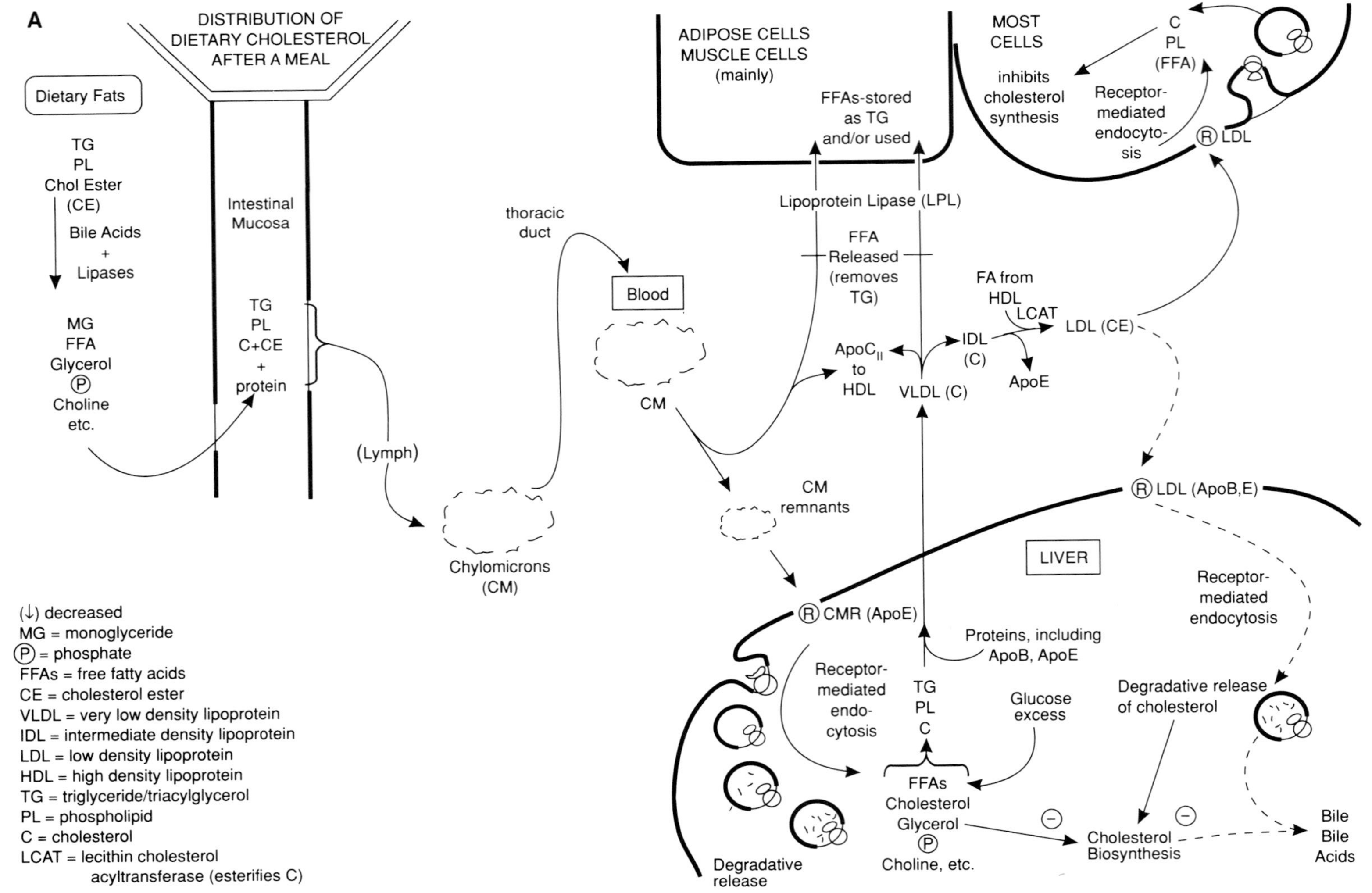

Figure 3.12. Distribution and disposal of cholesterol. **(A)** Uptake and distribution of dietary cholesterol and cholesterol coming from the liver, including feedback regulation of liver cholesterol synthesis by dietary cholesterol (entering through chylomicron remnant receptors that recognize apoprotein E), and expression of HMG-CoA reductase and LDL receptors (recognizing apoproteins B and E). [Feedback regulation also occurs in peripheral cells, as instituted by incoming LDL cholesterol.] See Figure 3.8 for other abbreviations.

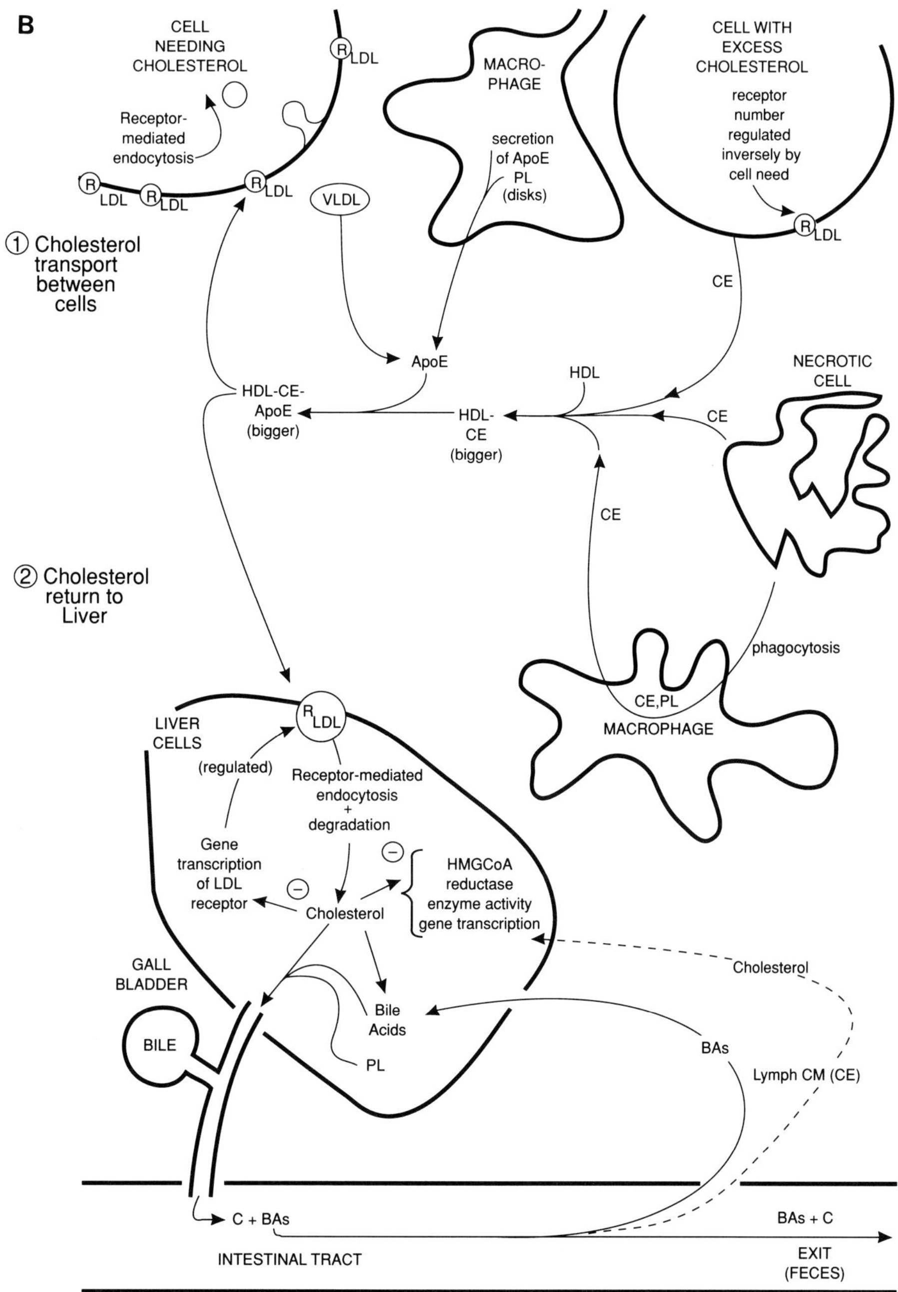

Figure 3.12. (*continued*) **(B)** Transfer of cholesterol ester from one cell to another, involving HDL and apoprotein E, and including return of peripheral cholesterol to the liver via liver LDL receptors, its partial conversion to bile acids, and secretion into the bile and small intestine. Abbreviations: Most are as in Figure 3.8; R refers to cell surface receptors that recognize specific apoproteins in the lipoproteins, as indicated (subscript); BAs = bile acids. [Major reference: Mahley (1988).] See text for further explanation.

ripheral LDL receptors are absent or impaired. The level of receptors on peripheral and hepatic cells can also be influenced by other factors, such as hormones (especially thyroxine), dietary cholesterol intake, and dietary fiber or nonabsorbable bile-acid-binding resins (given as part of therapy) (Table 3.4).

Disposal of serum cholesterol secreted by the liver on VLDL also depends on esterification of cholesterol with unsaturated fatty acids (from lecithin) (LCAT) to form LDL (Figures 3.8 and 3.9). Conversely,, overproduction (or overrelease) of cholesterol by (from) the liver may also be responsible for some of the hypercholesterolemia in our population. This could result from an altered structure or regulation of HMG-CoA reductase (so that cholesterol feedback inhibition is less effective); or overproduction of triacylglycerol, apoprotein B, or other factors leading to increased synthesis and release of liver VLDL. Decreased production and excretion of bile acids and cholesterol through the bile can also lead to hypercholesterolemia. Although (as already indicated) these are largely reabsorbed, there is sufficient loss to account for the needed daily production and/or absorption from the diet of about 1.1 g cholesterol/day (Brown et al., 1981). An average of about 50 mg of bile acids, formed from cholesterol (Figure 3.3), is irreversibly lost daily, although the amount depends on the fiber content of the diet (see below). The production of steroid hormones and vitamin D from cholesterol takes another 20 mg or so [6–29 mg are used for glucocorticoids alone per day (Briggs and Brotherton, 1970)], and small amounts are lost from the sloughing of cells from the skin and gastrointestinal tract.

The reabsorption of bile acids and cholesterol from the gastrointestinal tract depends, in part, on the degree of binding to dietary fiber. Pectins, carrageenan (Figure 2.1), and soluble fibers, but not cellulose and lignin, bind and increase the

Table 3.4. LDL Receptors on Liver and Other Cells

Characteristic	Extrahepatic LDL receptors	Hepatic LDL (Apo B/E) receptors	Hepatic Apo E receptors
Binding properties exhibited by both receptors in vitro	Affinity for apoE > apoB Binding abolished by: Ethylenediaminetetraacetic acid Modification of lysine or arginine residues of apoproteins Pronase treatment of membranes Antibody against LDL receptor of bovine adrenal cortex Receptor initiates endocytosis		Apo E
Major lipoproteins bound in vivo	LDL	LDL, IDL, VLDL	VLDL remnants, Chylomicron remnants and LDL
Factors that increase	(↑) or decrease (↓) receptors		
Genetic	(↓) Familial hypercholesterolemia (humans, WHHL rabbits)	(↓) Familial hypercholesterolemia (humans, WHHL rabbits)	
Hormonal	(↑) Thyroxine (↑) Insulin (↑) Platelet-derived growth factor (↑) ACTH in adrenal cortex	(↑) Thyroxine (humans)	
Nutritional	(↑) Cholesterol deprivation (↓) Excess cellular cholesterol	(↓) Cholesterol feeding (rabbits)	
Pharmacologic		(↑) 17α-Ethinylestradiol (rats) (↑) Bile-acid-binding resins (humans, dogs, rabbits)[a] (↑) Inhibitors of cholesterol synthesis (dogs)[b]	

Source: Modified from Brown et al. (1981) (see Figure 3.12).

[a] Cholesterol or cholestyramine.
[b] Mevinolin or compactin.

fecal excretion of bile acids and cholesterol (Huang et al., 1978; Story, 1980; see references, Chapter 2; see also Chapters 15 and 16). Other fiber may also enhance fecal sterol excretion by reducing the transit time of food passing through the small intestine. Increased rates of fecal bile acid or cholesterol loss can result in reduced levels of plasma cholesterol (on the order of 10%–25%). Indeed, hypercholesterolemia is often treated by administering nonabsorbable bile acid and cholesterol-binding resins, such as cholestyramine (see Chapter 15). Fiber will also enhance production of propionate by bacteria in the lower intestinal tract, which may inhibit liver cholesterol synthesis (Illman et al., 1988) after its absorption into the blood. The administration of clofibrate, a thyroxine analog, was also used in the past to aid hypercholesterolemia by inhibiting endogenous cholesterol synthesis without providing cholesterol (see Chapter 15). Mevinolin or Mevacor/Lovastatin have the same effect, thereby increasing hepatic apoprotein B/E (LDL) receptors for enhanced removal of cholesterol from the blood. (The latter medications are now widely used to correct certain hereditary hypercholesterolemias.)

Apart from heredity and dietary fiber, a major factor to influence serum cholesterol concentrations is the type *and amount* of fat in the diet. In general, a high fat intake goes with a tendency toward elevated blood cholesterol, although there are significant exceptions (see Chapter 15). Similarly, intake of more saturated fat, and a lower polyunsaturated to saturated fat (P/S) ratio (as in Western-style diets) tends to be associated with hypercholesterolemia. The actual type of fatty acid (rather than saturation versus polyunsaturation per se) is also important. The effects of different dietary fats seem to fall into three groups: (1) those high in stearate (18 : 0) or oleate (18 : 1) cause lower levels of blood cholesterol than those high in palmitate (16 : 0) (Bonanome and Grundy, 1988) or short-chain saturated acids (laurate and myristate; 12 : 0 and 14 : 0, respectively) (Kritchevsky et al., 1988); (2) stearate and oleate are not as effective as polyunsaturated fish oils (see below); and (3) fats high in linoleic acid (the essential n-6 fatty acid used for synthesis of arachidonate; Figure 3.2A) fall between oleate/stearate and the fish oils, or are closer to the latter. Representative data supporting these findings are shown in Table 3.5. Peanut oil and cocoa butter (or palm oil) (Table

Table 3.5. Effects of Type of Dietary Fat on Fasting Serum Cholesterol and Triglyceride

Diet high in	Triglyceride (mg/dl)	Cholesterol (mg/dl)		
		Total	LDL	HDL
I. Normal subjects				
Palmitate (16 : 0)	78	201	139	42
Stearate (18 :)	79	174*	108*	39
Oleate (18 : 1) (n-9)	74	181*	120*	42
II. Normal subjects				
American diet equiv.	76–80	185–191	127–129	40–53
Linoleate	75	174*	115*	54
EPA/DHA	45–50*	126–170*	94–111*	32–54
III. Normal subject				
American diet equiv.	76–88	199	128	54
Oleate	83	171*[a]	105*[a]	49
Polyunsaturated	73	178*[a]	111*[a]	52
IV. Type IIb Hyperlipidemia				
American diet equiv.	334	324	220	41
Linoleate	258*	235*	149*	44
EPA/DHA	118[0]	236*	194	34*
V. Type V Hyperlipidemia				
American diet equiv.	1432	377	77	31
Linoleate	841*	264*	79	31
EPA/DHA	282	195*	110	35

Source: I. Bonanome and Grundy (1988); II. Harris et al. (1988); III. Mensink and Katan (1989); IV and V. Phillipson et al. (1985). Data for (I) recalculated from mM.

* Within groups (I, II, etc), different symbols (or symbols vs. no symbols) mean significant differences between Means ($p < 0.02$–< 0.05).

[a] Male subjects responded more than females.

3.6) do not follow these "rules," the former being more and the latter being less cholesterolemic than might be predicted from their compositions. It is possible that other (nonfatty acid) factors may be involved (possibly plant sterols or tocotrienols; see below).

The reasons for the differences in the effects of these fatty acids are under active investigation and are beginning to become known. As already indicated under the section on essential fatty acids, part of the mechanism has to do with the formation of different prostanoids and leukotrienes (Figure 3.5), that have differential regulating effects on many aspects of metabolism and physiological function. (See also next section, Fish Oils.)

Other effects of these oils may be ascribable to changes in intestinal absorption. Specifically, evidence from studies with rats (as well as monkeys and humans) indicates that glycerides high in stearate (18:0) are digested and absorbed more slowly and less efficiently than those with other fatty acids (Krichevsky, 1988; Krichevsky et al., 1987), although this may not be the case in man (Bonamone and Grundy, 1988). Also, plant sterols (Table 3.6) (which are not well absorbed) inhibit absorption (or reabsorption) of cholesterol (see above). The length of the dietary fatty acids, which determines whether they travel on chylomicrons (or intestinal VLDL) entering the lymph as opposed to attaching to albumin in the blood, will also alter triglyceride distribution and metabolism. [Short-chain fatty acids (14 carbons and below), prevalent in coconut and breast milk, will follow the albumin/blood route.] Recent studies in hamsters suggest that saturated shorter chain fatty acids (mostly C8 and C10, as triglyceride) enhance, and medium-chain fatty acids (coconut oil) depress, uptake of LDL (Woollett et al., 1989), when fed with cholesterol; the medium-chain saturated fatty acids also enhanced liver cholesterol production. [Similar earlier studies with coconut (versus corn) oil, in monkeys, increased plasma LDL only when fed along with cholesterol (Ershow et al., 1981).] Finally, cholesterol absorption per se, while never that efficient, will be af-

Table 3.6. Fatty Acid Composition of Oils and Fats (Percentage)

	Capric/lauric and myristic	Palmitic	Stearic	Oleic	Linoleic	Linolenic	Arachidonic	EPA + DHA	Total sterols (mg/100 g)
Butter	10	21	10	25	2	1	—	—	0
Palm kernel oil[a]	69	8	2	13	2	—	—	—	80
Coconut	62	9	2	7	1	—	—	—	100
Cocoa butter	—	25	33	32	3	0.5	—	—	0
Lard (pork)	1	29	14	46	9	0.5	—	—	0
Mutton fat	2	19	22	32	3	—	—	—	0
Chicken fat	1	19	8	47	22	1.5	—	—	0
Peanut oil	0.2	8	4	55	26	—	2.2	—	240
Olive oil	—	11	2	72	8	1	—	—	110
Margarine	—	9	5	39*	25	1	—	—	?
Soybean oil	—	10	4	22	53	8	—	—	340
Corn oil	—	10	2	31	39	1	—	—	850
Cottonseed oil	1	21	5	18	47	0.4	—	—	327
Palm oil	1	38	5	38	11	—	—	—	?
Wheat germ oil	—	13	3	27	42	—	—	1	553
Sesame seed oil	—	8	4	40	42	0.4	—	—	865
Sunflower seed oil	—	5	4	22	55	0.5	—	—	350
Safflower seed oil	—	6	2	11	74	0.5	—	—	444
Linseed oil	—	6	3	17	13	55	—	—	430
Rapeseed oil[b]	0.7	3	2	24	15	5.2	—	7.4	250
Cod liver oil	3	10[c]	2	23	2	1	0.7	19	0
Herring oil	26[d]	15	1	3	14	—	—	18	0
Shark oil	6	28	4	16	0.3	—	5	20	0

Source: Mostly Souci et al., 1981/82. The most abundant fatty acid is underlined. *Partly translated.

[a] Not to be confused with palm oil (further down on list).
[b] 49% erucic acid (22:1, n-9).
[c] Palmitoleic = 8% (16:1).
[d] Mostly capric, butyric, and lauric acids.

fected by the quantity of fat consumed, being enhanced when intake is high (Linscheer and Vergroesen, 1988), as in the Western diet. An increased intake of saturated fat (at least as coconut oil, and with some cholesterol) may also enhance production of cholesterol and LDL, and depress LDL uptake, as indicated by studies in hamsters (Spady and Dietschy, 1989). [One wonders whether perhaps this happens because less substrate for prostaglandin production is being supplied (see next section).]

Apart from fiber and cholesterol intakes. Trace elements and other micronutrients may also play a role in determining cholesterol status. Specifically, it appears that copper and chromium deficiencies result in hypertriglyceridemia and hypercholesterolemia (see Chapter 7); the mechanisms are still unknown. Earlier studies, which have not been pursued, have suggested that vanadium, and possibly chromium, may reduce endogenous cholesterol biosynthesis (Underwood, 1977), perhaps by an effect on squalene synthetase (Curran and Burch, 1968). Intake of pharmacologic doses of niacin (3–9 g/day) can also reduce serum cholesterol (Kane et al., 1981), through a reduction in synthesis of VLDL. Niacin is also thought to enhance HDL synthesis, both of which factors are of interest in the reduction of atherosclerosis risk. Also of potential interest are tocotrienols, first isolated from barley but widely present in plants. These appear to be potent inhibitors of cholesterogenesis at levels of 2.5–20 ppm in the diet (determined in chicks) (Qureshi et al., 1986). Tocotrienols are almost identical in structure to vitamin E (tocopherols) (Figure 5.32), differing only in having an isoprenoid rather than a saturated side chain. These various matters require further experimental evaluation to determine their significance in preventing hypercholesterolemia and/or atherosclerosis (see Chapter 15).

In summary, cholesterol biosynthesis, distribution, and disposal from the body are influenced by a variety of factors, both hereditary and dietary. Alterations in one or more aspects of cholesterol metabolism can result in hypercholesterolemia. This is a "risk factor" that has been linked to atherosclerosis. Dietary manipulation of cholesterol intake will have only small effects on serum cholesterol unless coupled with increased intake of certain forms of fiber and/or bile-acid-binding resins. The potential benefits of certain trace elements, omega-3 (n-3) fatty acids, plant sterols, tocotrienols, and niacin remain to be explored.

Fish Oils and Omega-3 Fatty Acids

Interest in fish oils, high in EPA and DHA, stems from the observation that the Inuit (Eskimo people) on their traditional high fat and cholesterol diets did not generally suffer from atherosclerosis. We now understand that at least some of this has to do with the preferential formation of certain prostaglandins, thromboxanes, and leukotrienes from EPA (Figure 3.5) over those produced from arachidonic acid (AA). It is thought that the relative preponderance of AA over EPA/DHA (or vice versa) determines what products are formed by the cyclooxygenase and lipoxygenase initiated pathways. Various direct and indirect effects of the several products are summarized in Figure 3.13. One of the major effects appears to be on synthesis of VLDL, which is reduced by EPA. This has been studied mainly in the liver, but the effect may also occur in the intestine (Harris et al., 1988), since the increase of triglyceride (and perhaps cholesterol) in the blood after a meal is slower and less pronounced in individuals on a high fish oil diet. "Fat tolerance" curves that illustrate this point are given in Figure 3.14. As shown in part A, the rise in plasma triglyceride after a test meal of saturated fat was dramatically reduced in individuals on a fish oil diet. [This was not the case with those on an unsaturated plant fat diet.] However, it should also be noted (Figure 3.14B) that a fish oil test meal given to individuals on nonfish oil diets did not have the same effect. An adaptation to the fish or fish oil diet is thus required. Fish oils may also depress liver cholesterol synthesis, per se, as well as enhance the activity of LDL receptors, as suggested by studies in rats (Ventura et al., 1989). Presumably, the effect of the fish oil diet is due to production of more thromboxanes of the B series (Figure 3.13) (Lee et al., 1986) and/or prostaglandins of the 3 series (versus A thromboxanes and prostaglandins of the 2 series), due to substrate competition. However, substrate competition may not be the only determinant. Formation of PGI_2, for example, may not be decreased when PGI_3 formation is enhanced by fish oil ingestion, as suggested by data (from humans) on quantities of their urinary metabolites.

Evidence mainly from animal studies indicates that liver synthesis of fatty acids (and activity of acetyl-CoA carboxylase) is reduced by EPA and DHA, and this may also be the case for liver apoprotein B (needed for VLDL) and intestinal A-I (needed for chylomicrons) (Lakshman et al., 1988). In contrast, β-oxidation of fatty acids in liver peroxisomes (but not mitochondria) is en-

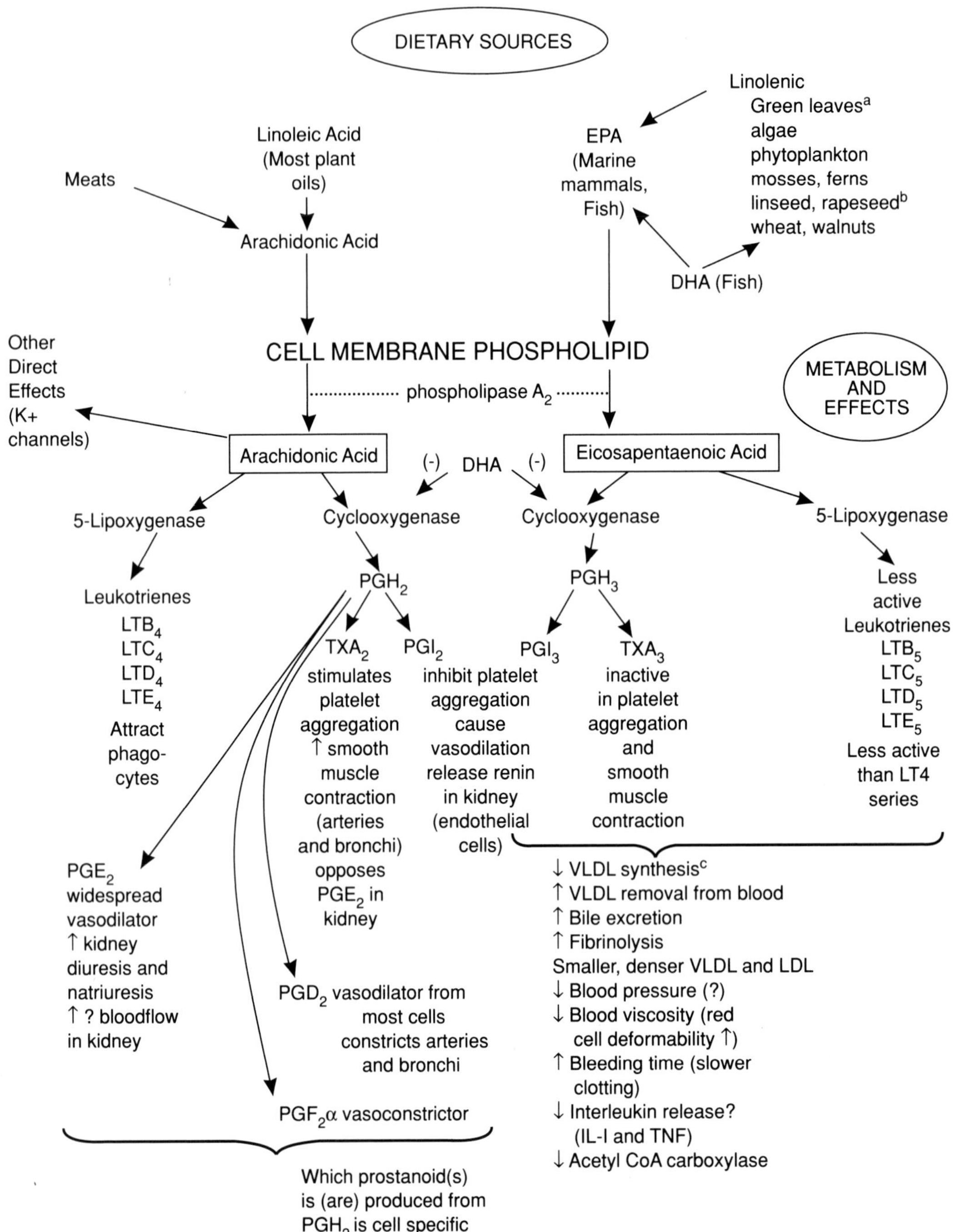

Figure 3.13. Dietary sources. (−) inhibits reaction; ↑ increases/stimulates; ↓ decreases. [*Source:* based on Leaf and Weber (1988) and others.]

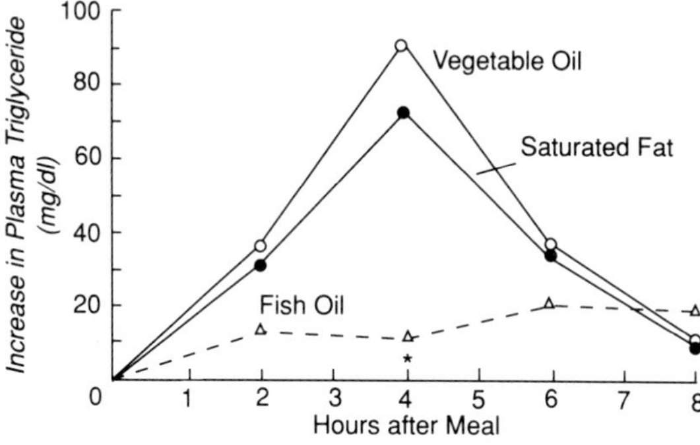

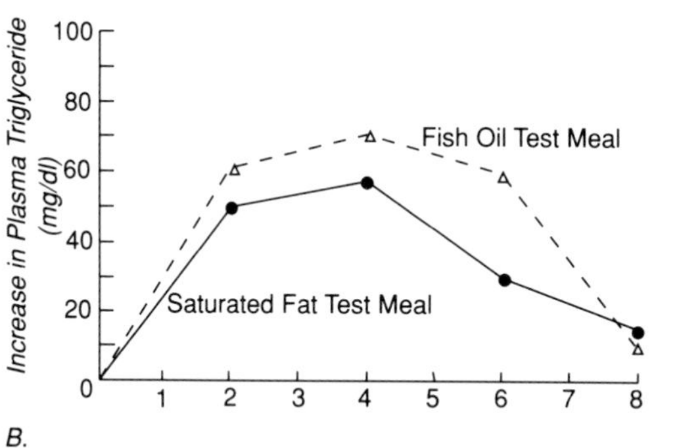

Figure 3.14. Fat tolerance curves in subjects on different diets given various test meals of triglyceride. **(A)** Time course of response of plasma triglyceride to ingestion of 50 g fat as vegetable oil, saturated fat (a mixture of peanut oil and cocoa butter), and fish oil (salmon oil), in individuals on diets containing these fats for 4 weeks. Dietary fat was 30–40% of calories. **(B)** Response of individuals on a saturated fat diet for 4 weeks to a test dose of fish oil or saturated fat. [*Source:* Reprinted by permission from Harris et al. (1988).]

hanced (Yamazaki et al., 1987), as is ketogenesis (Bergseth et al., 1986; Wong et al., 1984) and mitochondrial oxygen consumption. This suggests that in liver (and perhaps also in the intestinal mucosa) EPA and DHA cause the diversion of fatty acids from formation of triacylglycerol to enhanced utilization as fuel. β-oxidation in peroxisomes results in enhanced formation of more oxidized fatty acid fragments (and perhaps also acetyl-CoA), which may then be fed into the Krebs cycle and into ketone production within the mitochondria, after cross-membrane transport (Wong et al., 1984).

The actual weight of the intestinal mucosa (Thomson et al., 1988) and of the liver (Yamazaki et al., 1987) also increases in animals on a high fish oil diet, which may reflect an increased retention of fat and decreased release of VLDL and chylomicrons. Under these conditions, the end product of VLDL release (LDL) in the blood is smaller and has a lower melting temperature (Parks and Bullock, 1987).

The type of fat ingested can *also* influence the activity of the Δ^6- and Δ^5-desaturases, at least in the liver of the rat (Garg et al., 1988), as can the intake of cholesterol, when on a nonfish oil diet. Fish oils (presumably because of EPA and DHA) decrease the activities of both liver desaturases (Figure 3.6), which might be viewed as a kind of feedback control on their synthesis from linolenic acid. Thus, EPA and DHA inhibit formation of AA (from linoleic acid). In contrast, oils high in linoleic acid (like those of corn or safflower), *stimulate* desaturase activities. (Presumably, linolenic would have the same effect.)

Because of their effects on fatty acid and cholesterol synthesis and VLDL release, fish oils tend to lower not just serum triglyceride, but also cholesterol (Table 3.5). In general, the effects seem to be at least as good as (or better than) diets high in linoleate. This appears to be the case also for individuals with hereditary hyperlipidemias types V and IIb. In placebo trials, however, fish oil supplementation has not been uniformly successful (Demke et al., 1988), and it is clear that much more work will be required to determine the reasons for response variability.

Although most of the studies to date suggest that fish oil intake may be beneficial for a variety of reasons—including its potential effects on serum triglyceride, cholesterol, atherogenesis, and even blood pressure (Knapp et al., 1989; Schiff et al., 1989) (Figure 3.13)—they may not always be helpful and in some instances may be detrimental. Fish oils diminish the inflammatory response (Virella et al., 1989), and particularly the release of interleukin-1 (β and α) and tumor necrosis factor (Endres et al., 1989), which are important for the immune system. They prolong blood clotting time by reducing platelet activity; and they may reduce renin release, which helps to control kidney function and might be critical in patients where function is already impaired, as suggested by studies with rats (Scharschmidt et al., 1987). At the same time, fish oils may be more useful than aspirin (and other cyclooxygenase inhibitors) in suppressing chronic inflammation (also in rheumatoid arthritis; Kremer et al., 1989; Cleland et al., 1988), and better than cyclosporine in suppressing the immune response during organ transplantation without the concomitant nephrotoxicity (kidney damage) that is thought to be mediated by macrophage TXA_2 (Rogers et al., 1988).

Fish are not uniformly good sources of EPA and DHA (Table 3.7). In general, there is a connection to fat content, those like herring, mackeral, and salmon (with more fat) having more of the n-3 fatty acids than those lower in fat, like flounder and haddock. The others are mostly in between, and it is noteworthy that shellfish and other seafood also have some of these fatty acids (as do marine mammals), all of which are ingested directly or indirectly from phytoplankton (Leaf and Weber, 1988). The "effective" doses of EPA/DHA for various responses are still uncertain, although Gorlin (1988) has summarized the data, indicating 2–4 g/day for platelet/antithrombotic effects; 4 g/day for suppression of inflammation; and 4–24 g/day for the lowering of plasma lipids. [Harris et al. (1990) report 4.5 g is effective for the latter.] The various effects take up to 4 weeks to manifest. [Additional discussions of the effects of fish oils are given in Chapter 15.]

Trans Fatty Acids in the American Diet

It has been estimated that about 5.5% (or 8.3 g/day) of the fat presently eaten by Americans is in the form of *trans* fatty acids (see above, Structure of Fat in the Diet) (National Research Council, 1989). (Surveys of actual consumption suggest a lower intake.) The most common form of *trans* fatty acid is monounsaturated oleate (also designated 18 : 1t). The question arises as to whether this has any deleterious consequences. Although some aspects have been investigated, this question still cannot be fully answered, and some concern remains. What has been shown is that, at least in rats, these *trans* fatty acids cannot fulfill the role of essential fatty acids. There is evidence they can interfere with the conversion of normal linoleic acids (*cis*) to AA (Privett and Blank, 1964) through competition for Δ^5 and Δ^6 desaturases (Homan, 1981), and can interfere with the desaturation of stearic acid to oleic and palmitic acids (Homan, 1981), presumably by competition. Although *trans* fatty acids can be readily utilized for fuel, they can also accumulate in the phospholipid fractions of cells (Alfin-Slater and Aftergood, 1980), although they may not be incorporated as well as *cis* fatty acids into the C-2 position (see Emken, 1983). Data from month-long feeding trials in growing rats suggest that triacylglycerol enriched with *trans*-, as compared with *cis*-octodecanoate (but with the same amounts of linoleate), leads to an enhancement of liver fatty acid oxidation, especially in peroxisomes (Ide et al., 1987). Another report (Egwim and Kummerow, 1972) suggests that hydrogenated fat (45% of calories), containing 48% *trans* fatty acids, induces the accumulation of lipids in the heart, liver, and other organs of the rat over periods of 10–20 weeks, but Alfin-Slater et al. (1973) failed to find any obvious effects, when they fed rats with lesser amounts of margarine (25% of calories) containing 35% *trans* fatty acids over many generations. Krichevsky (1982), Krichevsky et al. (1984), and others have shown that *trans* fatty acids are hypercholesterolemic in rabbits but not in monkeys (at levels of 6% in the diet for long periods) and that they do not influence the incidence of atherosclerosis in these animals. There have also been reports of a higher content of *trans* fatty acids in adipose tissue from subjects that died of coronary heart disease as compared with other causes (see Booyens et al., 1988), although the studies were not controlled for diet, and much further work will be required to ascertain whether any long-term danger exists to man. However, in a recent Dutch study of normal young men and women, LDL cholesterol levels increased (and HDL cholesterol declined) when they were on diets with trans (versus cis) oleic acid (33 g/day) (Menink and Katan, 1990).

Table 3.7. Sources of Omega-3 (n-3) Fatty Acids (Eicosapentaenoic and Docosahexaenoic Acids)

Source	Amount (g/1/2 lb)	Amount (g/100 g)
Mackeral (Atlantic)	5.0–6.0	2.5
Salmon	4.0–4.4	1.2–1.4
Sardine (canned)	3.8	1.7
Eel	3.8	1.7
Bluefish	2.9	1.2
Herring	2.6–3.2	1.6
Whitefish (lake)	2.0	0.9
Squid	2.0	0.9
Striped bass	1.8	0.8
Trout (rainbow)	1.2–2.4	0.5–1.0
Oysters (Pacific)	1.2–2.0	0.5–0.9
Shrimp	1.0	0.4
Crab	0.9–1.0	0.4
Tuna	0.7	0.3
Cod	0.7	0.3
Carp	0.6	0.3
Lobster	0.5–0.6	0.3
Haddock	0.4	0.2
Clam	0.4	0.2
Flounder	0.4	0.2
Swordfish	0.4	0.2

Dietary Fat and Gallbladder Disease

Gallbladder disease arises from the formation of gallstones within the biliary tract. Most gallstones are comprised mainly of crystals of cholesterol (containing bile acids, variable amounts of bile pigments, sometimes calcium, and other substituents) (Figure 3.15). The secretion of bile is stimulated by the dietary intake of fats (see cholecystokinin; Chapter 1). Thus, the routine recommendation to patients with acute distress is to reduce fat consumption drastically (to 50 g or less) in order to prevent exacerbation of the problem. The specific origin of gallbladder disease is not well understood, although many possible aspects have been investigated (Dhar et al., 1980). Lowering cholesterol intake appears to be of no benefit. However, genetic hypercholesterolemia may increase the tendency to form gallstones. Increased dietary fiber does not necessarily have a favorable effect (Sylven and Borgstrom, 1969), although work by Thornton et al. (1983) on subjects with probable gallstones showed that these subjects produced a bile more supersaturated with cholesterol (and with higher saturation indices) when they consumed a refined diet, low in fiber, for 6 weeks, as opposed to when they consumed a diet high in whole grains, vegetables, and fruits for 6 weeks.

Cholesterol supersaturation of the bile is a requisite for gallstone formation, but is also prevalent in the normal population among people who do not develop stones (see Einarsson et al., 1985). Cholesterol saturation of the bile appears to increase with age (Einarsson et al., 1985), a phenomenon ascribable to decreased synthesis of bile acids and enhanced secretion of cholesterol by the liver. [No sex difference was observed.] Increased cholesterol saturation of bile (and a selective decrease in bile phospholipid) may also accompany ingestion of substantial amounts of beans, as by Native American groups (*Nutrition Reviews*, 1989; Nervi et al., 1989).

To avoid surgery for gallbladder stones, chenodeoxycholic acid supplementation (over months) may be useful in some cases, but the long-term effects of such treatment (if any) are unknown. [Bile acids can be promoters of carcinogenesis (see Chapter 16).] This bile acid is normally present in small amounts and is a better detergent than some of the other bile acids. Consequently, it may help to solubilize cholesterol stones. Aside from high fat intake, many patients with gallbladder problems cannot tolerate onions, curry, and other "gas-forming" foods, such as sauerkraut, radishes, cucumbers, and turnips (Dhar et al., 1980).

The incidence of gallstones is relatively high in Western populations, with their high calorie and high fat diets. Jews also have a high incidence, as do obese persons (Maclure et al., 1989). Tendencies to this disease are also generally hereditary and are more prevalent in women than in men, especially at menopause (Dhar et al., 1980).

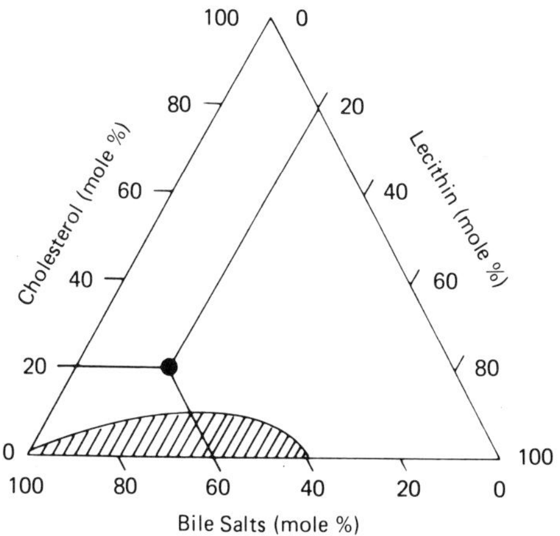

Figure 3.15. Solubility of cholesterol in bile. Cholesterol is present as a micellar liquid (shaded area) when in the presence of high concentrations of bile salts and lecithin. [*Source:* Reprinted with permission from Montgomery et al. (1983); modified from Small DM, N Engl J Med 279:488 (1968).]

Ethanol Metabolism, Diet, and Alcoholism

Ethanol is another energy-providing nutrient, produced from glucose through anaerobic microbial fermentation. In man, its metabolism is close to that of the fats and ketones. Its energy content is intermediate to that of fats and carbohydrates, at 7 kcal/g. Ethanol is absorbed efficiently from the gastrointestinal tract and metabolized primarily in the liver and mainly by a pathway shown in Figure 3.16: cytosolic alcohol dehydrogenase requires zinc and catalyzes production of NADH and acetaldehyde from ethanol and NAD^+. Further oxidation to acetate then occurs via a second (aldehyde) dehydrogenase. Most of this acetate in man enters the bloodstream and becomes a substrate for energy metabolism in other tissues (after activation to acetyl-CoA). (It should be noted that, normally, there is little acetate circulating as an energy source.) The rest of the acetate produced in the liver is mainly used for fatty acid synthesis in situ.

In the liver, ethanol oxidation by this route results in an increase in the cytoplasmic ratio of NADH to NAD^+, which enhances lactate production and secretion into the plasma (Figure 3.16). Lactate depresses urinary excretion of uric aid,

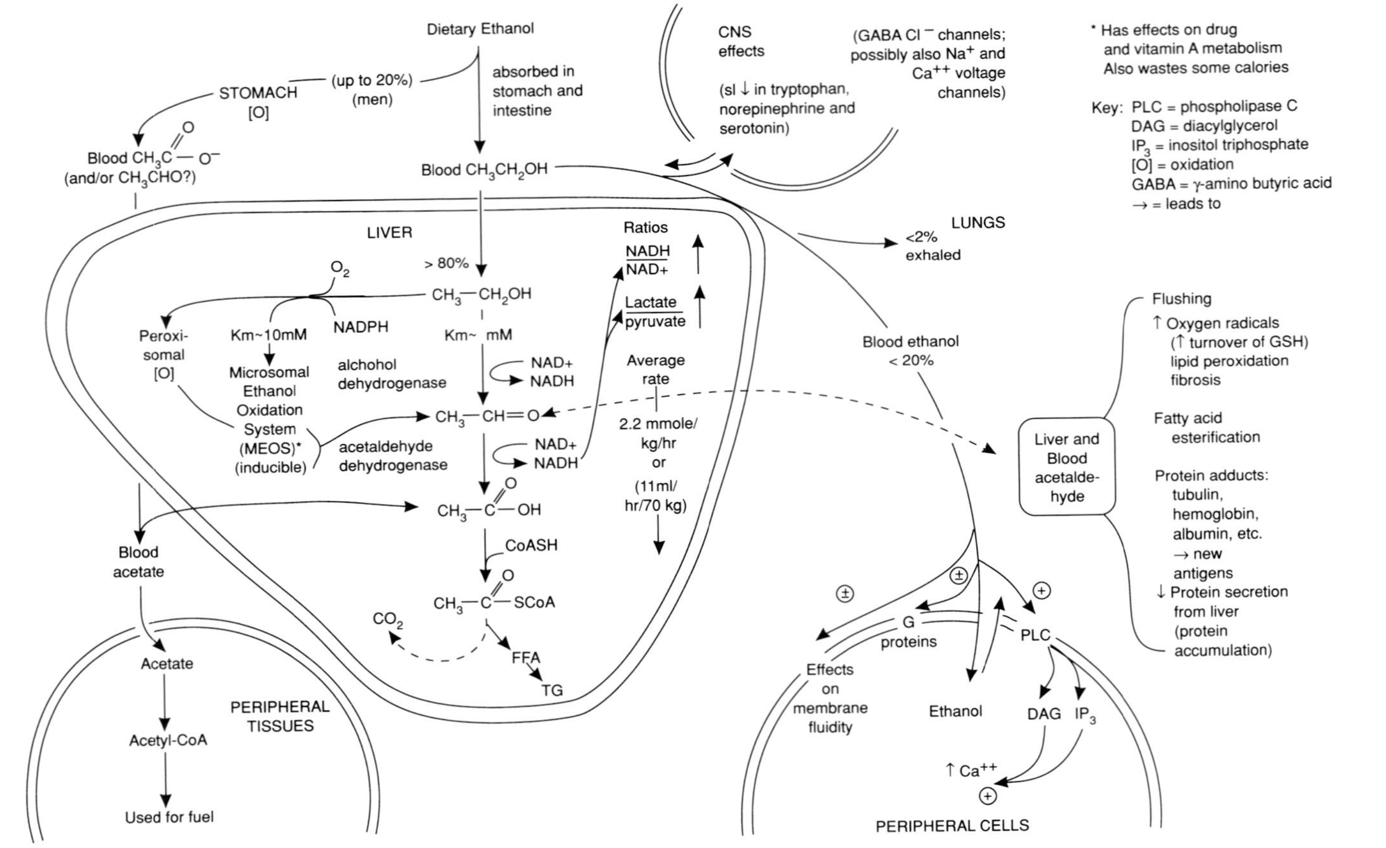

Figure 3.16. Ethanol metabolism and effects. Ethanol entering the liver is oxidized by up to 3 sets of enzymes, including the abundant zinc-dependent alcohol dehydrogenase and aldehyde dehydrogenase in the cytosol, peroxisomal enzymes, or the microsomal ethanol oxidation system (MEOS), the latter of which is ethanol inducible and also metabolizes many drugs and vitamin A. The overall effect is an increase in NADH/NAD+ ratios, and lactate to pyruvate concentrations in the liver, which results in increased lactate in the blood. Concentrations of acetate in the blood are also increased as are concentrations of uric acid (due to the elevated lactate). There are also increases in acetaldehyde in the liver and in the blood, resulting in adducts to proteins in the liver and circulation and various potential pathological consequences.

Ethanol directly enhances the activity of phospholipase C in various parts of the body and may also alter the response of membrane G proteins involved in second messenger production for hormones, neurotransmitters, etc. Effects on GABA-controlled chloride and voltage channels may also occur. A small proportion of ethanol entering the gastrointestinal tract is metabolized to acetate in the stomach lining itself, thus not entering directly into the blood. Blood ethanol: normal, about 0.02 mmole/L (0.1 mg/dl); intoxicated, 10–20 mmole/L (50–100 mg/dl); comatose, 90–130 mmole/L (400–600 mg/dl). [*Source:* Montgomery et al. (1983) and Lieber (1988a).]

thus also increasing plasma uric acid (Lieber et al., 1962). As a consequence of the increased synthesis of fatty acid from acetate, ethanol consumption also results in increases in liver and plasma triglycerides (Alfin-Slater and Aftergood, 1980).

Additional complexities in ethanol metabolism have more recently become apparent. First, the gastric mucosa also participates significantly in ethanol oxidation (Figure 3.16), and may in fact deflect up to 20% of ingested ethanol from the circulation (Caballeria et al., 1987), providing a kind of ethanol "barrier." This barrier is not present in alcoholics (with chronic excessive ethanol consumption) (Leiber, 1988*a*). It also appears to be much less active in women than in men, which (along with a lower body weight) would help to explain the greater susceptibility of women to ethanol intoxication.

Second, it has become evident that hepatocytes oxidize ethanol in three different places, one of which is an ethanol inducible system in the microsomes and involves a new form of cytochrome P450 (P450 IIEI, for "ethanol inducible"). The microsomal ethanol oxidation system (MEOS) (Figure 3.16) has a higher K_m for ethanol than alcohol dehydrogenase (about 10–15 m*M* versus 0.2–2 m*M*) and only becomes really important in individuals with a chronic high alcohol intake (Lieber, 1988*a*). The presence of this system explains several of the alterations in metabolism that occur in alcoholics, including the enhanced degradation of certain drugs (acetaminophen, CCl_4, cocaine, pentobarbital, and others, some of which form toxic metabolites) and the decrease in concentrations of hepatic vitamin A (through enhanced retinol degradation) (Leiber, 1988*a*, *b*). It also explains the increase in microsomal membranes induced by chronic ethanol ingestion.

One of the important aspects of the MEOS system is that it causes ethanol oxidation without formation of NADH that could form ATP. In fact, it will *draw* on NADH, because NADPH is required for the reaction and H_2O is produced. Thus, induction of ethanol oxidation by the MEOS should somewhat lower the cytosolic ratio of $NADH/NAD^+$, while also diverting ethanol calories to energy-wasteful oxidation. [The second oxidation step (that of acetaldehyde) would still produce NADH, and thus some energy.] The phenomenon of apparent wastage of ingested calories by heavy drinkers and alcoholics has been noted for a long time (Shaw and Leiber, 1980). It was known to be accompanied by an enhancement of oxygen consumption which we now can explain by the MEOS reaction. A third ethanol oxidizing system appears to be present in peroxisomes and also probably requires O_2.

The reasons for the toxicity of ethanol are also becoming clearer. Some of it is ascribable to acetaldehyde and some to ethanol per se. In the liver, increasing concentrations of acetaldehyde can result in the formation of various adducts to proteins and fatty acids. Acetaldehyde interacts with lysine ε-amino groups (and presumably also accessible N-terminal amino groups) to form Schiff base adducts that appear to alter protein function. Proteins thought to be targets include those of the intracellular microtubules that are involved in protein secretion, leading to intracellular protein accumulation and hepatomegaly (liver enlargement) which can be very extreme (see Lieber, 1988*a*); other intracellular and membrane proteins, some of which may now become antigenic; and even hemoglobin and albumin in the blood circulation.

Another effect of acetaldehyde is to enhance oxidative processes within the cell. This may partly result from an enhancement of the turnover of glutathione (see Figure 4.5, Chapter 4). [The tripeptide, or the cysteine used to form it, may react with acetaldehyde.] A production of radicals may also accompany the enhanced activity of the MEOS. This is thought to trigger increased collagen synthesis and other aspects of the beginning of liver fibrosis. It also can result in damage to liver mitochondria, with swelling, disorganization, and reduced oxidative phosphorylation and fatty acid oxidation (β-oxidation). Acutely, acetaldehyde in the circulation is thought to be responsible for the flushing that may accompany consumption of alcohol. Asians who tend to have less liver aldehyde dehydrogenase (and are thus more likely to accumulate blood acetaldehyde), are more susceptible to flushing at lower intakes of ethanol.

Ethanol itself can alter general membrane fluidity, leading to altered membrane function and signaling in many cells, including those of the brain. Some of these responses to ethanol are mediated by G proteins such as those involved in insulin action. [This may account for the insulin resistance induced by acute intoxication (Shelmet et al., 1988).] Ethanol effects on G proteins may also be a factor in platelet action (Tabakoff et al., 1988). Other effects may be mediated by phospholipase C (in plasma membranes) which is activated by ethanol, enhancing the release of inositol phosphates (IP_3) and diacylglycerol (DAG) (Figure 3.16). The latter are second messengers that stimulate (a) release of Ca^{2+} to the cytosol from the endoplasmic reticulum and (b) influx of extracellular Ca^{2+} through channels in the cell membrane, resulting in further changes in cell metabolism and physiology (Hoek and Taraschi, 1988). [For further details on the regulatory inositide system, see Chapter 5.] In the brain, this apparently interferes with GABA (γ-aminobutyric acid) regulation of central nervous system signals (Harris and Allan, 1989). Ethanol effects on the central nervous system have been reviewed by Charness et al. (1989).

In the liver, ethanol also induces the increased synthesis of some proteins, including the cytochrome P450 IIEI, already mentioned (as part of the MEOS), but especially also the so-called intracellular fatty-acid-binding protein (FABP). FABP normally is already 3%–4% of the protein in the cytosol of hepatocytes, and ethanol raises this even higher (Pignon et al., 1987). [Other inducers of this FABP are estrogens, fatty acids, and peroxidation (Clarke and Armstrong, 1989), the latter suggesting that acetaldehyde rather than ethanol might actually be the trigger.] Increased FABP may also contribute to (or indeed be a response to) the accumulation of liver lipid (or the fatty liver of alcoholics). Finally, ethanol actually forms esters with fatty acids in many tissues, including the tissues most likely to be damaged by alcoholism (liver, pancreas, heart, and fat) (see Lieber, 1988*a*). Whether this contributes to the damage is still unclear, but it might be a factor in suppressing fatty acid oxidation.

The alcoholic obtains a large proportion of his or her energy from ethanol. This commonly results in a decreased intake of nonalcoholic foods that contain the other nutrients necessary for normal health and causes a spectrum of varieties of malnutrition (Lieber, 1988b; Shaw and Lieber, 1980). The most common forms of malnourishment in alcoholics include deficiencies of folic acid, thiamin, and pyridoxine, as well as lower blood levels of manganese, calcium, zinc, and lower liver stores of vitamin A, even with adequate intake. [As already mentioned, vitamin A catabolism is thought to be enhanced by the MEOS.] Earlier studies in monkeys suggesting that folate deficiency results from impaired absorption and/or enhanced turnover and excretion (Tamura and Halsted, 1983) have not been confirmed (Lieber, 1988*b*). There are some reports that alcoholics tend to have greater than normal stores of iron. It is thought that this may occur via stimulation (by ethanol) of gastric acid secretion, resulting in enhanced iron absorption due to its greater solubilization and reduction (Turnbull, 1974). Enhanced losses of urinary nitrogen are also observed (Lieber, 1988*b*), suggesting a general enhancement of protein catabolism. Recent studies have verified that ethanol abuse even in asymptomatic alcoholics is associated with decreased skeletal and heart muscle strength (Urbano-Marquez et al., 1989).

The cirrhosis and liver damage that accompany chronic alcoholism are probably due to a combination of malnutrition and a direct toxic effect of the alcohol consumed. The latter is indicated by studies in humans (Shaw and Lieber, 1980) and in baboons (Rubin and Lieber, 1974), rats, and other animals in which a balanced diet did not or could not prevent cirrhosis and fatty liver induced by consumption of alcohol (Roe, 1979). As already indicated, acetaldehyde has been incriminated in the pathogenesis of most of the effects of alcohol abuse.

The question arises whether nutrient deficiency might encourage alcoholism. Information on such possibilities is extremely scanty. However, there is one study by Roger et al. showing that alcoholic rats greatly reduce their intake of alcohol when treated with the amino acid, glutamine (Rogers et al., 1955, 1956) and do not respond in the same way to any other amino acid administered. A small case study by Rogers and Pelton (1957) on 10 human alcoholics also suggested some correlation between glutamine intake and alcohol dependence. This has not been pursued.

Ethanol has been clearly implicated in the development of birth defects. Apparently the most critical period is at conception and during early embryogenesis, and the degree of teratogenicity is dose-dependent (Ernhart et al., 1987). Mental retardation has also been attributed to ethanol ingestion during pregnancy and ethanol is in fact considered a major cause of mental retardation in the West (Rosett and Weiner, 1985). Again, the most active component is probably acetaldehyde, which the fetus can acquire in at least two ways: (a) from the maternal circulation; and (b) from the placenta, where ethanol is also oxidized (Karl et al., 1988). Clearly, fetal exposure to acetaldehyde will occur under "social drinking" circumstances, and it has been advised that pregnant women (or those working to conceive) abstain from alcoholic beverages. A safe level of intake has not been established (National Research Council, 1988).

Traces of any ethanol consumed by the mother

will also be transferred to the nursing infant. While this appears not to alter mental development, it does seem to slightly (but significantly) impair the development of motor functions, as measured at 1 year of age (Little et al., 1989). Whether this persists into later life is unknown.

References

Alfin-Slater RB, Aftergood L (1980): *In* Alfin-Slater RB, Krichevsky D, eds: Human nutrition, a comprehensive treatise, vol 3A. New York: Plenum, p 117.

Alfin-Slater RB, Aftergood L, Melnick D (1973): J Am Oil Chem Soc 50:479.

Berdanier CD (1988): Nutr Rev 46:145.

Bergseth S, Christiansen EN, Bremer J (1986): Lipids 21:508.

Bergstrom JD, Robbins KA, Edmond J (1982): Biochem Biophys Res Commun 106:856.

Bergstrom JD, Sonnenberg N, Edmond J (1981): Biochem Soc Trans 9:292P.

Bonanome A, Grundy SM (1988): N Engl J Med 318:1244.

Booyens J, Louwrens CC, Katzeff IE (1988): Med Hypotheses 25:175.

Briggs MH, Brotherton J (1970): Steroid biochemistry and pharmacology. New York: Academic.

Brown MS, Goldstein JL (1979): Harvey Lect 73:163.

Brown MS, Kovanen PT, Goldstein JL (1981): Science 212:628.

Burgoyne RD, Cheek TR, O'Sullivan AJ (1987): TIBS 12:332.

Buzzard M, McRoberts MR, Driscoll DL, Bowering J (1983): Am J Clin Nutr 36:94.

Caballeria J, Baraona E, Lieber CS (1987): Life Sci 41:1021.

Cahill GF Jr, Aoki TT, Ruderman NB (1973): Trans Am Clin Climatol Assoc 84:184.

Carlson SE, Carver JD, House SG (1986): J Nutr 116:718.

Chan BL, Lisanti MP, Rodriguez-Boulan E, Saltiel AR (1988): Science 241:1670.

Charness ME, Simon RP, Greenberg DA (1989): N Engl J Med 321:442.

Circulation (1988): II-385.

Clarke SD, Armstrong MK (1989): FASEB J 3:2480.

Cleland LG, French JK, Betts WH, Murphy GA, Elliott MJ (1988): J Rheumatol 15:1471.

Colditz GA, Bonita R, Stampfer MJ, Willett WC, Rosner B, Speizer FE, Hennekens CH (1988): N Engl J Med 318:937.

Curran GL, Burch RE (1968): *In* Humphill DD, ed: Trace substances in environmental health. Columbia: University of Missouri Press, p 96.

Demke DM, Peters GR, Linet OI, Metzler CM, Klott KA (1988): Atherosclerosis 70:73.

Dhar P, Zamchek N, Broitman S (1980): *In* Goodhart RS, Shils ME, eds: Modern nutrition in health and disease. Philadelphia: Lea & Febiger, p 953.

Eckel RH (1989): New Engl J Med 320:1060.

Egwim PO, Kummerow FA (1972): J Nutr 102:783.

Einarsson K, Nilsell K, Leijd B, Angelin B (1985): N Engl J Med 313:277.

Eisenberg S (1980): Ann NY Acad Sci 348:30.

Emken EA (1983): J Am Oil Chem Soc 60:995.

Endres S, Ghorbani R, Kelley VE, Georgilis K, Lonnemann G, van der Meer JWM, Cannon JG, Rogers TS, Klempner MS, Weber PC, Schaefer EJ, Wolff SM, Dinarello CA (1989): N Engl J Med 320:265.

Ernhart CG, Sokol RJ, Martier S, et al. (1987): Am J Obstet Gynecol 153:33.

Ershow AG, Nicolosi RJD, Hayes KC (1981): Am J Clin Nutr 34:830.

Flynn MA, Nolph GB, Sun GY, Krause G, Dally JC (1986): J Am Diet Assoc 11:1541.

Garg ML, Thomson ABR, Clandinin MT (1988): J Nutr 118:661.

Goodknight SH Jr (1988): Semin Thromb Hemost 14:285.

Gorlin R (1988): Arch Intern Med 148:2043.

Grinker J, Hirsch J (1972): Ciba Found Symp 8:350.

Hamosh M, Klaeveman HL, Wolf RO, Scow RO (1975): J Clin Invest 55:908.

Hansen HS (1986): TIBS 11:263.

Hardie DG, Carling D, Sim ATR (1989): TIBS 14:20.

Harris RA, Allan AM (1989): FASEB J 32:1689.

Harris WS, Connor WE (1989): Am J Clin Nutr 51:399.

Harris WS, Connor WE, Alam N, Illingworth DR (1988): J Lipid Res 29:1451.

Hegsted DM, Nicolosi RJ (1987): Proc Natl Acad Sci USA 84:6259.

Hoek JB, Taraschi TF (1988): TIBS 13:269.

Homan RT (1981): *In* Beers RF Jr, Bassett EG, eds: Nutritional factors: Modulating effects on metabolic processes. New York: Raven, p 523.

Huang CTL, Gopalakrishna GS, Nichols BL (1978): Am J Clin Nutr 31:516.

Hwang DH, Boudreau M, Chanmugam P (1988): J Nutr 118:427.

Ide T, Watanabe M, Sugano M, Yamamoto I (1987): Lipids 22:6.

Illman RJ, Topping DL, McIntosh GH, Trimble RP, Storer GB, Taylor MN, Cheng B-Q (1988): Ann Nutr Metab 32:97.

Iso H, Jacobs DR Jr, Wentworth D, Neaton JD, Cohen JD (1989): N Engl J Med 320:904.

Jandacek RJ, Whiteside JA, Holcombe BN, Volpenhein RA, Taulbee JD (1987): Am J Clin Nutr 45:940.

Kane JP, Malloy MJ, Tun P, Phillips NR, Freedman DD, Williams ML, Rowe JS, Havel RJ (1981): N Engl J Med 304:251.

Karl PI, Gordon BHJ, Lieber CS, Fisher SE (1988): Science 242:273.

Katan MB, Beynen AC (1987): Am J Epidemiol 125:387.

Katan MB, Beynen AC, DeVries JHM, Nobels A (1986): Am J Epidemiol 123:221.

Kim D, Clapham DE (1989): Science 244:1174.

Knapp HR, FitzGerald GA (1989): N Engl J Med 320:1037.

Knittle JL, Hirsch J (1968): J Clin Invest 47:2091.

Kremer JM, Lawrence DA, Jubiz W (1989): NATO ASI Series (Series A) 171:343.

Krause MV, Mahan LK (1979): Nutrition and diet therapy (6th ed). Philadelphia: WB Saunders.

Krichevsky D (1982): Fed Proc 41:2813.

Krichevsky D (1988): Nutr Rev 46:177.

Krichevsky D, Davidson LM, Weight M, Kriek NP, Du-Plessis JP (1984): Atherosclerosis 51:123.

Krichevsky D, Tepper SA, Klurfeld DM, Fehr WR, Hammond EG (1987): Nutr Rep Intl 35:265.

Krichevsky D, Tepper SA, Lloyd LM, Davidson LM, Klurfeld DM (1988): Nutr Res 8:287.

Lakshman MR, Chirtel SJ, Chambers LL (1988): J Nutr 118:1299.

Lands WEM (1979): Annu Rev Physiol 41:633.

Leaf A, Weber PC (1988): New Engl J Med 318:549.

Lee TH, Israel E, Drazen JM, Leitch AG, Ravalese J III, Corey EJ, Robinson DR, Lewis RA, Austen KF (1986): J Immunol 136:2575.

Levine L, Moskowitz MA (1979): Proc Natl Acad Sci USA 76:6632.

Lieber CS (1988a): N Engl J Med 319:1639.

Lieber CS (1988b): Nutr Rev 46:241.

Lieber CS, Jones DP, Losowky MS, Davidson CS (1962): J Clin Invest 41:1963.

Linscheer WG, Vergroesen AJ (1988): *In* Shils ME, Young V, eds: Modern nutrition in health and disease. Philadelphia: Lea & Febiger, p 72.

Little RE, Anderson KW, Ervin CH, Worthington-Roberts B, Clarren SK (1989): N Engl J Med 321:425.

McClead Jr RE, Meng HC, Gregory SA, Budde C, Sloan HR (1985): J Pediatr Gastroenterol Nutr 4:234.

Maclure KM, Hayes KC, Colditz GA, Stampfer MJ, Speizer FE, Willett WC (1989): N Engl J Med 321:563.

Mahley R (1988): Science 240:622.

Marston R, Raper N (1987): Natl Food Rev Winter-Spring 36:18.

Mattson FH, Grundy SM, Crouse JR (1982): Am J Clin Nutr 35:697.

Mead JF (1980): *In* Alfin-Slater RB, Krichevsky D, eds: Human nutrition, a comprehensive treatise, vol 3A. New York: Plenum, p 213.

Mensink RP, Katan MB (1989): N Engl J Med 321:436.

Merrill AH Jr (1989): Nutr Rev 47:161.

Metzler DH (1977): Biochemistry. New York: Academic.

Montgomery R, Dryer RL, Conway TW, Spector AA (1983): Biochemistry, a case oriented approach (4th ed). St Louis: CV Mosby, p 453.

Morton RE (1988): J Biol Chem 263:12235.

Murphy RC, Mathews R, Pickett W (1981): *In* Beers RE Jr, Bassett EG, eds: Nutritional factors: Modulating effects on metabolic processes. New York: Raven, p 495.

National Research Council (1976): Fat content and composition of animal products. Washington, DC: National Research Council.

National Research Council (1989): Diet and health. Implications for reducing chronic disease risk. Washington DC: National Academy Press.

Nervi F, Covarrubias C, Bravo P, et al. (1989): Gastroenterology 96:825.

Neuringer M, Anderson GJ, Conner WE (1988): Ann Rev Nutr 8:517.

Nutrition Reviews (1987a): 45:232.

Nutrition Reviews (1987b): 45:246.

Nutrition Reviews (1988): 46:198.

Nutrition Reviews (1989): 47:369.

Ordway RW, Walsh JV Jr, Singer JJ (1989): Science 244:1176.

Parks JS, Bullock BC (1987): J Lipid Res 28:173.

Phillipson BE, Rothrock DW, Connor WE, Harris WS, Illingworth DR (1985): N Engl J Med 312:1210.

Pignon JP, Bailey NC, Baraona E, Lieber CS (1987): Hepatology 7:865.

Porter MW, Yamanaka W, Carlson SL, Flynn MA (1977): Am J Clin Nutr 30:490.

Privett O, Blank ML (1964): J Am Oil Chem Soc 41:292.

Qureshi AA, Burger WC, Peterson DM, Elson CE (1986): J Biol Chem 261:10544.

Read MH, Fisher KA, Bendel R, et al. (1989): J Am Diet Assoc 89:830.

Recht L, Helen P, Rasmussen JO, Jacobsen J, Lithman T, Schersten B (1990): J Int Med 227:49.

Roe DA (1979): Alcohol and the diet. Westport, CT: AVI.

Rogers LL, Pelton RB (1957): Q J Stud Alcohol 18:581.

Rogers LL, Pelton RB, Williams RJ (1955): J Biol Chem 214:503.

Rogers LL, Pelton BB, Williams RJ (1956): J Biol Chem 220:321.

Rogers TS, Elzinga L, Bennett WM, Kelley VE (1988): Transplantation 45:153.

Rosett HL, Weiner L (1985): Annu Rev Med 36:73.

Rubin E, Lieber CS (1974): N Engl J Med 290:120.

Ruderman NB, Aoki TT, Cahill GF Jr (1976): *In* Hanson R, Mehlman MA, eds: Gluconeogenesis. New York: Wiley, p 515.

Salomon RG, Jireusek MR, Ghosh S, Sharma RB (1987): Prostaglandins 34:643.

Scanu AM (1978): Ann Clin Lab Sci 8:79.

Scharschmidt LA, Gibbons NB, McGarry L, et al. (1987): Kidney Int 32:7000.

Schiff E, Peleg E, Goldenberg M, Rosenthal T, Ruppin E, Tamarkin M, Barkai G, Ben-Baruch G, Yahal I, Blankenstein J, Goldman B, Mashiach S (1989): N Engl J Med 321:351.

Shaw S, Lieber CS (1980): *In* Goodhart RS, Shils ME, eds: Modern nutrition in health and disease. Philadelphia: Lea & Febiger, p 1229.

Shelmet JJ, Reichard GA, Skutches CL, Hoeldtke RD, Owen OE, Boden G (1988): J Clin Invest 81:1137.

Souci SW, Fachmann W, Kraut H (1981): Food composition and nutrition tables 1981/82. Stuttgart: Wissenschaftliche Verlagsgesellschaft mbH.

Spady DK, Dietschy JM (1989): J Lipid Res 30:559.

Stein EA (1986): *In* Tietz NW, ed: Textbook of clinical chemistry. Philadelphia: WB Saunders, p 829.

Stolz A, Takikawa H, Ookhtens M, Kaplowitz N (1989): Annu Rev Physiol 51:161.

Story JA (1980): *In* Brewster MA, Naito HK, eds: Nutritional elements and clinical biochemistry. New York: Plenum, p 383.

Sylvén C, Borgstrom B (1969): J Lipid Res 10:351.

Tabakoff B, Hoffman PL, Lee JM, Saito T, Willard B, De Leon-Jones F (1988): N Engl J Med 318:134.

Tamura T, Halsted CH (1983): J Lab Clin Med 101:623.

Thomson ABR, Kellen M, Garg M, Clandinin MT (1988): Can J Physiol Pharmacol 66:985.

Thornton JR, Emmett PM, Heaton KW (1983): Gut 24:2.

Tietz NW (1976): Fundamentals of clinical chemistry. Philadelphia: WB Saunders, p 529.

Tofler GH, Brezinski D, Schafer Al, Czeisler CA, Rutherford JD, Willich SN, Gleason RE, Williams GH, Muller JE (1987): N Engl J Med 316:1514.

Turnbull A (1974): *In* Jacobs A, Worwood M, eds: Iron in biochemistry and medicine. London: Academic, p 370.

Underwood EJ (1977): Trace elements in human and animal nutrition. New York: Academic, p 370.

Urbano-Marquez A, Estruch R, Navarro-Lopez F, Grau JM, Mont L, Rubin E (1989): N Engl J Med 320:409.

van den Reek MM, Craig-Schmidt MC, Weete JD, Clark AJ (1986): Am J Clin Nutr 43:530.

Ventura MA, Woollett LA, Spady DK (1989): J Clin Invest 84:528.

Virella G, Kilpatrick JM, Eugeles MT, Hyman B, Russell R (1989): Clin Immunol Immunopathol 52:257.

Welin L, Svardsudd K, Wilhelmsen L, Larsson B, Tibblin G (1987): N Engl J Med 317:521.

Wong M, Nestel PJ, Trimble RP, Storer GB, Illman RJ, Topping DL (1984): Biochim Biophys Acta 792:103.

Woollett LA, Spady DK, Dietschy JM (1989): J Clin Invest 84:119.

Yamazaki RK, Shen T, Schade GB (1987): Biochim Biophys Acta 920:62.

Maria C. Linder, Ph.D.*

4

Nutrition and Metabolism of Proteins

Introduction to Protein

Consumption

The average American (and Western) adult consumes between 80 and 125 g of protein per day (average, 101 g/day in the United States). This is approximately twice the requirements set by United States and other health organizations (see below). Consequently, protein provides about 12% of the daily energy need. In the United States, the intake of protein has remained quite constant since 1900, but the proportion of protein from animal foods has more than doubled, to 70%. Protein malnutrition, also known as Kwashiorkor ("the evil spirit which infects the first child when it is born," in Ghanaian) (Whitney and Hamilton, 1981), is a common problem in Third World nations, where meat, fish, and other sources of protein are more scarce. From a world viewpoint, the protein consumption on the part of the West above what is required, and the preferential consumption of animal over vegetable protein, might thus be regarded as wasteful, especially in view of the cost of animal protein production. It is estimated, for instance, that the production of 1 kg of edible beef protein requires the feeding of 17 kg grain (or other) protein (Blaxter, 1977). However, conversion of fed protein to chicken meat, egg, or milk protein is three to four times more efficient. Also, ruminants (like sheep, goats, and cattle) can subsist largely on grasses and other plant materials inedible to other animals and humans, and this is advantageous to world protein production.

* California State University, Fullerton, CA.

Nutrition

Essential Amino Acids

The dietary protein requirement is based on the need for amino acids that are not synthesized by the body. Eight amino acids (Table 4.1) are definitely essential in the human diet (Irwin and Hegsted, 1971*a*). Within this group, much of the requirement for methionine can be substituted by cysteine (or cystine) and phenylalanine by tyrosine, and vice versa, as pathways for the formation of cysteine and tyrosine (from met and phe) exist in human tissues. For the infant, histidine is an essential amino acid, and there is also recent evidence of some need by the adult for total parental nutrition (TPN) (see Chapter 14). [The amino acid is essential for adult rats.] In earlier short-term (7–10 days) nitrogen balance studies there may have been a sufficient reserve of histidine available from the breakdown of hemoglobin (and other nonmuscle endogenous proteins) to cover this need (Irwin and Hegsted, 1971*a*). Also, there is evidence that the liver can synthesize histidine. Arginine is an amino acid formed by the liver (and to some extent by the kidney) through

Table 4.1. Essential and Nonessential Amino Acids

Essential amino acids[a]

Branch Chain AAs	$(CH_3)_2CH—CH(COO^-)(NH_3^+)$	Valine[G]
	$(CH_3)_2CH—CH_2—CH(COO^-)(NH_3^+)$	Leucine[K]
	$CH_3—CH_2—CH(CH_3)—CH(COO^-)(NH_3^+)$	Isoleucine[G, K]
Aromatic AAs	$C_6H_5—CH_2—CH(COO)(NH_3^+)$ (phenyl)	Phenylalanine[G, K]
	indolyl$—CH_2—CH(COO)(NH_3^+)$	Tryptophan[G, K]
Basic AAs	$^+H_3N—CH_2—(CH_2)_3—CH(COO^-)(NH_3^+)$	Lysine[K]
	imidazolium (N, NH_2^+)$—CH_2—CH(COO^-)(NH_3^+)$	Histidine[G b]
Other AAs	$HO(H_3C)CH—CH(COO)(NH_3^+)$	Threonine[G, K]
	$CH_3—S—(CH_2)_2—CH(COO)(NH_3^+)$	Methionine[G, K]

Nonessential amino acids[a]

$^+NH{=}C(NH_2)—N(H)—(CH_2)_3—CH(COO)(NH_3^+)$	Arginine[G]
pyrrolidinium ring (NH_2^+)$—CH(COO^-)$	Proline[G]
$OOC—CH_2—CH_2—CH(COO)(NH_3^+)$	Glutamic acid[G]
$H_2N—C(=O)—CH_2—CH_2—CH(COO^-)(NH_3^+)$	Glutamine[G]
$OOC—CH_2—CH(COO^-)(NH_3^+)$	Aspartic acid[G]
$H_2N—C(=O)—CH_2—CH(COO^-)(NH_3^+)$	Asparagine[G]
$+H_3N—CH_2—CH_2—CH_2—CH(COO^-)(NH_3^+)$	Ornithine[G]
($HS—CH_2—CH(COO)(NH_3^+)$)[c]	(Cysteine[G])[c]
($HO—C_6H_4—CH_2—CH(COO)(NH_3^+)$)[c] (4-hydroxyphenyl)	(Tyrosine[G, K])[c]
$HO—CH_2—CH(COO)(NH_3^+)$	Serine[G]
$HCH(COO)(NH_3^+)$	Glycine[G]
$CH_3—CH(COO)(NH_3^+)$	Alanine[G]
$H_2N—C(=O)—N(H)—CH_2—CH_2—CH_2—CH(COO^-)(NH_3^+)$	Citrulline[G]

[a] G, glucogenic; K, ketogenic; G,K, both.
[b] May only be required in infancy.
[c] Produced from essential amino acids: phe → tyr; met → cys.

the utilization of enzymes associated with the "urea cycle." No need for arginine in the diet has been demonstrated for the human infant, child, or adult (Irwin and Hegsted, 1971*a*), although it may be necessary for the maximal growth rate of some animals (notably, rats).

Almost without exception, the essential and nonessential amino acids are utilized by the body mainly to build proteins and are alpha, with both the amino and the carboxylic acid groups attached to the α-carbon. They are also L-amino acids. Small amounts of D-amino acids are present in the human diet, especially in processed foods, where they have been formed (by racemization) during manufacture (Man and Bada, 1987). D-amino acids have also been detected in animal tissues (e.g., in mice) where metabolism may occur via a D-amino acid oxidase (Nagata et al., 1989). As D-amino acids can inhibit absorption of L-amino acids and may have other selective effects on amino acid metabolism, this will require further attention.

Sources of Protein and Protein Quality

Numerous studies have been carried out to determine the normal human requirement for individual essential amino acids. What has emerged is an attempted formulation of the "ideal protein" (FAO, 1957) (Table 4.2) in terms of its relative content of essential amino acids. The proportions of essential amino acids in the "ideal" protein mixture are similar to those of egg or milk protein (Table 4.2). In general, proteins from animals, fowl, and fish have good proportions of the essential amino acids (Table 4.2). With the exception of soybeans, vegetable proteins do not meet the ideal and are usually less than ideal in one or two essential amino acids (Table 4.2). It may also be noted that root vegetables and tubers (such as potatoes) have half of their nitrogen in the form of small peptides and free amino acids, especially glutamine and asparagine. Also, 20% of milk nitrogen is in the form of nonprotein substituents, like urea, and the same is true for fish. [In contrast, seeds and grains have 95% or more of their nitrogen as protein.] Grains and nuts tends to be low in lysine and sometimes also tryptophan; legumes, though important as concentrated protein foods, tend to be deficient in sulfur amino acids. Consequently, a mixture of vegetable proteins from different sources, each with a relative, but different, deficit in essential amino acid, can form a more wholesome, "complete," or ideal mixture.

Table 4.2. Amino Acid as Percent Protein in Foods

Protein food	Lysine	Sulfur AAs	Threonine	Tryptophan	Leucine
Ideal[a]	5.5	3.5	4.0	1.0	7.0
Egg 12.8% protein	6.4	5.5	5.0	1.6	8.8
Milk (cow) 3.5% protein	7.8	3.3	4.6	1.4	9.8
Beef (hamburger)	8.7	3.8	4.4	1.2	8.2
Chicken 20.6% protein	8.8	4.0	4.3	1.2	7.2
Soybeans 34.9% protein[b]	6.9	3.4	4.3	1.5	8.4
Black beans 23.6% protein[b]	6.4	2.6[d]	3.4	1.0	8.7
Lentils 25.0% protein	6.1	1.5	3.6	0.9	7.0
Cornmeal 9.2% protein[b]	2.9	3.2	4.0	0.6	3.0
Oatmeal 14.2% protein[b]	3.7	3.6	3.3	1.3	7.5
Spirulina plankton	4.0	2.8	4.2	1.1	5.8
Collagen[c]	3.4	0.9	1.8	0.0	3.0

Source: Data recalculated from Krause and Mahan (1979).

[a] From Munro and Crim (1980); recalculated from NAS (1978) for the preschool child.
[b] Beans and grains—data for dry, uncooked.
[c] From White et al. (1973).
[d] Limiting (deficient) amino acids are underlined.

Table 4.3. Consumption of Essential Amino Acids and Protein by Vegetarians in the United States (g)

Amino acid	Nonvegetarians	Lacto-, ovovegetarians	Pure vegetarians
Isoleucine	6.6	5.4	4.0
Leucine	10.1	8.2	6.0
Lysine	8.3	5.4	3.7
Phenylalanine and tyrosine	10.4	8.8	7.0
Methionine and cysteine	4.3	3.2	2.7
Threonine	5.0	3.8	2.9
Tryptophan	1.5	1.2	1.1
Valine	7.1	5.6	4.3
Total protein intake	121	97	82

Source: Reproduced by permission from Hardage et al. (1966).

The corn (maize) and black beans of the Native American represent such a "natural" combination.

The vegetarian should be aware of a possible need for combining of protein sources, especially if no egg or milk-derived proteins are consumed. However, in the United States, there is little evidence for protein deficiency, even among pure vegetarians, as they tend to eat considerably more protein than they require (Table 4.3) (and thus make up for any deficits in specific amino acids).

The protein content of whole grains is not inconsiderable (Table 4.2); however, it should be remembered that the data given are for the dry grain (and bean) and that there will be a substantial water gain in cooking; resulting in a "dilution" of the inherent protein on a weight basis.

Apart from the proportions of essential amino acids present, the quality of a protein is determined by its digestibility and, in general, by its capacity to support the growth of experimental animals. As shown in Table 4.4, the proteins in foods of animal origin are more digestible than those from plants. Even though the digestibility of food proteins is generally high, it averages well under 100%, especially for vegetable sources, and this must be considered in assessing the daily protein requirement. Various rating procedures for protein quality have evolved, including "amino acid score," "biological value," and "protein efficiency ratio." The first relates the content of the limiting amino acid to the ideal, with the limiting amino acid being that which comes least close to meeting the ideal proportion in a given food. For example, since the content of lysine is 2.9% in cornmeal protein and the ideal is 5.5% (Table 4.2) (and this is the amino acid most limiting in relation to the ideal mixture), the amino acid score is $2.9/5.5 \times 100$ or 53%.

The "biological value" of a protein is determined by measuring the change in nitrogen excretion, relative to nitrogen intake, when experimental animals or humans are switched from a diet with no protein to one containing a limiting amount of protein:

$$\text{Biological value} = \frac{\text{Dietary N} - \left(\text{Urinary N} - \text{Urinary } N_0\right) - \text{Fecal } N_0}{\text{Dietary N}}$$

where N_0 represents the N lost while on a protein-free diet.

The protein efficiency ratio is based on the growth of experimental animals (often rodents) and compares the weight gained to the grams of protein consumed. Protein efficiency ratios are thus automatically corrected for the digestibility of the proteins (Table 4.4).

Table 4.4. Digestibility of Food Proteins

Food	Digestibility of protein (%)
Eggs	97
Meats, poultry, fish	85–100
Milk	81
Wheat	91–95
Corn	90
Soybeans	90
Other legumes	73–85

Source: Reprinted by permission from Reed (1980).

Protein Requirements

The protein requirement of the adult has been set at 0.75 g/kg body weight by the WHO/FAO/UNO (1985) *for Western diets* and has been accepted by the U.S. and Canadian governments. [The official

U.S. RDA is 0.8 g/kg of desirable body weight (National Research Council, 1988.] This is less than the figure used by Germany and Australia (1.0 g/kg). These requirements translate into values of about 56 g for the U.S. and Canadian male adult (and about 44 g for women). On an average weight basis, the requirement per kilogram is much greater for infants and children (see Chapter 11) and during pregnancy, and declines considerably in passing from early infancy to 2 years of age. A slow decline probably also occurs during adulthood (Clifford, 1980). Protein requirements appear to be more consistent on a body weight basis than on the basis of surface area or utilization of calories (Irwin and Hegsted, 1971b).

Estimates of protein need have been based on (a) measurements of normal daily nitrogen losses (feces, urine, skin, sweat, hair) to estimate minimal requirements, and (b) balance studies where the relative intakes and losses of nitrogen are compared at different low levels of protein intake and the data used to extrapolate a minimal requirement (Figure 4.1). The latter is based on the concept that the fully grown adult on a protein-deficient diet will go into more positive nitrogen balance when fed a diet higher in protein (essential amino acids). As increasingly higher amounts of protein are consumed, a stage will eventually be reached where no further replenishment of lost body protein is required (at least by the adult, who is no longer growing), and output will now equal input (zero nitrogen balance). Some of the shortcomings of this approach are that protein requirements are dependent on caloric requirements; for example, adequate calories will reduce protein requirements, probably by providing more carbon for formation of nonessential amino acids (Munro and Crim, 1988) (and perhaps also for gluconeogenesis). Hormonal status is also a factor (growth hormone and testosterone enhance positivity, corticosteroids and thyroxine negativity) (Munro and Crim, 1988). In any event, both kinds of information on nitrogen needs are subject to considerable individual variation. The results of such studies, combined with estimates of average protein quality and digestibility, plus safety factors, have resulted in the various recommendations for protein intake by government agencies. Estimates of minimal nitrogen losses, determined by placing men or women on protein-free diets for 7–10 days (Clifford, 1980), indicate that most nitrogen is lost as urea, ammonia, creatinine, and nitrate in the urine (and feces), although significant amounts are also accounted for by the sloughing off of epithelial cells (skin and gastrointestinal), and by losses in sweat or hair. [Although there was some interest in the possibility that traces of nitrogen are lost as N_2 gas by exhalation, this has not been borne out (Herron et al., 1973); but traces of nitrogen are also lost as exhaled ammonia, and small amounts as nasal secretions, seminal fluid, and menstrual blood (Munro and Crim, 1988). These are not usually considered.] Skin losses are estimated at 5–8 mg N/kg/day, fecal losses at about 12, and urinary losses at about 37, amounting to a total of 54 mg or about 0.34 g of protein/kg/day. With 2 standard deviations added to the value, this comes to 0.45

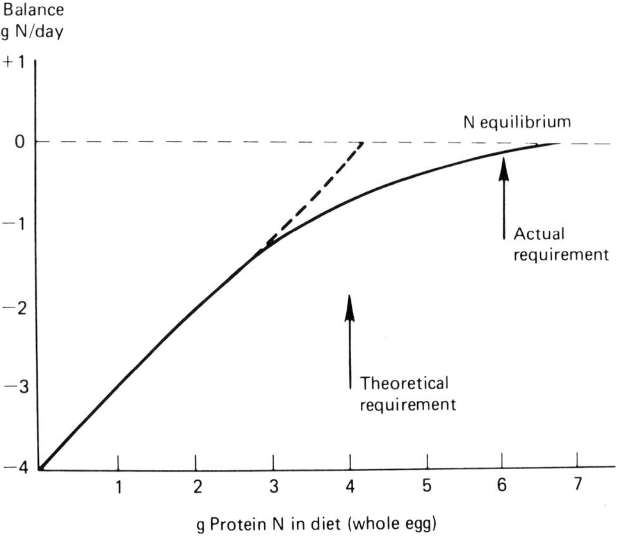

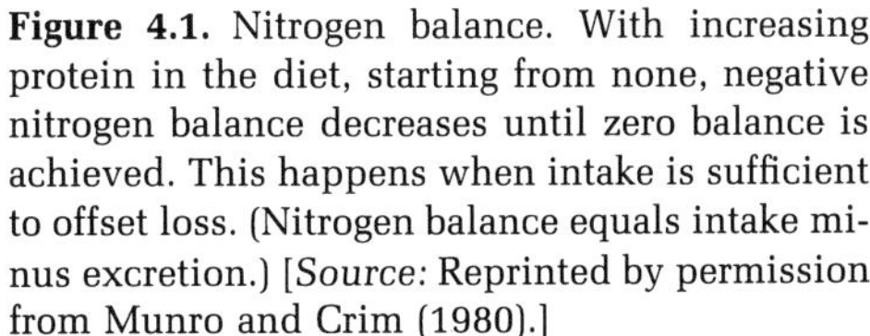
Figure 4.1. Nitrogen balance. With increasing protein in the diet, starting from none, negative nitrogen balance decreases until zero balance is achieved. This happens when intake is sufficient to offset loss. (Nitrogen balance equals intake minus excretion.) [*Source:* Reprinted by permission from Munro and Crim (1980).]

g of fully available/digestible, high-quality protein. [Safety margins for digestibility and quality bring the requirement into the region of 0.75 g/kg.]

Nitrogen balance (intake minus output) is positive in the growing infant or child, as well as in the pregnant or body-rebuilding adult and whenever there is tissue growth or replenishment (as during recovery from deficiency). Adults receiving a diet minimally or more than minimally adequate in protein will be in zero balance, where output equals intake. Negative balance occurs in fasting or starvation (where there is no intake) and also in pathologic situations (burns, injury, infections, fevers) and in severe psychologic stress. All are conditions where body function is diverted or activity reduced relative to the normal, as during bed rest or limb immobilization (when some muscle atrophy occurs), and/or in conditions where there is an abnormally high secretion of glucocorticosteroids. [The latter have catabolic effects on muscle protein (Goldberg et al., 1982).] In experimental animals, where one or more essential amino acids are deleted from the diet, it has been shown that negative balance will also occur; the other amino acids absorbed cannot be utilized for protein synthesis without the missing one, and there is a net (obligatory) loss of essential amino acids from endogenous protein on a daily basis (Munro and Crim, 1980). Thus, the physiological state greatly influences protein requirements, and hospitalized or ill patients may have different needs. Requirements may more than double, both acutely and in the long term, with injuries or burns so as to support the healing process. Requirements may also be increased in terminal cancer, and hyperalimentation of cancer patients is often instituted; however, there is no overall evidence that it prolongs life (see Chapter 14). Decreased protein intake is appropriate in treatment of diseases of the liver, kidney, and intestine, as these organs are especially involved in amino acid absorption, breakdown, and excretion of metabolites.

The adequacy of established requirements for protein and especially essential amino acids has recently been questioned by Young (1987) on the basis of apparent rates of oxidation established in in vivo kinetic studies. Using ^{13}C-labeled amino acids at different levels of intake, it appears that the body adapts to intake, and that higher requirements and a higher rate of muscle protein turnover may be associated with higher intakes. On this basis it is argued that the RDA for essential amino acids should be doubled or tripled. This goes against the general perception that a low but adequate protein intake (by standard measures) is satisfactory and perhaps even superior to an excessive intake of protein (as tends to exist in the Western world). The critical question is also whether (as postulated) a faster rate of muscle protein turnover is better than a slower one. More extensive and corroborating evidence is required if such a concept is to be considered further.

Functions of Amino Acids/Proteins in the Body

The consumption of protein is necessary to provide the body both with a source of nitrogen, for formation of nitrogenous constituents, and as a source of essential amino acids, those either not produced by the human organism or produced in insufficient quantities to provide for daily needs. The bulk of amino acids in the body is utilized for protein synthesis and is present in the body in the form of polypeptides and larger proteins. Nevertheless, significant quantities of amino acids are used in other ways (Table 4.5) and provide, among other things, nitrogen for the formation of nucleotides and nucleic acids. It is noteworthy that a coterie of amino acids is used for the formation of neurotransmitters and other nonpolypeptide hormones, as well as for polypeptide hormones, such as insulin and glucagon. Also, amino acids carry nitrogen from one tissue to another and even out of the organism (small amounts of amino acids are lost in the urine). Depending on amino acid intake, large quantities of nonessential amino acids may be produced from glucose, if and when needed for protein synthesis or other functions. Inorganic nitrogen, such as ammonium citrate, can serve as a nitrogen source for production of these amino acids (Irwin and Hegsted, 1971*a*). Protein can also be utilized for fuel—the carbon skeletons of the amino acids being converted either to glucose (glucogenic amino acids) and/or acetyl coenzyme A (acetyl-CoA) (ketogenic amino acids) (see Table 4.1) and stored as glycogen and/or triglyceride.

Protein Metabolism

Although, for the average American, the minimum intake of protein required is less than 60 g/day, she/he consumes about 80/100 g protein/day, based on intake data from food utilization (disappearance). Figure 4.2 provides an overview

Table 4.5. Functions of Amino Acids Other Than for Protein Synthesis and Energy Production

Amino acid	Function
Alanine	Glucogenic precursor; N-carrier from peripheral tissues to liver for N-excretion
Aspartate	Urea biosynthesis; glucogenic precursor; pyrimidine precursor
Cysteine	Precursor of taurine (used in bile acid conjugation and for other functions); reducing agent, also part of glutathione (important in the defense against oxygen radicals)
Glutamate	Intermediate in amino acid interconversions; precursor of proline, ornithine, arginine, polyamines, neurotransmitter α-aminobutyric acid (GABA); NH_3 source
Glutamine	Amino group donor to many nonamino acid reactions; N-carrier (crosses membranes easier than glutamate); NH_3 source
Glycine	Precursor in purine biosynthesis and for glutathione and creatine; neurotransmitter
Histidine	Precursor of histamine; donates to 1-C pool
Lysine	For cross-linking proteins (as in collagen); precursor of carnitine biosynthesis (used in fatty acid transport)
Methionine	Methyl group donor for many synthetic processes; cysteine precursor
Phenylalanine	Precursor of tyrosine, and via tyrosine, precursor of catecholamines, DOPA, melanin, thyroxine
Serine	Constituent of phospholipids; precursor of sphingolipids; precursor of ethanolamine and choline
Tryptophan	Precursor of serotonin; precursor of nicotinamide (B-vitamin)
Tyrosine	See phenylalanine

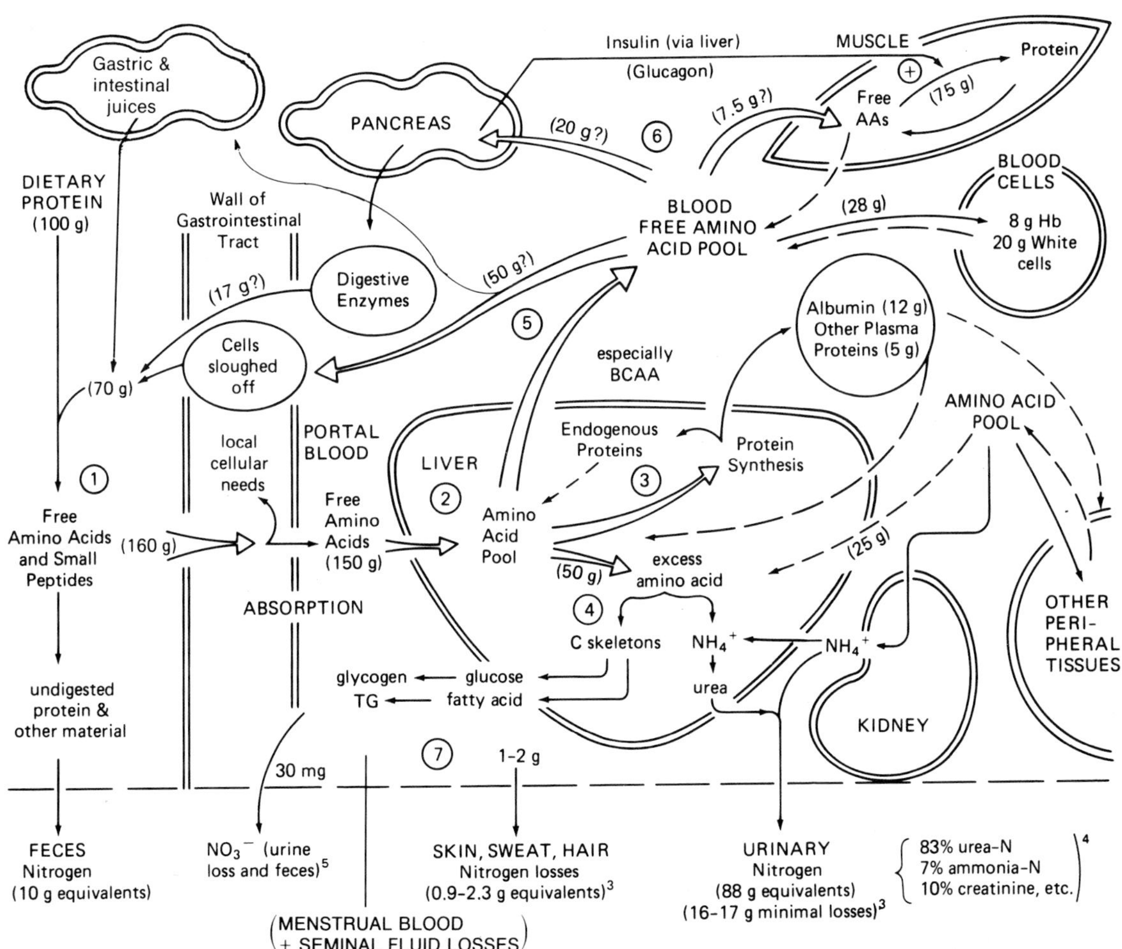

Figure 4.2. Human protein metabolism (62.5-kg person; 10,900 g protein[1]; 240 g synthesized and degraded daily[2]). Values shown are per day. Key: (1) Absorption of free amino acids and peptides after digestion; (2) uptake of dietary amino acids by the liver; (3) synthesis of liver and plasma proteins, especially albumin; (4) catabolism of excess amino acids; (5) distribution of amino acids to the rest of the body; (6) uptake by muscle, pancreas, epithelial cells; (7) excretion of amino acid nitrogen in various forms. Footnotes: [1]10,900 g protein, based on protein as 17.5% body weight. [2]240 g protein synthesis/degradation daily, based on calculations by Clifford (1980). [3]Based on a review by Irwin (1971b). [4]Data from Cahill (1973). [5]Calculated from Tannenbaum et al. (1978). [*Source:* Modified from Munro and Crim (1980, 1988).]

of the input, output, and turnover of nitrogen in the average American. The average American may contain 11 kg of protein, about 40% of which may be present in the muscles. About 2% (240 g) of this protein is degraded and resynthesized daily, requiring 260 g of amino acid for this process (10% H_2O is lost in peptide bonding). Of this amount, only about one sixth must come from the diet. This implies that only about one sixth of the amino acids released from degradation of endogenous proteins (260 g) are not recycled and are therefore lost and must be replenished from the diet. A major portion of the recycling of protein occurs through secretion of digestive enzymes, which are themselves degraded in the digestive tract and the amino acids reabsorbed. Also, roughly one quarter of the cells lining the gastrointestinal tract (lifespan 3–5 days) slough off daily, and the protein in these cells is also digested and mostly reabsorbed as amino acid. As already noted, the degradation and absorption of protein-derived amino acids from endogenous or exogenous sources is fairly efficient, with 70%–95% of plant and 85%–100% of animal (or human) protein being absorbed (Table 4.4). Probably about 6% of the nitrogen ingested and/or secreted into the gastrointestinal tract is ultimately lost through the feces (Figure 4.2). This is mainly in the form of bacterial and undigested protein. Thus, for an average American, about 170 g of protein enters the gastrointestinal tract, and almost all (160 g) is reabsorbed in the form of free amino acids and small peptides.

The digestion of protein begins in the stomach, with the combined denaturing (unfolding) action of HCl and the proteolytic action of pepsin (Figure 4.3). Further extensive digestion occurs in the upper small intestine, aided by various exo- and endopeptidases in the pancreatic and intestinal juices (Figure 4.3). In the process, proteins are fully degraded to free amino acids and small peptides.

The absorption of the digest is an energy-requiring process, involving several carrier systems for neutral, basic, and acid amino acids, as well as others for dipeptides. The relative rates of absorption of individual amino acids are as follows: branch chain amino acids and methionine > other essential amino acids > nonessential amino acids. Glutamate and aspartate are the least rapidly absorbed. The brush border of the intestinal epithelial cells contains oligopeptide hydrolases, and the cytosol contains other peptidases. Consequently, although substantial amounts of peptides may be absorbed into the epithelial cells (the exact proportion is unknown), only trace

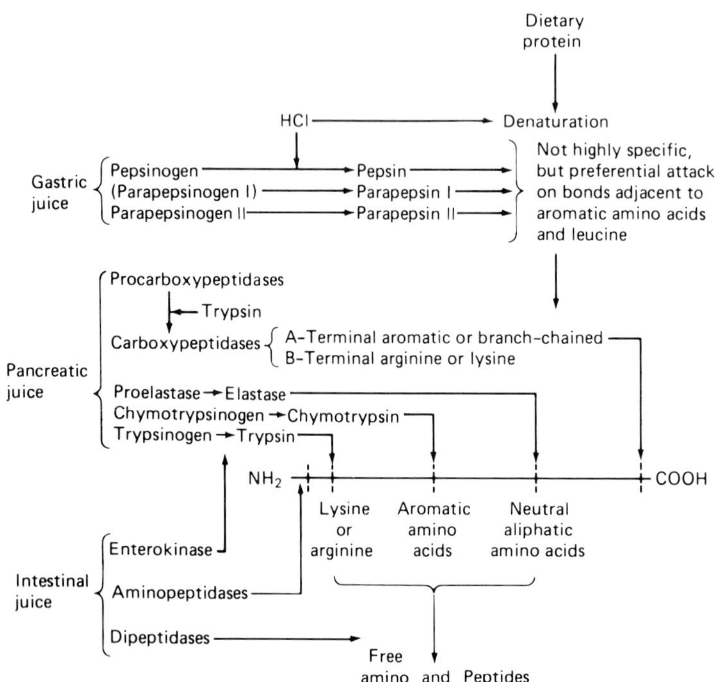

Figure 4.3. Proteolytic enzymes of the gastrointestinal tract. [*Source:* Modified from Gitler (1964).]

amounts enter the blood and are readily hydrolyzed by the liver and peripheral tissues. A significant portion of the absorbed amino acid is used by the intestine itself, for synthesis of its own proteins (including that for new cell production) and in part as an energy source. In the process, nitrogen—removed especially from incoming nonessential glutamate, glutamine, and aspartate—is released as alanine (formed from pyruvate via transamination). [Some is also released as citrulline and ornithine (see below).]

It should be noted that trace amounts of whole proteins are also absorbed through the intestinal wall and can enter the blood stream, as has been demonstrated by the recovery of ^{125}I-labeled proteins (for example, horse radish peroxidase) in peripheral blood after intragastric or intestinal administration (Gardner, 1988; Walker and Isselbacher, 1974; Warshaw et al., 1974). Some uptake of whole proteins appears to be part of the normal scheme of things, and may be important for the activity of the intestinal immune system, which secretes IgA as part of the body's defenses. Peyer's patches along the intestine appear to be "fed" foreign protein antigens via transcytosis across "M" cells which live in the villi of these areas (Gardner, 1988). In certain physiologic (including disease) states, the permeability of the intestine to whole proteins is enhanced, and transfer of whole proteins also occurs by passage *between* cells of the villus. This is also the case in infancy, especially if an infant is premature. The degree to which whole proteins pass beyond the mucosa and Peyer's patches into the circulation relates to the development of food allergies among individuals (see Food Allergies section below). Other possible associations are with autoimmune diseases, celiac and inflammatory bowel disease, toxigenic diarrheas, and chronic active hepatitis (Walker and Isselbacher, 1974).

Upon entering into the portal blood for distribution, the free amino acids encounter the liver, which is a major processor of the entering amino acid and, with muscle, is the major organ involved in the degradation of excess amino acids (Figure 4.2), as the average American consumes more than twice as much protein as needed to replenish the amino acids lost in normal body turnover. Some amino-acid-degrading enzymes in liver, such as tryptophan oxygenase and tyrosine aminotransferase, respond to the influx of amino acids by accumulating until the levels of their substrates again decline (Greengard et al., 1963; Schimke et al., 1965). This is particularly true when excess amino acid is consumed and more must be degraded (Munro and Crim, 1988). [The liver is the main (or only) site for degradation of most of the essential amino acids, except the branch chain amino acids, the catabolism of which mainly occurs in the muscles.] As concerns metabolism, protein synthesis in the liver, including the synthesis of albumin (Figure 4.4) and nucleic acid synthesis (Clifford, 1980; Munro and Crim, 1988), is very responsive to amino acid influx from the diet. Thus, after each protein-containing meal, there is a period of increased albumin and general protein synthesis (Clifford, 1980; Yap et al., 1978), which then tapers off and declines as amino acid influx declines between meals and overnight. The synthesis of muscle protein is also sensitive to amino acid influx and shows a similar variation related to eating patterns (Clifford, 1980). The effect on muscle protein synthesis, and part of the effect on liver pro-

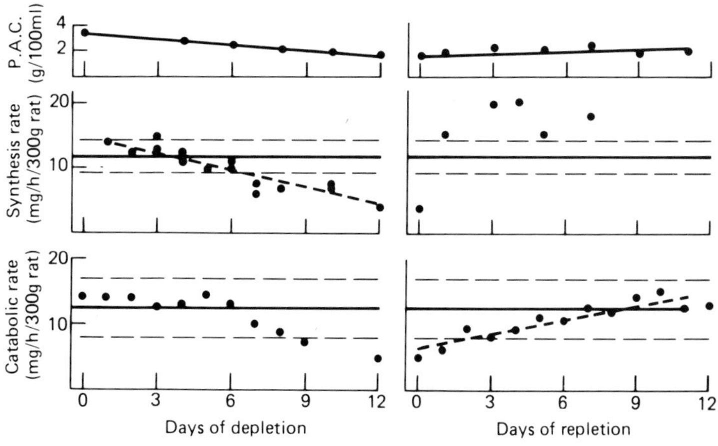

Figure 4.4. Adaptation of plasma albumin synthesis and catabolism to protein intake. Serial measurement of plasma albumin concentration (PAC), synthesis, and catabolic rates in rats during depletion and repletion of dietary protein. Mean control values ±2 SD are shown. [*Source:* Reprinted by permission from Hoffenberg (1970).]

tein synthesis, is mediated by insulin, which is secreted in response to amino acid (Rocha et al., 1972) and/or glucose influx. (Some amino acids also stimulate the release of pancreatic glucagon.) Insulin enhances transport especially of branch chain amino acids (the A system) and glutamine (Hundal et al., 1989), but has a more important effect on protein synthesis *per se*, probably at the initiation phase (Sato et al., 1981). Glutamine influx may also stimulate muscle protein synthesis (see Watford, 1989).

It is noteworthy that about one third of the amino acid required daily in the diet can be accounted for by the synthesis of albumin and other plasma proteins, which then enter the circulation. Most plasma proteins are degraded mainly by the liver, but this is not the case for albumin. The intestine accounts for some albumin uptake, but no single organ is considered a major source site for catabolism (Waldmann, 1977). Thus, it is tempting to think of albumin both as a temporary amino acid store and as a vehicle for transporting amino acids to peripheral tissues to replace daily losses. [Glutathione (Figure 4.5), a tripeptide and reducing agent, may also be viewed as having this function (see below).]

Based on nitrogen losses from muscles during fasting, approximately 75 g of protein is synthesized in the musculature daily. Estimates based on urinary excretion of methyl histidine are similar in adult men (Young and Munro, 1978). Histidine in muscle actin and myosin is methylated, and when degraded, the modified histidine is excreted and not recycled, thus giving a measure of actin/myosin catabolism. As the muscles account for about 40% of total body protein in the average individual (4.4 of 10.9 kg in the average adult), and 75 g of protein synthesis represents about 30% of the total protein synthesized in the body on a daily basis (Figure 4.2), muscle protein synthesis and turnover are somewhat slower than in the rest of the body, especially the epithelial and blood-forming tissues (see Chapter 1). Nevertheless, muscle protein represents the largest reserve from which amino acid may be drawn in times of need. This is important in fasting or starvation, when substantial portions of muscle protein are utilized for gluconeogenesis (see below). Production of new red and white blood cells (Figure 4.2) and replacement of epithelial cells lining the gastrointestinal tract and skin represent areas where body protein synthesis is especially active (also, the pancreas and intestinal mucosa, where significant amounts (about 7 g) of digestive enzymes are produced daily). As shown in Figure 4.2, total protein synthesis in liver, muscle, blood cells, pancreas, skin, and gastrointestinal tissue amounts to about 205 g, leaving 35 g of protein synthesis to take place in other organs of the body.

Most of the nitrogen from protein/amino acid catabolism is normally lost as urea through urinary excretion, though not inconsequential amounts are lost as urinary NH_4^+ and creatinine, skin and hair, and in miscellaneous forms (Figure 4.2). [Creatinine comes from creatine (and creatine phosphate) and is used as a high-energy phosphate reserve in muscles. Creatine, synthesized by liver and kidney, from arginine, glycine, and methionine (Figure 4.5), comprises 0.3%–0.5% of muscle weight, or about 1.2 kg/70 kg person.] Total nitrogen excretion will vary with the diet and physiologic state of the individual, being greater when protein consumption is high or fever is present and much less in fasting or when low protein diets are consumed (see more on fasting, below). For the normal American adult (in zero nitrogen balance), nitrogen excretion averages about 16 g/day (100 g protein $\div$ 6.25). It is noteworthy that about 0.03 g are lost as NO_3^- (Tannenbaum et al., 1978), and this appears to be independent of the presence of gut bacteria (Witter et al., 1981).

In summary, after a meal, especially one containing an amount of protein typical of Americans, the influx of amino acid results in surges in liver and muscle protein synthesis, the formation of increased amounts of serum albumin, and the degradation of excess amino acid to glucose precursors or acetyl-CoA. The latter substances are utilized for fuel or stored in the form of glycogen and triglyceride, whereas albumin continues to circulate and be degraded.

As absorption of amino acids from the intestine declines with time after a meal, synthesis of albumin and muscle protein slows and degradation continues. This can result in a net release of amino acid, especially from the muscle, as fasting begins and progresses. In long-term fasting, further adaptations occur in protein, amino acid, and overall fuel metabolism, reducing the need for muscle breakdown (see below).

Effects of Eating and Fasting on Blood Amino Acid Levels

The proportion of free amino acids in the body is only about 0.5% that of protein-bound amino acids (Munro and Crim, 1988). Intracellularly, concentrations of most nonessential amino acids

$H_3C-\overset{+}{N}(CH_3)_2-CH_2-CH(OH)-CH_2-COO^-$

Carnitine

γ-Glu Cys Gly

$^-OOC-CH(NH_3^+)-CH_2-CH_2-CO-NH-CH(CH_2SH)-CO-NH-CH_2-COO^-$

Glutathione (GSH)

$H_2N^+-CH_2CH_2SO_3^-$

Taurine

* SAM = S-adenosyl methionine

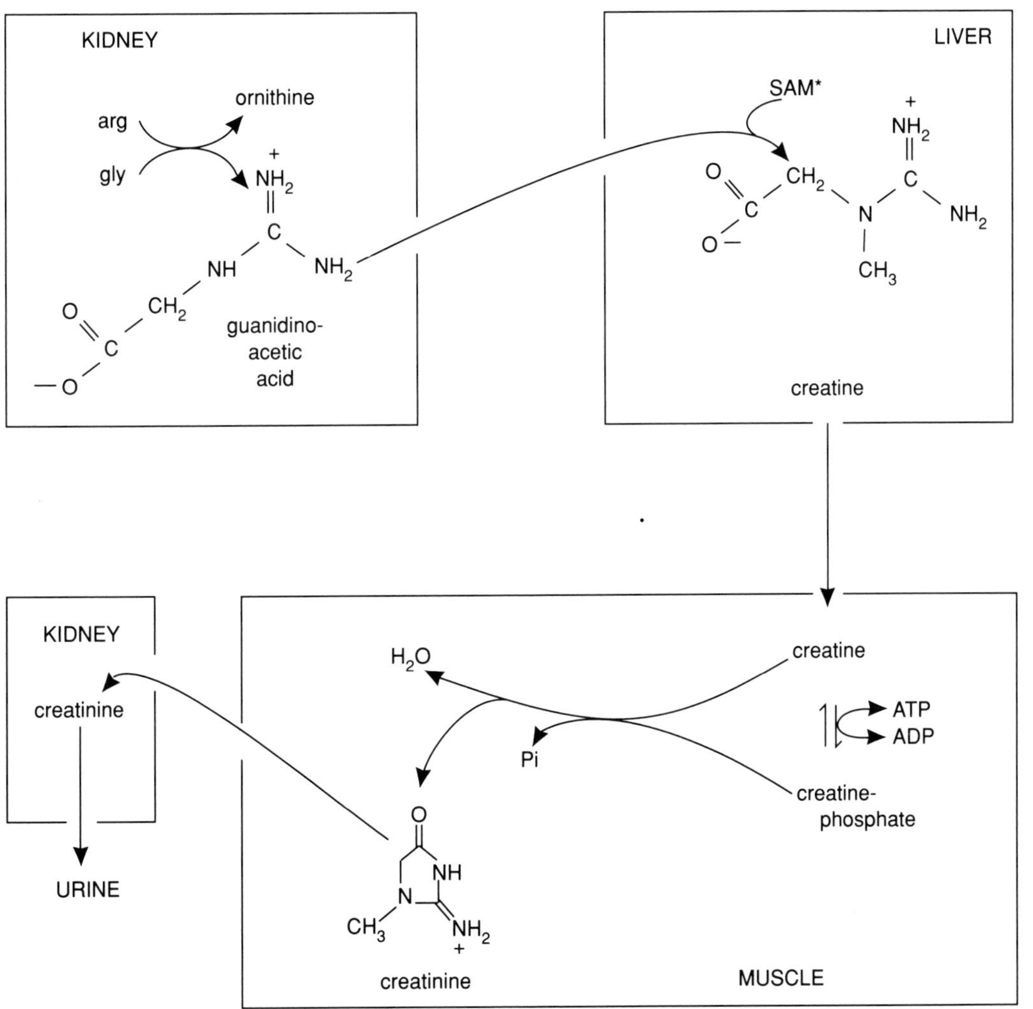

Figure 4.5. Structure and synthesis of various important amino-acid-derived substances found in the body. Pathways of creatine synthesis are based on Valgeirsdottir and Munro (1983).

(and particularly glycine, glutamine, glutamate, and alanine) are quite high relative to those of the essential amino acids (1000–3200 versus 20–24 μM, respectively). Concentrations of the former are lower in plasma (and interstitial fluid) and overlap more with concentrations of the essential amino acids (Table 4.6). In both compartments glutamine, glycine, and alanine predominate.

Concentrations of free amino acids in blood are not proportional to the general amounts found in food and tissue proteins (Table 4.6). This reflects differences in the transportability and variable metabolism of amino acids. Glutamic acid, with a net negative charge at physiological pH, is transported mainly in its amide form (as glutamine); glutamine and alanine play special roles in the shuttling of nitrogen and amino acid carbon between organs, resulting in their very high concentrations; branch chain amino acids (val, leu, ile) are not metabolized by the liver, accounting for their relatively high levels; and tryptophan and cysteine are actually largely bound to albumin during transport. As amino acids enter the intestinal epithelium after a protein-containing meal, some are utilized, and the mixture released into the portal blood contains a much smaller proportion of some amino acids, like glutamate and aspartate (Elwyn, 1970). Small amounts of amino acid are lost daily in the urine (Table 4.7).

Perhaps one third of the amino acids entering the liver from the portal blood are utilized for protein synthesis, as well as energy metabolism or gluconeogenesis (Yamamota et al., 1974), as previously noted (Figure 4.2). This helps to prevent drastic changes in peripheral blood amino acid concentrations. The effect of the liver (and some other adaptations) is such that overall amino acid nitrogen in peripheral blood only increases about 20% after a high protein meal (Figure 4.6), with little change in glycine and alanine

Table 4.6. Free Amino Acid Concentrations of Blood Plasma

	Venous[a] (μmol/L)	Arterial[b] (μmol/L)	Myoglobin (bovine) (residues/molecule)
Glutamine	265–490 (543)[c]	315–725[d]	3
Alanine	213–472	249 ± 36	10
Glycine	179–587	226 ± 13	9
Valine	168–317	222 ± 11	5
Proline	103–290	182 ± 18	3
Lysine	105–207	—	13
Threonine	76–194	124 ± 5	3
Serine	76–164	132 ± 8	4
Leucine	78–176	112 ± 6	11
Cysteine/cystine	70–108 (175)[e,g]	98 ± 5	0
Glutamate	51–181[d]	23–68[d]	8
Arginine	40–140	—	2
Taurine	32–138	43 ± 3	0
Isoleucine	40–99	53 ± 3	5
Phenylalanine	38–73	44 ± 2	5
Histidine	32–97	—	8
Tyrosine	22–83	41 ± 3	1
Ornithine	30–64 (65)[c]	—	0
α-Aminobutyrate	10–35	25 ± 3	0
Methionine	11–30	18 ± 1	2
Aspartate	1–11	20 ± 2	5
Tryptophan	6 (50–70)[c,f,g]	—	1
Citrulline	28[f]	36–2	0
Asparagine	?	?	2

[a] From Soupart (1961).
[b] Carotid artery; from Felig et al. (1973).
[c] Hill (1980).
[d] Marliss et al. (1971).
[e] Malloy et al. (1981).
[f] Ferenci (1978).
[g] Total free + bound (mainly bound to albumin).

Table 4.7. Urinary Output of Amino Acids

Amino acid	Urinary output (μmol/24 hr)[a]	Plasma clearance[b] (half-life)
Taurine	990	3 hr
Aspartic acid	60	3 hr
Histidine	900	6 hr
Glycine	1380	12 hr
Serine	400	17 hr
Methionine	50	24 hr (1 day)
Tyrosine	110	1.5 days
Threonine	150	2 days
Isoleucine	110	2 days
Phenylalanine	80	2 days
1/2 Cystine	120	2.5 days
Alanine	240	5 days
Leucine	809	5 days
Valine	90	9 days
Lysine	50	11 days
Proline	0	—

[a] Total output is 554 mg amino acid per day.
[b] Urinary output/plasma content (time necessary for excretion of amount normally present in plasma). From Soupart (1961).

concentrations and some increase in lysine levels. The branched chain amino acids increase much more markedly (Figure 4.6) and account for more than 70% of the amino acids released from the splanchnic bed (via the liver) to the rest of the body (versus about 20% of the amino acids ingested) (Munro, 1982; Wahren et al., 1976). This is because the liver does not contain appreciable amounts of branched chain amino acid transaminases [except for a small amount of leucine transaminase (Ogawa et al., 1970)], the enzymes necessary for the first step of their catabolism. These transaminases are located mainly in heart, skeletal muscle, and brain, with smaller amounts (but higher concentrations) in kidney and some in adipocytes. This underscores the importance of branched chain amino acids in muscle metabolism (see also below). Indeed, Wahner et al. (1976) have shown that these amino acids account for more than 50%–90% of muscle amino acid uptake in the 3 hr following a protein meal. As more branched chain amino acids enter than are needed for muscle protein synthesis, they also act as carriers of nitrogen to the muscles and in this capacity may serve to form some nonessential amino acids needed for muscle protein synthesis (Munro, 1982). In addition, they may inhibit influx of glutamine from the muscle by noncompetitive inhibition of a specific muscle cell membrane transporter (designated Nm) (Rennie et al., 1986). The increased intracellular glutamine may then stimulate muscle protein synthesis (Watford, 1989).

As mentioned earlier, influx of amino acids into the peripheral blood stimulates the release of insulin, which enhances muscle amino acid uptake by stimulating muscle protein synthesis. Certain amino acids (arginine and the branched chains, especially leucine) are better than others at causing insulin secretion (Rocha et al., 1972). Other amino acids (asparagine, glycine, serine, cysteine, etc.) stimulate secretion of glucagon, which serves to stimulate uptake of amino acids by the liver and also to prepare for gluconeogenesis and catabolism of the excess amino acid ingested. [Glucagon stimulates the synthesis of key gluconeogenic enzymes in the liver, such as phosphoenolpyruvate carboxykinase and pyruvate carboxylase (see Chapter 2, Figure 2.4a).] The concerted actions of both hormones thus serve to efficiently reduce plasma amino acid concentrations in the face of their influx from the gut. It may be noted that the level of protein intake also positively regulates liver levels of the urea cycle enzymes (Schimke, 1963), which are necessary for excretion of nitrogen derived from amino acid catabolism. This control may also involve glucagon (Snodgrass et al., 1978).

In contrast to the absorptive period after a protein-containing meal, the patterns of amino acid influx and efflux from different organs alter as dietary amino acid is disposed of in the postabsorptive state. In this case, insulin levels decline. Thus, the net influx of amino acid into muscle is reversed, especially as glycogen reserves are drawn upon and used up, and fasting (or starvation) sets in, requiring increased gluconeogenesis. As a result, skeletal muscles change to a net output of most amino acids (Figure 4.7). The largest proportion of the output is in the form of glutamine and alanine. Other researchers have shown that much of the nitrogen on these two amino acids has come from the deamidation of branched chain amino acids (Chang and Goldberg, 1978) and that alanine and glutamine serve as shuttles (to other tissues) of amino acid nitrogen and carbon. Almost all of the amino acid released is taken up by the splanchnic bed (Figure 4.7) (comprised of the intestine, liver, and other organs of the peritoneal cavity) and the kidney. The intestine and kidney (in acidosis) take a considerable portion of the glutamine and release alanine and serine (Matsutaka et al., 1973; Windmueller and Spaeth, 1974), with only small changes in the other amino acids. [Substantial

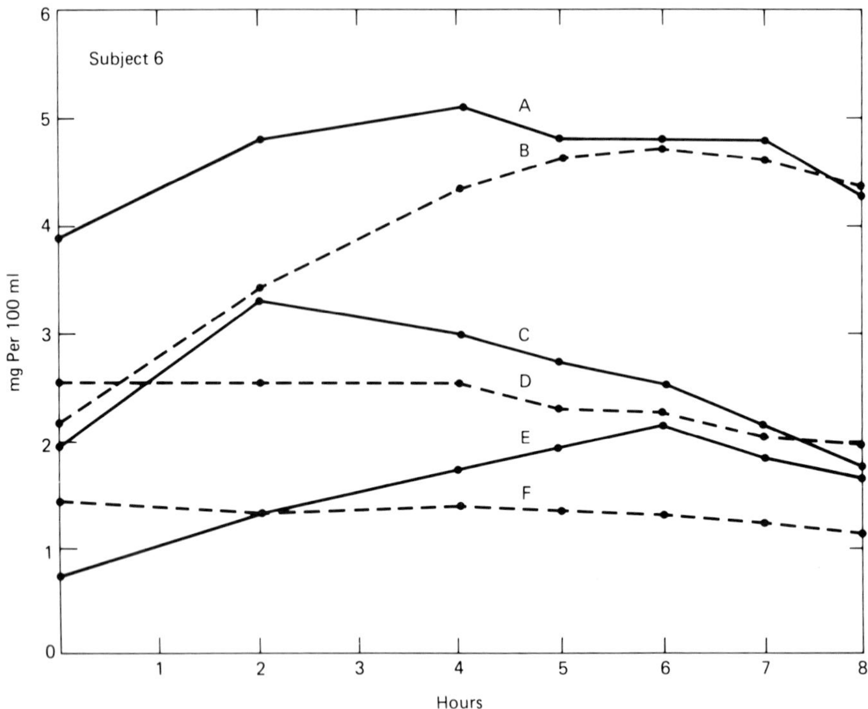

Figure 4.6. Plasma amino acid concentrations following a high-protein meal at zero time. Key: **(A)** total α-amino nitrogen; **(B)** valine; **(C)** lysine; **(D)** alanine; **(E)** isoleucine; **(F)** glycine (+ citrulline). [*Source:* Reprinted by permission from Frame (1958).]

amounts of citrulline are also released by the intestine (Windmueller and Spaeth, 1974).] The liver absorbs most of the alanine, glutamine, serine, and citrulline, as well as substantial amounts of the other amino acids present (Felig et al., 1973); these amino acids release their nitrogen directly or indirectly as ammonia (via glutaminase, glutamic dehydrogenase, and serine dehydratase) for incorporation into urea. [Citrulline enters the urea cycle directly and most other amino acids release their amino nitrogen by transamination with α-ketoglutarate, oxaloacetate, or pyruvate.] The carbon portions of the amino acids are used for glucose and ketone/fatty acid production. The glucose produced then exits the

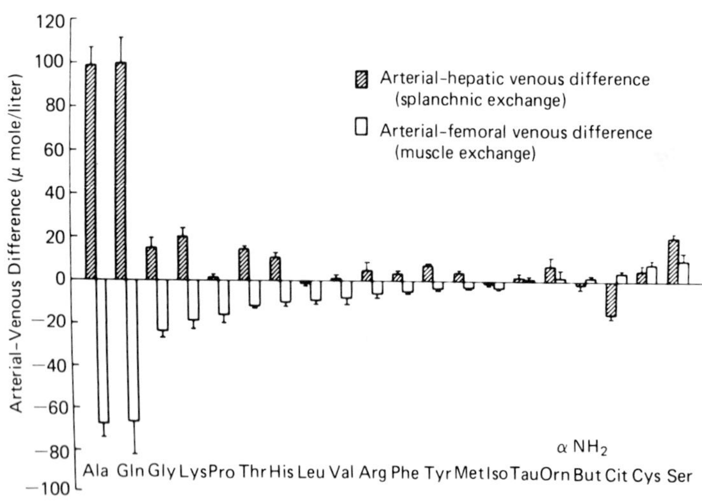

Figure 4.7. Muscle release of amino acid (□) and uptake by the splanchnic bed (■) during the postabsorptive period. [*Source:* Reproduced by permission from Felig (1975).]

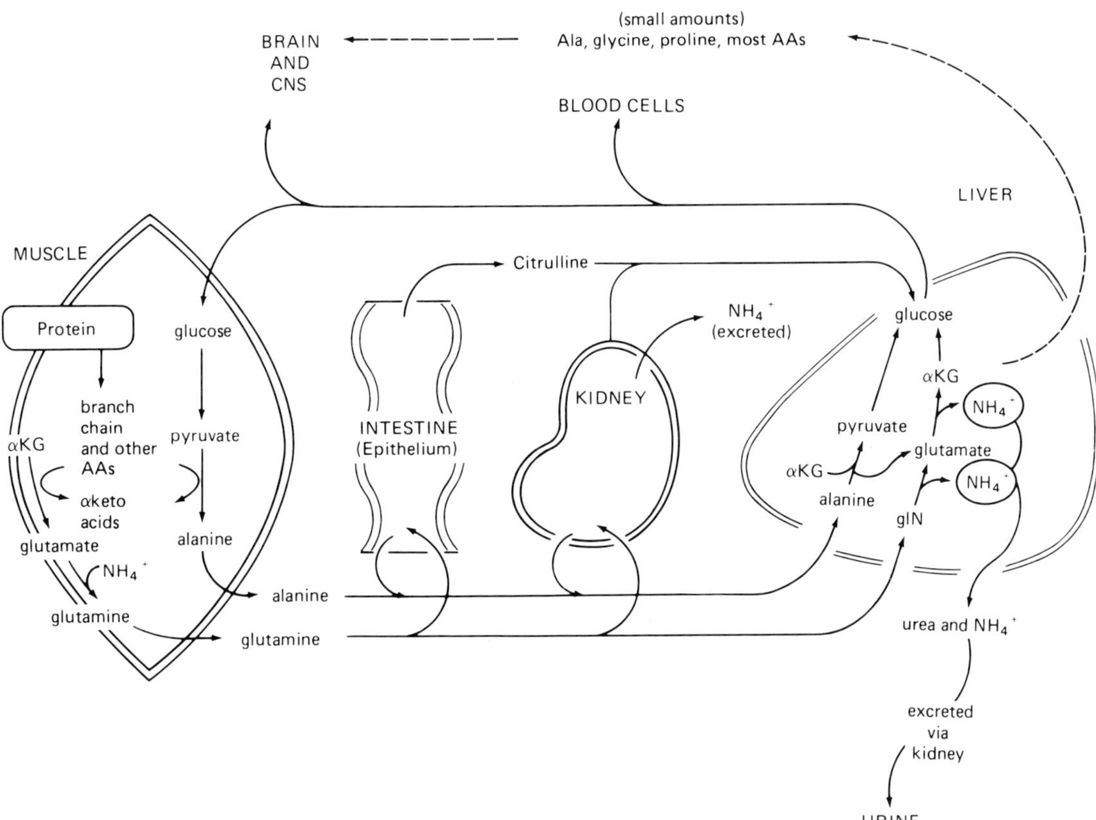

liver and becomes available to the glycolytic pathway, especially in blood cells and the central nervous system. Some of the glucose returns to the muscle, is broken down to pyruvate, reconverted to alanine, and reexits, de facto, creating a glucose–alanine shuttle between muscle and liver for amino acid nitrogen (Felig, 1975). Delivery of nitrogen (from amino acid breakdown) to the liver for urea and ammonia production is necessary for nitrogen excretion. [Nitrogen excretion is critical to survival; its hindrance (as in kidney malfunction) can lead to rapid death, with the buildup of potentially denaturing levels of urea.] The brain is not a part of the postabsorptive muscle–splanchnic interchange, but may participate by removing small amounts of most amino acids, especially alanine, glycine, and proline (Felig, 1975). A summary of these major organ interrelationships is given in Figure 4.8. The whole process of muscle protein catabolism and liver gluconeogenesis is regulated principally by secretion of glucocorticosteroids and glucagon and a relative lack of insulin.

Figure 4.8. Postabsorptive interorgan amino acid exchange. Release of amino acids (especially alanine and glutamine) from the muscle. Uptake of glutamine by intestine and kidney; output of alanine. Uptake of alanine and glutamine by the liver; output of glucose. Uptake of glucose by muscle. Uptake of glutamine, alanine, and branch chain amino acids by brain. Abbreviations: αKG, α-ketoglutarate (2-oxoglutarate); gln, glutamine; AAs, amino acids; ala, alanine. [*Source:* Based on references cited in the text.]

Protein and Energy Metabolism in Fasting, Starvation, and Low-Carbohydrate Diets

The response of protein metabolism to fasting, and starvation has been well studied, especially by Cahill and colleagues (1973) using obese patients receiving only water, vitamins, and minerals over periods of many weeks. Early in fasting (Figure 4.9), glycogen reserves are depleted, and protein (mainly from muscle) becomes the major source of carbon for glucose production (see

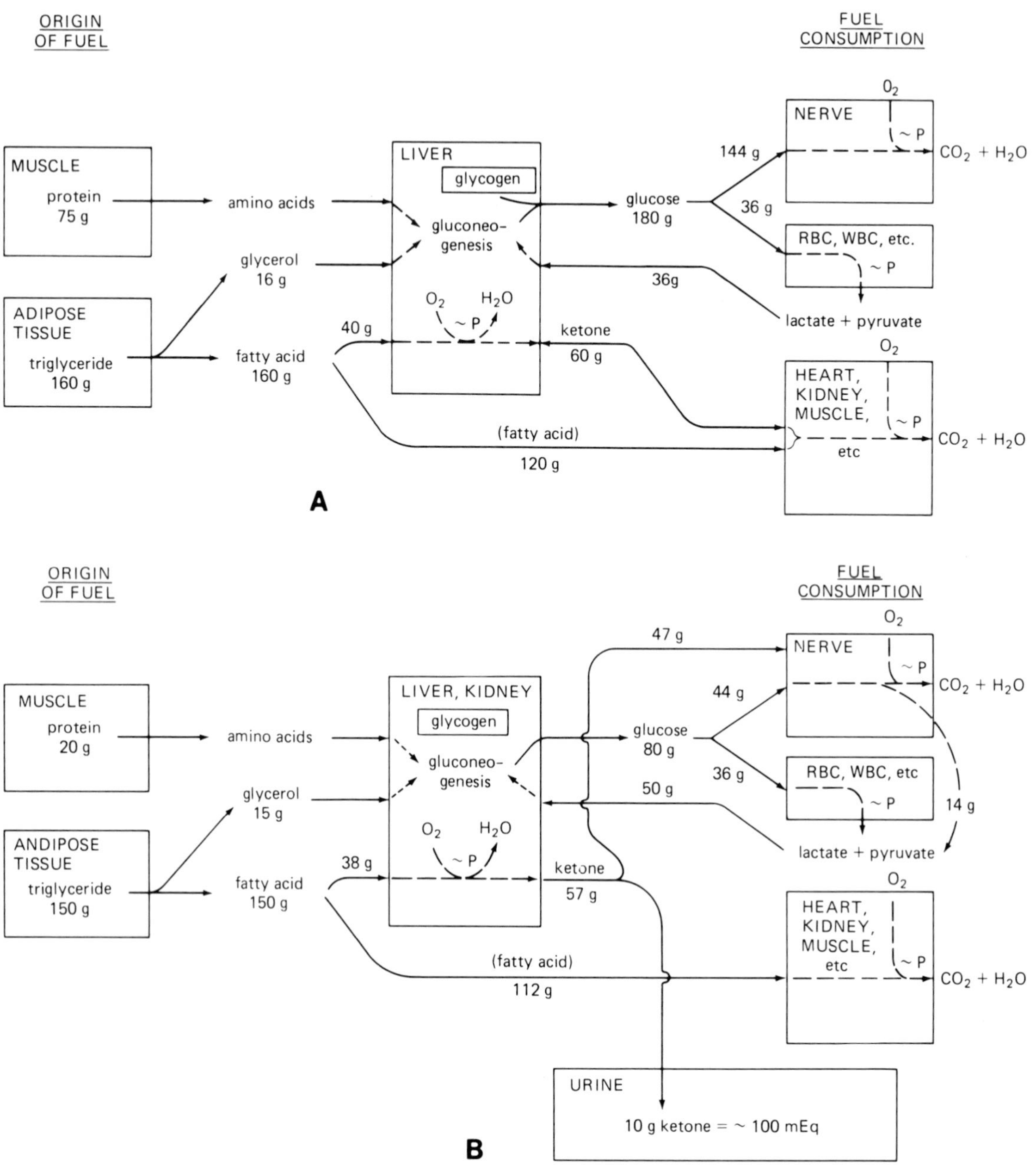

Figure 4.9. Fuel utilization and gluconeogenesis from muscle protein in early and prolonged fasting or starvation. **(A)** Adult man, after a 24-hr fast (24 hr basal = 1800 cal). **(B)** Adult man, after 5–6 weeks of fasting (24 hr basal = 1500 cal). Data show loss of muscle protein and adipose tissue triglyceride (main sources of fuel), their use in production of glucose and ketone bodies by the liver, and uptake of glucose, ketones, and fatty acids by organs requiring fuel for energy. Values given are grams per day, based on studies of numerous obese individuals fasting for various periods of time. [*Source:* Reprinted by permission from Cahill et al. (1973).]

Chapter 2). Some carbon for gluconeogenesis is also provided by the glycerol moiety of triglyceride, which is released from adipose cells into the circulation (see Chapter 3). Glucose is required in substantial amounts by blood cells and the central nervous system on a daily basis (Figure 4.9A). There is also an initiation of ketone body production by the liver (see Chapter 3) to provide a more water-soluble form of fat-derived fuel. A very similar adaptation of protein and energy metabolism occurs in persons consuming diets very low

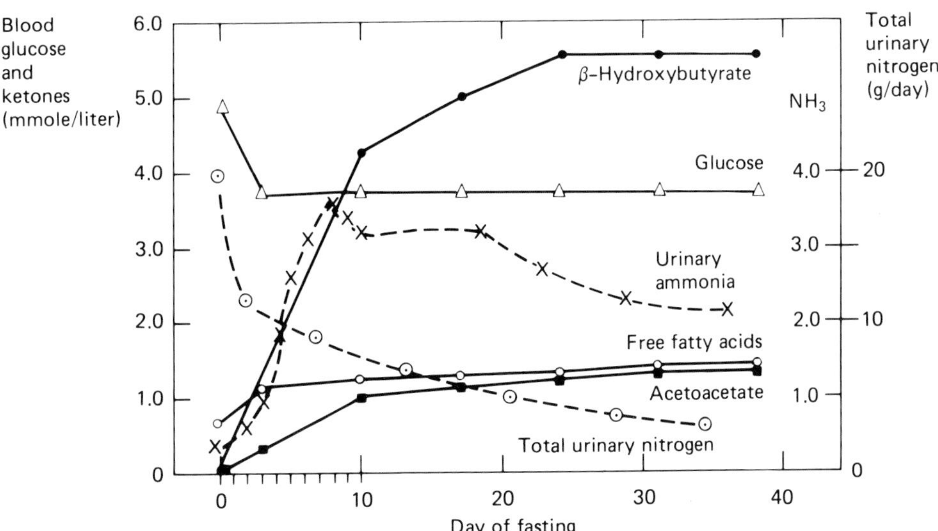

Figure 4.10. Blood glucose and ketones, urinary ammonia, and nitrogen during fasting. Graph depicts blood level of glucose and two forms of ketones (β-hydroxybutyrates and acetoacetate) as they change during fasting over 40 days. Also shown are amounts of urinary ammonia and total nitrogen excreted per day, during continuous fasting. [*Source:* Modified from Cahill and Aoki (1970); nitrogen data from Cahill et al. (1973).]

in carbohydrate, where there is little or no glycogen reserve. However, in this instance, dietary protein largely or fully substitutes for muscle protein in gluconeogenesis (see Chapter 8).

In continued fasting or starvation, if the degradation of muscle (and other) protein used in gluconeogenesis was to continue at the same rate as in early fasting, this would soon result in a life-threatening debilitation of muscle function. However, the body adapts to starvation and reduces the need for protein-dependent gluconeogenesis by boosting its production of ketones, a fuel alternate to glucose for most cells. Circulating ketones reach maximum levels after about 10 days of fasting (Figure 4.10) and now substitute for much of the glucose requirement of the central nervous system (Figure 4.9B). This drastically reduces the need for catabolism of muscle protein. With reduced protein catabolism, urinary nitrogen excretion also declines (Figure 4.10), and there is a shift from the excretion of urea to a predominance of ammonia loss. [Ammonia now accounts for 50% and urea 12% of the urinary nitrogen losses (Cahill et al., 1973).] This shift toward ammonia versus urea parallels the increased production (and excretion) of keto acids (Figure 4.10) and serves to maintain acid/base balance. Most ammonia production occurs in the kidney (Figure 4.8), through the action of glutaminase on glutamine, which, with alanine, is one of the two major amino acids carrying nitrogen from the muscles during muscle protein catabolism (see above).

The overall point is that muscle is a valuable reserve of carbons that can be utilized for glucose production when needed. However, the body prevents excessive losses of muscle proteins over long periods of fasting by adapting the central nervous system to utilization of ketone bodies for fuel. A parallel adaptation in the production and excretion of ammonium ions by the kidney neutralizes the increased ketone bodies (principally β-hydroxybutyric and acetoacetic acids). Without the latter adaptation, such large productions of keto acids would cause a severe ketoacidosis, as well as a loss of large quantities of sodium and potassium ions (accompanying ketones spilled into the urine).

The Role of Vitamin B_6 in Protein Metabolism

In the human, pyridoxine is intimately involved in the metabolism (especially catabolism) of amino acids, being a cofactor in the many transamination reactions that transfer the nitrogen moiety from one keto acid to another. This is the last step in synthesis of nonessential amino acids and the first step in amino acid catabolism (see Chapter 5). From this, it would appear that the requirement for vitamin B_6 must be related to the intake of protein, and thus, that those individuals consuming a great deal of protein will have a greater requirement for the vitamin than those ingesting less. Thus, the U.S. RDA for pyridoxine is related to the amount of protein consumed (0.02 mg B_6/g protein) (National Research Council, 1989). Appearance of homocystine in the urine may be evidence for pyridoxine insufficiency (see below and Chapter 5).

Protein and Disease

Homocystinuria

Homocystinuria usually refers to an inborn error of metabolism in which cystathionine synthetase is deficient or absent (Figure 4.11), resulting in the accumulation of a metabolite of methionine, homocysteine (see also Chapter 18), which is increased in the blood and excreted in large amounts in the urine, as homocystine (the dimer). A similar condition in otherwise normal people can result from deficiencies of vitamins B_6, B_{12}, or folate (see below), which are cofactors for enzymes that use homocysteine as a substrate (Figure 4.11). Homocystinurics usually die in late childhood or early adolescence, and autopsies have revealed that they suffer from advanced atherosclerosis. Indeed, homocystine has been found to be a potent atherogenic agent in animals (see Chapter 15). Children with this disease can be helped by limiting their methionine and protein intakes (Table 4.8), and some respond to a high intake of pyridoxine (vitamin B_6). More recently, it has been shown that they also respond to extra folate intake (Brattstrom et al., 1988*b*).

Homocystinuria can occur in normal individuals on high protein diets with a relative deficiency of vitamin B_6 as the cystathionine synthetase requires the vitamin as a cofactor. Deficiencies of cobalamin (vitamin B_{12}) (Brattstrom et al., 1988*a*; Stabler et al., 1988) or folate (Kang et al., 1987; Brattstrom et al., 1988*b*), both required for the reformation of methionine from homocysteine (Figure 4.11), also have this effect, and supplementation with one or both can reduce homocystinemia (elevated blood homocysteine)

Figure 4.11. Methionine catabolism. Methionine and cysteine metabolism including catabolism of methionine via homocysteine and cystathionine; catabolism of cysteine via taurine and hypotaurine; and the critical points where deficiencies of vitamins B_6, B_{12}, and folate would interfere with specific reactions. Asterisk (*) means this occurs in the absence of adequate vitamins B_6, B_{12}, or folate.

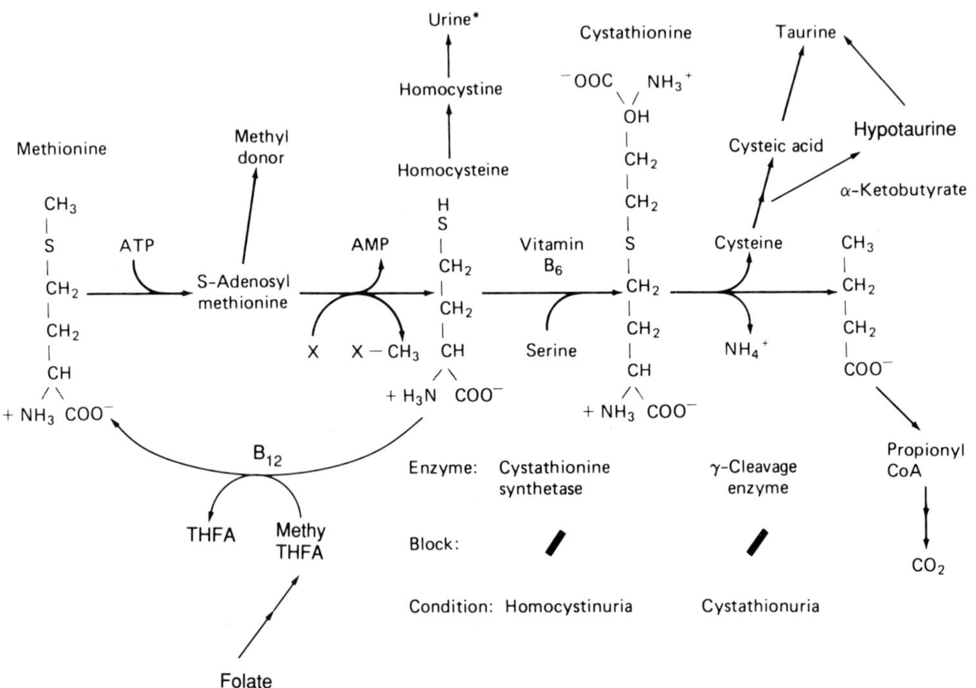

Table 4.8. Suggested Methionine and Protein Intakes in Homocystinuria[a]

Age (years)	Methionine (mg/kg/day)	Protein (g/kg/day)	Energy (kcal/kg/day)
0–0.5	42	2.00[b]	120
0.6–1.0	20	1.50	110
1–3	10–23	1.25	1300 total
4–6	10–18	1.00	1800 total
7–10	10–13	1.00	2400 total
Normal child			
10–12	22	0.81	1500–3000

Source: Data from Acosta and Elsas (1976).

[a] A high intake of vitamin B_6 is also recommended, at least on a trial basis (Spaeth and Barber, 1965).

[b] More is possible if low methionine mixtures are consumed.

(see also Chapter 5). It seems likely that such dietary deficiencies contribute to the development of atherosclerotic heart disease in the United States, where the ingestion of high-meat diets, often low in vitamin B_6 and folate, is very prevalent (see Chapter 15).

Phenylketonuria

This disease springs from a hereditary deficiency (or lack) of phenylalanine hydroxylase in liver (see diagram). This enzyme is needed for the conversion of phenylalanine to tyrosine and is also the route of breakdown for phenylalanine in

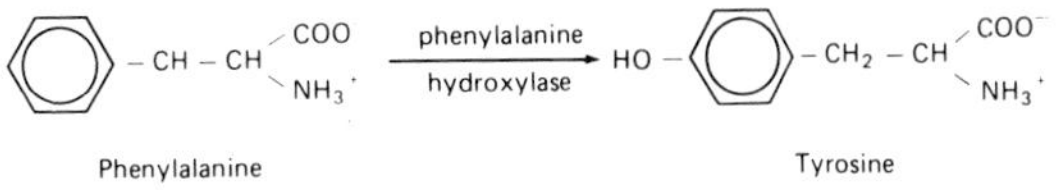

$$C_6H_5-CH_2-CH(NH_3^+)COO^- \xrightarrow[\text{hydroxylase}]{\text{phenylalanine}} HO-C_6H_4-CH_2-CH(NH_3^+)COO^-$$

Phenylalanine → Tyrosine

mammalian tissues. In the absence of this enzyme, phenylalanine accumulates in blood and tissues, and, in infancy and childhood, this has serious effects on brain function. Excess phenylalanine is converted to phenylpyruvic acid and is excreted in the urine, hence the phenylketonuria. If the defect is detected in time, infants and children can be raised quite normally by placing them on diets with a very low phenylalanine content (Table 4.9) (some phenylalanine is needed for protein synthesis) (Koch and Wenz, 1987).

The question is then whether and/or when it may be safe to discontinue rigid control of phenylalanine intake. Data suggest that the period before 6 years of age is particularly critical for IQ, but that it is best to continue on low phenylalanine through adolescence (and during pregnancy in later life). After 10 years of age and in adolescence, occasional "holidays" from the diet are allowed.

Tryptophan, Sleep, and Depression

The use of tryptophan supplements to aid in inducing sleep stems from the demonstration that this results in an increased uptake of the amino acid by the brain, which in turn induces an increased formation of 5-OH tryptamine (serotonin)

Table 4.9. Recommendations for Dietary Intakes in Phenylketonuria

Age (months)	Phenylalanine (mg/kg/day)	Protein (g/kg/day)	Energy (kcal/kg/day)	Protein from Lofenalac[a] (%)	Amount of Lofenalac (measure/kg)[a]	Amount of evaporated milk (oz)[b]
0–3	88	4.4	120	85	2.5–3	1–3
4–6	66	3.3	115	85	2–2.5	1–2.5
7–9	44	2.5	110	90	1.5–2	0.5–1.5
10–12	33	2.5	105	90	1.5–2	0.5–1
		(Total g/day)	*(Total kcal/day)*		*(Total measure/day)*	
13–24	25	25	1300	90	16	0–1
25–36	24	25	1300	90	16	None
37–48	20	30	1300	90	19	None
49–72	18	30	1800	90	19	None
73–96	17	35	2000	90	24	None
97–120	15	40	2200	90	28	None

Source: Reproduced by permission from Krause and Mahan (1979).

[a] Low phenylalanine commercial formula (1 measure equals 10 g, or 1 packed teaspoon).

[b] One ounce of evaporated milk contains 106 mg phenylalanine, 2.2 g protein, and 44 kcal.

(and probably also some other metabolites). Serotonin production in the brain is associated with drowsiness and is also increased by a high-carbohydrate meal. In contrast, intake of tryptophan as part of an amino acid mixture (derived from protein), and without carbohydrate, does not have this effect. The explanation is that uptake of tryptophan by the brain is dependent on the degree of competition exerted by neutral amino acids that use the same carrier in the blood–brain barrier (leu, val, ileu, phe, and tyr). With a high-carbohydrate meal, blood amino acid levels [especially of the branch chain amino acids (leu, val, ileu)] are reduced by insulin (see above), leaving less competition for entry of tryptophan into the brain. Hence, the tendency toward sleepiness that follows a meal. In the case of supplementation, increased tryptophan overwhelms the competition. [Unlike most other amino acids, most tryptophan in the blood is not free but carried by albumin (see Table 4.6).]

Numerous studies have shown that doses of 1–5 g of tryptophan are helpful in inducing sleep (Hartmann, 1977; Spinweber, 1986). (Doses of a gram are often sufficient, and 500-mg pills have been readily available in health food stores for some time.) Tryptophan supplementation (at 3–6 g/day) has also been used as an antidepressant (Prange et al., 1975; Thompson et al., 1982; Pollack and Kraritz, 1985) (in the United Kingdom, especially), although its effectiveness may be questioned (Chambers and Naylor, 1978; Mendels et al., 1975). Its effectiveness as a pain medication (Selzter et al., 1983) is also questionable, since studies supporting this were not double-blind. In general, it is recommended that tryptophan supplementation be accompanied by an increased intake of pyridoxine (vitamin B_6) to reduce accumulation of potentially deleterious tryptophan metabolites (see Chapter 5, Vitamin B_6).

Recently, a rash of cases of eosinophilia (high levels of eosinophils) and myalgia (muscle pain) was traced to the use of tryptophan supplements (Hertzman et al., 1990). Evidence obtained by the Center for Disease Control indicated that the eosinophilia–myalgia syndrome was due to a contaminant in some Japanese tryptophan preparations (*Wall Street Journal*, Jan 31, 1990; Belongia et al., 1990). [Others have speculated that changes in serotonin and other tryptophan metabolites (like quinolines) might be involved.] This remains to be resolved. More acutely, some subjects have reported nausea and vomiting (Greenwood et al., 1975) in response to doses of 5 g tryptophan, and rat studies indicate there can be liver pathology (accumulation of fat droplets) with a high intake. The molecular basis for these various phenomena, if indeed linked to tryptophan, remain to be elucidated.

Glutathione and Other S-Amino Acid Derivatives in Body Defenses

Glutathione (GSH) (Figure 4.5) is an important and abundant (~5 m*M*) constituent of most cells. As a strong sulfhydryl-reducing agent, it maintains many substances in the reduced state and takes part in the cell's defense against oxygen radicals (Beutler, 1989). (See also Chapter 5 and Figure 5.33.) This may occur directly by chemical reduction, or via catalysis involving several enzymes: GSH peroxidase (reacting with peroxides), thiotransulfurase (to reduce cysteine–SH groups on proteins), and glutaredoxin (which utilizes GSH for reduction of ribonucleotide reductase). More recent studies implicate it in the defense against cadmium (Singhal et al., 1987) and copper (Freedman et al., 1989) toxicity, and against the harmful effects of xenobiotic metabolites, such as N-acetyl-p-benzoquinonimine, formed (by mixed function oxidases and cytochrome P450) from acetaminophen (the active agent in Tylenol) (Smilkstein et al., 1988).

Still another function of GSH may be the transport of amino acids via the γ-glutamyl cycle described by Meister (1973), involving γ-glutamyl transpeptidase (GGT), a marker enzyme for liver damage and alcohol abuse. Finally, GSH is required in the synthesis of leukotrienes, again via GGT, from n-3 and n-6 polyunsaturated fatty acids (Hammarstrom, 1983) (see Chapter 3), which are important in the inflammatory response.

GSH is formed from glutamate, cysteine, and glycine, cysteine being the crucial (and only potentially limiting) amino acid. The availability of cysteine is determined by its content in food proteins and also the content of methionine, as methionine can be converted to cysteine. [Cysteine can substitute for much of the methionine requirement if choline is present in sufficient amounts to provide the methyl group (Figure 4.11) (Finkelstein et al., 1986).] Cysteine and hypotaurine (Figure 4.11), produced from cysteine, may be important in antioxidant defense (Canas et al., 1989). The availability of -SH groups directly from cysteine or indirectly from methionine thus plays a major role in the basic functioning and chronic health of the body.

Food Allergies

Food allergies (or hypersensitivities) appear to arise when very antigenic food proteins find their way past the immunological defenses of the digestive tract, past the "M" cells involved with the Peyer's patches, past the peptidases and other digestive enzymes in the intestinal lumen and intestinal mucosal cells, and into the blood (or lymph) circulation (Gardner, 1988; Walker, 1988) (Figure 4.12). [See also the earlier section on protein metabolism.] If very allergenic, these proteins (or parts of these proteins) elicit production of specific antibodies of the IgE and IgG classes, which can trigger hypersensitivity reactions that are harmful to the host (Aas, 1988). Less allergenic (or nonallergenic) proteins that may get into the blood will also elicit antibodies, but without inducing hypersensitivity (Walker, 1988). Hypersensitivity reactions include skin rashes and/or gastrointestinal responses, sneezing, and other nasal responses attributable to the release of histamine from mast cells, due to antigen–antibody complexation. [Recent data suggest that a propensity to food allergy is accompanied by a tendency of blood monocytes to secrete histamine-releasing factors, as well as the presence of a special form of IgE1, designated IgE+ (Sampson et al., 1989).]

Major food allergens for humans include ovalbumin (the major egg white protein), β-lactoglobulin and casein in cow's milk, as well as bovine albumin and γ-globulin (residual in beef meat) and certain proteins in fish, crustaceans, and nuts. A major food allergen is defined as a protein reacting with blood IgE in more than 50% of subjects allergic to the food in which the allergen is found (Aas, 1988). It is still unclear what determines the degree of hyperantigenicity of some proteins, although certain repetitive amino acid sequences within the same protein may be involved.

There are very few data available on the prevalence of food allergies in various population groups (Kjellman, 1988), although there is the general impression that the condition is common and widespread. Relationships between food allergies and infant diet have been studied more extensively, with the general finding of a positive correlation between early exposure to major allergens and the likelihood of developing hyperallergenic/hypersensitivity reactions (Jakobsson, 1988; Strobel, 1988; Walker, 1988). This relationship is ascribable to changes in the permeability of the intestinal mucosal barrier, which occur in the perinatal period, and the greater permeability of this barrier in newborn versus 9- to 20-week-old infants, or in premature infants versus those at term (Jakobsson, 1988). Recent studies on the appearance of maternal α-lactalbumin in the blood of infants soon after feeding indicated an almost exponentially decreasing relationship between stage of maturity and blood concentrations of the maternal protein, from 9 weeks before to 9–20 weeks after term (Jakobsson, 1988). [During this period, values fell from up to 12,000 ng/ml to less than 20!] The type of milk or formula, especially if fed to premature infants, may therefore make a difference to their development of food hypersensitivities. In general, human breast milk appears to protect against, and cow's milk formulas promote, the development of specific allergies. The allergen content of the mother's blood during gestation has little or no effect on the future development of allergies by the infant. In the case of the lactating mother, however, traces of some allergens in the mother's

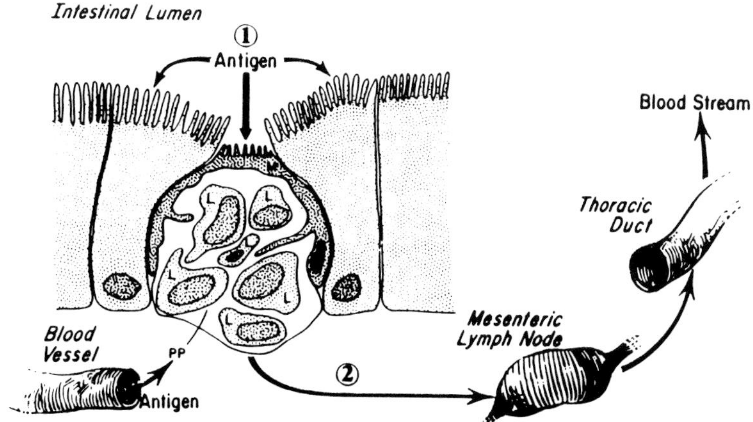

Figure 4.12. Transmucosal passage of whole proteins (antigens) via M cells (specialized epithelium), and potential interaction with lymphoid cells in Peyer's patches, before entry into the lymph and blood. [*Source:* Reprinted by permission from Walker (1988).]

blood may be transferred to the milk (Durand, 1988; Strobel, 1988; Vandenplas et al., 1988) and therefore enhance the development of hypersensitivity. Lactating mothers of infants at risk for developing allergy are therefore advised to stay away from foods rich in the most notorious allergens.

Protein Malnutrition

As mentioned earlier, kwashiorkor is a common problem in many Third World countries. It is often accompanied by a deficiency of calories as well as protein (marasmus), which will exacerbate the problem. In protein deficiency, there is a great deal of muscle wasting and a decrease in plasma protein concentrations, especially albumin. The latter causes a fall in plasma colloid osmotic pressure. Since colloid osmotic pressure is essential for the flow of water and metabolites from interstitial fluid back into the blood circulation, protein deficiency results in edema and in the distention of the belly seen in children with protein malnutrition. A deficiency in calories as well as essential amino acids will put further pressure on muscle and other body proteins, as they are a source of potential energy and may be needed for maintenance of blood glucose through gluconeogenesis (see Protein and Energy Metabolism in Fasting and Starvation and Low-Carbohydrate Diets). Either way, protein malnutrition results (by definition) in a negative balance (output > input), and this will be even more severe when caloric intake is also reduced. Indeed, even if essential amino acid intake in itself is marginally adequate, lack of calories will enhance body protein breakdown and create a negative nitrogen balance. [This may also occur when people go on certain weight-reducing diets (see Chapter 8).] Clearly, individuals with protein malnutrition are weakened and at risk with regard to all manner of diseases.

References

Aas K (1988): *In* Schmidt E, ed: Food allergy. New York: Raven Press, p 1.

Acosta P, Elsas L (1976): Dietary management of inherited metabolic disease. Atlanta: ACELMU.

Beutler E (1989): Annu Rev Nutr 9:287.

Blaxter KL (1977): *In* Proceedings of the 2nd International Symposium on Protein Metabolism and Nutrition, May 1977, The Netherlands, European Association for Animal Production, publication no 22.

Brattstrom LE, Israelsson B, Lindgarde F, Hultberg BL (1988a): Metabolism 37:175.

Brattstrom LE, Israelsson B, Jeppsson JO, Hultberg BL (1988b): Scand J Clin Lab Invest 48:215.

Canas P, Guerra R, Valenzuela A (1989): Nutr Rep Intl 39:433.

Cahill GF Jr, Aoki TT (1970): Med Times 98:106.

Cahill GF Jr, Aoki TT, Ruderman NB (1973): Trans Am Clin Climatol Assoc 84:184.

Chambers CA, Naylor GJ (1978): Br J Psychiatry 132:555.

Chang TW, Goldberg AL (1978): J Biol Chem 253:3677.

Clifford AJ (1980): *In* Alfin-Slater RB, Krichevsky D, eds: Human nutrition: A comprehensive treatise. New York: Plenum, p 183.

Elwyn DH (1970): *In* Munro HN, ed: Mammalian protein metabolism, vol IV. New York: Academic, p 523.

FAO (1957): Protein requirements, report on the FAO Committee, FAO Nutrition Studies no 16, Rome, October 24–31, 1955.

Felig P (1975): Annu Rev Biochem 44:933.

Felig P, Wahren J, Ahlborg G (1973): Proc Soc Exp Biol Med 142:230.

Ferenci P (1978): *In* Wewalka F, Dragosics B, eds: Ammoniak, und Hepatische Enzephalopathie. Stuttgart: Gustav Fischer.

Frame EG (1958): Clin Invest 37:1710.

Freedman JH, Ciriolo MR, Peisach J (1989): J Biol Chem 264:5598.

Gardner MLG (1988): Annu Rev Nutr 8:329.

Gitler C (1964): *In* Munro HN, Allison JB, eds: Mammalian protein metabolism, vol 1. New York: Academic, p 35.

Goldberg AL, Tischler M, DeMartino G, Griffin G (1982): Fed Proc 41:31.

Greengard AL, Smith MA, Acs G (1963): J Biol Chem 238:1548.

Greenwood MH, Lader MH, Kantameneni BD, Curzon G (1975): Br J Clin Pharmacol 2:165.

Hammarstrom S (1983): *In* Larsson A, Orrenhius S, Holmgren A, Mannervik B, eds: Functions of glutathione: Biochemistry, physiological, toxicological, and clinical aspects. New York: Raven, p 149.

Hardage MG, Crooks H, Stare F (1966): J Am Dietetics 48:25.

Hartmann E (1977): Am J Psychiatry 134:4.

Herron JM, Saltzman HA, Hills BA, Kylstra JA (1973): J Appl Physiol 35:546.

Hertzman PA, Blevins WL, Mayer J, Greenfield B, Ting M, Gleich GJ (1990): N Engl J Med 322:869.

Hill D (1980): Clin Chem 26:983.

Hoffenberg R (1970): *In* Rothschild MA; Waldmann T, eds: Plasma protein metabolism. New York: Academic.

Hundal HS, Rennie MJ, Watt PW (1989): J Physiol 408:93.

Irwin IM, Hegsted DM (1971*a*): J Nutr 101:539.

Irwin IM, Hegsted DM (1971*b*): J Nutr 101:385.

Jakobsson I (1988): *In* Food allergy, D Reinhardt, E Schmidt, eds: New York: Raven, p 243.

Jepson MM, Bates PC, Broadbent P, Pell JM, Millward DJ (1988): Am J Physiol 255:E166.

Kang SS, Wong PWK, Norusis M (1987): Metabolism 36:458.

Kjellman N-IM (1988): *In* Schmidt E, ed: Food allergy. New York: Raven, p 119.

Koch R, Wenz E (1987): Annu Rev Nutr 7:117.

Krause MV, Mahan LK (1979): Nutrition and diet therapy (6th ed). Philadelphia: WB Saunders.

Malloy MH, Rassin DK, Gaull GE (1981): Am J Clin Nutr 34:2619.

Man EH, Bada JL (1987): Annu Rev Nutr 7:209.

Marliss EB, Aoki TT, Pozefski T, Most AS, Cahill GF Jr (1971): J Clin Invest 50:814.

Matsutaka H, Aikawa T, Yamamota H, Ishikawa E (1973): J Biochem (Tokyo) 74:1019.

Meister A (1973): Science 180:33.

Mendels J, Stinnett JL, Burns D, Frazer A (1975): Arch Gen Psychiatry 32:22.

Morris IG (1968): *In* Code CH, ed: Handbook of physiology, section 6, vol III. Washington DC: American Physiological Society, p 1491.

Munro HN (1969): *In* Mammalian protein metabolism, vol III. New York: Academic, p 133.

Munro HN (1982): Parent Enteral Nutr 6:271.

Munro HN, Crim M (1980): *In* Shils ME, Goodhart RS, eds: Modern nutrition in health and disease (6th ed). Philadelphia: Lea & Febiger, p 51.

Munro HN, Crim M (1988): *In* Shils ME, Young VR, eds: Modern nutrition in health and disease (7th ed). Philadelphia: Lea & Febiger, p 1.

Nagata Y, Konno R, Yasumura Y, Akino T (1989): Biochem J 257:291.

NAS (1978): Nutritional evaluation of foods. Washington, DC: NAS.

National Research Council (1989): Diet and health: Implications for reducing chronic disease risk. Washington, DC: National Academy Press.

Ogawa K, Yokojima A, Ichihara A (1970): J Biochem (Tokyo) 68:90.

Pollack RL, Kravitz E (1985): J Nutr 117:1314.

Prange AJ Jr, Wilson IC, Lynn CW, Alltop LB, Stikeleather RA (1974): Arch Gen Psychiatry 30:56.

Reed PB (1980): Nutrition, an applied science. New York: West Publishing.

Rennie MJ, Hundal HS, Babij P, MacLennan P, Taylor PM, Watt PW, Jepson MM, Millward DJ (1986): Lancet 2:1008.

Rocha DM, Faloona GR, Unger RH (1972): J Clin Invest 51:2346.

Sampson HA, Broadbent KR, Bernhisel-Broadbent J (1989): N Engl J Med 321:228.

Sato F, Ignotz GG, Ignotz RA, Gansler T, Tsukada K, Lieberman I (1981): Biochemistry 20:5550.

Schimke RT (1963): J Biol Chem 238:1012.

Selzter S, Dewart D, Pollack RL, Jackson E (1983): J Psychiatr Res 17:181.

Singhal RK, Anderson ME, Meister A (1987): FASEB J 1:220.

Smilkstein MJ, Knapp GL, Kulig KW, Rumack BH (1988): N Engl J Med 319:1557.

Snodgrass PJ, Lin RC, Muller WA, Aoki TT (1978): J Biol Chem 253:2748.

Soupart P (1961): *In* Holden JT, ed: Amino acid pools. New York: Elsevier, p 232.

Spaeth GL, Barber GW (1965): Trans Am Acad Ophthalmol Otolaryngol 69:912.

Spinweber CL (1986): Psychopharmacology (Berlin) 90:151.

Stabler SP, Marcell PD, Podell ER, et al. (1988): J Clin Invest 81:466.

Strobel S (1988): *In* Schmidt E, ed: Food allergy. New York: Raven, p 89.

Tannenbaum SR, Fett D, Young VR, Land PD, Bruce WR (1978): Science 200:1487.

Thomson J, Rankin H, Ashcroft GW, Yates LM, McQueen JK, Cummings SW (1982): Psychol Med 12:741.

Valgeirsdottir K, Munro HN (1983): *In* Fischer JE, ed: Surgical nutrition. Boston: Little, Brown, p 129.

Vandenplas Y, Deneyer M, Sacre L, Loeb H (1988): *In* Schmidt E, ed: Food allergy. New York: Raven, p 257.

Wahren J, Felig P, Hagenfeldt J (1976): J Clin Invest 57:978.

Waldmann TA (1977): *In* Rosenoer VM, Oratz M, Rothschild MA, eds: Albumin structure, function, and uses. New York: Pergamon.

Walker WA (1988): *In* Schmidt E, ed: Food allergy. New York: Raven, p 15.

Walker WA, Isselbacher KJ (1974): Gastroenterology 67:531.

Warshaw AL, Walker WA, Isselbacher KJ (1974): Gastroenterology 66:987.

Watford M (1989): TIBS 14:1.

Windmueller HG, Spaeth AE (1974): J Biol Chem 249:5070.

Witter JP, Gatley SJ, Balish E (1981): Science 213:449.

White A, Handler P, Smith EL (1973): Principles of biochemistry (5th ed). New York: McGraw-Hill.

Whitney E, Hamilton EM (1981): Understanding nutrition. St Paul: West Publishing.

WHO/FAO/UNO (1985): Energy and protein requirements, WHO Technical Report Series no 724. Geneva: WHO.

Yamamoto H, Aikawa T, Matsutaka H, Okuda O, Ishikawa E (1974): Am J Physiol 226:1428.

Yap SH, Strair RK, Shafritz DA (1978): J Biol Chem 253:4944.

Young VR, Bier DM (1987): Nutr Rev 45:289.

Young VR, Munro HN (1978): Fed Proc 37:2291.

Maria C. Linder, Ph.D.*

5

Nutrition and Metabolism of Vitamins

Historical Introduction

Connections among dietary habits, specific diseases, and the special curative effects of certain foods have been recorded throughout history, beginning with Hippocrates' observation in Ancient Greece that liver could cure nightblindness. In England in 1757, James Lind noted that only fresh fruits and vegetables were effectual in curing scurvy; in Italy in 1810, Marzari first made a connection between maize diets and pellagra. In 1893, a Dutch physician in Java, named Eijkman, produced a paralysis in chickens, similar to that suffered by many humans in Asia for centuries, by feeding them the local polished rice. More importantly, he showed that the symptoms could be relieved by an extract from the polishings (bran and germ). These and further experimental observations, especially on beriberi, prompted Casimir Funk, in Poland, to formulate the "vitamin theory" of disease. He proposed that the four diseases, scurvy, rickets, pellagra, and beriberi, were due to a lack of four different vital "amines" in the diet. In the same year, in England, F.G. Hopkins reported that tiny amounts of certain factors from milk were necessary for the growth of rats on purified diets. (Funk and Hopkins received the 1929 Nobel Prize in medicine for these discoveries.) In the United States, McCollum and Davis at the University of Wisconsin demonstrated the need for a fat-soluble factor "A" from butterfat and egg yolk, and a heat-labile water-soluble factor "B" in wheat germ for the growth of young rats. The latter was found to cure beriberi. Further research showed that wheat germ contained several more, water-soluble, vital growth factors. All water-soluble vitamins, except C, are now considered B vitamins.

Nomenclature, Properties, and Sources of Vitamins

The vitamins known to be essential for human growth, maintenance, and health are listed in Table 5.1, along with information on their isolation, function, tissue distribution, and origin in nature and the food supply. It may be noted that, by definition, a vitamin is a complex organic substance, required in very small quantities in the diet relative to all other nutrients save the trace elements. Vitamins are essential (Table 5.1) in that they cannot be produced by our own tissues at all or in sufficient quantities to supply our needs under normal circumstances. Also shown in Table 5.1 are a few vitaminlike substances that are not considered essential, as they are usually produced by our own tissues in sufficient amounts or are part of other vitamins or nutrients we ingest (vitamin D, choline, lipoic acid, *p*-aminobenzoic acid, and inositol).

* California State University, Fullerton, CA.

Table 5.1. The Vitamins: Nomenclature, Distribution, Sources, and Deficiency Diseases

Vitamin	Deficiency disease	Discovery (isolation)	Enzyme cofactor	Cell/tissue distribution	Origins	Good food sources
B Vitamins						
Thiamin[a] B_1	Beriberi	Jansen and Donath (1926)	√	All	Plants, some yeasts, molds, bacteria	Seeds, nuts, wheat germ, legumes, lean meat
Riboflavin[a] B_2	(Pellagra)	Kuhn et al. (1933)	√	All	Plants, bacteria, fungi	Milk, organ meats, eggs, nuts, and seeds
Niacin[a] B_3 (nicotinic acid)	Pellagra	Elvehjem et al. (1937)	√	All	Plants, some bacteria, fungi, yeast[b]	Meats, nuts, legumes (not corn)
Pantothenic[a] acid, B_5		Williams (1939) (yeast)	√	All	Plants, some bacteria[c]	Yeast, grains (widespread), Royal jelly, egg yolk, liver
B_6[a] pyridoxine		Szent-Györgyi and other groups (1938)	√	All	Many bacteria, yeasts, fungi, plants[c]	Yeast, liver, wheat germ, nuts, beans, avocados, bananas
Folic acid[a] folacin, B_c vitamin M	(Anemia)	Stokstad; Pfiffner et al. (1943)	√	All	Plants, some bacteria[c]	Yeast, liver, alfalfa, spinach
B_{12}[a] cobalamin	Pernicious anemia	Rickes et al.; Smith and Parker (1948)	√	All	Fungi, some bacteria (not plants)	Liver, kidney, egg, cheese
Biotin,[a] H	Egg white injury	Kögl (1948)	√	All	Bacteria, yeasts, fungi[c] (plants may not make)	Yeast, liver, egg yolk, tomato, soybeans, rice, bran
Choline	Fatty liver		—	All	Some bacteria, plants[b] (animal tissues)	Egg yolk, meat, cereals, legumes, lecithin
Inositol	Fatty liver		—	All	Some bacteria, yeasts, plants[b]	Meat, milk, fruits, nuts, grains (oils), citrus, legumes
Lipoic acid			√	All	Some bacteria, plants[b]	Yeast, liver
PABA (p-amino benzoic acid)			√	All	Plants, bacteria	Vegetables?, fruits?, yeast, liver
Vitamin C[a] (ascorbic acid)	Scurvy	Zilva et al. (1917); Szent-Györgyi et al., King et al. (1928–1932)	√	All	Plants, most animals (except when young), some bacteria	Citrus, rosehips, acerola berries, cranberries, tomato, cabbage, fruits and vegetables in general
Fat-soluble vitamins						
A[a] retinoids	Night blindness	McCollum (1916); Karrer et al. (1931)	√	Selected tissues (especially liver)	Plants (carotenes)	Precursor in yellow-orange vegetable plants, carrots, liver, fish liver oils

Table 5.1 *(continued)*

Vitamin	Deficiency disease	Discovery (isolation)	Enzyme cofactor	Cell/tissue distribution	Origins	Good food sources
D[a] calciferols	Rickets	Mellanby and McCollum (1919–1922); Askew et al. (1931)	—	Selected tissues (especially liver)	Plankton; irradiation in animals, man (UV light)[b]	Fish liver oils (eggs)
E[a] tocopherols	(Sterility, rats)	Evans and Bishop (1922); Fernholz (1938)	√ ?	Most tissues	Plants	Vegetable and seed oils, green leaves
K[a] phylloquinones and menaquinones	Lack of blood clotting	Dam (1929); Doisy (1939)	√	Selected tissues	Bacteria, plants[c]	Green leafy vegetables, egg yolk, cheese

[a] Established as essential for humans.
[b] Some production in human tissues.
[c] Human gut bacteria are a significant source.

The most convenient way to classify the vitamins is by their solubility. There are much fewer fat-soluble vitamins than water-soluble vitamins (Table 5.1). The solubility of a vitamin influences its mode of action, storage, and toxicity. Generally speaking, and with the exception of B_{12}, water-soluble vitamins are not stored. They enter the body freely, are present in the intra- and extracellular fluids, and generally exit the body easily via the urine, relatively unchanged. Most water-soluble vitamins function as coenzymes in energy and protein/amino acid and nucleic acid metabolism. Alternatively, they are cosubstrates in enzymatic reactions, such as ascorbic acid in oxidation/reduction, or are structural components and latent regulatory agents, such as choline and inositol in phospholipids.

Fat-soluble vitamins have more individualized actions with the exception of vitamin E (a broad-spectrum, lipid antioxidant). They are readily stored, and again, with the exception of vitamin E, are not absorbed or excreted as readily as the water-soluble vitamins. With the exception of vitamin K, they are not coenzymes in the sense of the B vitamins. Indeed, two of them (vitamins A and D) may be viewed as hormones.

The capability for storage is related to vitamin toxicity. Those vitamins stored in liver, such as A and D, can be quite toxic if present in large amounts. This is not true of E or K, or of the vitamin A precursor carotenes, which like E are stored in adipose tissue. (Adipose tissue is a much larger and metabolically less active "reservoir.") In contrast, the water-soluble vitamins are quite nontoxic, although it cannot be excluded that prolonged overdosing with such vitamins may lead to long-range aberrations in metabolism (see below).

Most vitamins that find their way into our food supply are directly or indirectly synthesized by plants (Table 5.1). The exceptions are vitamin D, which can be produced in adequate amounts in our own bodies with the help of ultraviolet light, and vitamin B_{12}, the product of fungi, actinomycetes (soil microorganisms), and some bacteria. (Vegetarians must be alert for deficiencies in these two vitamins.) Foods of bird, animal, or fish origin contain the various vitamins mainly because they have themselves ingested plants. Our own gut bacteria normally also provide a sizeable portion of our vitamin K, as well as smaller amounts of some other (B) vitamins (Table 5.1). Food sources particularly rich in various vitamins are indicated in Table 5.1. In general, it may be stated that seeds of all kinds, including whole grains, nuts, and eggs (which are the "seeds" of the fowl), are especially rich in vitamins, particularly in the germ that will develop into the new plant or fowl. Yeast and yeast extracts are also excellent supplemental sources, as are liver and some other organ meats that tend to concentrate the vitamins in animal systems. Vegetables and fruits are essential contributors of vitamins in a well-rounded diet, being especially important for vitamins C and A, the latter in the form of its precursor, β-carotene.

The tendency in our society to refine whole grains and other carbohydrate sources, our dietary emphasis on muscle meats, and methods of food preparation that overcook or leach the vita-

Table 5.2. Effects of Milling and Processing on Vitamin Content of Grains

Food	Vitamin concentration (μg/g)					
	Thiamin	Riboflavin	Niacin	Pyridoxine	Folacin	Vitamin E
Whole wheat	3.5	1.5	50	1.7	0.3	16
Patent flour	0.8	0.3	9.5	0.5	0.1	2.3
Germ	22.0	5.5	80	12	1.5	125
Brown rice	3.4	0.5	47	10.3	0.2	
Polished rice	0.7	0.3	16	4.5	0.2	
Corn (whole kernel)	3.8	1.1	20			
Corn meal	1.4	0.5	9.9			

Source: Data from Schroeder (1975).

mins from foods are the main factors responsible for the existence of vitamin deficiencies within the U.S. population. Table 5.2 summarizes the effects on vitamin content of refining whole wheat, rice, and corn. The effects of various methods of food preparation on vitamin content are addressed in Chapter 10. As shown, the removal of the germ and the bran covering from these various grains (Figure 5.1) also removes most of the vitamin content. The same is true for the trace elements (Chapter 6). Most of the vitamins are present in the germ (the plant embryo), and this makes wheat germ an attractive and inexpensive vitamin supplement, especially if untoasted (to avoid heat destruction of some vitamins). Wheat flour, which is pervasive in our foods (from breads, rolls, and cakes, to pizza and spaghetti) is a staple consisting mainly of starch with the bran and germ removed. When "enriched," some of the nutrients removed in the milling have been added back to the level originally present, and this must be specified on the label. Fortified or supplemented foods contain nutrients added beyond the level originally present. Only foods labeled as "whole grain" or "whole wheat" contain the unrefined ingredients. [Refining of flour does have one advantage that should not be ignored, that is, whole grain flour is harder to ship and store long-term because the oils from the germ (not present in regular flour) can turn rancid.] Information on the structure, function, requirement, absorption, excretion, and metabolism of individual vitamins follows below.

Figure 5.1. Structure of the whole grain: wheat. Partial cutaway illustration. Components present on each part are indicated.

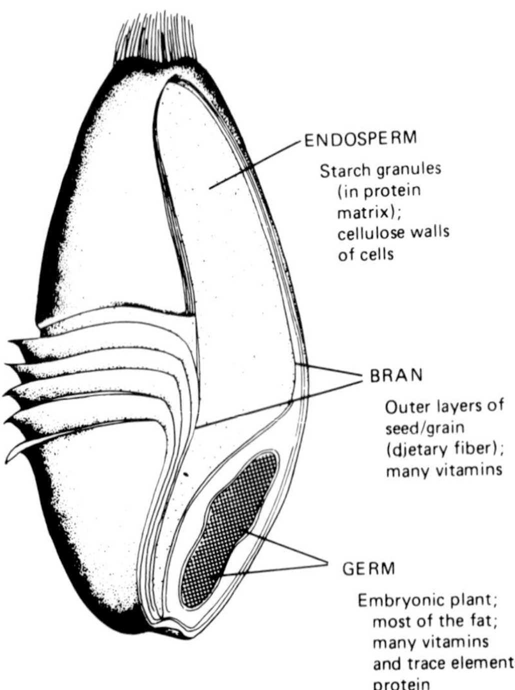

The B Vitamins Involved in Intermediary Metabolism: Thiamin, Riboflavin, Niacin, Pantothenic and Lipoic Acids, and Biotin

These vitamins are central to the metabolism of all cells, as they are coenzymes in specific reactions along the glycolytic, tricarboxylic acid (Krebs cycle), and pentose pathways (Figure 5.2), as well as in pathways subsidiary to energy metabolism. The vitamins associate with their cognizant enzymes through covalent or noncovalent bonds in the area of the active site. The tightness of the associations is dictated by the nature of the individual enzyme and is highly variable; for example, a given vitamin may be loosely associated

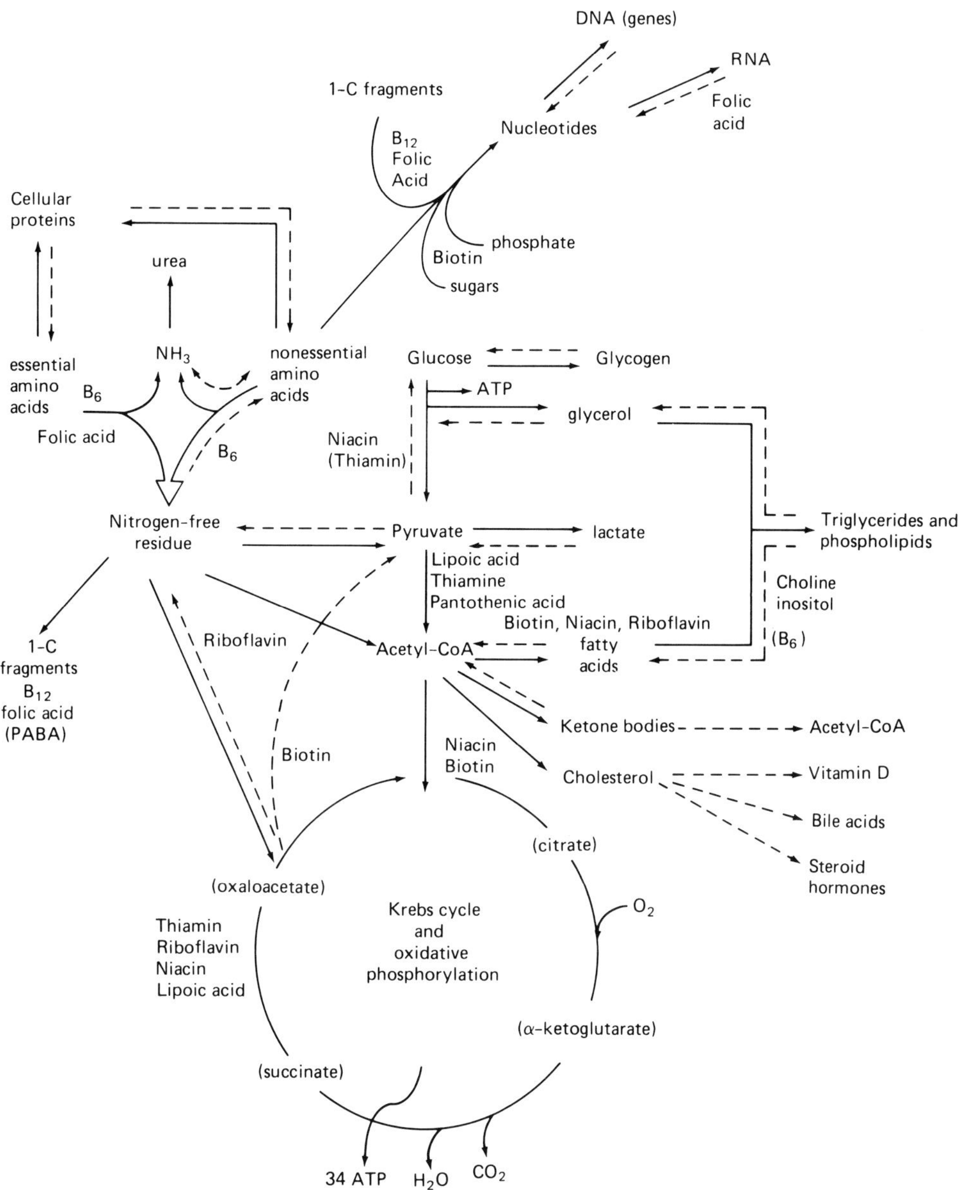

Figure 5.2. Involvement of water soluble B vitamins in intermediary metabolism.

with one enzyme and tightly with another at a given ambient vitamin concentration. The structure and metabolism of each of these vitamins is shown in Figures 5.3–5.9, along with summaries of their requirements and peculiarities of function.

Thiamin

This vitamin was first crystallized by Jansen and Donath in 1926 and first synthesized by Roger R. Williams and his colleagues in 1936 (Figure 5.3) (Neal and Sauberlich, 1980). The three known enzyme reactions in animals and man involving thiamin pyrophosphate as a coenzyme are pyruvate decarboxylase, α-ketoglutarate decarboxylase (in the Krebs cycle), and transketolase (in the pentose-phosphate shunt). (The latter is also very important in the "dark reactions" of photosynthesis in plants, during the conversion of CO_2 to carbo-

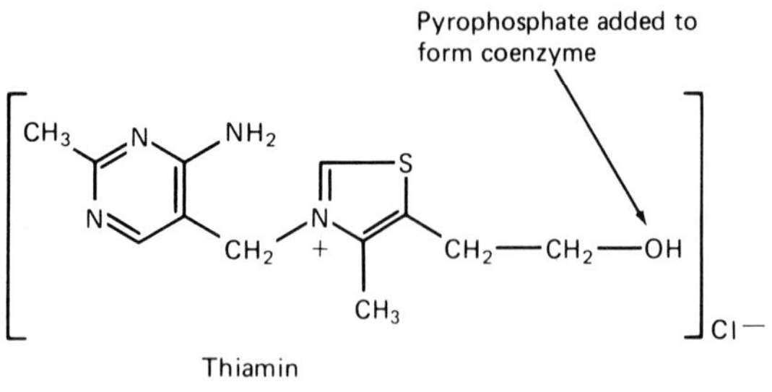

Pyrophosphate added to form coenzyme

$$\left[\ \text{CH}_3\text{-pyrimidine(NH}_2\text{)-CH}_2\text{-N}^+\text{(thiazole: CH}_3\text{, S)-CH}_2\text{—CH}_2\text{—OH}\ \right]\text{Cl}^-$$

Thiamin

Figure 5.3. Thiamin.

Functions and effects: Coenzyme for reactions central to intermediary metabolism in all cells (including the brain):

Decarboxylation reactions (pyruvate and α-ketoglutarate).

Transketolase reaction. (Erythrocyte activity used to determine status).

Requirements: 0.5 mg/1000 kcal (related to energy requirements)

Av. RDA: Women 1.0–1.1 mg/day (+0.4–0.5 in pregnancy and lactation)

Men 1.2–1.5 mg/day

(The presence of thiaminases or thiamine antagonists in tea, coffee, rice bran, and other foods, may increase requirements.)

Total in body: about 30 mg (80% as thiamin pyrophosphate).

Absorption: by active transport and passive diffusion.

Storage: none (except in the sense of being attached to enzymes).

Toxicity: very low; LD_{50} 125–350 mg/kg body weight (i.v.) mice-dogs; no ill effects in man, up to 200 × RDA.

Excretion: Thiamin and multiple metabolites excreted in urine.

Gross deficiency in man: peripheral neuropathy most marked in most actively used extremities. Leads to weakness, tenderness and atrophy of muscles, fatigue, decreased attention span, and amnesia. The heart is often affected (enlargement; tachycardia with physical effort). In Western societies, gross deficiency is mainly associated with alcoholism.

Good food sources: see Table 5.1.

[*Source:* Information from Neal and Sauberlich (1980), Gibbs and Seitchik (1980), McCormick (1988*d*), and Haas (1988).]

hydrates.) The first two of these reactions also require lipoic acid, NAD^+ (from niacin), and coenzyme A (from pantothenic acid) (Figure 5.2). Enzyme-bound thiamin pyrophosphate forms a substrate intermediate in these reactions. Some thiamin triphosphate is also formed and may play a separate role in brain cell viability, as suggested by data from patients with subacute necrotizing encephalomyelopathies (Leigh's syndrome) (Pincus et al., 1976).

Severe thiamin deficiency results in the disease known as "beriberi," which is characterized by peripheral neuropathy (dry beriberi), especially in the limbs used most frequently, accompanied by tingling, numbness, tenderness, and weakness, and/or cardiovascular problems (wet beriberi) (Figure 5.3) made worse by physical exertion and carbohydrate utilization for energy. Marginal thiamin deficiency may be quite common, especially among the elderly in our society who may have a low intake exacerbated by poor absorption, and in alcoholics (with poor nutrition and malabsorption). [Marginal deficiency may occur in 17%–27% of Americans (see Haas, 1988).] Thiaminases that destroy the vitamin (present in raw fish and shellfish; as in sushi), as well as tannins and other factors (in tea and coffee) which oxidize the vitamin, can decrease its content in the diet. Thiamin's considerable heat lability (see Chapter 10) and the refining of whole grains also contribute to a lower diet content. Deficiency is best judged by measuring erythrocyte transketolase or urinary thiamin excretion (see Chapter 12). Requirements are greater for women during pregnancy and lactation. Good food sources are meat, legumes, whole grains, and seeds.

Riboflavin

Further studies on the antiberiberi substance of McCollum in the 1920s, along with quite separate work on the properties of naturally occurring flavins, culminated in the discoveries of a substance, later called riboflavin, which could cure some of the symptoms of pellagra (Horwitt, 1980*a*). Riboflavin (Figure 5.4) was first isolated from milk in 1933 by Kuhn, Szent-György, and Wagner-Jauregg and was first synthesized in 1935. It functions as part of the two coenzymes, flavin adenine dinucleotide (FAD) and riboflavin-5′-phosphate (FMN), in various oxidation/reduction reactions, most notably, succinic dehydrogenase (which links the Krebs cycle directly to oxidative phosphorylation), and in the pathways for synthesis and oxidation of fatty acids (Figure 5.2). Flavins are especially useful in biologic systems, in that they are stronger oxidizing agents than NAD^+ (thus fitting in further along the e-transport chain). They can participate in one or two electron processes (and thus reactions with free radicals or metal ions), and in reduced form, they can react directly with O_2 (as in hydroxylation reactions) (Metzler, 1977). Riboflavin is thus an enzyme cofactor, or cosubstrate, fundamental

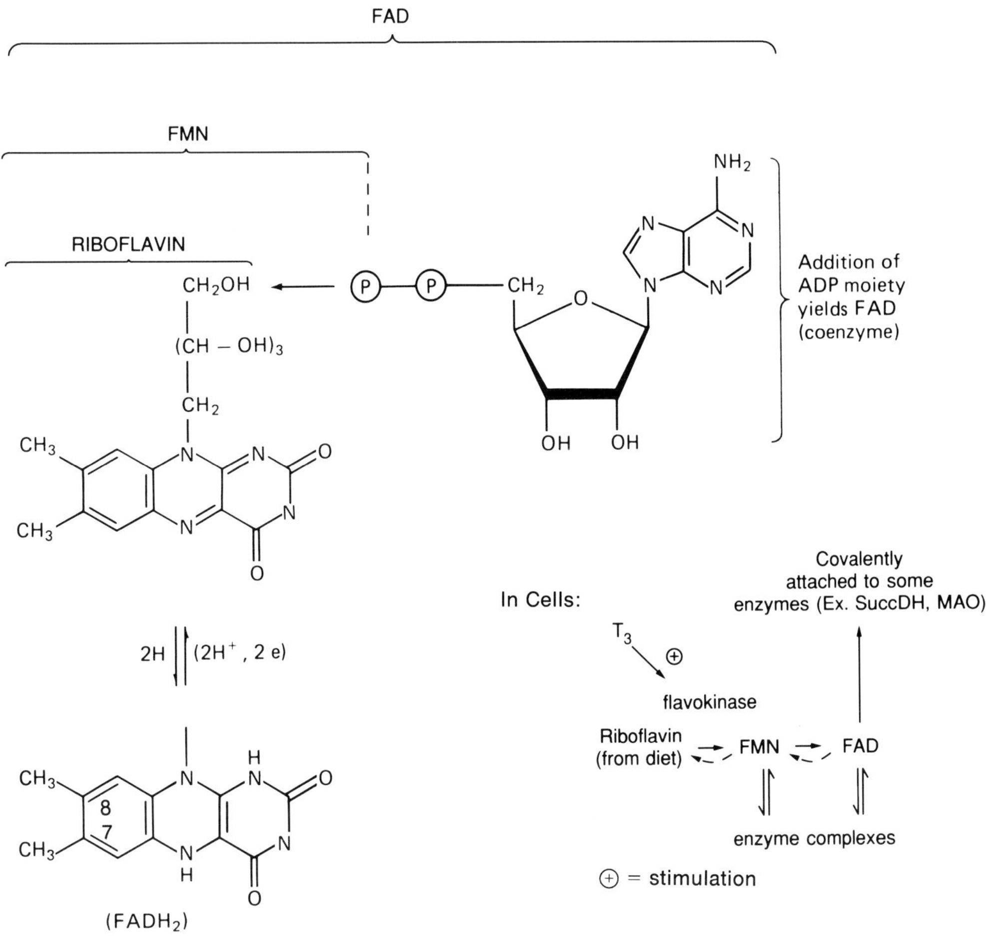

Figure 5.4. Riboflavin.

Functions and effects: Coenzyme in oxidation/reduction reactions involving:
electron transport (oxidative phosphorylation) (succinic dehydrogenase; succDH)
fatty acid synthesis and oxidation
amino acid oxidases
monoamine oxidase (MAO)
xanthine oxidase
glutathione reductase (erythrocyte) (used as a measure of riboflavin status).*

Requirements: men 1.4–1.7 mg/day
women 1.2–1.3 mg/day (+0.3–0.5 in pregnancy and lactation) related to and varies with protein requirements.

Total in body: 15 mg?? (mainly as FAD and FMN)

Absorption: occurs with ease, in upper small intestine, by energy-dependent process.

Storage: none

Toxicity: very low; LD_{50} 560 g/kg (i.p.) in rats; 2 g/kg (orally) in dogs caused no ill effects.

Excretion: riboflavin is lost mainly as its 7- or 8-hydroxymethyl derivatives in the urine (about 30% is lost as riboflavin per se). Small amounts are also lost in the bile.

Gross deficiency in man: vascularization of cornea
magenta tongue
seborrheic dermatitis (nose and scrotum)
Treat with oral 6 mg doses or 25 mg injection, i.m.

[*Source:* Information mainly from Horwitt (1980*a*),* McCormick (1988*a*), and Tietz (1976).]

to all areas of metabolism and intimately involved in the processes by which the oxidation of glucose and fatty acid is utilized for production of adenosine triphosphate (ATP) and the support of anabolic processes. Riboflavin coenzyme formation (and trapping in cells) is initiated through phosphorylation, by a flavokinase positively regulated by thyroid hormone (T_3) (Figure 5.4). Most riboflavin coenzymes associate and dissociate freely, but some are covalently bound to cysteinyl or histidinyl side chains of their enzymes via the methyl (C-8) carbon (McCormick, 1988*a*). Absorption occurs mainly in the proximal small intestine and most probably by a carrier-mediated process (Rose, 1987). Excretion is mostly as the 7- or 8-hydroxymethyl derivatives, in the urine, after microsomal oxidation by mixed function oxidases.

Gross human deficiencies of riboflavin are quite rare in Western countries, but are characterized by vascularization of the cornea, a magenta tongue (glossitis), inflammation of the mucous membranes at the corners of the mouth (angular stomatitis), and moist (seborrheic) dermatitis in the areas of the scrotum and nose (Figure 5.4). It is noteworthy that, in contrast to other vitamins, milk is a major source of riboflavin in the Western diet (as is animal meat); due to its light lability it should not be stored in clear glass bottles.

Table 5.3. The Content of Niacin-Equivalents in Various Foods

Food	Niacin (mg/1000 kcals)	Tryptophan (mg/1000 kcals)	Niacin-equivalent/ 1000 kcals
Cow's milk	1.21	673	12.4
Human milk	2.46	443	9.84
Beef, round	2.47	1280	46.0
Whole eggs	0.60	1150	10.8
Salt pork	1.15	61	2.17
Wheat flour	2.48	297	7.43
Corn grits	1.83	70	3.00
Corn	4.97	106	6.74

Source: Reprinted by permission from Horwitt (1980*a*).

Niacin

The disease pellagra was known to western Europe from the time of the introduction of maize (corn) as a food plant in the early 1700s. Confusion about the connection between this disease and a deficiency in nicotinic acid (niacin) persisted until 1937, despite preparation of the crude vitamin in 1867 and its isolation by Funk from rice polishings in 1911 (Federation Proceedings, 1981; Horwitt, 1980*b*). In retrospect, the confusion stemmed from the facts that (a) this vitamin can be produced in our own tissues from another essential nutrient, tryptophan (less available in corn and corn products), and (b) an imbalance of essential amino acids, such as found in corn protein, sorghum, or gelatin (see Chapter 4), could exacerbate the deficiency (Krehl, 1981), because of a relative lack of tryptophan in these sources, compounded by competitive effects (e.g., by leucine) on tryptophan absorption by the small intestine. It is now generally accepted that about 1/60 of the tryptophan in the diet is converted to nicotinic acid and nicotinamide (Figure 5.5) and that the rate of this conversion is enhanced in pregnancy or with the ingestion of oral contraceptives. Requirements for the vitamin are thus inexorably linked to intake of this essential amino acid and must be given in terms of niacin "equivalents." Indeed, as seen from the data in Table 5.3, even in some plant-derived foods (and more so in animal-derived foods), the tryptophan content is *more important* than the niacin content in providing niacin "equivalents." Thus, food tables based purely on niacin content are useless in estimating whether individuals are meeting their niacin requirements. Comparisons of pellagra-inducing diets on the basis of niacin equivalents per calories consumed indicates that as with thiamin, calories are an important parameter, with greater physical activity and/or caloric intake being related to a greater need for niacin (Horwitt, 1980*b*). Tryptophan metabolism is also dependent on vitamin B_6 (see below). This must be considered especially in pregnant women and those taking oral contraceptives.

Nicotinamide (niacinamide) is a substituent of perhaps the most central electron carrier substances in living cells (NAD^+/NADH; $NADP^+$/NADPH) and functions in many metabolic pathways, especially those of (a) anaerobic glycolysis, (b) Krebs cycle–oxidative phosphorylation, and (c) fatty acid synthesis and oxidation (Figure 5.2). Gross deficiency results first in weakness (lassitude), indigestion, and a lack of appetite, and later in the classic pellagra "3 Ds": *dermatitis* (in exposed or more mechanically used areas of the body), *diarrhea* (in most cases, sometimes with vomiting), and *dementia* (irritability, sleeplessness, confusion, and eventually even delirium and catatonia) (Horwitt, 1980*b*).

Like most of the other B vitamins, niacin is not stored and appears to be nontoxic in large doses (such as the 3–6 g/day nicotinic acid sometimes used to help lower serum cholesterol in hypercholesterolemia) (see Chapters 3 and 15). In such quantities, nicotinic acid has the pharmacologic effect of inhibiting liver very low-density lipoprotein (VLDL) production and producing peripheral vasodilation and flushing; after a few days of treatment, flushing usually no longer occurs. Administration of nicotinamide does not have the flushing (or cholesterol lowering) effect and is thus more commonly used to correct niacin deficiency (in therapeutic doses of 50–250 mg/day).

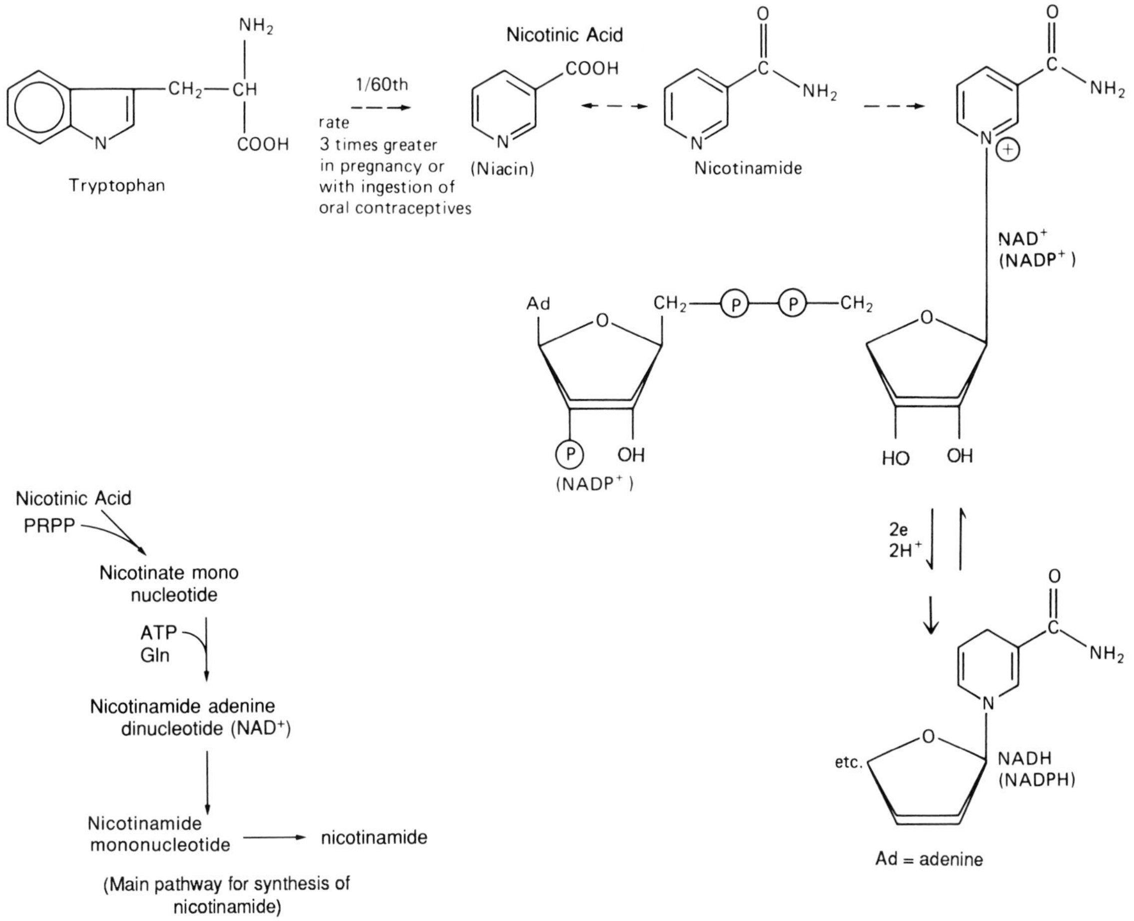

Tryptophan —— 1/60th rate, 3 times greater in pregnancy or with ingestion of oral contraceptives ——→ Nicotinic Acid (Niacin) ←——→ Nicotinamide ——→ NAD^+ ($NADP^+$)

Ad = adenine

2e, $2H^+$ ⇌ NADH (NADPH)

Nicotinic Acid
PRPP
↓
Nicotinate mono nucleotide
↓ ATP, Gln
Nicotinamide adenine dinucleotide (NAD^+)
↓
Nicotinamide mononucleotide ——→ nicotinamide

(Main pathway for synthesis of nicotinamide)

Figure 5.5. Niacin.

Food sources: whole grains (germ); seeds, nuts*; high protein foods: 60 g complete protein = 600 mg tryptophan = 10 mg niacin (equivalents), corn 0.6% tryp, other grains 1.0%, animal foods 1.4% of protein.

Function: coenzyme (e-carrier) in [O]/[H] reactions, including intermediary metabolism and oxidative phosphorylation, as well as glutamate dehydrogenase and glutathione reductase. Large doses: vasodilation (10 × RDA+); flushing; used to lower serum cholesterol (3–6 g/day).

Storage: none.

Excretion: main urinary metabolites are 1-methylnicotinamide and 1-methyl-3-carboxamido-6-pyridone, lost at an average rate of 3 mg/day.

RDA: 5–6 mg niacin equivalents for infants; 20 mg niacin equivalents for lactating women. Adult: 6.6 mg/1000 kcal; 15–20 mg men; 13–15 mg women.

* Some forms of niacin in cereal are less available, partly because of amide-linkage to ε-amino groups of lysine side chains of proteins (Narasinga et al., 1984).

The amide form of the vitamin is the predominant one normally circulating in the plasma.

Pantothenic Acid

Work by Roger R. Williams first indicated that pantothenic acid was an essential growth factor for yeast and before 1939, he and his coworkers isolated and synthesized the material, which was later shown by Elvejhem, Jukes, and others to be necessary for the growth of chicks, rats, and many other animal species (Sauberlich, 1980). Pantothenic acid is found largely as part of two coenzymes (coenzyme A and phosphopantetheine; Figure 5.6) in food sources as well as animal tissues. The exception is blood plasma where it is found primarily as pantothenic acid. Although not much is known about its absorption and metabolism, the fact that plasma contains the vita-

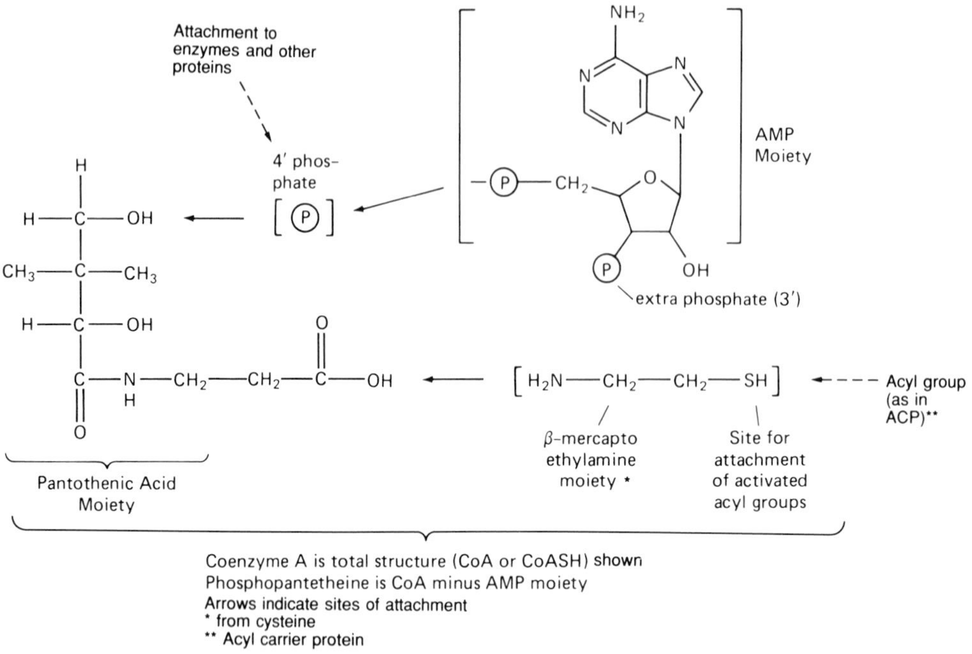

Coenzyme A is total structure (CoA or CoASH) shown
Phosphopantetheine is CoA minus AMP moiety
Arrows indicate sites of attachment
* from cysteine
** Acyl carrier protein

Figure 5.6. Pantothenic acid.

Functions: as part of coenzyme A and phosphopantetheine

Reactive –SH group serves as a carrier (and activator) for acyl groups, most notably in degradative energy-yielding pathways in mitochondria:

a. First step in Krebs cycle (transfer of acetyl group to oxaloacetic acid)

b. β-oxidation of fatty acids (recipient of acetyl units removed from FA chain; carrier of fatty acid moiety)

also synthesis of fatty acids, ketones, cholesterol, acetylcholine, porphyrin, sphingosine; also transfer of FAs or acetate to polypeptides, including some enzymes, receptors, hormones, histones, tubulin.

Storage: none

Requirements: 4–7 mg/day (safe and adequate intake; RDA not established); some increased need in pregnancy and lactation.

Sources: widely distributed but richest in whole grains (germ), legumes, liver, kidney, egg yolk.

Deficiency symptoms: irascibility, postural hypotension, anorexia, constipation, weakness and tingling of fingers and feet, tachycardia with physical effort.

Excretion: mainly as pantothenic acid in the urine. Less than 1 mg/day excreted suggests (implies) deficiency.

Toxicity: very low. No adverse effects of ingesting 10–100 g except occasional diarrhea.

[*Source:* Information mainly from Sauberlich (1980), Plesofsky-Vig and Brambl (1988), and McCormick (1988c).]

min in noncoenzyme form implies that the coenzymes in food are broken down before or during their absorption. Also, the vitamin is lost from the blood, mainly as pantothenic acid, via the urine.

The important coenzyme functions of intracellular pantothenic acid derivatives are numerous and quite well understood, especially the central roles of coenzyme A (CoA or CoASH) in the pathways of energy metabolism, and that of pantetheine-4′-phosphate as part of acyl carrier protein (ACP), in the synthesis of lipids: fatty acid, glycerides, cholesterol, ketone bodies, and sphingosine (Figure 5.7). Less well known is its role as an acyl carrier in fatty acid activation for synthesis of storage triglyceride (Figure 5.7), and in acetylation or acylation of various proteins to alter their activities, stability, and/or determine their cellular location or assembly (Plesofsky-Vig and Brambl, 1988). In each case, the peptide-linked β-mercaptoethylamine unit, with its high-energy SH group, serves as the site for acyl attachment and activation (with ΔG^0 in the range of 12,000 kcal for the acyl-CoA compounds). This directly or indirectly provides the impetus for synthetic reactions: (1) in the pathways of lipid synthesis and even degradation (e.g., the formation of citrate from acetate and oxaloacetate in the Krebs cycle); (2) in the N-terminal acetylation of numerous proteins/enzymes (which may influence their degradation via the ubiquitin path-

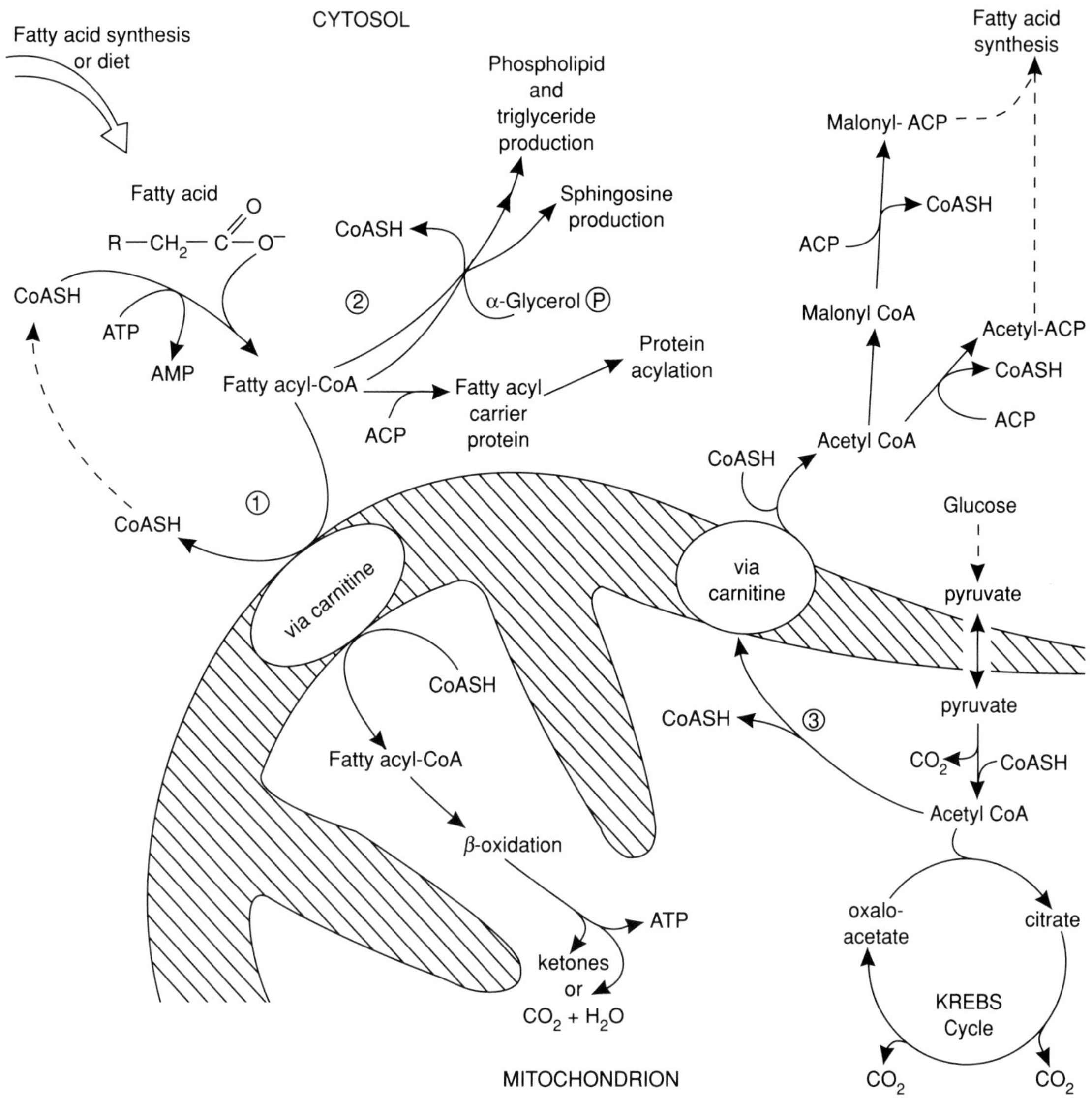

Figure 5.7. Functions of pantothenic acid as CoA in energy and fat metabolism. *Key:* (1) Delivery of fatty acids to mitochondria for beta oxidation (degradation). (2) Synthesis of triglyceride and phospholipid pathway. (3) Transfer of acetate units from mitochondria to cytosol and synthesis of fatty acids therefrom. CoASH refers to reduced CoA: ACP is acyl carrier protein; P is phosphate group.

way); (3) in the ε-amino acetylation of lysines in histones, tubulin, and some other proteins (influencing their stability and function); and (4) in the N-terminal myristylation (14-carbon fatty acid) or palmitic acid esterification of proteins (the latter to internal serine or perhaps threonine residues), which enhances or inactivates certain polypeptide hormones and may target other proteins to certain membranes or aid in their assembly (Plesofsky-Vig and Brambl, 1988).

Gross deficiency in pantothenic acid is thought to be extremely rare, except as an accompaniment of general malnutrition. When deliberately induced in humans, deficiency symptoms include vomiting, malaise, abdominal distress, and burning cramps, followed by tenderness in the heels, weakness and cramps in the legs, insomnia, fatigue, etc. (Sauberlich, 1980). The National Research Council (NRC) has not set an RDA (Recommended Daily Allowance), but considers that 4–7 mg/day should be adequate for children as well as adults (Figure 5.6). In the late 1940s and early 1950s, there was some interest in this vitamin as a factor in the healing of burns and other skin lesions, as well as in curing postoperative paralysis of the ileum, and even preventing the graying of hair (RB Rucker, personal communication). No further work has been published that confirms or refutes these initial claims. As with other B vitamins, the greatest concentrations are found in the germ of whole grains and nuts, as well as egg yolk, liver, kidney, heart, and soybeans.

Lipoic Acid

Lipoic acid, the only known function of which is in the oxidative decarboxylations of α-ketoacids, principally pyruvate and α-ketoglutarate (Figure 5.2), has not been shown to be essential as a dietary component for man or animal. As such minute amounts are needed, and because some lower organisms do require it as a growth factor, the question of whether it is produced in the tissues of man and other higher organisms or is acquired in sufficient quantities through the food supply remains unanswered (Reed, 1980). Lipoic acid (Figure 5.8), like thiamin and biotin, contains sulfur and has been isolated from liver and yeast (Reed, 1980). It is covalently linked to the enzymes that require it through a peptide bond with the ε-amino group of lysine.

Biotin

The structure of biotin was elucidated by du Vigneaud and coworkers in 1942, after its isolation by Kogl. It functions as the site for formation of a carboxylated intermediate (Figure 5.9), bound firmly to the enzyme by a peptide bond involving the ε-amino group of lysine side chains for at least four "CO_2-fixing" enzymes in animal cells: acetyl-CoA carboxylase (fatty acid synthesis), pyruvate carboxylase (formation of oxaloacetate and the reversal of glycolysis), propionyl-CoA carboxylase (disposal of odd chain length fatty acids and parts of the carbon skeletons of valine, isoleucine, threonine, and methionine, as well as pyrimidines), and β-methylcrotonyl CoA carboxylase (leucine degradation). Thus, biotin is intimately involved in energy metabolism, including gluconeogenesis. During digestion, biotin is initially

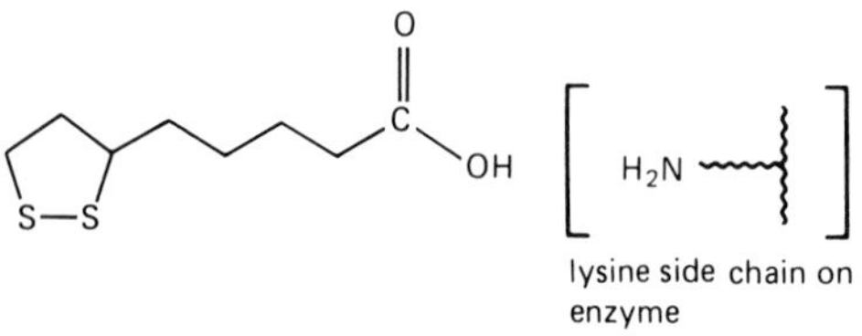

Figure 5.8. Structure of lipoic acid.

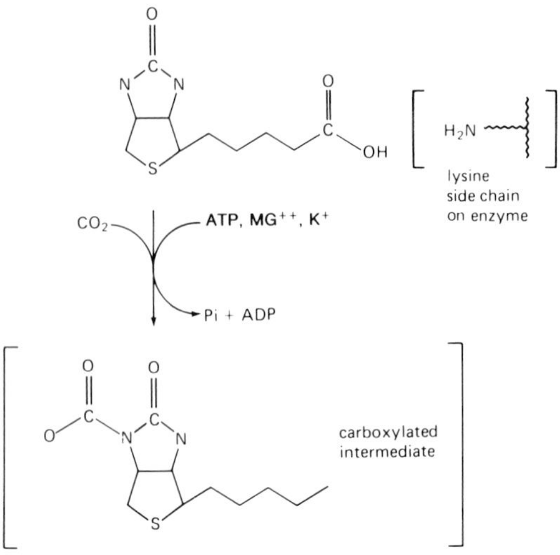

Figure 5.9. Biotin.

Requirements: probably 100 μg/1000 kcal/day (30–100 μg is safe and adequate intake).

Function: "fixation" of CO_2 in animal cells, e.g., carboxylation of pyruvate in the formation of oxaloacetate (and phosphoenolpyruvate) from pyruvate; and utilization of amino acid carbons (val, ile, leu, thr, met); carboxylation of acetyl-CoA to yield malonyl-CoA, used in FA synthesis.

Total in body: 1 mg??

Absorption: probably by facilitated diffusion at low concentrations and by simple diffusion of high concentrations in small intestine, especially jejunum (inhibited by avidin).

Storage: some, in the liver.

Toxicity: most probably low, since 5–10 mg injected daily into infants appeared to have no adverse effects.

Excretion: primarily free biotin in the urine.

Gross deficiency: scaly dermatitis and skin dryness; atrophy of the lingual papillae; graying of mucous membranes; depression, lassitude, muscle pain, and many more nonspecific symptoms. Induced by raw egg diets (avidin) or high doses of some antibiotics (or some anticonvulsive drugs).

Sources: foods (Table 5.1) and intestinal bacteria.

[*Source:* Information mainly from Appel and Briggs (1980*a*) and Dakshinamurti and Chauhan (1988).]

released from dietary protein as the lysine-adduct (biocytin) and either further digested to free biotin or absorbed as such and hydrolyzed within the intestinal mucosa, or elsewhere. [The biotinidase involved may also be the carrier protein for the vitamin in cells, as well as serum (Dakshinamurti and Chauhan, 1988).] A deficiency of biotin can be produced by an excessive intake of raw egg white, hence the association of this vitamin with "egg white injury" disease (Table 5.1). The reason is that raw egg white contains the 68,000-dalton glycoprotein, avidin, which tenaciously binds biotin at four sites. This prevents its absorption from the digestive tract (unless avidin is predenatured by cooking). Since a significant but variable proportion of our biotin is produced by endogenous bacteria (Swenseid et al., 1965) treatment with large doses of antibiotics can decrease biotin levels in human subjects (notably 6 g of streptomycin taken daily for 10–20 days). [In experimental animals, large antibiotic treatments routinely have this effect (Appel and Briggs, 1980*a*).] However, the doses of antibiotics commonly used by man over a week or less probably have relatively little influence (Appel and Briggs, 1980*a*).

Biotin deficiency results in a variety of symptoms of a general type, involving skin and mucous membranes, muscles, general lassitude, etc. (Figure 5.9). These symptoms are alleviated by injected daily doses of 150–300 μg over 3–5 days (Appel and Briggs, 1980*a*). Biotin, like other B vitamins, is not thought to be toxic, and initial studies by Paul et al. (1973, 1976), which suggested toxic effects with 5–100 mg/kg body weight in pregnant rats, have not been confirmed by others (Mittleholzer, 1976).

Choline and Inositol

These substances are normally produced in human tissues in sufficient amounts to meet our needs: choline from serine, via phosphatidylethanolamine and with the help of methyl groups from methionine (Figure 5.10); and myoinositol from glucose-6-phosphate by cyclization (Figure 5.11). (*Myo*inositol is a particular stereöisomer.) The need for dietary choline is thus dependent on the availability of dietary methionine, an essential amino acid found in relatively low quantities in proteins (especially the proteins of legumes; see Chapter 4). The quantitative relationships between methionine and choline intakes to cover the needs for both nutrients have not been worked out in the way they have been for niacin and tryptophan (Snyderman, 1980). Because of the relationship to 1-C metabolism (Figure 5.19, see p. 142), vitamin B_{12} and folic acid are also required for choline production.

In humans, no deficiency has yet been produced by an absence of choline or inositol in the diet, although there is the suggestion that choline deficiency may occur in subjects on total parenteral nutrition (TPN; total intravenous feeding) (Zeisel, 1988) and diet is a factor in the level of body inositol (Holub, 1986). (Blood choline levels fall, and fatty livers have been observed in TPN.) Rats and mice do rely on dietary sources of choline and develop fatty livers (accumulation of neutral lipids) when deprived of it. The form of fatty liver occurring differs from that found in alcoholics (accumulation of phospholipids), which is not cured by choline (Snyderman, 1980).

Inositol deficiency has also been associated with fatty liver in rodents (Gavin and McHenry, 1941) and chickens (Wright, 1970). In gerbils (especially female gerbils), there can also be hypercholesterolemia, accumulation of fat in the intestinal mucosa (lipodystrophy), and other major complications (Hoover et al., 1978). However, dietary deficiency does not necessarily produce these symptoms in other species, nor indeed does it necessarily produce any deficiency symptoms (Appel and Briggs, 1980*b*). As with choline, the induction of deficiency would appear to depend on other dietary factors, including intake of choline and total fat and the composition of the fatty acids ingested (Appel and Briggs, 1980*b*). Thus, at least in animals and under certain conditions, synthesis by liver, kidney, and other tissues is not sufficient to keep up with body needs. Both choline and inositol have been referred to as "lipotropic substances," meaning that they are required for the removal of fats from the liver.

Much of the choline and inositol in human tissues is part of the phospholipid (and sphingomyelin) present in the intracellular and plasma membranes of all cells. Phosphatidylcholine (lecithin) is most abundant in the plasma membrane, as is phosphatidylinositol and its di- and triphosphoinositide forms (extra phosphate groups on carbons 4 and 5 of the inositol moiety) (Figures 5.11 and 5.12).

Inositides are especially rich in the brain, where they may be involved in neurotransmission (see below). Free inositol is also found in high concentrations in some tissues, such as the lens (Appel and Briggs, 1980*b*) and epididymus (Morris and Collins, 1971), and is present (at 4.3–4.6 μg/ml) in normal human plasma as a nutrient source for cells that cannot make it. It is related in

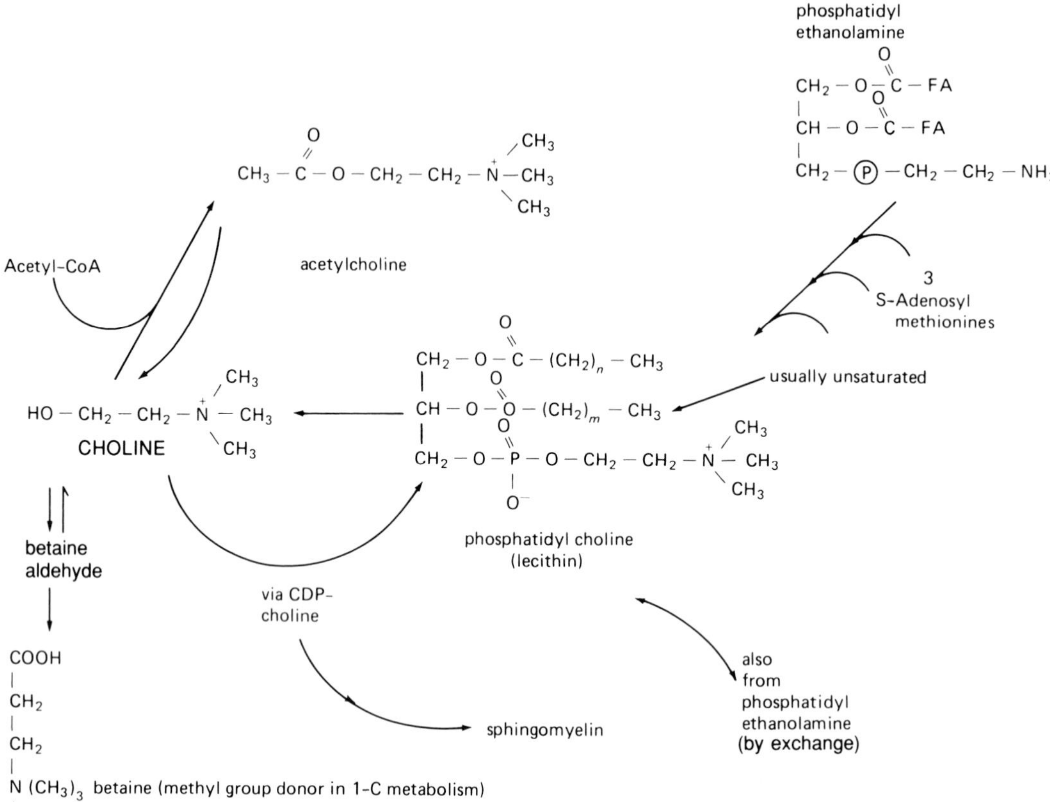

Figure 5.10. Nutrition and metabolism of choline.

Function:

a. major substituent of phospholipids in cell membranes, serum lipoproteins, and bile (emulsifier);

b. donor of fatty acid to cholesterol in formation of LDL from IDL (L-CAT);

c. source of methyl groups for synthesis of methionine;

d. substrate for formation of neurotransmitter, acetylcholine.

Toxicity: not well studied, but 20 g doses (20 × average intake) can cause dizziness, nausea, and diarrhea in some patients, and a fishy odor (due to bacterial breakdown to trimethylamine in the intestine).

Key: DAG, diacylglycerol; P, phosphate group.

[*Source:* Information mainly from Metzler (1977), Appel and Briggs (1980c), and Zeisel (1988).]

structure to phytic acid (phosphorylated at all six positions). Phytic acid (especially abundant in grains) is found in most plant cells and is implicated in the inhibition of intestinal calcium, iron, and zinc absorption (see Chapter 6).

Choline is widespread in the food supply, though relatively low in fruits and vegetables. It is estimated that the average American consumes between 0.4 and 0.9 g/day, largely as lecithin. Absorption is probably carrier-mediated, as well as by simple diffusion, and occurs all along the small intestine (and even in the colon), at least in rodents (Zeisel, 1988). Most choline is transported as part of lecithin phospholipid in chylomicrons and lipoproteins; but some also travels as free choline in the blood. This may come partly from the intestine but also from other tissues, though its exact origin is still unclear. Aside from its structural role as lecithin in cell membranes, choline is required for synthesis of acetylcholine, as a source of fatty acid for esterification of cholesterol by lecithin cholesterol acyl transferase (L-CAT) (see Chapter 3, Figure 3.8), as a component of all lipoproteins, and also as a source of methyl groups in 1-C metabolism when insufficient methionine is present in the diet. This accounts for the development of fatty livers in animals on a choline-deficient diet and insufficient methionine and/or vitamin B_{12} and folic acid, for adequate choline (and lecithin) synthesis. Degradation of choline is via oxidation (to betaine) and demethylation (Figure 5.10).

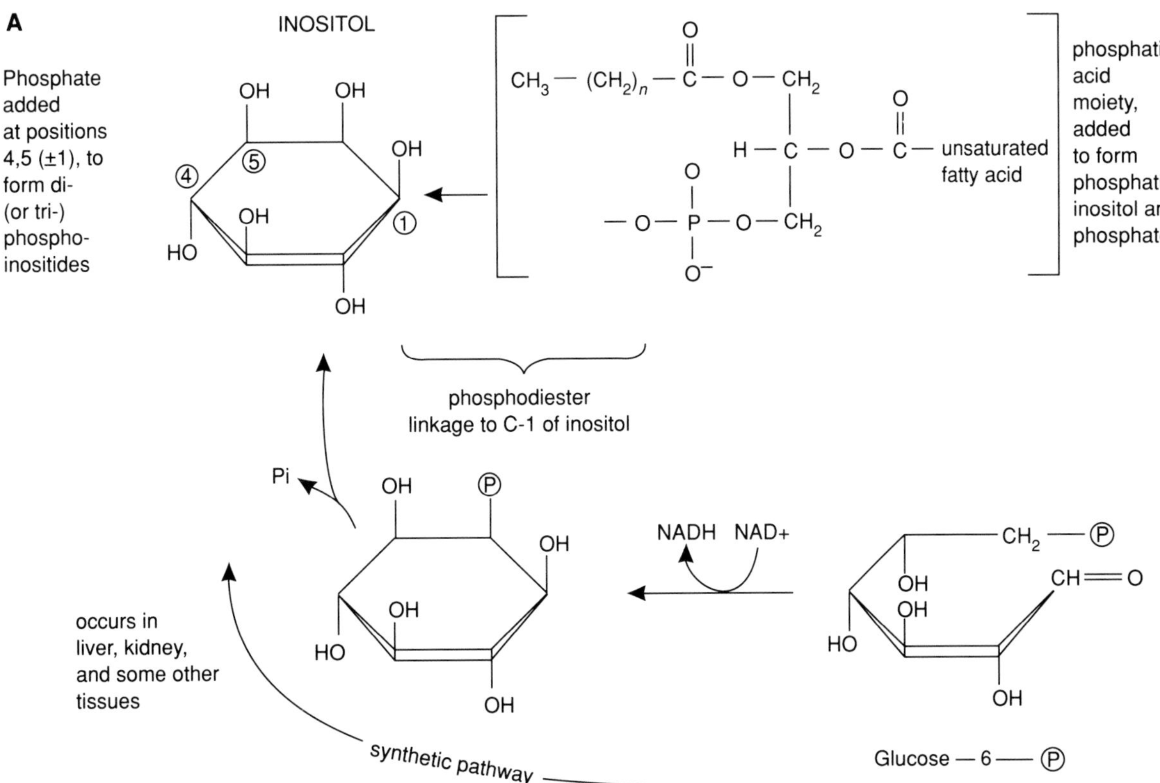

Very preliminary studies suggest that there may be a relationship between the availability of choline to the brain and some symptoms of memory or cognition loss in a few elderly persons with various forms of senility (but not Alzheimer's disease) (Wood and Allison, 1981; Zeisel, 1981). [An effect on memory has also been reported in mice (Bartus et al., 1980).] A high choline or lecithin intake will increase blood choline concentrations, and this is thought by most to lead to increased levels of choline within brain neurons, which in turn could result in increased formation of acetylcholine (see Zeisel, 1988). [In rats, a high choline intake can lead to increases in brain acetylcholine concentrations (Cohen and Wurtman, 1976; Zeisel, 1981), but not in all cases (Wecker, 1986).] In a few cases, large doses of pure lecithin (30 g; about 6 g choline), with or without anticholinesterase drugs, have improved memory in humans, presumably because of increases in brain acetylcholine concentrations (Growdon and Wurtman, 1979). A "cholinergic hypothesis" relating to geriatric memory dysfunction has even been postulated (Bartus et al., 1982). However, others have found no correlation between serum

Figure 5.11. Nutrition and metabolism of inositol. **(A)** Synthesis of phosphatidylinositides. **(B)** Nutrition, transport, and metabolism: central role of the kidney in inositol production; dietary sources and uptake, including transport via chylomicrons; catabolism via pentose shunt.

Function: found mainly as a component of the inositides in most cell plasma membranes, and as free inositol or inositol phosphates in cell cytoplasm. Turnover of these inositides is associated with the response of cells to various stimuli and the transfer of information, including nerve impulses in the central nervous system (Figure 5.12).

Tissue distribution: (phosphoinositides)[a]

Human	Liver	Heart	Spleen	Kidney	Skeletal Muscle	Lung	Rat Brain
Inositide (mg/g tissue)	3.02	1.05	0.93	0.85	0.85	0.16	0.98
Percent P in total phospholipid	8.6	6.1	4.4	5.5	6.0	3.2	—

[a] Based on Hawthorne and White (1975), Tables I and III, assuming an average phosphate content of 3.8% for the inositides.

Food sources: see Table 5.1.

Toxicity: very low; no obvious effects with 1 g injection i.v. into humans, or 3 g taken orally.

[*Source:* Based on Holub (1986).]

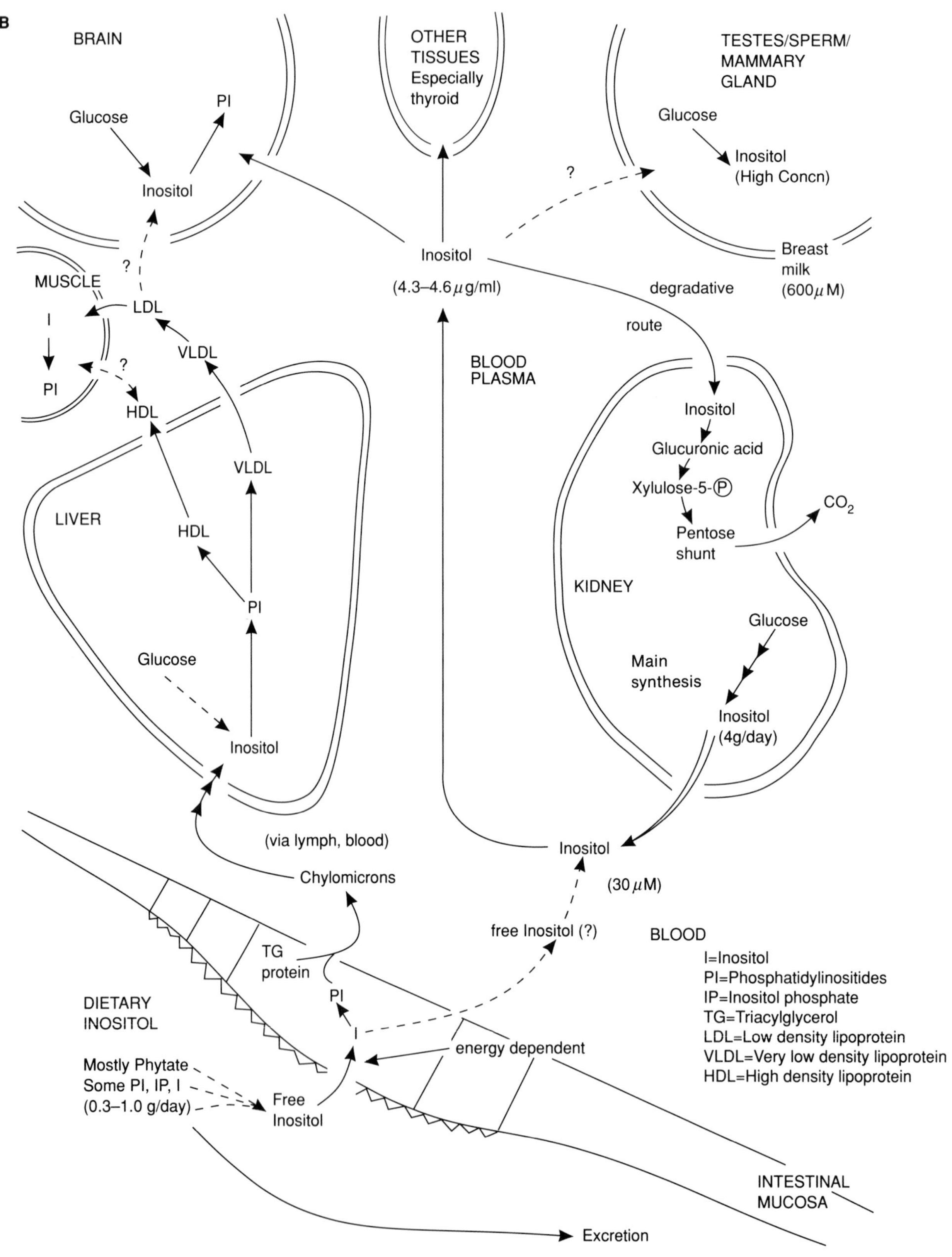
B
BRAIN
Glucose
PI
Inositol
OTHER
TISSUES
Especially
thyroid
TESTES/SPERM/
MAMMARY
GLAND
Glucose
Inositol
(High Concn)
?
Breast
milk
(600μM)
MUSCLE
?
LDL
I
PI
?
HDL
VLDL
Inositol
(4.3–4.6μg/ml)
degradative
route
BLOOD
PLASMA
Inositol
Glucuronic acid
Xylulose-5-Ⓟ
Pentose
shunt
CO_2
LIVER
HDL
VLDL
PI
Glucose
Inositol
KIDNEY
Glucose
Main
synthesis
Inositol
(4g/day)
(via lymph, blood)
Chylomicrons
Inositol
(30μM)
free Inositol (?)
BLOOD
TG
protein
PI
I
energy dependent
DIETARY
INOSITOL
Mostly Phytate
Some PI, IP, I
(0.3–1.0 g/day)
Free
Inositol
Excretion
INTESTINAL
MUCOSA
I=Inositol
PI=Phosphatidylinositides
IP=Inositol phosphate
TG=Triacylglycerol
LDL=Low density lipoprotein
VLDL=Very low density lipoprotein
HDL=High density lipoprotein

choline concentrations and cognitive function, in the elderly as a whole (Sanchez et al., 1984). It should be noted that federally regulated food standards allow the "lecithin" sold on the commercial market to be a mixture of various phospholipids and to contain less than 50% of actual lecithin (R. Wurtman, personal communication). Efforts are currently underway to make pure lecithin more available. Choline itself (and lecithin in very high doses) cannot be administered without some potential side effects (see Figure 5.10); and the possibility of depression/supersensitivity of dopamine receptors and disturbance of neurotransmitter balance remains a concern where prolonged intake of large doses is involved (Wood and Allison, 1981). Much further work is required before potential choline/lecithin treatment is generally applied.

As concerns inositol, myoinositol is formed from glucose-6-phosphate by cyclization, when required. Myoinositol is plentiful in foodstuffs, and estimates of average daily intake range from 0.3–1.0 g/day (Figure 5.11). In plant foods much of it is in the form of the hexaphosphate (phytic acid) hydrolyzable to inositol by a phytase in digestive juices (Broquist, 1988*a*) or in the intestinal brush border (Holub, 1986). Absorption is probably by active transport. Much of the dietary inositol is transported as phospholipid to liver and other tissues via chylomicrons and liver VLDL. Some occurs as free inositol in the blood and mainly derives from synthesis in the kidney. The brain, and to some extent the liver, are also active in synthesis of inositol, and the same may be true in tissues with a high inositol content (Figure 5.11). Catabolism probably occurs via reconversion of inositol to glucose or glucuronic acid (Lewin et al., 1976) via glycolysis and the Krebs cycle (as for glucose) or through the pentose shunt. The kidney is a major organ for catabolism, as plasma levels of inositol are greatly increased in rats and humans with nephrectomy or renal disease (Appel and Briggs, 1980*b*). Decreased kidney catabolism and increased plasma inositol concentrations also occur in diabetes, partly because the excess glucose in plasma may suppress uptake of inositol by the brain and central nervous system. Both a relative lack of inositol for the nervous system, or the opposite (namely, a high blood level of inositol), might be responsible for some of the impairment in motor nerve conduction associated with diabetes and kidney diseases (see Broquist, 1988*a*). However, inositol intake is not acutely toxic to humans at levels of 3 g given orally or 1 g by injection (Appel and Briggs, 1980*b*).

A large variety of cells, especially in tissues under neural control, have been found to respond to stimuli by enhancing the phosphorylation or dephosphorylation of inositides and by splitting inositol phosphate from the phosphoinositides in cell membranes (Michell, 1975). Indeed, it is now clear that hydrolysis of phosphatidylinositol phosphates initiates a "second messenger" system that causes changes in cell function in response to humoral agents interacting with cell surface receptors. This system is active not just in the central nervous system but in other cells all over the body. A summary of the steps involved is given in Figure 5.12. Phosphatidylinositides phosphorylated at positions 4 and 5 are formed in the cell membrane. Hydrolysis to inositol triphosphate (IP_3) and diacylglycerol (DAG) is catalyzed by a local phospholipase C, after activation of the latter by G proteins that respond to neurotransmitter/hormone-receptor interactions. [There are many forms of phospholipase C (Rhee et al., 1989).] (The humoral agents implicated are given in the legend to Figure 5.12.) The two products have different effects. DAG stimulates *protein kinase* C in the membrane (see left side of Figure 5.12), which then phosphorylates (and activates) a spectrum of cell-specific enzymes, transporter proteins, and/or receptors in a manner reminiscent of that "original" second messenger, cAMP (see Chapter 2). In contrast, IP_3 (the other product) mobilizes intra- and extracellular calcium from the endoplasmic reticulum and plasma (Figure 5.12, right side). The resulting increase in cytoplasmic Ca^{2+} concentrations affects a variety of enzymes and other protein activities involved in nerve conduction, muscle contraction, etc. Both types of second messengers are rapidly recycled, to allow for fine control of the responses. The unsaturated fatty acid (usually arachidonate) on the central carbon of the DAG can also be converted to prostaglandins (or other eicosanoids) to trigger additional responses. Membrane phosphoinositides, long ignored, have thus emerged as a central control point for regulation of cell function and growth.

Vitamin B_6

History and Deficiency Symptoms

The name of this vitamin was bestowed by Szent-György in 1934 on a factor (isolated in 1938) that prevented dermatitis in rats. The dermatitis is similar to that seen in essential fatty acid deficiency. In humans and other species, moist skin

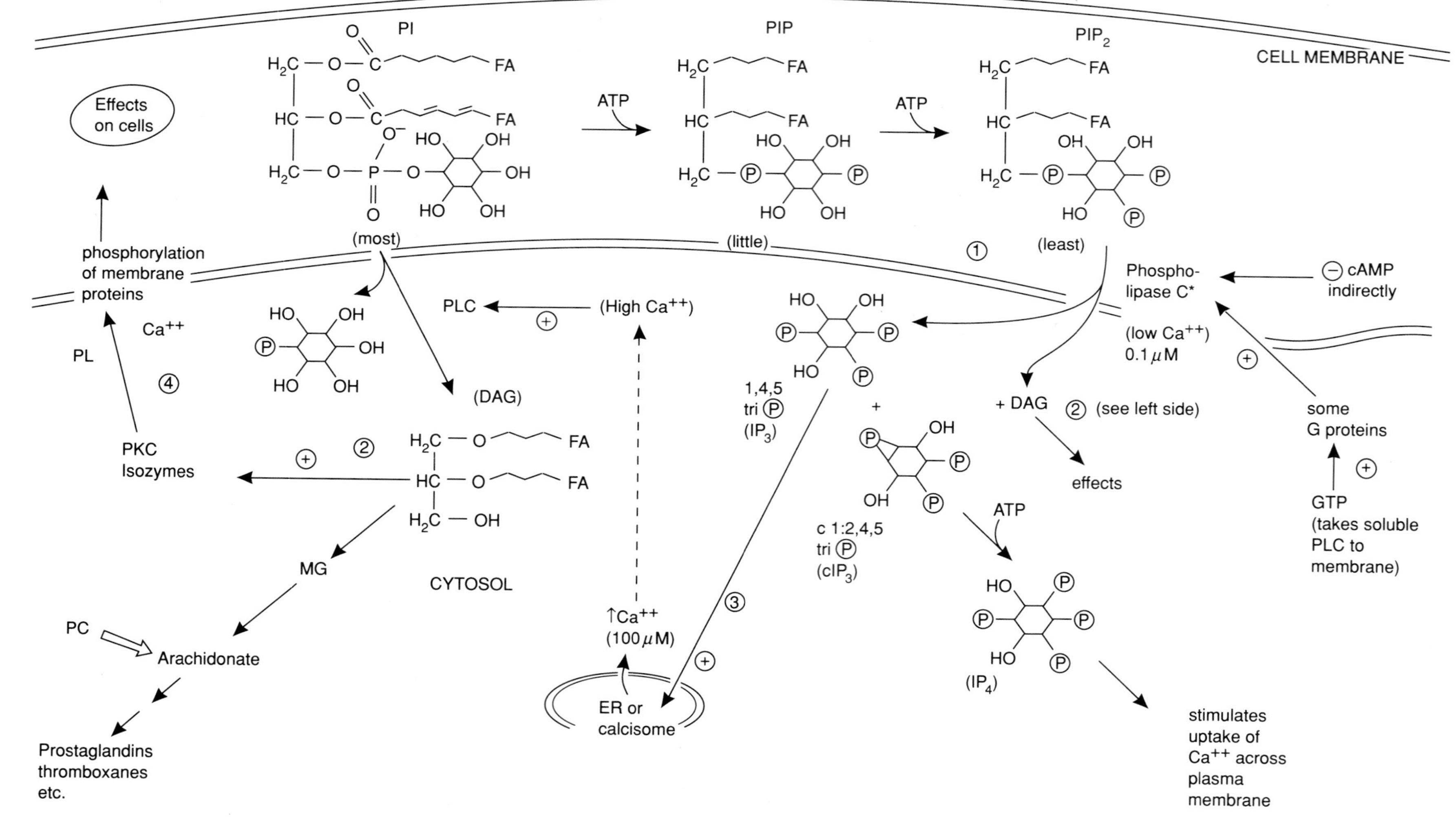
CELL MEMBRANE
PI
PIP
PIP_2
ATP
ATP
Effects on cells
(most)
(little)
(least)
1
Phospho-lipase C*
⊖ cAMP indirectly
phosphorylation of membrane proteins
PLC
(High Ca^{++})
(low Ca^{++}) 0.1 μM
Ca^{++}
PL
4
(DAG)
1,4,5 tri Ⓟ (IP_3)
+ DAG
2 (see left side)
effects
some G proteins
GTP (takes soluble PLC to membrane)
PKC Isozymes
2
c 1:2,4,5 tri Ⓟ (cIP_3)
ATP
MG
CYTOSOL
3
↑Ca^{++} (100 μM)
(IP_4)
PC
Arachidonate
ER or calcisome
stimulates uptake of Ca^{++} across plasma membrane
Prostaglandins thromboxanes etc.

lesions (seborrheic) also occur, along with a microcytic (small cell), hypochromic (pale) anemia, weakness, irritability, nervousness, and insomnia (Sauberlich and Canham, 1980). Infants may have convulsions, and, in adults, there may be increased urinary levels of urea, as well as trytophan, methionine, and glycine metabolites (kynurenine, xanthurenic and oxalic acids, and homocystine; see below). Although the molecular connections between seborrheic dermatitis and B_6 deficiency are not obvious, the involvement of this vitamin in amino acid and lipid metabolism may be a factor (see below). The hypochromic anemia may be explained by a decreased rate of porphyrin biosynthesis; the mental symptoms, insomnia, and convulsions may be related to the reduced formation of brain neurotransmitters, including γ-aminobutyric acid (GABA) and serotonin (5-OH tryptamine), as well as the accumulation of tryptophan metabolites (3-OH-kynurenine) that require B_6 for catabolism. The increased urinary levels of amino acid metabolites may be ascribed to the involvement of this vitamin in a host of degradative (and biosynthetic) reactions concerned with amino acid metabolism. Details of these matters follow in the section on "Function."

Figure 5.12. Phosphoinositides in cell regulation.

Key: PI = phosphatidylinositol
PA = phosphatidic acid
IP_2, IP_3, IP_4 = inositol di-, tri-, and tetraphosphates
DAG = diacylglycerol

Interaction of the stimulating agent with the cell membrane receptor initiates hydrolysis of phosphorylated PI by phospholipase C (1), forming DAG and various inositol phosphates. The DAG stimulates protein kinase C, resulting in phosphorylation of specific proteins and their activation (2). The inositol phosphates (possibly including cyclic forms) stimulate release of Ca^{2+} ions from the endoplasmic reticulum (or "calcisomes") (3), and then from the outside of the cell (4), increasing intracellular Ca^{2+} concentrations, which in turn activate another set of proteins/enzymes, etc. Different cells have different stimuli, as well as different proteins to be regulated within them.

Stimuli include the following: cholinergic (muscarinic), adrenergic (α_1), histamine (H_1), 5-hydroxytryptamine (5-HT_1), vasopressin (V_1), pancreozymin, substance P, bombesin, angiotensin II, bradykinin, thyrotropin, nerve growth factor, f-met-leu-phe, phagocyticable particles, secretagogues (antigen, etc.), thrombin, collagen, ADP, membrane depolarization, glucose, mitogenic stimuli (lectins, antisera, serum factors, transforming viruses, etc.).

Tissues affected include the following: smooth muscle, brain, liver, pancreas, parotid, hypothalamus, kidney, endothelia, thyroid, ganglia, pineal, neutrophils, mast cells, platelets, islets of Langerhans, cells in culture.

[*Sources:* Mitchell (1975); and others (see text).]

Terminology, Catalysis, and Absorption/Distribution

Vitamin B_6 is the collective term for pyridoxine, the form of the vitamin most prominent in plants, and for the phosphorylated forms, pyridoxal and pyridoxamine phosphate, which are most common in animal tissues (Figure 5.13). In the human, the vitamin is absorbed and transported mainly in the unphosphorylated form, and upon entering cells, is phosphorylated, thereby allowing its attachment to a variety of different enzymes. Here it functions as the active site for a host of reactions. Chemically, the capacity of the aldehyde group on pyridoxal phosphate to form a Schiff base with various amino groups, especially the α-amino groups of amino acids, is at the base of its catalytic properties. The classic "transamination" reaction between α-amino and α-keto acids is the prime example. In this instance, the vitamin first becomes an acceptor for the α-amino groups (forming pyridoxamine phosphate), and then through a reversal of the Schiff base process (Figure 5.13), it donates the amino group to an α-keto acid.

The vitamin is absorbed from the diet by diffusion mainly in unphosphorylated form (Figures 5.13 and 5.14), after dephosphorylation with the digestive tract. [A portion of the vitamin may also come from endogenous gut bacteria (McCormick, 1988*b*).] It was thought until recently that uptake into the mucosa was by simple diffusion, but evidence in rats suggests a saturable process is actually (or also) involved (Middleton, 1985). From the mucosa, most of the vitamin (pyridoxine from plants, with some pyridoxal from animal tissues/foods) is transported to the liver, where it is phosphorylated (Figure 5.14). There the phosphorylated pyridoxine is oxidized to pyridoxal phosphate (the most common and active coenzyme form of the vitamin), with the help of an FMN-requiring oxidase not found in most other tissues, except the brain (Leklem, 1988). Some of the pyridoxal phosphate is used for hepatic enzymes; some is dephosphorylated and released to the blood as pyridoxal, along with smaller amounts of the phosphorylated form; and some may be

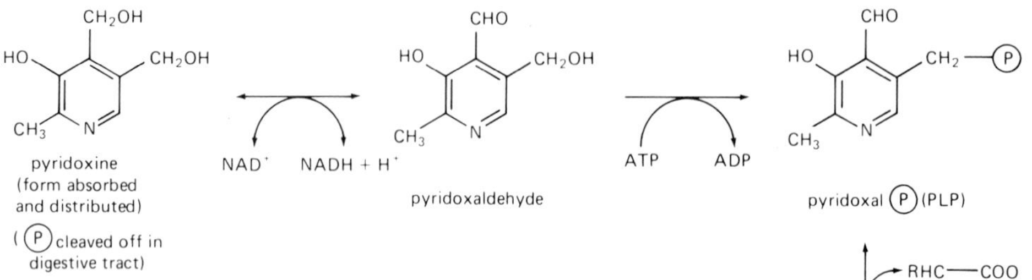

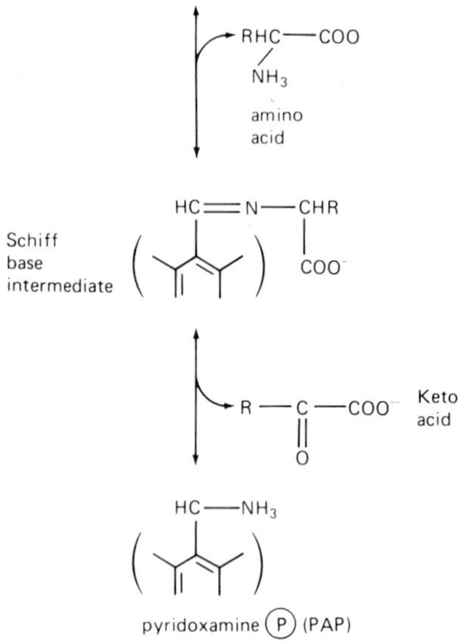

Figure 5.13. Vitamin B_6.

Functions: coenzyme in more than 100 enzyme reactions, in many areas of metabolism, but especially amino acid synthesis/catabolism/transport (intestinal). Also porphyrin synthesis, phospholipid and sphingolipid synthesis, taurine production; attached to phosphorylase.

Requirements: 1.6–2.0 mg/day RDA (U.S.)

Extra requirements in pregnancy/lactation, persons on oral contraceptives, hyperthyroidism, carpal tunnel syndrome, high protein diets, stress, hyperoxaluria.

Toxicity: acute very low; 1 g/kg tolerated well (PAP can be hypnotic). Toxicity may occur with chronic daily doses of 500 mg or more. (Am J Psychiatry 127:1091, 1971)

Absorption, metabolism, and excretion: absorbed mainly as pyridoxine and excreted as pyridoxic acid via the urine (see Figure 5.15).

Food sources: see Table 5.1.

[*Source:* Information mainly from Mahan et al. (1980) and Leklem (1988).]

converted to the degradation product, 4-pyridoxic acid. In subjects with alcoholic liver cirrhosis, blood pyridoxal phosphate levels are low, probably because of increased hepatocyte alkaline phosphatase activity, which converts it to pyridoxal (Merrill and Henderson, 1987).

Pyridoxal the major transport form available to cells from blood is about 30% of the vitamin in plasma but four- to fivefold more concentrated in red cells, where it is bound mainly to hemoglobin (as pyridoxal). [It may enhance O_2 binding (Benesch et al., 1977).] Sixty to seventy percent of the plasma vitamin is normally pyridoxal *phosphate,* bound mostly to albumin, and has a slower turnover. After diffusion into cells, pyridoxal is phosphorylated and used therein. (In muscle, most is bound to glycogen phosphorylase.) Ultimately, it is oxidized to pyridoxic acid and lost in the urine.

Functions

Until recently, vitamin B_6 was one of the most neglected vitamins in terms of studies of its metabolism and function in many important areas. We know it is a cofactor for more than 100 enzyme reactions, many of which occur in all cells, and some of which are only present in the liver (and kidney), the main site for amino acid catabolism and gluconeogenesis. (Consequently, liver is a good food source of the vitamin.) The majority of the reactions are concerned with amino acid metabolism:

1. Transamination, in synthesis of nonessential amino acids and as the first step in the catabolism of amino acids. It is noteworthy that some of the transaminases are rate-limiting for the breakdown of specific amino acids in the liver, like tyrosine, and that the concentrations of these enzymes may be regulated according to need by glucocorticosteroids, glucagon, and substrate concentrations (Figure 5.15). The liver enzyme, tyrosine aminotransferase, is the most well-known case in point and has served as a prototype for the study of enzyme regulation (Knox and Greengard, 1967).
2. Decarboxylation, employed in the synthesis of several important substances, such as the neuroactive amines [serotonin, tyramine, histamine, and γ-amino butyric acid (GABA) (Ta-

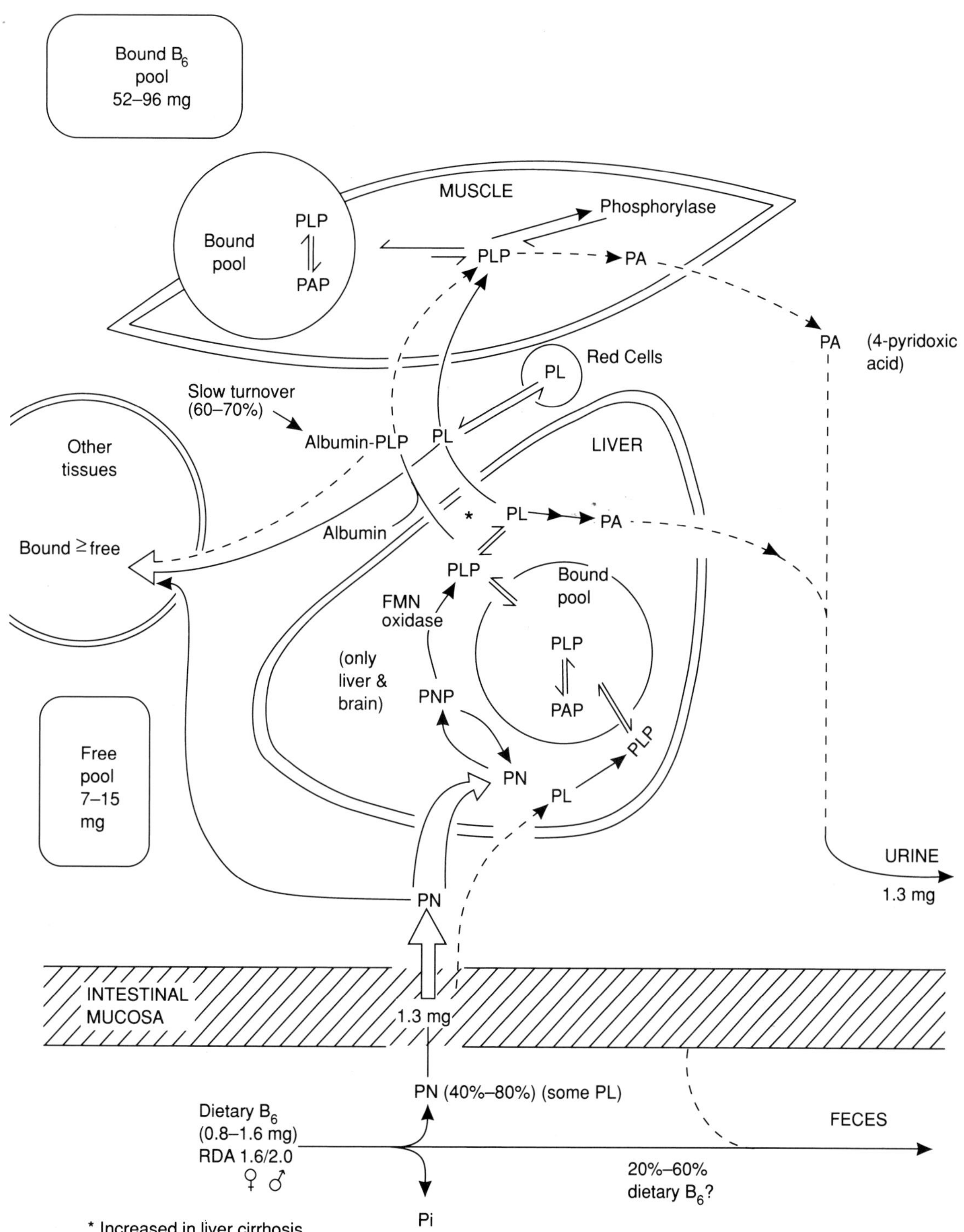

Figure 5.14. Vitamin B_6 nutrition/metabolism. *Abbreviations:* PN, pyridoxine; PL, pyridoxal; PLP, pyridoxal P; PAP, pyridoxamine P. Most B_6 is absorbed as pyridoxine and converted to pyridoxal and PLP in the liver. Some PLP exits the liver and travels in the blood on albumin, turning over slowly. PL is the form most actively transported to other cells from the liver. The main excretory form is pyridoxic acid, lost in urine. [*Sources:* Mehansho et al. (1980), Lim (1982), Shane (1982*a*), and Leklem (1988).]

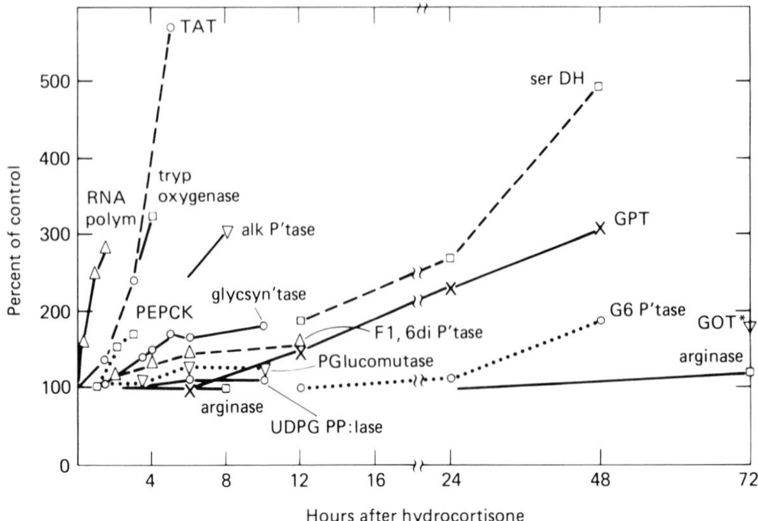

Figure 5.15. Response of enzymes to administration of glucocorticosteroids. Changes in various liver enzyme activities with time, following one i.p. injection of hydrocortisone into adult albino rats at doses from 1–10 mg/100 g body weight. Results for intact or adrenalectomized rats, male or female, fasted or fed, have not been differentiated. Key: RNA polymerase (△———△, RNA polym); tyrosine aminotransferase (O—O, TAT); tryptophan oxygenase (□———□, tryp oxygenase); phosphoenolpyruvate carboxykinase (□···□, PEPCK); alkaline phosphatase (▽———▽, alk, P'tase); glycogen synthetase (O———O, glyc syn'tase); fructose 1,6-diphosphatase (△—△, F1,6diP'tase); phosphoglucomutase (▽···▽, PGlucomutase); UDPG-pyrophosphorylase (O———O, UDPG PP'lase); arginase (□———□); serine dehydratase (□—□, ser DH); glutamic-pyruvic transaminase (x———x, GPT); glucose-6-phosphatase (O···O, G6P'tase); glutamic-oxalictransaminase (▽*, GOT) at very high doses of hydrocortisone. [*Source:* Reprinted by permission from Linder (1978).]

ble 5.4)]; δ-amino levulinic acid (the first step in porphyrin synthesis); and intermediates in the synthesis of sphingomyelin, phosphatidylcholine (lecithin), and taurine [important as a conjugator of bile acids and probably also in brain and eye function (see below).] Decarboxylation also comes into play in the breakdown and desulfuration of cysteine (Table 5.4).

3. Dehydratase reactions, where serine and threonine are converted to their α-keto acids through the oxidative removal of the amino group as ammonia (Table 5.4).
4. Side chain cleavage reactions, as in the formation of glycine (and formate) from serine (Figure 5.16), the splitting of alanine from kynurenine and 3-OH kynurenine (Figure 5.16) (in tryptophan degradation), and splitting of cystathionine (Figure 5.16) in methionine degradation.

Thus, vitamin B_6 is intimately involved with all phases of amino acid metabolism and also plays a central role in porphyrin and lipid metabolism. A considerable portion of the vitamin is also attached to glycogen phosphorylase and may even have a role in this reaction (see below). Apart from these actions, vitamin B_6 deficiency may depress uptake of amino acids by muscle cells (as demonstrated in rats with amino isobutyric acid), an effect that may be mediated by decreased secretions of growth hormone and/or insulin (Nutr Rev, 1979*a*). Furthermore, it may be necessary for the return (and thus inactivation) of steroid receptor complexes to the cytosol from the nucleus after they have promoted the transcription of certain genes (Compton and Cidlowski, 1986); and thus assume a regulatory function in steroid hormone action.

Consumption and Requirements

The U.S. RDA is set at between 1.6 and 2.0 mg for adults, with somewhat more recommended for women during pregnancy and lactation consuming about 100 g protein a day. [The milk content of B_6 is dependent on B_6 status (Sauberlich and Canham, 1980).] Requirements are dependent on protein intake (at 0.016 mg/g protein consumed), which makes a deficiency more likely among

Table 5.4. Other Enzyme Reactions Involving B_6

(serine dehydratase)
Serine ——→ pyruvate (− NH_3)
pyruvate ——→ glycolysis; gluconeogenesis

Serine ←——(THFA (tetrahydro folic acid))——→ glycine; 5, 10-methylene THFA
5, 10-methylene THFA ——→ 1-C metabolism

Serine[a] (+ palmitoyl-CoA, − CO_2) ——→ $CH_3—(CH_2)_{14}—C(=O)—CH(NH_3)—CH_2OH$
——→ sphingosine

phosphatidylserine ——→ phosphatidylethanolamine (− CO_2)
phosphatidylethanolamine ——→ choline

glycine + succinyl CoA ——→ δ-amino-levulinic acid (− CO_2)

glycogen + Pi ——(phosphorylase)[b]——→ glucose-1-phosphate (+ glycogen)

cysteine ——(+ O_2)[c]——→ cysteine sulfinic acid ——(− CO_2)——→ hypotaurine
hypotaurine ——→ taurine

glutamic acid ——→ γ-amino butyric acid (GABA) (− CO_2)
(GABA) ——→ brain function

[a] Information from Krishnankura and Sweeley (1976).
[b] B_6 does not participate in reaction.
[c] Step doesn't involve B_6: next step does.

Westerners on a typical high-protein diet. Whether the American diet, and even the RDA, is sufficient to meet the needs of 95% of the population probably requires some review, in that there are many conditions in which an increased intake of pyridoxine may ameliorate symptoms of deficiency and even more serious health conditions (Figure 5.13); from glucose intolerance to carpal tunnel syndrome and overall stress (see below). [The latter may be explained on the basis that glucocorticosteroids, secreted at higher levels in certain forms of stress, enhance protein and amino acid catabolism and induce increased synthesis of B_6-requiring enzymes (Figure 5.15).] Treatments with a variety of drugs, from isoniazid (used against tuberculosis) to penicillamine (used to relieve copper overload in Wilson's disease), also increase requirements by binding to, and thus inactivating, the vitamin, or (as with oral contraceptives) by increasing the synthesis and activity of enzymes requiring the vitamin. These matters are not widely known. Coupled with the fact that the best sources of B_6 are not meats (other than liver) but rather whole grains, legumes, and nuts (along with avocados and bananas) (Table 5.5), and that most B_6 is routinely removed from

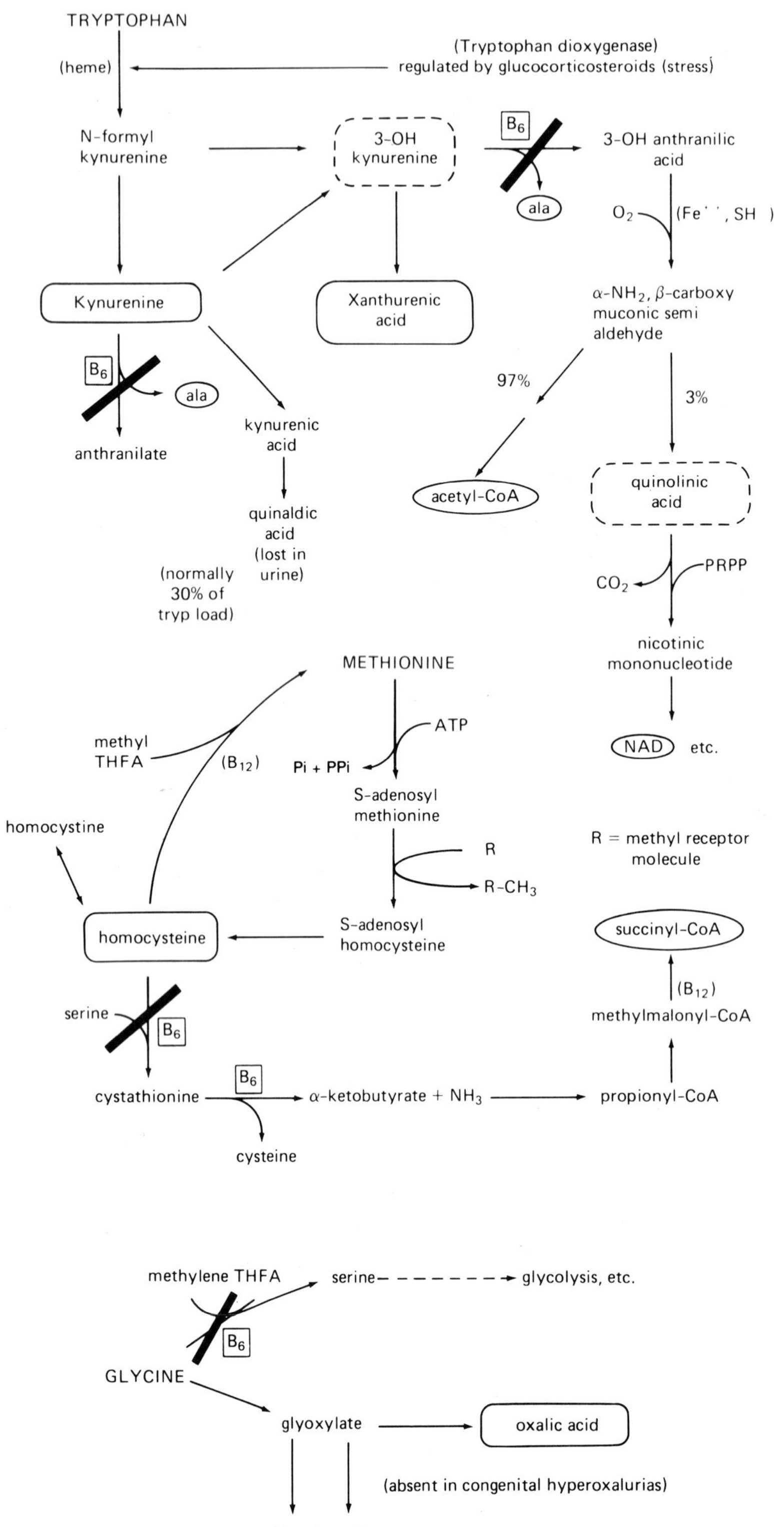

Figure 5.16. Effects of B_6 status on urinary excretion of tryptophan and methionine metabolites. Key: ○ Useful products of metabolism; ▬ blocked in B_6 deficiency; □ rising urinary excretion in B_6 deficiency.

Table 5.5. The Vitamin B_6, Thiamin, and Pantothenic Acid Contents of Common Foods[a]

Food	B_6	Thiamin	Pantothenic acid
Liver	6.5–8.4	2.5–3.0	64–77
Steak (raw round)	3.3	0.9	4.7
Fish (raw or canned)	2.3–4.3	0.3–1.0	2.8–5.5
Chicken (raw)	3.3–6.8	0.5–0.8	8–10
Eggs (raw)	1.1	1.1	16
Milk	0.4	0.4	3.1
Whole wheat bread	1.8	2.6	7.6
Cornmeal (dry enriched)	2.5	4.4	5.8
Soybean flour	7.2	1.1	22
Peanuts	4.0	3.2	21
Walnuts	7.3	3.3	9
Avocados	4.2	1.1	11
Bananas	5.1	0.5	2.6
Potatoes (raw)	2.5	1.0	3.8
Squash (raw)	0.8	0.5	3.6
Apples	0.3	0.3	1
Oranges	0.6	1.0	2.5
Tomatoes (raw)	1.0	0.6	3.3
Peas (raw)	1.6	3.5	7.5
Spinach (frozen)	1.5	1.0	1.5
Lettuce	0.6	0.6	2

Source: Adapted from Sauberlich and Canham (1980).

[a] Quantities in μg/g. It should be noted that bioavailability of B_6 may vary considerably, from 40%–100%, and that average availability is about 70% (Gregory and Kirk, 1981).

the whole grain during milling and processing (Table 5.2) and *not usually replaced* when flour is enriched, it seems likely that the average American may be suffering from a marginal B_6 deficiency. Vitamin B_6 deficiency is also commonly found in the chronic alcoholic.

The toxicity of excess vitamin B_6 in all of its forms is generally low (Figure 5.13), except when taken chronically, in very large doses. At chronic doses of 500–6000 mg/day (250–3000× the RDA), it can cause a loss of peripheral (and possibly central) nerve axon function leading to loss of sensation in hands and feet, difficulties in walking, etc. (Dalton, 1985; Foca, 1985; Parry and Bredesen, 1985; Schaumburg, 1983; Schaumburg and Berger, 1988). This appears to be only partly reversible. (It is noteworthy that B_6 *deficiency* causes a somewhat similar neuropathy.) There is no evidence that lower doses (on the order of 50–100 mg, or 30–60× the female RDA) cause any damage, and the acute toxicity of isolated large doses is minimal, although it can reduce prolactin secretion (via increased dopamine) and thus lower milk production in lactating women (Audon et al., 1985). Even with 500-mg doses, toxicity symptoms take several years to develop. The mechanism of the toxic effect is unknown, although it appears to involve axonal degeneration of dorsal root ganglion cells in the brain, which are not protected by the blood–brain barrier (Schaumburg and Berger, 1988). Because of several factors, including a structural similarity to dihydropyridine (used in controlling hypertension), it has been proposed that excess pyridoxine acts as a blocker of calcium channels (Leklem and Reynolds, 1988).

Symptoms of B_6 Deficiency: Urinary Amino Acid Metabolites

Due to its importance in amino acid catabolism, a deficiency of vitamin B_6 results in excretion of increased levels of some amino acid metabolites which are normally degraded further, specifically, metabolites of tryptophan, methionine, and glycine. Urea excretion is also enhanced, perhaps because of a decreased capacity to synthesize nonessential amino acids, resulting in decreased reutilization of ammonia and amino nitrogen. As shown in Figure 5.16, B_6 enzymes are in key positions along the pathways of degradational utilization of tryptophan, methionine, and glycine. (Other amino acid pathways are not as affected, presumably because the enzymes involved have a higher affinity for the vitamin.) B_6 deficiency results in an increased urinary excretion of xanthurenic acid, kynurenine, and hydroxykynurenine (from tryptophan). Indeed, the effect of a 2-g tryptophan load on excretion of these metabolites is commonly used to determine B_6 deficiency. Increased excretions of oxalic acid (due to a decreased capacity to convert glycine to serine) and homocystine (due to a block in cystathionine synthesis) (Figure 5.16) also can occur. The lack of B_6 will thus also reduce the formation of nicotinic acid (niacin) from tryptophan (see section on "Niacin," above) and can, in effect, cause a homocystinuria and oxaluria that may have serious consequences.

Hyperoxaluria may result in the formation of calcium oxalate stones in the kidney and/or throughout the urinary tract system. Congenital hyperoxalurias, due to a deficiency in enzymes allowing utilization of glyoxalic acid in energy metabolism (which also result in overproduction of oxalic acid), cause severe genitourinary problems and sometimes early death.

Homocystinuria, due to a congenital deficiency of cystathionine synthetase (Figure 5.16), results in severe growth abnormalities, mental retardation, and early death, probably from extensive atherosclerotic lesions throughout the vascular system (McCully and Wilson, 1975) (see Chapters 4, 15, and 18). It has been postulated that in many normal individuals, increased levels of homocystine in the blood, due to a relative deficiency of vitamin B_6, may contribute to the development of atherosclerosis in our society as a whole, since homocystine is a potent atherogenic agent in experimental animals. The evidence for this possibility is described in some detail in Chapter 15.

Involvement of B_6 in Glucose Metabolism

As already mentioned (Chapter 2), pyridoxal phosphate is also found firmly attached to the abundant liver and muscle enzyme, glycogen phosphorylase, which catalyzes the breakdown of carbohydrate stores to maintain blood glucose concentrations and to provide immediate energy to muscle cells when needed (see Chapter 2, Figure 2.2). Krebs and Fischer (1964) have estimated that half of the vitamin B_6 in the body and most of that in muscle is normally found on phosphorylase, due to the relatively large amounts of this enzyme versus other B_6 enzymes. Although not essential for enzyme activity it may play a modulating role in catalysis (Helmreich and Klein, 1980; Takagi et al., 1982). Krebs and Fischer have postulated that phosphorylase is a B_6 repository, or storage site. Evidence that vitamin B_6 status can influence glucose/glycogen metabolism springs from observations in rats and mice that B_6 deficiency reduces muscle glycogen phosphorylase levels as much as 65% and also lowers liver glycogen phosphorylase (Black et al., 1978; Krebs and Fischer, 1964). Conversely, high intake may increase it (Black et al., 1977). This knowledge has not been tested in the human.

The possibility of a different involvement of B_6 in glucose metabolism stems from observations of the occurrence of a pyridoxine-responsive glucose intolerance in some individuals, especially pregnant women (see Chapter 2, Figure 2.5). Women with pregnancy-associated glucose intolerance tend to excrete large quantities of xanthurenic acid (see above) when given a tryptophan load. Excretion of xanthurenic acid is greatly reduced upon treatment with 100 mg pyridoxine/day. Reduced xanthurenic acid excretion is accompanied by a marked improvement, or even normalization, of glucose tolerance curves in half or more of the individuals tested (Coelingh-Bennink and Schreurs, 1975). Similar results were reported by Spellacy et al. (1977) who found that blood insulin levels (after oral glucose) were not altered. Other reports indicate that 15%–20% or more of *oral contraceptive* users have decreased plasma concentrations of the vitamin (Miller, 1986), or less than fully active red cell aspartate aminotransferase activity (Salkeld, 1986), as well as xanthurenic aciduria after a tryptophan load, all of which respond to 10–20 mg doses of pyridoxine (Henderson and Hulse, 1978; Leklem et al., 1975; Rose, 1978). (This may mean they also have marginal glucose intolerance.) McCann and Davis (1978) have reported that patients with severe diabetes (and neuropathy) have reduced blood levels of pyridoxine and an increased urinary excretion of xanthurenic acid, both of which could be ameliorated with daily 100-mg doses of B_6. A substantial proportion of the patients tested also showed a marked improvement in glucose intolerance (as well as peripheral neuropathy) (Bernstein and Lobitz, 1988). The metabolic and molecular relationships between glucose intolerance and B_6 deficiency are unknown, although preliminary work suggests xanthurenic acid can form a tight complex with insulin and might reduce its biological activity (Spellacy et al., 1977). The incomplete degradation of tryptophan, more likely to occur in individuals on a high-protein diet, may thus result in inactivation of some of the circulating insulin secreted in response to glucose intake. The connection between oral contraceptive use (estrogens and progestogens) and the development of B_6 deficiency symptoms is not well understood. It is the *glucocorticosteroids*, and not the estrogens or progestogens, that induce increases in B_6-dependent transaminases (tyrosine aminotransferase, etc.; Figure 5.15) above normal levels. However, estrogens may reduce kynureninase (Bender et al., 1982), leading to diversion of tryptophan to xanthurenic acid.

Therapeutic Uses of B_6

Doses of B_6 (2.5 mg/day) have been used successfully against a certain form of sideroblastic anemia refractory to iron, B_{12}, or folate (Sauberlich and Canham, 1980); against dystonia (altered muscle tone) in Parkinson's patients treated with L-DOPA (Ebadi, 1978; Sauberlich and Canham, 1980); against convulsive seizures in newborn infants (Sauberlich and Canham, 1980; Waldinger and Berg, 1963) (2-mg doses) where the active (proconvulsive) agent may be 3-OH-kynurenine (Guilarte and Wagner, 1987); and in Huntington's chorea (Crow, 1974; Sauberlich and Canham, 1980). In the latter two conditions, a lack of GABA may also be a problem, as chorea patients appear to have abnormally low levels of this neurotransmitter in the basal ganglia of the brain (Crow, 1974) and because GABA antagonists (like bicuculline) cause convulsions (Metzler, 1977). Larger doses of B_6 (50 mg) have been used somewhat successfully against carpal tunnel syndrome (or tenosynovitis) in middle-aged and elderly patients (Ellis et al., 1979; Leklem and Reynolds, 1988). This use of B_6 was accidentally discovered by a rural Texas general practitioner, John M. Ellis, who was faced with many cases of gnarled, curled-up hands among his patients (Ellis and Presley, 1973). In his experience, other forms of arthritic and rheumatic disorders may also respond to the vitamin. Carpal tunnel syndrome is still generally treated with surgery, and the potential usefulness of B_6 has remained unknown and unexploited. There are reports that very large (potentially dangerous) doses ($\geq$500 mg/day) will help most women suffering from premenstrual syndrome (Abraham and Hargrove, 1980; Williams et al., 1985), but that lower doses (50–500 mg) will not (Hagan, 1985; Stokes and Mendels, 1972). Smaller daily doses (50 mg) have been used to enhance immune function in the elderly (Miller and Kerkvliet, 1988). Finally, B_6 deficiency has also been implicated in "Chinese restaurant syndrome" (Folkers et al., 1981), where large amounts of sodium glutamate are ingested and must be disposed of through transamination.

Vitamin B_{12} and Folic Acid

Vitamin B_{12} or Cobalamin

In the early 1800s, it was recognized by Combe, a Scottish physician, that a certain form of anemia [later characterized as megaloblastic anemia (enlarged red cells and marrow reticulocytes)] was probably due to a "disorder of the digestive and assimilative organs" (Herbert et al., 1980). In 1926, Minot and Murphy determined that this condition could be reversed and controlled by eating half-pound quantities of raw or lightly cooked liver daily (for which they received a Nobel Prize in medicine). In 1929, Castle and his colleagues postulated the existence of an "intrinsic factor" in gastric juice which, combined with an "extrinsic factor" in meat, would bring about the absorption of the "antipernicious anemia factor." The extrinsic factor was first isolated by groups of scientists at pharmaceutical houses in both the United States and Great Britain in 1948, and at about the same time, it was demonstrated that actinomycetes (soil bacteria) (also the source of most antibiotics) are the foremost synthesizers of this material in nature. Vitamin B_{12}, along with D, is the only vitamin generally absent from plant and vegetable foods, and consequently, the only vitamin that tends to be lacking in the diets of strict vegetarians. [A recent study reported that 92% of vegetarians had serum B_{12} levels below the normal range (<200 pg/ml; Dong and Scott, 1982).] It is found in eggs, dairy products, and of course, also in meats, especially liver (Table 5.1), as well as in fish, poultry, and seafoods (especially bivalves, such as clams which filter microorganisms). Fermented soybean foods have trace amounts (2–7 μg/100 g, dry) as do some legumes and seaweeds, which have symbiotic microorganisms (as in their root nodules) (Herbert et al., 1988). [Blue-green algae (including spirulina) can also be a good source.] However, there is evidence that strict vegetarians can acquire the vitamin from intestinal microorganisms; intestinal bacteria are good producers of the vitamin (Albert et al., 1980); strict vegetarians are not necessarily deficient in it (Satyranarayana, 1963); and bacterial microflora can be quite abundant in the lower *small* intestine of vegetarians (see Chapter 1), where B_{12} is best absorbed (Figure 5.17). [However, B_{12} is <u>not</u> abundant in the small intestine of omnivorous people (see Chapter 1).]

The structure of cobalamin (Figure 5.17) was the largest determined by x-ray diffraction in its time, and consists of the "corrin ring" (a more hydrogenated form of the porphyrin ring with differences also in the side chains of the ring), the presence of Co^{3+} (versus Fe^{2+}), and, most importantly, the presence of a dimethylbenzimidazole ring involved in cobalt chelation and attached to the corrin ring through a complex linkage involving an unusual ribose–phosphate moiety. The cobalt ion is at the active center of the ring—the site for attachment of alkyl groups during their transfer (presently the only known function of this trace element in human and animal tissues).

The absorption of cobalamin is more complex than that of other vitamins (Figure 5.17), involving binding to a carrier protein [or proteins, possibly transcobalamin III (TCIII), also known as R-binders]) in the saliva and gastric juices, and transport to the duodenum, where the complex is digested and the B_{12} is released to a 50,000 dalton glycoprotein ("intrinsic factor") secreted by cells in the stomach wall. (Here, B_{12} from the bile also

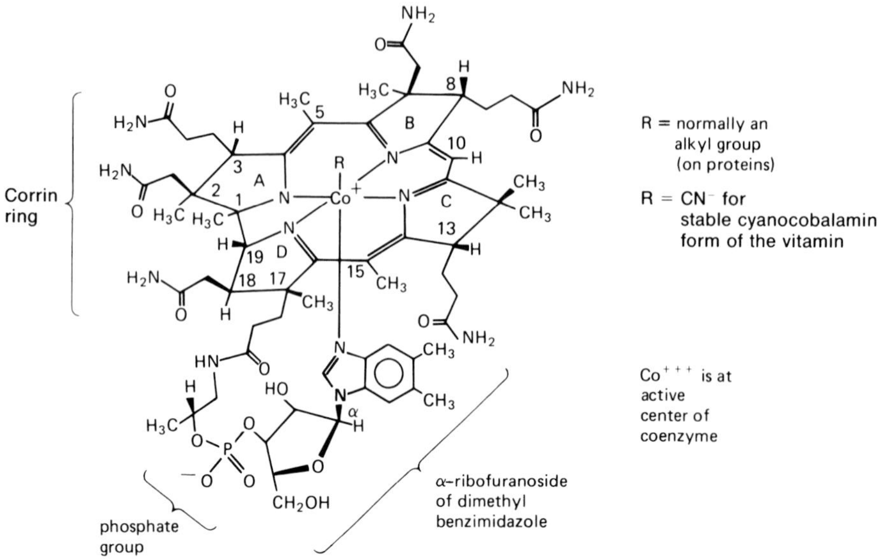

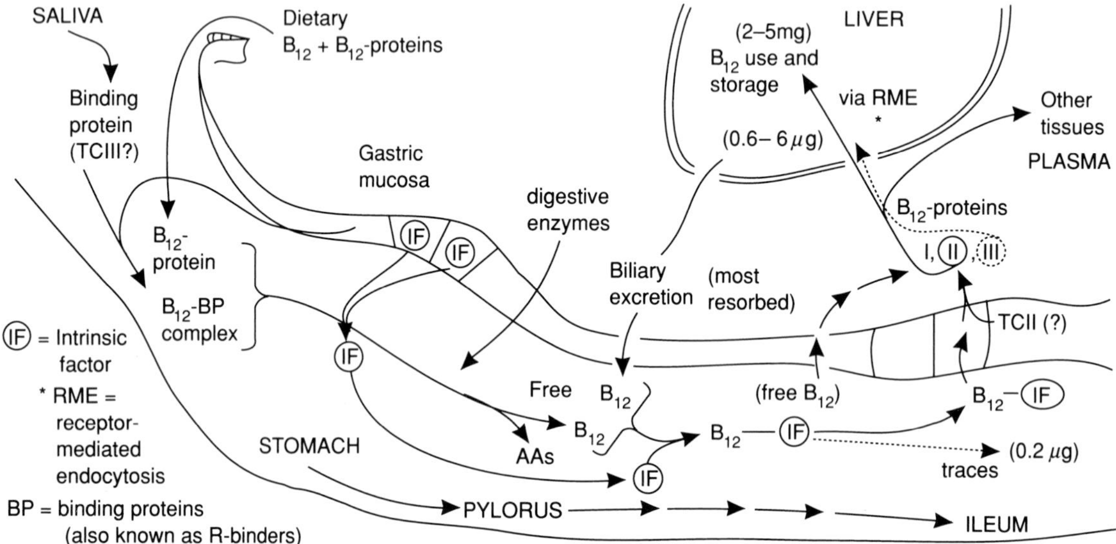

Figure 5.17. Vitamin B_{12} (cobalamin).

Functions: (as coenzyme)

To reform tetrahydrofolate from methylfolate (prevent trapping of folic acid as methylfolate).

To allow catabolism of odd chain length fatty acids and some amino acid carbons.

(May also aid in production of reduced glutathione.)

Requirements: 2 μg/day (NRC); 1 μg/day (FAO/WHO); 0.2 μg/day = MDR (minimal daily requirement).

Sources: liver, kidney, heart, clams, oysters (>10 μg/100 g); dry milk, some fish, egg yolks, crabs (3–10 μg/100 g); milk, cheese (1–3 μg/100 g).

Toxicity: nil, except that allergic reactions are sometimes produced at high doses.

Deficiencies due to the following:

Lack in the diet (occurs most often in vegans and alcoholics).

Absorption problems (genetic/other); lack of intrinsic factor and/or ileal disturbances.

Problems with utilization; antagonists in the diet; congenital enzyme deletions.

Increased excretion, e.g., liver disease.

Increased requirements: pregnancy, hyperthyroidism, increased hematopoiesis, parasites.

[*Source:* Information mainly from Herbert et al. (1980, 1988) and Cooper and Rosenblatt (1987).]

rebinds to the intrinsic factor.) Most food cobalamin is released to the R-binders during protein digestion in the stomach. Intrinsic factor allows binding of the vitamin to the brush border of mucosal cells in the ileum, and through this, an efficient absorption into the mucosa and blood. It is thought that from 1.5–3 μg of B_{12} can be bound to the intrinsic factor and absorbed in this way, per day, in the normal adult. In the blood, B_{12} is attached to three different proteins, TCI, II, and III. TCII is the most abundant and the most important for transport and uptake of B_{12} by the liver and other tissues (Herbert et al., 1988). A β-globulin of about 50,000 daltons, synthesized by a variety of tissues, it may pick up B_{12} within cells of the intestinal mucosa (Cooper and Rosenblatt, 1987). TCIII may also carry some B_{12} to the liver (Herbert et al., 1988). TCI and III are heterogeneous glycoproteins of about 60,000 daltons (also known as "R binders") produced mainly by granulocytic white blood cells. Delivery by these various carriers appears to involve receptor-mediated endocytosis (and protein digestion in lysosomes). Of the 1–10 mg vitamin B_{12} present in normal individuals, 50%–90% is located and stored in the liver; irrespective of the amount stored, 0.1%–0.2% is lost in the bile per day, although almost all is reabsorbed. Doses of 0.1–0.2 μg/day are probably sufficient to meet the minimal needs of individual adults, although the RDA is set at 2 μg (Figure 5.17). Consequently, when there is little or no B_{12} in the diet, it takes 3–6 years or more to develop a functional deficiency (Herbert et al., 1988). This is also why stores of the vitamin tend to increase with age in the average (omnivorous) person. [There is no evidence of toxicity associated with this accumulation (Herbert et al., 1988).]

Cobalamin analogs (inactive as B_{12}) apparently also exist in foods and are absorbed and excreted, using the same R binders and other mechanisms. The functions and effects of these are unknown, although it has been postulated that R binders exist partly to rid the body of these analogs (Cooper and Rosenblatt, 1987) and that the analogs may be responsible for some of the neurologic abnormalities that occur in B_{12} deficiency (Carmel et al., 1988*a*, 1990).

In pernicious anemia, a hereditary condition that tends to develop in later years (after 60) but has also been detected in younger people, the intrinsic factor is not produced and/or secreted at all, or it is secreted in quantities insufficient to assure the efficient absorption of the vitamin. In this condition, the vitamin can either be injected (generally in doses of 100 μg about once a month) or given orally in large amounts (30 μg), 0.1%–1% of which will be absorbed by diffusion through all parts of the small intestine (Cooper and Rosenblatt, 1987). Partial gastrectomy will also reduce the availability of intrinsic factor, and thus, the availability of B_{12} to the body. It may also reduce release of food-bound cobalamin to R binders in the stomach (Carmel et al., 1988*c*; Carmel, 1990). Other more rare conditions (Figure 5.17) can affect B_{12} status; in chronic alcoholism, a lack of B_{12} from deficient intake and alcohol antagonism to uptake is very common. Increased needs for the vitamin occur in pregnancy, hyperthyroidism, and in situations where hematopoiesis is enhanced. Increased excretion and loss of the vitamin may occur in liver disease. Based on preliminary studies in rats, large amounts of pectin and other soluble fibers may reduce absorption (Cullen and Oace, 1989*a*,*b*), although the mechanism and relevance to human nutrition is unknown. The claim that vitamin B_{12} is destroyed by excess ascorbic acid (vitamin C) is without convincing foundation (Newmark et al., 1976), having been based on inadequate assays of the vitamin in food preparations stored with and without various concentrations of vitamin C (Herbert and Jacob, 1974).

Only two enzymatic reactions in animals and humans have so far been found to require the services of vitamin B_{12} (Figure 5.17). These are: (1) methylmalonyl-CoA mutase, in the rearrangement of methylmalonyl to succinyl-CoA, necessary for the disposal of odd-numbered fatty acids (ending with a propionyl versus acetyl-CoA group) and parts of the carbon skeletons of valine and some other amino acids; (2) methionine synthetase, in the transfer of a methyl group from methyltetrahydrofolic acid (methyl THFA) to homocysteine in order to form methionine, necessary for the interconversion of sulfur amino acids (cys to met) (Banerjee and Matthews, 1990); and more importantly, to reform THFA that might otherwise become trapped as methyl THFA (see more below). The metabolism and function of B_{12} is thus intimately entangled with that of another vitamin, folic acid, and both vitamins are fundamental to what is known as 1-C metabolism, involved in the transfer of various 1-C units in biosynthetic reactions (see below).

Other actions of the vitamin, as a coenzyme or otherwise, cannot be excluded at this time. For one, there may be an involvement in synthesis of either the lipid or protein part of myelin, independent of the methylmalonyl-CoA reaction (Herbert et al., 1988). This would explain the demyelination (or lack of myelination) and nerve degeneration observed in B_{12} deficiency. It may also be the basis for the development of neuropsychiatric disorders in some individuals with only mild B_{12} deficiency (homocysteinemia but no anemia) (Lindenbaum et al., 1988). [Alternatively, the accumulation of odd chain length fatty acids in nerve cells (Barley et al., 1972) might be at fault.] B_{12} deficiency also appears to result in a loss of tissue carnitine, perhaps in the form of a propionic acid adduct entering the blood and urine (Brass and Stabler, 1988). Presumably, this would occur because of methylmalonate and propionate accumulation due to their lack of conversion to succinate via methylmalonyl-CoA mutase (see section on Carnitine). Less carnitine could have consequences for the shuttling of fatty acids between mitochondria and the cytosol, and for fatty acid (beta) oxidation. Of additional interest are recent observations that the release of alkaline phosphatase and osteocalcin from osteoblasts (symptomatic of bone mineral building activity) is dependent on vitamin B_{12} status (Carmel et al., 1988*b*). The metabolic and molecular basis of this dependence is unknown. Finally, there has been some popular interest in the possibility that pharmacologic (1–5 mg) doses of B_{12} might be used to improve the well-being of patients claiming tiredness, for which other reasons have been eliminated. Several studies on physical performance, strength, and endurance lend no support to this hypothesis (Than et al., 1978). One controlled study of 28 patients receiving 5 mg twice weekly did record an effect (Ellis and Nasser, 1973).

Folic Acid

In contrast to vitamin B_{12}, folates are most abundant in plant food sources, especially when raw or relatively unprocessed, as the vitamin is susceptible to heat destruction. Whole grains, yeast preparations, and liver are especially rich sources (Table 5.1). Most of the folic acid in food is attached to a polymer of glutamic acid. This polyglutamate "tail" must be split off, down to the mono- (or di-) glutamate form, at the brush border during absorption in the small intestine (by active uptake). Folate binding proteins in milk may enhance absorption efficiency by delivering it to mucosal carriers while protecting it from loss to intestinal bacteria (Said et al., 1986), and folate may be absorbed even more readily by the jejunum than the duodenum (Tani et al., 1983). Upon distribution through the blood circulation (partly attached to plasma proteins), about 50% of the total body folate is stored in polyglutamate form by the liver (Figure 5.18). Recent studies indicate that these polyglutamate forms are active forms of the vitamin, and that addition of polyglutamate "tails" is a way of keeping the vitamin in cells (Brody et al., 1982; Shane and Stokstad, 1985). For use as a coenzyme in various reactions folic acid is reduced with the aid of NADPH to tetrahydrofolic acid (THFA) (Figures 5.18 and 5.19). Excretion occurs via the bile and the urine, with little or no catabolism of the vitamin.

Minimal daily requirements are geared to growth and to absorbability of the vitamin and are thought to be about 50 μg for the average, nonpregnant, normal adult. Allowing for 50% efficiency of absorption, the FAO/WHO (and now the NRC) have set the RDA at 180–200 μg (Figure 5.18).

Insufficiency in the diet may become evident in pregnancy and usually occurs in alcoholics. Insufficient absorption and utilization of folates occur in individuals taking a variety of drugs, including the anticonvulsant, Dilantin, barbiturates, antimalarials, and chemotherapeutic agents (methotrexate and aminopterin). The latter are direct chemical analogs of the vitamin (pteroylglutamate) (Figure 5.18) and have been used to inhibit tumor cell proliferation by interfering with 1-C metabolism and thus DNA synthesis (see below). Inadequate utilization of folates may also occur in vitamin B_{12} deficiency, when a large percentage of the folic acid may be trapped as methylfolate (see below); the same can occur when diets contain large amounts of glycine and methionine. Oral contraceptives also prevent adequate utilization, possibly by interfering with the addition and cleavage of the polyglutamate "tail" during storage and utilization of the vitamin (Herbert and Jacob, 1974). Increased losses of the vitamin occur in liver disease, via the bile, and in kidney dialysis. Increased requirements occur during infancy, in the hyperthyroid individual, and in individuals with stimulated hematopoiesis. Exposure to strong sunlight or long-term phototherapy may cause vitamin destruction (Branda and Eaton, 1978) and thus also increase requirements.

Functions of B_{12} and Folic Acid

The main functions of these two vitamins are so interconnected that it is difficult to distinguish a deficiency in one from that in the other without extensive testing. Nevertheless, folate deficiency is usually associated with wasting of body tissue,

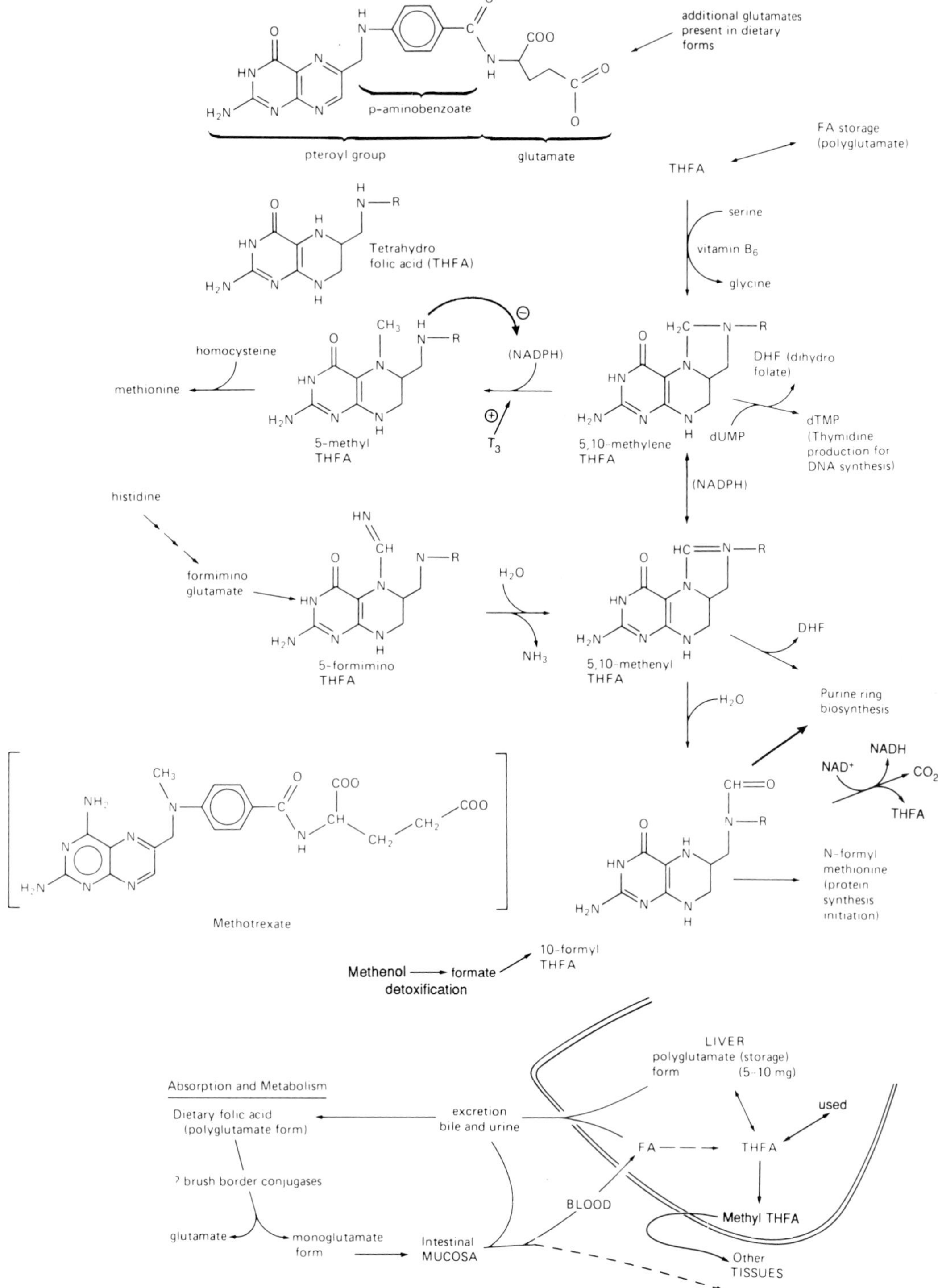

Figure 5.18. Folic acid.

Functions: coenzyme in 1-C donating/receiving reactions, in amino acid, purine, and nucleic acid metabolism.

Requirements: RDA 180–200 μg (3 μg/kg body weight); MDR 50 μg.

Toxicity: nil

Deficiency: due to dietary lack or inadequate absorption (congenital, or due to food or drug antagonists, or general malabsorption).

[*Source:* Information mainly from Herbert et al. (1980, 1988), and Metzler (1977).]

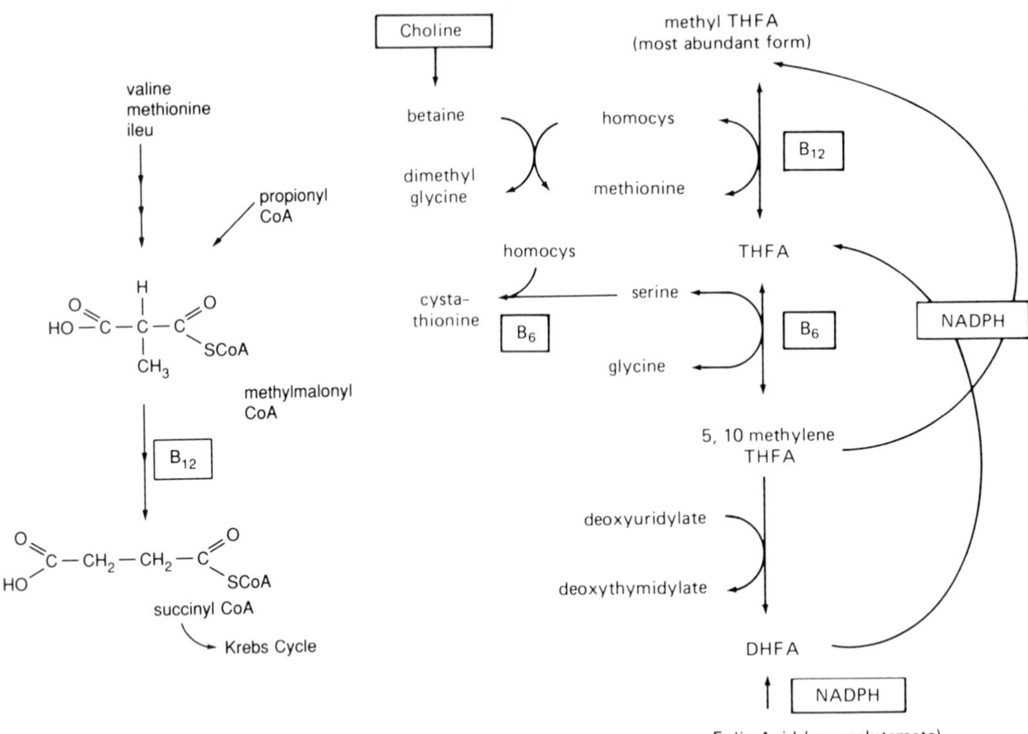

Figure 5.19. Interactions of vitamins in one-carbon (and three-carbon) metabolism.

	Plasma Concentration	Liver Concentration	Total in Body
B_{12}, normal adults[a]	200–900 pg/ml	~1 μg/g	1–10 mg
moderate deficiency	80–130 pg/ml	~0.16 μg/g	0.25 mg
Folate, normal adults	5–16 ng/ml	~0.7 μg/g	2.5–5 mg

[a] Herbert et al. (1980).

while B_{12} deficiency may occur in individuals of normal and excess body weight. Deficiency in B_{12} is also associated with more severe neurologic symptoms (and even neuropsychiatric disorders; Lindenbaum et al., 1988). Figure 5.19 illustrates the important interactions of these two vitamins, and with Figure 5.18, indicates the basis for the effects of deficiencies of these vitamins on tissue metabolism. At any instant in the mammalian cell, the majority of the active folate is in the form of methyltetrahydrofolic acid (5-methyl THFA) (Figures 5.18 and 5.19). THFA, however, is required in a number of different forms (Figure 5.18) in order to perform its duties as a coenzyme: (a) in the formation of thymidylate (the rate-limiting step in DNA synthesis), (b) in catabolism or interconversion of some amino acids, (c) in purine, and (d) in protein synthesis. To prevent "trapping" of folic acids as methyl THFA, a B_{12}-requiring transmethylase catalyzes the methylation of homocysteine to form methionine (needed for S-adenosylmethionine, the most common methyl-group donor in vertebrate cells) and regenerates THFA, to be used in DNA synthesis, etc. In the absence of sufficient B_{12}, folic acid accumulates in the methyl THFA form and is unable to support synthesis of DNA, thus reducing cell proliferation. This is because of the irreversibility of the NADPH-dependent dehydrogenase reaction converting 5,10-methylene THFA to methylfolate. In this condition, the ingestion of larger amounts of folic acid can partially relieve a THFA lack by directly providing more, as yet "untrapped," folic acid. Thus, excess folate intake can mask a deficiency in B_{12}, permitting the neurologic deterioration characteristic of chronic B_{12} deficiency to continue. It is for these reasons that the FDA has limited the content of folate to 250 μg/multivitamin tablet.

Those tissues (like the hematopoietic bone marrow) most dependent on cell proliferation will be the first affected by a deficiency of THFA. In the absence of sufficient B_{12}, there will be too little thymidylate for hematopoietic DNA synthesis. This results in the formation of megaloblastic ("giant") cells in the marrow (with sufficient cytoplasm but insufficient chromatin to divide). A similar situation arises in folic acid deficiency, where DNA synthesis is also reduced due to a lack of methylene THFA for thymidylate synthesis, and methenyl and formyl THFA for purine biosynthesis (Figure 5.18). An excess of dietary glycine and methionine may also reduce the availability of methylene THFA by working against the "forward" reactions from homocysteine to methionine, and serine to glycine (Figure 5.19). The interactions of 1-C metabolism with vitamin B_{12}, choline, and other vitamins ($NADP^+$) are also illustrated in Figure 5.19.

B_{12} and folate may also have other, as yet undiscovered metabolic functions. B_{12} may aid in the retention of folate by cells, and deficiency may decrease folate retention (Shane and Stokstad, 1985), perhaps because the methyl THFA that accumulates in deficiency is not a good substrate for the folylpolyglutamate synthetase. B_{12} is also necessary (in some situations or tissues) for formation of methionine and cysteine (Figure 5.19), and thus reduced glutathione (see also Chapter 4 and Figure 4.11). Therefore, in B_{12} and/or folate deficiency, one of the symptoms is accumulation of homocysteine, and homocystinuria. (Homocysteine is an atherogenic agent; see Chapter 15.)

Vitamin C

History

Scurvy is a disease known since ancient times and was a particular scourge to sailors on long voyages in the 15th through 19th centuries. The symptoms of scurvy, which reflect a gross deficiency of ascorbic acid (the "a-scorbutic" vitamin), are swollen legs with puffed sinews, blotched with capillary hemorrhages, and decaying peeling gums and loose teeth; there is also decreased capacity to heal wounds, depression, and fatigue.

Since the 16th century, many reports attributed the cure of scurvy to the ingestion of fruits, vegetables, grasses, berries, and even spruce leaves and green bark (Hodges, 1980). However, the initial discovery by Sir Richard Hawkins in the 16th century, that oranges and lemons were particularly effective in curing British sailors of the disease, had to be repeated in the 18th century, by James Lind before the British Admiralty decreed the prescription of lemon juice for all British sailors, in 1795 (Hodges, 1980). Even so, scurvy killed many soldiers in the American Civil War; and as late as 1912, the team of Captain Robert Scott exploring the South Pole met with death by scurvy. Based on observations on the treatment of scurvy in Norwegian sailors, Holst and Frolich (in 1909) first formally proposed that this disease was a dietary deficiency. In 1928, actual isolation of "hexuronic acid" from oranges, cabbages, and adrenal glands was accomplished by Szent-Györgyi (who later received the Nobel Prize for this work), and by King and Waugh from lemon juice. The vitamin was first synthesized in 1933 by Reichstein (Hodges, 1980).

A requirement for this substance is unique to man, other primates, fish, flying mammals, passeriformes birds, and the guinea pig; in other animals it is synthesized from glucose. The structure of ascorbic acid (Figure 5.20) is that of an oxidized form of glucose, and the more oxidized dehydro form also has antiscorbutic activity. [In primates, the next oxidation state (di-ketogulonic acid) does not).] In primates and presumably also in humans, the last step in synthesis of ascorbate from glucose (via D-glucuronic acid) is absent. This is the step in which L-gulonolactone is dehydrogenated prior to enolization (Metzler, 1977).

Functions

At the molecular level, ascorbic acid (and dehydroascorbate), like vitamin E, is a powerful reducing agent, and as such, has a general importance as an antioxidant, affecting the body's "redox potential" (the relative states of oxidation/reduction of other water-soluble substances inside and outside of the cells). As in the case of vitamin E, it is thought that ascorbic acid functions as a general source of reducing equivalents throughout the body. [Indeed, there is evidence that vitamin C can regenerate oxidized vitamin E (Niki, 1987).] But only a few enzyme reactions are thought to specifically require the vitamin. The reactions especially involving ascorbate are hydroxylations using molecular oxygen, and have Fe^{2+} or Cu^{2+} as a cofactor. Here, ascorbate is thought to play either of two roles: (1) as a direct source of electrons for reduction of O_2 (e.g., as a cosubstrate), or (2) as a protective agent for maintaining the Fe (or Cu) in a reduced state. Most notable among these hydroxylations are the formation of hydroxyproline

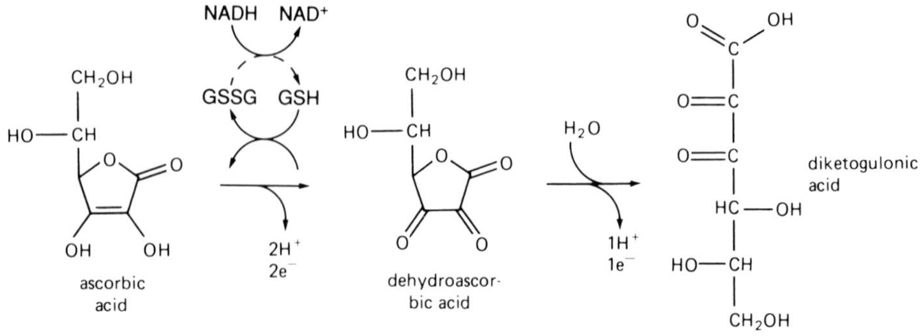

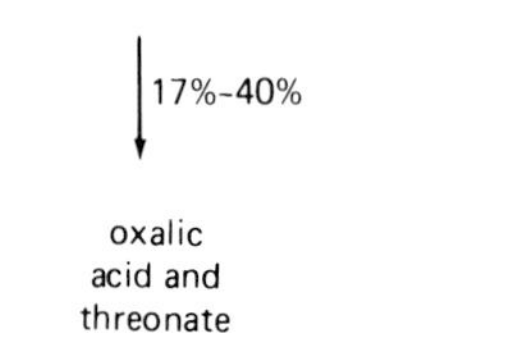

NADH NAD+
GSSG GSH
ascorbic acid
2H+ 2e−
dehydroascorbic acid
H2O
1H+ 1e−
diketogulonic acid
17%–40%
oxalic acid and threonate

Figure 5.20. Vitamin C.

Urinary excretion: ascorbate, dehydroascorbate, diketogulonate, and oxalic acid.

Functions: involved in hydroxylation reactions (often with Fe^{2+} or Cu^{2+}), such as proline and lysine, in procollagen synthesis; dopa and tyr (to neurotransmitters); C-terminal amidation of some neurohypophyseal hormones; also general antioxidant; transport/absorption of Fe^{2+} and $SO_4^{=}$.

RDA: 60 mg for adults; more in smoking, pregnancy, and lactation; 35–45 mg for infants and children; increased requirements may occur with wound healing, oral contraceptive use, and stress.

Food sources: fresh fruits and vegetables, especially citrus.

Toxicity: very low, except large doses may obscure some clinical tests.

and hydroxylysine during synthesis of procollagen on the endoplasmic reticulum of connective tissue cells (Figure 5.21); synthesis of carnitine from lysine (see end of chapter), carnitine being important in the transport of fatty acids into mitochondria for oxidation; the hydroxylation of dopamine (and perhaps also tyrosine and tryptophan) in the formation of catecholamines (and perhaps serotonin–5-OH tryptamine); the hydroxylation of 4-OH-phenylpyruvate (in the major route for tyrosine degradation); and probably the hydroxylation of steroid hormones, aromatic drugs, or carcinogens through the microsomal monooxygenase systems of the liver endoplasmic reticulum. An additional (Cu-dependent) reaction involving the amidation of the C-terminal glycine residue of some polypeptide hormones (including corticotropin and growth hormone-releasing factors, calcitonin and MSH) also depends on vitamin C (England and Seifter, 1986). The involvement of ascorbate in these reactions would appear to be the basis for its importance to connective tissue, steroid, drug, and endocrine metabolism.

The formation of collagen is especially important during growth and development, when collagen fibers are constantly being laid down and also removed. Once physical maturity is achieved, there is relatively little turnover of collagen itself, one of the few proteins in the body for which this may be said. (Whether this is true for all areas of the body is not clear.) Injury always requires the production of additional connective tissue and collagen fibers (scar tissue). Procollagen is produced on the rough endoplasmic reticulum of connective tissue fibroblasts (Figure 5.21), where microsomal Fe^{2+}-dependent enzymes also hydroxylate specific proline and lysine residues prior to secretion of the protein. In the extracellular space, procollagen is cleaved to tropocollagen and selected lysine residues are oxidized by the Cu enzyme—lysyl oxidase. This allows polymerization and crosslinking to form collagen fibers. Lysyl oxidase is also active in the crosslinking of elastic fibers (elastin) and may have a similar role in maturation of complement factor C1q (England and Seifter, 1986). It is thought that the function of ascorbate here is to reduce enzyme Fe which becomes oxidized to Fe^{3+} rather than to participate directly in the enzymatic reaction or as a factor affecting synthesis of collagen protein per se (England and Seifter, 1986).

Ascorbic acid may have another function in connective tissue metabolism as a carrier for sulfate groups (see Figure 6.2) needed in the formation of glycosaminoglycans (chondroitin sulfate, dermatan sulfate, etc.; Figure 2.7). (These are part of the gel matrix of the "ground substance" between cells in all organs.) There would seem to be an obvious connection between these needs for ascorbic acid in connective tissue metabolism

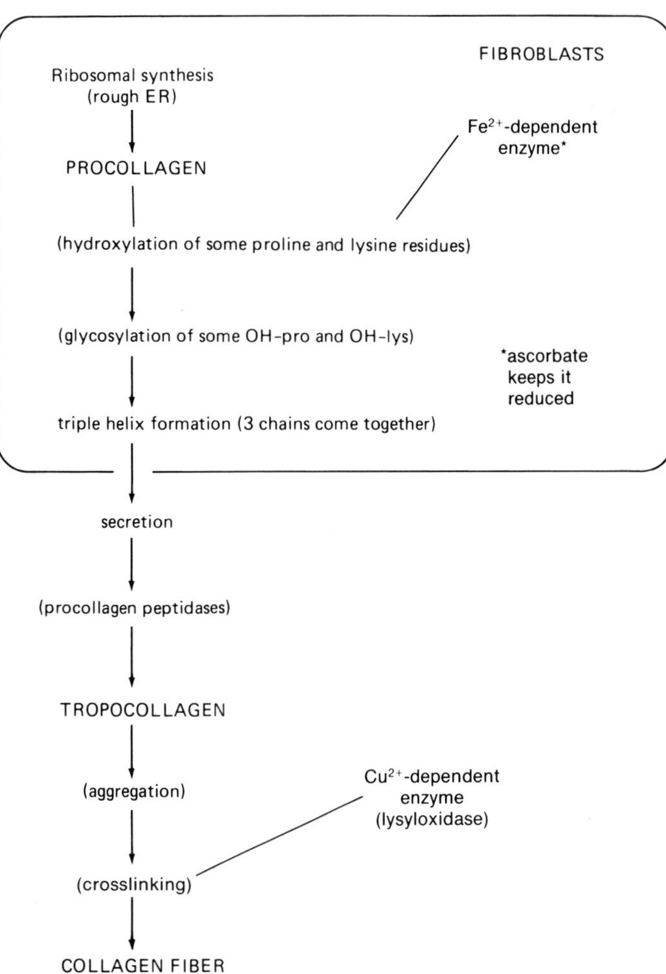

Figure 5.21. Functions of ascorbic acid in collagen production and secretion by fibroblasts. ER, endoplasmic reticulum. [*Source:* adapted from Pott and Gerlach (1980).]

and the symptoms of scurvy: capillary hemorrhage, bleeding and peeling gums, impaired wound healing, and a "dissolving away of ground substance" (Anderson, 1977), although other (still unknown) aspects of ascorbate metabolism may also be involved.

As concerns the microsomal "drug metabolizing" enzymes, where ascorbate may also be active, these are required for the normal inactivation and excretion of steroid hormones, all save the estrogens. The same enzymes are capable of acting on alien synthetic substrates, such as drugs and carcinogens (barbiturates, methylcholanthrene, etc.). The resulting hydroxylation makes them more water soluble and thus more likely to be excreted from the body through the urine. In this regard, it has been shown in rats that exposure to polychlorinated biphenyls (PCBs) greatly increases their need for vitamin C (Kato et al., 1981). The increased need for ascorbic acid in conditions of stress (where glucocorticosteroid synthesis and secretion are enhanced), as well as in users of oral contraceptives [which contain progestogens and/or increase the levels of microsomal hydroxylases (Briggs and Briggs, 1972; McLeroy and Schendel, 1973)], must be related to the role of this vitamin in microsomal hydroxylation reactions (see more below). The microsomal hydroxylation of cholesterol derivatives, on the pathway to bile acid synthesis (the major pathway of bile acid degradation), probably also involves ascorbic acid, as ascorbate deficiency decreases bile acid production in guinea pigs (Orten and Neuhaus, 1975).

Another area of hydroxylation reactions where ascorbate is clearly required is in the synthesis of biogenic amines in the central nervous system and adrenal medulla (Linder, 1991). The highest tissue concentrations of the vitamin, by far, are in these two tissues. The involvement of vitamin C as a cosubstrate in the hydroxylation of dopamine (and perhaps even tyrosine) on the pathway to norepinephrine, and in the adrenal medulla on the pathway to the other catecholamine, epinephrine, is crucial for the normal function of the nervous system, for production/availability of epinephrine in the "fright/flight" mechanism, or more generally, in connection with stress. [The release of epinephrine serves to stimulate the breakdown of glycogen and triglyceride, for an immediate availability of reserve energy. These hormones act through the cAMP–protein kinase system, in target tissues (see Chapters 2 and 3).] Stress or fear can trigger the pituitary–adrenal axis and cause a simultaneous secretion of epinephrine (adrenaline) and vitamin C into the blood circulation. (The degradation of tyrosine via 4-hydroxylphenylpyruvate hydroxylase also requires the services of a reducing agent like ascorbic acid, as may the hydroxylation of tryptophan on the pathway to serotonin production in the brain. Here the involvement of ascorbate is not as clear.) Another cosubstrate role for hormone synthesis in the brain is in the amidation of C-terminal glycine residues, already cited, by a Cu-dependent enzyme also especially present in the neurohypophysis (see Linder, 1991). And recent studies also suggest that ascorbate itself (released with catecholamines) is necessary for the evocation of increased numbers of cell surface acetylcholine receptors by muscle cells responding to nerve stimuli (Horovitz et al., 1989).

Other functions of vitamin C (Figure 5.20) include a role in iron metabolism, especially the enhancement (through chelation) of intestinal iron absorption and transfer into the blood (see Chapter 7). Ascorbate may also be involved in the mobilization of stored iron, especially from hemosiderin, in the spleen. The capacity of this vitamin to chelate calcium may mean it has a function in bone mineral metabolism as well. [Classic animal experiments point to a role in tooth formation (Hodges, 1980).] Also, the vitamin is used up more rapidly in persons smoking tobacco, probably because the smoke contains components that promote oxidation reactions.

A less well-defined molecular action of ascorbic acid may be to suppress the production of fecal mutagens (Bruce, 1983; Dion et al., 1982). Using the Ames test, it has been shown that moderate supplementation of the diet with 120 mg vitamin C markedly reduces the concentration of mutagens in human feces. This was especially so if 50–100 IU of vitamin E was also given (see Chapter 16). Some effects of large doses of vitamin C on the immune system have also been reported (Anderson et al., 1980), specifically the enhanced response of neutrophils to chemotactic stimuli and enhanced proliferation of lymphocytes in response to mitogens. Indeed, leukocytes accumulate high concentrations of ascorbate, and this may prevent autooxidation of the oxygen radical-forming system integral to their function (Anderson and Lukey, 1987), as well as modulate their production of leukotrienes (Steinhilber et al., 1987). The mechanisms of these effects remain to be explained and explored, but may be related to the occasional positive responses of individuals with colds to megavitamin C intake (see below). In this regard, the vitamin appears also to be an antihistamine (Clemetson, 1989; see more below).

Metabolism and Toxicity

Ascorbate is very rapidly and efficiently absorbed from the diet by an energy-dependent process. After absorption, it rapidly equilibrates in intra- and extracellular compartments, although it is concentrated in some specific cells (notably those of the adrenal medulla and neurophypophysis, as well as in leukocytes). Thus, intake of large doses will increase concentrations of the vitamin in tissues as well as blood plasma. One report indicates that absorption of large doses can be markedly diminished by concurrent intake of ethanol (Fazio et al., 1981). The significance of this, if any, remains to be evaluated. Although not widely discussed, there is good evidence of a "ceiling" to absorption of ascorbate when taken in high doses. This has been estimated to be about 3000 mg (per day) in the adult (Rivers, 1987).

As with the B vitamins, ascorbic acid is at least acutely very nontoxic. This has been amply demonstrated through self-experimentation in our population. It does not exclude the possibility that problems may arise in long-term use. Indeed, there is one case in the literature linking iron overload to excessive vitamin intake, and another unpublished case is known to this author. Although iron overload is rare (see Chapter 7), it is a very serious disease. However, long-term studies of individuals taking megadoses of vitamin C suggest there is no general risk of acquiring excess iron (Cook et al., 1984). Thus, it would seem prudent to monitor serum ferritin levels in individuals consuming megadoses of ascorbate (over months and years) only if they are at risk for iron overload (see Chapter 7).

Other areas where excessive C intake can create problems are (a) in the diabetic who relies on at-home urinary glucose tests to determine insulin needs [assays may be off in the false-positive or false-negative direction (Herbert, 1979)]; (b) in assays of serum B_{12} (Herbert et al., 1978); and (c) in patients on certain anticoagulants, such as dicumerol (Herbert, 1979). There may also be some interference with copper absorption or metabolism (Finley and Cerklewski, 1983; see Chapter 7).

On a theoretical basis, there has been concern about increased serum and urinary levels of uric acid (precipitating gout) and increased production of oxalic acid (producing calcium oxalate stones in the kidney and uritogenital systems). However, no cases of gout or stones have as yet materialized that could be ascribed to excessive ascorbate intake even with enormous doses (White, 1981), and except for occasional individuals (who seem to overrespond with oxalate production) or those with a tendency toward oxalate urinary stones, megadoses of C should not be a problem (Rivers, 1987). Nevertheless, the connections between ascorbate and oxalate metabolism are of interest and may require more investigation.

A major pathway of ascorbic acid catabolism is to oxalate (Figure 5.22). It has been estimated that one third to one half of urinary oxalate is derived from ascorbate in normal adults and that 17%–40% of C-1-labeled ascorbate (at normal doses) is excreted as oxalate (Hodgkinson, 1977). Based on studies with monkeys (Tillotson and McGown, 1981), a much lower percentage is converted when there is excessive ascorbate intake (10 versus 0.5–1 mg/kg). The rest is excreted mainly as urinary ascorbic acid; the capacity of kidney tubules for reabsorption saturates at plasma concentrations of 8–9 μg/ml (0.8–0.9 mg/dl) (Rivers, 1987). With excessive intake, intestinal absorption also decreases from 90% to 50% or less (Hodges, 1980; Rivers, 1987) and most is lost in the urine, within 24 hr (Hodges, 1980; Anderson, 1977). In the normal-to-deficient intake range, however, a rather constant 3% is lost per day (Hodges, 1980), and significant portions are lost in the feces and as CO_2.

The latter results and others have been used to estimate at what intake rates blood and tissue "saturation" with vitamin C will normally occur: 45 mg/day (the 1974 U.S. RDA) should maintain a normal 1500 mg body pool (well above the 300 mg cut off for scurvy); intakes of 120 mg (twice the current U.S. RDA) should normally maintain full tissue "saturation" (or a 4000 mg body pool). Others estimate that the "saturable" pool is much smaller (20 mg/kg body weight; Rivers, 1987), and that a maximum of about 3000 mg can be absorbed per day by the average adult (see above). Individuals will vary in their metabolism. Presumably, the excess vitamin is rapidly unloaded; indeed, it is difficult to raise blood levels beyond a certain point even with very large doses (Figure 5.23). Concern that sudden cessation of megadosing, after the body has adjusted to the high intake, could result in a precipitous fall of serum (and leukocyte) ascorbate concentrations (Figure 5.23) and even produce scurvylike symptoms may be without experimental foundation (Rivers, 1987).

Vitamin C, the Common Cold, and the Immune Response

Ever since Nobel Laureate, Linus Pauling, first launched his campaign for the use of high doses of ascorbic acid to combat the common cold, there has been much public interest in this idea, and numerous investigative studies have been launched. In the early ones, groups of individuals, usually in institutions like boarding schools, were/were not supplemented with relatively small daily doses (100–200 mg). More recently, in response to Pauling's criticism, experimental protocols have called for supplementation with 1–2 g/day (Table 5.6). Overall, these studies do not show that vitamin C has a clear-cut and consistent effect on either cold prevention and/or duration. The success rate for high doses of vitamin C does not appear to be any better than for the lower doses. Some studies were entirely negative, others showed overall statistically significant changes in cold incidence or duration of 15%–30%. Results from a sampling of well-controlled studies are shown in Table 5.6.

Susceptibility to viral infections, such as colds, must involve many other factors, including initial vitamin status (Anderson, 1977). Thus, intake of increased amounts of vitamin C will not predictably be of any help. On the other hand, it would appear that under certain conditions, some individuals do respond favorably to increased vitamin C intake. A favorable response may be related to effects of ascorbic acid on the immune

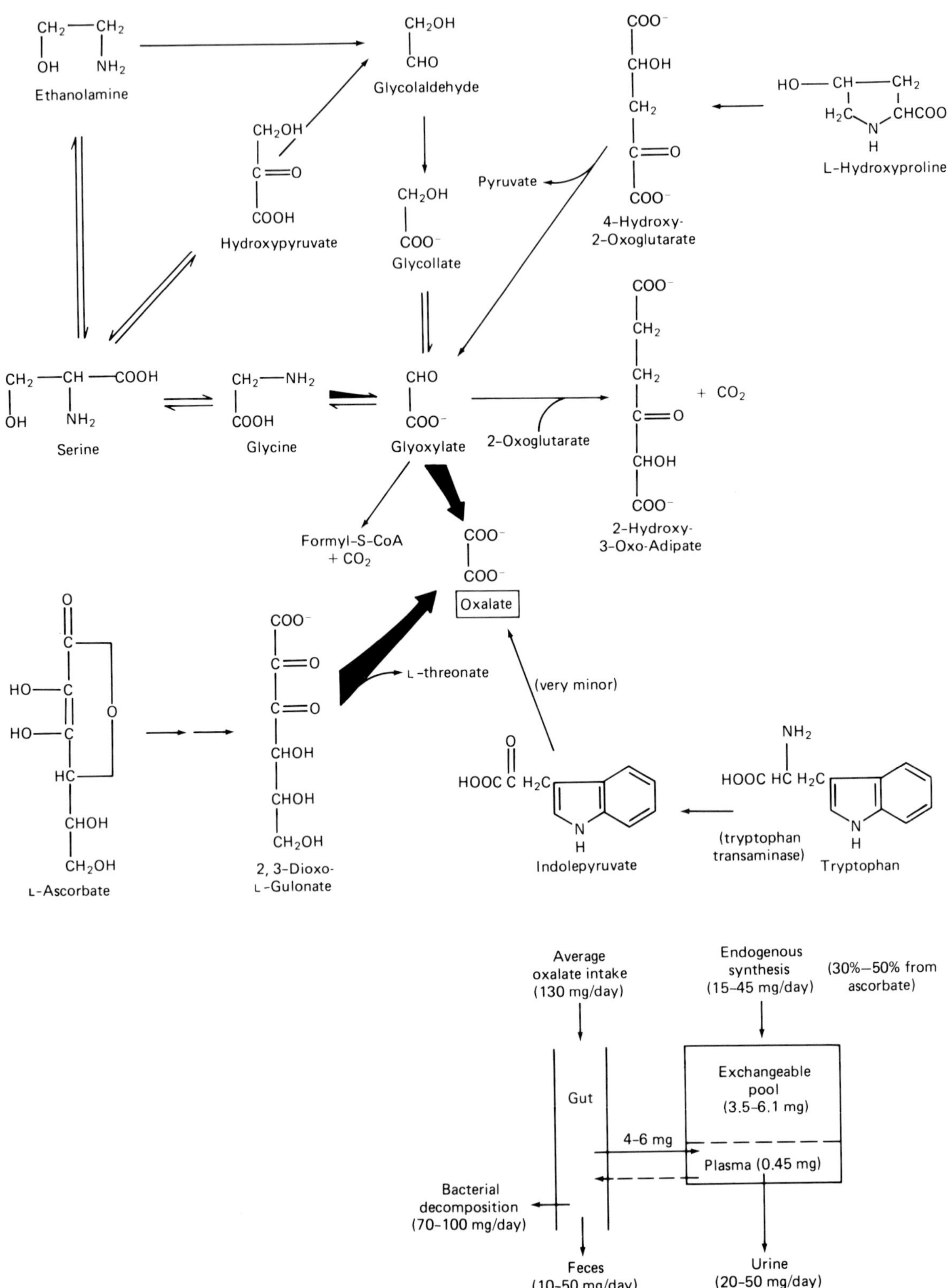

Figure 5.22. Oxalic acid production and balance in humans. [*Source:* After Hodgkinson (1977).]

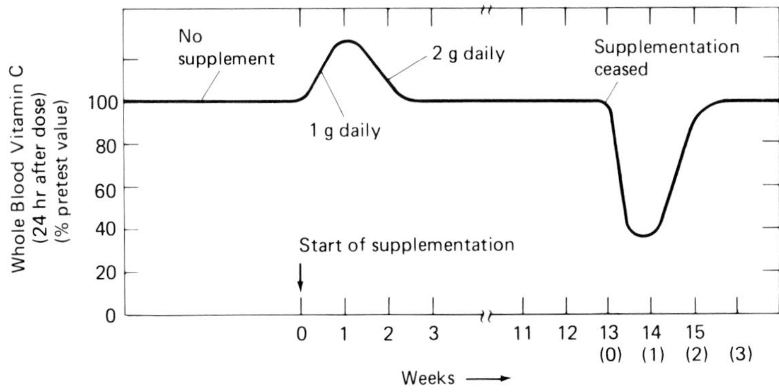

Figure 5.23. The effect of megadoses of ascorbic acid on resting blood vitamin levels. [*Source:* Modified from Anderson (1977).]

system and leukocyte function, previously mentioned (Anderson et al., 1980).

In only a few studies has the effect of increasing C intake upon onset of illness been tested (therapeutic versus prophylactic treatment; Table 5.6). Moreover, very few have recorded information on cold severity and the number of days a person stays home from work (disability). This was examined in a series of studies by Anderson et al. (Table 5.6). In the first and third of these studies there were marked, highly significant, 20%–30% reductions in disability when individuals took increased doses of C (versus placebo) at the onset of and during the illness. Specifically, in the first study, patients went from 1 to 4 g/day; in the third, from 500 mg once a week, to 1500 mg and 1000 mg per day. Anderson concludes that the main effect is on the "malaise" that accompanies the illness (Anderson, 1977). This may well be the result of the antihistamine effect of the vitamin, since Clemetson (1980) has shown (a) an inverse relation between blood ascorbate and histamine concentrations, (b) that histaminemia (elevated blood histamine) occurs in ascorbate deficiency, and (c) that doses of 1 g/day dramatically lower blood histamine levels. With high doses of C, there is also a depression of 5-lipoxygenase activity and less production of LTB_4 (leukotriene B_4) (Steinhilber et al., 1987). [LTB_4 produced from arachidonic acid and other eicosanoid fatty acids is involved in the inflammatory response (see Chapters 3 and 15).] More of these kinds of studies are necessary to fully assess these matters.

Other investigators have shown that, upon onset of a cold, blood leukocyte ascorbate levels fall (Figure 5.24) and that only high doses are able to restore them before the illness is overcome. Leukocyte ascorbate levels are commonly used as an index of ascorbate status and may or may not be useful in this regard (Hodges, 1980) (see Chapter 13). Various (often contradictory) effects of ascorbate status on cellular immunity and leukocyte function have been reported (Anderson et al., 1980; see above), including inhibition of bacteriocidal action at high doses (Shilotri and Bhat, 1977), increased neutrophil activity in response to endotoxin (Anderson et al., 1980), better maintenance of oxygen radical production (Anderson and Lukey, 1987), and a better functioning of complement C1 (England and Seifter, 1986; Ramachandran, 1978). An inhibition of bronchial constriction by high levels of ascorbate (perhaps via reduction of histamine release) would also ameliorate the symptoms of upper respiratory infection, asthma, or exposure to oxidants, such as ozone (Chatham et al., 1987; Mohsenin and DuBois, 1987). The mechanisms of these effects are still unknown, although eicosanoids could be involved.

In his book, *Vitamin C and the Common Cold*, Pauling (1970) gives other reasons for favoring a greatly increased intake of vitamin C. Rats, he says, produce 25–58 mg ascorbate/kg body weight/day. Extrapolated to a 70-kg human, this would mean 2–4 g. This argument fails to take into consideration the relative metabolic rates and lifespans of the rat and the human, the exact ratios of which are difficult to define, but probably lie somewhere between 10 and 30. A linear extrapolation from rodent experiments, based on body weight, will thus give a very exaggerated value for human intake. Pauling also explains that gorillas (which of course are much more like the human) eat about 4.5 g ascorbate/day in their natural habitat. However, just because these vegetarian animals eat so much ascorbate does not mean that they need it. [Indeed, there may be a 3 g

Table 5.6. Effect of Vitamin C on Upper Respiratory Illness[a]

Reference	Total cases	Study duration	Dose of ascorbate (g/day)	
			Prophylactic	Therapeutic
Anderson et al. (1972)	818 (adults)	3–4 months	1	4 (3 days)
Anderson et al. (1974)	3520 (adults)	3 months	0.25–1.0	4–5 (1 day)
Anderson et al. (1975)	622 (adults)	3.5 months	0.5	1–1.5 (4 days)
Coulehan et al. (1974)	644 (children)	3.5 months	1–2	—
Coulehan et al. (1976)	868 (children)	3.5 months	1	—
Karlowski et al. (1975)	311 (adults)	9 months	1	3 (1 day)
Miller et al. (1977)	88 (children twins)	5 months	0.5–1.0	—
Pitt and Costrini (1979)	674 (adults)	2 months	2	—

[a] The above studies were double-blind. NS = statistical difference is not significant ($p > 0.05$).

"ceiling" to ascorbate absorption (Rivers, 1987).] An additional, perhaps more persuasive argument for increased intake is suggested by studies with rats in which cold exposure resulted in increased ascorbate synthesis.

Figure 5.24. Leukocyte ascorbic acid levels during cold illness, with and without ascorbate supplementation. [Source: Anderson (1977). Reprinted by permission from Nutrition Today magazine, P.O. Box 1829, Annapolis, MD 21404. January/February 1977.]

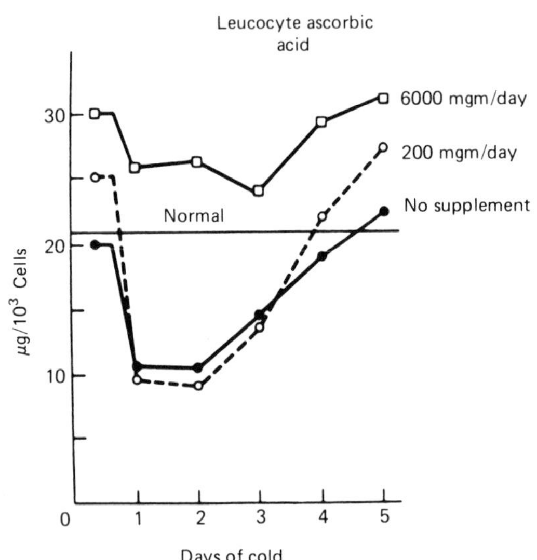

Vitamin C Intake and Other Diseases

Three epidemiologic studies, one in 1955, the others more recent, have indicated a higher incidence of atherosclerosis and heart disease in persons consuming less than versus more than 50 mg ascorbate/day (see Gey et al., 1987; Knox, 1973; Krumdieck and Butterworth, 1974). In another report (Ramirez and Flowers, 1980), 150 patients with proven cardiac atherosclerosis were found to have significantly lower leukocyte levels of ascorbic acid (averaging less than 50%) as compared to controls without coronary artery disease. This was true both for patients who smoked and for those who did not. There has also been some evidence that massive doses of the vitamin may lower serum cholesterol (Hodges, 1980; Spittle, 1971), especially in cardiac patients (Anderson, 1977), perhaps through a stimulation of cholesterol conversion to bile acids (see above). Other studies have failed to confirm, and sometimes even contradict, this idea (Anderson, 1977; Hodges, 1980). The relationship between vitamin C and atherosclerosis thus remains unclear.

The original studies that were carried out on cancer patients, with massive intakes (10 g/day) of ascorbate, suggested that this treatment prolongs the life of terminal patients with all kinds of cancer two- to sevenfold (Cameron and Pauling, 1978; see Chapter 16). However, the studies suffered from the serious drawback of a lack of con-

Table 5.6 *(continued)*

Change with ascorbate (%)		
Incidence	Duration	Other
7% ↓	12% ↓	30% ↓ (days at home)
NS	NS	$p < 0.001$
0%–10% ↓	0%–11% ↓	10%–20% ↓ (days at home) (5 g)
NS	NS	0%–10% ↓ (days at home) (4 g)
3%–8% ↓	7%–9% ↓	25% ↓ (days at home)
NS	NS	$p < 0.05$
0%	28%–32% ↓	—
	$p < 0.001$	
0%	43% ↑	—
	$p < 0.05$	
19% ↓	6% ↓	17% ↓ (duration, with therapeutic dose)
NS	NS	($p < 0.001$)
0%	1% ↓	0% days in bed
	NS	
0%	2% ↓	Colds "less severe"
	NS	

trols with no placebo treatment. Moreover, double blind repetitions of such studies, at the Mayo Clinic, failed to show a specific ascorbate (versus placebo) effect. (See Chapter 16 for further details and other aspects.)

Other health effects involving vitamin C may include a deficiency in leukocyte ascorbate concentrations in diabetics, leading to a decreased capacity for wound repair and response to infection (Pecoraro and Chen, 1987). It has been speculated that this could arise from increased competition for entry through a membrane transport system shared by glucose. A propensity of cataracts to form may also be linked to low ascorbate (and vitamin E) availability (Lohmann, 1987; Varma, 1987), perhaps from a relative lack of reducing equivalents. In general, exposure to oxidizing agents (including cigarette smoke; Keith and Mossholder, 1986) in the diet or air, remains a factor in determining ascorbate status and has been recognized as such in setting the new U.S. RDAs for this vitamin.

Consumption and Requirements

Over the past 80 years, and especially since 1939, there has been a marked reduction in the consumption of fresh fruits and vegetables by Americans (Labuza and Sloan, 1979), amounting to about 50% and 30%, respectively. Nevertheless, the estimated average daily intake of vitamin C is in the 80–100-mg range based on "market basket" surveys by the USDA (National Research Council, 1989). On the basis that averages are meaningless where the individual is concerned, a large percentage of the American population is consuming amounts of the vitamin well below the present U.S. RDA of 60 mg. It should be noted that this RDA value has been among the most controversial and most debated by the NRC, for reasons that should be apparent from the preceding sections. With some possible exceptions, the controversy is over intakes in the low (30–120 mg) range, and not over the use of megadoses. One of the problems has been to define symptoms of deficiency other than by the extreme symptoms of scurvy. It is fair to say that a number of factors may increase our requirements for the vitamin to above 60 mg/day, including smoking, the use of oral contraceptives, and wound healing. This has been recognized in the current U.S. RDA requirements (Figure 5.20). The most concentrated sources of the vitamin are citrus fruits, rose hips, black currents, cranberries, broccoli, Brussels sprouts, kale, and collard and turnip greens. Good sources also are other members of the cabbage family, beet greens, strawberries, and watercress; even potatoes contain sufficient C to prevent scurvy. The vitamin is quite unstable at neutral or alkaline pH, especially upon heat exposure (see Chapter

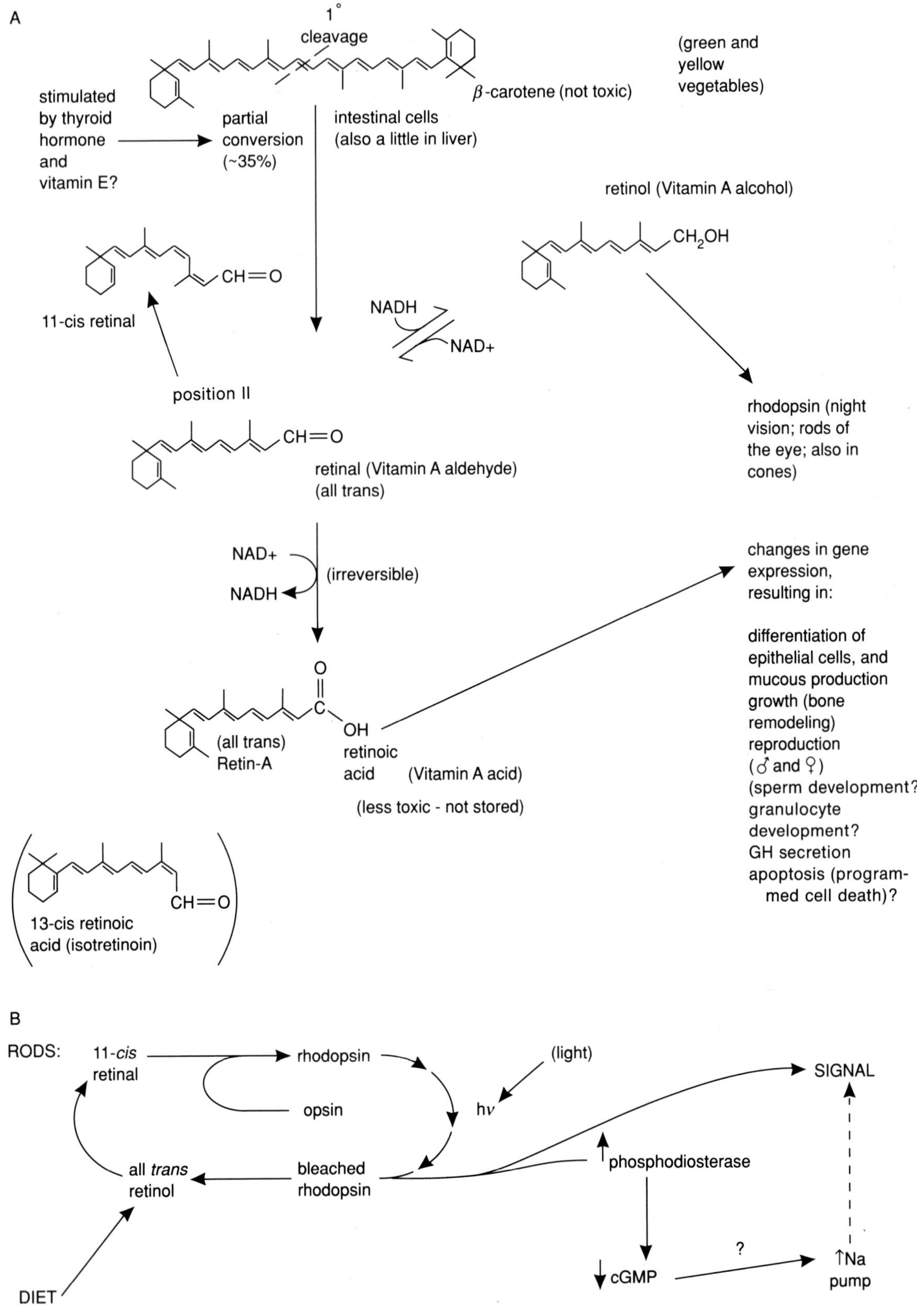

A
1°
cleavage
β-carotene (not toxic)
(green and yellow vegetables)
stimulated by thyroid hormone and vitamin E?
partial conversion (~35%)
intestinal cells (also a little in liver)
retinol (Vitamin A alcohol)
CH2OH
CH=O
11-cis retinal
NADH
NAD+
position II
rhodopsin (night vision; rods of the eye; also in cones)
CH=O
retinal (Vitamin A aldehyde) (all trans)
NAD+
NADH
(irreversible)
changes in gene expression, resulting in:
differentiation of epithelial cells, and mucous production
growth (bone remodeling)
reproduction (♂ and ♀)
(sperm development?)
granulocyte development?
GH secretion
apoptosis (programmed cell death)?
O
C
OH
(all trans) Retin-A
retinoic acid
(Vitamin A acid)
(less toxic - not stored)
CH=O
13-cis retinoic acid (isotretinoin)
B
RODS:
11-cis retinal
rhodopsin
opsin
(light)
hν
SIGNAL
all trans retinol
bleached rhodopsin
↑phosphodiosterase
DIET
↓cGMP
?
↑Na pump

10), but it is quite stable in acid (as in many juices) and fairly stable during its temporary cool storage in fresh produce.

Vitamin A

History and Structure

In 1909, Strepp recognized that egg yolk contained a fat-soluble material essential for life. In 1919, this material, as well as that extracted from animal fats and fish oil by McCollum, was named fat-soluble "A" by the latter (McCollum et al., 1922) and, in 1920, "vitamin A" by Drummond (Pawson, 1981). The alcohol form of the vitamin was purified and its structure proposed by Karrer et al. in Basel, Switzerland, in 1931; synthesis was accomplished in 1947 at the pharmaceutical firm of Hoffmann-La Roche (also in Basel). The plant form of this vitamin, β-carotene, isolated 100 years earlier, was shown by Steenbock to have high vitamin A activity in 1919, and in the mid-1930s, Wald made his electrifying discoveries of the direct molecular role of this vitamin in the visual process (for which he received the Nobel Prize in 1967).

Vitamin A exists in three oxidation states (the alcohol, aldehyde, and acid), which are thought to carry out its various functions; these are retinol, retinal, and retinoic acid (Figure 5.25). β-Carotene contains the carbons and ring structure for two molecules of the vitamin and is cleaved to the vitamin mainly by the intestine during its absorption. [Other less active carotenoids are also present in foods (see below).] As a group, the various forms of vitamin A, as well as synthetic analogs and metabolites, are called retinoids, stemming from the importance of the vitamin to the retina. In metabolism, *cis* and *trans* forms may have different roles (e.g., the 11-*cis* and all-*trans*; see below). In the mammalian organism, interconversion of retinol and retinal occurs, but oxidation of the aldehyde to retinoic acid is an irreversible process (Figure 5.25).

Figure 5.25. Vitamin A.

Functions: Structural: vision. Humoral: epithelial cell differentiation and mucous production; fertility; bone growth (reshaping); certain functions in other cells.

Requirements: 800 (women), 1000 (men) μg retinol equivalents (= 4–5000 IU) (1 retinol equivalent = 6 μg carotene); increased requirements during pregnancy and hypothyroidism (?).

Deficiency: affects epithelia, night vision, growth, and fertility (atrophy of gonads); keratinization.

Toxicity: occurs with prolonged high dosing (20–30 × RDA).

Storage: yes; up to 1 year's supply.

Functions

The functions of this vitamin have been under intensive study in recent years, and this has lead to considerable information on its modes of action. There are four main areas of involvement (Figure 5.25): vision, differentiation of epithelial cells, growth, and reproduction. The main role of vitamin A in vision revolves around the fact that the rods of the eye contain membranous discs consisting of lipid that is embedded primarily with the ~30,000 dalton protein, opsin. This protein combines with 11-*cis* retinaldehyde to form rhodopsin (visual purple), the direct recipient of light energy during vision in dim light (noncolored, gray-black vision). Many of the steps leading from "activation" of rhodopsin by light to the visual signal in the brain via the optic nerve have now been elucidated. When light strikes, the 11-*cis* retinal part of rhodopsin is isomerized and reduced to all-*trans* retinol, and released (Figure 5.25, bottom). This triggers a decrease in the permeability of rod cell membranes to Na^+, which results in increased polarization and thus a nerve impulse to the brain (Metzler, 1977; Stryer, 1987). The impulse to close multiple Na^+ channels (obtainable with a single photon of light) occurs via activation of "transducin" [a GTP-binding ("G") protein] which, in turn, activates a phosphodiesterase that cleaves cGMP in the cytosol. (cGMP keeps Na^+ channels open.) After the all-*trans* retinol is split off (Figure 5.25), a few seconds are required for spontaneous recombination of opsin with the 11-*cis* aldehyde (formed from all-*trans* retinol or retinol-ester). Most of the vitamin is recycled, although a small portion must be replaced daily. The cones of the eyes, used in normal (colored) vision also contain some retinaldehyde, combined with "cone opsin" to form porphyropsins, which absorb light of lower energy (Metzler, 1977). Similar steps may be involved in this process. However, vitamin A deficiency has a much more marked effect on night vision, and a diminution of this capacity is one of the first symptoms of deficiency.

In contrast to the "structural" roles of vitamin A in visual excitation is its apparently humoral role in other physiologic functions, especially in epithelial, osteoid (bone), and gonadal tissues.

This accounts for its maintenance of epithelial cell differentiation and mucous production, and its roles in bone remodeling during growth and in support of male and female fertility. Roles in myeloid cell differentiation (to granular leukocytes) and macrophage activity are also apparent (see below). Retinoic acid appears to be the active (or most active) agent in these effects, although retinol has not been excluded as a slower-acting (or delivery) form of the vitamin/hormone. Several distinct carrier proteins and receptors are involved. Mechanisms of action are under active study and suggest the following sequence of events (Figure 5.26): retinol, retinol-ester, and/or retinoic acid enter the cell and either bind to specific carrier proteins found in most tissues (Chytil and Ong, 1987) or (in the case of retinoic acid) to a specific receptor which belongs to the thyroid and glucocorticoid hormone receptor family (Umesono et al., 1988). These proteins carry the hormone-vitamin to the nucleus, where they activate transcription of specific proteins through effects on the promoter regions of their genes. In the case of retinoids delivered to the nucleus by cellular retinol and retinoic acid-binding proteins (CRBP and CRABP), the hormone-vitamin is transferred to another/other (receptor) protein(s) to cause gene activation. In the case of retinoic acid bound to its hormone receptor, this complex itself becomes associated with the DNA.

It is of great interest that the complex of thyroid hormone (triiodothyronine; T_3) with its receptor will bind to the same promoter regions of some of the same genes (Bedo et al., 1989). The production of certain proteins is thus under dual control by vitamin A and T_3. In this connection it is also of interest that plasma retinol (bound to RBP, see below) is carried by transthyretin (TTR), the protein that carries thyroid hormone, although the two hormones are independently regulated.

It seems likely that some (or even most) of the retinoic acid that acts on gene transcription arrives as retinol (on RBP) and is oxidized to retinoic acid in the target cells, before binding to its receptor and acting in the nucleus. How the vitamin-hormone forms are delivered to cells still has not been completely worked out, although retinol (on RPB-TTR) and retinoic acid (on albumin) may enter via membrane receptors (Chytil and Ong, 1987). [Apparently the retinol-ester in chylomicron remnants is also capable of entering some cells (Wathne et al., 1988). This would probably occur by diffusion, since only hepatocytes have "remnant" receptors (see Chapter 3).]

As concerns specific functions, it has been known for a long time that deficiency of the vitamin leads to a reduction in mucous-secreting cells and a replacement of columnar epithelial cells by thick layers of horny, stratified epithelium in many parts of the body (Lui and Roels, 1980). This includes keratinization of the corneal epithelium, lung, skin, and intestinal mucosa, and a drastic reduction in goblet cells within the intestinal crypts and villus surfaces. The rates of columnar cell proliferation and migration along the villus are not altered (Olson et al., 1981), but the synthesis of specific glycoproteins and protein glycosylation in the intestinal mucosa and in liver can be markedly depressed (Chan and Wolf, 1987; DeLuca et al., 1969). In cultured cells of many kinds, effects on morphology, cell adhesion, and growth rate are observed, as well as a modulation of the forms of glycosaminoglycan produced (DeLuca and Shapiro, 1981). These various changes may be partly explained by a dependence on vitamin A for gene expression of glycosyltransferases (Chan and Wolf, 1987) and fibronectin (Kim and Wolf, 1987), possibly even transglutaminases (see below). [Excluding effects on reproduction and vision, the retinoic acid form of A would appear to be able to support all/almost all of the A functions (Dowling and Wald, 1960).]

A third functional area for vitamin A is in growth, specifically in modulating the growth of bones through remodeling. Vitamin A is essential for the activity of cells in the epiphyseal cartilage, which must undergo a normal cycle of growth, maturation, and degeneration to permit normal bone growth, which is controlled at the epiphyses (Shaw and Sweeney, 1980). (In deficiency, bone resorption is retarded, although there is no defect in the normal calcification process.) The mechanism may involve control of 1,25-dihydroxy vitamin D receptors on the surface of osteoclasts (which demineralize the bone) (Petkovich et al., 1984). [Vitamin *D* is also necessary for demineralization (see below).]

Another function of retinoic acid, with potentially wide-ranging consequences, is as an inducer of transglutaminases. These enzymes catalyze the crosslinking of proteins by amidating the γ-carboxyl group of a glutamate residue with an ε-amino group of lysine (or spermine, spermidine, etc.). This reaction is thought to be necessary for macrophage function, blood clotting, and cell adhesion and also in apoptosis (or programmed cell death) which may be the mechanism by which most adult tissues and organs

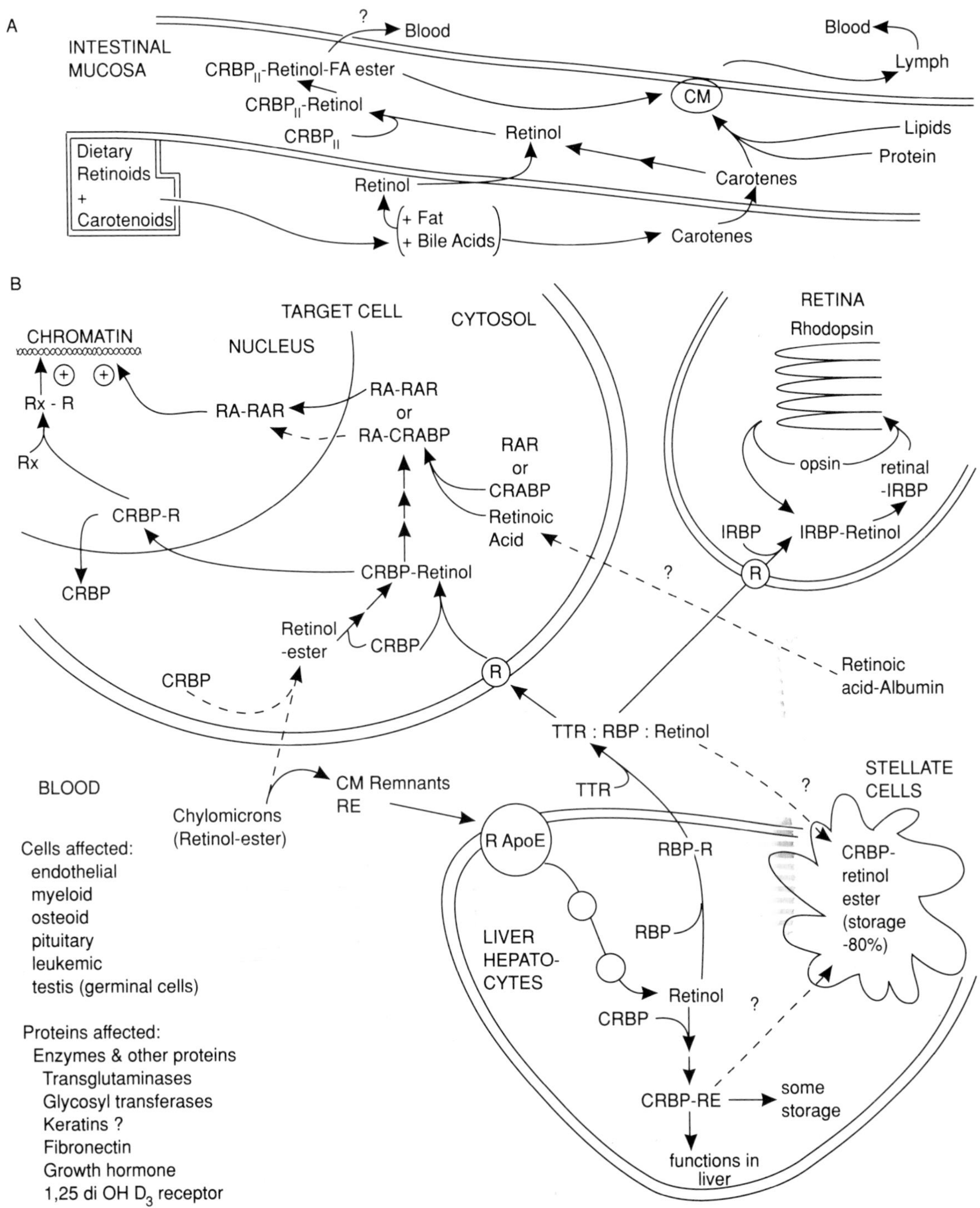

Figure 5.26. Mechanism of vitamin A absorption and hormone action. **(A)** Processing of retinol and carotenes during intestinal absorption. **(B)** Retinoid binding proteins in liver and other tissues, involved in storage and transport of retinoids; action of retinoic acid (and perhaps other retinoids) on cells via increased gene transcription, following binding to receptors and promoter regions of specific genes. *Key:* RBP, retinol binding protein; CRBP, cellular retinol binding protein; CRABP, cellular retinoic acid binding protein; Rx, retinoid receptor (form of vitamin unknown); RAR, retinol (or retinoid) receptor; IBRP, retinoid binding protein in retina; CM, chylomicrons; RApoE, receptor for CM remnants; TTR, transthyretin; +, stimulates transcription.

maintain a constant cell number (Davies, 1989). It has been studied most extensively in macrophages in connection with the soluble cytosolic transglutaminase (Chiocca et al., 1988).

Finally, vitamin A (acid and/or alcohol) plays a role in fertility. In vitamin A deficiency, spermatogenesis is arrested at the spermatid stage in rats, chickens, and cattle and is reversed with vitamin treatment. Deficiency also interferes with the estrus cycle, placental development, and other aspects of female reproduction in the rat and chick, causing fetal resorption. [For further review, see Wolf (1980) and Goodman (1984).] Little is known about the molecular events involved except that retinoic acid acts on gene transcription in the nucleus of germinal cells of the testis and that CRBP is present in high concentrations in the epididymus (Chytil and Ong, 1987). Evidence from several animal studies also suggests a role in the formation of adrenal progesterone (and androgen derivatives) from pregnenolone (Grongaud et al., 1969) (and cholesterol). Progesterone is the precursor steroid hormone from which all other steroids are synthesized, including androgens and estrogens (see Figure 5.29, p. 162). There are favorable effects of β-carotene feeding on fertility of cattle, and the corpus luteum may store and cleave this vitamin A precursor in connection with luteal function (Sklan, 1983).

Absorption, Metabolism, and Excretion

Dietary vitamin A is ingested mainly in the form of its β-carotene precursor, or as retinol, from plant and animal foods, respectively. [Plant foods also contain many other carotenoids, only some of which have provitamin activity (see below).] Efficient absorption, especially of β-carotene, requires release from endogenous proteins, or deesterification, and the presence of other dietary fats and secreted bile acids (Figure 5.27). Within the intestine (but also a little in the liver), a portion of the β-carotene is split into two retinal units (and perhaps also into retinoids with longer side chains; Figure 5.28), and these are incorporated into chylomicrons for transport to the liver (and other organs), via the lymph and blood. The remaining carotenes are also transported this way and eventually delivered to adipose cells via chylomicrons, very low-density lipoproteins and low-density lipoproteins (Blomhoff, 1987). While in mucosal cells, retinol is bound to a special binding protein (CRBPII; Figure 5.26B). There is a limit to the convertibility of β-carotene to vitamin A. Excessive carotene intake appears to have no serious consequences, whereas excessive retinol or retinol intake is quite toxic. Serum carotene levels are highly variable and generally reflect recent intake, while retinol concentrations are determined by the rate of liver secretion and are maintained at a fairly constant level except in deficiency or toxicity (Figure 5.27). Excess vitamin A absorbed is stored mostly as palmityl (and some other) fatty acid esters of retinol, in the liver; excess carotene is stored in fatty tissues. Of recent interest is the finding that with normal or excess intake, most liver retinol is not stored in hepatocytes but rather in adjacent stellate cells in the space of Disse (Blomhoff, 1987). [This is not the case, however, when liver reserves are low (Batres and Olson, 1987).] The manner by which transfer occurs between these cells is still unknown but could involve RBP.

For secretion into the plasma from the liver, retinol (or other retinoids) combine with RBP which is synthesized there (Figure 5.27). (Zinc and an adequate intake of protein are required for normal production of RBP. Thus, a deficiency of zinc or protein malnutrition will interfere with vitamin A function by preventing its normal rate of release from liver stores.) Upon leaving the liver, vitamin A–RBP forms a 1 : 1 complex with TTR (also previously known as "prealbumin") in the plasma, presumably to prevent loss of the vitamin through glomerular filtration. This complex transports the vitamin to its various target cells, where a receptor on the cell surface mediates its uptake and transfer to intracellular RBPs (Goodman, 1981). Some retinoic acid may also enter from albumin, and some retinol from chylomicron remnants (presumably by diffusion; see above).

Oxidation of retinol to retinaldehyde requires NAD^+ and is reversible. The second step, to retinoic acid, is not reversible in animal tissues. Thus, only the intake of retinol or retinal (or precursors) results in storage of the vitamin. Retinoic acid has a rapid turnover, and a number of its metabolites have been isolated from bile and urine, including the 5,6-epoxide, 4-hydroxy, 4-oxo, and more polar derivatives (which may have additional hydroxylations and/or side chain cleavage) (DeLuca and Shapiro, 1981; Roberts, 1981). These are not thought to possess significant biologic activity (DeLuca and Shapiro, 1981; DeLuca et al., 1981). In the human, the excretion is probably 2 : 1 via the bile versus the urine, based on studies with the close analog of retinoic acid, etretine (Paravicini et al., 1981). At least in the rat, only a small proportion of the biliary excretion is as glucuronide derivatives (DeLuca et

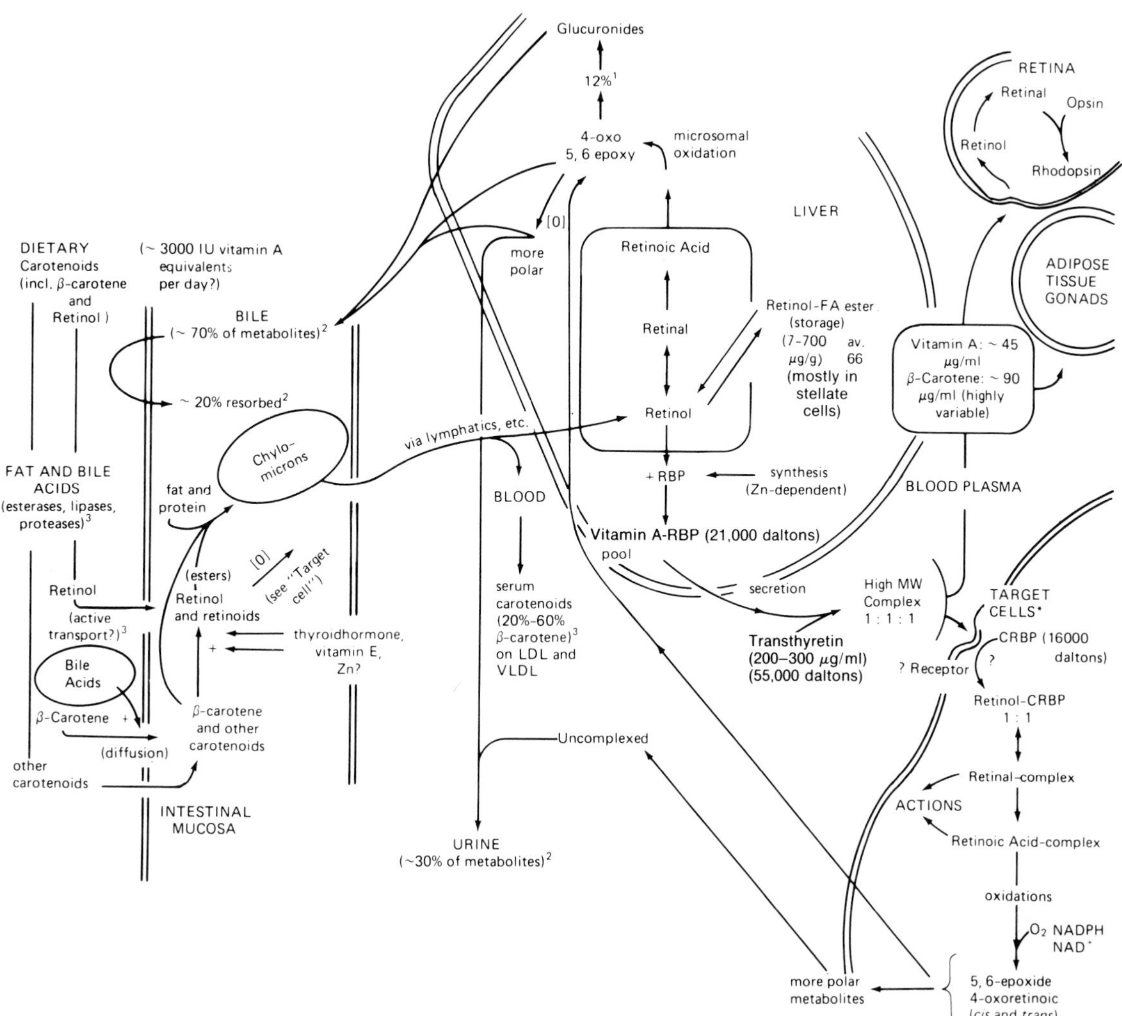

Figure 5.27. Nutrition and metabolism of vitamin A: Overview. Dietary vitamin A (and carotenoids) (left) are absorbed into the intestinal mucosa with the help of bile acids. Here, some of the retinol is oxidized and utilized locally, and the rest is transported to the liver, after incorporation into CM. (Some carotene is split to retinol in the intestine, a process regulated in part by thyroid hormone and other factors. Other aspects of the fate of carotenoids are described in another section.) Most vitamin A is stored in the liver, mainly in stellate cells, after esterification with palmitate in hepatocytes. A certain proportion is released from the liver attached to RBP, and combines with plasma TTR (formerly known as prealbumin) for circulation and distribution to target cells: retina, epithelia, kidney, intestine, liver, gonads, etc. In the retina the vitamin becomes part of rhodopsin, involved in vision; in other cells, it combines with CRBP and as such (or after oxidation to retinoic acid, bound to CRABP) fulfills its hormone actions via effects on transcription of specific genes (see Figure 5.26). Inactivation of the vitamin-hormone occurs by further oxidation, and the metabolites are ultimately transported to the liver and lost mainly through the bile. Footnotes: [1]DeLuca et al. (1969). [2]Based on studies with etretine (Bollag and Matter, 1981). [3]Simpson and Chichester (1981). [4]Rodriguez and Irwin (1972). Other references: Roberts (1981), Frolik (1981), Goodman (1981), Blomhoff (1990).

al., 1981). About 20% of the material lost in the bile would appear to be reabsorbed (Paravicini et al., 1981) (including any retinyl or retinoyl glucuronides).

Excess β-carotene that is not converted to retinol has a different pattern of tissue accumulation and toxicity than does vitamin A, with the largest portion being stored in adipocytes all over the body. In man, this accounts for the yellowish tint of fatty tissue layers. It is hypothesized that β-carotene is slowly lost from tissues and body fluids via the bile.

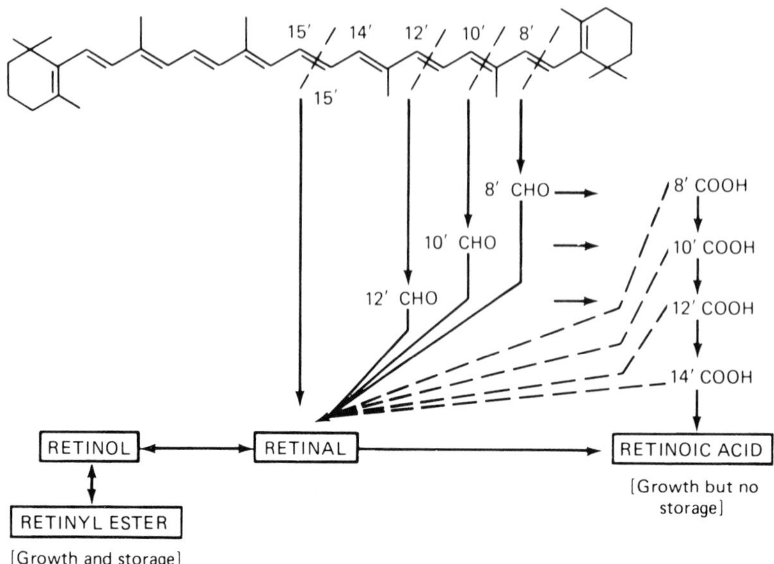

Figure 5.28. Conversion of β-carotene to retinol: possible mechanisms. [*Source:* Reprinted with permission from the Annual Review of Nutrition, Volume 1. © 1981 by Annual Reviews Inc.]

Requirements and Toxicity

As vitamin A is ingested in two main forms, the requirement is calculated on the basis of retinol equivalents, and is 4000/5000 IU (or 800/1000 μg) of retinol for women/men, respectively (Figure 5.25). An additional 1000 IU is recommended during pregnancy and lactation. Estimates vary on the amounts of β-carotene that are equivalent to retinol (see below). The rates of conversion to retinol depend, in part, on thyroid hormone, Zn, Fe, and vitamin E status (Figure 5.27) (see below).

The toxicity of retinol and retinal is well known, although only occasional cases of hypervitaminosis are encountered. These are usually among persons who have ingested megadoses of vitamins in general, or among patients who have received large doses over long periods of time in the treatment of dermatological disorders. It is thought that the toxic symptoms (skin erythema and desquamation, increased liver size, abdominal pain, nausea, headache, and appetite loss) result from damage to membranes of liver and various other cells by free retinol, present in amounts above those which can be bound by RBPs (Roberts, 1981). The lysosomal membranes of the liver would appear to be especially affected (Roels, 1967), resulting in increased lysosome fragility. (How all this relates to stellate cells has not been explored.)

There is also a positive association between excessive intake of vitamin A (18,000 IU+) in early pregnancy and the development of birth defects (Olson, 1990) that may be related to the special sensitivity of cells of the neural crest to excess retinol. Retinoic acid, which is not stored, is less toxic than retinol and retinal, but not without serious bone effects when taken in large doses over time (Pittsley and Yoder, 1983).

Food Sources, Consumption, and Deficiency

Vitamin A is present in provitamin carotenoid forms, principally as β-carotene, in most plant and vegetable foods, and mainly as retinal (esters) in foods of animal, bird, and fish origin. Carotenoids are perhaps the most prevalent pigments in the plant kingdom and are also responsible for the red-pink colors of salmon flesh, lobster shells, and flamingo feathers. Only some of these carotenoids possess provitamin A activity (Table 5.7).

There is considerable confusion about the actual provitamin A content of vegetables and fruits and about the degree to which the provitamins are converted to active derivatives in the gut and elsewhere. The first reflects methodological problems in assaying α- and β-carotenes; more recent HPLC procedures give values that are up to 17 times lower than those of the old AOAC assay (Simpson and Chichester, 1981). Consequently,

Table 5.7. Food Carotenoids with Provitamin A Activity

Carotenoid	Structure	Relative pro-A activity (%)
β-Carotene	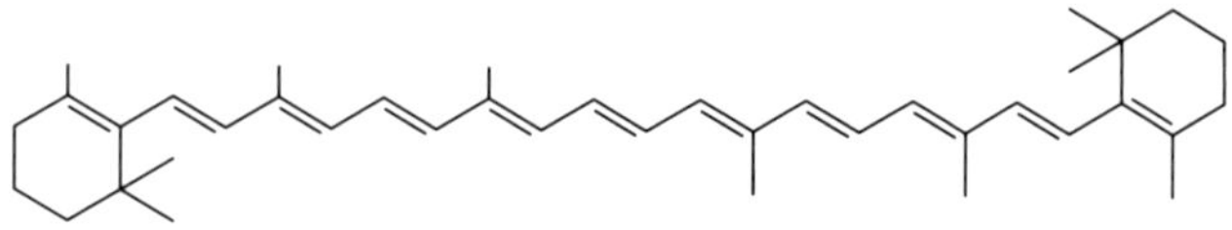	100
α-Carotene	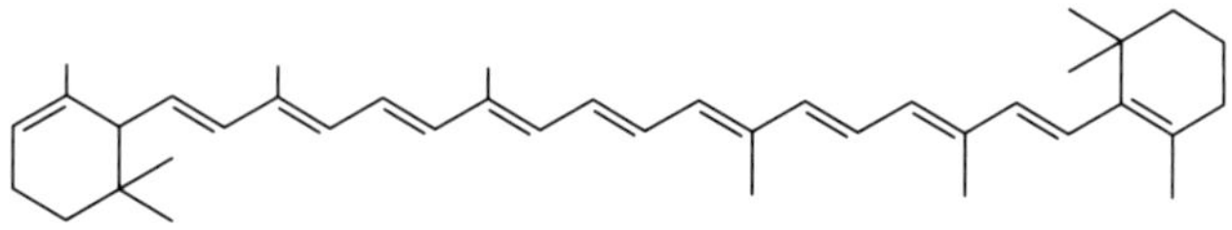	50 – 54[a]
γ-Carotene	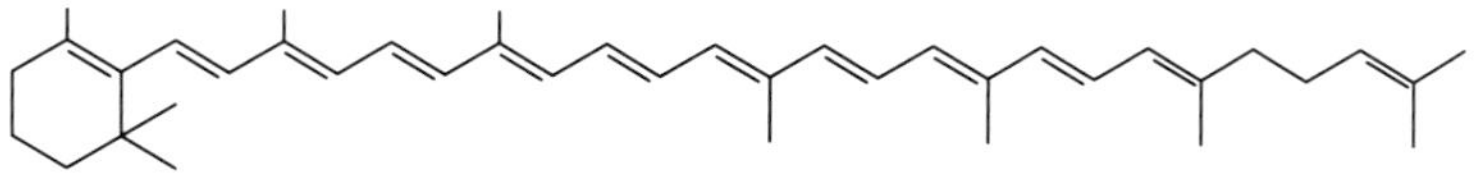	42 – 50
β-Zeacarotene	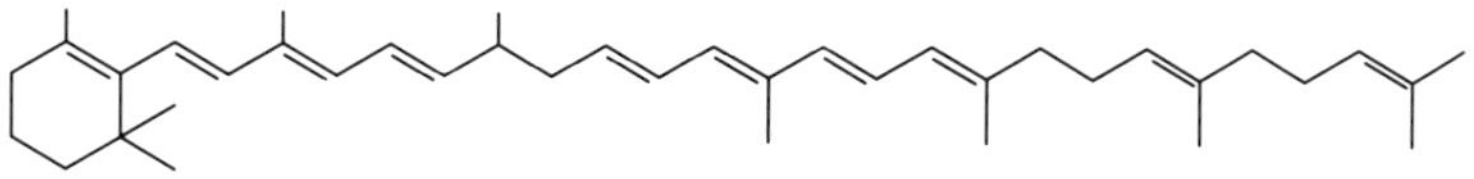	20 – 40
β-Carotene-5, 6-mono-epoxide	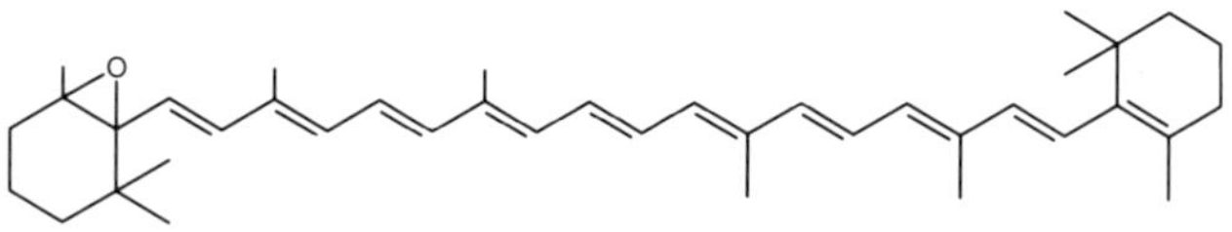	21
3,4-dehydro-β-Carotene	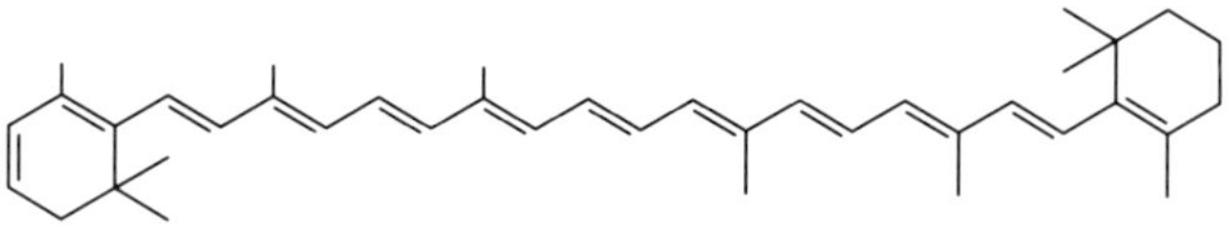	75
Lutein	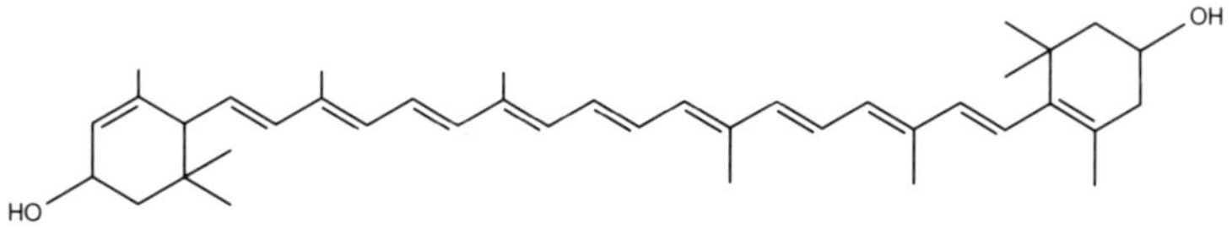	0

Source: Data from Simpson and Chichester (1981).

[a] Vitamin A sparing; it does not combine with RBP to be distributed to tissues by that mechanism.

we have no reliable values for vegetables and only some for fruits (Table 5.8).

In the intestinal mucosa (Figure 5.27) and also to some extent in the liver, carotenoids are converted to retinoids with various degrees of vitamin A activity. [The corpus luteum can also split the provitamin (Skylan, 1983).] β-Carotene itself can either be split into two units of retinol or into one unit with different side chain lengths (Figure 5.28) by dioxygenase(s). This process may be stimulated by thyroid hormone, Zn (Simpson and Chichester, 1981), vitamin E, and dietary unsaturated fatty acids (Rodriguez and Irwin, 1972). (In the corpus luteum it varies with ovulation.) As a result, the relationship between carotenoid intake (even β-carotene intake) and vitamin A equivalents is highly variable and experimentally tenuous, averaging from 2 : 1 to 4 : 1 or more. For this reason, the NAS has set a 6 : 1 ratio of β-carotene to retinol (Figure 5.25) for safety.

Retinoids are particularly concentrated in liver, egg yolk, milk fat, and fish oils. (Polar bear liver may, in fact, contain toxic amounts; on the order of 2×10^6 IU/100 g.) Yellow, orange, and green vegetables are apt to contain large quantities of β-carotene, especially pumpkins and carrots (11,000 and 7500 IU/serving, respectively, AOAC measurements) (Table 5.8). In the United States and the West, vitamin A deficiency is not very common, but may occur in children with

Table 5.8. Carotene and Provitamin A Contents of Fruits and Vegetables

	Total carotenes[a] (μg/g)	β-Carotene[b] (μg/g)	Total carotene per serving (approx μg)
Apples			
Whole	55–126	2–76	4000
Peeled	1–5	(0.2)[c]	132
Apricots	35	21	1700
Avocados	6	0.5	260
Beans (green)	—	(3.6)	—
Beet greens	100	(36)	4400
Blackberries	6	0.6	260
Broccoli	52	(15)	2300
Carrots	110	(66)	4800
Collards	200	(56)	8800
Grapes	2	0.6	90
Melons			
Cantaloupe	21–62	0.4–6	5500
Watermelon	21–62	0.4–6	5500
Oranges (pulp)	24–27	0.1–0.3	1100
Papaya	11–30	(11)	1500
Peaches	27	2.7	1200
Peas	—	(3.8)	—
Pepper (green)	9–11	1.2–1.5	440
Spinach	200	(49)	8800
Squash			
Acorn	39	(7)	1700
Butternut	177	(38)	7800
Yellow	14	(3)	600
Zucchini	9	(2)	400

[a] Data from Goodwin and Goad (1970), with the exception of values for vegetables, which are from *Nutrition Action*, February 1982.

[b] Usually multiplied by 1.67 to get IU of vitamin A.

[c] Values in parentheses are calculated from vitamin A values in food tables (Handbook of the Nutritional Contents of Foods, prepared for the USDA. New York: Dover Publications, 1975) divided by 1.67.

severe cystic fibrosis or malnutrition, or in alcoholics (who may have impaired night vision). If so, it may generally be treated by giving 30,000 IU or more of retinol orally, for several days, along with some oil (as for example in the form of cod or halibut liver oil). (For symptoms of deficiency, see above.) In Third World countries, such as India, parts of Africa, the Middle East, Southeast Asia, and South America, deficiency is more common, as evidenced by the frequency of xerophthalmia (an extreme dryness, keratinization, and cloudiness of the eyeball) in infants and young children.

It should be mentioned that vitamin A status is also very dependent on adequate intake of protein, calories, and Zn. The levels of RBP (and prealbumin) in plasma have even been used as indicators of protein-calorie malnutrition (among dieters), and the synthesis of RBP is Zn-dependent (Figure 5.27). RBP synthesis is also reduced in various forms of liver disease (including alcoholic cirrhosis), and this reduces availability of the vitamin to nonhepatic cells. Growth hormone may also play a role in the synthesis or secretion of RBP-vitamin-A from the liver (Ahluwalia et al., 1980, 1981).

Vitamin A and Disease

Vitamin A and thyroid status. Interrelations between retinoids and thyroid function appear to be of three kinds: (1) those relating to the conversion of carotenes to retinoids (ie, dioxygenase activity); (2) those relating to the plasma circulation of the two factors, both of which are bound to TTR (this binding is not competitive); and (3) a potential synergism between their actions on gene transcription in some cells. Stimulation (or regulation) of dioxygenase activity would appear to be one of the roles of thyroid hormone, in that hypercarotenemia tends to occur in the hypothyroid state, and similarly, symptoms of night blindness are often associated with a lack of thyroid function (Rodriguez and Irwin, 1972). On the other side of the coin, vitamin A deficiency can increase plasma thyroxine concentrations, but not result in hyperthyroid symptoms (Nutr Rev, 1979b). Also, supplemental intake of retinoids appears to decrease plasma levels of thyroid hormone in hyperthyroid individuals (Rodriguez and Irwin, 1972); it also lowers serum protein-bound iodine in rats. The exact relationships here remain to be elucidated, but may involve a derangement of thyroid gland feedback regulation by thyroid-stimulating hormone (Nutr Rev 1979b). Another factor may be that retinoic acid and thyroid hormone receptor complexes both bind to the same promoter sites of certain genes, as appears to be the case for that of growth hormone in the pituitary (Bedo et al., 1989). Indeed, interactions of these hormones at the growth hormone promoter site may be important in controlling body growth in relation to nutrient availability.

Vitamin A and cancer. In the 1920s, it was recognized that vitamin A deficiency could result in changes in the morphology of epithelial tissues that were reminiscent of those seen in precancerous conditions (Bollag and Matter, 1981). It has since been shown that the induction of skin, lung, bladder, colon, and mammary tumors can be inhibited by the vitamin and that transformed cells in tissue culture can respond by becoming more differentiated when treated with the vitamin. (Actual regression has been seen with skin papillomas.) It is thought that the mechanism of action must be related to the essential effects of the vitamin on epithelial cell differentiation involving gene transcription. Because prolonged use of vitamin A at high doses may be toxic, a great deal of effort has been expended to develop less toxic analogs of 13-*cis* retinoic acid (which is not stored) for use against the cancer cell (Figure 5.26). A full discussion of these matters is given in Chapter 16.

Serum vitamin A and other disease states. Serum levels of vitamin A appear to decrease during periods of infectious illness, especially when accompanied by fever (Rodriguez and Irwin, 1972); and a recent report indicates that supplementation with extra vitamin A is beneficial in the treatment of children severely ill with measles (Hussey et al., 1990). Serum retinol levels also decrease with physical exercise and with prolonged sun exposure, but on a yearly basis, tend to be at their lowest in mid-winter in cold climates. The meaning of these changes remains to be determined. Vitamin A storage levels in liver tend to be decreased by ethanol intake, as well as by certain xenobiotics, which may be ascribed at least partly to increased retinoid oxidation by the microsomal ethanol-oxidizing system or similar P450 drug-metabolizing enzymes (see Chapter 3, Ethanol Metabolism, Diet, and Alcoholism), and a redistribution of the vitamin to other tissues (Leo et al., 1988).

Retinoic acid and wrinkles. As already indicated, retinoids are especially important in the maintenance and differentiation of epithelial tissues, which includes the skin. Indeed, the all-*trans* retinoic acid form of the vitamin (also known as tretinoin or Retin-A) and, more recently, the analog 13-*cis* retinoic acid (isotretinoin; Figure 5.25) have been used successfully in the treatment of skin problems, especially severe acne. [Another analog, etretinate, has been used against psoriasis (Coble et al., 1987; Groenhoej-Larsen et al., 1988; Teelman and Bollag, 1990).] Typically, an oral intake of isotretinoin for 20 weeks results in prolonged remission of the skin condition. More recently, it has been claimed (and publicized) that topical treatment of the skin can remove or lessen wrinkles. This claim is currently being examined by the FDA and its veracity has been questioned. It is clear, however, that there is some kind of skin cell response, which can be ascribed to humoral effects on gene transcription. This should also involve a "push" toward developmental differentiation and full secretory activity, along with a diminution in the rate of cell proliferation and tendency toward cancer (Kraemer et al., 1988). Diminished synthesis of keratins is also likely to be involved (DeLuca, 1988). Taking this vitamin analog is not without side effects, however, even if the acid forms are not stored (the main reason for toxicity of excess vitamin A). At high doses, tretinoin and isotretinoin (and etretinate) are teratogenic, making them quite unsafe for pregnant women (Kraft et al., 1989; Stern, 1989). It is also not clear what the effects of long-term use of isotretinoin on skin might be; long-term oral intake can result in skin and bone problems (Roe, 1988; see Chapter 19). Use of these substances should therefore be approached with caution and only instituted with good reasons.

Vitamin D

History, Structure, and Biosynthesis

By 1919, Sir Edward Mellanby in England had succeeded in inducing rickets in dogs through dietary manipulation, which could be cured with cod liver oil (Mellanby, 1919). In 1922, McCollum et al. (1922) reported that the factor responsible was not vitamin A, but vitamin "D," as the growth and xerophthalmic (dry eyeball) activity of the former could be destroyed by mild oxidation of cod liver oil, leaving the antirachitic activity intact (Schnoes and DeLuca, 1980). One form of the vitamin was first isolated from food sources in 1931, another in 1936, and synthesis was accomplished in 1936 (Schnoes and DeLuca, 1980).

Vitamin D is not a true vitamin in many respects. It is not required from the diet, except under certain conditions, and is normally produced in our own tissues. It is generally not produced by plants and microorganisms, and its mechanism of action is primarily that of a steroid hormone. Vitamin D_3 (cholecalciferol) is made in our skin from 7-dehydrocholesterol (Holick and Clark, 1978; Schnoes and DeLuca, 1980) by a nonenzymatic process, catalyzed by ultraviolet (UV) light energy (Figure 5.29) to form the previtamin. The latter, by thermal activation, slowly rearranges to D_3 (cholecalciferol) and is then released to the vitamin D binding protein (DBP) in plasma for transport, distribution, and storage. The dis-

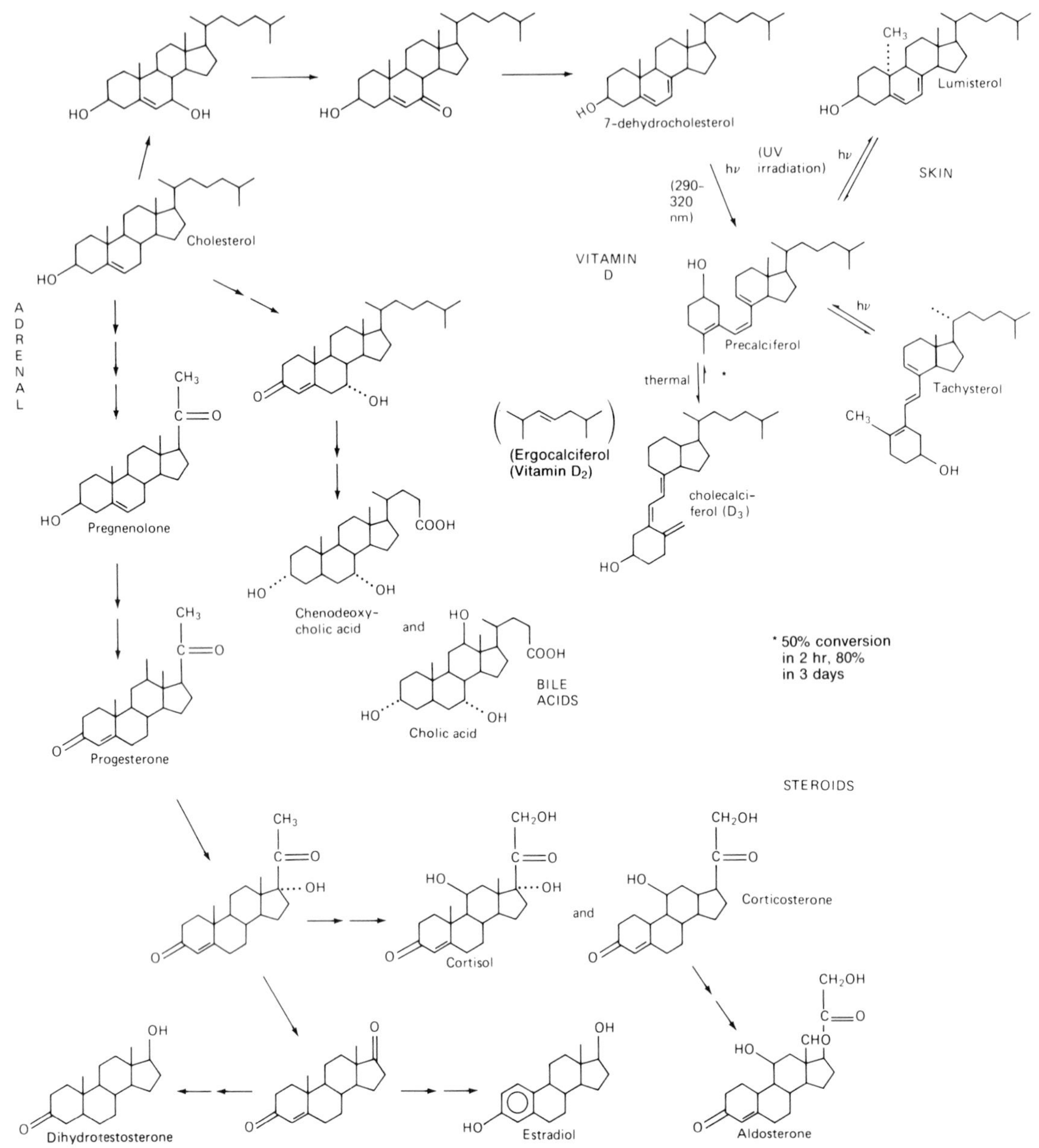

Figure 5.29. Synthesis of vitamin D and other compounds from cholesterol.

covery that UV irradiation was necessary for this process was first made by Huldschinsky in 1919, who found that exposure of children to sun or UV light would cure rickets. The molecular step was then pinpointed by Steenbock and Black in 1924. Moreover, these authors discovered that irradiation of foods could have the same effect. Thus, the treatment of milk, containing ergosterol (with an extra unsaturated bond at C-22 on the side chain), produces vitamin D_2 (ergocalciferol) (Figure 5.29). (Vitamin D_1 turned out to be an impure preparation of vitamin D_2.) As the vitamin is not very abundant in our food supply, it is generally added to the milk (or produced in situ through UV irradiation) in the United States and Canada. This is not the case in many other countries, and parts of Europe, where winter comes with long periods of gray weather; vitamin D deficiency is not uncommon in growing children.

Food Sources, Consumption, Absorption, and Metabolism

As already indicated, most of the vitamin comes to us through the milk and other fortified (supplemented) processed foods. Fish oils and egg yolks are naturally rich sources, but otherwise, raw foodstuffs contain little or no vitamin D. (Animal liver is not even a rich source.) Intestinal absorption requires the presence of bile acids. Absorption occurs in the jejunum and/or ileum, and the vitamin absorbed into the intestinal mucosa is transported to the liver via the chylomicron–lymph system, as in the case of triglycerides and cholesterol (Figure 5.30). The vitamin is released from chylomicrons and lipoproteins in the liver, with the help of a specific DBP (DeLuca, 1980). A portion of all vitamin D reaching the liver (from exogenous or endogenous sources) is 25-hydroxylated and released for circulation in the plasma. Thus, plasma levels of 25-OH-D_3 are related to the size of the liver stores. In the plasma, it circulates on another DBP (an α_1-globulin), also known as the group-specific component (Gc) (Schoentgen et al., 1986). The 25-OH form of the vitamin is then activated by the kidney in response to changes in blood calcium concentrations (see below). The rest of the vitamin is stored for future use. After activation, the vitamin is metabolized and excreted from the body via the bile; 3% may be lost through the urine.

Functions

The only clearly defined function of vitamin D so far is in the maintenance of plasma calcium homeostasis, in conjunction with parathyroid hormone (Figure 5.30). This is essential for long-term bone metabolism and structure and for the maintenance of cellular and neural functions that in-

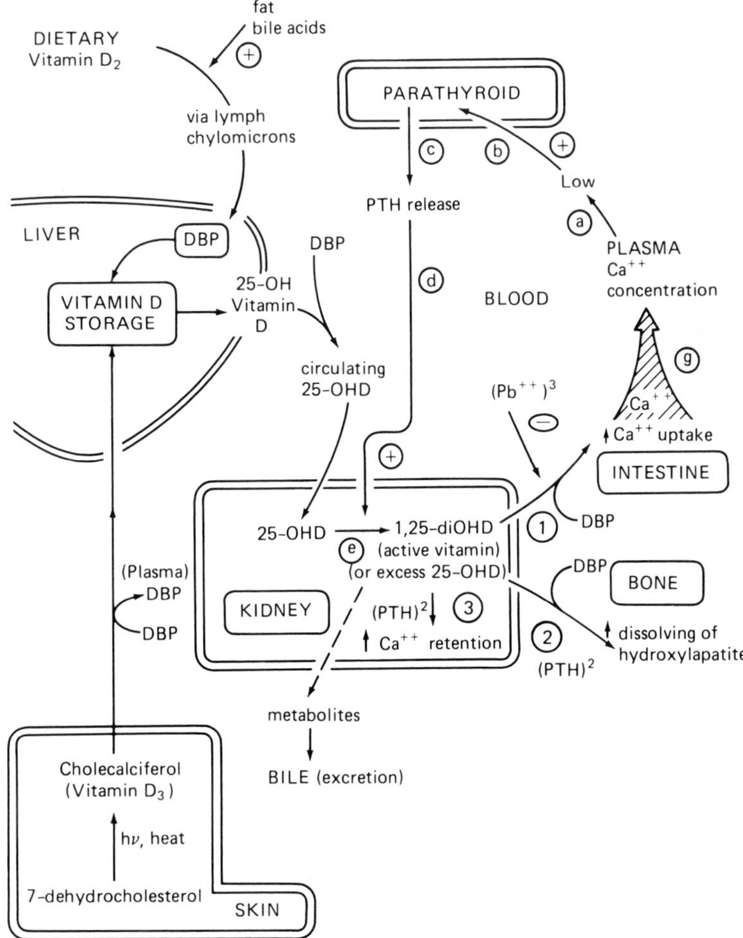

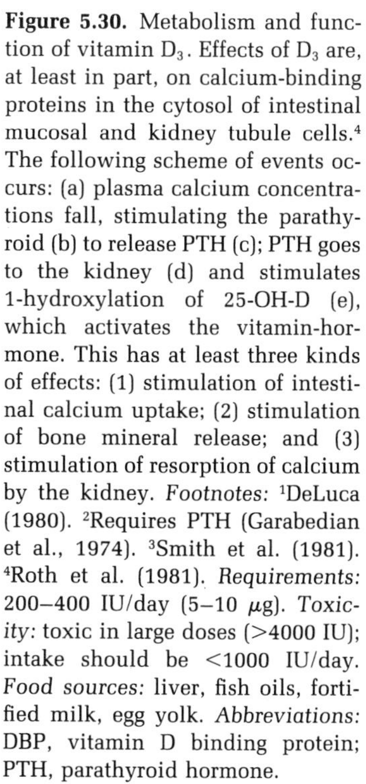

Figure 5.30. Metabolism and function of vitamin D_3. Effects of D_3 are, at least in part, on calcium-binding proteins in the cytosol of intestinal mucosal and kidney tubule cells.[4] The following scheme of events occurs: (a) plasma calcium concentrations fall, stimulating the parathyroid (b) to release PTH (c); PTH goes to the kidney (d) and stimulates 1-hydroxylation of 25-OH-D (e), which activates the vitamin-hormone. This has at least three kinds of effects: (1) stimulation of intestinal calcium uptake; (2) stimulation of bone mineral release; and (3) stimulation of resorption of calcium by the kidney. *Footnotes:* [1]DeLuca (1980). [2]Requires PTH (Garabedian et al., 1974). [3]Smith et al. (1981). [4]Roth et al. (1981). *Requirements:* 200–400 IU/day (5–10 μg). *Toxicity:* toxic in large doses (>4000 IU); intake should be <1000 IU/day. *Food sources:* liver, fish oils, fortified milk, egg yolk. *Abbreviations:* DBP, vitamin D binding protein; PTH, parathyroid hormone.

volve fluxes of Ca ions across intra- and extracellular membranes. [These fluxes are part of the mechanisms by which the actions of some hormones are carried out and are necessary for the generation of some nerve impulses and muscle contractions (see Choline and Inositol and Chapter 6).] Indeed, vitamin D deficiency and hypocalcemia can result in convulsive seizures.

When blood calcium concentrations begin to fall (Figure 5.30a and b), increasing amounts of parathyroid hormones are released (Figure 5.30c). This causes the activation of 25-OH vitamin D in the kidney by a second hydroxylation at C-1 (Figure 5.30d and e), forming the active vitamin or hormone. This has three effects: (1) it signals cells of the intestinal mucosa to increase calcium (and phosphate) absorption; (2) there is an immediate flux of Ca^{2+} from the fluid compartment of the bone to the plasma; and (3) it signals the distal kidney tubule cells to retain (resorb) more calcium, which is otherwise lost in the urine. Thus, an immediate increase in plasma Ca concentrations is achieved (Figure 5.30g). The last two effects (on bone and kidney) require the simultaneous presence of parathyroid hormone (PTH) (Figure 5.30) and are thus generally more fleeting. In the intestine, the effect on Ca^{2+} absorption is slower to peak and much more sustained, being maximal 6 hr after 1,25-diOH-D administration to rats; a second phase of increased Ca^{2+} absorption occurs by 24 hr, if the rats have been deficient in the vitamin. All of the effects are thought to occur at least partly through a steroid hormone-like mechanism, which induces the increased transcription, and thus translation, of mRNAs coding for proteins involved in calcium and phosphate absorption. By such mechanisms, the steroid vitamin crosses the cell membrane and binds to cytosol receptor proteins (sedimentation coefficient 3.2–3.7 S). In calcium deficiency, the concentration of these receptors in mucosal cells increases (Favus et al., 1988). Activation of this complex within the cytosol allows its entry into the nucleus and binding to the chromatin, resulting in increased formation and transfer into the cytosol of mRNA for calcium and phosphate transport proteins. The hormone–receptor complex binds to a vitamin D regulatory element in the promoter region of specific genes via "zinc fingers" (Morrison et al., 1989). The result is an enhanced rate of synthesis of proteins involved in calcium and phosphate absorption, or resorption.

The nature of these proteins is only just beginning to emerge, and their mechanisms of action are still unclear. In the intestinal mucosa, the best known protein induced is known as a calbindin D_{9K}, which belongs to the family of calmodulins that regulate other enzymes and proteins through calcium binding (Reichel et al., 1989). [Different (larger) calbindins (like D_{25K}) are found in other tissues, including kidney and brain, not all of which are regulated by active vitamin D (Varghese et al., 1988).] It is thought that another protein (or proteins) is involved in enhancing the intestinal calcium uptake and transport (DeLuca, 1988), which results in the release of Ca^{2+} into the plasma/interstitial fluid at the serosal surface. A more rapid, nontranscriptionally initiated enhancement of Ca^{2+} absorption may also be triggered by the hormone (Nemere et al., 1984). In the bone, the active vitamin induces at least two proteins secreted by osteoblasts: "bone and matrix Gla proteins" (BGP and MGP). The former is also known as osteocalcin and may promote Ca^{2+} release by inhibiting bone mineralization (Price, 1988). (It binds very tightly to hydroxylapatite.) Glucocorticoids (binding to another promoter site) inhibit osteocalcin gene expression (Morrison et al., 1989). MGP is much more widely distributed in tissues and has some as yet unknown extracellular function (for details, see Vitamin K). Both of these proteins need γ-carboxylation for normal function, a process dependent on vitamin K. A more long-term (and less direct) effect of 1,25-diOH-D_3 may be to increase the number of osteoclasts (Reichel et al., 1989). (Osteoclasts are involved in demineralization.) In the kidney, calbindin and other proteins are induced, but the mechanisms leading to enhanced Ca^{2+} (and phosphate) resorption are again unclear. The end result is nevertheless that blood calcium concentrations are restored.

If sufficient calcium is available in the lumen of the small intestine (see Chapter 6), the ultimate effect of vitamin activation is to increase the amount of calcium in the body, in part to replace what may have been taken from the bone for maintenance of blood concentrations. In the absence of sufficient calcium in the diet, blood calcium concentrations are maintained, but at the expense of bone, leading to osteoporosis (see Chapter 6). In the total absence of vitamin D, a more severe lack of bone mineralization results, called osteomalacia or rickets. Here, calcium and phosphate, though perhaps available in the diet, are not absorbed in sufficient amounts. In low concentrations, the active vitamin also appears to be necessary for *mineralization* of the bone (the laying down of bone mineral) possibly through regulation of osteoblast receptors for growth factors (Wozney et al., 1988), effects on alkaline phosphatase (implicated in the mineralization process; see Chapter 6, Calcium), and/or other "morphogenic proteins" (Reichel et al., 1989; Turner et al., 1988).

Based on observations that receptors for 1,25-diOH-D are found in most cells of the body, including the heart, pancreas, and skin (Haussler, 1986; Stumpf et al., 1979), and cells of the immune system (Yousefi et al., 1989), the vitamin may have other, as yet undiscovered, functions, including effects on the development of muscle strength (DeLuca, 1980); immunity (Manolagas et al., 1985; Quesada et al., 1989); and differentiation, maturation, and even deactivation of hematopoietic myeloid and/or epidermal cells (Reichel et al., 1989). Secretion of several hormones (including prolactin and calcitonin) is also affected at the transcriptional level. Some of these effects may be mediated by changes in Ca^{2+} uptake (Walters et al., 1987).

Perhaps most exciting of all has been the discovery that, at least for osteocalcin, the promoter site to which the D hormone–receptor complex binds in the osteoblast nucleus is the same as that to which the estrogen–receptor complex binds (estrogen regulatory element) (Komm et al., 1989). This may be an important clue to the origin of postmenopausal osteoporosis and the connections between estrogen, vitamin D, and calcium metabolism.

Hypocalcemia can thus occur either through insufficient dietary uptake or kidney retention of calcium (Figure 5.30), through deficiency of vitamin D, or in the hypoparathyroid state (see also Chapter 6). Because kidney activation of the vitamin-hormone is central to vitamin D action and the regulation of blood calcium concentrations, loss of kidney function or absence of kidneys will produce hypocalcemia and severe bone disease. Frequent dosing of dialysis patients without kidney function with small amounts of 1,25-diOH-D will alleviate hypocalcemia and bone disease (DeLuca, 1982). *Hypercalcemia*, on the other hand, can occur in hyperparathyroidism (Figure 5.30, step c) and under conditions of excessive intake of vitamin D. In this latter condition, there is an increase in the circulation of 25-OH-D, which, though not doubly hydroxylated, substitutes for the active hormone vitamin at high concentrations.

Hypovitaminosis D either results from insufficient vitamin production, plus dietary lack, or from malabsorption of fats. Individuals affected have low serum calcium (and phosphate) concentrations and high levels of alkaline phosphatase, reflecting increased osteoblastic and osteoclastic activity but without mineralization. Levels of circulating PTH are also increased, which enhance urinary excretion of phosphate and further reduce bone calcification. Plasma citrate concentrations are also depressed, probably reflecting the relative lack of bone calcification activity (see Chapter 6). Rickets is usually diagnosed based on bone deformities and serum chemistry. A vitamin-D-resistant form of rickets is known, which is characterized by a disturbance of phosphate transport and resorption (DeLuca, 1980, 1988). It may or may not also involve an alteration of vitamin D metabolism. Treatment with the active vitamin-hormone, and oral phosphate appears to have had some success.

Inactivation of the hormone-vitamin occurs (as with most steroids) principally through further hydroxylation at C-24, C-26, and perhaps other sites, in the kidney and other tissues (DeLuca, 1980; Schnoes and DeLuca, 1980). (C-24 hydroxylation also routinely occurs to 25-OH-D.) All but 3% of the metabolites are returned to the liver and excreted in the bile. None of these metabolites are thought to be active.

Requirements, Toxicity, and Possible Connection to Atherosclerosis

The RDA for adult men and women, as well as infants and children, is 200–400 IU or 5–10 μg (1 μg = 40 IU). Daily doses greater than 1000 IU (or 25 μg) are not recommended, and doses greater than 10 times the RDA can be toxic. The symptoms of toxicity include hypercalcemia (serum calcium above 12 mg/dl), a deposition of calcium in soft tissues (especially the kidney, heart, lung, and vasculature), hypercalciuria, and possible kidney stones. As already alluded to, the resulting hypercalcemia and hypercalciuria are thought to occur through overproduction of 25-OH-D, which substitutes for the 1,25-diOH form at high concentrations. Mild hypervitaminosis is treated with abstention; more severe cases are given glucocorticosteroids or calcitonin (Milhaud, 1968) to decrease plasma Ca^{2+} concentrations.

It had been suggested that chronic overconsumption of vitamin D is a contributing factor to the development of atherosclerosis, citing vitamin D_3 "disappearance" data (the amount of vitamin being added to the U.S. food supply). Among the arguments was that clear-cut hypervitaminosis D results in cardiac myopathy and atherosclerotic lesions of the vasculature, where calcium deposits cause damage especially to elastic tissues and, eventually, also to smooth muscle cells. Also, chronic intakes of vitamin D_3 at levels five to 10 times the RDA for monkeys (with or without cholesterol) readily induces arterial damage and atherosclerosis in these animals and other species. (It is noteworthy that vitamin D_2 does not have the same effect as D_3 in the squirrel monkey.) Arterial thromboses can also be induced with excessive vitamin D. Although these findings have relevance for persons consuming excessive amounts of vitamin D, direct analysis of the foods eaten by Americans does not support the concept of excessive intake. With very few exceptions, foods are low in this vitamin (it takes 1 quart of milk to obtain the RDA), and the "disappearance" data may probably be explained on the basis that most of the manufactured vitamin goes into animal feeds. Conversely, however, 1,25-diOH-D appears to be needed for normal cardiac muscle contraction (Weishaar and Simpson, 1989) and (less directly) for regulation of blood pressure (via effects on calcium homeostasis) (McCarron et al., 1987).

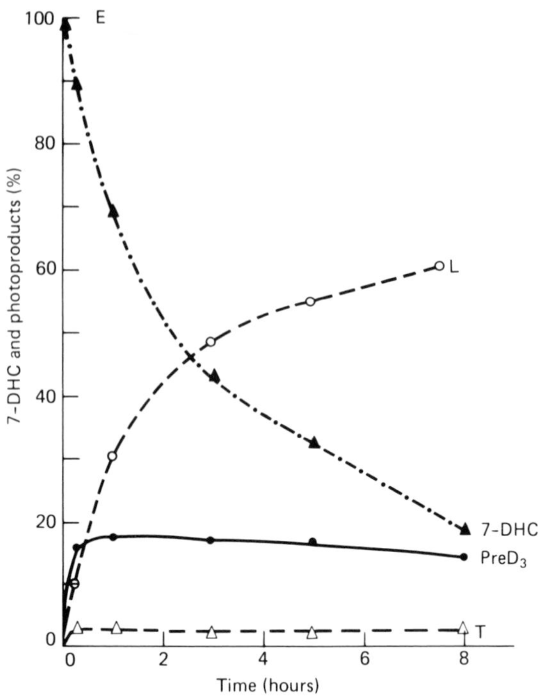

Figure 5.31. Synthesis of previtamin D_3 and other photoproducts in skin during prolonged intense light exposure. An analysis of the photolysis of 7-dehydrocholesterol (7-DHC) in the basal cell layer and the appearance of the photoproducts previtamin D_3 ($PreD_3$), lumisterol$_3$ (L), and tachysterol$_3$ (T) with increasing time of exposure to equatorial-simulated solar ultraviolet radiation. Bars above data points show the standard error of the mean of three determinations. [*Source:* Reprinted by permission from Holick et al. (1981).]

Climate, Tanning, and Vitamin D Production

As excessive accumulation of vitamin D is toxic, and because exposure to sunlight (or other UV radiation) stimulates endogenous vitamin production, it has been postulated that the function of melanin in the skin (as in tanning or in African blacks living in equatorial regions) evolved to protect man from vitamin D toxicity. In vitro work on samples of human skin lends support to these suppositions (Holick et al., 1981; Webb and Holick, 1988). Exposure to equatorial versus Boston sunlight conditions doubled the initial rate of pre-D production. [Indeed, winter sunlight in Boston was unable to promote formation of vitamin D (Webb et al., 1988).] The amount of light exposure required to achieve maximum synthesis of previtamin D_3 increased over a five- to sixfold range with increasing melanin content. Consequently, total pre-D_3 synthesized per 3 hr of exposure was much less in dark versus light skin. However, another protective mechanism was also operative (Figure 5.31). With continued exposure, previtamin D_3 production ceased and increasing proportions of the dehydrocholesterol substrate were converted to biologically inactive photoproducts, especially lumisterol. This occurred because (a) the nonenzymatic isomerization of the previtamin (to cholecalciferol; Figure 5.29) is a very slow process (requiring several days to complete), and (b) the sun will photodegrade some of the previtamin that accumulates (to lumisterol and tachysterol), thus preventing overproduction of the potentially toxic vitamin (Webb and Holick, 1988).

Interactions of Vitamin D, Ca, and Pb

Apart from high levels in blood and tissue, lead (Pb) intoxication in man is characterized by (a) decreased serum 1,25-diOH-D (and 25-OH-D) concentrations (Rosen et al., 1980); (b) a lower intestinal absorption of calcium; and (c) increased serum concentrations of PTH. The same symptomology is seen in rats on diets of 0.82% Pb, as lead acetate (Smith et al., 1981), and a low intake of calcium or phosphorus. From the animal experiments it appears that Pb interferes with the increased intestinal uptake of calcium stimulated by active vitamin D. [It does not interfere with the bone and kidney actions of the hormone, except perhaps hydroxylation of the 25-OH vitamin to the 1,25-diOH vitamin (Figure 5.30) (Rosen et al., 1980; Smith, 1981).] At the same time, administration of oral vitamin D in the diet, with or without added Pb, enhances the accumulation of Pb in blood, bone, and tissues (Smith, 1981), because it uses the same intestinal transport system (see Chapter 6). Thus, Pb blocks intestinal absorption of calcium, but vitamin D stimulates Pb uptake. [The effects of Pb are much greater on low calcium or low phosphate diets.]

Vitamin D and Ca Metabolism in Pregnancy and Lactation

During gestation, 25–30 g of calcium are transferred from mother to fetus, and intestinal calcium absorption (and bone loss) is increased (see Chapter 6). As might be expected, serum levels of 1,25-diOH-D are also elevated in pregnancy and in lactation (when calcium continues to be transferred to the infant via the milk) (Kumar et al., 1980). However, at least in rats, vitamin D deficiency does not substantially inhibit calcium transfer to the fetus (Halloran and DeLuca, 1979). Also, the increased circulation of 1,25-diOH-D does not relate to an increased level of circulating PTH (Kumar et al., 1980). This has caused speculation that other hormones, such as estrogens, may enhance the rate of hydroxylation of the 25-OH vitamin (Kumar et al., 1980) and/or that factors other than vitamin D can determine the availability of calcium to the fetus.

Vitamin E

History and Structure

A component of vegetable oils essential for female reproduction in rats fed a rancid lard diet was first identified by Evans (and Bishop) in 1922 and named tocopherol ("to bring forth offspring"). This factor was also present in wheat germ, alfalfa, and lettuce (and was distinct from vitamins A and D), prevented fetal resorption, and was named vitamin E by Sure in 1924 (Scott, 1980). Evans isolated the vitamin in 1936, and the structure of α-tocopherol was elucidated by Fernholz in 1938 (Horwitt, 1980*b*).

Studies by Pappenheimer and Goetsch, in 1931, also implicated vitamin E in the prevention of encephalomalacia in chicks (a softening of brain tissue) and in nutritional muscular dystrophy in rabbits. Failure to cure similar human symptomologies (especially muscular dystrophy) with the vitamin, and further confusion about the true origins of these and other symptoms, lead to a feeling that vitamin E had little or no function in human metabolism. An excellent, detailed accounting of these historic ups and downs and the discoveries that lead to a recognition of the interactions between vitamin E and other nutrients in diet and metabolism (see below) has been presented by Milton Scott (1980).

There are at least eight forms of tocopherol (vitamin E) produced by plants that enter our food supply. These various forms are distinguished by the placement of various methyl groups, both on the phenyl ring and on the side chain of the molecule, as well as the state of unsaturation of the side chain (Figure 5.32). Based on assays in rodents and chicks, the most active (and most abundant) form in foodstuffs is a particular stereoisomer of α-tocopherol (although corn oil, for example, contains 90% γ-tocopherol, which is only 7.4% as active in the rat fertility test). The stereoisomer of α-tocopherol, previously known as "d," is now referred to as RRR-α-tocopherol (2R, 4′R, 8′R). This is more active than the 8 stereoisomer racemic mixture (all-rac-α-tocopherol) (see Figure 5.32 for values). The most important configuration for activity is that surrounding carbon 2. The reactive hydroxyl group on the phenyl ring can be esterified, but deesterification is necessary for activity. "DL"-α-Tocopherol acetate (a particular racemic mixture no longer available), used to establish international units, was given the value 1.0/mg. All-rac-α-Tocopherol acetate is currently being tested as a substitute and should be very similar. As a result, 1 mg of all-rac-α-tocopherol (nonesterified) is probably equivalent to about 1.36 IU, and 1 mg RRR-γ-tocopherol is equivalent to 1.49 IU (Figure 5.32). Other forms appear to be less active in animal studies but still contribute to "α-tocopherol equivalents." RRR-α-tocopherol (and the man-made stereoisomer of the α-form; SRR) appear not to be distributed as readily as RRR-α-tocopherol. The available human and monkey data indicate that all are incorporated into chylomicrons by the intestine, but that the liver preferentially puts the RRR-α form into secreted very low-density lipoproteins (Traber and Kayden, 1989; Traber et al., 1990*a*, *b*). Some α-tocopherol is transferred to cells (and

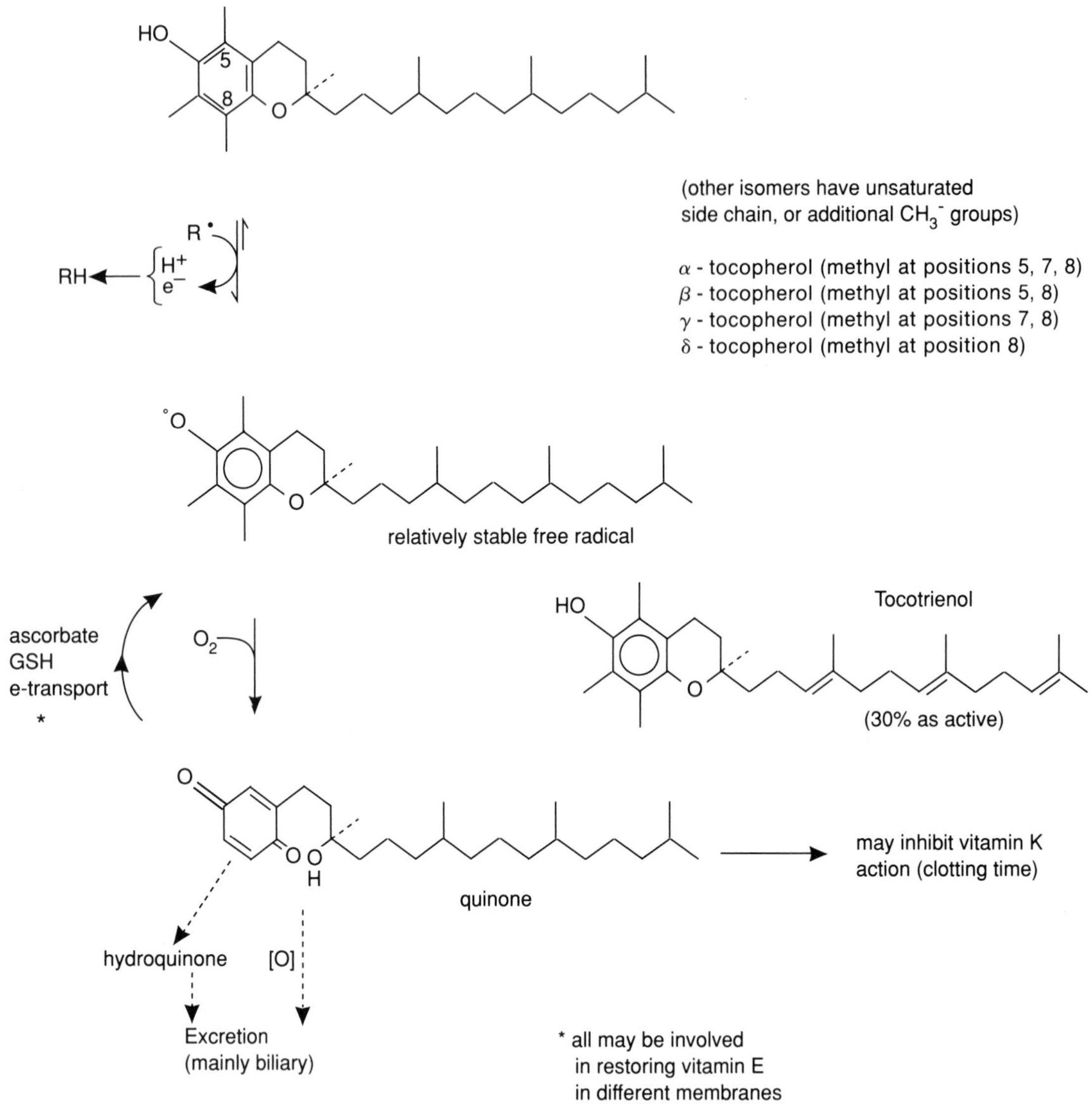

HO 5 8 O

(other isomers have unsaturated side chain, or additional CH_3^- groups)

R• RH ← {H^+, e^-}

α - tocopherol (methyl at positions 5, 7, 8)
β - tocopherol (methyl at positions 5, 8)
γ - tocopherol (methyl at positions 7, 8)
δ - tocopherol (methyl at position 8)

°O O

relatively stable free radical

ascorbate
GSH
e-transport
*

O_2

HO O Tocotrienol

(30% as active)

O O O H

quinone

may inhibit vitamin K action (clotting time)

hydroquinone [O]

Excretion (mainly biliary)

* all may be involved in restoring vitamin E in different membranes

Figure 5.32. Vitamin E.

Functions: primarily is an antioxidant, especially to prevent oxidation and peroxidation of polyunsaturated fatty acid units of membrane phospholipid (within and on the plasma membrane of cells). This works against injury to cell membranes, as in red blood cell fragility (man) and probably the muscular dystrophy of animals. It also prevents/reduces the accumulation of ceroid pigment granules in soft tissues, which normally increases with age. In animals, effects are also on fertility:

1. normal functioning of the seminiferous epithelium and sperm production.
2. implantation and sustaining the fetus in the uterus.

Finally, suppression of the production of fecal mutagens.

Toxicity: nil, 800 IU/day for 3 years.

Requirements: 8–10 mg/day (adults); 3–4 mg (infants); linked to intake of polyunsaturated fatty acids.

1 mg DL-α-tocopherol acetate = 1.0 IU = 1.0 all rac-α-tocopherol acetate

1 mg DL-α-tocopherol = 1.1 IU = 1 mg all rac-α-tocopherol

1 mg D-α-tocopherol acetate = 1.36 IU = 1 mg RRR-α-tocopherol acetate

1 mg L-α-tocopherol = 1.49 IU = RRR-α-tocopherol

α and γ forms also have some activity (α, 40%–50%; γ, 10%–30%; δ, ~1%).

[*Source:* Farrell (1988).]

high-density and low-density lipoproteins) from chylomicrons (or its remnants) in the plasma, but the liver may dispose of the rest through the bile (along with much of the SRR and γ-isomers). Whether the particular assays used to assess biologic activity of the various isomers are entirely appropriate for evaluation of human needs is not that clear (Bland, 1980), in view of species differences which occur in the symptomology of deficiency (Farrell, 1988). The distribution, availability, and "vitamin E" contributions of tocotrienols (with the side chain unsaturated; Figure 5.32) in foods (especially grains) are also uncertain. [Indeed, these may have independent effects, as suggested by their potential to lower serum cholesterol (see Chapters 3 and 15).] Thus, it is possible that γ-tocopherols are just as important in the human diet (Bland, 1980).

Sources

Tocopherols are found in conjunction with plant oils, especially those with polyunsaturated fatty acids. Grains and other seeds mainly concentrate these oils in the germ. As if by design, there appears to be a relationship between the concentration of linoleic acid in various plant oils and the concentration of tocopherols; the latter are able to preserve and prevent the oxidation of the relatively unstable fatty acids. Depending on the method of extraction of the oils from the seeds and the refining processes superimposed, various amounts of the tocopherols will be retained in the oils actually consumed by the public. Typically, about two thirds of the vitamin may be lost during production of commercial vegetable oils. Processing of wheat into ordinary flour removes most of the vitamin through separation of the germ, and most of the rest is destroyed by bleaching. With the possible exception of liver, animal foods are poor sources. Depending on the source, plant oils will contain quite varied proportions of the various tocopherols (Table 5.9). As already stated, the nutritional significance of this for man is unclear. Americans are thought to consume between 4 and 13 mg/day (or 7–9 IU), the average being close to the RDA. If the contributions of other tocopherols are counted in, the intake of equivalents is probably considerably higher (Farrell, 1988). Needs will depend especially on intakes of polyunsaturated fatty acids. [They will also depend to some extent on the availability of reducing equivalents from other sources (see below).]

Absorption, Storage, and Excretion

Vitamin E is absorbed in conjunction with fatty acids and triglycerides. As for the other fat-soluble vitamins, its absorption requires the presence of some fat in the diet and the action of bile acids. Malabsorption (e.g., if the bile duct should be blocked) is the most common reason for gross deficiencies. On average, about 20%–40% is absorbed (Sokol, 1988). Vitamin E is initially distributed from the intestine through the lymphatic circulation, as a part of the chylomicrons, from where it also "rubs off" on cells, such as erythrocytes. From the liver onward, its distribution follows that of triglyceride and other lipids, via lipoproteins (VLDL and LDL, and perhaps HDL) to adipose tissue and intra- and extracellular membranes. As a result, vitamin E becomes more evenly distributed around the body than the other fat-soluble vitamins, with highest concentrations normally in plasma, liver, and adipose tissue (especially brown fat). Plasma levels of vitamin E are related to the level of circulating lipid and are thus in themselves a poor measure of vitamin status. (The ratio of E to plasma lipid is the best measure.) Turnover of tocopherols in adipose tissue and the brain is much slower than in other tissues, which mitigates against calling fat tissue a store of the vitamin (Farrell, 1988). Nevertheless, the large capacity of fat tissue to hold tocopherols accounts for the nontoxicity of vitamin E (relative to that of vitamins A and D). [In adipocytes, 99% of the vitamin is with the bulk lipid (triglyceride) of the cell (Traber and Kayden, 1987).] Little is known about the metabolism and excretion of this vitamin in man, although it is thought that further oxidation to the quinone (and hydroquinone) may occur, leading primarily to biliary excretion of these and perhaps other metabolites (Figure 5.32). (A small portion is also lost in the urine.)

Toxicity

Human studies in which megadoses of 600–800 IU α-tocopherol were supplied to adults daily for 4 weeks to 3 years have resulted in no long- or short-term health problems or changes in blood chemistry. Two exceptions, for which the implications are unknown, were a lowering of serum thyroid hormone levels and a slight increase of fasting triglyceride concentrations for young women (Tsai et al., 1978). Parenteral hyperdosing, at least in premature infants, may also not be without side effects (Phelps, 1984; Sobel et al.,

Table 5.9. Tocopherol Content (mg/100 g) of Common Foodstuffs

Food	α	β	γ	δ	Total
Oils					
Safflower	34–46	—[b]	7–19	24	
Sunflower	49	—	5	0.8	
Corn	5–26	5	44–70	1–14	
Soybean	3–12	—	32–63	5–25	56–109
Nuts					
Almonds	23–32	0.3	0.9 (0.5[a])	—	
Walnuts, pecans	0.4–1.2	—	16–20	—	
Peanuts	10–11	—	7–8	1–2	
Grains					
Oats, whole	1.5–2.1	—	0.05	—	
Wheat, whole	1.0–1.4	0.7–0.8 (2.5–3.3)[a]	—	—	0.3–0.5
Rice, brown	0.3–1.4	—	0.3–0.4	—	
Fruits/vegetables					
Muskmelon	10	—	—	—	
Canteloupe	0.1	—	—	—	0.14
Bananas	0.2–0.5	—	—	—	0.4
Orange juice	0.04	—	—	—	0.18
Carrots	0.5–0.6	0.01–0.02	—	—	
Broccoli	0.5	—	0.2	—	
Tomatoes	0.4	—	—	—	0.85
Beans (cooked)	0.02–0.3	—	0.1–7.1	tr-0.5	
Cauliflower	0.04	—	0.05	—	
Meats, fish, etc.					
Butter	1.7–3.3	—	0.14	—	1–3.2
Milk	0.04	—	—	—	0.1
Eggs	0.5	—	—	—	1.4
Hamburger	0.3–0.4	—	—	—	0.5–0.6
Haddock	0.4–0.6	—	—	—	1.2
Liver	0.5–0.6	—	—	—	1.6
Margarine	3.0–33	—	29±	8±	

Source: Data from Bauerfeind (1977) (determinations from 1965–1975).

[a] Trienol form.
[b] Not determined or detected.

1982) and megadoses of E antagonize the action of coumarin anticoagulants in patients requiring these drugs. (See Chapter 19 for details.)

Functions

The most obvious function of vitamin E is as an antioxidant and anti-free radical agent, especially for unsaturated fatty acids in the phospholipid of cell membranes. The reactive hydroxyl group on the phenyl ring is capable of oxidation and loses either an electron or a hydride ion. In the latter case, it forms a fairly stable free radical (Figure 5.32). This can later be oxidized further to the quinone and/or hydroquinone and be lost in the bile and urine. The prevention of lipid oxidation, specifically the peroxidation of unsaturated fatty acids and cholesterol, in cell membranes and in other sites of fat accumulation probably accounts for most, if not all, of the symptoms associated with vitamin E deficiency in animals and humans (Table 5.10). In humans, the most clear-cut example is enhanced erythrocyte fragility (tested in vitro with H_2O_2 or oxygen/light exposure), as observed in adults on different diets and in newborn infants, especially those of low birth weight (<1500 g) and/or prematurity. In deficiency, the erythrocytes are more easily destroyed and also exhibit a marked change in morphology, probably due to a crosslinking of membrane proteins

Table 5.10. Conditions Responding to Treatment with Vitamin E in Experimental Animals

Condition	Experimental animal	Tissue affected	PUFA[a] influence	Prevented by: Vitamin E	Se	Antioxidants in general	ami
		REPRODUCTIVE FAILURE					
Embryonic degeneration							
Type A	Rat, hamster, mouse, hen, turkey	Vascular system of embryo	X	X		X	
Type B	Cow, ewe			—[b]	X[c]		
Sterility (male)	Rat, guinea pig, hamster, dog, cock, rabbit, monkey	Male gonads		X			
		LIVER, BLOOD, BRAIN, CAPILLARIES, PANCREAS					
Necrosis	Rat, pig	Liver		X	X		
Fibrosis	Chick, mouse	Pancreas	X	X		X	
Erythrocyte hemolysis	Rat, chick, man (premature infant)	Erythrocytes	X	X		X	
Plasma protein loss	Chick, turkey	Serum albumin		X	X		
Anemia	Monkey	Bone marrow		X		X	
Encephalomalacia	Chick	Cerebellum	X	X		X	
Exudative diathesis	Chick, turkey	Vascular system		X	X		
Kidney degeneration	Rat, mouse, monkey, mink	Kidney tubular epithelium	X	X	X		
Steatitis (ceroid)	Mink, pig, chick	Adipose tissue	X	X		X	
Depigmentatior	Rat	Incisors	X	X		X	
		NUTRITIONAL MYOPATHIES					
Type A (nutritional muscular dystrophy)	Rabbit, guinea pig, monkey, duck, mouse, mink	Skeletal muscle		X		?	
Type B (white muscle disease)	Lamb, calf, kid	Skeletal and heart muscles		—[b]	X[c]		
Type C	Turkey	Gizzard, heart		—[b]	X[c]		
Type D	Chicken	Skeletal muscle	—[d]	X			X

Source: Reproduced with permission from Scott (1980).

[a] Polyunsaturated fatty acids.
[b] Not effective in diets severely deficient in selenium.
[c] When added to diets containing low levels of vitamin E.
[d] A low level (0.5%) of linoleic acid is necessary to produce dystrophy; higher levels did not increase vitamin E required for prevention.

n reports
ts may
amin
(Bland,
be the case
itical nature of
evention of antiox-
s is without dispute

s to be particularly critical
elopment and maintenance of
cle function. From experience with
ith cholestasis (bile duct obstruction)
ne other conditions leading to poor ab-
ion of the vitamin, it has become clear that
eficiency results in neuromuscular damage (to Schwann cells, dorsal root ganglia, and muscle enervation) that can be helped by parenteral treatment with the vitamin (Sokol, 1988). [In adults with a low E intake, a decreased concentration of the vitamin in peripheral nerves precedes the degeneration that accompanies severe deficiency (Traber et al., 1987).] Even more dramatic effects have been observed in some animal species (see below). Again, the mechanism is thought to involve protection against oxygen radical damage.

Other problems of the premature infant seem also to be abolished by vitamin E, namely, bronchopulmonary dysplasia (abnormal development of the lungs), and retinopathy (pathology of the retina; retinal fibroplasia), which can occur upon exposure to high oxygen pressure. Several clinical studies have indicated that vitamin E administration during development or in the acute phase, can alleviate pulmonary distress (Ehrenkranz et al., 1978) and cure the retinopathy (Bieri et al., 1983; Johnson et al., 1974). However, the treatment of infants with large parenteral doses may not be entirely benign and must be further studied (Phelps, 1984; Sobel et al., 1982). Low E has been implicated in sudden infant death (Money, 1978). Again, it is thought that protection against oxidation is the basis for the vitamin's action. In young men and women, very low serum levels of this vitamin have been found in cystic fibrosis and may be responsible for the spinocerebellar disorders that occur in these conditions (Elias et al., 1981). Long-term intake by adults of 600 mg vitamin E per day prevents the otherwise severe photooxidation damage to red cell membranes that occurs when their cells are exposed in vitro. It is also implicated in preventing photooxidative damage to the lens (and thus in preventing cataract formation) (Taylor, 1989) and seems important for the maintenance of the photosensitive outer segments and pigment epithelium of the retina (Dratz et al., 1989).

The mechanism through which the tocopherols are thought to act is illustrated in Figures 5.32 and 5.33. Superoxide anion radicals ($.O_2^-$) and peroxide (H_2O_2), produced through the oxidation of endogenous or exogenous substrates (A^1H; A^2H_2) and partly catalyzed by membrane enzymes like cytochrome P450 oxidase and xanthine oxidase, interact (or react) with other proteins to produce hydroxyl free radicals (King et al., 1975) or similar radical species. These, in turn, can oxidize unsaturated fatty acids of the phospholipid of mitochondrial, microsomal (endoplasmic reticulum), and plasma membranes via peroxidation in a chain reaction (Bland, 1980). (Cholesterol can also be oxidized.) The result is a mixture of oxidized and cleaved products that alters the stability of the membrane. Similar oxidations can occur in lipid droplets in adipocytes and other cells.

It is the attacks on polyunsaturated fatty acid units and cholesterol that are prevented by the tocopherols present in the cell membranes and lipid droplets. In the process, the vitamin is oxidized. The muscular dystrophylike symptoms of vitamin E deficiency encountered in rodents, rabbits, and even monkeys probably result from damage to cell membranes, in this case in the muscle, and this may also be true of the hemorrhagic processes encountered in the cerebellum of animals and children suspected of extreme vitamin E deficiency.

Another outcome of the lack of antioxidant action of vitamin E, and which occurs in its deficiency, is the accumulation of "lipofuscin" or "ceroid pigment" granules in many tissues, including the central nervous system, lungs, kidneys, adipocytes, and muscle (Horwitt, 1960*b*) (Table 5.10, steatitis). These granules contain oxidized unmetabolizable lipids that have partially crosslinked with protein or peptides to form a hard globule that cannot be disposed of by the body. It has been speculated that the accumulation of such granules may contribute to the aging process. The granules normally accumulate with age, and this accumulation is inhibited by a high vitamin E intake, at least in mice (Tappel, 1968). Also, the results of one study have suggested that antioxidants prolong the lifespan of mice (Tappel, 1968).

Although the only clear-cut symptoms of induced vitamin E deficiency in adult humans are those involving red cell membrane stability, substantial evidence of other effects in animals (in-

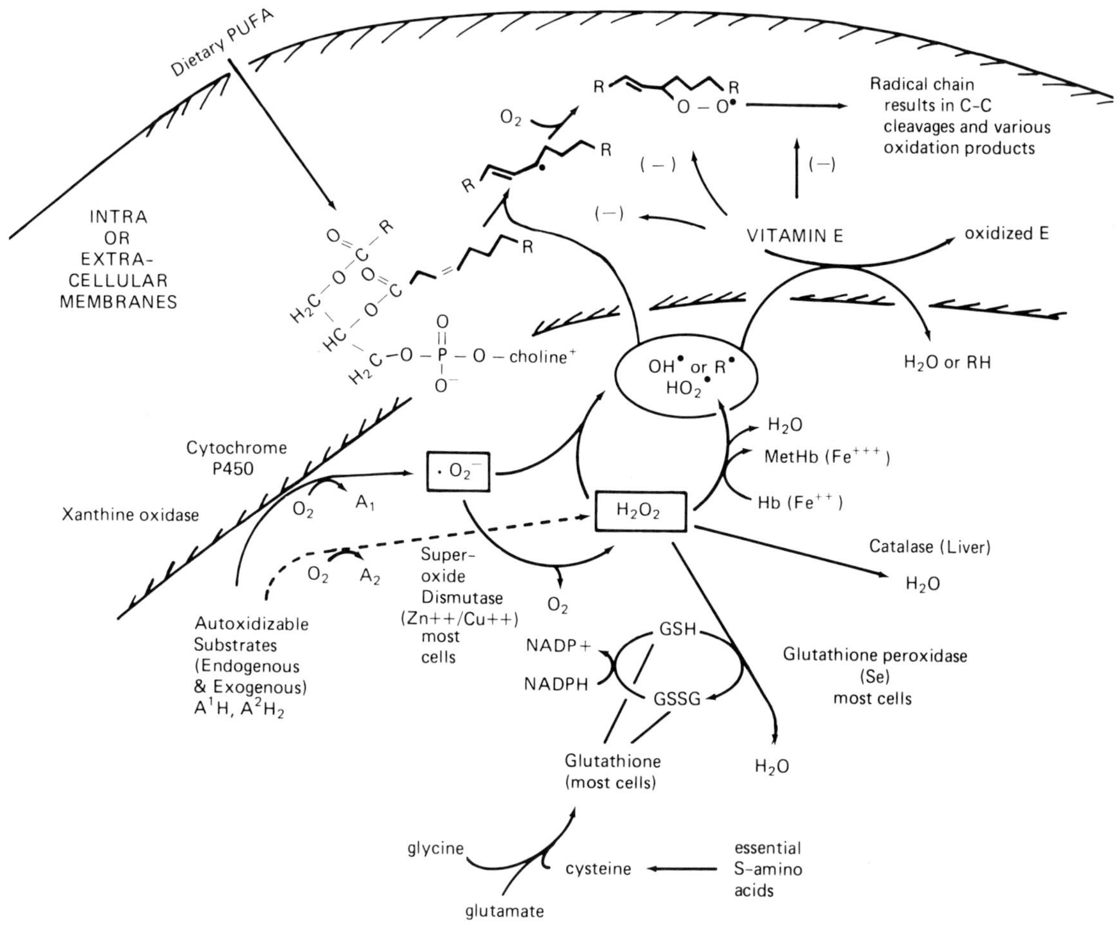

cluding primates) and children attest to the likelihood that vitamin E is important to adult humans. Among the possibilities are roles in female and male reproductive function (Table 5.10 and Figure 5.32) and the prevention of various forms of organ degeneration (Table 5.10). All of these may eventually be explained by a prevention of oxidation and peroxidative damage to cellular membranes and/or inhibition of the accumulation of ceroid pigment granules. As concerns reproduction, studies in several animal species have clearly shown that in males, vitamin E deficiency results first in sperm immotility, then in degeneration of the semeniferous epithelium, and thus a cessation of sperm production. It is also necessary for the normal *development* of full male gonadal function and fertility and its lack during early life and puberty has irreversible effects (at least in rats). The exact roles of vitamin E in these pro-

Figure 5.33. Superoxide anions ($\cdot O_2^-$) are produced by the interaction of various oxidizable substrates and molecular oxygen, partly with the involvement of xanthine oxidase and cytochrome P450. Superoxide is either converted to peroxide (H_2O_2), with the help of the enzyme superoxide dismutase (copper- and zinc-dependent), or interacts with peroxide to form radicals such as OH· or $HO_2\cdot$. [Peroxidase also forms radicals by interacting with hemoglobin (Hb) or other substrates.] These radicals can initiate chain reactions within cell membranes involving the unsaturated fatty acid moieties of the phospholipids. Vitamin E inhibits these processes. Peroxide can also be dissipated to H_2O via reactions involving catalase or glutathione peroxidase (a selenium-dependent enzyme). Through glutathione, this also involves the metabolism of sulfur-containing amino acids. Symbols: GSH, glutathione (reduced); GSSG, glutathione (oxidized); $NADP^+$/NADPH, oxidized/reduced nicotinamide adenine dinucleotide phosphate; MetHb, methemoglobin. [*Source:* Based on information from King et al. (1975), Metzler (1977), and Scott (1980).]

cesses are still a mystery, although the most obvious have been ruled out by recent studies in rats: the effects on follicle-stimulating hormone, luteinizing hormone, testosterone, or inhibin (Cooper et al., 1987). In females, there is probably a failure of uterine function in vitamin E deficiency, with a lack of development of the vasculature that would allow the conceptus to implant in the uterine walls. This may result in resorption of the fetus if implantation does not go forward.

As concerns muscle function, diseases such as muscular dystrophy and myasthenia gravis in man have not been cured by increasing vitamin E intake and are thought to be of genetic origin. Strangely enough, these human diseases are accompanied by other symptoms normally seen in vitamin E deficiency: ceroid pigment deposition, low plasma and adipose tissue vitamin E concentrations, creatinuria, muscle weakness, and increased plasma creatine phosphokinase activity (all indicative of muscle cell damage). The same symptomology is seen in conditions where there is intestinal malabsorption of fat and steatorrhea (loss of fat in the feces) (Bland, 1980): cystic fibrosis of the pancreas, biliary atresia or cirrhosis, sprue, and chronic pancreatitis. Only the creatinuria, in some cases, has responded to α-tocopherol treatment (Horwitt, 1980*b*).

Another possible function for vitamin E, also probably related to its antioxidant capacity, may be suppression of the production of fecal mutagens within the intestinal tract, especially the colon. Using the Ames test, Bruce (1983) found that the level of mutagens in feces of humans varies greatly and is dependent on their dietary intake of vitamins E and C. Moreover, in individuals with high fecal mutagen concentrations, supplementation with 120 mg ascorbate plus 50–100 IU vitamin E greatly lowered or eliminated the mutagen content of the feces. Intake of the vitamin above what is presently recognized as necessary may thus serve a protective function against carcinogenesis.

Another area of action/function that may be emerging is that of inhibiting and modifying prostaglandin formation. In platelets, vitamin E may reduce thromboxane A_2 formation from arachidonic acid (Karpen et al., 1982) and enhance production of prostaglandin I_2, which normally inhibits platelet aggregation (Panganamala and Cornwall, 1982). The response to E can be biphasic, with enhanced synthesis of particular prostaglandins at lower doses and inhibition at high doses (Diplock et al., 1989; Buttriss and Diplock, 1988). The vitamin also has potential inhibitory effects on the 5-lipoxygenase which initiates production of leukotrienes (Redanna et al., 1989). Thus, vitamin E may modulate an important aspect of cell regulatory cascades.

Interactions with Selenium, Unsaturated Fat, Sulfur Amino Acids, and Other Antioxidants

It is now clear that the need for vitamin E is influenced quite strongly by other dietary factors, especially those noted above (Table 5.10). Our present conceptions of how these interdependencies arise is illustrated in Figure 5.33. Apart from the inhibition by tocopherols of unsaturated fatty acid peroxidation by free radicals, superoxide anion radicals and peroxides can be inactivated by three other enzyme systems: Cu/Zn superoxide dismutase, a zinc- and copper-dependent enzyme in the cytosol that converts $.O_2^-$ to H_2O_2; glutathione (GSH) peroxidase, a Se-dependent enzyme designed to dispose of H_2O_2 that is present in most tissues; and the heme-enzyme, catalase, which is found mainly in the liver. (A Mn-dependent superoxide dismutase in mitochondria will also play a role in antioxidant metabolism.) The involvement of GSH peroxidase explains the sparing of vitamin E both by Se (part of the enzyme) and sulfur amino acids (necessary for GSH substrate production) (Figure 5.33). The interrelationship of intakes of polyunsaturated fatty acids (PUFAs) and vitamin E (Table 5.10) is based on the fact that these fats are the ones most readily oxidized both in the food itself, within cell membranes, and in the body's fat stores.

Recent work suggests that vitamin E intake is spared also by other means. At least in the retina, oxidized vitamin E can be regenerated by electrons from ascorbic acid (vitamin C) despite their differential compartmentation (aqueous versus lipid) (Niki, 1987). Similarly, GSH may regenerate oxidized vitamin E in microsomal membranes (McCay et al., 1989), and preliminary evidence suggests that electron transport can regenerate reduced tocopherols in mitochondrial membranes (see Packer et al., 1989). These regenerations are possible because of the relative stability of the vitamin E radical formed upon oxidation, and this may also explain why vitamin E is only needed in rather small amounts.

Requirements and Consumption

The NAS-NRC has recommended that adult men and women consume between 8 and 10 mg of α-tocopherol equivalents per day (for infants 3–4 mg/day and children and teenagers doses in between). This is, of course, a compromise and is subject to the intake of other nutrients (see above). It is based primarily on the long-term studies of Elgin (Horwitt, 1980*b*) and the effects of tocopherol intake on plasma tocopherol concentrations. It is supported by evidence extrapolated from animal experiments. However, it may not normally be optimal for suppression of fecal mutagen production (Bruce, 1983; Dion et al., 1982).

Although it has been established that about 15 mg of α-tocopherol is available for consumption by the average American (Table 5.11), other evidence indicates that intake is highly variable and that there is considerable deficiency in the North American population (Bland, 1980; Horwitt, 1980*b*; Scott, 1980). On the basis that deficiency is defined by a plasma serum concentration of less than 0.50 mg/dl, the average citizen of Pittsburgh and New York City is deficient at 0.37–0.51 mg/dl (Bland, 1980). This may, in part, reflect our high intake of PUFAs, decreased intake of lard, and the overall high intake of dietary fat versus carbohydrates, along with a reliance on processed versus whole grain cereal products and a relatively low intake of Se.

Table 5.11. α-Tocopherol Available for Consumption from Various Foods in the United States (1960)

		D-α-Tocopherol	
	Total fat (g/day)	Content (mg/100 g fat)	Amount (mg/day)
Visible fats			
Butter	7.19	1.6	0.115
Lard	9.55	2.3	0.220
Margarine	9.42	10.2	0.961
Shortening	15.62	10.0	1.562
Other fats and oils	14.15	50.0	7.063
Total	55.92		9.921
Other food fats			
Dairy products	23.31	1.6	0.378
Eggs	5.33	10.7	0.572
Meats, etc.	52.08	1.7	0.893
Beans, peas, nuts, etc.	5.33	9.3	0.496
Fruits and vegetables	1.74	91.7	1.597
Grain products	2.23	48.9	1.092
Total	90.02		5.028
Totals	145.94		14.949

Source: Reproduced by permission from Harris and Embree (1963).

Vitamin E and Miscellaneous Health Problems

Vitamin E and aging. The theory that vitamin E may inhibit the aging process has to do with its effects on ceroid granule formation, which normally occurs with aging and in some forms of degenerative diseases and is reduced by vitamin E intake (see above section, Functions). Nevertheless, at present, there is no consistent evidence that prolonged feeding of high doses of vitamin E (or other antioxidants, such as BHA) increases the lifespan (Tappel, 1968).

Vitamin E and fat malabsorption. As cited earlier, malabsorption of fat that is induced by a variety of other problems and leads to steatorrhea also results in malabsorption of this fat-soluble vitamin, and in vitamin E deficiency (see section on Functions for details).

Vitamin E and blood circulation in the elderly. Although the mechanism is unclear, controlled studies have shown that large doses of the vitamin (300–600 mg/day over at least 3 months) can significantly increase peripheral blood circulation and increase the walking capacity of elderly patients with thrombophlebitis and/or intermittent claudications (reduced blood supply) (Boyd et al., 1949; Livingstone and Jones, 1958; Haeger, 1982). Further work is required to confirm and clarify the nature of these effects.

Vitamin E and other diseases. Vitamin E may be beneficial in the recovery from ischemic conditions, such as after coronary bypass surgery or brain injury (see Diplock et al., 1989*a*), when suppression of damage due to aspects of the inflammatory response may be helpful. Similarly, in osteoarthritis, treatment with vitamin E may improve mobility and diminish pain (Blankenhorn, 1986; Machtley and Ouaknine, 1978). Although a variety of claims have been made for effects of E on other disorders (from ulcers to cancer), the evidence available is not sufficient to support them at this time.

Vitamin E and other toxins. Several animal studies indicate that ozone, nitrogen oxides, and other constituents of smog (or cigarette smoke) injure the lungs and that this damage can be averted or hindered by increased intake of vitamin E, even at doses in the range of the RDA (Tappel, 1980). Also, initial studies in rats have shown that increased vitamin E intake can protect against lipid peroxidation in the lung (Sevanian et al., 1982) and against liver damage by carbon tetrachloride (CCl_4) (Tappel, 1980).

Vitamin K

History, Structure, and Sources

A fat-soluble factor necessary for blood clotting in chicks was discovered in Germany in 1929 by Heinrik Dam (a Dane) and later named vitamin K, the K standing for "koagulation" (coagulation) (Olson, 1980). The pure vitamin (K_1) was first obtained from alfalfa in 1939, and later, it became clear that bacteria synthesized another form (K_2), with a more unsaturated side chain (see Figure 5.34). The two forms, phylloquinones and menaquinones, provide roughly half each of the amounts absorbed into the human body and stored in the liver (Olson, 1980). Menadione, a water-soluble form (without the side chain) synthesized commercially, is also active. All forms can undergo a reversible reduction to the hydroquinone (Figure 5.34).

The fat-soluble vitamin Ks are obtained from plant, animal, and bacterial sources. This is one of the vitamins where an appreciable quantity of the human requirement is obtained from synthesis by endogenous bacteria, as menaquinone. Phylloquinone (vitamin K_1) is especially abundant in alfalfa, cabbages, and leafy vegetables (Table 5.12) and probably accounts for most of the vitamin obtained from the diet by the average American. Meats, especially liver, eggs, and cheese, also provide some menaquinone. Sterilization of the digestive tract with antibiotics results in a loss of about half of the daily intake. This can be significant, if there are no body stores. It can be critical for the newborn infant, born with an unpopulated, sterile, digestive tract and very little in the way of stores. (As a precaution, newborn infants are usually given vitamin K to prevent the acute consequences of vitamin K deficiency.)

Figure 5.34. Vitamin K.

Functions: cofactor for enzymes that catalyse the γ-carboxylation of specific glutamate residues on proteins involved in Ca^{2+} binding, including four blood clotting factors, osteocalcin, and a renal protein.

Requirements: 60–80 μg/day, adults.

Deficiencies: extremely rare except in some newborns and in persons on long-term, strong, antibiotic treatment.

Toxicity: little known, except for menadione which is fairly toxic.

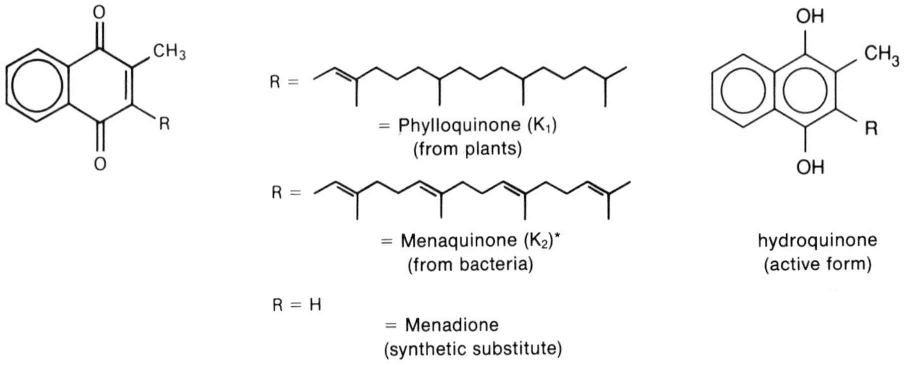

O
CH3
R
O
R =
= Phylloquinone (K1)
(from plants)
R =
= Menaquinone (K2)*
(from bacteria)
R = H
= Menadione
(synthetic substitute)
OH
CH3
R
OH
hydroquinone
(active form)

Antagonists:

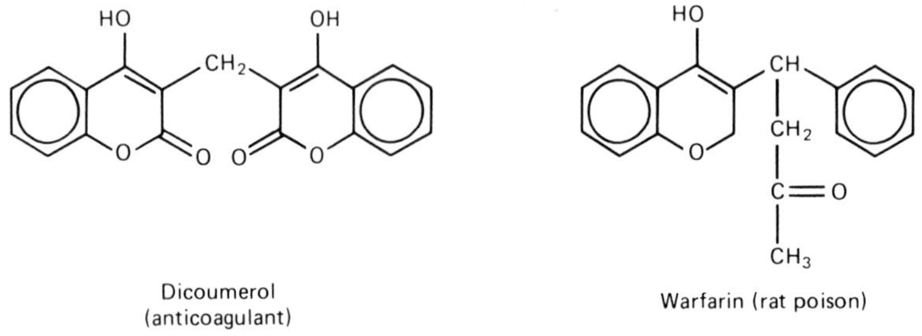

HO
OH
CH2
O
O O
O
Dicoumerol
(anticoagulant)

HO
CH
CH2
C=O
CH3
O
Warfarin (rat poison)

Table 5.12. Phyllo- and Menaquinone Content of Selected Foods (average values)

Food	Vitamin K (μg/100 g)
Green tea (dry)	712
Turnip greens	650
Broccoli and cabbages	125–200
Lettuce	120
Spinach	89
Peas and beans	14–19
Cereal grains	4–20
Fruits and berries	<8
Liver	
Beef	92
Chicken	7
Ham, ground beef	7–15
Eggs (whole)	11
Cheese	35
Milk	3

Source: Data from Olson (1980).

Functions

For many years, the only known function of vitamin K was in blood clotting, although the mechanism remained obscure. More recently, there has been an explosion of knowledge in this area, due to the reports by Stenflo, Nelsestuen, Magnussen, and their colleagues in 1974 that a fragment of prothrombin contained γ-carboxyglutamate acid (Olson, 1980). Soon after, it was shown that vitamin K is a cofactor in the γ-carboxylation of glutamic acid residues on several of the blood clotting factors of the coagulation cascade (Figure 5.35) (Esmon et al., 1975; Olson, 1980). An involvement of this vitamin in the γ-carboxylation of several other, quite different proteins has also been shown, proteins that are involved in bone metabolism (hydroxylapatite dissolution), and in connective tissue and kidney function. In all cases, the vitamin appears to be required for the γ-carboxylation of specific glutamic residues, which in turn, allows a firm binding of Ca^{2+}.

In bone, the 49- or 50-amino acid protein, osteocalcin (or "bone Gla protein"; BGP), which has three γ-carboxyglutamate residues (Gla) is involved in the action of vitamin D in bone Ca^{2+} mobilization (Price, 1988; Price and Baukol, 1980). Active diOH-D acts on osteoblasts to increase synthesis and secretion of osteocalcin, which then binds tightly to hydroxyapatite, thus perhaps preventing further mineralization (Price, 1988). (Binding of this very soluble protein is dependent on Gla residues.) Some osteocalcin also escapes into the plasma, especially if vitamin K status is compromised (so it cannot be γ-carboxylated). Conditions like Paget's disease and hyperparathyroidism, characterized by an enhanced bone mineral turnover, thus also show increases in serum osteocalcin concentrations (Nutr Rev, 1981*b*).

Another well-characterized (extracellular) Gla protein, matrix Gla protein (or MGP), is also regulated by active vitamin D (Price, 1988). Highly insoluble (due to aggregation) and with about 80 amino acids (5 Gla residues), its mRNA is expressed in most body tissues, and especially in the lung, heart, and kidney (Fraser and Price, 1988) (with very little in the liver and brain). In terms of actual protein, however, there is very little except in bone, cartilage, and dentin (with just a little in lung, heart, and kidney). The function of this protein is uncertain but may relate to the extracellular matrix. Homologies among parts of MGP, BGP, and the various (γ-carboxylated) clotting proteins probably reflect their communal substrate recognition by the vitamin K-dependent γ-carboxylase.

The kidney also contains a Gla protein that may be involved in resorption of Ca^{2+} by the kidney tubules (Lian et al., 1978) (a function also related to vitamin D action). In addition, Gla proteins have been found in calcium-containing human kidney stones, and increased urinary excretion of free and protein-bound Gla occurs in some patients with kidney stones and in others with pathologic subcutaneous calcification (scleroderma and dermatomyositis) (Lian et al., 1978).

The tissue distributions of vitamin K, vitamin K epoxidase, and epoxide reductases also suggests that the action of the vitamin is more general and not confined to a few tissues (Bell, 1978). Uptake by the spleen equals that of the kidney, at least in rats, and is exceeded by that of the lungs, skin, and muscle. [γ-Carboxylation of ribosomes may also occur, at least in liver, and the vitamin may play a role in electron transfer, at least in bacteria (Olson, 1980).] Thus, it is likely that we are just beginning to understand the full functions of the phyllo- and menaquinones.

Absorption, Transport, and Excretion

Vitamin K is absorbed with variable efficiency (10%–80%), depending on the amount of accompanying fat in the diet and help of bile acids. It is distributed like other lipids, initially on chylomicrons, and then on VLDL and LDL (see Chapter 3). The liver is the main repository, although

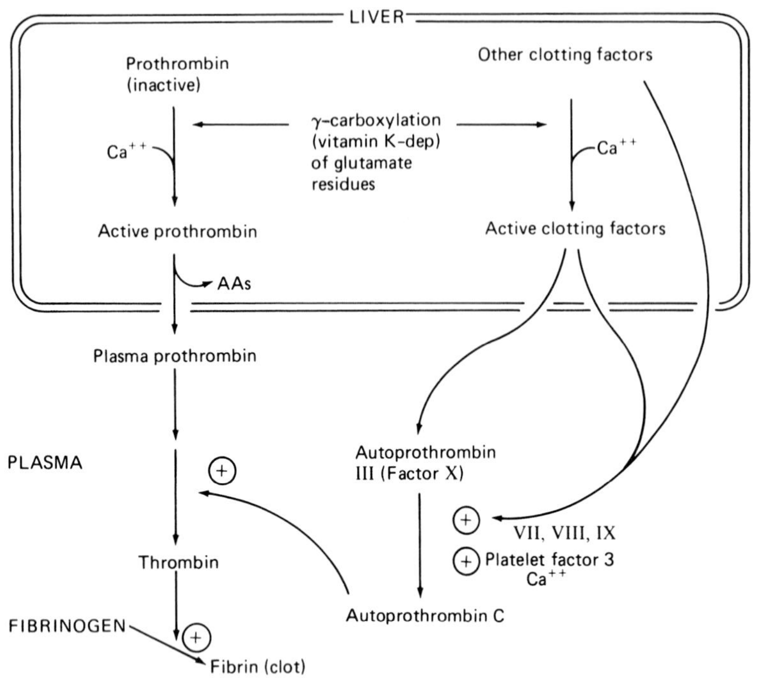

Prot.〰C(=O)—CH(CH$_2$CH$_2$COO$^-$)—N(H)—C〰 $\xrightarrow[\text{γ-carboxylase, NADH (microsomes)}]{CO_2,\ O_2,\ \text{Vitamin K}}$ 〰C(=O)—CH(CH$_2$CH(COO$^-$)COO$^-$)—N(H)—C〰Prot. Ca^{++}

Figure 5.35. Involvement of vitamin K in blood clotting and γ-carboxylation. *Key:* AAs are amino acids. Vitamin K-dependent γ-carboxylation of glutamate residues results in a high affinity of the latter proteins for Ca^{2+}. The resulting Ca^{2+} binding is important for the function of these proteins.

there appears to be a rapid turnover, and average body pools are probably very small (on the order of 50–100 μg; with total turnover in about a day) (Olson, 1988). (This supports the need for a constant supply from gut bacteria.) Liver vitamin K is usually half in the form of phylloquinone and half as bacterial menaquinones. Serum, however, contains mostly phylloquinones, suggesting that one might be converted to the other. Vitamin K and its oxidized metabolites are lost mainly in the bile but also partly in the urine.

Requirements and Toxicity

The NAS has advised a daily dietary intake of 60–80 μg by adults (Figure 5.34), and the average intake by Americans on a mixed diet is thought to be 300–500 μg daily. These amounts should be more than adequate, particularly as gut bacteria supply a substantial fraction. Indeed, evidence of overt vitamin K deficiency in humans is quite rare. Exceptions are the newborn infant (already cited) and persons with warfarin poisoning (warfarin is used as rat poison) or those on dicoumerol therapy for thromboembolic disease. Both of the latter substances (Figure 5.34) are potent inhibitors of vitamin K action, probably via effects on the reductases that regenerate the active hydroquinone (Olson, 1988). Although vitamin K is fat soluble, there are no known cases of toxicity in man. Indeed, little is known about the toxicity of the vitamin even in animals. The exception is the synthetic form, menadione, which appears to react with sulfhydryl groups on proteins and can be quite toxic (Mezick et al., 1970).

Other Vitaminlike Substances

Carotenes

Until recently, carotenes in nutrition have been considered only in relation to their role as precursors of vitamin A (Table 5.7). Now, however, the possibility of some additional independent role in health maintenance no longer seems far-fetched. The stimulus for such thinking has come first from epidemiological data showing a more significant inverse correlation between carotene intake and the incidence of certain forms of cancer than for retinoids; and animal studies in which regression of certain tumors has been demonstrated with β-carotene; a similar response has been obtained with canthaxanthin, a carotenoid that cannot be converted to vitamin A (see Chapter 16 for details). Of additional interest is the fact that carotenes are powerful antioxidants (Dimitrov, 1986), and thus may belong to the group of nutrients generally recruited to prevent inappropriate oxidations. One example of this has been the successful treatment of photosensitivity conditions with excess carotene (Mathews-Roth, 1982), where singlet oxygen production by light can lead to cell damage (as in certain porphyrias) (Goodwin, 1986). The differential handling of carotenes and retinoids by the mammalian organism, and a considerable capacity of the body for nontoxic carotene storage, both speak to a need for these components independent of vitamin A. Relatively little is known about the absorption, transport, and metabolism of carotenes or of their mechanisms of action (Goodwin, 1986). What is known is covered under the section on vitamin A.

Bioflavonoids

The possibility that flavonic compounds might be necessary in the prevention of capillary permeability or fragility was introduced in 1936 by Szenti-György, who later named these substances vitamin P. In 1950, this term was discontinued in favor of "bioflavonoids," to indicate that, although they might have biologic activity, this was more in the nature of nonspecific preventative effects and not essential for life.

Typical flavonoids are shown in Figure 5.36. They are colorful antioxidants, found mostly as glycosides, capable of chelating metal ions, and responsible for the colors of berries (red/blue). Most are in cytosolic cell vacuoles in the skin of citrus (yellow/colorless) and other fruits and vegetables. Some (free) flavonoids may also be on cell surfaces (Wollenweber, 1988). It is estimated that about one half of our normal daily average intake of 1–2 g is absorbed (Weininger and Briggs, 1980), mostly in the form of quercetin and kaempferol (Bokkenheuser and Winter, 1987) after hydrolysis of rutin, quercitrin, and robinin (glycosidic forms). In plants, they are thought to function var-

Figure 5.36. Some bioflavonoids.

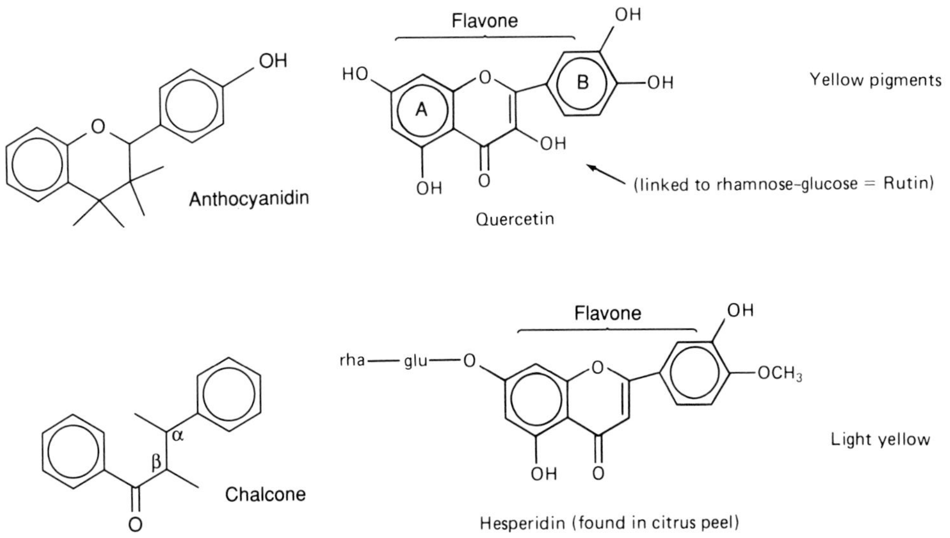

iously as insect attractants, repellants, and antifungal agents. Many have been identified as the active ingredients of folk medicines (see Cody et al., 1988).

Apart from antioxidant actions, certain bioflavonoids inhibit aldose reductase, which converts glucose and galactose to their polyols. [These polyols have been implicated in the neuropathy of diabetes and in the cataract formation that accompanies diabetes and galactosemia (see Chapter 2).] Flavonoids, like quercetin, also inhibit phosphodiesterases (which break down cyclic nucleotides) and thus affect smooth muscle relaxation.

Numerous therapeutic uses have been claimed which are considered controversial (Weininger and Briggs, 1980). Nevertheless, it should be noted that there are many reports of beneficial effects including prevention of stillborn births or neonatal deaths due to erythroblastosis (Jacobs, 1965), reduced red blood cell aggregation and reduced bleeding associated with capillary fragility (Miner, 1955), as well as cholesterol lowering, antihypertensive, antiallergic, antiviral, anticancer, and even contraceptive effects (Cody et al., 1988; Gabor, 1988). Some of the studies are recent and sophisticated, but their overall relevance to everyday nutrition and health is still uncertain. One study reports, that together with large doses of vitamin C, they may have a beneficial effect on the incidence of cold sores due to herpes infection (Terezhainy et al., 1978); although the individual contribution of the flavonoids and C were not evaluated. This is supported by other evidence of antiviral activity (Vlietinck et al., 1988). In general, food flavonoids would appear to be quite nontoxic, but frequent therapeutic use of certain forms may not be entirely benign (Jaeger et al., 1988).

Carnitine (Vitamin B_t)

This substance is a dietary essential only for the mealworm larva, a characteristic that lead Fraenkel to its discovery in 1947. It may, however, also be required by premature human infants and newborn rats (Hahn, 1982). It is synthesized from lysine and methionine in animal tissues (kidney and liver) by a pathway containing two steps that require Fe^{2+} and ascorbate for hydroxylation (Figure 5.37). From these tissues it travels to other cells via the blood. It is present in large quantities in muscle meats [where it represents 0.1% of tissue dry matter (Metzler, 1977)], milk, liver, and yeast. [Concentrations are also especially high in the epididymus (Broquist, 1988*b*).] In contrast, there appears to be very little carnitine in plant-derived foods. Since carnitine is formed from amino acids, protein malnutrition will lower carnitine production and tissue concentrations, a phenomenon that may have adverse consequences for fatty acid transport and oxidation (see below).

At this time, the only clear (but important) biochemical functions of carnitine are in lipid metabolism, as a carrier of acyl acids across cell membranes (Figure 5.37). Carnitine is mandatory for transport of long-chain fatty acids into mitochondria for β-oxidation (Broquist and Borum, 1982). This is particularly important for tissues, like muscles, which depend a great deal on fatty acids for energy, and may be considered the most central role of this factor. Brown adipose tissue is also highly dependent on carnitine to aid in the heat-producing β-oxidation of fatty acids. Ketogenesis (in liver and kidney) also depends on this carrier function of carnitine, for which carnitine is bound to a membrane acyltransferase.

More recent work indicates that carnitine (and its transferases) may also play other roles, including the transfer of acetyl and short-chain acyl units back to the cytosol (to form acyl-CoAs). Perhaps even more importantly, it may serve as a blood-borne carrier of odd carbon pieces for excretion in the urine (Bleber, 1988). An example of this would be the transport and excretion of propionyl-carnitine in B_{12} deficiency states (Brass and Stabler, 1988), where conversions of propionyl-SCoA (formed in degradation of isoleucine and some other amino acids) is blocked (see section on vitamin B_{12}). Certain drugs may also be detoxified and removed in this manner (Bieber, 1988), which may account for the presence of carnitine in peroxisomal and microsomal (ER) membranes. In animals, a marginal carnitine deficiency (achieved by feeding a low lysine diet) resulted in fatty liver, which was relieved by giving carnitine (Broquist and Borum, 1982). It is possible that similar defects in lipid metabolism could occur in subjects suffering from protein deficiency.

Tissue carnitine concentrations appear to be depressed in certain lipid storage diseases of the muscle, in diabetes, muscular dystrophy, and hyperthyroidism, and sometimes in pregnancy and with physical exertion (Bray and Briggs, 1980). Whether this represents a basic defect, or secondary response to any of these conditions is unclear at this time. Congenital carnitine deficiency has been reported in humans, with evidence of cytoplasmic lipid vacuole accumulation within weak muscle cells (Dickerson and Timkovitch, 1975).

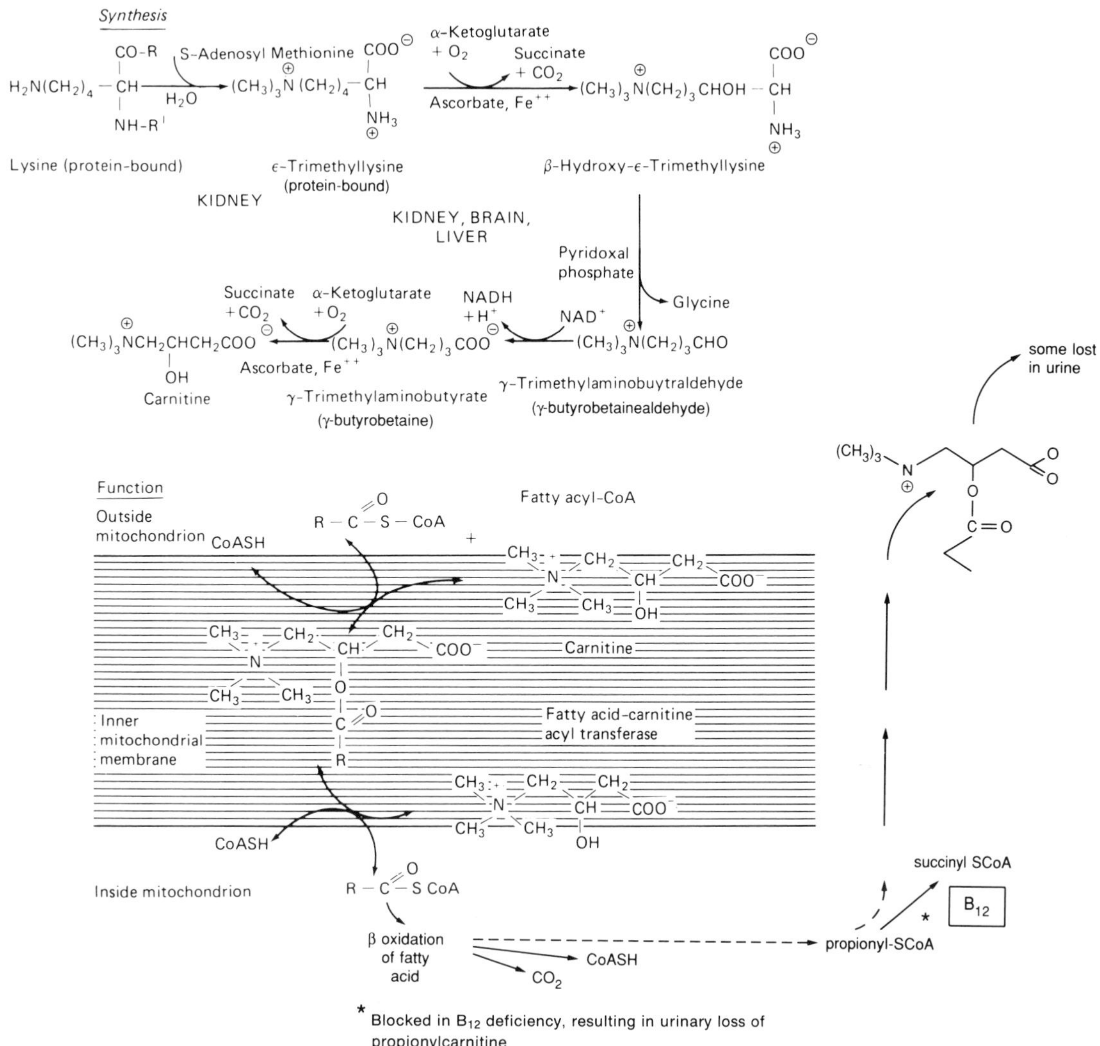

Figure 5.37. Synthesis and functions of carnitine. The upper part of the figure shows the synthetic pathway for synthesis of carnitine from lysine and S-adenyl-methionine, via steps involving several vitamins. Lower half shows involvement of carnitine in transfer of fatty acids across the mitochondrial membrane for β-oxidation (left), and potential "spillage" of propionyl carnitine out of mitochondria and the cell into the urine, in B_{12} deficiency (right). [*Source:* Nutr Rev (1978, 1981*a*), Bieber (1988), and Brass and Stabler (1988).] See also Figure 5.7.

Pyrroloquinoline Quinone (PQQ) or 6-OH Dopa

PQQ (Figure 5.38) was first identified in 1979 as a cofactor for the methanol dehydrogenase of bacteria (Duine and Frank, 1980) and has since been thought to be associated with more than 15 other enzymes in many organisms (including plants), and at least six in animal tissues (also referred to as quinoproteins). A spectrum similar to that of pyridoxine (or pyridoxal phosphate; Figure 5.13) was a confounding factor in the identification of PQQ as a necessary component for lysyl oxidase and dopamine-β-hydroxylase, and some confusion still reigns. Indeed, Klinman and her colleagues, working with amine oxidase (Janes et al., 1990), have concluded that the actual factor is 6-OH dopa (topa), which (in the quinone form) could oxidize and cyclize to a substance resembling PQQ (Figure 5.38). Either way, the cofactor may (like B_6) participate in Schiff-base type reactions (Duine and Jongejan, 1989). Like riboflavin and nicotinamide cofactors, it also functions as an intermediate in hydride extraction/dehydrogenase reactions, and most of the mammalian enzymes with which it is involved also have Cu^{2+} in the active site.

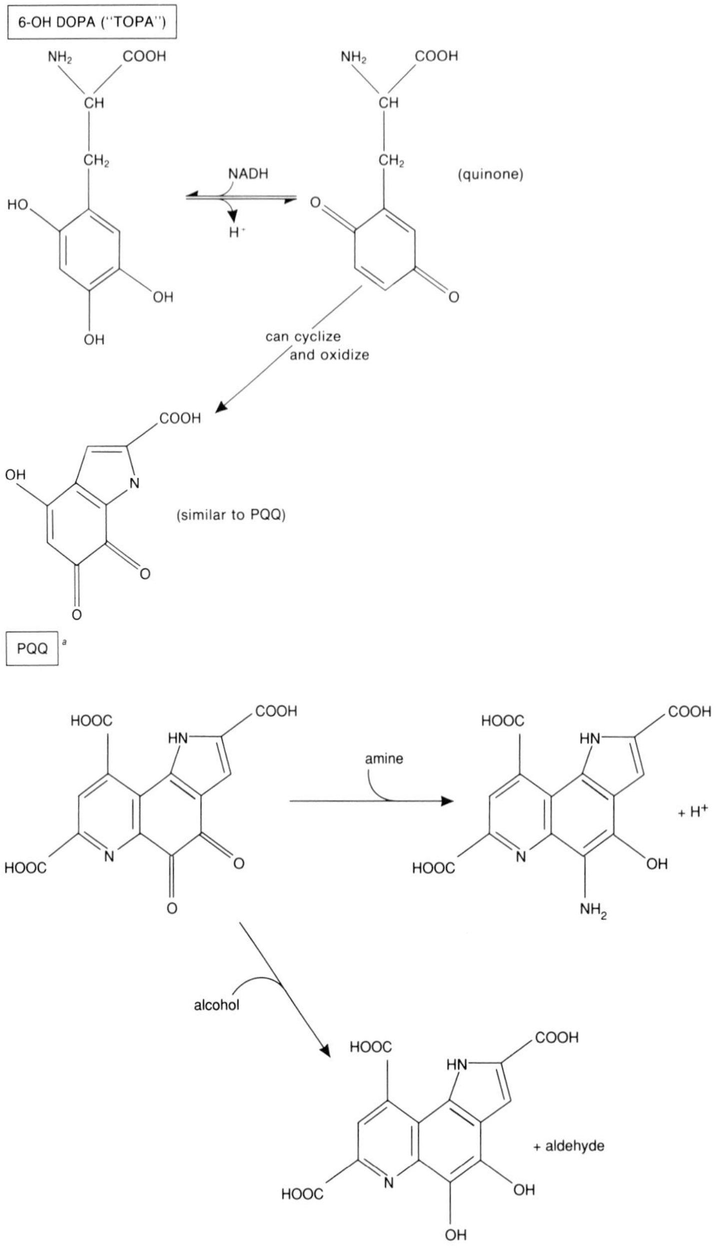

6-OH DOPA ("TOPA")

NH_2 COOH CH CH_2 HO OH OH

NADH

H⁻

NH_2 COOH CH CH_2 O O

(quinone)

can cyclize and oxidize

COOH OH N O O

(similar to PQQ)

PQQ [a]

HOOC COOH HN HOOC N O O

amine

HOOC COOH HN HOOC N OH NH_2

$+ H^+$

alcohol

HOOC COOH HN HOOC N OH OH

+ aldehyde

Probable cofactor for:
- Lysyl oxidase (Cu^{2+})
- Dopamine-/β-hydroxylase (Cu^{2+})
- Amine oxidase (Cu^{2+})
- Diamine oxidase (Cu^{2+})
- DOPA decarboxylase
- Choline dehydrogenase
- [several bacterial, plant and fungal enzymes, including galactose oxidase (fungi) and lipoxygenase (soybeans).]

[a] Based on Duine and Jongejan (1989).

Figure 5.38. Structure and function of 6-OH dopamine and/or pyrroloquinoline quinone. [*Source:* mainly Janes et al. (1990), Duine and Jongejan (1989), Linder (1990), and Nutr Rev (1988).]

Little is known about the synthesis, nutrition, and metabolism of either PQQ or 6-OH dopa except that they are produced by bacteria, are ubiquitous in foods, and may be essential in the diet. Evidence for the latter stems from studies with mice on defined diets devoid of PQQ (and on antibiotic treatments), which resulted in a modest reduction in skin lysyl oxidase (Killgore et al., 1989). It seems likely we will soon know more about these factors.

Nonvitamins

Pangamic Acid (Vitamin B_{15})

This rather mysterious material was patented by Krebs (of Laetrile fame). It was first prepared from apricot pits in 1951 and later from rice, liver, blood, and yeast, and proposed for treatment of cardiovascular and rheumatic diseases. Its apparent common presence in foods and physiologic effects lead to its designation as a B vitamin by some investigators (Kraushaar et al., 1963), a designation that has been soundly rejected by most others. There is no evidence that its lack in the diet results in a deficiency disease; nor is it even known whether the human (or animal) body can produce it. The designation B_{15} comes from speculation that pangamate is the same as a liver factor given that name by some Japanese researchers (Kraushaar et al., 1963).

Studies on pangamate preparations in the 1960s indicated the material was a mixture of diisopropylammonium dichloroacetate (DIPA, the "active ingredient") and gluconic acid and glycine (Fig. 5.39) (Bigi, 1966). Since then, Stacpoole (1977) reports that the structure of "pangamate" has been clarified as D-gluconodimethylaminoacetic acid (Figure 5.38), and a more reliable assay has been developed that confirms its general presence in cereal grains (Kraushaar et al., 1963). Sale of "pangamate" has been a fad in the health food industry. Some of the pills sold in the United States are listed as containing equimolar amounts of calcium gluconate and N-dimethylglycine. This would appear to be another in the series of formulations given the name.

Little is known of the functions and effects of pangamate at the molecular level, but European and Russian researchers have recorded consistent effects of enhanced O_2 uptake, more rapid adaptation to strenuous exercise (less lactate production, more glycogen, and muscle creatine phosphate), and better adaptation to hypoxia in animals and humans (Kraushaar et al., 1963). Less consistent effects on cardiovascular function and

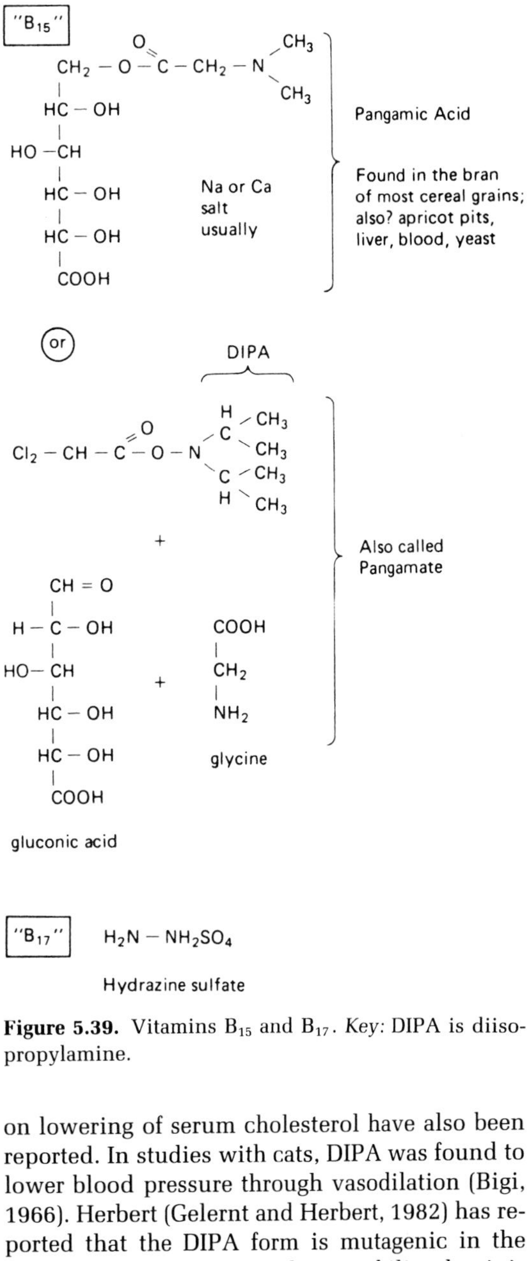

"B_{15}"

$CH_2-O-C(=O)-CH_2-N(CH_3)_2$, HC–OH, HO–CH, HC–OH, HC–OH, COOH

Na or Ca salt usually

Pangamic Acid

Found in the bran of most cereal grains; also? apricot pits, liver, blood, yeast

or

DIPA

$Cl_2-CH-C(=O)-O-N$ [$CH(CH_3)_2$]$_2$

+

CH = O, H–C–OH, HO–CH, HC–OH, HC–OH, COOH

gluconic acid

+

COOH, CH_2, NH_2

glycine

Also called Pangamate

"B_{17}" $H_2N-NH_2SO_4$

Hydrazine sulfate

Figure 5.39. Vitamins B_{15} and B_{17}. *Key:* DIPA is diisopropylamine.

on lowering of serum cholesterol have also been reported. In studies with cats, DIPA was found to lower blood pressure through vasodilation (Bigi, 1966). Herbert (Gelernt and Herbert, 1982) has reported that the DIPA form is mutagenic in the Ames assay, which raises the possibility that it is also carcinogenic. In summary, though the material is perhaps a natural product present in foodstuffs, there is no evidence that pangamate (D-gluconodimethylaminoacetic acid) is a nutrient, much less a vitamin, and, if anything, it should be considered a drug. The DIPA form may in fact be toxic.

Hydrazine Sulfate (Vitamin B_{17})

This man-made material has been applied by some physicians and researchers (in the United

States and the Soviet Union) to the treatment of cancer. Some studies of terminal cancer patients have claimed a significant effect on cancer cachexia (lack of appetite), leading to weight gain, which may be useful in prolonging life (Gold, 1981). The potential mechanism of this effect is not clear but may involve inhibition of gluconeogenesis. Clearly, the material is not a vitamin.

Laetrile

Laetrile itself is not considered a vitamin even by the individuals who favor its use as drug against cancer. A full discussion of this material and its effects is found in Chapter 16.

References

Abraham GE, Hargrove JT (1980): Infertility 3:155.

Ahluwalia GS, Kaul L, Ahluwalia BS (1980): J Nutr 110:1185.

Ahluwalia GS, Kaul L, Ahluwalia BS (1981): Nutr Rev 39:139.

Albert MJ, Mathan VI, Baker SJ (1980): Nature 283:781.

Anderson R, Lukey PT (1989): Ann NY Acad Sci 498:229.

Anderson R, Oosthuizen R, Maritz R, Theron A, Van Rensburg AJ (1980): Am J Clin Nutr 33:71.

Anderson TW (1977): Nutr Today (January/February):1.

Anderson TW, Beaton GH, Corey PN, Spero L (1975): Can Med Assoc J 112:823.

Anderson TW, Reid DBW, Beaton GH (1972): Can Med Assoc J 107:503.

Anderson TW, Suranyl O, Beaton GH (1974): Can Med Assoc J 111:31.

Andon MB, Howard MP, Moser PB, Reynolds RD (1985): Pediatrics 76:769.

Appel JA, Briggs GM (1980*a*): *In* Goodhart RS, Shils ME, eds: Modern nutrition in health and disease (6th ed). Philadelphia: Lea & Febiger, p 274.

Appel JA, Briggs GM (1980*b*): *In* Goodhart RS, Shils ME, eds: Modern nutrition in health and disease (6th ed). Philadelphia: Lea & Febiger, p 286.

Appel JA, Briggs GM (1980*c*): *In* Goodhart RS, Shils ME, eds: Modern nutrition in health and disease (6th ed). Philadelphia: Lea & Febiger, p 282.

Banerjee RV, Matthews RG (1990): FASEB J 4:1450.

Barley FW, Sato GH, Abeles RH (1972): J Biol Chem 247:4270.

Bartus RT, Dean RL, Goas AJ, et al. (1980): Science 209:301.

Bartus RT, Dean RL, Beer B, Lippa AS (1982): Science 217:408.

Batres RO, Olson JA (1987): J Nutr 117:874.

Bauernfeind JC (1977): Crit Rev Fd Sci Nutr 9:337.

Bedo G, Santisteban P, Aranda A (1989): Nature 339:231.

Bell RG (1978): Fed Proc 37:2599.

Bender DA, Tagoe CE, Vale JA (1982): Br J Nutr 47:609.

Benesch R, Benesch RE, Edalki R, Suzuki T (1977): Proc Natl Acad Sci USA 74:1721.

Bernstein AL, Lobitz CS (1988): *In* Leklem JE, Reynolds RD, eds: Clinical and physiological applications of vitamin B-6. New York: Alan R Liss, p 415.

Bieber LL (1988): Annu Rev Biochem 57:261.

Bieri JG, Corash L, Hubbard VS (1983): N Engl J Med 308:1063.

Bigi B (1966): Arch Biochem Cosmetol 9:62.

Black AL, Guirard BM, Snell EE (1977): J Nutr 107:1962.

Black AL, Guirard BM, Snell EE (1978): J Nutr 108:670.

Bland J (1980): *In* Brewster MA, Naito HK, eds: Nutritional elements and clinical biochemistry. New York: Plenum, p 139.

Blankenhorn G (1986): Z Orthop Ihre Gvenzgeb 124:340.

Blomhoff R (1987): Nutr Rev 45:257.

Blomhoff R, Green MH, Berg T, Norum KR (1990): Science 250:399.

Bokkenheuser VD, Winter J (1987): *In* Cody V, Middleton E Jr, Harborne JB, Beretz A, eds: Plant flavonoids in biology and medicine II. New York: Alan R Liss, p 143.

Bollag W, Matter A (1981): Ann NY Acad Sci 359:9.

Boyd AM, Ratcliffe AH, Jepson RP, James GWH (1949): J Bone Joint Surg [Br] 31:325.

Branda RF, Eaton JW (1978): Science 201:625.

Brass EP, Stabler SP (1988): Biochem J 255:153.

Bray DL, Briggs GM (1980): *In* Goodhart RS, Shils ME, eds: Modern nutrition in health and disease (6th ed). Philadelphia: Lea & Febiger, p 291.

Briggs M, Briggs M (1972): Nature 238:277.

Brody T, Watson JE, Stokstad EL (1982): Biochemistry 21:276.

Broquist HP (1988*a*): *In* Shils ME, Young VR, eds: Modern nutrition in health and disease (7th ed). Philadelphia: Lea & Febiger, p 459.

Broquist HP (1988*b*): *In* Shils ME, Young VR, eds: Modern nutrition in health and disease (7th ed). Philadelphia: Lea & Febiger, p 453.

Broquist HP, Borum PR (1982): Adv Nutr Res 4:181.

Bruce WR (1983): Progr Clin Biol Res 132D:131 (Proceedings of the 13th International Cancer Congress, Seattle, September 8–15, 1982: Part D).

Burton GW, Ingold KU (1989): Ann NY Acad Sci 570:7.

Buttriss JL, Diplock AT (1988): Biochim Biophys Acta 963:61.

Cameron E, Pauling L (1978): Proc Natl Acad Sci USA 75:4538.

Carmel R (1990): Am J Hematol 34:108.

Carmel R, Karnaze DS, Weiner JM (1988*a*): J Lab Clin Med 111:57.

Carmel R, Lau K-HW, Baylink DJ, Saxena S, Singer FR (1988*b*): N Engl J Med 319:70.

Carmel R, Sinow RM, Siegel ME, Samloff M (1988*c*): Arch Intern Med 148:1715.

Chan VT, Wolf G (1987): Biochem J 247:53.

Chatham MD, Epler JH Jr, Sauder LR, Green D, Kulle TJ (1987): Ann NY Acad Sci 498:269.

Chiocca EA, Davies PJA, Stein JP (1988): J Biol Chem 263:11584.

Chytil F, Ong DE (1987): Annu Rev Nutr 7:321.

Clemetson CAB (1980): J Nutr 110:662.

Coble BI, Dahlgren C, Stendahl O (1987): Acta Derm Venereol (Stockh) 67:481.

Cody V, Middleton E Jr, Harborne JB, Beretz A, eds (1988): Plant flavonoids in biology and medicine II. New York: Alan R Liss.

Coelingh-Bennink HJT, Schreurs WHP (1975): Br Med J 3:13.

Cohen EL, Wurtman RJ (1976): Science 191:561.

Colman N, Hettiarachchy N, Herbert V (1981): Science 211:1427.

Compton MM, Cidlowski JA (1986): Endocr Rev 7:140.

Cook JD, Watson SS, Simpson KH, Lipschitz DA, Skikne BS (1984): Blood 64:721.

Cooper BA, Rosenblatt DS (1987): Annu Rev Nutr 7:291.

Cooper DR, Kling OR, Carpenter MP (1987): Endocrinology 120:83.

Coulehan JL, Eberfard S, Kapner L, Taylor F, Rogers K, Garry P (1976): N Engl J Med 295:973.

Coulehan JL, Reisinger KS, Rogers KD, Bradley DW (1974): N Engl J Med 290:6.

Crow TJ (1974): Nature 252:634.

Cullen RW, Oace SM (1989*a*): J Nutr 119:1115.

Cullen RW, Oace SM (1989*b*): J Nutr 119:1121.

Dakshinamurti K, Chauhan J (1988): Annu Rev Nutr 8:211.

Dalton K (1985): Lancet 2:1168.

DeLuca HF (1980): *In* Goodhart RS, Shils ME, eds: Modern nutrition in health and disease (7th ed). Philadelphia: Lea & Febiger, p 160.

DeLuca HF (1982): Biochem Soc Trans 10:147.

DeLuca HF (1988): *In* Shils ME, Young VR, eds: Modern nutrition in health and disease (7th ed). Philadelphia: Lea & Febiger, p 313.

DeLuca HF, Zile M, Sietsema WK (1981): Ann NY Acad Sci 359:25.

DeLuca LM, Shapiro SS (1981): Ann NY Acad Sci 359.

DeLuca LM, Little EP, Wolf G (1969): J Biol Chem 244:701.

Dickerson RE, Timkovich R (1975): *In* Boyer PD, ed: The enzymes (3rd ed), vol 11. New York: Academic, p 397.

Dimitrov NV (1986): *In* Bland J, ed: A year in nutritional medicine (2nd ed). New Canaan, CT: Keats Publishing, p 167.

Dion PW, Bright-See EB, Smith CC, Bruce WR (1982): Mutat Res 102:27.

Diplock AT, Xu G-L, Yeow C-L, Okikiola M (1989*b*): Ann NY Acad Sci 570:72.

Dong A, Scott SC (1982): Ann Nutr Metab 26:209.

Dowling JE, Wald G (1960): J Biol Chem 146:587.

Dratz EA, Farnsworth CC, Loew EC, Stephens RJ, Thomas DW, Van Kuijk FJGM (1989): Ann NY Acad Sci 570:46.

Dubick MA, Rucker RB (in press): Manuscript submitted.

Duine JA, Frank J (1980): Biochem J 187:221.

Duine JA, Jongejan JA (1989): Annu Rev Biochem 58:403.

Ebadi M (1978): *In* Proceedings of a workshop on vitamin B_6. Washington, DC: National Academy of Sciences, p 129.

Ehrenkranz RA, Bonita BW, Ablow RC, Warshaw JB (1978): N Engl J Med 299:564.

Elias E, Muller DPR, Scott J (1981): Lancet 2:1319.

Ellis ER, Nasser S (1973): Br J Nutr 30:277.

Ellis JM, Presley J (1973): Vitamin B_6, the doctor's report. New York: Harper and Row.

Ellis J, Folkers K, Watanabe T, Kaji M, Saji S, Caldwell JW, Temple CA, Wood FS (1979): Am J Clin Nutr 32:2040.

England S, Seifter S (1986): Annu Rev Nutr 6:365.

Esmon CT, Sadowski JA, Suttie JW (1975): J Biol Chem 250:4744.

Farrell PM (1988): *In* Shils M, Young V, eds: Modern nutrition in health and disease. New York: Plenum, p 340.

Favus MJ, Mangelsdorf DJ, Tembe V, Coe BJ, Haussler MR (1988): J Clin Invest 82:218.

Fazio V, Flint DM, Wahlquist ML (1981): Am J Clin Nutr 34:2394.

Federation Proceedings Symposium (1981): Conquest of pellagra 40:1519.

Fesus L, Vilmos T (1988): Adv Exp Med Biol 231:119.

Fesus L, Vilmos T, Autuori F, Ceru MP, Tarcsa E, Piascentini M (1989): FEBS Lett 245:150.

Finley E, Cerklewski F (1983): Sci News 124:281.

Foca FJ (1985): Arch Phys Med Rehabil 66:634.

Folkers K, Shizukuishi S, Scudder SL, Willis R, Takemura K, Longenecker JB (1981): Biochem Biophys Res Commun 100:972.

Fraser JD, Price PA (1988): J Biol Chem 263:11033.

Frolik CA (1981): Ann NY Acad Sci 359:37.

Gabor M (1987): *In* Cody V, Middleton E Jr, Harborne JB, Beretz A, eds: Plant flavonoids in biology and medicine II. New York: Alan R Liss, p 1.

Garabedian M, Tanaka Y, Holick MF, DeLuca HF (1974): Endocrinology 94:1022.

Gavin G, McHenry EN (1941): J Biol Chem 139:485.

Gerlernt MD, Herbert V (1982): Nutr Cancer 3:129.

Gey KF, Stahelin HB, Puska P, Evans A (1987): Ann NY Acad Sci 498:110.

Gibbs CE, Seitchik J (1980): *In* Goodhart RS, Shils ME, eds: Modern nutrition in health and disease (6th ed). Philadelphia: Lea & Febiger, p 743.

Gold J (1981): Nutr Cancer 3:31.

Goodman DS (1981): Ann NY Acad Sci 359:69.

Goodman DS (1984): The retinoids. New York: Academic.

Goodwin TW (1986): Annu Rev Nutr 6:273.

Goodwin TW, Goad LJ (1970): *In* Hume AC, ed: The biochemistry of fruits and their products, vol 1. London: Academic, p 305.

Gregory JF III, Kirk JR (1981): Nutr Rev 39:1.

Groenhoej Larsen F, Jakobsen P, Groenhoej Larsen C, Kragballe K, Nielsen-Kudsk F (1988): Pharmacol Toxicol 62:159.

Grongaud R, Nichol M, Desplanques D (1969): Am J Clin Nutr 22:991.
Growdon JH, Wurtman RJ (1979): Nutr Rev 37:129.
Guilarte TR, Wagner HN Jr (1987): J Neurochem 49:1918.
Haas RH (1988): Annu Rev Nutr 8:483.
Haeger K (1982): Ann NY Acad Sci 393:369.
Hagan I (1985): Acta Obstet Gynecol Scand 64:667.
Hahn P (1982): Nutr Res 2:201.
Halloran BP, DeLuca HF (1979): Science 204:73.
Harris PL, Embree ND (1963): Am J Clin Nutr 13:385.
Haussler MR (1986): Annu Rev Nutr 6:527.
Hawthorne JN (1982): Nature 295:281.
Hawthorne JN, White DA (1975): Vit Horm 33:529.
Helmreich EJM, Klein HW (1980): Agnew Chem (Engl) 19:441.
Henderson LM, Hulse JD (1978): *In* Human vitamin B_6 requirements, proceedings of the workshop, June 1976. Washington, DC: National Academy of Sciences, p 21.
Herbert VD (1979): *In* Labuza PT, Sloan AE, eds: Contemporary nutrition controversies. Los Angeles: West Publishing, p 223.
Herbert V, Jacob E (1974): JAMA 230:241.
Herbert V, Coleman H, Jacob E (1980): *In* Goodhart RS, Shils ME, eds: Modern nutrition in health and disease (6th ed). Philadelphia: Lea & Febiger, p 229.
Herbert V, Coleman H, Jacob E (1988): *In* Shils ME, Young VR, eds: Modern nutrition in health and disease (7th ed). Philadelphia: Lea & Febiger, p 388.
Herbert VE, Jacob E, Wong K-T, Scott J, Pfetter RD (1978): Am J Clin Nutr 31:253.
Hodges RE (1980): *In* Goodhart RS, Shils ME, eds: Modern nutrition in health and disease (6th ed). Philadelphia: Lea & Febiger, p 259.
Hodgkinson A (1977): Oxalic acid in biology and medicine. London: Academic.
Holick MF, Clark MB (1978): Fed Proc 37:2567.
Holick MF, MacLaughlin JA, Doppelt SH (1981): Science 211:590.
Holub BJ (1986): Annu Rev Nutr 6:563.
Hoover GA, Nicolosi RJ, Corey JE (1978): J Nutr 108:1588.
Horovitz O, Knaack D, Podleski TR, Salpeter MM (1989): J Cell Biol 108:1823.
Horwitt MK (1980*a*): *In* Goodhart RS, Shils ME, eds: Modern nutrition in health and disease (6th ed). Philadelphia: Lea & Febiger, p 197.
Horwitt MK (1980*b*): *In* Goodhart RS, Shils ME, eds: Modern nutrition in health and disease (6th ed). Philadelphia: Lea & Febiger, p 204.
Hussey GD, Klein M (1990): N Engl J Med 323:160.
Jacobs WM (1965): Am J Obstet Gynecol 25:648.
Jaeger A, Walti M, Neftel K (1988): *In* Cody V, Middleton E Jr, Harborne JB, Beretz A, eds: Plant flavonoids in biology and medicine. New York: Alan R Liss, p 379.
Janes SM, Mu D, Wemmer D, et al. (1990): Science 248:981.
Johnson L, Schaffer D, Boggs TR (1974): Am J Clin Nutr 19:147.
Karlowski TR, Chalmers TC, Freunkel CO, Kapikian AZ, Lewis TL, Lynch JM (1975): JAMA 231:1038.
Karpen CW, Pritchard KA Jr, Arnold JH, Cornwall DG, Panganamala RV (1982): Diabetes 31:947.
Kato N, Kawai K, Yoshida A (1981): Am J Clin Nutr 11:1727.
Keith RE, Mossholder SB (1986): Intl J Vitam Nutr Res 56:363.
Killgore J, Schmidt C, Duich L, et al. (1989): Science 245:850.
Kim HY, Wolf G (1987): J Biol Chem 262:365.
King MM, Lai EK, McCoy PB (1975): J Biol Chem 250:6496.
Knox EG (1973): Lancet 1:1465.
Knox WE, Greengard O (1967): Adv Enzyme Regul 4:247.
Komm BS, Ternpening CM, Benz DJH, et al. (1988): Science 241:81.
Kraemer KH, DiGiovanna JJ, Moshell AN, Tarone RE, Peck GL (1988): N Engl J Med 318:1633.
Kraft JC, Nau H, Lammer E, Olney A (1989): N Engl J Med 321:262.
Kraushaar AE, Schunk RW, Thym HF (1963): Arzneimittelforsch 13:109.
Krebs E, Fischer EH (1964): Vitam Horm 22:399.
Krehl WA (1981): Fed Proc 40:1527.
Krishnankura K, Sweeley CC (1976): J Biol Chem 151:1597.
Krumdieck C, Butterworth CE Jr (1974): Am J Clin Nutr 27:866.
Kumar R, Cohen WR, Epstein FH (1980): N Engl J Med 302:1143.
Labuza TP, Sloan AE (1979): Contemporary nutrition controversies. Los Angeles: West Publishing.
Leklem JE (1988): *In* Leklem JE, Reynolds RD, eds: Clinical and physiological applications of vitamin B-6. New York: Alan R Liss, p 3.
Leklem JE, Reynolds RD (1988): *In* Leklem JE, Reynolds RD, eds: Clinical and physiological applications of vitamin B-6. New York: Alan R Liss, p 437.
Leklem JE, Brown RR, Rose DP, Linkswiler H, Arend RA (1975): Am J Clin Nutr 28:146.
Leo MA, Kim C-L, Lieber CS (1988): Drug–Nutrient Interact 5:227.
Levander OA, Welsh SO, Morris VC (1980): Ann NY Acad Sci 355:227.
Lewin IM, Yannai Y, Sulimovici S, et al. (1976): Biochem J 156:375.
Lian J, Hauscha PV, Gallop PM (1978): Fed Proc 37:2615.
Lim KL, Young RW, Palmer JK, Driskell JA (1982): J Chromatogr 250:86.
Lindenbaum J, Healton EB, Savage DG, et al. (1988): N Engl J Med 318:1720.
Linder MC (1978): *In* Schaefer KW, Hildebrandt G, Macbeth N, eds: A new image of man in medicine, vol II. Mt. Kisco, NY: Futura, p 109.

Linder MC (1991): The biochemistry of copper. New York: Plenum, in press.

Livingstone PD, Jones C (1985): Lancet 2:602.

Lohmann W (1987): Ann NY Acad Sci 498:307.

Lui NST, Roels OA (1980): *In* Goodhart RS, Shils ME, eds: Modern nutrition in health and disease (6th ed). Philadelphia: Lea & Febiger, p 142.

Machtey I, Ouaknine L (1978): J Am Geriatr Soc 26:328.

Mahan R (1980): *In* Goodehart RS, Shils ME, eds: Modern nutrition in health and disease (6th ed). Philadelphia: Lea & Febiger.

Manolagas SC, Provvedini DM, Tsoukas CD (1985): Mol Cell Endocrinol 43:113.

Mathews-Roth MM (1982): Oncology 39:33.

McCarron DA (1987): J Lab Clin Med 110:663.

McCay PG, Brueggemann G, Lai EK, Powell SR (1989): Ann NY Acad Sci 50:32.

McCollum EV, Simmonds N, Becker JE, Shipley PG (1922): J Biol Chem 53:293.

McCormick DB (1988*a*): *In* Shils ME, Young VR, eds: Modern nutrition in health and disease (7th ed). Philadelphia: Lea & Febiger, p 362.

McCormick DB (1988*b*): *In* Shils ME, Young VR, eds: Modern nutrition in health and disease (7th ed). Philadelphia: Lea & Febiger, p 376.

McCormick DB (1988*c*): *In* Shils ME, Young VR, eds: Modern nutrition in health and disease (7th ed). Philadelphia: Lea & Febiger, p 383.

McCormick DB (1988*d*): *In* Shils ME, Young VR, eds: Modern nutrition in health and disease (7th ed). Philadelphia: Lea & Febiger, p 355.

McCully KS, Wilson RB (1975): Atherosclerosis 22:215.

McLeroy VI, Schendel HE (1973): Am J Clin Nutr 26:191.

Mehansho H, Buss DD, Hamm MW, Henderson LVM (1980): Biochim Biophys Acta 631:112.

Mellanby (1919): J Physiol 52:1 iii.

Merrill AH Jr, Henderson JM (1987): Annu Rev Nutr 7:137.

Metzler DA (1977): Biochemistry. New York: Academic.

Meydani SN, Barklund MP, Liu S, et al. (1990): Am J Clin Nutr 52:557.

Mezick JA, Settlemire CT, Briekley GP, Barefield KP, Jensen WN, Cornwell DG (1970): Biochim Biophys Acta 219:361.

Michell RH (1975): Biochim Biophys Acta 415:81.

Middleton HM (1985): J Nutr 115:1079.

Milhaud G (1968): *In* Talmage RV, Belanger LF, eds: Parathyroid hormone and thyrocalcitonin (calcitonin). New York: Excerpta Medica, p 86.

Miller JZ, Nance WE, Norton JA, Wolen RL, Griffith RS, Rose RJ (1977): JAMA 237:248.

Miller L (1986): J Nutr 116:1344.

Miller LT, Kerkvliet NI (1988): *In* Leklem JE, Reynolds RD, eds: Clinical and physiological applications of vitamin B-6. New York: Alan R Liss, p 133.

Miner RW (1955): Ann NY Acad Sci 61:637.

Mittleholzer E (1976): Int J Vitam Nutr Res 46:33.

Mohsenin V, DuBois AB (1989): Ann NY Acad Sci 498:259.

Money DFL (1978): N Z J Sci 21:41.

Morris RN, Collins AC (1971): J Reprod Fertil 27:201.

Morrison NA, Shine J, Fragonas J-C, Verkest V, McMenemy ML, Eisman JA (1989): Science 246:1158.

Narasinga Rao BS, Gopalan C (1984): Niacin. *In* Olson RE, et al., eds: Present knowledge in nutrition (5th ed). Washington: The Nutrition Foundation.

National Research Council (1989): Diet and health: Implications for reducing chronic disease risk. Washington, DC: National Academy Press.

Neal RA, Sauberlich HE (1980): *In* Goodhart RS, Shils ME, eds: Modern nutrition in health and disease (6th ed). Philadelphia: Lea & Febiger, p 191.

Nemere I, Yoshimoto Y, Norman AW (1984): Endocrinology 115:1476.

Newmark HL, Scheiner J, Marcus M, Prabhudesal M (1976): Am J Clin Nutr 29:645.

Niki E (1987): Ann NY Acad Sci 498:186.

Nutr Rev (1978): 36:305.

Nutr Rev (1979*a*): 37:90.

Nutr Rev (1979*b*): 37:300.

Nutr Rev (1981*a*): 39:24.

Nutr Rev (1981*b*): 39:282.

Nutr Rev (1988): 46:139.

Olson JA, Rojanapo W, Lamb AJ (1981): Ann NY Acad Sci 359:181.

Olson RE (1980): *In* Goodhart RS, Shils ME, eds: Modern nutrition in health and disease (6th ed). Philadelphia: Lea & Febiger, p 170.

Olson RE (1988): *In* Shils ME, Young VR, eds: Modern nutrition in health and disease (7th ed). Philadelphia: Lea & Febiger, p 328.

Olson RE (1990): UC Berkeley Wellness Lett 6(5).

Orten JM, Neuhaus OW (1975): Human biochemistry. St. Louis: CV Mosby.

Pacht ER, et al. (1986): J Clin Invest 77:789.

Packer L, Almada AL, Rothfuss LM, Wilson DS (1989): Ann NY Acad Sci 570:311.

Panganamala RV, Cornwall DG (1982): Ann NY Acad Sci 393:376.

Paravicini V, Stockel K, MacNamara PJ, Hanni R, Bussinger A (1981): Ann NY Acad Sci 359:54.

Parry G, Bredesen DE (1985): Neurology 35:1466.

Pascoe GA, Olafsdottir K, Reed DJ (1987*a*): Arch Biochem Biophys 256:150.

Pascoe GA, Reed DJ (1987*b*): Arch Biochem Biophys 256:159.

Paul PK, Duttagupta PN (1976): J Nutr Sci Vitaminol 222:181.

Paul PK, Duttagupta PN, Argarwal HC (1973): Curr Sci 42:623.

Pauling L (1970): Vitamin C and the common cold. San Francisco: WH Freeman.

Pawson BA (1981): Ann NY Acad Sci 359:1.

Pecoraro RE, Chen MS (1988): Ann NY Acad Sci 498:248.

Petkovich PM, Heersche JNM, Tinker DO, Jones G (1984): J Biol Chem 259:8274.

Phelps DL (1984): Pediatr 74:1114.

Pincus HJ, Solitare GB, Cooper JR (1976): Arch Neurol 33:759.

Pitt HA, Costrini AM (1979): JAMA 241:408.

Pittsley RA, Yoder FW (1983): N Engl J Med 308:1012.

Plesofsky-Vig N, Brambl R (1988): Annu Rev Nutr 8:461.

Pott G, Gerlach U (1980): Enzyme 25:394.

Price PA (1988): Annu Rev Nutr 8:565.

Price PA, Baukol SA (1980): J Biol Chem 255:11660.

Quesada JM, Solana R, Serrano I (1989): N Engl J Med 321:833.

Ramachandran GN (1978): Quantum Chem: Quantum Biol Symp 5:15.

Ramirez J, Flowers NC (1980): Am J Clin Nutr 33:2079.

Redanna P, Whelan J, Burgess JR, Eskew ML, Hildenbrandt G, Zarkower A, Scholz RW, Reddy CC (1989): Ann NY Acad Sci 570:136.

Reed PB (1980): Nutrition, an applied science. Los Angeles: West Publishing, p 272.

Reichel H, Koeffler HP, Norman AW (1989): N Engl J Med 320:980.

Rhee SG, Suh P-G, Ryo S-H, Lee SY (1989): Science 244:546.

Rivers JM (1987): Ann NY Acad Sci 498:445.

Roberts AB (1981): Ann NY Acad Sci 359:45.

Rodriguez MS, Irwin MI (1972): J Nutr 102:75.

Roels DA (1967): *In* Sebrell WH Jr, Harris RS, eds: The vitamins. New York: Academic.

Rose DP (1978): *In* Proceedings of a workshop on vitamin B_6. Washington, DC: National Academy of Sciences, p 193.

Rose RC (1987): *In* Johnson LR, ed: Physiology of the gastrointestinal tract. New York: Raven, p 1581.

Rosen JF, Chesney RW, Hamstra A, DeLuca HF, Mahaffey KR (1980): N Engl J Med 302:1128.

Roth J, Thorens B, Hunziker W, Norma AW, Orci L (1981): Science 214:197.

Said HM, Horne DW, Wagner C (1986): Arch Biochem Biophys 251:114.

Salkeld RM (1986): Clin Chim Acta 49:195.

Sanchez CJ, et al. (1984): J Am Geriatr Soc 32:208.

Satyanarayana NS (1963): Ind J Med Res 51:380.

Sauberlich HE (1980): *In* Goodhart RS, Shils ME, eds: Modern nutrition in health and disease (6th ed). Philadelphia: Lea & Febiger, p 209.

Sauberlich HE, Canham JE (1980): *In* Goodhart RS, Shils ME, eds: Modern nutrition in health and disease (6th ed). Philadelphia: Lea & Febiger, p 216.

Schaumburg HH (1983): Neurology 29:429.

Schaumburg HH, Berger A (1988): *In* Leklem JE, Reynolds RD, eds: Clinical and physiological applications of vitamin B-6. New York: Alan R Liss, p 403.

Schaumburg HH, Kaplan J, Windebank A, Vick N, Rasmus S, et al. (1983): N Engl J Med 309:445.

Schnoes HK, DeLuca HF (1980): Fed Proc 39:2723.

Schoentgen F, Metz-Boutigue M-H, Jolles J, Constans J, Jolles P (1986): Biochim Biophys Acta 871:189.

Schroeder HA (1975): The trace elements and man. Old Greenwich, CT: Devin-Adair.

Scott ML (1980): Fed Proc 39:2736.

Sevanian A, Hacker AD, Elsayed N (1982): Lipids 17:269.

Shane B (1982*a*): Ann NY Acad Sci 393:111.

Shane B, Stokstad ELR (1985): Annu Rev Nutr 5:115.

Sharma RV, Mathur SN, Dmitrovskii A, Das RC, Ganguly J (1977): Biochim Biophys Acta 468:183.

Shaw JH, Sweeney EA (1980): *In* Goodhart RS, Shils ME, eds: Modern nutrition in health and disease (6th ed). Philadelphia: Lea & Febiger, p 855.

Shilotri PG, Bhat KS (1977): Am J Clin Nutr 30:1077.

Simpson KL, Chichester CO (1981): Annu Rev Nutr 1:351.

Sklan D (1983): Int J Vitam Nutr Res 53:23.

Smith CM, DeLuca HF, Tanaka Y, Mahaffey KR (1981): J Nutr 11:1321.

Snyderman SE (1980): *In* Goodhart RS, Shils ME, eds: Modern nutrition in health and disease (6th ed). Philadelphia: Lea & Febiger, p 753.

Sobel S, Gueriguian J, Troendle G, Nevins E (1982): N Engl J Med 306:867.

Sokol RJ (1988): Annu Rev Nutr 8:351.

Spellacy WN, Buhi WC, Birk SA (1977): Am J Obstet Gynecol 127:599.

Spittle CR (1971): Lancet 2:1280.

Stacpoole PW (1977): World Rev Nutr Diet 27:145.

Steenbeck H, Black A (1924): J Biol Chem 61:405.

Steinhilber D, Moser U, Roth RJ, Schmidt KH (1987): Ann NY Acad Sci 498:522.

Stern RS (1989): N Engl J Med 320:1007.

Stokes J, Mendels J (1972): Lancet i:1177.

Stryer L (1987): Sci Am 257:42.

Stumf WE, Sar M, Reid FA, Tanaka Y, DeLuca HF (1979): Science 206:1188.

Swenseid ME, Schick G, Vinyard E, Drenick EJ (1965): Am J Clin Nutr 17:272.

Takagi M, Fukui T, Shimomura S (1982): Proc Natl Acad Sci USA 79:3716.

Tani M, Fushiki IT, Iwai J (1983): Biochim Biophys Acta 757:274.

Tappel AL (1968): Geriatrics 23:97.

Tappel AL (1980): Executive Health 26.

Taylor AT (1989): Nutr Rev 47:225.

Teelmann K, Bollag W (1990): Dermatologica 180:30.

Terezhainy GT, Bottompey WK, Pelleu GH (1978): Oral Surg Oral Med Oral Pathol 45:56.

Than T-M, May M-W, Aung K-S, Mya-Tu M (1978): Br J Nutr 40:269.

Tietz N (1976): Fundamentals of clinical chemistry. Philadelphia: WB Saunders, p 559.

Tillotson JA, McGown EL (1981): Am J Clin Nutr 34:2397; 2405.

Traber MG, Kayden HJ (1987): Am J Clin Nutr 46:488.

Traber MG, Kayden HJ (1989): Ann NY Acad Sci 570:95.

Traber MG, Sokol RJ, Ringel SP, Neville HE, Thellman CA, Kayden HJ (1987): N Engl J Med 317:262.

Traber MG, Burton GW, Ingold KU, Kayden HJ (1990*a*): J Lipid Res 31:675.

Traber MG, Rudel LL, Burton GW, Hughes L, Ingold KU, Kayden HJ (1990*b*): J Lipid Res 31:687.

Tsai AC, Kelley JJ, Peng B, Cook N (1978): Am J Clin Nutr 31:831.

Turner RT, Farley J, Vandersteenhoven JJ, Epstein S, Bell NH, Baylink DJ (1988): J Clin Invest 82:212.

Umesono K, Giguere V, Glass CK, Rosenfeld MG, Evans RM (1988): Nature 336:262.

Varghese S, Lee S, Huang Y-C, Christakos S (1988): J Biol Chem 263:9776.

Varma SD (1987): Ann NY Acad Sci 498:280.

Vlietinck AJ, Berghe DAV, Haemers A (1988): *In* Cody V, Middleton E Jr, Harborne JB, Beretz A, eds: Plant flavonoids in biology and medicine II: Biochemical, cellular, and medicinal properties. New York: Alan R Liss, p 283.

Waldinger C, Berg RB (1963): Pediatrics 32:161.

Walters MR, Ilenchuk T, Claycomb WC (1987): J Biol Chem 262:2536.

Wathne KO, Norum KR, Smeland E, Blomfoff R (1988): J Biol Chem 263:8691.

Webb AR, Holick MF (1988): Annu Rev Nutr 8:375.

Webb AR, Kline L, Holick MF (1988): J Clin Endocrinol Metab 67:373.

Wecker L (1986): Can J Physiol Pharmacol 64:329.

Weininger J, Briggs GM (1980): *In* Goodhart RS, Shils ME, eds: Modern nutrition in health and disease (6th ed). Philadelphia: Lea & Febiger, p 279.

Weishaar RE, Simpson RU (1989): Endocr Rev 10:351.

White JD (1981): N Engl J Med 304:1491.

Williams MJ, Harris RI, Dean BC (1985): J Int Med Res 13:174.

Wolf JD (1980): *In* Alfin-Slater RB, ed: Nutrition of the adult: Micronutrients. New York: Plenum, p 97.

Wollenweber E (1987): *In* Cody V, Middleton E Jr, Harborne JB, Beretz A, eds: Plant flavonoids in biology and medicine II: Biochemical, cellular, and medicinal properties. New York: Alan R Liss, p 45.

Wood JL, Allison RC (1981): Effects of consumption of choline and lecithin on neurological and cardiovascular systems. Washington, DC: US Department of Commerce Technical Information Service.

Wozney JM, Rosen V, Celeste AJ, et al. (1988): Science 242:1528.

Wright KN (1970): Nutr Rep Int 2:209.

Yousefi S, Vu G, Carandang G (1989): Cancer Res 49:5083.

Zeisel SH (1981): Annu Rev Nutr 1:95.

Zeisel SH (1988): *In* Shils ME, Young VR, eds: Modern nutrition in health and disease (7th ed). Philadelphia: Lea & Febiger, p 440.

Zipursky A, Brown EJ, Watts J, Milner R, Rand C, Blachette VS, Bell EF, Paes B, Ling E (1987): Pediatrics 79:61.

Maria C. Linder, Ph.D.*

6

Nutrition and Metabolism of the Major Minerals

After carbon, hydrogen, oxygen, and nitrogen, those elements required in greatest abundance in the daily diet are calcium, phosphorus, sulfur, potassium, sodium, chlorine, and magnesium (Table 6.1). With the exceptions of sulfur and phosphorus, these minerals are largely present in foods as inorganic substituents; whereas sulfur is present in sulfur amino acids and sulfated glycosaminoglycans, and phosphate mainly in nucleotides, nucleic acids, and phospholipids.

The largest quantities of calcium, phosphorus, and magnesium are found in bone, as part of the minerals that provide bone structure and density. Bone also serves as a storage pool for these elements, from which the rest of the body can draw. The exact role of magnesium in bone mineral structure is not clear. Calcium and phosphorus form the crystalline and amorphous hydroxylapatite (see below).

The role of these three elements outside of bone is just as important. Details on the roles of calcium in nervous function, hormone action, blood clotting, etc., are given later in this chapter, along with further information on phosphate, magnesium, and other major minerals.

* California State University, Fullerton, CA.

Phosphorus

The adult human body contains two thirds of a kilogram of phosphorus (Table 6.1), of which 85% is in bone. Otherwise, phosphorus is mainly involved in energy metabolism, as part of adenosine triphosphate (ATP), which is the "energy currency" of the body, and as part of other nucleotides, nucleic acids, and various phosphorylated compounds. It participates in activation reactions in all areas of metabolism (Figure 6.1) to form high energy intermediates, such as those involved in intermediary metabolism or as part of the regulation of metabolism, including phosphorylation/dephosphorylation of enzymes, phosphoinositides/inositol phosphates, and so on. Intracellular concentrations of phosphate are much higher than extracellular ones, as phosphorylated compounds do not easily cross cell membranes. Inorganic phosphate is present probably in 5–20 m*M* quantities within various cell compartments, on its way on and off nucleotides and other metabolic substituents. As a result, it is the main intracellular buffer. As part of phospholipids, it is also responsible for the charge that renders them detergents and allows the formation of a bilayer (membrane) structure in aqueous solutions.

Phosphate is very abundant in processed foods, colas, and other soft drinks. It is also generally abundant in foods with a high protein content, such as meats. It is very prevalent in the American diet, where its preponderance over calcium is of some concern (see below). Phosphorus

Table 6.1. Summary of the Nutrition and Functions of the Major Minerals and Simple Macronutrients

Element	Average amount (70-kg man)	Primary functions	Good food sources	Average intake (mg/day)	RDA (U.S. adult)
Calcium (Ca^{2+})	1200 g	Bone and tooth structure; transmission of nervous/mechanical/hormonal impulses; enzyme regulation; blood clotting	Milk, cheese, shellfish	500–1200	800
Phosphorus ($HPO_4^{=}$, $H_2PO_4^-$)	660 g	Bone and tooth structure; part of ATP, etc., and RNA/DNA; intimately involved in energy metabolism, storage, and regulation; intracellular buffer; part of membrane phospholipid	Colas, foods rich in protein, whole grains, meat	1000–1500	800
Sulfur ($S^=$ or $SO_4^=$)	200 g	Large amounts as part of S-containing amino acids in proteins; also part of important coenzymes (vitamins) in enzyme reactions; part of keratan (mucopolysaccharide) and other glycosaminoglycans in skin, cartilage, and connective tissue	High protein foods, eggs	See essential amino acids	
Potassium (K^+)	149 g	Intracellular electrolyte/cation, cellular osmotic pressure; its relation to Na^+ and Cl^- outside the cell results in cell membrane potential and charge, allowing nerve impulses, heart beats, etc.	Vegetables, fruits, meats, milk	2000–5000	2500
Sodium (Na^+)	99 g	Extracellular electrolyte/cation, osmotic homeostasis of extracellular environment (body fluids) (see above); regulates blood volume; 30%–45% present in bone	Processed foods, table salt	3000–7000 (range 6000–18,000)	2500
Chlorine (Cl^-)	99 g	Main extracellular anion; accompanies Na^+ in body fluids (almost exclusively extracellular)	Processed foods, table salt	3000–9000	2000
Magnesium (Mg^{2+})	26 g	Sixty percent + in bone; the rest is involved in important enzyme reactions, including those utilizing or forming ATP (protein synthesis, energy metabolism, muscle contraction, etc.)	Nuts, cocoa, whole grains and seeds, molasses	180–480	300–350

is readily absorbed from the diet in the form of free inorganic phosphate, after digestive hydrolysis and release from most foodstuffs. Only the phosphorus that is part of dietary phytic acid or phytates (Figure 6.1) and is especially prevalent in cereal grains is not well hydrolyzed and therefore unavailable. [Indeed, phytic acid forms insoluble Ca^{2+}, Mg^{2+}, and Fe^{2+} salts, preventing absorption of the latter substituents (see below).] Some other dietary factors (including Fe^{2+}, Mg^{2+},

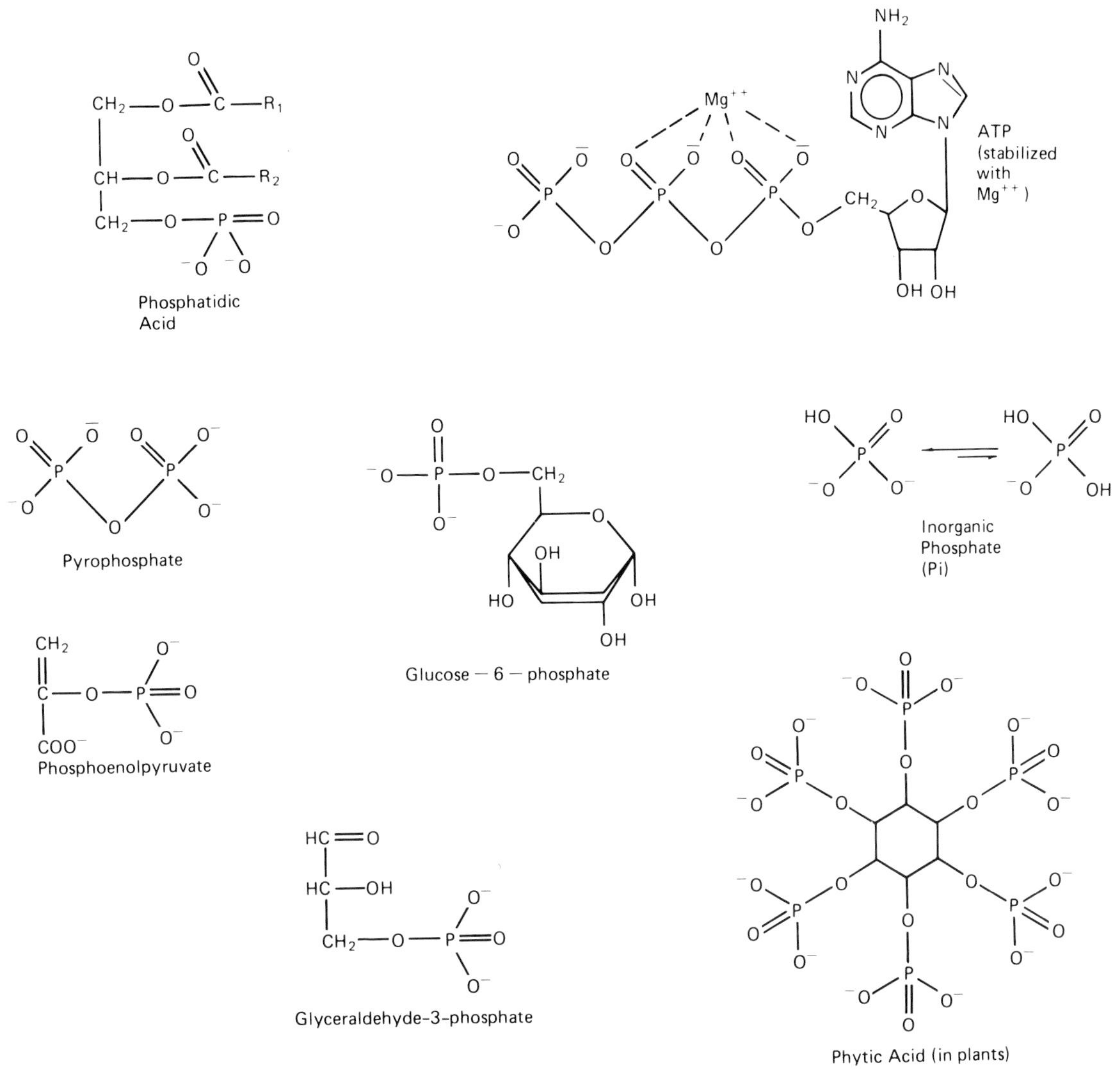

Phosphatidic Acid

ATP (stabilized with Mg^{++})

Pyrophosphate

Glucose — 6 — phosphate

Inorganic Phosphate (Pi)

Phosphoenolpyruvate

Glyceraldehyde-3-phosphate

Phytic Acid (in plants)

Figure 6.1. Representative phosphates found intracellularly.

unsaturated fatty acids, and Al-based antacids) will also inhibit phosphate absorption by forming insoluble salts (Avioli, 1988). Some food phosphate is hydrolyzed by the action of alkaline phosphatase in the brush border of intestinal mucosal cells, and absorption (70%–90% of intake) occurs both by an energy-dependent process (involving a saturable carrier) and by passive diffusion (Avioli, 1988). The energy-dependent process relies on counter transport of Na^+, and in animals (but perhaps not in man) may be enhanced by the active hormone form of vitamin D (Avioli, 1988; DeLuca, 1974). Most phosphorus is carried in the blood mainly as inorganic phosphate or as part of phospholipid.

Phosphorus homeostasis appears to be achieved mainly by regulating excretion via the urine, although about one third (about 0.4 g) of the daily intake is secreted into the digestive tract and lost in the feces. (Daily intake is quite varied, but in the range of 1.2 g/day.) Urinary phosphate excretion shows diurnal variations and a positive relation to exercise, being lowest shortly after waking (Avioli, 1980). This rhythm may be related to the activity of the adrenal cortex, which determines the diurnal variation in cortisol secretion and has its apex in the early morning (before awakening), enhancing phosphate resorption by the kidney tubules. [Acute doses of corticosteroids also depress urinary phosphate (and

Na^+) excretion by stimulating tubular resorption (Avioli, 1988).] The renal resorption of phosphate (normally 85%–95%) is increased as well by activated vitamin D and by short-term treatment with growth hormone; it is decreased by parathyroid hormone (PTH) and estrogen, long-term glucocorticosteroids, thyroid hormone, and elevated plasma Ca^{2+} (or Mg^{2+}) concentrations (Avioli, 1980, 1988). A high intake of phosphate relative to calcium (especially if the latter is low), resulting in high P:Ca ratios in serum, will trigger PTH release and enhance phosphate losses despite an activation of vitamin D_3. [Further details on this (and other calcium-related aspects of phosphate metabolism) are described in the section on Calcium, and in Chapter 5, Vitamin D.]

Magnesium

Sixty percent or more of the magnesium in the body is located in the bone, as part of the crystalline mineral (70%) and the hydrated crystal surface (30%). The rest of the body's magnesium is mainly within the cells of soft tissues (20% in muscle), where its major function may be to stabilize the structure of ATP in ATP-dependent enzyme reactions (Figure 6.1). (Intracellular concentrations are about 6–10 m*M* and are mostly in complex form.) Numerous (>300) enzymes throughout metabolism are involved, including several in glycolysis and the Krebs cycle, adenyl cyclase (which forms cAMP), various phosphatases, and reactions in protein and nucleic acid synthesis. Mg^{2+} also plays a role in neuromuscular transmission and activity, acting in concert with, or against, the effects of calcium (Hubbard et al., 1969). As a consequence, one effect of magnesium deficiency is to enhance muscle irritability and, if the deficiency is sufficiently severe, to induce tetany. Conversely, excessively large doses of magnesium, especially when coupled with renal insufficiency (preventing adequate excretion), can cause central nervous system depression, anesthesia, and even paralysis (Shils, 1980, 1988). Mg^{2+} and Ca^{2+} in the plasma also have effects on vascular smooth muscles, causing relaxation and constriction, respectively (Avioli, 1988). (This could have implications for blood pressure.) Some of the effects of magnesium are thus on calcium metabolism, and there seems to be an important role for this mineral in reaction to bone mineral mobilization and PTH function. Shils (1980) has postulated from the evidence available in humans that magnesium is necessary for the actions of PTH and activated vitamin D in bone calcium mobilization (see Calcium, below, and Chapter 5). Low levels of magnesium may enhance PTH production and secretion, whereas higher levels mimic Ca^{2+} and suppress secretion. Thus, Mg is intimately involved with other major minerals in the metabolism of bone, as well as the soft tissues. However, the mechanisms involved in all these actions are very poorly understood, and the various possible clinical symptoms attributed to magnesium deficiency by researchers still present a rather incoherent picture (Shils, 1980, 1988).

Magnesium is present in variable amounts in foods (Tables 6.1 and 6.2) and in lower quantities overall today than in 1909; whole grains, nuts, seeds, and cocoa are especially rich sources; it is also part of the chlorophyll in leafy plants. Intake is highly variable (130–500 mg) and absorption averages 30%–40% of dietary intake (Shils, 1988) being inversely related to the amount present. Like phosphate, Mg^{2+} is probably absorbed both by an active saturable carrier mechanism and by diffusion. Dietary calcium and phosphorus do not affect absorption, and it is unlikely that the active hormone form of vitamin D plays a role in regulating uptake (Shils, 1988). In the blood, most of the magnesium is in the form of the free ion, or complexed to small molecules. As with phosphorus, homeostasis occurs mainly via adjustment of urinary excretion (tubular resorption), although about 25% of the 130 mg absorbed daily (from an average intake of 300 mg) is secreted as part of the digestive juices (Shils, 1988). As with phosphate, magnesium excretion is enhanced by thyroid hormones as well as by acidosis, aldosterone, and by depletion of phosphate and potassium. It is reduced by stimulatory effects of calcitonin, glucagon, and PTH on tubular resorption, as well as in hypocalcemia (low plasma calcium), hypomagnesemia, and metabolic alkalosis (Shils, 1988). As measured by hypomagnesemia, magnesium deficiency occurs principally as a complication of other disease states, involving intestinal malabsorption and/or decreased renal function (requiring dialysis). It generally results in abnormally low plasma Ca^{2+} and K^+ (as well as Mg^{2+}) concentrations, leading to neurologic symptoms and even tetany. Many individuals consume much less magnesium than the RDA: 280 mg for women and 350 mg for men. Recent animal studies have linked a low intake of magnesium to high blood pressure (Weaver, 1987) and cardiovascular disease (Altura and Altura, 1987). Magnesium deficiency may be treated orally (various Mg salts) or

Table 6.2. Concentrations of Phosphorus, Calcium, Magnesium, and Oxalate in Representative Foods[a]

Food	P	Ca	Mg	Oxalate
Milk	93	115–118	10–13	0.5–0.9
Cheeses (cheddar)	479	750	45	0
Yogurt	79	111		
Eggs, whole	183	48	11	0–0.9
Hamburger, cooked	214	8–12	28	0.4
Haddock (fish)	197	17–23	28	0.2
Sole (fish)	64	4	30	
Oysters, raw	143	94	24	
Chicken, roasted	169	9	19	0.3–1.9
Oatmeal, dry	406	53	144	1.0
Cornflakes	45	9–17	16–36	5.6
Bread				
White	87	70–108	24	4.9
Whole wheat	228	99	78	
Apple	2	2–3	5	1.5
Orange	15	3–30	11–14	6.2
Strawberries	20	16–20	11	1.9
Tomato	27	10–13	10	5.3
Broccoli	61	80	24	Low?
Cabbage	26	44–65	20	1.0
Peas, boiled	66	20	20	0.8–1.3
Cauliflower	56	24	15	1.0
Kale	60	160	37	Low
Onion	33	28	12	3.0
Potato	43	6–9	34(22)[b]	23
Lettuce	21	20–26	10	17
Rhubarb	8	12–43	10	260
Beets	23	11–19	37	122
Spinach	51	93–111	76	779
Ovaltine, powder		126	33	46
Tea (in 100 ml water)				
1 g infused 2 min	0	2.8	0.6	46
1.5 g infused 6 min	0	5.2	2.5	83
Chocolate, bitter	385	78	292	124

Source: Oxalate values from Hodgkinson (1977). Other values mainly from Handbook of the Nutritional Contents of Foods (prepared for USDA) (1975) but also from Hodgkinson (1977).

[a] mg/100 g, fresh unless indicated otherwise.
[b] Peeled.

The nutrient content of common Nigerian vegetables, high in oxalates, is (% dry weight): 27% protein, 2.4% Ca, 1.7% Mg, 0.019% Fe, 11.3% total oxalates (10.8 soluble) for *Celosia argenta;* 30% protein, 2.1% Ca, 1.6% Mg, 0.03% Fe, 11.5% total oxalates (5.9 soluble) for *Amaranthus caudatus* (Oke, 1979).

by injection (i.v. or i.m.; up to 2 g $MgSO_4$, over 1–2 hr).

Sulfur

Sulfur is present in the diet mainly in the form of cysteine and methionine, but it is also a major substituent of the glycosaminoglycans, chondroitin sulfate, dermatan sulfate, and hyaluronic acid (Table 6.1). These latter are the "gels" of the interstitial "ground substance" of tissues (found in greater or lesser amounts) but are present especially in cartilage and skin, where there is a high connective tissue content. Sulfur is absorbed either as part of amino acids or as inorganic sulfate, with equally good efficiency. Apart from an important structural role in intracellular proteins, where it can form crosslinkages through disulfide bonds, sulfur is the site for attachment and transfer of 1-C methyl groups, via S-adenosylmethionine (see Chapter 4). It is also part of the important reducing agent, glutathione (Figure 4.2), and various important coenzymes and vitamins, including coenzyme A (Figure 5.6). In oxidized (sulfate) forms, sulfur is associated with the

"Activated" forms of $SO_4^{=}$

$^{-}O-S(=O)_2-O-P(=O)_2-O-CH_2$ – ribose (Ⓟ) – Adenine

3′-phosphoadenosine-5′-phosphosulfate

$HC=O$ / $HC-O-S(=O)_2-O^{-}$ / $HO-CH$ / $HC-OH$ / $HC-OH$ / COO^{-}

Ascorbic acid-2-sulfate

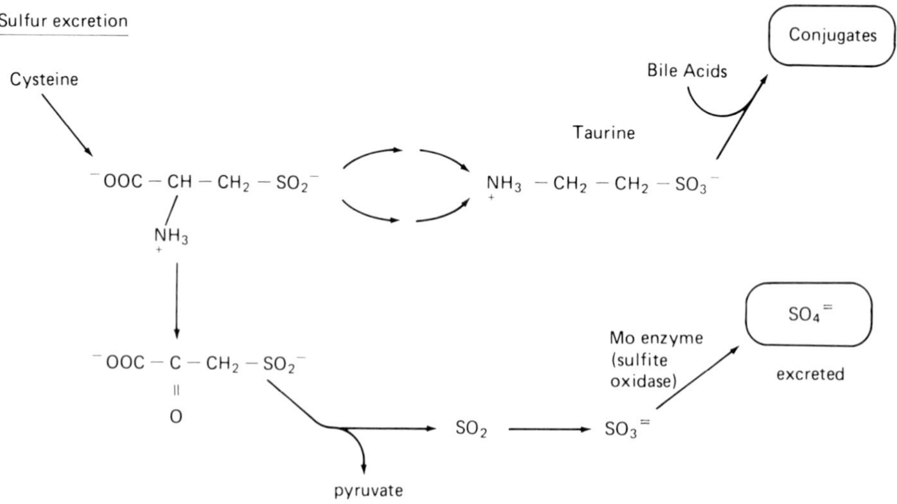

Glycosamino glycans:

$R-NH-SO_3^{-}$

(sulfatases) → $SO_4^{=}$

polysaccharide (aminoglycan)

Figure 6.2. Aspects of sulfur metabolism. Important sulfur compounds include thiamin, biotin, lipoic acid, coenzyme A, glutathione, Fe-S (electron transport), methionine, cysteine. Hereditary absence of sulfatases: excretion of heparin–SO_4 in urine, mental retardation. [*Source:* Information from Metzler (1977).]

mucopolysaccharides already cited and is used to render metabolites more water-soluble for urinary excretion (notably, metabolites of steroid hormones and certain drugs). For formation of mucopolysaccharides or steroid metabolites, sulfate is transferred on 3′,5′-adenosine diphosphate (Figure 6.2). Mucopolysaccharide production is especially important during growth and development, and upon injury, when connective tissue metabolism becomes active in wound repair.

Whereas most of the sulfur is ingested as amino acid, most is lost in the urine after oxidation to sulfate and is lost mainly as the free ion, $SO_4^{=}$ (Figure 6.2). (The rest is attached to urinary and fecal metabolites.) Sulfate is also one of the intracellular electrolytes and is found in the plasma in low concentrations (Figure 6.3). Production of sulfate, from either methionine or cysteine, proceeds through cysteine sulfonic acid to sulfinyl pyruvate, SO_2, and finally $SO_4^{=}$. Sulfite oxidase (a molybdenum-dependent enzyme) is

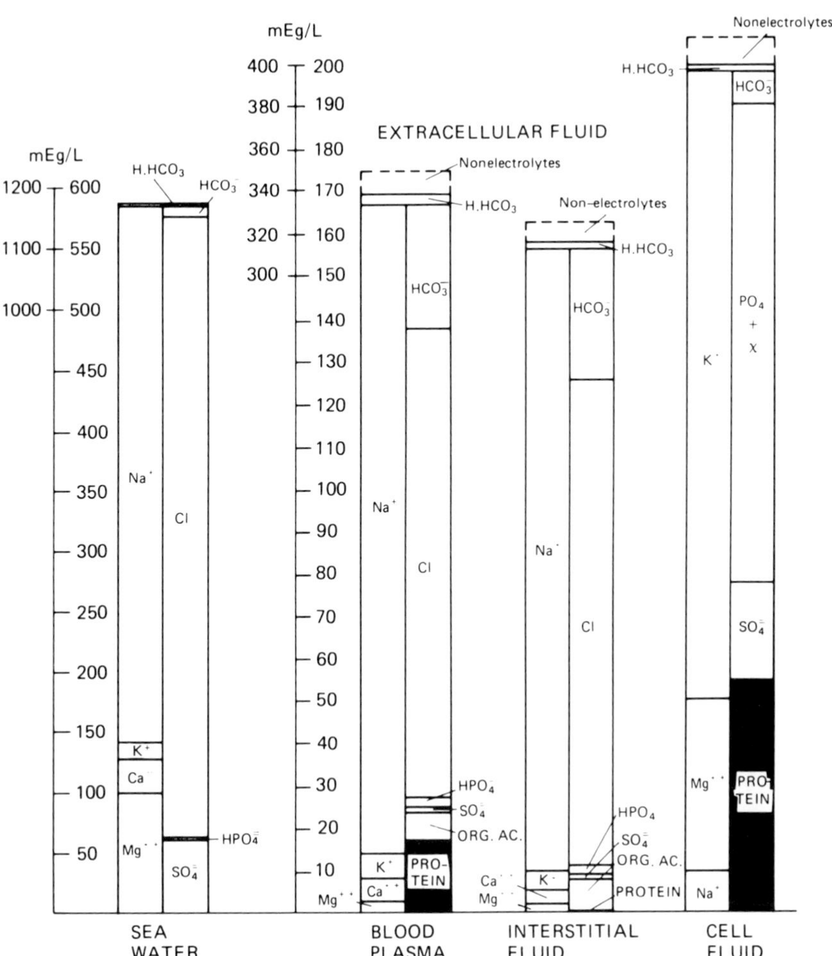

Figure 6.3. Distribution of electrolytes in intra- and extracellular fluids and in comparison with seawater. Scale is in milliequivalents of cations or anions per liter of water. Note scale difference for sea water. [*Source:* Reprinted by permission from Gamble (1958).]

the last step in this process (Figure 6.2). (Another branch of this pathway is to taurine, also used to conjugate bile acids.) Sulfatases remove $SO_4^=$ from mucopolysaccharides during their normal turnover, for excretion. Congenital deficiencies in sulfite oxidase and such sulfatases have been observed and are associated with mental retardation (Metzler, 1977) (see Chapter 18).

Sodium, Potassium, and Chloride

These ions are the most abundant electrolytes in the human and animal body. Present as fully dissociated ions, they are the main particles responsible for fluid osmolarity (osmotic pressure); they also influence ionic strength and, thus, the solubility of proteins and other substituents. The osmotic pressure of the intracellular and extracellular environment is very rigidly controlled, largely through energy-dependent regulatory mechanisms that determine the rate of resorption of sodium ions and water by the kidney.

Sodium, potassium, and chloride ions are present on either side of the cell plasma membrane, in quite different concentrations (Figure 6.3), resulting in some very steep chemical gradients. The series of events that gives rise to this differential disposition of ions and the resulting membrane and cell phenomena may be described as follows. (1) All plasma membranes, including nerve axon membranes, contain an energy-dependent Na^+ pump (also known as Na^+/K^+ ATPase), which actively transfers Na^+ from the intracellular to the extracellular environment. (2) As Na^+

exits, K^+ enters, which results in high concentrations of Na^+ extracellularly and high K^+ intracellularly. (3) Chloride ions remain mainly extracellular, as the intracellular fluid already contains sufficient anions ($HPO_4^=$, $SO_4^=$, and protein) to balance the K^+ and Mg^{2+} within. ($HPO_4^=$, Mg^{2+}, protein, etc. have difficulty crossing cell membranes.) In the interest of maintaining osmotic balance across the cell membrane, there are more divalent ions within the cell which, with the larger number of intracellular protein particles, balance the larger number of monovalent electrolytes (and lesser numbers of protein particles) extracellularly. (4) The steep K^+ gradient from inside to outside the cell (produced and maintained by the sodium pump) is the main factor responsible for the membrane potential and membrane charge of mammalian cells. One explanation is that as K^+ efflux occurs along the chemical gradient, the available counter ions, which could accompany the K^+, are limited to Cl^- and some OH^-. These latter tend to remain intracellular because of counteracting chemical gradients. As a result, there is a slight charge separation, which, at the level of the cell membrane, results in a 0.10-V membrane potential. It is this potential that is affected (depolarized) during the conduction of nerve impulses or contraction impulses within heart muscle. Depolarization travels down the nerve axon and triggers release of neurotransmitters; in muscle cells it results in further changes in intracellular ions that trigger contractions; in all cells, the increased intracellular Na^+ enhances pump activity to restore the intra- and extracellular Na^+ and K^+ imbalance. Any substantial increase in the extracellular concentration of potassium (as such a momentary reduction in the activity of the sodium pump) will lower the chemical gradient for K^+ and, thus, the membrane potential, causing a depolarization of the membrane. If extracellular K^+ concentrations rise too far, this will interfere with normal heart and nervous function. [Extracellular (plasma) K^+ concentrations greater than 7.5 m*M* are dangerous; 10 m*M* K^+ can be fatal (Tietz, 1976).]

A generalized model for the structure of the sodium pump is given in Figure 6.4. Much has been learned about its disposition in different cells and its regulation (Rossier et al., 1987). Most of the activity resides in the longer (α) subunit, which has Na^+- and ATP-binding sites on portions that extend into the cytoplasm and K^+ (and ouabain) sites on the exterior. The pump is immediately activated by an increase in intracellular Na^+ concentrations. (Variations in extracellular

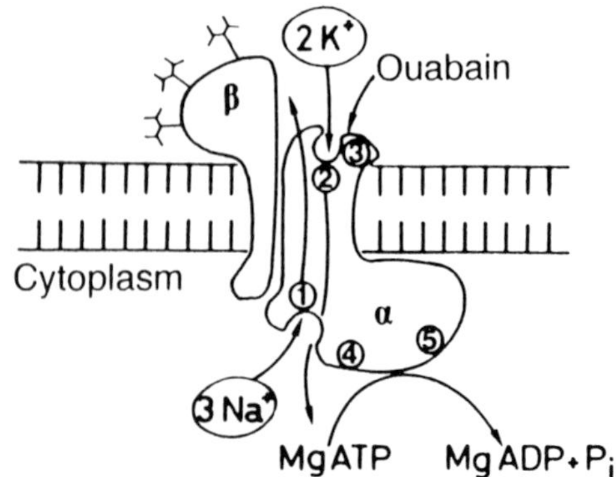

Figure 6.4. The Na^+/K^+ ATPase in cell membranes and its regulation. The enzyme is comprised of two subunits: α, with intra- and extracellular binding sites for Na^+ (1), K^+ (2), ouabain (3), ATP (5), and for phosphorylation (4); and β, with carbohydrate on the exterior and the N-terminal part of the peptide on the interior. Hormones that modulate activity in various cells include: aldosterone, catecholamines, EGF, cortisol, glucagon, insulin, progesterone, thyroid hormone, and vasopressin. [*Source:* Reprinted by permission from Rossier et al. (1987).]

K^+ have little effect.) Regulation of Na^+/K^+ ATPase activity by hormones occurs either by direct action via cell surface receptors and second messengers specific for different types of cells, or by enhancement of transcription of genes for subunits of the enzyme. [At least five variants of the α subunit are known.] The direct hormonal effects are rapid, the transcriptional effects slower and more long-term; different groups of hormones are involved (Figure 6.4). Some cells do not have hormone-responsive systems.

Potassium ions are readily lost through the kidneys (no resorption by tubules), and this process is enhanced (by Na^+/K^+ exchange) through aldosterone. [Aldosterone controls Na^+ resorption (see below).] Potassium is readily available in unprocessed foodstuffs, but is especially rich in nuts, whole grains, meats, and fruits (particularly avocados and bananas; Table 6.3). Dietary potassium deficiency is probably rare, although intake may often be suboptimal, especially with diets high in processed foods. (See more below, in relation to hypertension.) Hypokalemia (low serum K^+) is rare, but may occur in aciduria, Cushing's disease (hypersecretion of adrenal steroids), and with vomiting or diarrhea. Hyperkalemia is clinical evidence for tissue damage (as in myocardial infarction) or renal failure (Figure 6.5).

Whereas potassium is distributed in response to energy-dependent forces that manipulate the

Table 6.3. Sodium and Potassium Content of Representative Foods[a]

Food	Sodium	Potassium
Apples, raw, pared	1	110
Asparagus	4	207
Avocados, raw	4	604
Bananas, raw	1	370
Beans, green, cooked	4	151
canned (solids and liquid)	236	95
Berries (black, blue, boysen)	1	81–170
Broccoli	13	464
Cabbage, raw, red, green	20–26	233–268
Celery, raw	132	344
Kale	42	490
Lettuce	15	224
Oranges, raw, peeled fruit	1	200
Olives, Greek style	3288	—
Papaya	3	211
Pineapple	2	173
Potatoes, cooked	3	262
Watermelon	1	158
Pretzels	1680	130
Bread, whole wheat	527	273
white, enriched	507	105
Almonds, dry raw	4	773
Oatmeal, before cooking	2	352
after cooking with salt	218	61
Bacon, cured, fried cooked drained	1021	236
Hamburger, cooked, prepared (fast food)	47	450
Chicken, light or dark, roasted	64–86	321–411
Halibut, broiled	134	525
Tuna, canned, in water	41	279
in oil (solids and liquid)	800	301
Eggs, raw, whole	122	129
Milk, whole	50	144
Cheeses, cheddar/Swiss	700–710	82–104
Soups, commercial, tomato, prepared	396	94
Tomato catsup, regular	1042	363

Source: Data from Krause and Mahan (1979) and Souci et al. (1981).

[a] mg/100 g.

distribution of Na^+, and Cl^- is passively distributed in response to "vacancies left by other anions," the concentration of sodium ions in body compartments is carefully controlled. The osmolarity of blood and interstitial fluids is directly regulated by the kidney through manipulation of water and sodium excretion. The governing standard is a constancy of extracellular (and intracellular) osmolarity. If additional sodium is absorbed from the diet and enters the extracellular fluid, extra water must be retained to keep the sodium diluted. At the same time, the kidney will enhance the rate of sodium excretion by depressing reabsorption. If water alone is ingested and absorbed, an immediate (slight) dilution of the plasma is sensed, and the kidney immediately retains additional sodium to maintain the osmolarity of the plasma. With water intake, there is also an immediate increase in the rate of diuresis. If sodium and water are absorbed at the same time, depending on the osmolarity of the absorbed fluid relative to that of the body, there may be no immediate change in the rate of water or sodium resorption by the kidney (see Chapter 1, Figure 1.7), and the extra sodium and water will gradually be lost over the ensuing hours and days.

These various adaptations are regulated by steroids and natriuretic/antidiuretic hormones. For Na^+ (Figure 6.5), the rate of resorption is sensed by the juxtaglomerular apparatus, which, if blood concentrations fall, releases angiotensinogen. The latter is converted to angiotensin in the blood and stimulates secretion of aldosterone from the adrenal cortex. This steroid, in turn, stimulates the resorption of Na^+ by kidney tubules (and enhances K^+ loss). A higher Na^+ concentration is countered by less resorption plus natriuresis, involving atrial natriuretic factor (ANF).

Sodium, Potassium, and Hypertension

Hypertension is a disease that affects a substantial proportion of the population of Western industrialized nations. Hypertension, characterized by a consistent abnormally high diastolic and/or systolic blood pressure (>99 and >150 mm Hg, respectively), in theory can arise through an increase in blood volume and/or a constriction of the vasculature, as well as through factors which affect cardiac output, heart rate, and so on. The question is whether sodium intake plays a role in the development of hypertension and/or in exacerbating/ameliorating the condition once it has arisen.

There are three types of evidence relating sodium intake to hypertension (Altschul et al., 1982): (1) epidemiologic studies showing a positive relationship between intake and incidence of hypertension in population groups around the world or within subpopulations of one group; (2) observations that therapeutic management of hypertension is made easier by lowering sodium intake; and (3) experimental evidence of abnormal sodium handling in individuals with a family history of hypertension or in genetically hypertensive animals. Epidemiologic data have often been

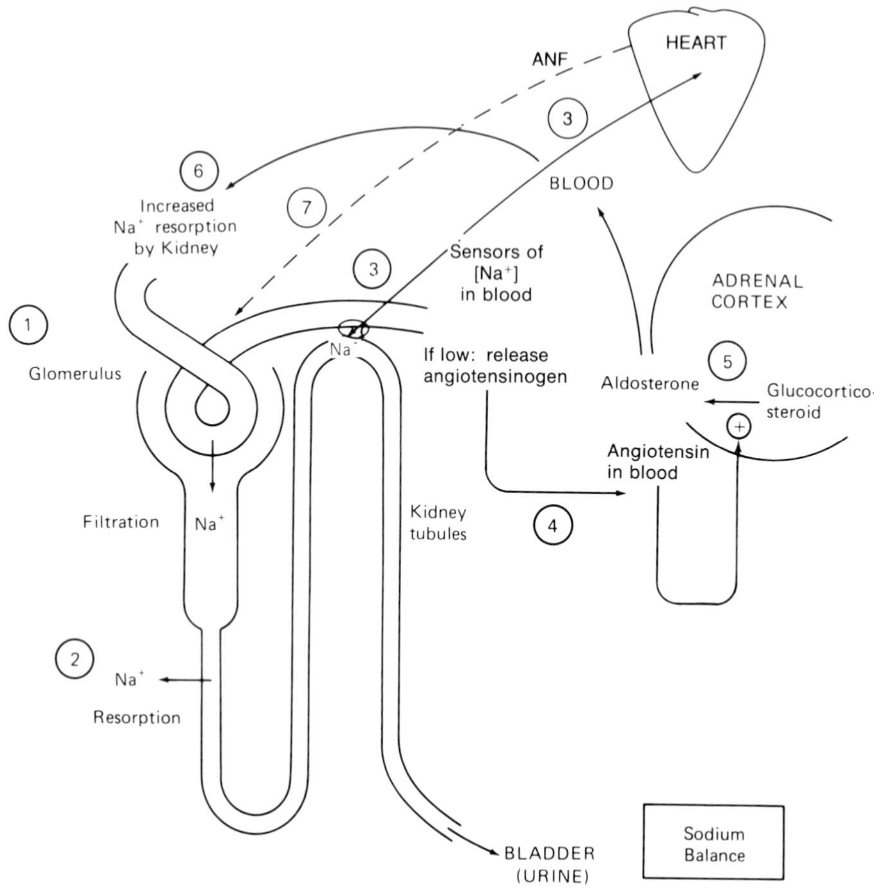

Figure 6.5. Sodium balance. Sodium is filtered efficiently through the glomerulus (1) and resorbed by the kidney tubules (2). The degree of resorption is dependent on blood concentrations, as sensed by the juxtaglomerular apparatus (3) and the heart. If plasma concentrations decrease, angiotensinogen is released from the kidney, leading to angiotensin which activates production and secretion of aldosterone by the adrenal cortex (5). Aldosterone (a steroid hormone) acts on the kidney tubules to increase Na^+ resorption (6). Also, atrial natriuretic factor (or peptide; ANF) released by the heart (7) promotes Na^+ diuresis (loss through the kidney). If Na^+ concentrations rise above normal, no aldosterone is released and resorption is rapidly reduced. Effect on K^+ is opposite to that on Na^+ (aldosterone). Normally, K^+ is easily lost from kidneys. Conditions in which changes in plasma Na^+ and K^+ may occur are indicated to the right.

Hyponatremia	*Hypokalemia*
Polyuria, diarrhea	Diarrhea, vomiting
Aciduria (uncompensated)	Aciduria
Addison's disease (aldosterone)	Cushing's disease (excess steroids)
Renal tubule disease	Dietary K^+ deficiency

Hypernatremia	*Hyperkalemia*
Cushing's disease	Tissue damage (MI), etc.
Brain injury	Renal failure
Excess Na^+ ingested/ dehydration	

Key: MI, myocardial infarction (heart attack).

impressive cross-culturally, but, within a given homogeneous population, repeated studies have usually failed to show strong correlations between sodium intake and hypertension. These findings have been confirmed once again in the massive prospective "Intersalt" study (involving 52 different population centers worldwide) in which 24-hr sodium excretion (a measure of intake) was compared with blood pressure (Intersalt Cooperative Research Group, 1988). Intracenter, there was a positive correlation only with systolic pressure (after correction for body mass index and high alcohol use), whereas intercenter, there appeared to be no correlations between sodium and blood pressure (except if four, very low Na^+, "outlier" groups were included). [Body mass index (a measure of obesity) and alcohol abuse were much more important factors (see below).] The exception appears to be that segment of a population with a family history of hypertension, within which a relation between sodium intake and hypertension reemerges on a statistical basis. In such "salt-sensitive" individuals (Fujita et al., 1980; Kurtz et al., 1987) increased NaCl intake has clear (enhancing) effects on blood pressure, although initial studies suggest this may not be the case with other sodium salts (such as Na citrate) (Kurtz et al., 1987). Regardless of salt-sensitivity, experience shows that the need for intake of hypotensive drugs may be reduced when sodium intake is decreased in individuals afflicted with hypertension.

Studies with strains of hypertensive rats and other sodium-sensitive animals suggest that there is an inability of the kidney to excrete sodium adequately at low renal perfusion pressures, so that higher (hypertensive?) pressures are required to achieve adequate Na^+ output. The question is whether this is a defect in kidney function and/or an abnormality imposed by an increase in blood fluid volume (the latter from too much sodium and fluid intake and retention). From the manipulations previously described, it seems clear that individuals who ingest more Na^+ will retain more water to keep this electrolyte diluted. Since NaCl remains extracellular, interstitial fluid may accumulate and plasma volume grow. An increased plasma volume may result in increased blood pressure, especially if the flexibility of the vasculature has been reduced by atherosclerosis. Either way, a decrease in sodium intake should be beneficial.

Of special interest is more recent evidence that hypokalemia, and the ratio of Na^+/K^+ intake, may be more important determinants of blood pressure than Na^+, even with salt-sensitivity. Population studies have shown that ratios of Na^+/K^+ were better correlated with high blood pressure than either Na^+ or K^+ alone (Intersalt Cooperative Research Group, 1988; Khaw and Barrett-Connor, 1988; Tobian, 1988). Moreover, several studies have indicated that potassium supplements can lower blood pressure in groups of hypertensive subjects (Iimura et al., 1981; Tobian, 1988), although this is not always the case (Grimm et al., 1990). Even more importantly, it now appears that dietary depletion of potassium will raise blood pressure even in normotensive subjects (Krishna et al., 1989), and that salt-sensitive rats on a high NaCl diet show fewer lesions of the kidney and less hypertrophy of their artery walls when supplemented with K^+ (Tobian, 1988). In human potassium depletion, the enhancement of blood pressure may be mediated at least partly by a decreased capacity for Na^+ excretion (and diminished levels of aldosterone) (Krishna et al., 1989). Moreover, potassium-depleted subjects became "salt-sensitive," responding to NaCl intake with a significant increase in blood pressure. All of this suggests that a deficiency of potassium, especially in the face of a high sodium intake, is an important determinant of hypertension. Indeed, Tobian (1988) points out that the average potassium intake of the U.S. population (on the order of 65 mequivalents or 2500 mg/day) is only about one quarter of that of hunter-gatherers, and that many other populations with a low potassium intake, notably Chinese, Japanese, Tibetan (and southeastern U.S. Blacks) (averaging 20–45 mequivalents), have a particularly high prevalence of hypertension and stroke. [Increased potassium ingestion would come especially from intake of certain vegetables, fruits, and fish (see Table 6.3).]

Salt-sensitivity appears to be enhanced not only by potassium depletion, but also by obesity. Recent studies have demonstrated that weight reduction will result in a lowering of blood pressure, irrespective of sodium intake (Rocchini et al., 1988, 1989; Tuck et al., 1981), and that the salt-sensitivity observed in obese subjects can be lost with weight reduction (Rocchini et al., 1989). [In the obese, blood levels of aldosterone, insulin, and norepinephrine did not decrease with an increase of Na^+ in the diet.]

Other factors that can induce hypertension include alcohol consumption (Friedman et al., 1988; Intersalt, 1988) (above 2–3 drinks a day), and the degree of release of natriuretic hormone (ANF). Sodium intake causes the release of ANF, which inhibits Na^+/K^+ exchange not just in the kidney (preventing Na^+ resorption) but also in smooth muscle cells of the arteries, causing them to contract (Groban et al., 1989; Marx, 1981). Though much remains to be learned, it is clear that sodium and potassium intake can both perturb blood pressure when genetic and other predisposing factors are present. Moreover, a significant portion of the American population is probably sodium-sensitive, due to genetics, obesity, or hypokalemia. Therefore, a movement toward reduction of sodium intake and increased potassium intake would appear to be advisable. The great preponderance of sodium intake is nondiscretionary (Altschul et al., 1982); that is, it is not added in the kitchen or at the table, but is inherent in the food or added during processing. A reduction in the use of sodium in food processing would thus seem a prudent public health measure, as would the intake of more fruits and vegetables where ratios of K/Na are high.

Dietary Sodium

Sodium in the diet is mainly in the form of NaCl, present naturally within the food or deliberately added as a flavor enhancer (Table 6.3). The average American consumes about 15 lbs of NaCl per year, which has been added to processed foods. Monosodium glutamate is also a major sodium source in processed foods. For individuals who should cut down on sodium intake, flavoring with garlic and other spices is recommended. Some KCl (which has a different, more bitter taste) may be substituted, but large doses must be avoided (see Hyperkalemia and Figure 6.5). Nutritional sodium deficiency does not occur in our society, but deficiency may be induced by various abnormal conditions, including Addison's disease (Figure 6.5), where there is a loss of adrenal function and aldosterone production. Hypernatremia may occur temporarily upon eating large amounts of NaCl, especially when unaccompanied by fluid intake. Cushing's disease, where excessive corticosteroid production results in sodium retention (as with aldosterone) has a similar consequence.

Calcium

This is the fifth most abundant element in the human and animal body (Table 6.1). Ninety-nine percent is present in the skeleton, primarily as hydroxylapatite $[3Ca_3(PO_4)_2 \cdot Ca(OH)_2]$. Bone density (and calcium deposition) vary with age, increasing in the first part of life and decreasing gradually with age from early adulthood onward (see Figure 6.6). The rest of body calcium is intra- and extracellular, where it plays an extremely vital role in directing cell function and nerve impulses. Calcium is also an integral component of the blood clotting mechanism (see Vitamin K, Chapter 5). The concentration of calcium in plasma, especially the concentration of free calcium ions, is carefully maintained so as to provide the Ca^{2+} necessary in transmission of nerve impulses and muscle contractions and to carry out regulatory functions initiated by some hormones, as illustrated in Figure 6.7. Fluxes of Ca^{2+} across endoplasmic reticulum (or "calcisome") and the plasma membranes are integral to nervous and muscular function, and different mechanisms for altering internal (intracellular) Ca^{2+} concentrations are operative in different cells. Fluxes of Ca^{2+} across intra- and extracellular membranes also mediate the actions of many hormones, growth factors, and neurotransmitters in many kinds of cells (Figure 6.7), and especially those in which inositol phosphates are released from plasma phosphatidylinositides (see Chapter 5, Inositol, Figure 5.12). Important to these processes is the high extracellular to intracellular (cytosol) Ca^{2+} concentration gradient and a consistent extracellular Ca^{2+} concentration. Substantial changes, such as a fall in extracellular free Ca^{2+}, will result in neuromuscular irritability (muscle cramps and inadvertent contractions) and even tetany.

On an acute basis, blood calcium concentrations are homeostatically controlled by a combination of Ca^{2+} fluxes into and out of the blood from the bone and/or intestine, and urinary Ca^{2+} resorption. The major control is on the flux of Ca^{2+} out of the fluid compartment of the bone, where it is in equilibrium with amorphous calcium phosphate (Figure 6.8; top panel). This occurs through the action of the PTH, which in turn controls the activation of 25-OH vitamin D to its hormonal form (1,25 di-OH-D_3), and both hormones interact to increase blood calcium concentrations. Through activated vitamin D, PTH rapidly increases bone calcium resorption, and the resorption of calcium by kidney tubules. It also stimulates intestinal absorption of dietary calcium (an effect that is slower and more lasting). The actions of 1,25-diOH-D involve changes in the transcription of specific genes within osteoblasts, including that for osteocalcin (or bone Gla protein; BGP) (Komm et al., 1988) and probably some calbindins. The physiological effect of the vitamin-hormone via BGP also depends on γ-carboxylation of certain glutamate residues, which may be important for binding of BGP to hydroxylapatite. [γ Carboxylation is dependent on vitamin K.] The vitamin D hormone has a slower secondary effect on the proliferation and differentiation of osteoclasts (Holtrop et al., 1981; McSheehy and Chambers, 1987). (For further details on the actions of vitamin D hormone, see Figure 5.30, Chapter 5.)

Thyroid secretion of calcitonin tends to lower blood calcium concentrations by having the op-

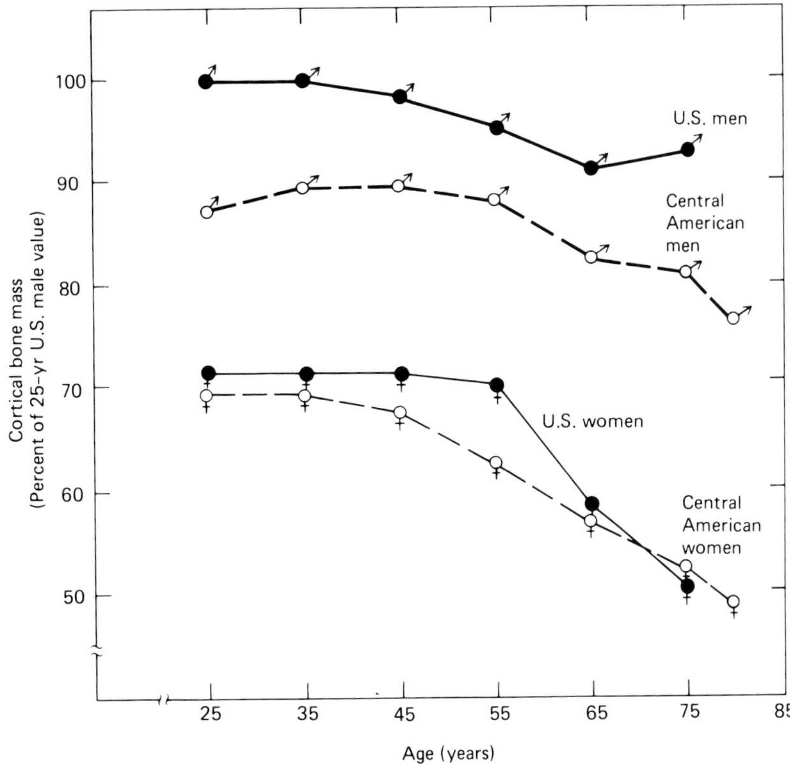

Figure 6.6. Age-related changes in cortical bone mass. (*Source:* Data recalculated from Garn et al. (1969).]

posite effect on bone calcium flux and causing increased deposition of bone mineral. Overall, this regulation is less important than that of the parathyroid–vitamin D-hormone system. Indeed, thyroid removal seems to have little or no effect on skeletal mass (Hurley et al., 1987). [Other hormones that can influence mineralization to some extent include thyroxine, growth hormone, estrogens, androgens, and insulin (Avioli, 1988; see below).]

For mineralization, crystals of hydroxylapatite are deposited within the matrix of collagen and elastic fibers that comprise the bone framework. The initial nucleation site for the crystals appears to be related to the structure of the collagen fibers with a 600 Å spacing, and may require collagen phosphorylation (Avioli, 1988). Crystallization probably involves the transformation of amorphous calcium phosphate, which makes up about 4% of the total bone mineral and is in a form of equilibrium with the Ca^{2+} and inorganic phosphate (or phosphorylated collagen) in the extracellular fluid of the bone. Various factors must influence both the "equilibrium" between amorphous and crystalline hydroxylapatite and between the former and "free" calcium (and phosphate) concentrations. For example, it is thought that the concentrations of certain metabolites, such as phosphocitrate (Lehninger, 1981), will influence the crystallization rate. On the surface of the crystalline hydroxylapatite are found various concentrations of citrate, carbonate, 30% of the magnesium in bone, and other ions, all of which may play a role in the process. Also, it is thought that the deposition of amorphous calcium phosphate is at least partly controlled by the concentration of inorganic phosphate, which, in turn, may be dependent on the rate of cleavage of Pi from glucose-1-phosphate by the alkaline phosphatase of osteoblasts (Krause and Mahan, 1976). Serum alkaline phosphatase is elevated in infants and children, especially during growth spurts, and also increased in adults with disturbances of bone growth (such as Paget's disease, involving increased osteoblast activity). Inappropriate deposition of calcium phosphate crystals may occur in soft tissues and joints in conjunction with high concentrations of inorganic pyrophosphate, causing arthritis (Lust et al., 1981), or in heart, kidney,

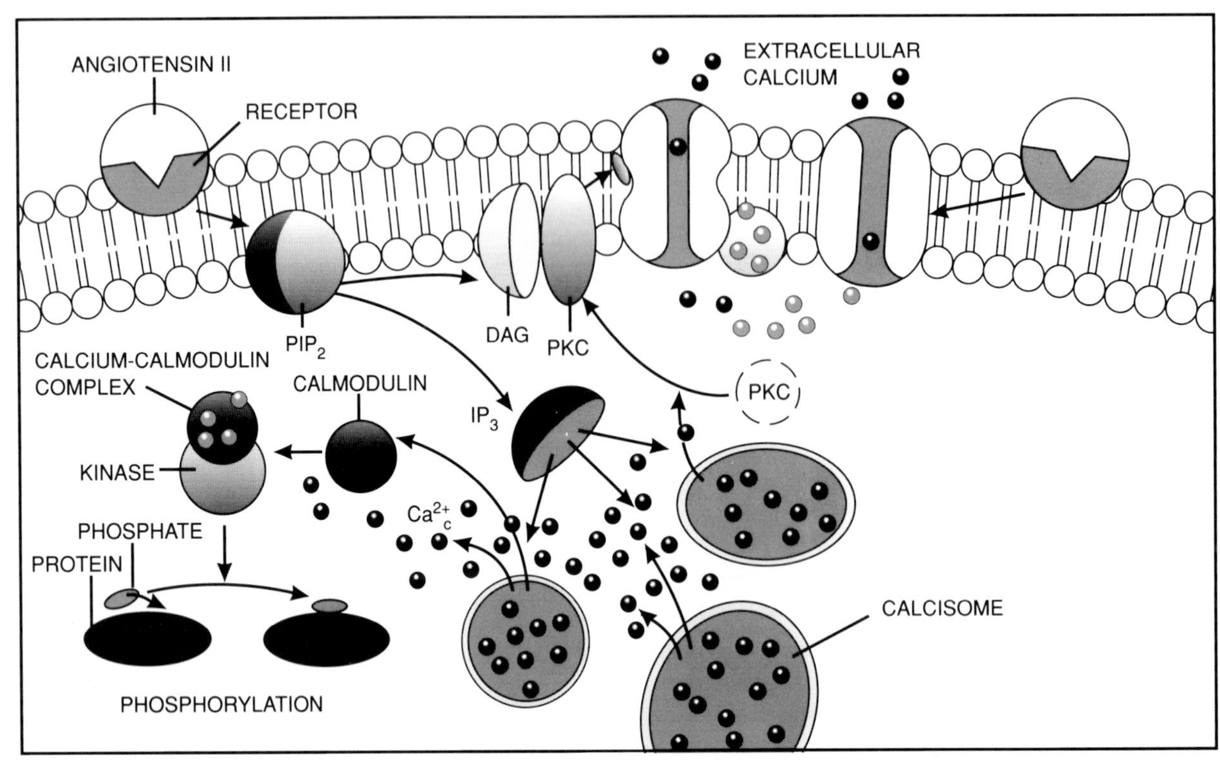
ANGIOTENSIN II
RECEPTOR
EXTRACELLULAR
CALCIUM
PIP$_2$
DAG
PKC
CALCIUM-CALMODULIN
COMPLEX
CALMODULIN
IP$_3$
PKC
KINASE
PHOSPHATE
PROTEIN
Ca^{2+}_c
CALCISOME
PHOSPHORYLATION

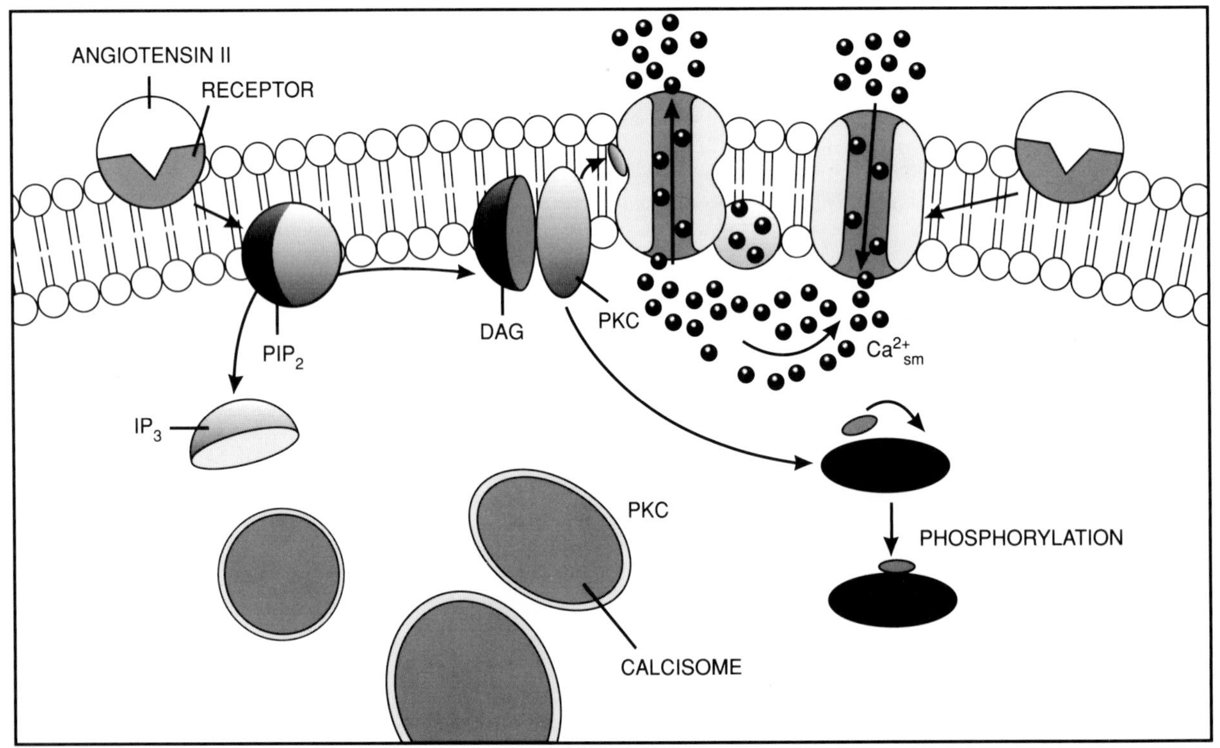
ANGIOTENSIN II
RECEPTOR
PIP$_2$
DAG
PKC
Ca^{2+}_{sm}
IP$_3$
PKC
PHOSPHORYLATION
CALCISOME

and blood vessels when magnesium concentrations are inadequate (Seelig and Haddy, 1980).

The availability of other minerals (see top right, Figure 6.7) will also influence the degree of mineralization, although the molecular events involved are still not clear. Most of these minerals (except Mg^{2+}) can replace Ca^{2+} or $PO_4^{=}$ in the apatite (e.g., fluorohydroxyapatite lending strength to the bone). Some may also act directly on the osteoblasts or osteoclasts: fluoride can enhance osteoblast cell proliferation (Lau et al., 1987); manganese may be essential for the function of both cell types (Strause and Saltman, 1989; see Chapter 7, Manganese).

Calcium is found in three forms in the plasma: as the free ion (about 47%); in chelated nonprotein-bound form, primarily complexed with citrate and other organic acids (6.5%); and bound to proteins, especially prealbumin (46%) (Avioli, 1988). There appears to be no direct relationship between total plasma Ca^{2+} and the critical free Ca^{2+} concentration, although about equal proportions are normally found in the free and bound compartments. The free Ca^{2+} fraction is the one considered to be readily accessible to cells and is the one monitored by the parathyroid and thyroid glands. (In interstitial fluid, almost none of the Ca^{2+} is protein-bound.) As blood calcium (and interstitial fluid) concentrations fall, increased PTH is secreted (see Chapter 5, Figure 5.30). This results in an increased rate of 1-α-hydroxylation of 25-OH cholecalciferol (from the plasma) by the kidney, to form 1,25-dihydroxylcholecalciferol (active vitamin D), also referred to as "calcitriol." This signals the kidney tubules to enhance their rate of calcium resorption, stimulates increased efflux of calcium from the bone fluid compartment (and dissolution of hydroxylapatite), and stimulates intestinal absorption of calcium from the diet. Conversely, as blood calcium concentrations increase, less PTH is secreted, and these changes are reversed. With increasing plasma Ca^{2+} concentrations, increased calcitonin is also secreted (by the thyroid). This enhances the rate of bone mineralization, perhaps partly by stimulating the osteoblasts.

Another factor that influences plasma calcium concentrations is the proportion of calcium to phosphorus in the diet. Diets with a disproportionately high ratio of P : Ca (or an acute high intake of phosphate) can enhance the secretion of PTH and, thus, bone demineralization. This could be a factor in the development of osteoporosis, the phenomenon of decreased bone density and mineralization that commonly occurs with age, especially in women after menopause. Further aspects of this phenomenon are discussed below.

Figure 6.7. Calcium fluxes involved in regulation of cell function and hormone action, as illustrated for angiotensin II affecting adrenal cells. Calcium acts as a "messenger" in at least two different ways (top and bottom). **Top:** Binding of hormone to receptor causes the breakdown of membrane phosphatidylinositide diphosphate (PIP_2) into inositoltriphosphate (IP_3) and diacylglycerol (DAG). The IP_3 results in release of Ca^+ from internal membranous vesicles ("calcisomes"), increasing concentrations of calcium in the cell fluid (Ca^+). This binds to calmodulin, enhancing the activity of protein kinases and thus the phosphorylation of specific enzymes/proteins that carry out the responses of the cell to the original hormone (in this case, synthesis and release of aldosterone). The increased Ca^+, plus the DAG, also activate (and bring to the plasma membrane) protein kinase C (PKC). **Bottom:** In the more sustained phase of the response, hormone-receptor binding also directly activates calcium channels in the membrane, causing increased influx and efflux of extracellular Ca^+, and the phosphorylation of further enzymes/proteins by PKC. [*Source:* Reprinted by permission from Rasmussen (1989).]

Calcium Absorption, Metabolism, and Excretion

The amount of calcium absorbed from the diet per day is dependent on (a) the relative proportions of chelating and precipitating agents in the diet, which determine the amount of calcium actually available for absorption, and (b) the degree of activated vitamin D stimulation of the apparatus for absorption in the intestinal mucosa, which determines the rate of calcium uptake (left and bottom, Figure 6.8). [This involves synthesis of specific proteins in the mucosal cells (see Chapter 5).] The average American diet contains 500–1200 mg calcium/day. Individuals, especially adults, show enormous variations in calcium intake. This is partly because calcium is distributed unevenly in foodstuffs (Table 6.2). It is very high in milk and dairy products, including cheeses, and is also quite high in nuts and whole grains; however, it is relatively low in most other products. [In the United States, dairy products account for 72% or more of dietary calcium (Avioli, 1988; Marston and Welsh, 1983).] Some plant foods may have quite high total concentrations, but the calcium may be unavailable because of the high concentrations of oxalate (Table 6.2) or phytates (and possibly other parts of the bran in whole grains).

This is especially so for spinach, rhubarb, and beets (oxalates), and sometimes so for cereal grains (phytates, etc.). In the English diet, the oxalate contributed by tea is thought to be a factor in determining calcium status (Hodgkinson, 1977). Also, in Nigeria and other parts of central Africa, plants with a high oxalate content are staple sources of carbohydrate and protein (see footnote to Table 6.2), and this may contribute to nutritional deficiencies in these regions. The presence of oxalate in the diet also decreases the availability of dietary Mg and Fe. Oxalic and phytic acids render all these minerals less available by forming water-insoluble salts. Under normal dietary conditions in the United States, however, these dietary substituents may not be important factors in determining calcium absorption (Greger, 1988). In general, plant foods have less available calcium, but there are exceptions, including kale (Weaver et al., 1987), which has a fairly high calcium content (Table 6.2) with an availability apparently as high as that of milk and cheese, and broccoli, which is likely to be similar in this regard.

Working in the opposite direction, namely to increase the availability of dietary Ca^{2+} (and other minerals), are chelating agents that retain the mineral in water-soluble form. For the mineral calcium, lactose, citrate, H^+, certain amino acids, and even glucose (Knowles et al., 1988) and sucrose (Ambrecht and Wasserman, 1976) serve this function. In general, a meal will tend to enhance absorption of supplemental calcium, perhaps by enhancing release of stomach acids (Heaney et al., 1989). Calcium is about equally available from various supplements, including the carbonate, lactate, or gluconate (in which calcium is 40%, 13%, and 9% of the pill weight, respectively).

Only 30%–50% of dietary calcium is normally absorbed, with a much higher proportion in the case of growing children (drinking milk). The capacity for absorption decreases substantially with age and is greater in men than in women at all ages (Avioli, 1980). The amount of calcium excreted in the urine reflects the amount of calcium absorbed from the diet, and not necessarily the total consumed. Urinary calcium losses are enhanced by acidosis, a high protein intake (Hegsted and Linkswiler, 1981) (although this may depend upon the type of protein, duration of intake, and its phosphate content) (Howe, 1985), and a high phosphate intake (especially if calcium intake is low). An approximately equal proportion of calcium is lost through secretions that enter the gastrointestinal tract (mainly in the small intestine) and are only partly reabsorbed (Figure 6.8) (Avioli, 1988). Sweat losses can also be significant. During pregnancy and lactation, additional (large) quantities are transferred (lost) on a daily basis.

Calcium Requirements

For adults, the RDA for calcium in the United States is 800 mg, with larger amounts for pregnant and lactating women. Large quantities are required during growth for infants and children. (Indeed, it should be stressed that at least two to three glasses of milk a day are required to meet the optimal needs of the growing child or teenager.) The RDA varies considerably from country to country, partly because there is some adaptation of the body to low or high calcium intake, as shown by balance studies on different populations. Also, balance studies are not likely to be very accurate in determining calcium absorption and retention (Avioli, 1980). Thus, official requirements range from 400–1000 mg/day around the world. Nevertheless, it should be stressed that the calcium requirement does not diminish with age, and there has been a great deal of debate about whether a much higher intake shouldn't be recommended for the elderly (National Institute of Arthritis, Diabetes and Digestive and Kidney Diseases, 1983; National Research Council, 1989). Certainly, surveys of elderly populations indicate that a low calcium intake is very common (especially among women), which may be ascribed partly to the fact that milk and milk products, the best sources of calcium, are shunned for their fat and cholesterol contents. [See also Chapter 12, and next section in this chapter, on osteoporosis.]

In summary, calcium status is determined by a combination of nutritional and hormonal factors, which, by complex interactions, determine the amount of calcium available for absorption, the intestinal capacity for absorption, and the extent of calcium losses via the urine, sweat, and feces. Of primary importance are the calcium content of the food and inherent factors, like lactose and oxalate, which determine availability; parathyroid and thyroid functions, which act through vitamin D and other hormones; and finally, phosphorus and protein metabolism. Further aspects of these interactions are described below.

Aging, Bone Demineralization, Osteomalacia, and Osteoporosis

As already mentioned, bone mineral content is at its height in early adulthood and then gradually declines with age (Figure 6.6). This decline cannot be prevented, although the rate of decline can be slowed. The rate of decline is particularly rapid in women after menopause and can lead to osteoporosis, a common problem among elderly women.

Osteomalacia and osteoporosis are both conditions in which bone mineral content (and density) is decreased, with or without a concomitant decrease in the organic bone elements, respectively. (Organic bone elements are collagen, osteoblasts, osteoclasts, and connective tissue.) Osteomalacia usually occurs at younger ages (e.g., in the calcium deficiency of pregnancy). Osteoporosis also affects the loss of trabecular bone (in the torso) more severely than it does peripheral (cortical) bone. Both conditions reflect a decrease in bone hydroxylapatite content and are thus forms of calcium deficiency of the bone. ("Osteopenia" is a more general term for lack of bone mineral.)

Osteoporosis, and the resulting fragility of bones enhancing their breakage, is a major public health problem in the United States and most "Western" nations. Perhaps ironically, it is most common in countries that (on average) also have a relatively high calcium (and protein) intake (Hegsted, 1986). In the United States, 2.3 million fractures occur per year in individuals over 45 years of age, most of which are made more likely by a low bone density, and most of which occur in women. Currently, there is still a great deal of debate about the nature, origins, and optimal treatment of this disease. This is not surprising in view of the complex nature of the process of bone mineralization, and the maintenance of calcium homeostasis. Nevertheless, some consensus is emerging on many aspects of this problem, and new and exciting observations have been made (also through the application of molecular biology) that will help to resolve some of the fundamental remaining questions.

The main risk factors for osteoporosis are summarized in Table 6.4. At least four types of factors are involved: genetics, estrogens/androgens, physical activity, and diet/dietary history. Blacks have a higher bone density than whites, and this may be due to a decreased turnover of the mineral of the bone (Weinstein and Bell, 1988). The finding that postmenopausal women are especially susceptible to bone demineralization implies that the process tends to accelerate with a decline in estrogen secretion. At menopause, there tend to be changes in calcium metabolism (Table 6.5). These changes are often exaggerated in women with osteoporosis: intestinal absorption of calcium may be less, although even with osteoporosis, many individuals have a normal absorption

Table 6.4. Risk Factors in Osteoporosis and Changes in Bone and Calcium Metabolism with Menopause[a]

I. Risk factors in osteoporosis (in approximate decreasing order of importance)
Female sex
Caucasian or Oriental ethnicity
Positive family history
Low calcium intake (lifelong)
Early menopause (or hysterectomy)
Not physically active
Many children
Alcohol abuse
Cigarette smoking
High caffeine intake
High protein intake
High phosphate intake
II. Changes that occur with menopause
Decreased estrogen production
Enhanced rates of bone loss
Enhanced excretion of calcium in the morning urine
Slight increase in serum ultrafiltrable calcium
Decreased intestinal absorption of calcium at low calcium intakes
III. Changes with menopause that can be associated with osteoporosis
Decreased intestinal absorption of calcium
Decreased activation of 25-OH vitamin D_3
Decreased responsiveness of the parathyroid to low plasma calcium
Increased urinary excretion of hydroxyproline
Increased serum levels of HCO_3^-
Increased serum levels of IL-1 (interleukin-1)

[a] Modified from Thorneycroft (1989).

rate. Losses of calcium in the morning urine (after an overnight fast) tend to be greater. There is slightly but significantly more nonprotein-bound Ca^{2+} in the blood plasma, an increase in HCO_3^- (that may or may not be related), and an increase in plasma interleukin-1 (IL-1) which is implicated in bone resorption (Pacifici et al., 1989). (IL-1 secretion is enhanced by inflammatory processes, which are more prevalent in the elderly.)

There can also be a decreased capacity to make vitamin D_3 (Holick, 1986) or to activate it to the hormone, 1,25-dihydroxycholecalciferol (Ramazzato et al., 1986); a decreased responsiveness of the parathyroid to changes in serum phosphate (or calcium); and a concomitant enhanced excretion of hydroxyproline in the urine. The latter is a breakdown product of collagen and elastin fibers (an important part of the bone matrix), and its increased secretion is consistent with enhanced

Table 6.5. Changes in the Parameters of Calcium Metabolism at Menopause and with Osteoporosis[a]

Parameter	Older women, postmenopause	Younger women, premenopause	Women with osteoporosis	Reference
Calcium absorption				
Fractional rate per hr	0.75	—	0.56[d]	Nordin et al. (1985)
	0.67	0.66	(Some are normal)	Nordin (1986)
mmol/hr[b]				
low Ca diet	0.23[d]	0.37	—	Ireland and Fordtran (1973)
high Ca diet	0.18	0.23	—	
Urinary				
OH–Pro : creatinine (× 1000)	19.3	—	22.3[d]	Nordin et al. (1985)
Ca : creatinine	0.25	—	0.32[d]	Nordin et al. (1985)
a.m.	0.13[d]	0.05	—	Gallagher and Nordin (1973)
p.m.	0.17	0.14	—	
Serum				
Ultrafiltrate Ca	1.60[d]	1.56	—	Nordin et al. (1989)
Complexed Ca	0.40[d]	0.36	—	
Protein-bound Ca	0.83	0.83	—	
HCO_3^-	29.1[d]	28.2	—	
PTH response to phosphate intake[c]	Acute 26%–43% increase	—	0%–19%[d] increase	Silverberg et al. (1989)
diOH-D response to phosphate intake[c]	No change	—	50% decrease (5 days)	Silverberg et al. (1989)
Urinary calcium losses (day 3 vs day 1)[c]	57% decrease	—	53% decrease	Silverberg et al. (1989)

[a] Within 10 years of menopause.
[b] At 4 mM Ca^{2+}.
[c] 2 hr after 1 g phosphate.
[d] $p < 0.01$ for difference from value on same line.

bone destruction. Some of the data supporting these points are given in Table 6.5.

What the data suggest overall, is that depending upon family history and genetics (as well as lifelong dietary and exercise habits), an individual woman will arrive at menopause with a greater or lesser propensity toward osteoporosis. This propensity will be exaggerated if there are additional genetic defects, involving calcium absorption and bone remineralization. The same will be true for older men, except that they need not contend with the acute loss of estrogen.

For individuals who do not have a major defect in calcium absorption, calcium supplements can make an important difference in the rate of bone loss (Table 6.6) especially in women more than 5 years postmenopause (Dawson-Hughes et al., 1990). If the capacity for calcium absorption is defective, this could be due to a reduced capacity to activate vitamin D (via 1-α-hydroxylation; see Chapter 5) or a defect in the responsiveness of genes for the proteins that carry out the actions of this vitamin-hormone. If the former is true (which will be the case in some individuals), treatment with the preactivated hormone (also known as "calcitriol") should and can be successful. Indeed, several studies indicate a positive response in subjects with osteoporosis (Table 6.6; Caniggia et al., 1988; Gallagher et al., 1988; Nordin et al., 1988). Negative studies (such as those of Ott et al., 1989) could be explained on the basis that the subjects studied did not have a defect in the enzymes for vitamin D activation but rather in the receptor for the hormone-vitamin, or in enzymes/proteins responsive to the hormone-vitamin.

What is also clear is that, at least in women, loss of estrogen can play a role, and that estrogen replacement seems to be especially effective in reducing bone mineral losses (Table 6.6). Recent findings from molecular biology would appear to shed some exciting new light on the mechanism involved. First, osteoblasts (responsible for bone mineralization) have estrogen receptors, thus

Table 6.6. Effects of Calcium Supplementation, Estrogen or 1,25-DiOH Vitamin D Replacement on Parameters of Calcium Metabolism in Women with Postmenopausal Osteoporosis[a]

Parameter	Percent change with treatment: Calcium supplement	Estrogen	diOH vitamin D	Reference
Loss of bone mineral				
Forearm (18 mo) (mg/cm)	50% less loss	—	—	Polley et al. (1987)
Forearm (24 mo)				
proximal	47% less loss	100% less loss	—	Schwartz et al. (1985)
distal	No difference			
Total body (24 mo)	44% less loss	87% less loss	—	Schwartz et al. (1985)
Metacarpal cortical bone area (mm^2)	65% less loss	100% less loss	—	Horsman et al. (1977)
Calcium absorption				
Fractional	—	—	24% more	Riggs et al. (1987)
Units	No difference	No difference	—	Schwartz et al. (1985)
Urinary/OH pro : creatinine				
Those with normal absorption	31% less	—	—	Horowitz et al. (1984)
Those with reduced absorption	No difference	—	29% less[b]	Need et al. (1985)
Those with normal absorption	No difference	37% less	—	Schwartz et al. (1985)
Serum				
Alkaline phosphatase	No difference	24% less	—	Schwartz et al. (1985)
Bone Gla protein	No difference	47% less	—	Schwartz et al. (1985)
IL-1	—	Much less	—	Pacifici et al. (1989)

[a] Long-term treatments.
[b] Plus Ca.

linking estrogen to the stimulation of activity in these cells (Eriksen et al., 1988; Komm et al., 1988). [Steroid hormones (like estrogens and activated vitamin D) act by binding to cytosolic or nuclear receptor proteins, and after modification these complexes bind to specific portions of the DNA in the promoter regions of specific genes, to initiate or enhance gene transcription.] Second, and perhaps even more importantly, it has been discovered that the hormone-receptor complex for estradiol may interact with the same regulatory elements in the promoter regions of certain genes as the receptor complex for 1,25-dihydroxycholecalciferol (calcitriol; the active vitamin D hormone). This appears to be the case at least for one vitamin D-responsive protein, osteocalcin (BGP) (Komm et al., 1988). If this were also the case for the genes most critical to intestinal calcium absorption and osteoblast bone mineralization, it would explain the effectiveness of estrogen in these processes. Moreover, it would explain why estrogen is effective when other conditions underlying aging and osteoporosis are impaired (such as the capacity to activate vitamin D and/or the effectiveness of the vitamin-hormone). (It would also explain why estrogen depletion at menopause does not necessarily pose a problem for older women, since active vitamin D can substitute for the estrogen.) Assuredly, much more will soon be discovered about this bihormonal regulation of genes involved in calcium metabolism.

Returning to the matter of estrogen replacement, however, an acute loss of estrogen underlies many or most of the changes in calcium metabolism that may occur at menopause. Nevertheless, only a portion of postmenopausal women will actually develop a dangerous loss of bone mineral, greatly increasing the likelihood of fracture. For these, estrogen replacement therapy could be important. Increasingly, all women at menopause are strongly encouraged to accept estrogen replacement, especially for the first 5–10 years. In one study of women at high risk, the rate of hip fracture was reduced about threefold by this treatment (Kiel et al., 1987). Even quite low doses of estrogen (0.3–0.6 mg/day) as available from "skin patches" appear to be effective (Ettinger et al., 1987; Linsday et al., 1984). However, there is a "downside," which is that hormonal replacement (estrogen ± progestins) leads to some increase in the risk of endometrial (Persson et al., 1989) and breast cancer (Bergkvist et al., 1989; Key and Pike, 1988). (Also, there is the continued bother of menstruation.) These aspects must also be considered.

With regards to other factors, physical activity throughout life is an important stimulus for the laying down and maintenance of dense bone. Thus, continued physical activity (against resistance) throughout life will tend to slow down the loss of bone mineral (Lane et al., 1986). Conversely, lack of physical activity, as occurs in the bedridden or in gravity-free conditions, can result in bone demineralization. The mechanisms by which these effects occur is unclear, but would appear to involve the thyroid and parathyroid glands (Bergstrom, 1978), which affect the flux of calcium in and out of the bone fluid compartment (Figure 6.8). It is noteworthy that even exercise in bed does not prevent calcium efflux from the bone and that, in this case, a loss of bone matrix as well as mineral is involved (osteomalacia). Weight-bearing exercise appears to be the most effective, as long as it is also not overdone (Avioli, 1988; Marcus et al., 1989).

Throughout life (also for the elderly), the amount of calcium in the diet and the ratio of phosphate to calcium in the diet plays an important role. The U.S. RDAs for calcium and phosphorus are both 800 mg for adults. Ideally, the intake of calcium should be in the same range as the intake of phosphorus, although ratios of 1.5 : 1 (P : Ca) may be acceptable. A high phosphate intake enhances the secretion of PTH in part at least by lowering serum calcium concentrations. This is particularly the case in subjects where the ratio of P : Ca is high (>2 : 1), as illustrated by data in Figure 6.9. The increased PTH activates vitamin D and induces the usual three phenomena (see Figure 5.30; Chapter 5), including bone demineralization if there is insufficient calcium relative to phosphorus available for absorption. Thus, bone demineralization can result from a diet very high in P : Ca and, perhaps, even when "sufficient" calcium is present (according to the RDA). [Processed food diets (not uncommon in Western countries) tend to be high in phosphorus, and ratios can easily reach 2.5 or more (Draper and Bell, 1980).] The situation of the Canadian Eskimo is another illustration. These Eskimo abandoned their traditional diet (which included soft bones from fish and land animals along with the meat) for a diet very high in meat without the bone component (hence with little calcium). Compared with the average Canadian non-Eskimo population, intake of calcium has been 12%–60% less at all ages. As a result, serum calcium concentrations have been lower and serum phosphate concentrations much higher, again at all ages (Draper and Bell, 1980). Another factor that exacerbates the problem is the high protein content of the diet, as this enhances urinary calcium excretion (see above). This population has had an unusually high incidence of osteoporosis in both men and women.

Although there is a great deal of individual variation, the "average" American diet with its high meat, high processed food, and high carbonated beverage content has a P : Ca ratio and protein intake that tend to be in the same direction as those of the Canadian Eskimo. The carbonated beverage and processed food components alone can easily add 1000 mg P to a diet (Draper and Bell, 1980). It should be stressed that failure in early life to lay down sufficient bone mineral will exacerbate the problem in later life, as there will be less mineral to lose in the aging process.

Several other dietary components may also play a role in osteoporosis or its potential consequences. Fluoride can lend strength to bones and teeth by forming fluoroapatite; it may also stimulate the proliferation and activity of osteoblasts (Dandona et al., 1988; Farley et al., 1983). Fluoride also increases levels of alkaline phosphatase and osteocalcin in blood plasma (Dandona et al., 1988; Kanwar and Dhar, 1989; Wergedal et al., 1988), which are symptoms of osteoblast activity. All of these phenomena can also result from the actions of activated vitamin D (1,25-dihydroxycholecalciferol). Thus, fluoride may directly or indirectly stimulate a similar set of genes at least in bone cells, and thus may work against the fragility of bones (and bone breakage) in osteoporosis. Indeed, fluoride supplements (50 mg/day) have been used for some time, to stimulate bone formation and retard bone mineral losses (Jowsey et al., 1972; Riggs et al., 1983; Spencer et al., 1985). A more recent 4-year, double-blind, prospective study of women with osteoporosis and vertebral fractures, however, suggests that fluoride treatment may not always be helpful: Supplements of 75 mg F^-/day (with 1500 mg Ca) did not reduce the incidence of vertebral fractures, as compared with that of the placebo group, and in fact *increased* the incidence of nonvertebral fractures (suggesting that extra fluoride had enhanced fragility) (Riggs et al., 1990). Densities of cancellous bone in the spine and neck were significantly enhanced by the treatment, but densities of radial (cortical) bones were slightly but significantly decreased. It is possible that these doses of fluoride

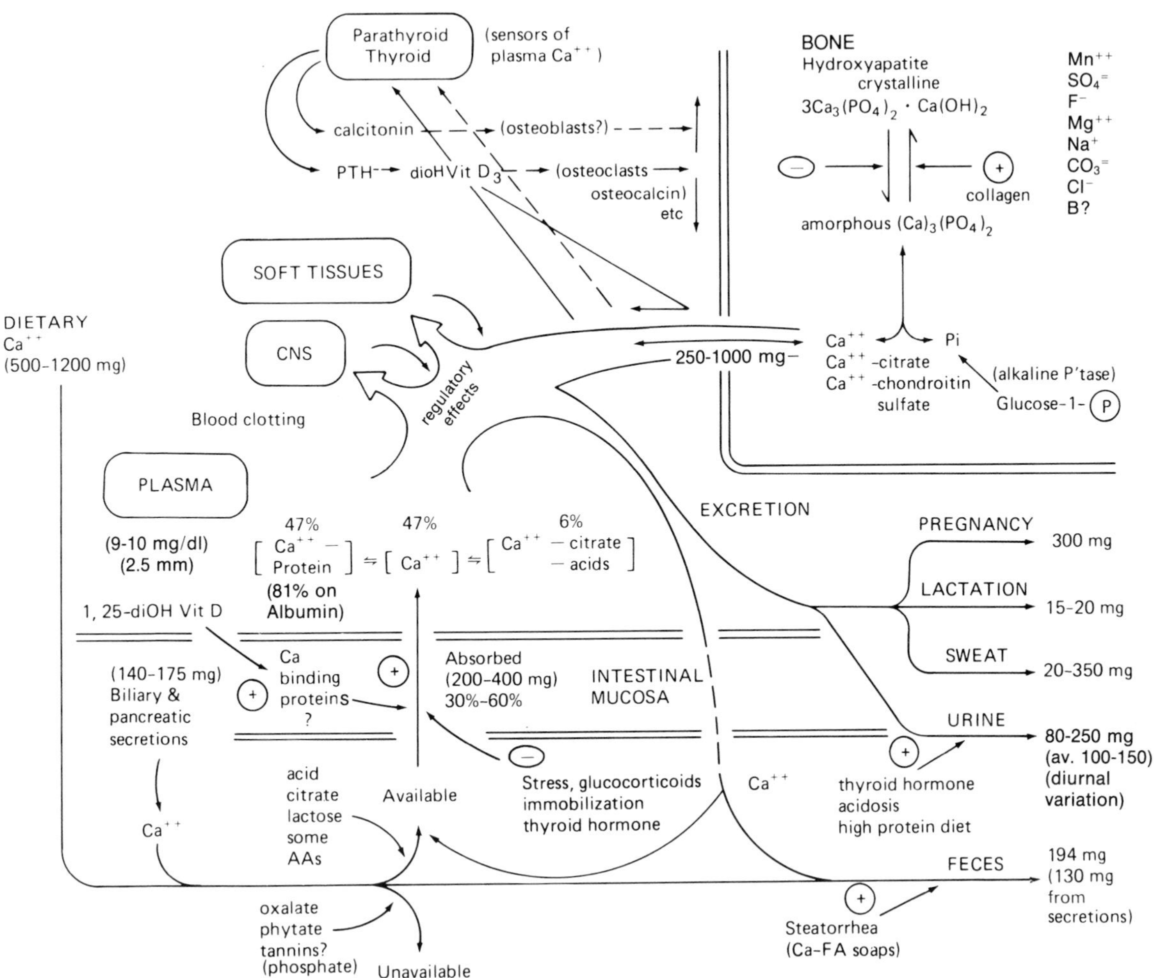

Figure 6.8. Nutrition and metabolism of calcium. Total in the body about 1200 g. Hypocalcemia (<7 mg/dl plasma), tetany. Hypercalcemia (<12 mg/dl plasma), nonspecific symptoms. + indicates stimulation; – indicates depression. Calcium in the diet is only partly available, and availability and absorption are modulated by other food factors. Absorption is promoted by vitamin D-hormone, probably via calcium-binding proteins. Transport via the blood is to all cells (where it participates in regulatory aspects) and especially to the bone (where it becomes part of the skeletal mineral). Blood Ca^+ concentrations are kept within certain limits, mainly through regulation by PTH (and active vitamin D), but also by thyroid-derived calcitonin. Mineralization and demineralization of bone involves activation of osteoblasts and osteoclasts, respectively, and production of inorganic phosphate (Pi) via alkaline phosphatase. Losses of calcium from the body are mainly via urine and feces. Amounts are mg/day.

may have been too high, for this particular population group (naturally exposed to a certain level of fluoride). It is quite clear that too high concentrations of fluorine are dangerous to bone (see Chapter 7; Krishnamachari, 1990; Riggs et al., 1987). Alternatively, the increased bone density induced by fluoride treatment may not be effective in preventing fractures, and/or that lower doses would be more effective, especially if F^- intake is already in the normal range.

Sufficient availability of vitamin B_{12} (cobalamin) may also be critical to osteoblast activity (and osteocalcin production) (Carmel et al., 1988). Moreover, there is recent interest in the possibility that boron plays a role in bone mineralization: It tends to concentrate in bone; and a study in which postmenopausal women were supplemented with this trace element indicated

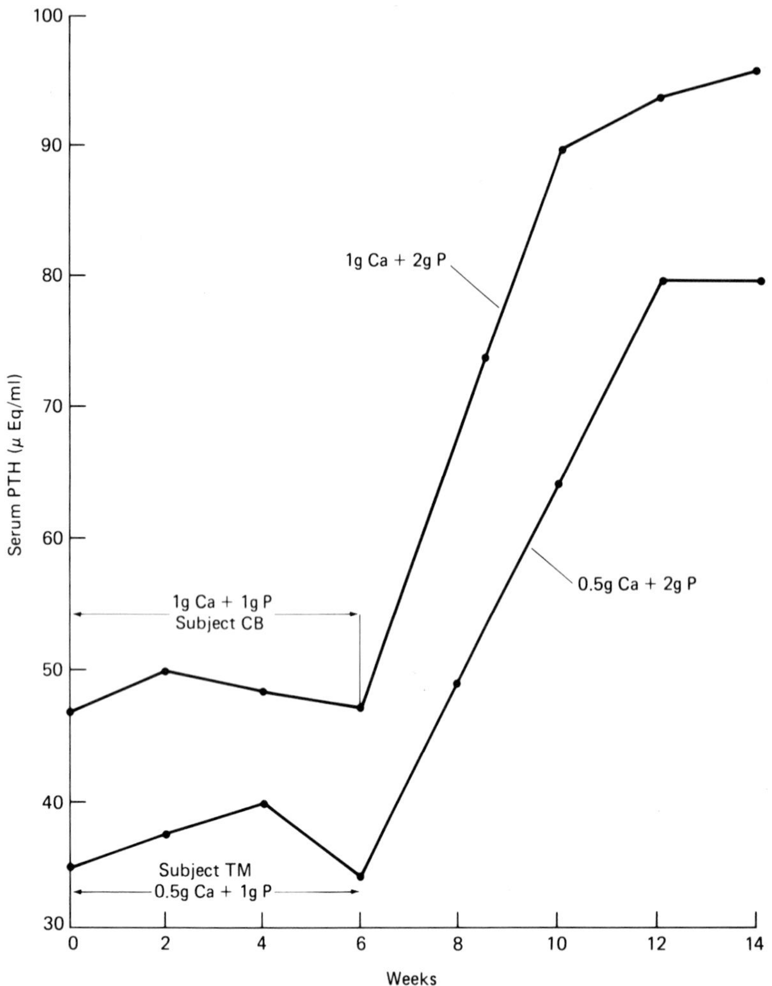

Figure 6.9. Effect of dietary phosphorus on concentrations of parathyroid hormone in serum. PTH, immunoreactive parathyroid hormone in adults on various diets. [*Source:* Reprinted by permission from Draper and Bell (1980).]

that it lowered their urinary calcium losses, and raised endogenous serum levels of estrogen (see Chapter 7, Table 7.14).

Finally, a high caffeine intake has been found to increase loss of calcium in the urine (calciuria) of humans (Massey and Wise, 1984) and rats (Whiting and Whiting, 1987). How caffeine has this effect is still unclear, although it is well-known that caffeine (and theophylline) inhibit the phosphodiesterase that inactivates cAMP (to form AMP). [At least in rats, theophylline was even more effective in promoting calciuria than caffeine (Whiting and Whitney, 1987), consistent with its superior capacity to inhibit phosphodiesterase.] Also, rat studies with indomethacin (Whiting and Whitney, 1987) and human studies with aspirin (Hollingbery et al., 1985) suggest that prostaglandin (or thromboxane) production is involved, as both these inhibitors of the cyclooxygenase (that initiates eicosanoid synthesis) inhibited the calciuria. (For details on prostanoid synthesis, see Chapter 3.) Thus, caffeine (or theophylline) may enhance the effects of certain hormones that act via cAMP to activate synthesis of prostaglandins, which promote excretion of calcium in the urine. Alternatively, eicosanoid synthesis may be enhanced by caffeine through other means; and the eicosanoids may enhance calcium excretion by stimulating a cAMP-dependent pathway. [Prostaglandins can stimulate adenyl cyclase in some tissues.] Apparently, caffeine is not promoting diuresis (Whiting and Whitney, 1987). Caffeine effects in humans occur with consumption of 200–399 mg/day (3–5 cups of coffee) (Nutr Rev, 1988).

References

Altschul AM, Grommetr KJ, Slotkoff L, Ayers WR (1982): *In* Beers RF Jr, ed: Nutritional factors: Modulating effects on metabolic processes. New York: Raven, p 45.

Altura BT, Altura BM (1987): Magnesium-Bull 9:6.

Ambrecht HJ, Wasserman RH (1976): J Nutr 106:1265.

Avioli LV (1980): *In* Goodhart RS, Shils ME, eds: Modern nutrition in health and disease (6th ed). Philadelphia: Lea & Febiger, p 294.

Avioli LV (1988): *In* Shils ME, Young VR, eds: Modern nutrition in health and disease. Philadelphia: Lea & Febiger, p 143.

Bergkvist L, Adami H-O, Persson I, Hoover R, Schairer C (1989): N Engl J Med 321:293.

Bergstrom WH (1978): Am J Dis Child 132:553.

Caniggia A, Nuti R, Lore F, Martini G, Righi G, Turchetti V (1988): Proceedings Workshop on Vitamin D, 7th (Vitamin D: Cell Clin Endocrinol), p 807.

Carmel R, Lau K-H, Baylink DJ, Saxena S, Singer FR (1988): N Engl J Med 319:70.

Dandona P, Coumar A, Gill DS, Bell J, Thomas M (1988): Clin Endocrinol 29:437.

Dawson-Hughes B, Dallal GE, Krall EA, Sadowski L, Sahyoun N, Tannenbaum S (1990): N Engl J Med 323:878.

DeLuca HF (1974): Fed Proc 32:2211.

Draper HF, Bell RR (1980): Adv Nutr Res 2:90.

Eriksen EF, Colvard DS, Berg NJ, Graham ML, Mann KG, Spelsberg TC, Riggs BL (1988): Science 241:84.

Ettinger B, Genant HK, Cann CE (1987): Ann Intern Med 106:40.

Farley JR, Wergedal JE, Baylink DJ (1983): Science 222:330.

Friedman GD (1988): Prev Med 17:387.

Fujita T, Henry WL, Bartter FC, Lake CR, Delea CS (1980): Am J Med 69:334.

Gallagher JC, Nordin BEC (1973): *In* van Keep PA, Lauritzen C, eds: Ageing and estrogens. Basel: Karger, p 98.

Gallagher JC, Goldgar D, O'Neill J (1988): Proceedings Workshop Vitamin D, 7th (Vitamin D: Mol Cell Clin Endocrinol), p 836.

Gamble JL (1958): Chemical anatomy, physiology, and pathology of extracellular fluid. Cambridge: Harvard University Press.

Garn SM, Rohmann CG, Wagner B, Davila GH, Ascoli W (1969): Clin Orthop 65:51.

Greger JL (1988): Cereal Foods World 33:796.

Grimm RH, Neaton JD, Elmer PJ, et al. (1990): N Engl J Med 322:569.

Groban L, Ebert TJ, Kreis DU, Skelton MM, Van Wynsberghe DM, Cowley AW Jr (1989): Am J Physiol 256:F780.

Heaney RP, Gallagher JC, Johnson CC, Neer R, Parfitt AM, Whedon GD (1982): Am J Clin Nutr 36(Suppl):986.

Heaney RP, Smith KT, Recker RR, Hinders SM (1989): Am J Clin Nutr 49:372.

Hegsted DM (1986): J Nutr 116:2316.

Hegsted M, Linkswiler HM (1981): J Nutr 111:244.

Hodgkinson A (1977): Oxalic acid in biology and medicine. New York: Academic.

Holick MF (1986): Clin Nutr 5:121.

Hollingbery PW, Bergman EA, Massey LK (1985): Fed Proc 44:1149.

Holtrop ME, Cox KA, Clark MB, Holick MF, Anast CS (1981): Endocrinology 108:2293.

Horowitz M, Need AG, Philcox JC, Nordin BEC (1984): Am J Clin Nutr 39:857.

Horsman A, Gallagher JC, Simpson M, Nordin BEC (1977): Br Med J 2:789.

Howe (1985): *In* Kies C, ed: Nutritional bioavailability of calcium. Washington, DC: American Chemical Society, p 125.

Hubbard JL, Llinas R, Quastel DMJ (1969): Electrophysiologic analysis of synaptic transmission (Monograph, 19, Physiol Soc London). London: Edward Arnold.

Hurley DL, Tiegs RD, Wahner HW, Heath H III (1987): N Engl J Med 317:537.

Iimura O, Kijima T, Kikuchi K, Miyama A, Ando T, Nakao T, Takigami Y (1981): Clin Sci 61(Suppl):77S.

Intersalt Cooperative Research Group (1988): Br Med J 297:319.

Jowsey J, Riggs BL, Kelly PJ, Hortenan DL (1972): Am J Med 53:43.

Kanwar KC, Dhar S (1989): Fluoride 22:128.

Key TJ, Pike MC (1988): Eur J Cancer Clin Oncol 24:29.

Khaw K-T, Barrett-Connor E (1988): Circulation 77:53.

Kiel DP, Felson DT, Anderson JJ, Wilson WF, Moskowitz MA (1987): N Engl J Med 317:1169.

Knowles JB, Wood RJ, Rosenberg IH (1988): Am J Clin Nutr 48:1471.

Komm BS, Terpening CM, Benz DJ, Graeme KA, Gallegos A, Korc M, Greene GL, O'Malley BW, Haussler MR (1988): Science 241:81.

Krause MV, Mahan LK (1979): Food, nutrition, and diet therapy (6th ed). Philadelphia: WB Saunders.

Krishna GG, Miller E, Kapoor S (1989): N Engl J Med 320:1177.

Krishnamachari KAVR (1990): 7th international symposium on trace element metabolism in man and animals (TEMA-7), Dubrovnik, May.

Krook L, Whalen JP, Lesser GV, Lutwak L (1972*a*): Cornell Vet 62:371.

Krook L, Lutwak L, Whalen JP, Hendrikson PA, Lesser GV, Uris R (1972*b*): Cornell Vet 62:32.

Kurtz TW, Al-Bander HA, Morris RC Jr (1987): N Engl J Med 317:1043.

Lane NE, Bloch DA, Jones HH, Marshall WH, Wood PD, Fries JF (1986): JAMA 255:1147.

Lau KHW, Farley JR, Freeman TK, Baylink DJ (1989): Metab Clin Exp 38:858.

Lehninger A (1981): Lecture at California State University, Fullerton.

Linsday R, Hart DM, Clark DM (1984): Obstet Gynecol 63:759.

Lust G, Faure G, Nettier P (1981): Science 214:809.

Lutwak L, Krook L, Hendrikson PA, Uris R, Whalen JP, Coulston A, Lesser G (1971): Isr J Med Sci 7:504.

Marcus R (1989): Arch Intern Med 149:2170.

Marston RM, Welsh C (1983): Nat Food Rev 21:17.

Marx JL (1981): Science 212:1255.

Massey LK, Wise KL (1984): Nutr Res 4:43.

McSheehy PMJ, Chambers TJ (1987): J Clin Invest 80:425.

Metzler DA (1977): Biochemistry. New York: Academic.

National Institute of Arthritis, Diabetes, Digestive and Kidney Diseases (1983): Osteoporosis: Cause, treatment, prevention (NIH publication no 83-2226). Bethesda, MD: US Department of Public Health and Human Services.

National Research Council (1989): Diet and health. Washington, DC.

Need AG, Horowitz M, Philcox JC, Nordin BEC (1985): Miner Electrolyte Metab 11:35.

Nordin BEC (1986): J Food Nutr 42:67.

Nordin BEC, Morris HA (1989): Nutr Rev 47:65.

Nordin BEC, Robertson A, Seamark RF, et al. (1985): J Clin Endocrinol Metab 60:651.

Nordin BEC, Need AG, Morris HA, Horowitz M (1988): Proceedings Workshop on Vitamin D, 7th (Vitamin D: Mol Cell Clin Endocrinol), p 826.

Nordin BEC, Need AG, Hartley TF, Philcox JC, Wilcox M, Thomas DW (1989): Clin Chem 35:14.

Nutr Rev (1988): 46:233.

Oke OL (1979): Amaranth Proc, vol 22.

Ott SM, Chestnut CH III (1989): Ann Intern Med 110:267.

Pacifici R, Rifas L, McCracken R, Vered I, McMurtry C, Avioli LV, Peck WA (1989): Proc Natl Acad Sci USA 86:2398.

Persson I, Adami H-O, Bergkvist L (1989): Br Med J 298:147.

Petkovich PM, Wrana JL, Grigoriadis AE, Heersche JNM, Sodek J (1987): J Biol Chem 262:13424.

Polley KJ, Nordin BEC, Baghurst PA, Walker CJ, Chatterton BE (1987): J Nutr 117:1929.

Ramazzotto LJ, Curro FA, Gates PE, Paterson JA (1986): Gerontology 5:159.

Rasmussen H (1989): Sci Am 262:62.

Riggs BL, Nelson KI (1985): J Clin Endocrinol Metab 61:457.

Riggs BL, Baylink DJ, Kleerkoper M, Lane JM, Melton LJ (1987): J Bone Min Res 2:123.

Riggs BL, Hodgson SF, O'Fallon WM, Chao EYS, Wahner HW, Muhs JM, Cedel SL, Melton LJ (1990): N Engl J Med 322:802.

Riggs BL, Seeman E, Hodgson SF, Tanes DR, O'Fallon WM (1983): N Engl J Med 306:446.

Rocchini AP, Katch V, Anderson J, et al. (1988): Pediatrics 82:16.

Rocchini AP, Key J, Bondie D, Chico R, Moorehead C, Katch V, Martin M (1989): N Engl J Med 321:580.

Rossier BC, Geering K, Kraehenbuhl JP (1987): TIBS 12:483.

Schwartz M, Anwah I, Levy R (1985): Clin Orthop 192:180.

Seelig MS, Haddy FJ (1980): *In* Cantin MR, Seelig MS, eds: Magnesium in health and disease. Lancaster, UK: MTP Press, p 605.

Shils ME (1980): *In* Goodhart RS, Shils ME, eds: Modern nutrition in health and disease (6th ed). Philadelphia: Lea & Febiger, p 310.

Shils ME (1988): *In* Shils ME, Young VR, eds: Modern nutrition in health and disease. Philadelphia: Lea & Febiger, p 159.

Silverberg SJ, Shane E, de la Cruz L, Segre GV, Clemens TL, Bilezikian JP (1989): N Engl J Med 320:277.

Souci SW, Fachmann W, Kraut H (1981): Food composition and nutrition tables 1981/82. Stuttgart: Wissenschaftliche Verlagsgesellschaft.

Spencer H, Kramer L, Osis D, Wiatrowski E (1985): J Environ Pathol Toxicol Oncol 6:33.

Strause LG, Saltman P (1987): *In* CAS Symposium Series 354. Washington, DC: American Chemical Society, p 46.

Thorneycroft IH (1989): Am J Obstet Gynecol 160:1306.

Tietz N (1976): Fundamentals of clinical chemistry (2nd ed). Philadelphia: WB Saunders.

Tobian L (1988): Nutr Rev 46:273.

Tuck ML, Sowers J, Dornfeld L, Kledzik G, Maxwell M (1981): New Engl J Med 304:9300.

Walser M (1967): Ergeb Physiol 59:185.

Watkin (1980): *In* Goodhart RS, Shils ME, eds: Modern nutrition in health and disease (6th ed). Philadelphia: Lea & Febiger, p 781.

Weaver CM, Martin BR, Ebner JS, Krueger CA (1987): J Nutr 117:1903.

Weaver K (1987): Trace Subst Environ Health 22:136.

Weinstein RS, Bell NH (1988): N Engl J Med 319:1698.

Wergedal JE, Lau KHW, Baylink DJ (1988): Clin Orthop 233:274.

Whiting SJ, Whitney HL (1987): J Nutr 117:1224.

Maria C. Linder, Ph.D.*

7

Nutrition and Metabolism of the Trace Elements

Overview of Trace Element Nutrition and Function

Apart from the chemical elements already covered in previous chapters (from C, H, O, and N to Ca, P, and Na, down to Mg), the human body contains and incorporates trace quantities of most (or all) of the other elements in the periodic table. Iron is normally the most abundant of these remaining elements (Table 7.1), and at the other end of the spectrum are the almost undetectable amounts of chromium, cobalt, and even the precious metals silver and gold. Estimates of amounts present in the average 70-kg North American are available for many of these elements, based on analyses of organs, tissues, and body fluids (Table 7.1).

Many trace elements are known to be essential for life, health, and reproduction and have well-established functions, serving as cofactors in enzyme reactions, components of body fluids (electrolytes), sites for binding of oxygen (in transport), and structural components of nonenzymatic macromolecules. The importance of iron was established in the 17th century and that of iodine in the late 19th century. Many more discoveries were made in the 1920s, 1930s, and 1950s (Table 7.1) and further substantial additions to the list of essential elements have occurred in the 1970s and early 1980s by techniques which permit a sufficient purification of foodstuffs and the prevention of environmental contamination, to allow the effects of specific deficiencies to be examined in animal systems. As a result, elements that were originally noted only for their toxicity (such as Pb, As, and Se) have now been relegated to the "essential" category, at least for animals. (Obviously, the quantity required for life and health is less than the quantity required for toxic effects.)

Some trace element researchers, notably the late Klaus Schwarz, have speculated that probably all the chemical elements will eventually be shown to have a biologic role. Nevertheless, some of these (notably Cd, Pb, and As) will continue to be noted mainly for their nonessential detrimental influences on human metabolism.

With the exception of iron and iodine, the importance of trace elements to our diet is only just beginning to be acknowledged. Deficiencies of specific trace elements are beginning to be associated with the development of chronic health problems (e.g., fluorine and dental caries; chromium and glucose tolerance; copper and hypercholesterolemia). Consequently, the effects of food refining should be reassessed. As already indicated for the vitamins (see Chapter 5, Table 5.2), the preparation of patent flour from whole wheat (and perhaps other aspects of food processing) removes a large portion of the majority of the beneficial trace elements from the food (Table

* California State University, Fullerton, CA.

Table 7.1. Trace Elements in Humans: Their Absorption, Distribution, and Excretion

Element (in order abundance)	Average content in the 70-kg body (mg)	Ease of absorption from diet (%)	Approximate normal plasma concentration (ng/ml)	Binding to plasma components	Main organs of accumulation	Main route of excretion	Determination essential for man or animal (year)
Iron (Fe)[a]	3500–4500	5–15	1000 (500,000)[b]	Transferrin	Liver, spleen	Bile	17th century
Fluorine (F)[a]	2600–4000	40–100	200–1000	Albumin	Bone, teeth	Urine	1972
Zinc (Zn)[a]	1600–2300	31–51	1000	Albumin, α_1,α_2-globulins	Skin, bone	Pancreas, bile	1934
Silicon (Si)[a]	(1100)	30–50?	500[c]	Monosilicic acid	Skin, lymph node, bone epiphyses, tendons	Urine	1972
Zirconium (Zr)	250–420	0.01		(Like V?)	Fat?	Bile	
Strontium (Sr)	340	<20	13	Half bound; half chelated	Bone		
Rubidium (Rb)	320	90	930	Free ion (like K^+)	None		
Bromine (Br)	200	99	3500	Free ion (like Cl^-)	None		
Lead (Pb)[a]	122	5	1–8	Transferrin?	Bone	Bile	1979
Copper (Cu)[a]	110	30–60	1000	Ceruloplasmin, transcuprein alb, AAs	Liver	Bile	1928
Boron (B)	48	99	200	?	Bone	Urine	
Aluminum (Al)	45	1	5?	Transferrin	(Lung)[d]	Urine	
Cadmium (Cd)	30–38	6	1–2	Protein bound	Kidney, liver	Urine	(1976)
Barium (Ba)	22	1–15	10–100		Skin?	Urine	
Selenium (Se)[a]	21	35–85	100–130	Protein bound	Kidney?	Urine (bile, exhalation)	1957
Germanium (Ge)	(20)	Easy			Spleen	Urine	
Iodine (I)[a]	10–20	100	60	Mainly as T_3, T_4	Thyroid	Urine	
Tin (Sn)[a]	14	2	23		Liver, spleen, lung	Bile?	1970
Arsenic (As)[a]	8–20	(5)	4–6		Skin? hair?	Urine, bile	1975
Manganese (Mn)[a]	12–16	3–4	0.6–2	Transferrin, α_2M?	Liver, bone	Bile	1931
Molybdenum (Mo)[a]	9–16	40–100	2–6[c]	Protein bound	Liver? bone?	Urine (bile?)	1953
Mercury (Hg)	13	5–10	2–6	Complex?	Kidney		
Vanadium (V)[a]	10	0.1–1.5	5	Transferrin	Fat?	Urine	1971
Titanium (Ti)	9	1–2	21		(Lung)	Urine	
Nickel (Ni)[a]	5–10	3–6	0.2–2	Albumin, some free	Skin, liver (muscle)	Urine	1973
Tellurium (Te)	7	20–50			Bone		
Antimony	6	Poor	2		Spleen, liver, kidney		
Cobalt (Co)[a]	1.1–1.5	63–97	0.1–0.4	Albumin	Liver, fat	Urine	1935
Chromium (Cr)[a]	(?)	0.5–2	0.19	Transferrin	Spleen, heart	Urine	1959
Lithium (Li)	0.9?	High	11	Free ion?	Lymph nodes?	Urine	1978

Source: Modified from Linder (1978), with information from Iyengar and Woittiez (1988) and Davidson and Ward (1988), among others.

[a] Determined to be essential (at least in animals) (underlined).
[b] Value for whole blood.
[c] Mainly within red cells (in blood).
[d] Accumulation from airborne sources.

7.2). Although there are exceptions (Se, for instance), the trace elements tend to concentrate in the germ of seeds and grains, where the highest concentrations of B vitamins are also found. Typically, when processed foodstuffs, such as flour, are enriched, iron may be replaced, but other trace elements are not. As a consequence, the prominence of refined processed foods in our diet may be responsible for some of the trace element deficiencies in our society. Indeed, it has been repeatedly shown that actual intakes of many trace elements, such as zinc, copper, and chromium, fall below the RDA or what experimental work suggests would be optimal (see below). A summary of the nutrition and metabolism of individual trace elements, some of their interactions and relations to disease, follows.

Iron

Content in the Body and Functions

Iron (Fe) is the most abundant trace element in the human and animal body and one of the two most abundant in nature. The adult human body contains somewhere between 2.5 and 4 g of this element, with about 2.0–2.5 g circulating in red cells as a component of hemoglobin (Figure 7.1). Trace amounts (perhaps 300 mg in all) are associated with electron transport and with several enzymes—notably: the heme-containing cytochromes and iron-sulfur proteins of electron transport and oxidative phosphorylation in all cells, and the enzymes of "drug metabolism" (involving cytochromes P450 and b_5), principally in liver; also the widely distributed enzyme, ribonucleotide reductase (involved in the synthesis of deoxyribonucleotides for DNA); several enzymes involved in synthesis and degradation of biogenic amines (including tyrosine and tryptophan hydroxylases that initiate formation of dopa and serotonin); the myeloperoxidase of leukocytes involved in bacterial killing; and the liver heme enzymes, catalase and tryptophan oxygenase. Larger amounts of iron are found in the form of myoglobin in muscle cells, and highly variable amounts are stored in ferritin, a multisubunit protein present in all cells, but especially in the liver, spleen, and bone marrow. Iron is also stored in hemosiderin, thought to be a breakdown product of ferritin. From its association with these specific proteins, it is clear that the principal functions of iron in the body involve oxygen transport within

Table 7.2. Effects of Food Processing and Refining on Trace Element Content[a]

Food	Zinc	Copper	Manganese	Cobalt	Chromium[b]	Molybdenum	Selenium
Wheat							
Whole	32	4.1	49.0	0.75	1.75	0.79	0.31
Flour	8.9	1.5	6.0	0.36	0.23	0.32	
Germ	134	7.4	137	0.50	1.27	0.67	
Rice							
Whole (brown)	6.5	4.1	2.8	0.16	0.16		
Polished	1.6	3.0	1.5	0.10	0.04		
Sugar							
Cane	0.5	1.0	1.8	0.03	0.10	0.13	
Molasses	8.3	6.8	4.2	0.25	1.21	0.19	
White sugar	0.2	0.6	0.1	<0.05	0.02	0.0	
Vegetables							
Legumes	10.7	1.3	0.4	0.15	0.05	1.73	0.02
Roots	3.4	0.7	0.8	0.13	0.08	0.23	<0.02
Leaves and fruit	1.7	0.4	3.5	0.14	0.03	0.06	<0.02
Fruits	0.5	0.8	1.0	0.14	0.02	0.06	<0.02
Nuts	34	14.8	17.7	0.26	0.35		0.72
Condiments/spices	23	6.8	92	0.52	3.3	0.45	0.24
Meats	31	3.9	0.2	0.22	0.13	2.06	2.06
Seafoods	18	1.5	<0.1	1.56	0.17	0.10	0.57
Eggs	21	4.1	0.5	0.10	0.16	0.49	
Milk	3.5	0.2	0.2	0.06	0.01	0.20	0.02

Source: Data from Schroeder (1973).

[a] $\mu g/g$.

[b] Must now be considered approximate (see section on Chromium).

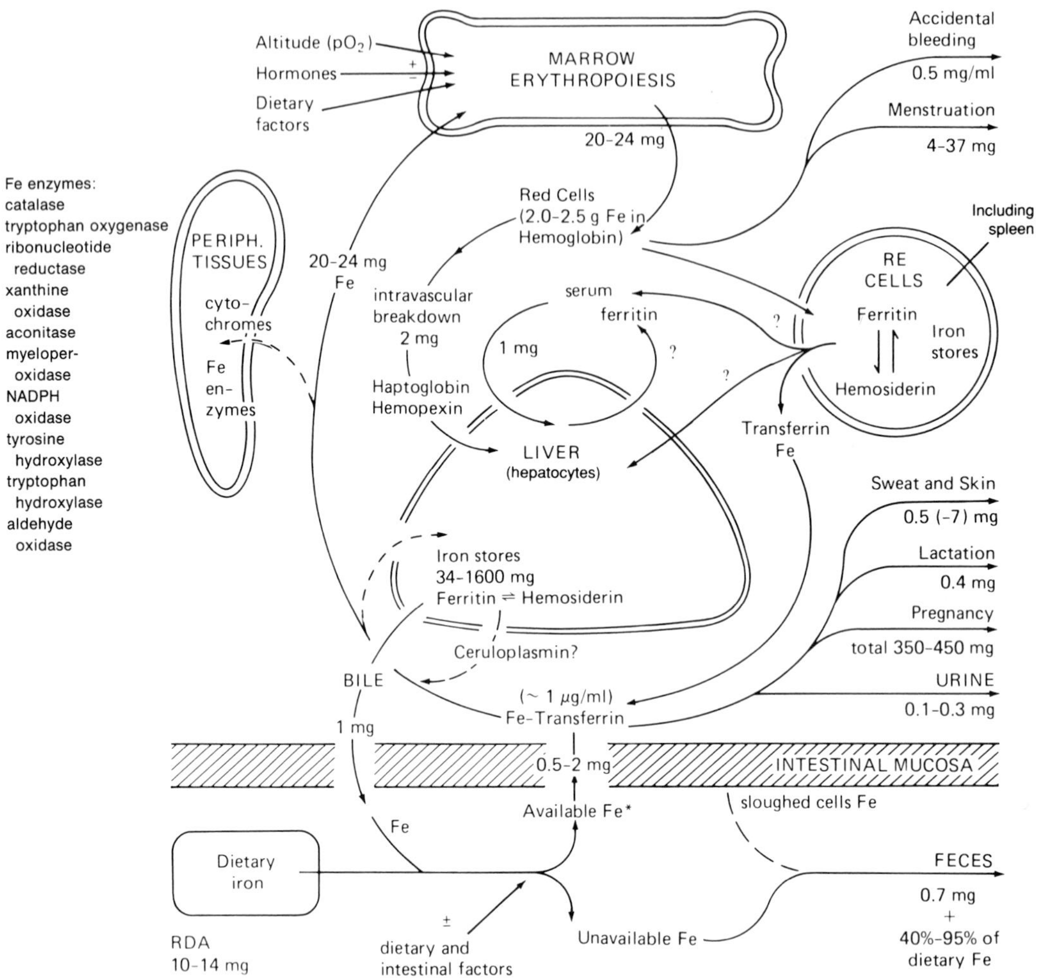

Figure 7.1. Nutrition and metabolism of iron. Quantities are average values per day. Total body iron 2.5–3.5 g. Dietary iron is made more or less available by various dietary factors, see text). About 1 mg is absorbed into the blood and carried on transferrin to liver and other tissues, including the bone marrow. Most iron is involved in red cell production and function (as hemoglobin), some 20–24 mg of iron turning over through red cell destruction and replacement daily, mainly via reticuloendothelial (RE) cells. Erythropoiesis is influenced by oxygen tension, altitude, and other factors. Excess iron is stored as ferritin and hemosiderin, especially in liver, spleen, and bone marrow. Tissues contain many iron enzymes, including the cytochromes. Iron is lost through the bile and in variable amounts through other routes shown by the arrows on the right. Asterisk (*) means: heme Fe is probably absorbed by a mechanism different from that for Fe^{2+}/Fe^{3+}; Fe^{2+} may be absorbed better than Fe^{3+}. Dagger (†) means: Fe is not readily lost from the body except by bleeding.

blood and muscle and electron transfer in relation to energy metabolism. It is also intimately involved in cell proliferation, the production and disposal of oxygen radicals (and peroxide), systemic hormone action, and in some aspects of immune defense.

Overview of Absorption, Metabolism, and Excretion

The average daily American diet contains 10–50 mg of iron. A substantial percentage of U.S. women probably do not receive the RDA (of 15 mg) in their diets, and only about 10%–15% of the iron is absorbed. The reason for the low absorption may be ascribed to the relative unavailability of the element in the diet and to endogenous control of the rate of uptake. The absorptive capacity of the intestinal mucosa is regulated according to the body's needs by mechanisms that have so far eluded investigators (see below). A larger proportion of dietary iron is absorbed in deficiency, and absorption into the body per se is greatly reduced when the body has large iron stores. Oxalates, phytates, tannins, and other phenolic compounds in the diet, all of which are present in various plant foods, tend to form insoluble iron precipitates that render the iron unavailable for absorption. A neutral or alkaline aqueous environment (high OH^- concentration), such as occurs in the upper small intestine and is accentuated in achlorohydria (a relative lack of HCl production in the stomach), promotes formation of insoluble hydroxides. Counteracting these effects are dietary iron-chelating and reducing agents, such as ascorbic acid, fructose, fumarate, citrate, and certain amino acids, which help retain the iron in solution and make it available for absorption. "Naturally" chelated iron in the form of heme groups, present in meats (and blood-containing tissues), is absorbed more readily (and by an independent mechanism) than iron found in plants. Consequently, iron is less available from plant foods, and vegetarians are more apt to develop iron deficiency (see below).

Food Sources

As already described, meats with residual blood or muscle cells are generally rich in iron and contain a form of iron chelate more available for absorption than nonheme iron or iron in plant- and animal-derived foods. The old adage that spinach is good for you because it is high in iron is only partly true: spinach does indeed contain a substantial amount (Figure 7.2), but this iron has a low availability due to the high oxalate content (see Chapter 6, Table 6.2). The same may be said for some other plant foods. Other factors (Table 7.3) that may reduce iron absorption include phytic acid (Figure 7.3) prevalent in grains, tannins present in tea and certain leafy vegetables (Disler et al., 1975; Torrance et al., 1982), bioflavonoids present in fruits, and possibly some forms of fiber. Although early data suggested legumes (and soybeans) might be a useful vegetarian source, more recent data indicate that this iron also has a low availability, although the reason is unclear (see Thompson, 1988). As in the case of calcium (see Chapter 6), broccoli may be an exception to the low content and availability of plant food iron, although this has not been tested. (It has a fairly good iron content and probably little oxalate or phytate.) Eggs are low in available iron because of

Figure 7.2. Bioavailability of iron in various foods. Iron absorption by adults from a range of foods. Absorption is given as percent of dose (mean ± SE) for the number of cases indicated. Note log scale. [*Source:* Reprinted from Layrisse and Martinez-Torres (1971).] (*) means that the seeming high availability of soy iron now appears to be incorrect (Lynch et al., 1984; Thompson, 1988).

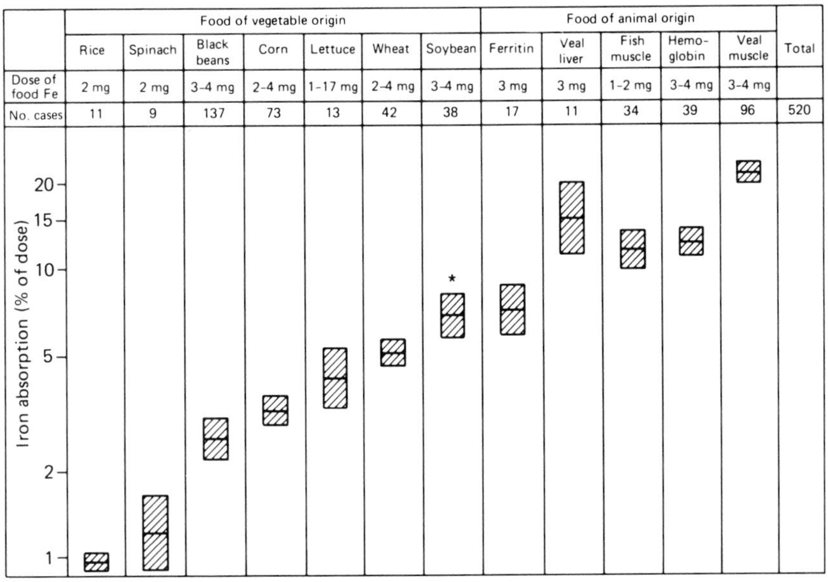

	Food of vegetable origin							Food of animal origin					
	Rice	Spinach	Black beans	Corn	Lettuce	Wheat	Soybean	Ferritin	Veal liver	Fish muscle	Hemo-globin	Veal muscle	Total
Dose of food Fe	2 mg	2 mg	3-4 mg	2-4 mg	1-17 mg	2-4 mg	3-4 mg	3 mg	3 mg	1-2 mg	3-4 mg	3-4 mg	
No. cases	11	9	137	73	13	42	38	17	11	34	39	96	520

Iron absorption (% of dose)

20
15
10
5
2
1
*

Table 7.3. Factors that Enhance and Hinder Intestinal Iron Uptake

Enhance iron uptake	
Nutrients (act directly)	Endogenous factors (probably act indirectly)
Ascorbic acid (vitamin C) Fructose Citric acid Dietary protein Lysine Histidine Cysteine Methionine (EDTA, NTA) (natural chelation, as in heme groups)	Enhanced erythropoiesis as with hypoxia (altitude), hemolysis, hemorrhage, androgens, cobalt salts (release of erythropoietin is usually involved) Low iron stores Idiopathic hemochromatosis (genetic defect)
Inhibit iron uptake	
Nutrients	Endogenous factors
Oxalic acid Tannins Phytate[a] Carbonate Phosphate Fiber[a] (not cellulose) Excess of other metal ions Co^{2+}, Cu^{2+}, Zn^{2+}, Cd^{2+}, Mn^{2+}, Pb^{2+} Lack of dietary protein	High iron stores (if also in marrow) Infection/inflammation Lack of stomach acid (achylia, achlorohydria)

Source: Based on Linder (1973, 1977).

[a] Effect is not always found.

the presence of phosvitin (Figure 7.2). [In general, factors that inhibit Ca^{2+} and Mg^{2+} absorption (Chapter 6) also inhibit iron absorption.] Milk and dairy products are low in iron, which makes them poor sources. [This has implications for pregnancy and the infant (see below).] Conversely, a variety of chelating agents in the diet enhance iron availability and absorption (Table 7.3), especially (plant-derived) ascorbic acid, some amino acids, and dietary protein (especially animal protein) in general. The presence of precipitating or chelating agents within a given food influences not only the availability of nonheme iron in that food, but also the availability of nonheme iron in other foods in the same meal. The ultimate availability of the iron in a given meal is thus determined by the mix of factors competing for iron binding.

Regulation of Iron Absorption

The degree to which available dietary iron is actually absorbed, first by entering the cells of the intestinal mucosa, then by being transferred to the blood (Figure 7.4), is largely regulated by the body's needs, with more entering the blood when stores are low, and vice versa. This means that iron homeostasis is largely controlled by regulation of absorption rather than excretion. The capacity of mucosal cells to take up iron appears to be determined by the number of iron receptors on the mucosal surface. Further transfer (across the serosal surface into the blood) is more stringently controlled and involves mechanisms as yet undetermined. The signal (or signals) that influences absorptive capacity is still unclear and all the obvious possibilities have been eliminated (Linder, 1978): mucosal cell ferritin, erythropoietin, transferrin, transferrin saturation, etc. Some recent evidence suggests that a humoral factor produced by reticulocytes may be involved (Finch, 1986; Raja et al., 1990). Almost without exception, processes that stimulate erythropoiesis (anoxia, loss of blood, etc.) and/or lower the iron content of the body (blood loss, iron deficiency) are associated with an enhanced capacity for intestinal iron absorption. The normal regulatory mechanisms present, together with the amounts of available dietary iron, determine just how much iron enters mucosal cells and is transferred further into the body. In this regard, it should be noted that, despite endogenous controls to the contrary, higher concentrations of available iron in the diet will result in greater absorption, even when the body's iron stores are high [e.g., endogenous controls can be overridden and continuous overconsumption of iron can result in iron overload (see below)]. Furthermore, a genetic defect in the "down-control" of iron absorption (idiopathic or familial hemochromatosis) will result in long-term overabsorption of dietary iron and parenchymal cell iron overload.

Iron Metabolism and Turnover

Roughly 1% of red blood cells (lifespan 120 days) are degraded and reformed daily, amounting to a turnover of 19–24 mg of hemoglobin iron per day in the adult (Figure 7.1). Aged red cells are phagocytosed by reticuloendothelial cells (RE), principally in the spleen and liver. Iron released from degraded hemoglobin and porphyrin rapidly appears on transferrin and in some ferritin in the plasma, probably within minutes of damaged red

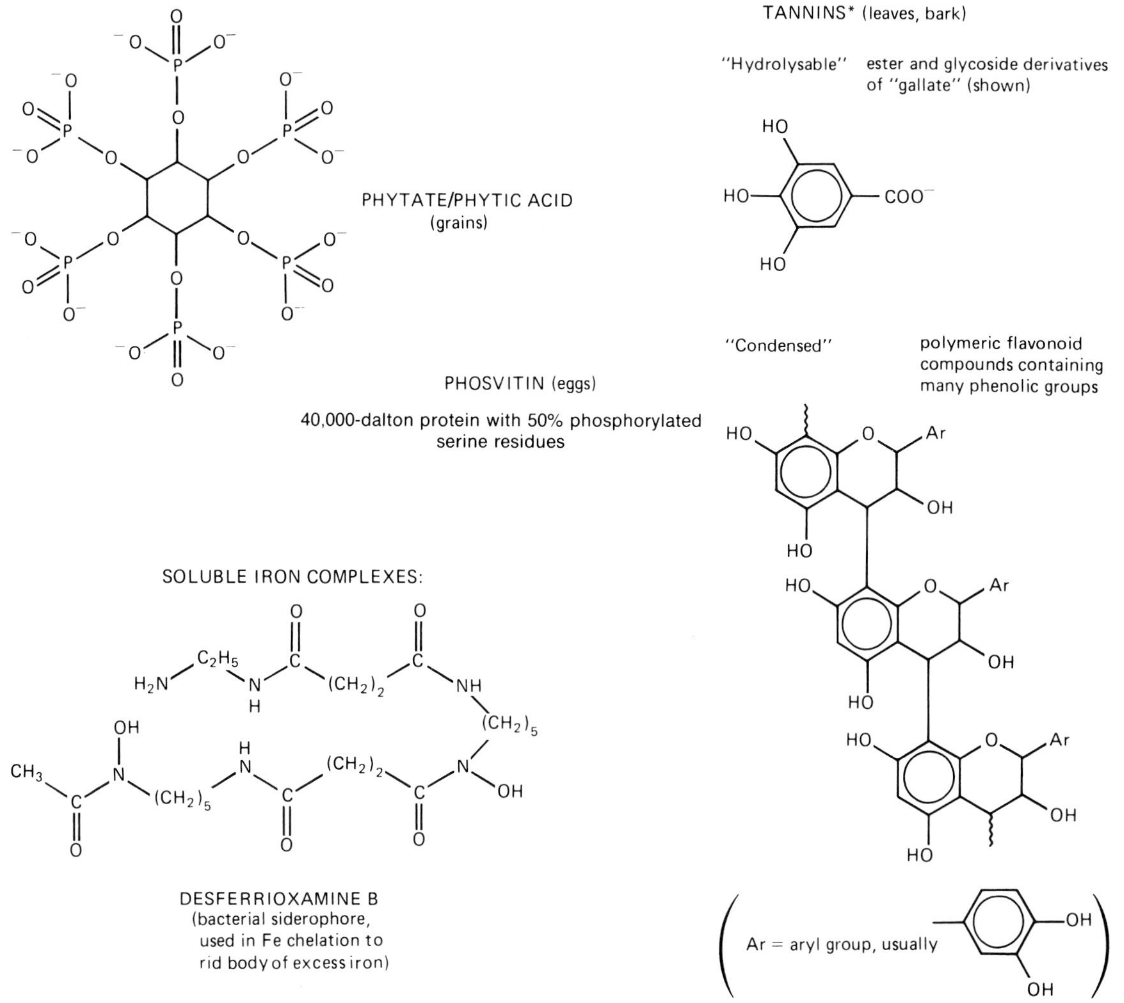

PHYTATE/PHYTIC ACID
(grains)

PHOSVITIN (eggs)
40,000-dalton protein with 50% phosphorylated serine residues

SOLUBLE IRON COMPLEXES:

DESFERRIOXAMINE B
(bacterial siderophore, used in Fe chelation to rid body of excess iron)

TANNINS* (leaves, bark)

"Hydrolysable" ester and glycoside derivatives of "gallate" (shown)

"Condensed" polymeric flavonoid compounds containing many phenolic groups

(Ar = aryl group, usually)

Figure 7.3. Substances that can form biounavailable (often insoluble) iron complexes. Asterisk (*) means darken when Fe^{3+} is added. [*Source:* Information partly from Mann (1978).]

cell uptake (Siimes and Dallman, 1974). Transferrin transports the iron back to the bone marrow for resynthesis of hemoglobin, or to wherever it is needed. Any high-iron ferritin in the serum is rapidly taken up by the liver hepatocytes (Mack et al., 1981; Sibille et al., 1989*a*, *b;* Siimes and Dallman, 1974) and perhaps also by some other cells. Some of the iron may be transferred locally as (high-iron) ferritin between Kupffer cells and hepatocytes (Sibille et al., 1988). If necessary, intracellular ferritin iron may also be mobilized (from these cells) for transport to the bone marrow. For mobilization, iron within the central $(FeOOH)_n$ core of ferritin must be reduced, chelated, and transferred to the plasma, where it must be reoxidized to Fe^{3+} for transport on transferrin. [It is still not clear whether or not this requires predigestion (degradation) of ferritin protein, or whether iron is mobilized from inside the intact ferritin molecule.] Studies from two laboratories indicate that the copper-containing plasma protein, ceruloplasmin, plays a role in iron mobilization (see Copper, below), although in free energy terms, it has been calculated that the "pull" of erythropoiesis (in the bone marrow) should be sufficient to cause the flow of iron out of storage into the bone marrow (May and Williams, 1977). Iron lost from red cells before their uptake by RE cells is transported as hemoglobin or porphyrin iron, on haptoglobin and hemopexin, respectively, and enters liver parenchymal cells for in-

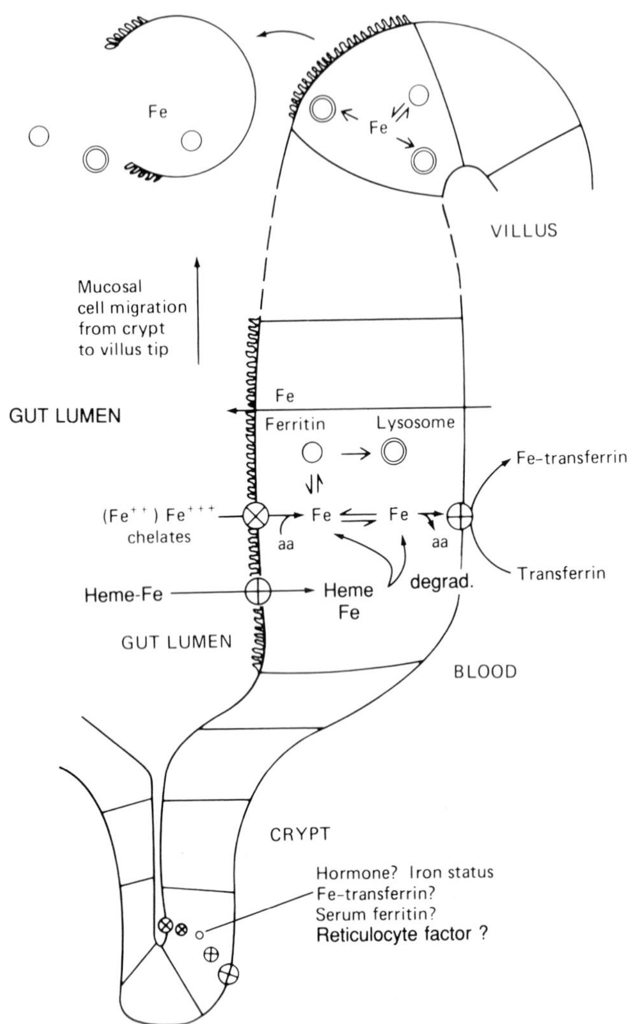

Figure 7.4. Composite picture of the mechanism of iron absorption. The picture shown is an attempt to assemble available evidence into a model. Ionic iron in the intestinal lumen adsorbs to specific receptors in the brush border of the cells lining the intestine. (Iron may be delivered to these receptors in chelated form.) From the receptors, the iron is transferred to the cytoplasm of the epithelial cells by an energy-dependent process. The newly absorbed iron appears to be present in the cytosol in low molecular weight form, possibly chelated with citrate, fructose, and amino acids, and in equilibrium with relatively unsaturated ferritin molecules. Upon reaching the serosal surface of the cell, the iron becomes attached to transferrin for transport in the plasma. The serosal transfer mechanism probably also involves receptors in the cell membrane and may be independent of cell energy. Iron in the mucosal cell that is not transferred to the plasma is retained in the cell, probably mostly as ferritin, until it is sloughed off at the tip of the villus and thus returns to the lumen of the gut. (In iron deficiency, especially, some iron may also migrate across the cytosol of the epithelial cell attached to a protein of similar size and structure to transferrin.) The iron status and erythropoietic needs of the individual, as well as some other factors, regulate iron absorption, particularly at the level of serosal transfer. It appears likely that homeostatic mechanisms within the body affect the populations of receptors at the time of mucosal cell formation in the crypts. This is an acceptable explanation in the case of the receptors on the brush border, which change slowly over several days in response to iron status. The intermediaries (humoral factors?) in these regulatory processes have not been identified, but a reticulocyte factor may be involved. Finally, iron can enter the mucosal cells from the plasma, especially their mitochondria, and can pass into the lumen by active extrusion, notably in the lower part of the small intestine. [*Source:* Modified from Linder and Munro (1977).]

corporation into hepatocyte ferritin. The release of hemoglobin iron, incorporated into ferritin and hemosiderin in the spleen, would also appear to depend on the availability of ascorbic acid, as, at least in the guinea pig, ascorbate deficiency reduces recycling of red cell iron, and this is associated with an enhanced proportion of iron in spleen hemosiderin (Lipschitz et al., 1971; H.P. Roeser, unpublished observations). In this regard, the fraction of stored liver iron in hemosiderin varies inversely with ascorbate (Lipschitz et al., 1971) and probably also with vitamin E (Golberg and Smith, 1958) status. Moreover, intake of large doses of ascorbate by iron-loaded individuals can result in severe toxicity due to iron release into the blood (Lipschitz et al., 1971; Nienhuis, 1978; Wapnick et al., 1968).

The contribution of ferritin to serum transport of iron is probably low (Munro and Linder, 1978), although it cannot be excluded that this kind of transfer may be significant at the local level in the liver (via interstitial fluid) and even between spleen and liver (via the blood), a transfer which is never "seen" by the peripheral circulation. High-iron (tissue) ferritins are very rapidly absorbed by hepatocytes (Mack et al., 1981; Simon et al., 1987), whereas the most common (normal) form of ferritin in serum has a much longer half-life (Worwood et al., 1983). The latter is also low in iron; it is at least partially glycosylated and may be a smaller molecule overall (Goode et al., 1991). The low-iron form of serum ferritin may also be deliberately secreted as an acute phase reactant (Campbell et al., 1989; Konijn et al., 1981; Linder et al., 1990; Schiaffonati et al., 1988). Thus, there may be two classes of "serum ferritin." At least in the absence of inflammation, cancer, and some other states (see below) the level of (one or both of) these "serum ferritins" is related to tissue iron stores and can be used to assess their size.

Iron Deficiency: Causes and Treatment

From the previous discussion it is clear that iron deficiency results from a relative lack of iron (or available iron) in the diet and/or substantial losses of iron from the body through bleeding, pregnancies, and other routes. The most overt symptom of iron deficiency is a hypochromic, microcytic anemia. This is associated with an increased concentration of circulating transferrin (and thus an increased total iron-binding capacity of serum), decreased transferrin saturation, and (unless masked) a decreased concentration of serum ferritin (to 12 ng/ml or less). Little or no stainable iron in bone marrow smears is the most unequivocal indicator of deficiency.

The relative lack of red cells associated with iron deficiency results in a decreased capacity for oxygen transport and thus puts a limit on oxygen-dependent energy metabolism. In skeletal muscle, this is exacerbated by reductions in myoglobin and cytochrome content, which lead to a greater reliance on glycolysis (and glucose) for energy (Brooks et al., 1987; Henderson et al., 1986). In deficiency, skeletal muscle, intestinal mucosa, and leukocytes are preferentially bereft of iron, whereas heart and brain are hardly affected (Dallman, 1986). (Liver and kidney lie in between.) The liver appears to adapt by increasing gluconeogenesis from lactate to supply more glucose.

The resulting reduction in the capacity of the intestinal mucosa for energy production and proliferation can have profound effects on nutrient absorption and on the integrity of the gastrointestinal tract. The capacities of leukocytes to kill bacteria can also be compromised. Here, killing occurs via the iron-dependent "respiratory burst" and myeloperoxidase, producing toxic, oxidized halogen compounds from peroxide and OH·. This capacity is reduced even in mild iron deficiency, as is the capacity of T cells to proliferate (Kuvibidila et al., 1983, 1990). Thus, two aspects of immune function are impaired by iron deficiency. Most of the effects on intestine and immune cells are probably caused both by a lack of energy and by a lack of active ribonucleotide reductase necessary for new cell formation (DNA synthesis).

During early infancy (or gestation), the development of brain function may also be particularly vulnerable, and, in children, deficiency will reduce binding of serotonin and dopamine to their ("D_2") receptors (Dallman, 1986). (It appears this may impair certain aspects of cognitive function.) Another potentially related syndrome of deficiency is an increase in the urinary excretion of norepinephrine. The reason for this is still unclear.

Most of the symptoms of iron deficiency are repaired quite rapidly, many even by simple restoration of a normal hematocrit (as by transfusion), although certain functional defects (e.g., in the brain) will take much longer and may even sometimes be irreversible.

Iron deficiency is the most common cause of anemia and a common problem in North America as well as in other parts of the world. Due to its multiple potential origins, it is difficult to say to what extent iron deficiency is due to dietary lack or excessive need on the part of individuals or the general population. Certainly, both play a role, as in the case of vegetarian women (more likely to be deficient because of their diets) and multiparous women (who needed to transfer extra iron to their offspring). Despite an enormous variability in iron status, iron deficiency appears to be more common in premenopausal women (who are subject to menstrual bleeding and pregnancies) than in men. Also, although pregnant women might not always require them, a lack of iron supplements can result in a dangerous depletion of iron stores (Taft et al., 1978). Consequently, it is recommended that all pregnant women partake of extra iron. (The RDA for pregnant women is 30 mg.) Although vegetarians are more likely to develop a deficiency, this is not commonly the case.

Deficiency is common in infancy, especially if the mother was deficient and/or the infant was born prematurely. Prematurity is a factor because the rate at which iron is assimilated and stored by the fetus is most rapid in the last weeks of pregnancy (Figure 7.5). It has been estimated that 20% of the iron store is accumulated in the last 2 weeks of gestation (Widdowson et al., 1974), and as milk is a poor source of iron this store is of great importance in the first 6 months of life when milk is the primary food. The early "anemia of infancy" reflects a change from production of fetal to adult hemoglobin. Only after 3–6 months of life does an anemia become apparent in infants with deficient iron stores.

Iron deficiency is commonly treated by giving oral iron supplements, for example, 250 mg iron as $FeSO_4$ to adults. For infants, formulas supplemented with ferric lactobionate and other chelates are also available, but should not be given indiscriminately, as iron supplementation can exacerbate infectious processes (see below). Daily iron absorption can be doubled or tripled by taking supplemental iron with orange juice or other ascorbate-containing foods (Cook, 1977).

Figure 7.5. Age changes in human liver iron, zinc, and copper concentrations. B = birth. [*Source:* Modified from Linder (1978).]

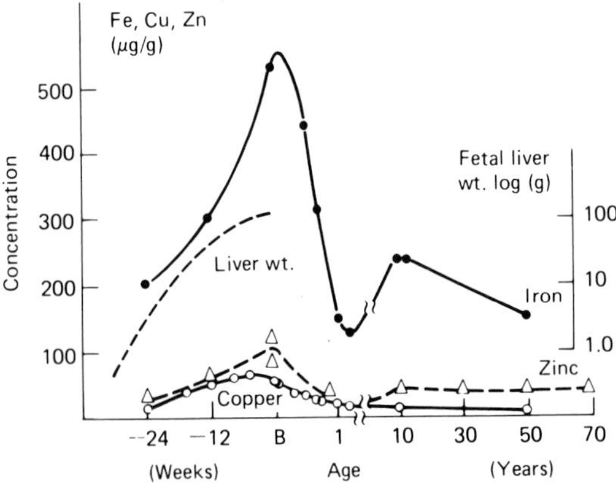

Iron Toxicity and Overload: Causes and Treatment

Although not as common as deficiency, iron overload is a dangerous debilitating condition that results in damage to the liver, heart, pancreas, and possibly other organs. Two forms are known: *genetic hemochromatosis,* resulting from inappropriately high absorption of dietary iron, and *acquired hemochromatosis,* a phenomenon secondary to (a) hypoplastic anemia (where blood transfusions introduce large amounts of iron); (b) conditions where erythropoiesis proceeds but is ineffective (causing excessive iron accumulation not just from transfusion, but from stimulation of intestinal absorption by the anemic state); (c) excessive long-term intake of iron, especially in connection with alcohol (as in the case of African Bantu tribesmen who brewed their beer in cast iron vessels); and (d) iron overload secondary to some forms of liver disease (porphyria cutanea tarda, alcoholic cirrhosis, following portocaval anastomosis) (Halliday and Powell, 1982; Powell and Halliday, 1982). In the genetic disorder, and ultimately also in the others, there is an accumulation of iron in the parenchymal (typical functional) cells of the various organs, leading to physical damage and functional impairment, including liver cirrhosis, heart failure, and diabetes (damage to the pancreas). Accumulation of excess iron in parenchymal cells occurs especially when iron enters by the dietary route [as in genetic (idiopathic) hemochromatosis and situations a, b, and c, above). Accumulation in RE cells (as is more likely to occur from blood transfusions) appears to be less damaging. Usually, both forms of accumulation occur in the acquired forms of hemochromatosis.

[Although vitamin C (ascorbate) enhances iron absorption, it does not appear that the consumption of megadoses significantly increases iron stores (assessed by serum ferritin) in normal individuals over a period of several years (see Chapter 5, Vitamin C), but individuals at risk for iron overload should probably be proscribed from taking large doses of the vitamin.]

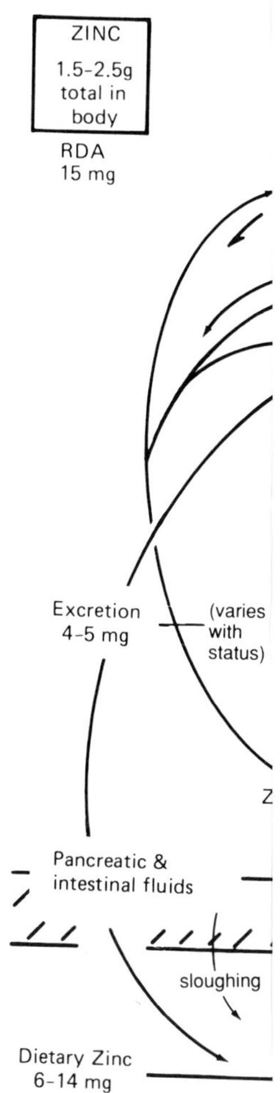

metabolism. As indicated in
necessary for the activity of
zymes associated with carbo
metabolism, protein degrada
nucleic acid synthesis, heme l
dioxide transport (carboni
many other reactions. Its mos
on the metabolism, function,
skin, pancreas, and male repr
though it plays essential role
deficiency will result in broad
diminished growth. In the pa
ciated with the abundantly
necessary for digestion. It is a
stored insulin, although it doe
a direct role in insulin action
for the development of male

Iron overload in early or later forms is mainly detected by measuring serum ferritin and finding consistent elevations (above 1000 ng/ml) (Powell and Halliday, 1978). In severe disease, levels of 4000–10,000 ng/ml are common. Iron overload is generally treated by phlebotomy, except when this is impossible (as in thalassemias, which require transfusions). Alternatively, desferrioxamine-B (Figure 7.3), a bacterial, high-affinity, iron-chelating agent from *S. pilosus*, can provide some relief by enhancing urinary iron losses (Bassett et al., 1980). Even with chelating agents, some of the injurious effects of excess iron at an advanced stage will not be reversed and may lead to early death (Bassett et al., 1980; Powell and Halliday, 1978).

Acute iron intoxication does occur in the United States, usually in children that get hold of adult iron supplements. This can result in severe necrotizing gastroenteritis, in which there is damage to the gastrointestinal tract (Thompson, 1988), presumably through the direct interference of iron with normal cell function, perhaps through enhancement of oxygen radical formation. Normally, such destructive effects are prevented by specific proteins that bind and sequester the iron inside and outside cells. When these are overwhelmed, membrane lysis and other destructive events occur. Sometimes death will result.

Iron and Disease

In infectious disease, serum iron concentrations (and transferrin iron binding) decrease (Figure 7.6) and intestinal iron absorption is reduced. [Most serum iron enters liver and spleen, and (low iron) serum ferritin is released.] It is thought that, at least in bacterial infections, these phenomena reflect an effort on the part of the body to reduce the availability of iron to bacteria, which require it for their own growth and proliferation. In support of this, it has been demonstrated that apotransferrin can inhibit bacterial cell proliferation (Weinberg, 1974) and the same is true for lactoferrin, an analogous protein found in milk (Bullen et al., 1972) (which may explain the anti-"cholic" effects of human breast milk compared to formula). [Along similar lines, apotransferrin (which binds serum iron) and haptoglobin (which binds hemoglobin) are bacteriostatic; the latter may be a factor in wound healing (Eaton et al., 1982).] Conversely, the administration of iron enhances the virulence of, or decreases bacteriostatic responses in, bacterial and other infections,

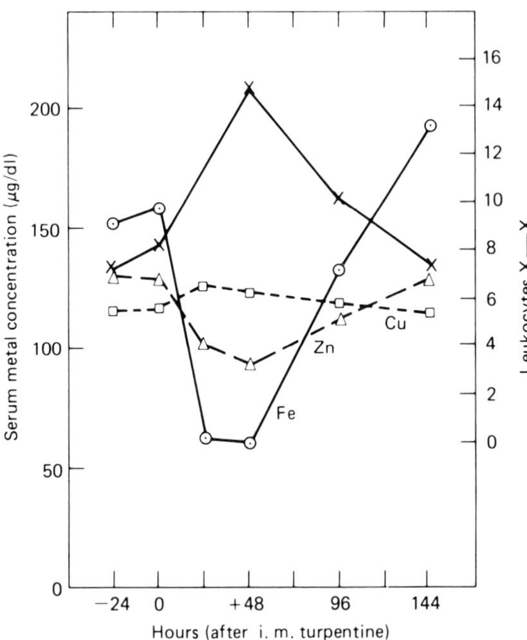

Figure 7.6. Reaction of serum trace elements to systemic inflammation. Plasma selenium may also be a negative acute phase reactant. [*Source:* Redrawn from Wolff (1956).]

as shown in animal studies (Holbein et al., 1979; Weinberg, 1974) and more recently in babies (Becroft et al., 1977; Webster et al., 1981) and adults (Oppenheimer et al., 1986*a*, *b*). [Iron fortification of milk formula has even been implicated in SIDS (sudden infant death syndrome) (Moore and Worwood, 1989).] Intake of high-iron foods or iron supplements during infections is thus not recommended. Indeed, nature appears to prepare the newborn infant to adjust more easily to the (1) accumulation (and residency) of gut bacteria by "preproviding" excess iron during gestation, so that it need not initially enter the digestive tract; and (2) by providing lactoferrin in milk which can keep any iron that does enter from bacteria and deliver it to lactoferrin receptors in the infant mucosal brush border. [Lactoferrin is not well-digested in the infant's digestive tract (Lonnerdal, 1988).]

Increases in serum ferritin concentrations are associated with several disease processes (Table 7.4), notably infections, liver disease, and cancer. As indicated earlier, the increase in infection/inflammation may reflect a deliberate secretion of (low iron) ferritin as an acute phase reactant (although its function here is still obscure). The releases associated with other diseases may reflect a

Table 7.4. Serum Ferriti

Gro
Normal subjects
Adult males
Adult females
Children
At birth
At 1 mo
At 6 mo–puberty
Pregnant women (32–40 v
Primary iron metabolism dis
Iron deficiency
Iron deficiency during the
Iron overload (siderosis ar
Precirrhotic familial hemo
Transfusion overload (thal
Thalassemia (no transfusic
Refractory anemia
Other diseases
Inflammation and infectio
Adult
Children
Liver disease
Rheumatoid arthritis
Renal disease
Malignancy
Early breast cancer
Hodgkin's disease
Acute leukocytic leukemia
Children
Under treatment
After treatment
Chronic leukemia
Granulocytic
Lymphatic
Myelomatosis

Source: Information summarized

[a] Mean value.
[b] 95% confidence limits.
[c] ↑ = increase.

leakage of cellular ferritir although deliberate secreti as a source at this time. In cesses can mask evidence increasing serum ferritin. T iron therapy for deficiency

Zinc

Abundance and Distribu

The average adult body cc 2.5 g zinc (Zn). A major po in bone and is unavailable t

levels of testosterone are reduced in zinc deficiency (Abbasi et al., 1980; Castro-Magana et al., 1981; Hambidge et al., 1986).] The role of zinc in skin and connective tissue metabolism involves effects on protein and collagen synthesis and degradation (collagenase is a zinc enzyme) and, perhaps, also on cell replication, although these are not as well defined (Solomons, 1981). Some of these effects are mediated by a need for zinc not just in DNA synthesis but in the structuring of chromatin (perhaps via phosphorylation of histone HI; Barrett, 1976), and for the regulatory actions of some proteins in gene transcription via "zinc finger" elements in their structure (Chesters et al., 1988; Klug and Rhodes, 1987; Sunderman, 1990).

Among the most abundant zinc enzymes is erythrocyte carbonic anhydrase, essential for acid–base balance. Superoxide dismutase (requiring Cu and Zn) in the cytosol of all cells and especially erythrocytes is thought to play a defensive role in the disposal of damaging superoxide anions (see Chapter 5, Figure 5.33). In its association with various dehydrogenases, zinc plays a role not only in intermediary metabolism, but also in alcohol detoxification and in vitamin A metabolism. Retinal dehydrogenase in the retina, involved in metabolism of vitamin A-containing visual pigments, is a zinc-dependent enzyme. Moreover, zinc is necessary for the synthesis of retinol binding protein in the liver (see Chapter 5), which is required for distribution of the vitamin via the plasma. The latter connection to vitamin A metabolism potentially links zinc availability directly or indirectly to various vitamin A-dependent functions. These include the general integrity of the retina (Leure-duPree and McClain, 1982) and skin, and perhaps also the expression/production of growth hormone (turned on by the retinoic acid-hormone receptor complex; see Chapter 5), as well as triiodothyronine (which shares aspects of transport with vitamin A).

Zinc may also be required for the activity of adrenocorticotropic hormone (ACTH) (Flynn et al., 1972), and for stability (against hydrolysis), and the capacity to secrete prostaglandins of red cell, platelet, and other plasma membranes (Bettger and O'Dell, 1981; Li and O'Dell, 1986; O'Dell et al., 1987). [Prostaglandin function (secretion?) but not synthesis may be impaired in zinc deficiency (Hambidge et al., 1986; O'Dell et al., 1983.]

Zinc is fundamental to T cell function in immunity (deficiency leading to thymic atrophy and/or decreased thymic hormone and lymphokine production); a depression of natural killer cell and lymphocyte activities; and delayed hypersensitivity (Fernandes et al., 1979; Fraker et al., 1982; Hambidge et al., 1986; Iwata et al., 1979). There may also be a direct action of zinc in antibody production by B cells. From these observations, it is evident that zinc is fundamental to growth and remarkable for its broad involvement in metabolism.

Intake, Absorption, Distribution, Excretion, and Storage

The average American consumes about 10 mg zinc/day, although this is quite variable and often lower. This should be compared to an RDA of 15 mg for the adult (Figure 7.7). Of this 20%–30% (2–5 mg) is absorbed. The rate of absorbance by the small intestine is somewhat related to zinc status, being greater than normal in zinc deficiency. The availability of dietary zinc is also a factor in determining absorption, although this is probably not as variable or as critical as for iron. Phytate and fiber, both of which are prevalent in whole grains, are probably the main factors lowering availability; at the same rate of intake, zinc balance may be slightly negative in persons on a high versus low fiber diet (Kelsay et al., 1979). However, vegetarians generally do not show evidence of zinc deficiency (Anderson et al., 1981), probably because vegetarian whole grain diets, as a rule, contain considerably more zinc and other trace elements than other American diets (Kelsay et al., 1979). Indeed, apart from muscle/organ meats (especially lamb and beef), the richest sources of dietary zinc are whole grains (the germ), seeds, nuts, eggs, and root and leafy vegetables (Solomons, 1988).

Joining dietary zinc in the digestive tract are about 4–5 mg zinc released from proteolytic enzymes originating in the pancreas, and some derived from the bile (Figure 7.7). Probably 20% of this zinc is also reabsorbed, but the pancreatic pathway is the major excretory route for zinc from the body. Overall absorption of zinc is by an energy-dependent process and is enhanced by citrate. [In milk, a significant protein of zinc is bound to citrate and more available than protein-bound zinc (Hurley, 1982; Lonnerdal, 1988).] Reports of the involvement of a pancreatic stimulatory factor, possibly picolinic acid (Evans, 1980), in intestinal zinc absorption would appear to be invalid (Hurley and Lonnerdal, 1982). Other factors that enhance absorption may be histidine and glutamate (Hambidge et al., 1986).

Zinc is absorbed by passive carrier-mediated

diffusion into mucosal cells and from there a portion is transferred across the basolateral membrane (to blood and interstitial fluid) by an energy-dependent process. The second step in absorption is the most critical and the one regulated by dietary need (Hambidge et al., 1986; Solomons, 1988). It is also the site where other metal ions (notably Cu^{2+} and Fe^{2+}/Fe^{3+}) will compete for uptake when present in excess amounts. Thus, large iron supplements (as taken in pregnancy) can inhibit zinc absorption (Solomons, 1988), whereas large zinc supplements can induce copper deficiency (Porter et al., 1977; Prasad et al., 1978). [This competition has been exploited as a means of lowering copper accumulation and intoxication in persons with Wilson's disease (Brewer et al., 1983) (see below Copper).]

Absorbed zinc retained by mucosal cells will be used for internal enzymes and the excess will induce and bind to metallothionein (a 6100 dalton, high-cysteine metal binding protein). Zinc reentering from the blood has the same fate. When the zinc content of the diet is high, more metallothionein is induced (by a direct effect on the metal regulatory element in the promoter region of the gene, enhancing transcription) (Hamer, 1986), and more zinc is retained by mucosal cells. This metallothionein may then become a "trap" for zinc (and other divalent metal ions) entering from the diet, thus working against too much absorption. As Cu^{2+} will displace Zn^{2+} from this storage protein, long-term excess intake of the latter will also reduce copper absorption by trapping it in the mucosa. Copper, and zinc thus retained, are lost to the feces when the mucosal cells are sloughed off at the tips of the villi (after their 2–4-day life/migration from the crypts). This sloughing of cells is probably the other major route for zinc excretion. Excretion (at least by the intestinal route) appears to adapt to the availability of zinc in the diet, over a broad range, thus making "balance studies" unreliable for the determination of zinc requirements. [King has proposed that the minimum requirement would be the amount of zinc needed to maintain the exchangeable body pool as determined kinetically (King et al., 1990).] Small amounts of zinc are also lost in urine, and through sweat, hair, and skin; lactation, pregnancy, and menstruation impose additional losses (Figure 7.7).

Following transfer to the plasma, zinc becomes bound to three components (Figure 7.7) in equilibrium with each other. The major portion is carried on albumin, although a sizeable amount is bound to the antiprotease, α_2-macroglobulin. From the blood, zinc is taken up by numerous tissues, in greater or lesser amounts, as needed. In contrast to iron, zinc is not really stored and is readily lost from the body.

Deficiency and Toxicity

Zinc is among the least toxic of trace elements. No adverse effects (other than on absorption of copper) have been noted after weeks of intake at more than 10 times the RDA (Venugopal and Luckey, 1978). (In animals, pancreatic damage has been observed with enormous doses.) However, ingestion of $ZnSO_4$ tablets (or other zinc supplements) can cause discomfort if taken without a meal. Zinc deficiency is not uncommon and may occur because of inadequate intake or availability, malabsorption, or increased rates of loss from the body (Table 7.5). Studies in the late 1950s and early 1960s revealed that symptoms of growth retardation, skin lesions, and impaired sexual development in adolescent malnourished boys in Iran and Egypt could largely be attributed to a deficiency of zinc (Halsted et al., 1972), probably exacerbated by intake of high phytate bread that is a staple in those areas (Hambidge et al., 1986). In 1973–1974, acrodermatitis enteropathica, with symptoms of severe skin lesions, diarrhea, and loss of hair (alopecia), was also recognized as a disease of zinc deficiency (Moynahan, 1974) due to an inborn defect in the capacity for zinc absorption (Lombeck et al., 1975). Other impairments include the loss of taste and smell acuity and impaired wound healing (Table 7.5). Henkin (1984) has suggested that, of the 7% of the U.S. population who have an impairment in taste/smell, about 25% may be suffering from marginal or gross zinc deficiency due to a decreased ability for zinc absorption. The mechanism of zinc involvement is unclear, but it is probably a preneural event (Hambidge, 1986) that may involve a lack of zinc attachment to "gustin," a salivary protein (Janjua and Ali, 1986).

Increased zinc losses occur in burn victims and patients with kidney damage. In the latter, glomerular leakage of zinc attached to albumin is the main factor. Similarly, patients may lose substantial amounts of zinc during kidney dialysis, and those on total parenteral nutrition (intravenous feeding) will receive less zinc than they require if the trace element has not been added to the fluids administered (see Chapter 14).

Zinc deficiency, at least at a marginal level, is probably quite common in our society and is likely to occur under the specific predictable conditions listed and described (Table 7.5). Zinc sta-

Table 7.5. Causes and Symptoms of Zinc Deficiency

Causes of zinc deficiency	Symptoms
Inadequate dietary intake	Anorexia
Protein-calorie deficiency	Impaired smell and taste
Patients on protein-restricted diets	Growth retardation
Synthetic diets	Hypogonadism
Intravenous feeding	Delayed wound healing
Malabsorption	Impotence in renal dialysis patients
Acrodermatitis enteropathica	Depression, mood lability, impaired concentration
Celiac disease and other enteropathies	Intention tremor
Pancreatic insufficiency	Nystagmus
Chronic inflammatory bowel disease	Dysarthria
Immaturity of absorptive systems	Jitteriness
Increased body losses	Photophobia, night blindness, blepharitis
Starvation	Skin lesions (digits, perineum, parietal, nasolabial folds)
Burns	Paronychiae with monilial superinfection
Diabetes mellitus	Nails (growth arrest, loss, Beau's lines)
Ketoacidosis	Hair growth arrest or alopecia
Diuretic treatment	Diarrhea
Kidney damage	Decreased cell-mediated immune function
Proteinuria	
Hepatic disease	
Intravascular hemolysis (e.g., sickle cell anemia)	
Porphyria	
Chelating agent therapy	
Chronic blood loss	
Parasitic infection	
Dialysis	
Exfoliative dermatitis	
Excessive sweating	

Source: Modified from Agget and Harries (1979).

tus, especially marginal deficiency, is not easy to assess. Serum/plasma zinc concentrations are still the most common measure, and plasma and/or hair concentrations of less than 50 μg/dl and 70 μg/g, respectively, may be indicative of deficiency. However, a variety of conditions and treatments, including inflammation, stress, cancer, smoking, estrogen or glucocorticoid disturbances or treatments, long-term fasting, hemolysis, or venous occlusion (Solomons, 1988), will affect the level in the serum. Many of these factors act by inducing liver metallothionein, which is thought to then withdraw some of the metal from the plasma (and hold it in the hepatocytes). This occurs as part of the acute phase reaction (Figure 7.6), and Sugarman et al. (1982) have proposed that (as with iron) this may help subdue bacterial infections. [Indeed, infusion of zinc into the blood of animals brought into an inflammatory state by endotoxin can enhance the virulence of the inflammatory process (Bremner, 1990).] Levels of erythrocyte carbonic anhydrase of serum alkaline phosphatase and salivary zinc concentrations may also be of some use in assessing zinc status, but Henkin (1984) has suggested that the only good way is to test absorption and retention of ^{65}Zn and calculate its storage, distribution, and turnover in the slow and fast turnover compartments of the body. The most promising new test on the horizon may, however, be erythrocyte or serum metallothionein, since the amounts of this protein in erythrocytes when corrected for the percentage of reticulocytes tends not to vary with the physiologic state (Bremner, 1990); the trace levels in serum generally reflect intracellular liver levels of zinc (Grider et al., 1989*a*, *b*; Bremner and Beattie, 1990), as well as whole body status. Zinc deficiency is commonly treated by administering 25–50-mg tablets of $ZnSO_4$. However, it should be noted that deficiency in the slow-turnover compartment may take weeks and even months to overcome because of the slow rate of influx/exchange of incoming zinc with this compartment (Henkin, 1984) (which includes the bone).

Zinc and Wound Healing

Zinc has a special promotional role in skin and connective tissue metabolism. This has indirectly been recognized since ancient Greek times, when calamine lotion ($ZnCO_3$) was first used on the skin (Agget and Harries, 1979). Part of the connection may also be the delivery of vitamin A (necessary for epithelial cell differentiation), and the fact that it is a cofactor for collagenase (Figure 7.7). The use of zinc to stimulate wound healing may be of some practical value in patients with evidence of zinc deficiency (Wacker, 1978). For example, treatment of surgical patients with three daily oral doses of 50 mg Zn (as $ZnSO_4$) has been shown to enhance the rate of wound closure (Pories et al., 1967; Underwood, 1977).

Copper

Abundance and Distribution

The average adult human body probably contains 100–120 mg of copper (Cu), an abundance considerably below that of iron or zinc. Except in certain disease states and in deficiency, the body's copper content is probably homeostatically controlled, and there is little storage of the excess, metabolically inactive metal ion. In man the highest concentrations of copper are in kidney and nails (Table 7.6). Concentrations are also high in liver, brain, heart, and skeleton, with lower amounts in other organs and tissues and the blood. In terms of masses, the skeleton and liver, brain, muscle, and blood account for much of the copper, although it is found in all cells and tissues.

Table 7.6. Iron and Copper Concentrations of Various Adult Organs

	Iron (μg/g)	Percent of body content	Copper (μg/g)	Percent of body content
Blood	500	70	1.1	6
Bone	<300	5?	>4	46
Liver	180	8	6.2	10
Kidney	16	0.1	12	3
Heart	20	0.1	4.8	2
Brain	33	1.4	5.2	9
Spleen	70	0.2	1.5	0.2
Lung	19	0.5	1.3	1
Muscle	9	6?	0.9	26
Hair	—	—	2	—
Nails	—	—	20	—

Source: Modified from Linder and Munro (1973) and Linder (1991).

Functions

Copper is associated with a discrete number of oxygenases, both intra- and extracellularly, including cytochrome oxidase, the terminal component of the electron transport chain in all mammalian cells. Apart from the latter, the most abundant copper-containing enzymes are cytosolic superoxide dismutase (Table 7.7), which also contains zinc and is concerned with the disposal of potentially damaging superoxide anions (see Chapter 5, Figure 5.33), and ceruloplasmin, which comprises about 60% (and not 90%–95%) of the copper in plasma and interstitial fluid (Wirth and Linder, 1985). Ceruloplasmin is a somewhat weak, broad-specificity oxidase. Its main functions are in copper transport and in antioxidant defense as an extracellular scavenger of superoxide and other oxygen radicals (Linder, 1991). It may also play a role in allowing the flow of iron from storage sites (in liver parenchymal cells) to transferrin, for transport to the bone marrow and other sites. Specifically, it has been postulated to be necessary for oxidation of Fe^{2+} (which leaves ferritin where it is stored) to Fe^{3+}, in order to allow attachment to transferrin (Frieden, 1971). This is based on observations that copper-deficient rats accumulate liver iron and that infusion (or liver perfusion) of ceruloplasmin causes an immediate release of liver iron to circulating transferrin (Osaki and Johnson, 1969; Roeser et al., 1970). Such a function of ceruloplasmin would help to explain the similar symptomatology of iron and copper deficiency anemias, although other connections may be critical: energy availability for hematopoiesis, through oxidative phosphorylation (and cytochrome c oxidase) may be rate-limiting; and Cu/Zn superoxide dismutase and another "pink" copper protein are necessary parts of the red blood cell (Linder and Munro, 1973).

Another important copper protein is lysyl oxidase (Table 7.7) secreted by connective tissue cells to aid in the crosslinking of elastin and collagen, a role that is integral to connective tissue and blood vessel maintenance (O'Dell, 1981). Other copper enzymes are as follows: dopamine-β-hydroxylase, necessary for catecholamine production in brain and adrenal (Table 7.7); amine (and certain diamine) oxidases, in plasma and some cells, involved in the inactivation of hista-

Table 7.7. Reactions Catalyzed by Some Mammalian Copper Enzymes

Ceruloplasmin

$$\frac{1}{2}O_2 + 2\,Fe^{++} \xrightarrow{2H^+} 2\,Fe^{+++} + H_2O$$

Cytochrome oxidase

$$\frac{1}{2}O_2 + 2e^- \begin{pmatrix} cyt \\ + \\ Cu^+ \end{pmatrix} \xrightarrow{2H^+} H_2O$$

Dopamine-β-hydroxylase

$$\frac{1}{2}O_2 + \text{dopamine (3,4-dihydroxyphenethylamine)} + 2e^-\ (\text{ascorbate}) \longrightarrow \text{norepinephrine}$$

Lysyl oxidase

$$O_2 + R\text{-CH(OH)-CH}_2\text{-NH}_2 + H_2O \xrightarrow{NH_3\ ?} H_2O_2 + R\text{-CH(OH)-CHO}$$

Superoxide dismutase

$$2O_2^{\overline{\cdot}} + 2H^+ \rightleftharpoons H_2O_2 + O_2$$

mine, polyamines, tyramine, and tryptamine (also in the intestine); tyrosinase, necessary for melanin production in skin; and an enzyme catalyzing α-amidation of some peptide hormones in the pituitary and other endocrine glands (Eipper and Mains, 1988). Lysyl oxidase, dopa-β-hydroxylase, amine oxidase (and possibly the α-amidating enzyme) also probably have another common cofactor, originally thought to be pyrroloquinoline quinone (Gallop et al., 1989), but more likely to be 6-OH dopa (see end of Chapter 5 and Figure 5.38). It is certain that the involvement of copper in the function of further enzymes will be discovered.

Apart from enzymatic functions, copper proteins and chelates probably have other, less understood, roles. Of particular interest are observations that antiinflammatory drugs (such as aspirin) have their actions as copper chelates (see more below), that copper deficiency decreases immune function (Prohaska and Lukasewycz, 1981, 1990; see Chapter 17), that numerous copper chelates have anticancer activity (see more below), and that copper plays a stimulatory role in angiogenesis (McAuslan et al., 1980; Raju et al., 1982).

Intake, Absorption, Distribution, Excretion, and Storage

The average American consumes 1.2–1.7 mg Cu/day, roughly half of which may be absorbed into the blood (Figure 7.8). In contrast to zinc and iron, the availability of dietary copper is quite good, although two of the same interfering parameters apply: (1) fiber tends to adsorb copper and enhance its fecal excretion; and (2) copper partially competes for absorption with Zn^{2+} (and some other transition metal ions, possibly includ-

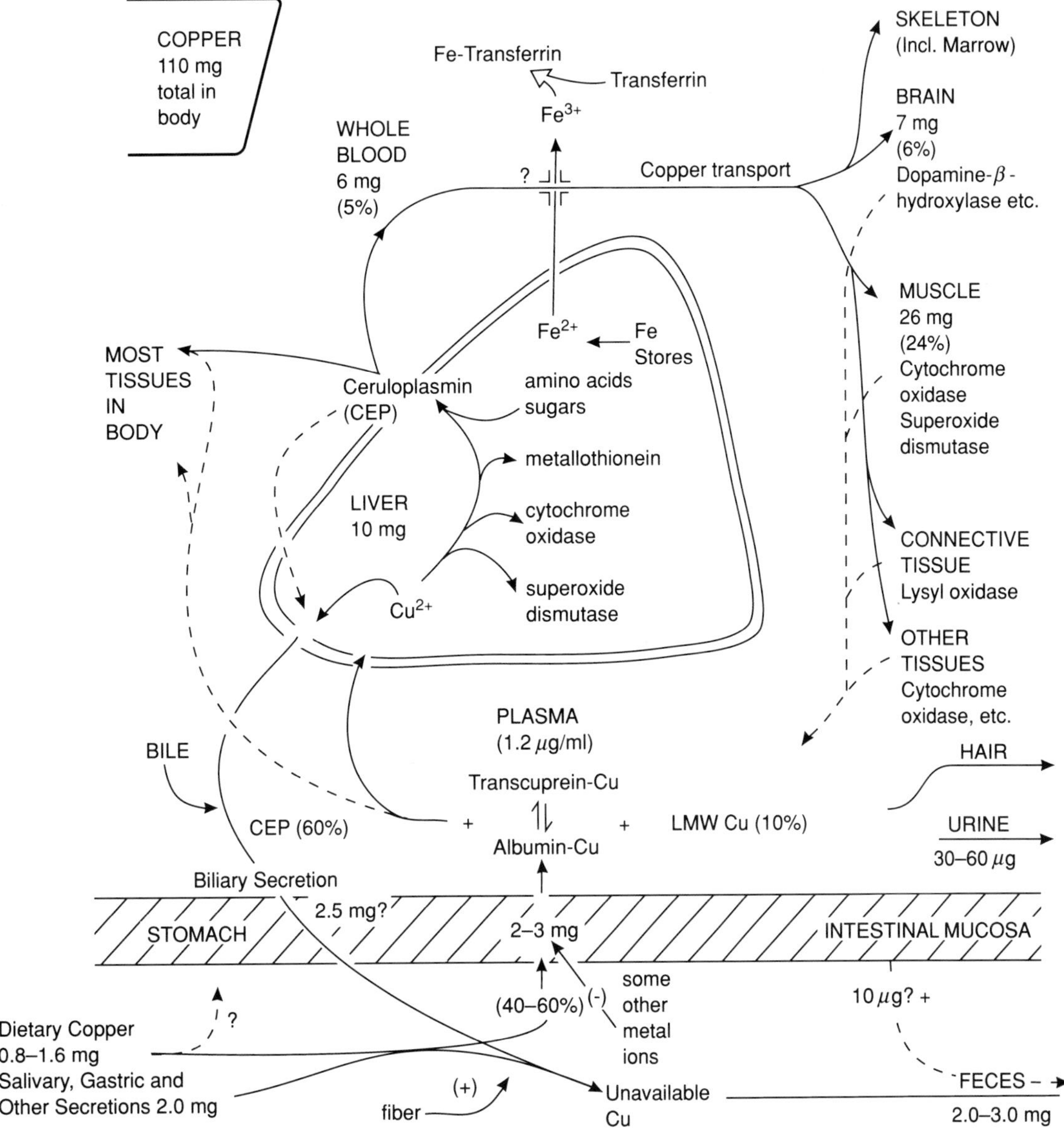

Figure 7.8. Copper metabolism and nutrition (100–120 mg total in body). Dietary copper is made more or less available by other dietary factors, including amino acids and fiber (see text). About 1 mg of dietary copper (plus 1–2 mg of the copper secreted into the digestive tract) is absorbed into the blood, mainly by the small intestine, and carried on transcuprein and albumin to the liver, where it is incorporated into liver enzymes and secreted into the blood on ceruloplasmin for transport to other tissues. Losses are mainly through the bile and through intestinal and gastrointestinal juices. Copper is used for a variety of enzymes, some ubiquitous to cells. Considerable copper is present in the skeleton (including the bone marrow).

Best food sources: whole grains, shellfish, legumes, liver, nuts.

Increased needs: may be present with total parenteral nutrition, premature birth.

Data are per day unless otherwise indicated.

[*Source:* Modified from Linder (1991).]

ing Fe^{2+}). As with zinc and iron, the enhanced percent loss of copper with higher fiber diets is mostly (or completely) compensated by a much higher dietary copper intake (Kelsay et al., 1979*a*, *b*).

Absorption of copper appears to be enhanced by dietary protein and amino acids and by other chelating agents, presumably acting to enhance water solubility (Linder, 1991). Some data have suggested that large doses of ascorbate (vitamin C) inhibit copper absorption, perhaps through reduction, but the weight of the evidence is against this (Jacob et al., 1987; Linder, 1991).

Copper, like zinc and many other trace elements, is most abundant in the germ of whole grains (see Table 7.2). Thus, vegetarians show little or no evidence of copper deficiency (Abdulla et al., 1981). Apart from whole grains and nuts, legumes, liver, and shellfish are good dietary copper sources, although it has been noted that the concentration of copper in foodstuffs has declined since 1942 (Klevay and Forbush, 1976). Copper is also abundant in molasses and Brewer's yeast. And among fruits, it is highest in avocadoes; it is least abundant in muscle meats (except duck), milk and dairy products, and in nonwhole grain cereals and baked goods. The U.S. adult recommendation for safe and adequate intake is 1.5–3.0 mg, but numerous studies indicate this is usually not met.

Overall, the absorption of copper is an energy-dependent process. Absorption, and particularly the transfer from intestinal mucosa to the blood, is a regulated process (Cohen et al., 1979) that is influenced by changes in physiologic state, such as estrogen levels and the presence of cancer in the host. Evidence from studies with rats suggests that the concentration of metallothionein in cells of the intestinal epithelium determines how much of the entering dietary copper is free to proceed into the blood or must stay behind attached to this small, high cysteine protein. Conditions that increase metallothionein (such as a high zinc diet or estrogen) decrease overall copper transfer to the blood, whereas in cancer, the opposite pertains (Sonsma et al., 1981).

In the blood plasma, copper is initially bound to albumin (Figure 7.8) and a new protein, "transcuprein," and carried to the liver where it is (1) incorporated into ceruloplasmin and specific liver protein/enzymes, or (2) lost via the bile. Ceruloplasmin is secreted into the plasma and, apart from its antioxidant and enzymatic functions, transports the copper to cells throughout the body (Campbell and Linder, 1981; Goode et al., 1990). [A smaller portion of the copper is transported via transcuprein and albumin; the low molecular weight copper pool in plasma (principally Cu-histidine$_2$) is probably not normally a direct cellular copper source (Linder, 1991).

Incorporation of copper into ceruloplasmin may be necessary for copper homeostasis and excretion from the body, as ceruloplasmin accumulates when excretion is blocked or reduced, and because copper accumulates in the liver (and the central nervous system) when there is inadequate ceruloplasmin synthesis (Wilson's disease). Excretion, especially in humans, is thought to be mainly via the bile, although a significant percentage is released into the gastrointestinal tract by other secretions and the sloughing off of cells (Figure 7.8) (Linder, 1991). Except for copper in bile, most is reabsorbed. Very small amounts are lost in the urine. Homeostasis is maintained mainly by regulating excretion; thus, "copper balance" (intake minus output) will adapt to high and low copper intakes (Milne et al., 1990; Turnlund and Keyes, 1990).

Except for the fetus in gestation (Figure 7.5), there is little storage of copper in body tissues, and liver concentrations are remarkably constant, except in disease conditions or deficiency. What copper is stored is attached to intracellular metallothioneins, the 6100-dalton, one-third cysteine proteins that also bind zinc, cadmium, mercury, and some other rare metal ions and can be induced in certain cells by many of these metals (including copper).

Deficiency and Toxicity

By the oral route, copper is generally quite nontoxic for humans and most animals, although there have been some rare instances of acute toxicity due to the consumption of acidic beverages (or water) with very high concentrations (Venugopal and Luckey, 1978). Tissue accumulation usually only occurs with diets containing copper concentrations 200–500 times the normal. Even then, the main problem may not be the toxicity of copper but rather its interference with the uptake and distribution of other metal ions, notably those of zinc and iron. Chronic excessive intake can, however, result in liver cirrhosis (especially in early childhood) when other conditions are also present, notably in the case of Indian infants who receive milk that has been boiled in brass vessels (Tanner, 1989, 1990). Acute toxicity is marked by hemolysis, with possible damage also to cells of the liver and brain. Toxic accumulations in liver and the brain occur in inherited Wilson's disease (see below).

Copper deficiency is not uncommon, as judged by the values for serum copper or ceruloplasmin measured in so-called "normal populations" (Linder et al., 1981). The level of ceruloplasmin (which comprises about 60% of serum copper) is very sensitive to copper status in the direction of deficiency (Linder et al., 1979). [Excess copper in the body in itself does not, however, increase levels of ceruloplasmin or serum copper.] Symptoms of copper deficiency include decreased levels of serum copper and ceruloplasmin, an anemia similar to that of iron deficiency, neutropenia, and a degeneration of the vasculature (with hemorrhage) ascribable to the lack of elastin (and perhaps also collagen) production. Depigmentation of skin, kinky hair, brain damage, hypotonia, and hypothermia may also occur, especially in children (Solomons, 1981). At least in rats, copper deficiency is also associated with hypercholesterolemia.

Copper deficiency is most likely to occur from lack of intake, as in the case of a deficient diet or parenteral feeding. Excess loss of copper, as through kidney dialysis, can also cause deficiency. There has been some recent interest in the findings in experimental (male) animals that fructose (or sucrose) intake may exacerbate copper deficiency (Fields et al., 1986*a*, *b*). The exact reason for this is yet to be determined but may involve alterations in sorbitol metabolism (see Chapter 2) (Fields et al., 1989). (Fructose consumption has been rising due to the increased use/availability of high fructose corn syrup.) Copper deficiency is not uncommon in premature or low birth weight infants on parenteral nutrition. Deficiency may partly be induced or enhanced by excessive urinary excretion when free amino acids are infused (Nutr Rev, 1981; Tyrala et al., 1982). In adults, deficiency can generally be reversed by oral supplementation with low doses (up to 2 mg/tablet). [Note that, at 25–40 mg, $CuSO_4$ is a potent emetic (Solomons, 1981).]

Disease Associations

Inborn diseases of copper metabolism. Menkes' and Wilson's diseases are inborn errors that effect copper status in opposite directions. Menkes', an X-linked defect characterized by all of the overt symptoms of gross copper deficiency save the anemia/neutropenia, is detected in infancy and involves a defect in copper absorption by the intestine and the liver (Danks, 1981; Solomons, 1981). Not only is little copper absorbed from the diet (it accumulates in the intestinal mucosa and is not transferred to the blood), but the liver appears refractory to uptake, even when copper is administered by injection. Copper accumulates in some cells, such as those of kidney, and in fibroblasts. These children usually die at a very early age. Only limited relief of the symptomatology (and limited prolongation of life) have been achieved with parenteral administration of copper salts (Williams, 1982) and Cu-histidine is currently being tested (B Sarkar, personal communication); few, if any, children normally survive beyond 3 years (Sass-Kortsak, 1965). The exact defects responsible have not yet been identified, but may involve expression of metallothioneins (Goode, 1991).

On the other side of the coin, Wilson's disease does not usually become evident until late adolescence, when the effects of reduced excretion of copper from the body begin to cause a toxic accumulation in the liver, kidney, cornea, and central nervous system. An incapacity of the liver to produce ceruloplasmin at normal rates may be part of the problem, as copper transport by ceruloplasmin may be related to the capacity for ridding the body of excess copper through the bile (see above). When the toxic effects have not progressed too far, Wilson's disease has been treated with chelating agents with some success and has resulted in a prolonged life expectancy. Usually, penicillamine has been used, which is a bacterial ionophore that increases urinary excretion of copper (and zinc as well as perhaps other trace elements). Excess oral zinc is now also given to avert zinc deficiency and reduce dietary copper absorption (see section on Zinc).

Copper and cancer. Cancer causes a profound alteration in the compartmentation and metabolism of copper in the body. Based on studies in animals and man, levels of serum ceruloplasmin and copper are increased; liver and kidney copper concentrations decline; there is a decrease in total body turnover of copper; and (at least in rats) an enhanced rate of intestinal copper absorption is observed (Linder et al., 1981). The rate of synthesis, and structure, of ceruloplasmin are altered, as are a variety of other aspects of copper distribution and metabolism. Of further interest are observations that dietary copper, and especially copper chelates, can inhibit chemical carcinogenesis in laboratory animals [see Linder et al. (1981) and Chapter 16], and that low Cu/Zn ratios may be associated with a higher incidence of stomach cancer in man (Stocks and Davies, 1964). The significance of these observations is not as yet clear, but Linder has hypothesized that ceruloplasmin and low molecular weight copper chelates might play opposite roles (promotional and inhibitory, respectively) in tumor growth and development. These roles may involve stimulation of tumor growth by ceruloplasmin, via provision of copper for new cells, and through stimulation of angiogenesis by other forms of copper (McAuslan et al., 1980; Raju et al., 1982; Wissler et al., 1986). Conversely, certain copper chelates could induce chromosomal damage in tumor cells, thereby inhibiting DNA/RNA synthesis (Marshall et al., 1981) and enhancing cell death (Petering, 1980). Effects on cell-mediated immunity (Koller, 1987; Mulhern and Koller, 1988; Prohaska and Lukasewycz, 1981) might also be involved.

Copper and inflammation. Serum copper concentrations and ceruloplasmin are often increased 20%–30% in inflammatory conditions (Table 7.8), suggesting a positive role for copper (as ceruloplasmin) in the healing process and in connective tissue repair. Many types of cell-mediated inflammatory processes are propagated by the production of superoxide anions (Salin and McCord, 1977) and other oxygen radicals. In the face of this, damage to normal tissues/cells may be minimized by extracellular ceruloplasmin playing the role of a radical scavenger (along with Cu/Zn superoxide dismutase and other components of the intracellular antioxidant defense system). [Plasma copper and ceruloplasmin concentrations rise in inflammation (Figure 7.6).] The same oxidative processes can also be inhibited by copper-amino acid chelates that have superoxide dismutase activity, and by antiinflammatory copper-binding agents, like salicylates (Richardson, 1976; Sorenson, 1982). Thus, copper would appear to play several central roles in the healing and repair process. [For further information, see Chapter 17, Nutrition and Infection.]

Ceruloplasmin and disease diagnosis. The importance of ceruloplasmin as a source of copper for cells and as a potential agent (1) in the pathway of iron flux from liver storage sites, (2) in angiogenesis (the laying down of blood vessels and capillaries), and (3) in biliary copper excretion has already been described. Clinical observations of the "ups and downs" of serum ceruloplasmin in various conditions must be related to the functions of this unusual α_2-glycoprotein, and it is unrewarding to dismiss ceruloplasmin as "just another acute phase reactant." In the case of cancer, we have already detailed possible ways in which ceruloplasmin function and cancer growth might be related (see above). With further observation, the apparent reasons for changes (especially increases) in other conditions may become apparent. Certainly, the increase observed in pregnancy appears to be related to the need for copper transfer to the fetus (Linder et al., 1990*b*).

Table 7.8 summarizes the conditions in which ceruloplasmin (and serum copper concentrations) are altered. It should be noted that the largest changes occur in cancer, pregnancy, and hepatobiliary disease, and that, at least in some forms of cancer, the degree of increase in ceruloplasmin is positively related to disease severity and the prognosis (Linder et al., 1981). A return of ceruloplasmin to normal (or near normal) levels accompanies cancer remission, and prolonged or recurrent increases are associated with progression of recurrence. Studied use of ceruloplasmin assays may thus help the physician in disease assessment. In this regard, assays of ceruloplasmin (based on enzyme activity or immunoassay) are preferable to measurements of total serum copper concentrations (Linder et al., 1981).

Copper and Cholesterol Metabolism

In the rat (Klevay, 1973) and probably also in man (Klevay et al., 1984; Reiser et al., 1985), there is an inverse correlation between levels of serum cholesterol [mainly low-density lipoproteins (LDL)] and copper deficiency. Moreover, in man there would appear to be a relationship between the ingestion of diets low in copper (and/or with a high ratio of zinc to copper) and hypercholesterolemia, and deficiency also causes diminished heart function (Prohaska and Heller, 1982) and hypertrophy. On the basis of these facts, Klevay (1985) proposed that copper deficiency may be contributing to the hypercholesterolemia, hypertriglyceridemia, and also to the atherosclerosis prevalent in our society today. Despite considerable work by several laboratories, the reasons for the hypercholesterolemia of copper deficiency (when it occurs) are still unclear. Investigations of potential changes in liver cholesterol and very-low density lipoprotein (VLDL) synthesis and secretion, activities of lipoprotein lipase (LPL) and lecithin: cholesterol acyl transferase (L-CAT),

Table 7.8. Serum Copper and Ceruloplasmin Concentrations in Various Conditions

Condition	Change in serum copper or ceruloplasmin[a]
Normal conditions	
Menstruation	
Proliferative phase	No change (Cu)
Luteal phase	No change (Cu)
Pregnancy	
Second trimester	90% (Cp)
Third trimester	135% (Cp)
Use of oral contraceptives	
With estrogen	74% (Cu)
With only progestogen	No change (Cp)
Smoking	21% (CpO)
Infectious disease	
Bronchitis	37% (CpO)
Hepatitis	
Acute	22% (Cp)
Chronic	No change (Cp)
Tuberculosis	47% (Cu)
Typhoid fever	33% (Cu)
Virus vaccine administration (equine)	27% (Cu)
Noninfectious disease	
Cancer	30%–82% (CpO)
Chronic obstructive lung disease	37% (CpO)
Epilepsy	14%–53% (Cu)
Fibroadenoma	52% (CpO)
Fibrocystic breast disease	54% (CpO)
Kidney dialysis (chronic)	No change (Cp)
Liver cirrhosis	
Biliary	69%–92% (Cp/Cu)
Nonbiliary	22% (Cp)
Multiple sclerosis	18% (CpO)
Myocardial infarction (acute)	22%–230% (Cu/CpO)
Psoriasis	29% (Cu)
Renal insufficiency	Little change (Cp/Cu)
Surgery (noncancer)	24% (Cu)
Ulcers/polyps	33% (CpO)
Wilson's disease	65% (Cp)
Drug-related disorders	
Alcohol withdrawal syndrome	15% (Cu)
Methadone therapy	91% (Cp)

Source: Modified from Linder et al. (1981).

[a] Cp is ceruloplasmin, measured immunologically. CpO is ceruloplasmin, measured as oxidase activity. Cu is serum copper concentration.

and turnover of LDL have yielded conflicting results (Linder, 1991). Dietary factors (such as the type of protein) may also modify the copper deficiency response, at least in rats (Stemmer et al., 1985). Further work will be necessary to establish the exact molecular events involved and their validity for man. A role for excess zinc in the development of copper deficiency hypercholesterolemia now seems doubtful, except as a means of exacerbating copper deficiency through competition for intestinal absorption.

Manganese

Like zinc, manganese (Mn) is associated with a large number of enzymes in many areas of metabolism, including pyruvate and acetyl-CoA carboxylases and isocitrate dehydrogenase in the Krebs cycle and mitochondria; the mitochondrial form of superoxide dismutase, where it may help to protect mitochondrial membranes (Hurley, 1982); arginase, the terminal enzyme in urea production; and other cytosol enzymes involved in the pentose phosphate shunt, glycolysis (glucokinase), and serine metabolism (hydroxymethyltransferase) (Linder, 1978). Of special interest is its association with some of the enzymes of mucopolysaccharide, glycoprotein, and lipopolysaccharide production, including galactose transferase and other membrane-bound glycosyltransferases. Indeed, manganese deficiency has substantial effects on the production of hyaluronic acid, chondroitin sulfate, heparin, and other forms of mucopolysaccharide that are important for growth and maintenance of connective tissue cartilage and bone (Cavalieri, 1980) (see Chapters 2 and 6). More recent work suggests an involvement also with γ-carboxylation of the glutamate side chains of certain (vitamin K-dependent) proteins (Gla proteins). These are important in blood clotting, but also in basic aspects of calcium metabolism involving intestine, kidney, and bone. Indeed, the connection of manganese to bone mineralization and demineralization has been clarified by recent studies in rats in which both osteoblast and osteoclast activities were reduced in deficiency, resulting in osteoporosis and osteopenia (reduced bone cell number) (Strause and Saltman, 1987). Manganese has also been implicated in melanin and dopamine production, in fatty acid synthesis, and in formation of membrane phosphatidylinositol. Apart from enzymes, it is associated with nucleic acids, and a portion is present in the mineral compartment of the bone. (Bone manganese is not an available store for use by soft tissues.) Deficiency results in hypocholesterolemia [which may be due to a need for manganese by cholesterogenic enzymes (Krishna et al., 1966)] and a "finely scaling," minimally erythematous "rash" (Friedman et al., 1987) (perhaps due to its function in connective tissue metabolism).

Although widely involved in metabolism, deficiency does not appear to have broad effects and is not very common, probably because the much more abundant ion, Mg^{2+}, can substitute for Mn^{2+} in many of its various enzyme-related functions. [e.g., Pyruvate carboxylase is just as active (and uses Mg^{2+}) in Mn^{2+} deficiency (Leach, 1974).] Judging from observations of the effects of manganese deficiency in animals, the roles of this element in mucopolysaccharide and lipopolysaccharide formation would appear to be the most vital. Normal growth of endochondral bone would appear to depend on the formation of manganese-dependent cartilage and connective tissue components and perhaps only indirectly on a manganese-dependent calcification.

Other effects of manganese deficiency are an impairment of glucose tolerance and β-cell granulation in the pancreas (observed in guinea pigs) and an impairment of lactation and fetal development (observed in rats). In this connection, some of the highest manganese concentrations are found in the lactating mammary gland; also, the developmental formation of the labyrinth of the ear appears critically dependent on this element (Cavalieri, 1980). [Expression of a genetic defect in otolith production (crystalline particles in the ear) in "pallid" rats is prevented by feeding the pregnant mothers extra manganese (Hurley, 1968), and otolith crystals are embedded in a mucopolysaccharide-rich matrix (Nutr Rev, 1988).] Manganese may also play a role in fertility, although the mechanism remains obscure (Nutr Rev, 1988). Protection of animals against chronic hydrazaline poisoning by manganese has caused speculation that similar symptoms seen in lupus erythematosus in man might be due to the same problem (Comens, 1960). This has not been followed up.

Manganese is considerably less abundant than Mg, Fe, Zn, or Cu in the body and is absorbed quite poorly (Table 7.1; Figure 7.9). The average American probably consumes 2–4 mg/day (Friedman et al., 1987; Schroeder, 1973), which is within the 2.5–5-mg range suggested by the NAS (Figure 7.9). Intestinal absorption is hindered by calcium, phosphate, iron, and phytate and aided by histidine and citrate (Garcia-Aranda et al., 1984). Blood distribution is probably via transferrin (see Iron, above), where concentrations are 1%–2% that of plasma Fe (or Zn or Cu). Major organs of accumulation are liver, kidney, and bone, although the highest concentrations are found in the pineal, pituitary, and lactating mammary glands. (Manganese is normally lowest in lung and muscle.) The pancreas is also avid for manganese uptake (Cavalieri, 1980). Liver concentrations are quite constant throughout life (Figure 7.10). As for Fe, Zn, and Cu, excretion is via the bile and pancreatic and intestinal fluids. Urinary losses are miniscule, but may reflect dietary status (Nutr Rev, 1988).

Rich food sources include nuts and whole grains, where the major portion is in the germ (Table 7.2); leafy vegetables are also good sources, where a Mn^{2+} component is part of the second electron transport chain of photosynthesis. (Mg^{2+} is part of the chlorophyll.) Meats, milk, poultry, and seafood are poor sources. Manganese is abundant in tea, but in a form that is even less available than otherwise (Kies et al., 1987).

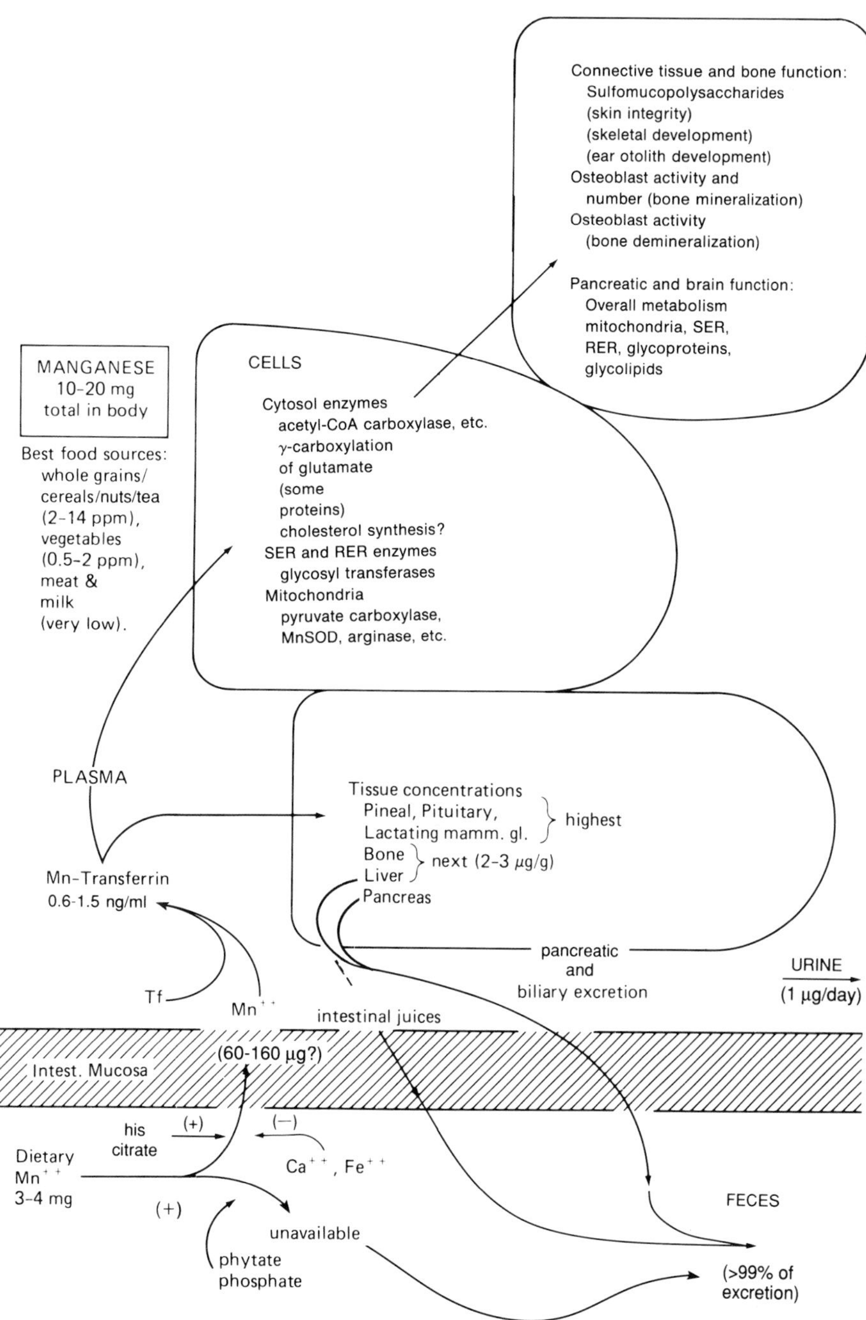

Figure 7.9. Manganese (10–20 mg total in body).

Best food sources: whole grains/cereals (2–14 ppm), vegetables (0.5–2 ppm), meat and milk (very low).

Key: SOD, superoxide dismutase; RER, rough endoplasmic reticulum; SER, smooth endoplasmic reticulum.

[*Source:* Based on Hurley (1982), Linder (1978), Garcia-Aranda et al. (1984), Friedman et al. (1987), Nutr Rev (1988), and Saltman (1989).]

Only one case of "spontaneous" manganese deficiency has been reported in humans (Doisy, 1972), although it has been demonstrated in numerous animal systems. Except when inhaled (as in the case of some miners), it is a very benign element and can be tolerated orally at very high doses with no apparent adverse effects. Over time, high doses can potentially interfere with the availability and metabolism of other transition

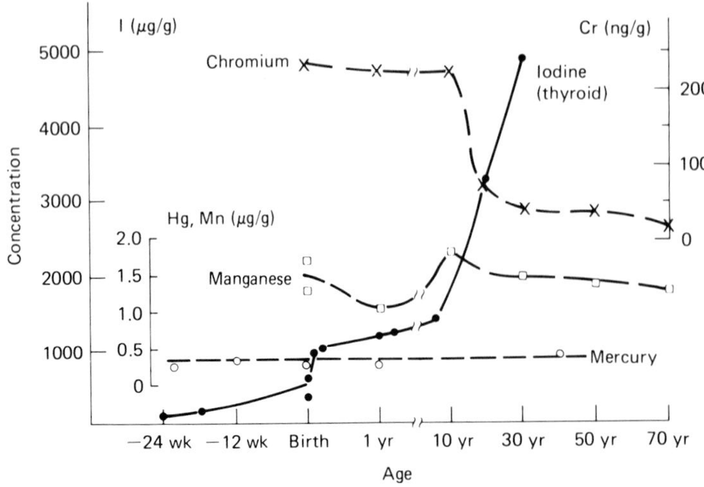

Figure 7.10. Age changes in human liver trace element concentrations: chromium, manganese, iodine, and mercury. B = birth; wk = week; yr = year. (Chromium concentrations are lower on the basis of current methods.) [*Source:* Modified from Linder (1978).]

metal ions, although this has not been adequately studied.

Molybdenum

Molybdenum (Mo) is notable for its interactions with sulfur, iron, and copper. Though probably required in smaller quantities than copper (the estimated range for safe and adequate intake is also 0.15–0.50 mg/day), until now, it has been found to be necessary for the function of only three mammalian enzymes: the xanthine, aldehyde, and sulfite oxidases (Figure 7.11). All three of these enzymes contain flavin and iron, the first two in the form of an Fe–S moiety similar to that of the ferredoxins. (Nitrate reductase in plants and bacteria, required for N-fixation, is also Mo and Fe–S-dependent.) Sulfite oxidase, necessary for the disposal and excretion of sulfur (as sulfate; see Chapter 6, Figure 6.2), contains an Fe-porphyrin instead of an Fe–S moiety. Molybdenum, in the +5/+6 oxidation states, is thought to function, with the other cofactors mentioned, in the transfer of electrons for the oxidation/reduction process. Xanthine oxidase, found in several tissues (liver, intestine, spleen, kidney, and others) as well as in milk, is necessary for the terminal oxidation of purines to allow their excretion as uric acid (Figure 7.11). It is also capable of oxidizing some aldehydes, pteredines, NADH, and some pyrimidines (Cavalieri, 1980). In a genetic deficiency of molybdenum metabolism, urinary uric acid excretion is decreased, and xanthine/hypoxanthine losses are enhanced (Rajagopalan, 1988). Aldehyde oxidase (in liver) can act on many of the same substrates as xanthine oxidase in the liver, and little is known about its actual function and further tissue distribution (Rajagopalan, 1988). Sulfite oxidase is necessary for the completion of S-amino acid catabolism (and S excretion) and for inactivation of the otherwise destructive sulfite ion.

In all three enzymes, molybdenum is present in the form of a pterin-derived cofactor (Figure 7.11), the exact structure of which is still uncertain because of its lability (Rajagopalan, 1988). A more stable form of this cofactor (not bound to enzyme) probably also accounts for a substantial proportion of the molybdenum in tissues (40% in rat liver).

Molybdenum salts are capable of inhibiting the intestinal absorption of iron and copper through mechanisms that are poorly understood but may involve competition for brush-border receptors and/or (in the case of copper) the formation of Cu-molybdate or thiomolybdate compounds that are poorly absorbed and do not render the copper available for incorporation into ceruloplasmin and other copper-containing proteins. In ruminants, excessive molybdate intake, especially when coupled with a high sulfur intake and low copper content of forage crops, produces a de facto copper deficiency, with its concomitant symptomatology (see Copper, above). This probably results from formation in the intestine of biologically unavailable cupric thiomolybdate complexes, such as CuMoS (Suttle, 1974*a*, *b*), and has been a problem in some areas of the world, notably Britain and New Zealand. The condition may occur even with a high copper intake (and liver copper accumulation) if tetra-

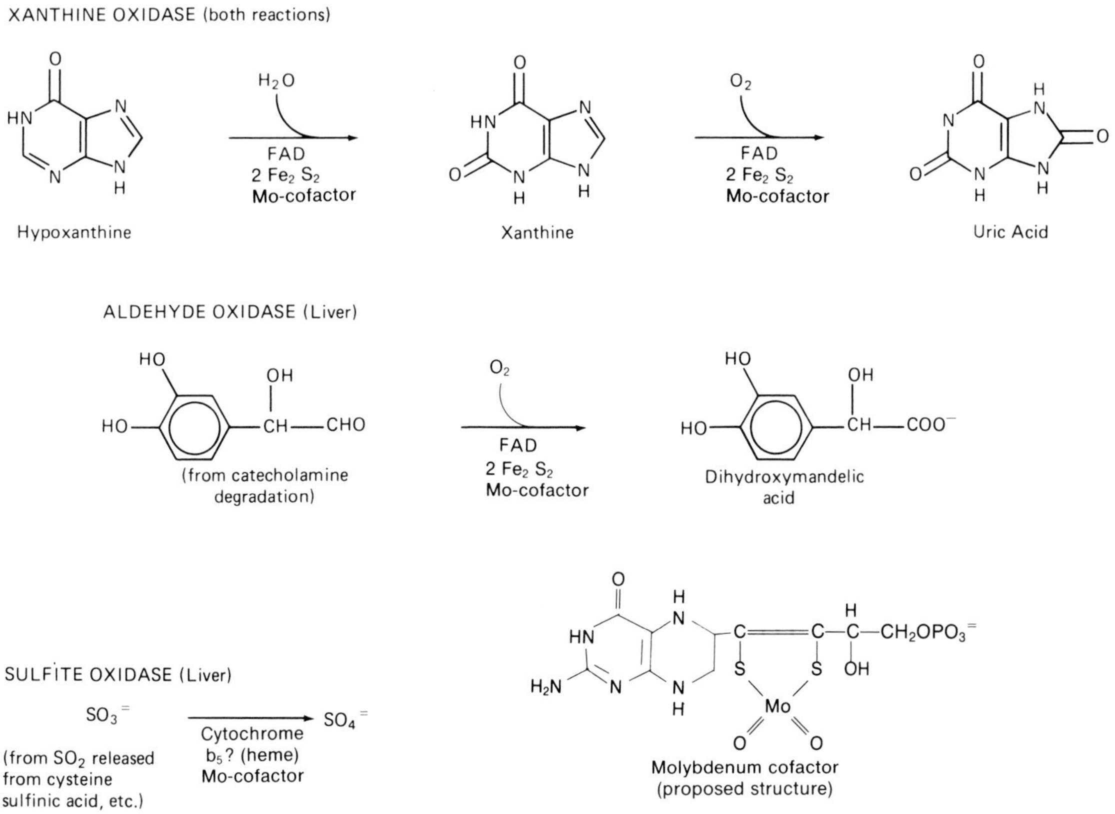

XANTHINE OXIDASE (both reactions)

Hypoxanthine → (H_2O; FAD, 2 Fe_2S_2, Mo-cofactor) → Xanthine → (O_2; FAD, 2 Fe_2S_2, Mo-cofactor) → Uric Acid

ALDEHYDE OXIDASE (Liver)

HO–C$_6$H$_3$(OH)–CH(OH)–CHO (from catecholamine degradation) → (O_2; FAD, 2 Fe_2S_2, Mo-cofactor) → Dihydroxymandelic acid (HO–C$_6$H$_3$(OH)–CH(OH)–COO^-)

SULFITE OXIDASE (Liver)

$SO_3^=$ (from SO_2 released from cysteine sulfinic acid, etc.) → (Cytochrome b_5? (heme), Mo-cofactor) → $SO_4^=$

Molybdenum cofactor (proposed structure)

Figure 7.11. Reactions of molybdenum-containing enzymes and potential structure of the molybdenum cofactor. [*Source:* From Rajagopalan (1988).]

thiomolybdate intake is also sufficiently elevated (Gawthorne et al., 1981). In humans and nonruminants, copper deficiency from excess molybdate intake is very rare, as the intake of copper usually exceeds that of molybdate. Indeed, a deficiency of molybdenum (from insufficient intake relative to copper) is more likely (Seelig, 1973). In animals, molybdenum deficiency reduces liver and intestinal xanthine oxidase activities, which can be reversed by giving oral molybdate salts. In chicks, a molybdenum deficiency has been produced with tungstates, resulting in enhanced urinary excretion of xanthine and hypoxanthine, as well as decreased excretion of uric acid. This results in growth retardation and death. Functional symptoms of molybdenum deficiency in man have only been reported in one case involving total parenteral nutrition (see Chapter 14) (Abumrad et al., 1981) and as a consequence of the genetic inability to form molybdenum cofactor (Rajagopalan, 1988).

Molybdenum is absorbed very readily from the diet (Table 7.1), except in the presence of $SO_4^=$, which competes with $MoO_4^=$ (Mills and Davis, 1987). Resorption of molybdate by kidney tubules is also affected, so that enhanced intake of S-amino acid-rich proteins will enhance urinary molybdenum losses. (Urine is the principal excretory route, although small amounts may also be lost in the bile.) The element is distributed by the blood plasma bound to protein and accumulates mainly in the liver, lung, bone, and skin (Table 7.1). Molybdenum is three to five times less abundant in the body than copper and only 1/500 as concentrated in the plasma. Schroeder (1973) had estimated a daily average U.S. intake of 300 μg (as compared with about 1000–1500 μg for copper), almost all of it from foodstuffs (versus water). As with many other trace elements, it is particularly abundant in the germ of grains, and much of it is lost during the processing of wheat into regular flour (Table 7.2; Schroeder, 1973). Good food sources are whole grains and probably legumes (beans), where the element is an active part of the nitrogen-fixing apparatus (nitrate reductase; nitrogenase).

Fluorine

Fluorine (F) is one of three halogens essential for the normal life, health, and reproduction of man and animal. It is normally present in the body in quantities comparable to those of iron, which is the most abundant trace element (Table 7.1). Despite its position in the periodic table, its functions would appear to be quite different than those of bromine and chlorine (which act in similar fashion). Most fluorine is found in bone, where it readily combines with calcium or hydroxylapatite to form fluorapatite. This is important for hardening the tooth enamel and contributes to the stability of the bone mineral matrix (Krishnamachari, 1987; Messer et al., 1974; Shaw and Sweeney, 1980). It may also provide "nucleation sites" for crystallization of the bone mineral and enhance bone density (Figure 7.12). These effects of fluorine on bones and teeth have been of great interest as a potential means of reducing dental caries and even osteoporosis (see below). However, numerous animal experiments have failed to show that a lack of fluorine intake results in obvious skeletal abnormalities.

Traces of inorganic and organic fluorine are found in most soft tissues and fluids. Plasma concentrations of both forms are variable, with the inorganic fluorine levels being related to dietary intake (in the range of 0.1–5 μg/ml). The levels of organic fluorine may be related to industrial exposure, as plasma from rural Chinese contains much lower levels than that from urban Chinese in industrialized areas (0.1 versus 0.2–0.85 μg/ml) (Belisle, 1981). Ingestion of diets low in fluorine by rats or mice has resulted in growth retardation, increasing infertility, and anemia, the latter two phenomena being progressively enhanced over several generations (presumably through progressive depletion of the element). These effects were partially (for growth) or completely (fertility and anemia) reversed by adding fluoride to the diet (Messer et al., 1974). The molecular bases for these potentially important actions of fluorine are unknown.

It is well established that the fluoride intake of children correlates inversely with their incidence of dental caries. Numerous epidemiologic studies have shown a negative correlation of the natural (or added) fluoride content of drinking water with the percentage tooth decay of the population (Figure 7.12), and a positive correlation of fluoride intake with bone density (Shaw and Sweeney, 1980). This suggests that the drinking water is the main source of fluorine, although the fluoride content of foodstuffs is in the same range, and very high concentrations are found in black tea

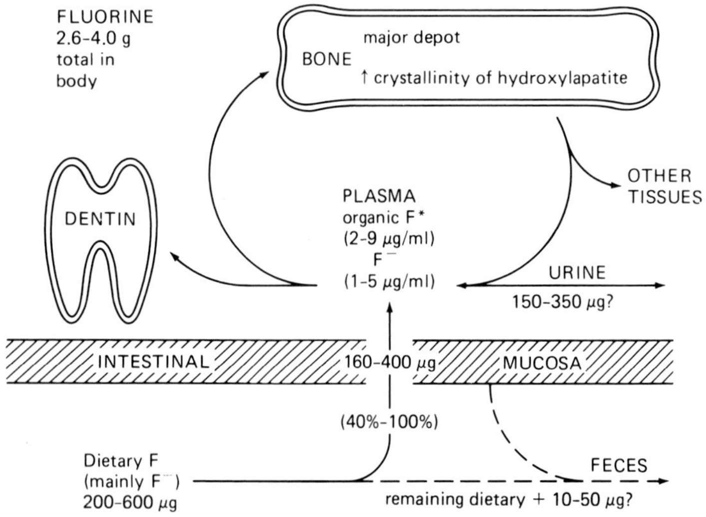

Figure 7.12. Nutrition and metabolism of fluorine (2.6–4.0 g total in body). Asterisk (*) means characteristic of all people in industrialized countries.

Food sources: most foods contain 0.2–1.5 μg/g (ppm); seafood 5–15 μg/g (ppm); tea leaves 75–100 μg/gh (1 cup ~ 0.1 mg). (Water and food concentrations are especially high in some parts of India.)

Needs: growth, fertility, prevention of anemia of pregnancy and infancy (rodents); important for teeth, especially during development; skeletal strength.

Toxicity: can be toxic, as in fluorosis (mottled teeth, skeletal abnormalities, including osteoporosis); potential effects on glycolysis (inhibits enolase) and adenyl cyclase (stimulates cAMP production).

City	Water F^- (μg/ml)	Tooth decay: Children (no.)	Tooth decay: No caries (%)
Colorado Springs CO	2.6	404	28.5
Gainsburg IL	1.9	273	27.8
East Moline IL	1.2	152	20.4
Pueblo CO	0.6	614	10.6
Marian OH	0.4	263	5.7
Middletown OH	0.2	370	1.9

Source: Data from Shaw and Sweeney (1980).

and seafoods (not consumed as much by growing children). [In China, plant foods rather than water have a very high fluoride content (Krishnamachari, 1987).] It is noteworthy that the largest differences in dental caries incidence (and bone density) occur in populations consuming less than 0.3 versus more than 1 ppm (Shaw and Sweeny, 1980; Figure 7.12). This has led to the recommendation that in areas of low water fluorine content, water be supplemented to 1 ppm (1 μg/ml), or that drops or tablets be given orally to children throughout the period of tooth development (from birth through the midteens). As shown in Figure 7.13, the recommendation of 1 ppm represents a compromise between maximal tooth hardening (caries prevention) and minimal fluorosis (the toxic and/or unsightly effects of excessive fluoride intake). During gestation, very little of the element is transferred to the fetus, although the barrier is not totally impermeable and traces find their way to the bones and teeth of the fetus (Cerlewski and Ridlington, 1988).

Fluorine is one of the few trace elements where doses for beneficial and toxic effects are not widely separated. However, acute toxic effects are rare. Chronic ingestion of 2.5 ppm or more by children will strengthen their teeth and bones, but also produce an unsightly and permanent mottling (of the teeth). At 3–5 ppm, toxic effects have been shown to occur in cattle, characterized by weakness, loss of appetite, gastroenteritis. The latter will occur in humans at higher levels. It has been estimated that an intake of 8 ppm over 35 years would exhaust the storage capacity of the skeleton for fluoride and result in a "spillover" of excess F^- into soft tissues, with similar toxic effects (Underwood, 1977). Chronic exposure to excess fluoride also produces skeletal changes, especially in the long bones, including

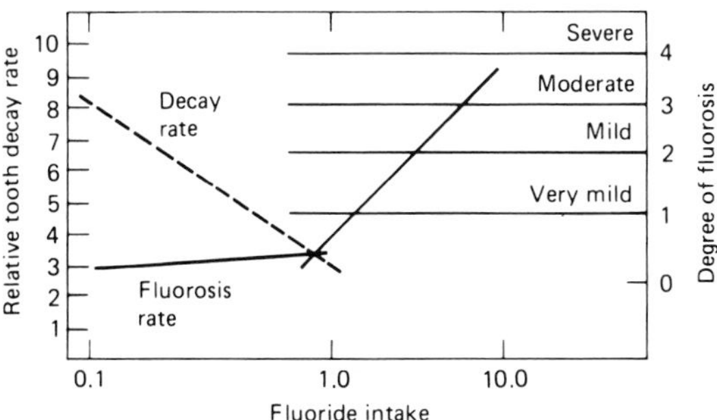

Figure 7.13. Effects of fluorine intake on tooth decay (---) and fluorosis (——). [*Source:* Modified from Hodge and Smith (1954).]

the thickening of cortical areas, osteoporosis and/or osteomalacia, calcification of tendons, ligaments, and interosseous membranes, and the development of bone spurs (Krishnamachari, 1987). At least partly, this reflects an increased turnover of the mineral of the bone, probably through a stimulation (by excess F^-) of parathyroid hormone secretion (Krishnamachari, 1990). It leads to osteolysis and an irreversible skeletal rigidity. The condition has been quite common in certain regions of India and China, where fluoride levels are high in soil and water. (Even here, use of fluoride toothpaste is sometimes inadvertently promoted!) The basis for F toxicity is unclear, although its affinity (and involvement with) calcium is part of the story. Millimolar concentrations of F are also inhibitory to enolase (Wang and Himoe, 1974) (one of the enzymes of glycolysis) in vitro and stimulate adenyl cyclase, producing cAMP, the "second messenger" for the action of numerous hormones (see Chapter 2, Figure 2.4). It seems unlikely that such high concentrations would occur in vivo, except perhaps locally in bone. Fluoride is readily absorbed from the diet and lost mainly in the urine.

Selenium

As with fluorine, selenium (Se) is an essential trace element, for which requirements and toxic doses are not widely separated. Until 1969, selenium was of interest mainly for its induction of the "blind staggers" and "alkali disease" in cattle and sheep, in seleniferous areas of the world, where certain plants have a high selenium content (Underwood, 1977). Its importance for human and animal metabolism has become apparent more recently, spurred by the discovery of a Se-dependent enzyme, glutathione peroxidase (widely distributed in tissues), and suggestive evidence that selenium plays a role in the prevention of certain forms of cancer (see Chapter 16).

The main reason for its late recognition as an essential element is the overlap of its actions with those of vitamin E. This began with the demonstration by Schwarz and Foltz (1958) that a form of liver necrosis in rats could be cured by administration of either factor. Retrospectively, the reason for the overlap and confusion is at least partly apparent: glutathione peroxidase and vitamin E both play a role in the detoxification of peroxides and free radicals, which have their most damaging effects on cell membranes in blood, liver, and other tissues. The interactions of these factors, along with Cu, Zn, and S-amino acids, are illustrated in Figure 5.33 (Chapter 5).

Glutathione peroxidase is a 4-subunit enzyme with one selenium per subunit in the form of Se-cysteine, required for activity. This Se-cysteine appears to be formed (pretranslationally) from a particular serine tRNA and an inorganic form of selenium (Figure 7.14) (Leinfelder et al., 1988; Sunde and Evenson, 1987). The resulting Se-cys-tRNA recognizes the codon, "UGA," which is also a termination codon for some polypeptides (especially in microorganisms). This exciting series of discoveries indicates there is a specific genetic code requiring insertion of Se-cysteine (rather than sulfur-containing cysteine) into certain proteins. Indeed, synthesis of glutathione peroxidase may be regulated transcriptionally by selenium (Smith et al., 1989; Sunde et al., 1989).

Other proteins that contain Se-cysteine include a certain selenoprotein "P" made by the liver, that may transport and/or store selenium (at least in rats) (Burk and Gregory, 1982); three selenoproteins in the testes (McConnell et al., 1979) and several in other mammalian tissues (Evenson and Sunde, 1988) (microorganisms), most notably, the deiodinase that converts thyroid hormone (T_4) to triiodothyronine (T_3; the active form of the hormone) (Arthur and Beckett, 1990). [This means that selenium deficiency will impinge on thyroid function.] It is possible that Se-methionine is also incorporated into proteins in place of sulfur-containing methionine, and perhaps this insertion is random and nonspecific. [Se-methionine may be the main form of selenium in plants (Hawkes et al., 1985; Waschulewski and Sunde, 1988).]

Figure 7.14. Proposed pathway for insertion of Se-cysteine into proteins via tRNA recognizing the UGA codon. [*Source:* Sunde et al. (1989) and R. Sunde, personal communication.]

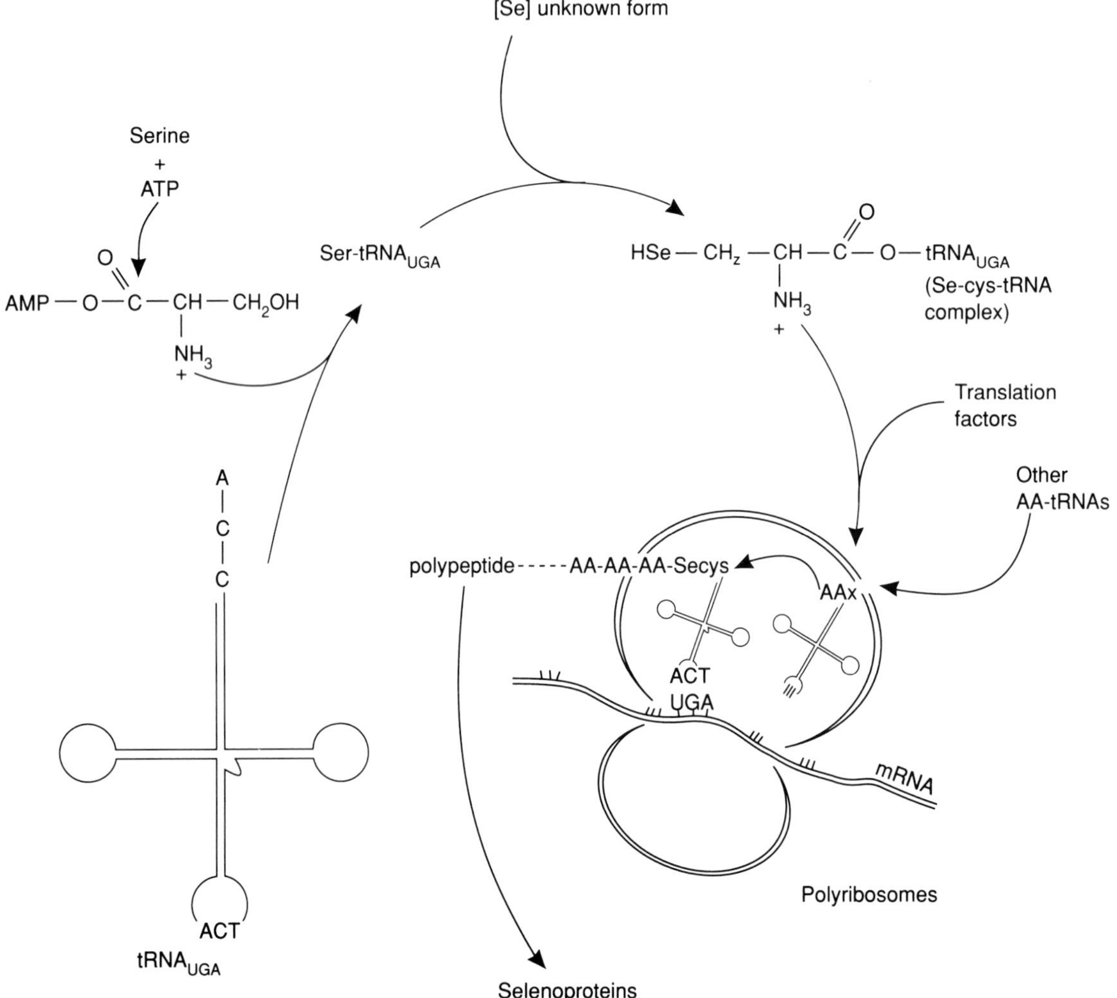

The basis for other metabolic effects of selenium is not clear at this time. Deficiencies produced in animals cause growth retardation, cataract formation, lack of spermatogenesis (and abnormal placental retention), as well as dystrophic and necrotic symptoms if vitamin E concentrations are also insufficient. The aspermatogenic effects may also be due to a lack of glutathione peroxidase (Pond et al., 1981), as well as other specific testicular selenoproteins (Evenson and Sunde, 1988). Deficiency has been reported in protein-calorie malnourished children, infants on various formula diets, and in children and adults on total parenteral nutrition. The latter resulted variously in cardiomyopathy, myositis (muscle inflammation), and lightening of the fingernail beds (Fleming et al., 1982; Kien and Ganther, 1983), or enhanced skin pallor and curling of scalp hair, all of which responded to selenium therapy (Vinton et al., 1987). Preliminary studies indicate a connection between selenium deficiency and Keshan disease, a childhood cardiomyopathy (necrotic disease of the cardiac muscle) prevalent in one area of China (Keshan Disease Group, 1979; Zhu, 1981). Disturbances in selenium metabolism also appear to be associated with Duchenne's muscular dystrophy (enhanced selenium excretion) and with some diseases in which ceroid pigment granules (oxidized lipids) accumulate in nervous tissue (Westermarck et al., 1981; Westermarck and Santavuori, 1984). Selenium deficiency has been assessed by low blood selenium concentrations and/or responses to selenium supplementation, specifically, an amelioration of anemia, growth retardation, and painful muscular symptoms (Smith et al., 1982), and the degree of positive response of blood glutathione peroxidase activity upon supplementation with 100+ μg daily doses of selenium, as selenomethionine or sodium selenite (Thomson et al., 1982).

Figure 7.15. Selenium nutrition and metabolism (quantities per day). Selenium (6–21 mg? total in body).

Best food sources: grains (depending on soil), possibly garlic, meat, and fish (higher concentrations, but generally less bioavailability).

Deficiency: in protein-calorie malnutrition, or total parenteral nutrition, results in growth retardation, aspermatogenesis, cataracts.

Toxicity: can be toxic (anti-S action); inhibits mitosis, "blind staggers," rough hair (in animals on high selenium forage).

[*Source:* Mason (1988) and Levander (1986).]

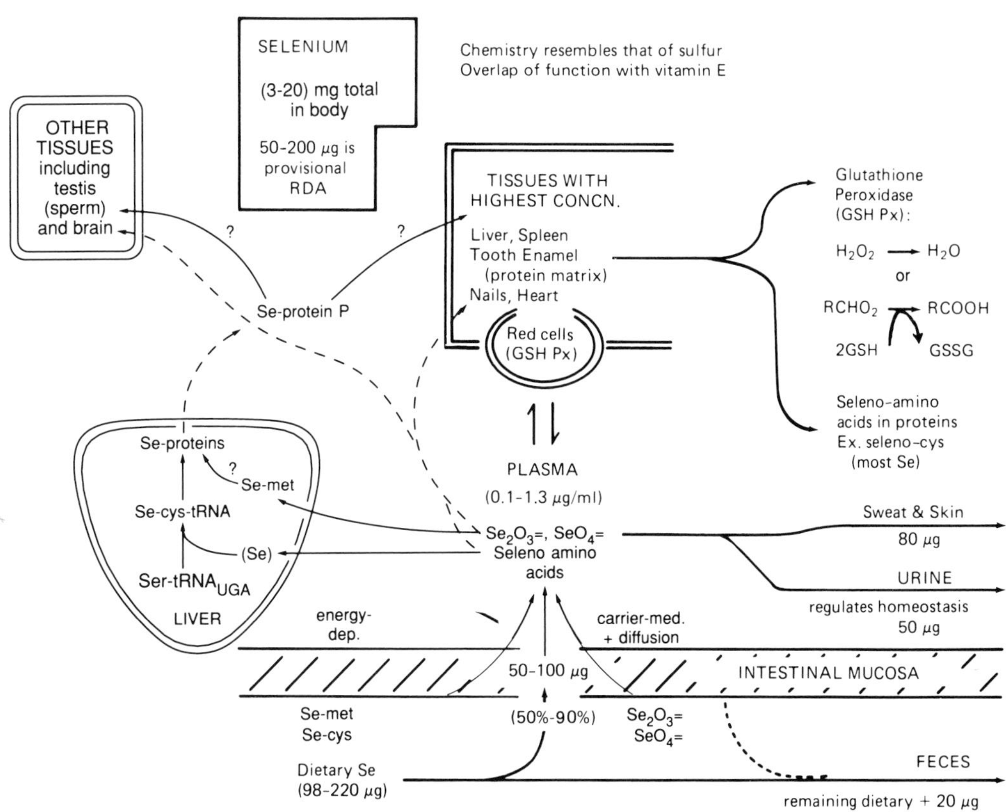

The NAS-NRC has advised that intakes of 50–200 μg Se/day are safe and adequate, but has most recently recommended adult intakes of 55 and 70 μg for women and men, respectively. (This does not fully address the problem of potential differences in bioavailability.) As already mentioned, protein-containing foods like meats and seafood, tend to be rich in selenium (mainly in the form of selenocysteine), but this selenium seems not to be as available (Mason, 1988). Levels of selenium in plant foods and grains will vary with soil content, and grains can be important sources. Garlic and mushrooms can also be high in selenium. With the exception of asparagus, vegetables and fruits are generally not good sources. In general, plant-derived selenium (perhaps as Se-methionine and Se_2O_3) may be more efficiently absorbed. Thus, the average American diet usually contains enough selenium, but may be deficient in certain circumstances.

Selenium is thought to be absorbed fairly readily (Figure 7.15), although bioavailability differs with the source. In some studies with selenium-deficient rats, the capacities of selenium from tuna, beef kidney, wheat, and selenite to restore glutathione peroxidase activity showed the selenite to be most effective and the tuna to be significantly inferior (Douglass et al., 1981). (As already mentioned, plant selenium may tend to be more available.) Selenium may be transported from the gut to the liver mainly on VLDL and LDL (Cavalieri, 1980) and achieves its highest tissue concentrations in red cells, liver, spleen, heart, nails, and tooth enamel (Figure 7.15). It also concentrates in the testes and sperm, which are also more refractory to dietary deprivation (Mason, 1988). Selenium is lost from the body mainly via the urine, following its metabolism (Figure 7.15), probably in the form of di- and trimethylselenonium compounds (Foster et al., 1986; Ganther, 1987; Sun et al., 1987). Traces are exhaled as dimethylselenide. In America, overt deficiencies occur primarily in infants or adults on artificial formula or parenteral diets. Toxic effects are probably extremely rare, since selenium intake is well below the levels required except perhaps in certain high soil selenium regions where levels in local foods may be high, or when supplementation has accidentally been excessive (Levander, 1986). However, as already mentioned, selenium is a potentially toxic trace element, and its toxic effects in cattle and sheep have been a problem in some countries. As exemplified by the "blind staggers," it causes damage to liver, and to skeletal and cardiac muscle. From animal studies it has been estimated that the long-term ingestion of 5 ppm Se (amounting to 2400–3000 μg/person/day) would lead to similar toxic effects in humans. This is roughly 25 times the average present consumption.

Selenium and Disease

The possibility that adequate selenium intake may prevent or retard tumor development (Chapter 16) suggests the need for an adequate selenium intake. Its importance in the genetic disorder leading to deposition of ceroid or lipofuscin granules in neurons has already been mentioned. [Here, degeneration of nerves and vision was retarded by oral supplementation with Na selenite (25–100 μg/kg) (Westermarck and Sandholm, 1977; Westermarck and Santavuori, 1984).] The cardiomyopathy of Keshan disease (in a certain part of China) has been linked to a severe local soil selenium deficiency, and its prevalence has been decreased by dietary supplements (Yang, 1987). In Finland, the severe soil deficiency is being corrected by application of the element to fertilizer (Tolonen et al., 1988). There may also be other connections between selenium deficiency and cardiovascular disease, as suggested by epidemiological studies in Finland (Salonen, 1985) and the United States (Levander, 1986; Moore et al., 1984). The mechanism may involve increased aggregability of platelets and production of thromboxane A_2, with less prostacyclin (PGI_2). (See Chapters 3 and 15 for more information on the functions of these substances.) In geriatric subjects, combined supplementation with vitamin E was also found to improve mental, emotional, and physical parameters of well-being, in a double-blind Finnish trial (Tolonen et al., 1985, 1987).

Silicon

Silicon (Si) is another recent addition to the roster of essential trace elements, as determined in chicks (Carlisle, 1974) and rats (Schwarz, 1974*a*, *b*) placed on diets containing only 1 ppm of the element on a dry weight basis. [Normally, foodstuffs average 20+ ppm (Schwarz, 1977).] Silicon deficiency resulted in growth retardation and a deformation and incomplete development of the skeleton. Further studies have indicated that the major defect is in connective tissue metabolism, specifically, the formation of glycosaminoglycans (Schwarz, 1974*a*, *b*, 1977) and collagen (Carlisle,

1982*a*, *b*) necessary for the formation of matrix and ground substance. Schwarz (1977) and others (Varma, 1974) have shown that silicon is found mainly in the skin and cartilage, but also in numerous other tissues associated with various glycosaminoglycans (from chondroitin sulfate, to heparan and hyaluronic acid) and attached to collagen. It is also associated with elastin and maintains the integrity of elastic tissues in animals fed an atherogenic diet (Loeper et al., 1979). Schwarz postulated that silicon acts at least partly as a cross-linking agent in these components, forming bridges with an ether (or ester) configuration (e.g., R-O-Si-O-R). The chemistry of this element is very similar to that of carbon and thus is ideally suited to this purpose (Schwarz, 1974*a*). Working with chicks and more recently with chondrocytes in culture, Carlisle has concentrated on the possibility that silicon acts on these cells by stimulating collagen and mucopolysaccharide production (Carlisle, 1982*a*, *b*, 1986). This view is not incompatible with the incorporation of silicon into these compounds. Because of its importance to connective tissue proteins and glycosaminoglycans, silicon helps to provide the organic matrix for the proper mineralization of bones and teeth and accumulates during the early phases of bone mineralization, especially in the epiphyses, where it is present in osteogenic cells (Carlisle, 1986). Its concentration decreases as bones mature, which helps to explain the decline in whole body (and connective tissue) content that occurs with age. In the skin it accumulates at the surface in the ceroid epidermis and also in the hair follicles. In blood vessels, it is concentrated in the intimal layer (see below). Whether all the functions of silicon in these tissues involve collagen, elastin, and mucopolysaccharide production remains to be determined.

The amount of silicon in the body is quite unclear (Table 7.1), although gram quantities are surely present. Schroeder (1973) estimated a concentration of 260 ppm (dry weight), which would suggest about 3 g/60-kg person (wet weight). As already mentioned, highest concentrations (100–500 μg/g) are in the skin, tendons, bone epiphyses, and artery walls. Very high concentrations are also found as microscopic silica crystals in the lymph nodes (Hamilton et al., 1972/1973). It is thought that these may arise from the filtration of SiO_2 crystallites (known as "phytoliths") absorbed from plant foods, as these pass through the barrier of the intestine and circulate in the lymph and blood, even being transferred to the fetus in pregnancy (Carlisle, 1986; Geissler and Gerloff, 1965). Whether this form of silicon has a function is unknown. In most soft tissues, concentrations of silicon (about 20–40 μg/g) are much lower than in skin, and they are even lower in blood and blood plasma (about 1 and 0.5 μg/ml, respectively) (Table 7.1). From the data available (Carlisle, 1986), it would seem, however, that all tissue concentrations in man are dramatically (20–40 times) higher than those of rats or monkeys! This will need to be confirmed. In body fluids and blood plasma, the main form of silicon is silicic acid (H_2SiO_3), which is freely diffusible and is the form excreted in the urine (the primary exit route). Other silicon is probably part of some extracellular substances.

Silicon is absorbed in variable amounts from the diet, probably depending on its form. (Aluminosilicates are very poorly absorbed, some organic forms are very easily absorbed.) Relatively little is known about these processes, although it has been estimated that intakes range from 20–46 mg/day of which 30%–50% may be absorbed (and lost in the urine) (Kelsay et al., 1979*a*; Nielsen, 1988). In the diet, silicon is most abundant in high fiber foods and husks of grains (Table 7.9). Within foods, it appears to be largely associated with the various kinds of fiber, and thus, is largely removed during refining (Table 7.9). In the plant it is thought to confer structural stability on cell walls and to modulate lignin biosynthesis (which may also explain its antifungal actions) (Marshner, 1986). Water may also be a significant source (in the range of 2–12 μg/ml) (Schwarz et al., 1977). Meats, fish, and dairy products are poor sources. As we presently have no concept of the silicon requirement of man, the question of whether the dietary intake of this element is optimal, and whether it is adversely affected by our low fiber diets, cannot as yet be answered.

The questions of dietary adequacy and the potential connection of silicon to development of atherosclerotic vascular disease were of special interest to Schwarz (1977). Loeper (1966, 1979) and others have shown an inverse relationship between the silicon content of the arterial wall and the degree of atherosclerosis present. Moreover, Schwarz and colleagues found that the normal arterial wall, especially the intima, contains exceptionally high concentrations of bound silicon. Some studies by DeFranciscis et al. (1974) have reported blood lipid lowering effects of large quantities of silicates administered in drinking water. Coupled with the epidemiologic correlations between fiber intake and reduced cardiovascular disease, these observations can be wielded

Table 7.9. Silicon Content of Some Foodstuffs

Foodstuff	Approximate average concentration (μg/g)			
	Whole	Refined/polished	Fiber/bran	Hulls
Grains				
Oats	4600	130		16,900
Barley	2000			
Sorghum	600			
Rice	360	70		22,500
Rye	70			
Wheat	65	30	230–1700 (3)	
Maize	40			
Vegetables				
Soybeans	1700	90		
Turnips	120			
Green beans	100			
Carrots	5			
Potatoes	2			
Cabbage	3			
Fruits/nuts				
Raisins	140		1100 (4)[a]	
Peanuts	50			
Other foods				
Sugar beets	2300			
Sugar cane	1100	<2		
Beer	45			
Beef	7			
Pork	7			
Fish	4			
Milk	1.4			

Source: Calculated from Schwarz (1977), Nielsen (1988), Nuurtamo et al. (1980), and Varo et al. (1980*a*, *b*, *c*).

[a] Pectin preparations.

into the argument that silicon deficiency (from lack of fiber intake) is a contributing factor in the development of atherosclerosis. The further observation that two populations of Finns with more than a twofold difference in the long-term rate of cardiovascular disease also imbibed water with almost a twofold difference in silicon content (the higher silicon group having less disease) lends further support to this contention, especially as other known risk factors were not adequate to explain the differences observed (Schwarz et al., 1977). Recent studies in rabbits support a connection between silicon intake and reduced formation of atheromatous plaque (Loeper et al., 1988). Also, the long-standing notion of an association between "hard" water intake and decreased atherosclerosis may be related to these matters. Obviously, much further work is required to clarify the possible interactions between these parameters and the whole matter of the molecular role(s) of this interesting trace element.

Chromium

Chromium (Cr) was first determined to be essential for animals by Schwarz and Mertz in 1959. Later on, chromium deficiency (and its symptomatology) was documented in humans, specifically in patients on long-term total parenteral nutrition (Jeejeebhoy et al., 1977, see Chapter 14). In both the animal and man, chromium deficiency appears to be characterized by glucose intolerance and elevated serum cholesterol and triglyceride. At least in animals, it may enhance the risk of developing sclerotic aortic plaques (Anderson, 1988). A persistent elevation of fasting insulin levels is also observed (Mertz, 1979). In biologic systems, chromium is found primarily in the +3 ionic state, although the +2 and +6 states also occur.

The most well-studied function of chromium is in the prevention of glucose intolerance. Earlier work led to the theory that chromium is part of, or necessary for, a glucose tolerance factor (GTF), a water-soluble component of liver, blood plasma, Brewer's yeast, and some other biologic extracts and cells. In early studies (Mertz, 1974), analysis of the semi-purified material from Brewer's yeast and liver suggested it was a complex of Cr^{3+} with two nicotinic acid moieties and three amino acids, especially glycine, glutamic acid, and cysteine. However, synthetic complexes of chromium made with mixtures of these components did not have the same degree of biologic activity as the material produced by living cells, such as the yeast. More tellingly, some GTFs isolated from yeast were found to contain no chromium (Haylock et al., 1983; Hwang et al., 1987), although others did (Tokuda et al., 1987). A 1 : 2 : 1 molar complex of Cr^{3+} : nicotinate : glutathione was also reported to have biologic activity (Nath and Sidhu, 1979). (Glutathione contains glycine, glutamate, and cysteine.) More recently, Yamamoto et al. (1987) have reported the isolation of an amino acid-containing (peptide?) component with chromium, from liver and milk (Mr 1500), which has biological activity, stimulating adipocytes to take up glucose and potentiating insulin action. The overall picture remains somewhat confused, although most everyone agrees that the element, at least indirectly, has a function in insulin action (and thus glucose tolerance) (Anderson, 1988; Offenbacher and Pi-Sunyer, 1988).

Indeed, it still seems likely that the direct or indirect action of chromium is to enhance the effectiveness of insulin. Evidence in support of this includes data from early studies with epididymal fat pads in which the insulin-stimulated uptake of glucose and galactose was enhanced by extracts from high chromium Brewer's yeast (Mertz and Roginski, 1963) by a mechanism that probably involves increased membrane recruitment of glucose transporters. Recent studies with human cells indicate that the density of insulin receptors is enhanced by chromium supplementation (presumably of deficient subjects) (Anderson et al., 1987). Also, supplementation of deficient total parenteral nutrition patients and other subjects has repeatedly shown the sparing of insulin needed for glucose tolerance (Anderson, 1988), and, concomitantly, that a high glucose intake increases concentrations of chromium in the plasma (especially in obese subjects with less glucose tolerance) (Earle et al., 1989) and stimulates loss of chromium from the body via the urine (Koslovsky et al., 1986). (Urine is the main excretory route.) This suggests that efflux of chromium into the blood enhances the effectiveness of insulin by increasing its binding to cells and the number of its receptors, but the molecular interactions that may be involved are still a mystery.

Chromium deficiency may also produce hypercholesterolemia, although the results of various studies have not been unequivocal (Offenbacher and Pi-Sunyer, 1988). All in all, the existing data suggest that when chromium deficiency is present, supplementation with high chromium Brewer's yeast or inorganic Cr^{3+} (versus low chromium Torula yeast) may improve not just glucose tolerance, but also serum lipids (see below). Here the mechanisms are even further from being understood. A possible clue may lie in the observations of Okada et al. (1983, 1984) and Ohba et al. (1986) that Cr^{3+} binds to chromatin in liver hepatocytes, enhancing gene expression, especially in the nucleoli. It is also remotely possible that in some form, chromium may normally inhibit liver hydroxymethylglutaryl-CoA reductase (the rate-limiting enzyme in cholesterol synthesis), in analogy with the action of vanadium (see below). However, in vitro, the effect of chromium can be stimulatory as well as inhibitory, depending on the concentration (Underwood, 1977).

Chromium levels in tissues and foodstuffs were first measured in the 1960s, but only quite recently did it become apparent that contamination readily occurs and that a host of precautions (including air filtration and siliconization of needles) must be taken to avoid it. As a result, we are somewhat in the dark about the actual chromium contents of most materials, and the earlier values are most clearly too high. Blood serum values, for example (now about 0.2 ng/ml) (Iyengar and Woittiez, 1988; Offenbacher and Pi-Sunyer, 1988), were previously thought to be eightfold higher (although some carefully validated recent values of 0.7–1.2 ng/ml have also been reported for subjects after a glucose load) (Earle et al., 1988). Either way, the concentration of chromium in blood is among the lowest (or the lowest) known for an essential trace element (Table 7.10).

In tissues (especially liver), chromium concentrations are probably much higher than in blood (on the order of 8 or more ng/g) (Iyengar and Woittiez, 1988). [Earlier values were in the same range (Table 7.10).] Recent analyses of hair have also given high values (45 ng/g), suggesting this as another route for chromium excretion (Grant et al., 1988). [Values for sweat were very low (0.05 ng/ml).] On the basis of recent data, chromium intakes range from 10–60 μg/day (averaging 25–30 μg) in self-selected American and European diets. This is one half to one third as much as earlier estimates (Kumpalainen et al., 1979). Ear-

Table 7.10. Possible Chromium Contents of Human and Animal Tissues[a,b]

Tissue	Adult man: American	Adult man: Nonindustrialized	Infants, American	Animals, wild and domestic	Male CD rats[c]	
Liver	0.02	0.04–0.17	0.54	0.16	0.009	
Kidney	0.03	0.10–0.72	1.6	0.18	0.006	
Heart	0.02	0.03–0.08	1.1	0.14	0.018	
Lung	0.20	0.17–0.32	0.85	0.24	0.009	
Spleen	0.02	0.09–0.22	1.0	0.48	0.031	
Aorta	(0.4)[d]	(0.13–0.6)[d]	0.4	—	0.029	(pancreas)
Muscle	0.03	—	—	0.11	0.030	(bone)
Stomach	0.03	—	—	0.07	0.14	(testis)

Source: Calculated from data of Schroeder (1973).

[a] μg/g, wet weight.
[b] Most of the values are probably much higher than actual but may still be qualitatively or relatively correct.
[c] Recent (more accurate) data from Verch et al. (1983). (Data for heart, pancreas, and testis were quite variable.)
[d] Numbers in parentheses were estimated, based on 2% dry/wet weight.

lier studies on human tissues (Table 7.10) suggested that intakes were much higher in nonindustrialized countries (and for wild animals). This must be reexamined, but is compatible with more recent data confirming the loss of chromium during refining of whole grains or sugar (from sugar cane) (Anderson, 1988), although the absolute values are lower. In a typical American diet (poor in whole grains), data suggest that cereal products, fruits and berries, milk and dairy products, and beverages (especially wine and beer) contribute equally to daily chromium intake, meats being a close second (Anderson, 1988). (Fish seems to have very little.) Data on Finnish foods (Anderson, 1985*b*) confirm earlier studies indicating that seeds (nuts, whole grains), raisins, Brewer's yeast, and some condiments (notably black pepper) are high in this element (Table 7.2). This again suggests that the earlier data are qualitatively and relatively correct. Levels may also be high (3–9 μg/g) in some plant parts and herbs (like blueberry leaves, artichokes, sage, and shepherd's purse) traditionally used against diabetes type II in herbal medicine (Muller et al., 1988). [Mushrooms, asparagus, and prunes also appear to be rich sources (Anderson, 1985*a*, *b*).] Vegetables and meats, as a whole, are not as concentrated in this trace element.

Inorganic chromium salts, even those containing Cr^{3+}, are absorbed very poorly (about 1%), and the same appears to be the case for dietary chromium. Amino acids, oxalate, and nicotinic acid (Urberg and Zemel, 1987) may enhance intestinal absorption. Chromium contamination (amounting to 12 μg/day) in some parenteral feeding solutions is probably more than sufficient to maintain normal glucose tolerance, even when losses are enhanced through trauma (Anderson et al., 1988). Urinary losses probably average about 0.2 μg/day (Anderson, 1988) (or less than 1% of an average intake of 30 μg). Supplementation increases urinary losses. Absolute daily body requirements may indeed be quite small, but dietary intakes may often still be insufficient. [It is one of the least toxic of trace elements (Venugopal and Luckey, 1978).]

Following absorption, chromium is probably transported on the iron-carrier protein of blood plasma, transferrin. In hemochromatosis (iron overload) when transferrin is saturated with Fe^{3+}, Cr^{3+} binding is reduced and the element is lost more readily in the urine (Offenbacher and Pi-Sunyer, 1988). The portion not binding to transferrin may partly be bound to albumin. Of added interest are observations that Cr^{3+} can complex with lactate (as well as HCO_3^- and citrate) (Wallaeys et al., 1988), which may explain the enhanced blood levels and urinary losses that accompany strenuous exercise (Anderson, 1988). From the intestine, most of the chromium proceeds to the liver, where some of it may be incorporated into a GTF. When blood glucose concentrations rise, and/or insulin is secreted, increased GTF and/or chromium flows into the plasma (Levin, 1983). This enhances the effect of the insulin secreted, and increased Cr^{3+} is lost in the urine.

The quantity of GTF or chromium released in response to an oral glucose load or glucose tolerance test (measured as serum chromium) may be a measure of nutritional chromium status (Canfield, 1979), although this remains to be established. Many individuals with marginal glucose intolerance (as well as many diabetics) display a reduced or absent release of chromium in response to oral glucose. Juvenile and adult-onset diabetics also generally have lower hair concentrations of chromium than normal adults. Whether or not responsive to chromium, diabetics may absorb chromium from the diet more rapidly than normal individuals and excrete it more rapidly in the urine.

Treatment of Glucose Intolerance with Chromium or GTF

By now, numerous studies indicate that, for individuals with various degrees of glucose intolerance, treatment with chromium (especially in the form of high chromium Brewer's yeast as compared with low chromium Torula yeast) has a significant ameliorating effect on glucose intolerance in a substantial proportion of cases (Canfield, 1979; Offenbacher, 1981). The results of three studies of normal and hyperglycemic women and of elderly men are summarized in Table 7.11. They show that supplementation with "GTF chromium" for 1–2 months significantly reduced glucose and insulin elevations. Inorganic chromium salts were usually less effective, perhaps because of a lower absorbability. [Parenteral Cr^{3+} works very well (see Chapter 14).] Alternatively, Brewer's yeast contains additional helpful factors. True diabetics, as defined by fasting blood glucose values of >140 mg/dl on more than one occasion, are just beginning to be tested (Levin, 1983) and the full story is not in. The initial studies indicate that type I diabetics (with a defect in insulin production/secretion) have elevated serum chromium concentrations, while type II diabetics (with impaired insulin action) are normal in this regard. The degree of postprandial increase in chromium was inversely related to fasting glucose levels in these patients, and in type II diabetics, there was some enhancement of insulin secretion upon long-term chromium supplementation. It should be stressed that, in the studies on glucose intolerance, not *all* subjects responded to chromium treatment. Moreover, in some studies (Offenbacher et al., 1985) most did not respond to chromium treatment, especially when their chromium intake was already greater than 50 μg/day (which is not surprising).

The most inexpensive means of treatment would appear to be the ingestion of 4–5 g of Brewer's yeast/day (about 45 μg Cr/g) (Anderson et al., 1983; Polansky et al., 1982). The effect is

Table 7.11. Effects of 1–2 Months of Brewer's Yeast (Chromium) Supplementation on Oral Glucose Tolerance and Serum Lipids: Sample Studies[a]

	Mean values			
Study/parameter	Before supplementation	After supplementation	Significance (p)	Percent improving
Total glucose[b]				
Normal women (15)	660	624	<0.05	73
Hyperglycemic women (12)	1065	982	<0.05	58
Total glucose[b,c]				
Normal subjects (17)	508	500	NS	
Possible diabetics (15)	648	551	<0.01	
Diabetics (38)	923	817	<0.001	
Intolerant elderly men (11)[d]				45–55
Plasma glucose (mg/dl)				
0 time	106	99	NS	
1 hr	201	162	<0.01	
2 hr	162	132	<0.001	
Insulin (μU/ml)				
1 hr	78	70	NS	
2 hr	118	83	NS	
Cholesterol (mg/dl)	245	205	<0.01	
Triglyceride (mg/dl)	121	112	NS	

[a] See Canfield (1979).
[b] Total blood glucose/dl at zero time and 4–5 additional times after 100-g oral intake, added together.
[c] Men and women.
[d] Men over 75 years of age with glucose intolerance.

not immediate and requires 1–6 months for a maximum response (Canfield, 1979). In contrast, the response to parenteral Cr^{3+} takes only a few days (Offenbacher and Pi-Sunyer, 1988), suggesting that absorption may be the limiting factor. Not only does a hyperglycemia tend to improve, but also a *hypo*glycemia, in terms of glucose tolerance (Anderson et al., 1983, 1987).

Chromium and Hypercholesterolemia

One of the symptoms of chromium deficiency in animals and man can be hypercholesterolemia, which can be reversed by refeeding the trace element. The mechanism of this effect is unknown. Several human studies (Canfield, 1979) indicate that supplementation with Brewer's yeast preparations (containing GTF chromium) lowers human serum cholesterol, usually by about 15%–17% (see Table 7.11). The effect appears to be greater among individuals with a plasma cholesterol exceeding 240 mg/dl (Canfield, 1979), and LDL cholesterol is reduced while high-density lipoprotein (HDL) cholesterol rises (Riales, 1979). Increased HDL and decreased LDL are associated with a decreased risk of atherosclerotic heart disease. Some experiments suggest that chromium deficiency in animals enhances atherosclerosis (Schroeder and Balassa, 1965). However, as with some of the other studies, interpretation of the results is confounded by the use of Brewer's yeast extracts that may contain other active factors, and by the need for really "clean" techniques leading to a better understanding of how tissue chromium levels correlate with, and respond to, such treatments.

Iodine

The importance of iodine (I) to human metabolism has been recognized since the last century (Table 7.1), although the helpful effect of eating seaweed or burnt sponges (rich in iodine) on goiter has been known since ancient times throughout the world (Cavalieri, 1980). Goiter, an enlargement of the thyroid gland (with hypertrophy and/or hyperplasia of the follicular epithelium), occurs in response to iodine deficiency. Even today, the only known role of iodine is in thyroid function, where it is part of tri- and tetraiodothyronines, which are the thyroid hormones (T_3 and T_4) (Figure 7.16). (Thyroxine is another name for T_4). However, the element is actively concentrated from the blood, not only by thyroid cells but also by those of the gastric mucosa, salivary glands, and choroid plexus (also lactating mammary gland) (Figure 7.17). This suggests other functions and may be especially interesting with regard to the brain, where the choroid plexus produces most of the "plasma" proteins destined for cerebrospinal fluid, and where transthyretin (the transport protein for T_3 and T_4) is abundant (see below).

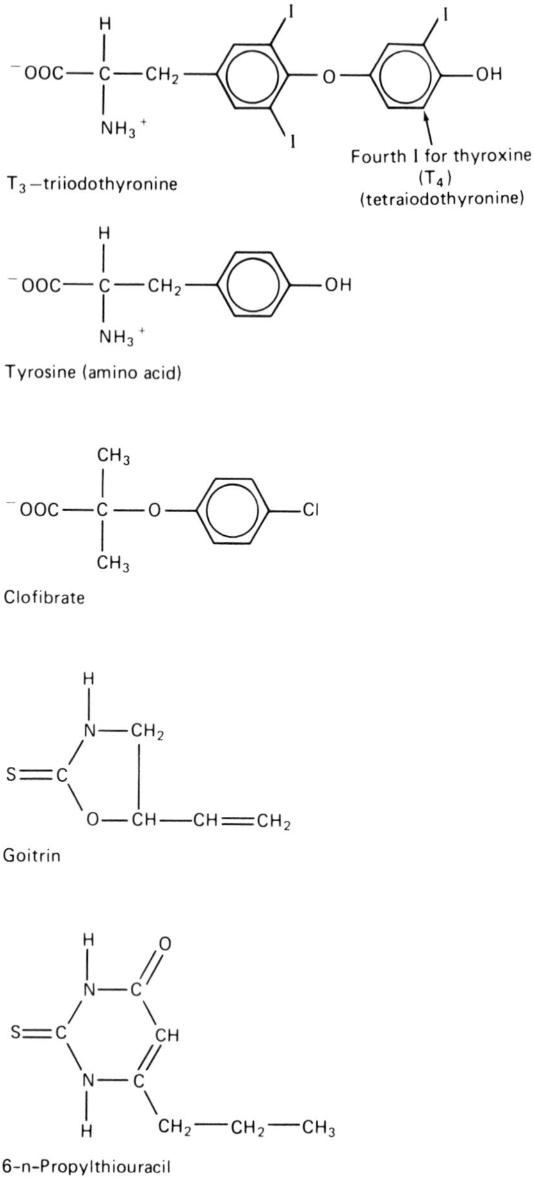

Figure 7.16. Structure of thyroid hormones and related substances.

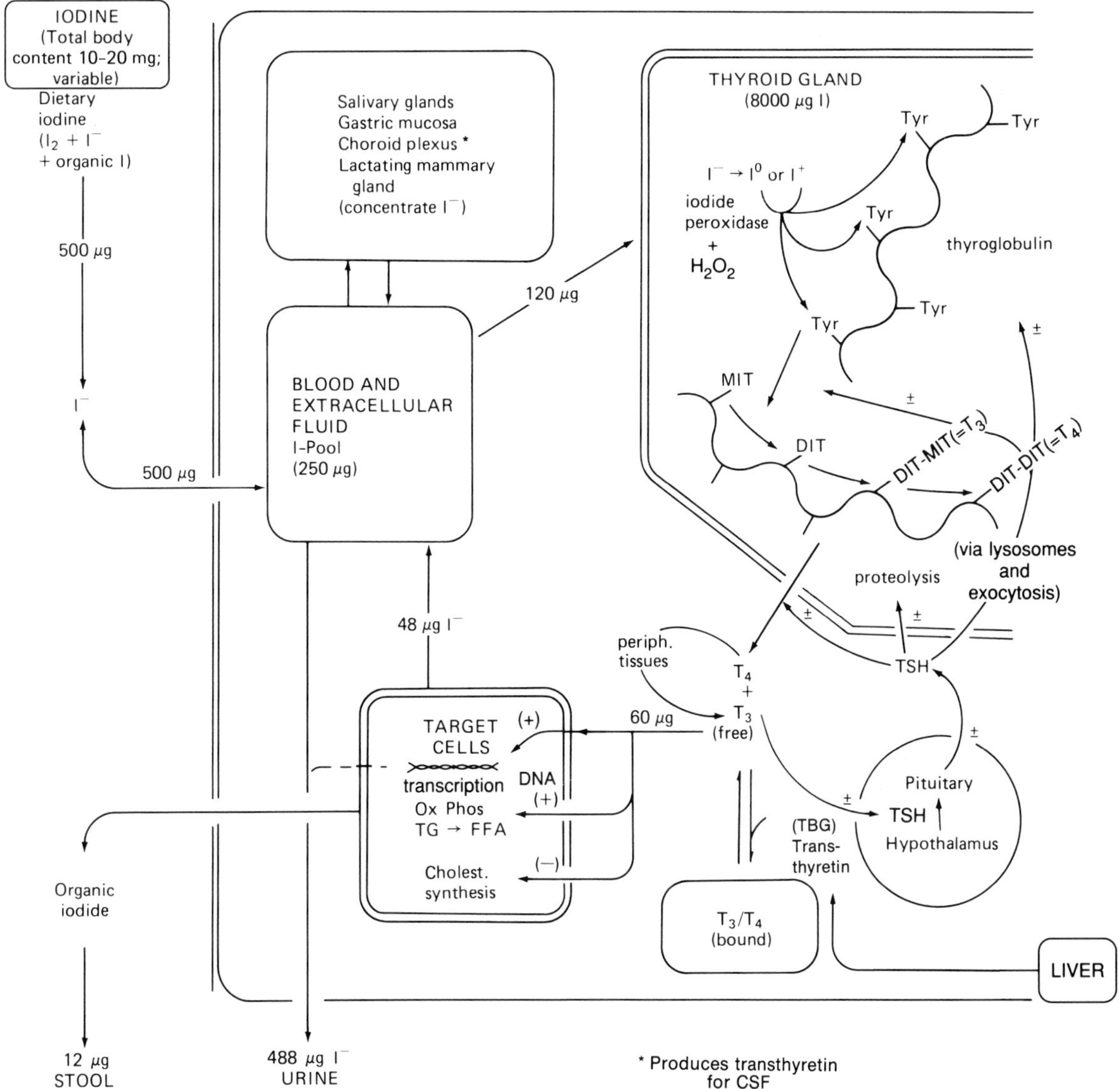

Figure 7.17. Nutrition and metabolism of iodine (total body content 10–20 mg, variable). Dietary iodine is efficiently absorbed and transported (mainly as I^-) in the blood plasma to several tissues that concentrate the element, including especially the thyroid gland. In the latter, I^- is oxidized and added to tyrosine residues on thyroglobulin, ultimately to form T_3 and T_4 for secretion into the plasma, where most becomes bound to transthyretin (made in the liver). T_4 is also converted to T_3 in peripheral tissues; and free T_3 in plasma is the active hormone form that acts on target tissues. Most metabolic effects of T_3 are probably mediated by enhanced transcription of specific genes.

Major food sources: marine fish and shellfish (0.8 μg/g), iodized salt. [Meat and vegetables are ~ 0.03–0.05 μg/g.]

Key: CSF, cerebrospinal fluid; T_3, triiodothyronine; T_4, tetraiodothyronine; TBG, thyroid-binding globulin; MIT, monoiodotyrosine; DIT, diiodotyrosine; TSH, thyroid-stimulating hormone; TRH, TSH-releasing hormone.

[*Source:* Based in part on Cavalieri (1980) and Hetzel and Maberly (1986).]

The specific functions of thyroid hormones are still not well understood, although it is clear that they do have effects on oxygen consumption and metabolic rate (see also Chapter 8). This has lead to the concept that they may be important in the regulation of basal metabolic rate (Chapter 8). The original observation of Lardy and Maley (1954), that at high concentrations thyroxine could uncouple oxidative phosphorylation in isolated mitochondria, and later observations on α-glycerol phosphate shunting (Lee and Lardy, 1965), suggested that the hormones might be acting directly or indirectly by decreasing the efficiency with which energy derived from catabolism could be harnessed to do anabolic work (production of heat versus ATP). At the same time, numerous studies have shown there is little or no change in the phosphate to oxygen ratio when whole cells or tissues are treated with iodine-containing hormones (Metzler, 1977; Oppenheimer and Surks, 1975). It is well established that thyroid hormones increase the number, size, and activity of mitochondria, in part by increases in the rate of synthesis of specific mitochondrial proteins (Oppenheimer and Surks, 1975). Total cellular protein synthesis can also be enhanced (Oppenheimer and Surks, 1975), although little is known about the specific proteins that are affected. The mechanism of many (or most) of these effects involves changes in transcription after binding of triiodothyronine to specific receptors in the nuclei of target cells (see below).

In parallel with those effects, thyroid hormones increase the utilization of ATP to accelerate transmembrane ion transport, especially that of Na^+. Oppenheimer and Surks (1975) have suggested that the actions of these iodine hormones on metabolic rate may indeed be only indirect, stimulating ATP use by membrane transport systems, which in turn creates an increased need for ATP production, for which the whole cell then mobilizes. This remains to be more fully explored.

Another effect of thyroid hormones may be to stimulate release of fatty acids from adipose tissue by enhancing local cAMP concentrations. This may result from an inhibition by T_3/T_4 of the cAMP-degrading enzyme, phosphodiesterase (also inhibited by caffeine and other methylxanthines). Similarly, thyroxine may inhibit the rate-limiting enzyme in cholesterol biosynthesis [hydroxymethylgutaryl-CoA reductase (HMG-CoA reductase); see Chapter 3]. This would explain why plasma cholesterol concentrations are influenced by thyroid (or iodine) status. [An analog of the thyronines, clofibrate (Figure 7.17), was used in the past to treat hypercholesterolemia in patients with advanced atherosclerosis (see Chapter 15).]

Consumption of iodine is highly variable in different parts of the world, but it is thought to average about 500 μg/day in the United States (about five times the RDA). (This is about the amount in 5 g of iodized salt, in the United States.) The richest food sources are seafoods (300–3000 ng/g), followed by vegetables, meats, and eggs (about 300 ng/g), dairy products and cereals (about 100 ng/g), and finally fruits (40 ng/g) (Cavalieri, 1980; Hetzel and Maberly, 1986). (These values are extremely variable and depend on soil, fertilizer, and food processing practices.) As a result of the abundance in seafood, the Japanese consume milligram quantities of iodine. In the United States and Canada, iodine is increasingly obtained through food supplementation (e.g., iodized table salt), as well as from medications and diagnostic agents.

In the gastrointestinal tract, dietary iodine is converted to I^- and is easily absorbed, where it is transported in the blood plasma and joins extracellular and intracellular iodide pools (Figure 7.17). Iodine enters the thyroid, where most of it is stored, and, after peroxidation, becomes attached to the tyrosine residues of thyroglobulin (670,000 daltons, containing 120 tyrosine residues). The hydroxyphenyl ring structure of a tyrosine residue is iodinated ortho to the OH group (Figure 7.16) to form mono and then diiodo tyrosine units (on thyroglobulin). These are eventually coupled to form triiodo and tetraiodothyronine units (still on the "mother" protein) that can be released as thyroid hormones (T_3 and T_4) by proteolysis (Figure 7.17). (T_4 is much more abundant than T_3). The "free" level of these hormones in the plasma is monitored by the hypothalamus, which then controls the rate of proteolytic cleavage of T_3/T_4 from thyroglobulin and release into the blood plasma, via thyroid-stimulating hormone (TSH). Plasma concentrations of T_4 greatly exceed those of T_3, and the latter is considered the active hormone. Most of the active T_3 is produced from T_4 by deiodination in non-thyroid tissues. Most of the T_4 and T_3 is bound to plasma proteins, mainly transthyretin (formerly known as thyroid-binding globulin or TBG), but the "free" T_3 is active on target cells, where it binds to nuclear receptors (Burnside et al., 1990; Bosselut et al., 1988). This stimulates transcription of certain genes, leading to cell responses that may explain many or most of the effects attributable to thyroid hormone. [Additional (extranuclear) interactions with cell structures/molecules may occur as well.] In target cells and liver, much of the hormone is then degraded and the I^- conserved for reuse, if necessary. As a consequence, a much lower intake of iodine than that practiced in the United States can be adequate for iodine and thyroid function.

Iodine deficiency reduces production of thyroid hormones, especially T_4, and reduces the rate of energy metabolism. Iodine deficiency (and the resulting reduction in available T_3/T_4) mobilizes the mechanisms for stimulating T_3/T_4 production (TSH) and iodine retention by the body. Concentrations of transthyretin, a prealbumin also involved in transport of vitamin A, are increased, and TSH stimulates synthesis of thyroglobulin. This directly or indirectly causes hypertrophy and/or hyperplasia of thyroid follicles. The resulting enlarged thyroid, or goiter, can usually be treated by giving dietary iodine. If longstanding, the only appreciable effect will be seen with thyroxine treatment (0.1–09.3 μg/day) (Cavalieri, 1980).

While iodine deficiency has always been present to some extent in goiter, it is not the only factor precipitating this disease. Genetic tendencies, including defects in enzymes involving iodine and thyroid metabolism, as well as intake of "goitrogens," also play a role. Goitrogens are present to a variable degree in many foodstuffs, notably rutabagas, turnips, and cabbages, and some of these have been isolated (Figure 7.16). They cause goiter by inhibiting the synthesis and secretion of thyroid hormones.

Iodine is a fairly benign trace element, which is thought to cause little or no apparent harm at 10–20 times the required daily doses (1–2 mg). Chronic doses tenfold or higher may be harmful, however, causing "iodine goiter" (Hetzel and Maberly, 1986). In animal studies, excessive amounts have been shown to inhibit thyroid hormone synthesis, and the same has been shown in humans with a hyperactive thyroid (Cavalieri, 1980). Thyroid necrosis has also been reported (India?) (Stanbury, 1988).

Vanadium

Vanadium (V) has long been considered a possible essential element (Curran and Burch, 1968; Hopkins and Mohr, 1974). This is partly because it does have pharmacologic effects at higher doses, but it is still quite uncertain that the element is required for normal health. Relatively little is known about its intake, functions, and metabolism. Available data suggest that at higher (probably unphysiological) concentrations it has inhibitory effects on a number of enzymes, notably ATP-hydrolyzing enzymes (including Na/K ATPases), glucose-6-phosphatase, alkaline phosphatase, and some enzymes of glycolysis (Nielsen, 1982, 1988). This might explain certain effects on bone and glucose metabolism that have been previously reported (see below). Orthovanadate $(VO_4^{3-})(V^{+5})$, formed from hydration of V_2O_3, has a similar chemistry to phosphate. Perhaps because of this, it accumulates at the sites of rapid mineralization of tooth dentin and bone, as shown by studies with $^{48}V_2O_5$ in mice (Soremark and Ullberg, 1962; Thomassen and Leicester, 1960). Indeed, it appears that vanadate may stimulate the activity of bone mineralization-promoting osteoblasts (Figure 7.18), possibly by enhancing the tyrosine kinase-mediated actions of other factors/hormones (see legend to Figure 7.18). [This might also explain some of its insulin-like effects (see below), and its potentiation of the action of certain growth factors (Carpenter, 1981).] Several studies in the 1950s indicated that V_2O_3, given orally or parenterally, would protect rats, guinea pigs, and hamsters against a cariogenic diet, but this was not confirmed by later work.

With regard to glucose metabolism, the vanadate ion $(H_2VO_4^-)$ would appear to be capable of mimicking most of the effects of insulin on adipocytes (Duckworth et al., 1988), although showing some preferential stimulation of the pentose phosphate shunt. As already mentioned, this may be related to a potentiation (or activation) of tyrosine kinase activity (Figure 7.18), induced by insulin in its receptors (or by other growth factors). (However, the effect may only occur at high concentrations.) The effects of insulin on *liver* enzymes and glucose metabolism appear also to be mimicked by vanadate (Gil et al., 1988), at least in rats and even in the absence of insulin. Specifically, normal glucokinase and phosphofructokinase concentrations (and activities) were restored in streptozotocin-treated diabetic rats by oral administration of sodium orthovanadate in isotonic NaCl (amounting to daily intakes of 77 mg/kg). (The hyperglycemia was also obliterated by this treatment.) This finding bears further study. Vanadium may also bind to glutathione (Degani et al., 1981); and Nielsen (1980) has reported that, in rats, vanadium deficiency symp-

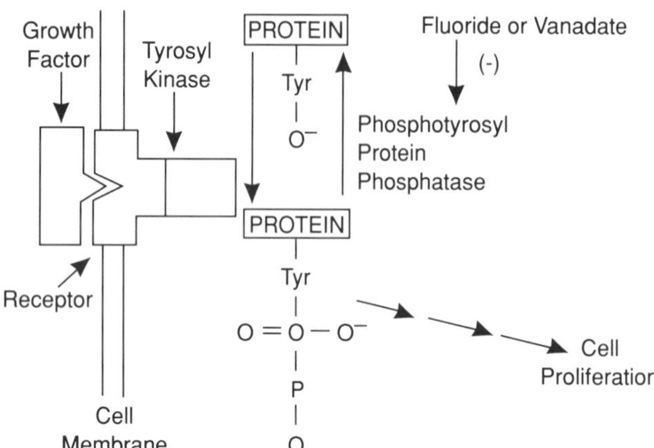

Figure 7.18. Possible mechanism of action of vanadate and fluoride on bone metabolism. Osteoblast activity is stimulated by growth factors enhancing tyrosine kinase activity and phosphorylation of specific proteins. This stimulus is counteracted by a phosphatase (phosphotyrosylprotein phosphatase) that removes the added phosphate. Vanadate (VO_4^{3-}) and F^- may inhibit this activity, thus potentiating the actions of growth/regulatory factors on the osteoblast. [*Source:* Modified from Lau et al. (1988).]

toms are alleviated by a high cysteine diet (cysteine is part of glutathione).

Another site of action may be inhibition of squalene synthetase, on the pathway of cholesterol synthesis (Curran and Burch, 1968). Further suppression of cholesterol synthesis may occur through stimulation by vanadium of acetoacetyl-CoA deacylase, diverting acetoacetate from cholesterol to keto acid production. In tune with this are observations that vanadium, given as vanadylate (VO^{2+}) or V^{5+}, suppresses liver cholesterol synthesis, in vivo and in vitro, in young rats and can lower plasma cholesterol in the same animals, as well as in rabbits and young human subjects. Vanadium is ineffective in older rats or humans with or without hypercholesterolemia (Curran and Burch, 1968; Underwood, 1977). A lowering effect on plasma phospholipid concentrations has also been observed (Dimond et al., 1963), and there may be a similar effect on plasma triglycerides, since vanadium-deficient chicks can display hypertriglyceridemia (Hopkins and Mohr, 1974). However, the overall effects of vanadium on lipid metabolism are not consistent, in that *increases* of total lipid and cholesterol have also been reported with vanadium supplementation in chicks (Hafez and Kratzer, 1976; Nielsen and Ollerich, 1973). (Is the chick different?) In any event, the various phenomena point to a role for vanadium in regulating aspects of lipid metabolism.

Finally, vanadium interacts with nonheme iron metabolism: as vanadyl (VO^{2+}), it binds to (and is carried by) plasma transferrin; as vanadate, it deposits in intracellular ferritin; but it does not interfere with iron absorption and is not incorporated into heme (Nielsen, 1987).

Our knowledge of vanadium has not progressed very much since the mid-1960s. From what little is known, the American food supply contains very low but variable quantities, about three orders of magnitude less than concentrations of copper or manganese (Table 7.1), most fruits and vegetables having less than 1 or 2 ng/g (wet weight) (Nielsen, 1987). Grains, meats, fish, and dairy products seem to have a bit more (5–40 ng/g) and a few more exotic foods and spices have higher quantities (dill seeds, parsley, black pepper, mushrooms, and shellfish, >100 ng/g). The efficiency of absorption may also be lower than that of manganese (which has a very low efficiency; Table 7.1). Little is known about our needs (if any) for vanadium, and whether the amount or type absorbed by Americans is adequate. Myron et al. (1978) estimate that institutional diets provide about 20 μg/day. Thus, it is impossible to say whether inadequate intake (of a certain form of vanadium) is a factor in the prevalence of hypercholesterolemia, hypertriglyceridemia, atherosclerosis, or any other disease.

Following its absorption from the gut, vanadium is probably first associated with low molecular components and later becomes attached to plasma transferrin (which also carries Fe^{3+}, Mn^{2+}, and Cr^{3+}) in the blood. Tissue concentrations are very low and almost impossible to interpret. Levels reported for human liver, for example, vary from 7.5–110 ng/g, those for brain from 30–130 ng/g (Nielsen, 1986; Schroeder, 1973; Sabbioni and Marafante, 1981). In the cell (e.g., in liver) some of the vanadium gradually becomes associated with ferritin, the major site for iron storage in cells (Sabbioni and Marafante, 1981). Some vanadium remains in low molecular weight form. Unlike iron, however, 80%–90% of vanadium is lost from the body through the urine.

Vanadium can also be absorbed through inhalation, a matter that has been studied in connection with the environmental impact of fuel combustion for production of electricity. This inhaled form of vanadium probably is also biologically available, and excessive exposure may be toxic. Potential toxicity from exposure to vanadium in industry has been of concern because the element is toxic at relatively low doses and because the element is so rapidly absorbed through the lungs and skin (Venugopal and Luckey, 1978). The importance of vanadium in various industrial processes, and its release into the environment, have resulted in many human cases of toxicity, involving sore eyes and bronchi, dermatitis, and other symptoms. Toxicity from diet is rare. However, 20–25 μg/g concentrations are sufficient to cause toxicity in experimental animals (Venugopal and Luckey, 1978).

An interesting aspect of vanadium toxicity is its depletion of ascorbic acid, and the counteraction of vanadium toxicity by this vitamin (Mitchel and Floyd, 1954). [Iron also can reduce toxicity (Nielsen, 1988).] Other aspects of its effects probably result from excessive inhibition of the various metabolic pathways already cited.

Tin

Tin (Sn) has been placed in the category of essential trace elements on the basis of its dramatic growth-enhancing effects when added to the purified "ultra-clean" diets of rats (Schwarz, 1974*a*, *b*; Schwarz et al., 1970). The basis for these or other effects of the element on metabolism is not known and has hardly been studied, although Schwarz had pointed out that tin is one of the few elements capable of forming truly covalent bonds and that it is well suited to forming coordination complexes with four to six ligands. As a result, it might be incorporated directly, or through complexion, into various biologic molecules, including proteins. The 0.13-V oxidation-reduction potential of Sn^{2+}/Sn^{4+} also puts it in the range of physiologically important components of electron transport, such as flavin-proteins/enzymes (Schwarz et al., 1970).

Schroeder (1973) has estimated that Westerners contain about 0.2 ppm of tin, or approximately 12 mg/60-kg body weight, with the highest concentrations in liver and spleen (Venugopal and Luckey, 1978). This amount is probably more than is found in persons from less industrialized countries, where there is less exposure to tin either from canned foods or the industrial environment (Venugopal and Luckey, 1978; Schroeder, 1973). In line with this, little or no tin has been detected in the fetus or newborn, though accumulation begins immediately after birth (Greger, 1988; Linder, 1978).

Americans probably consume between 1 and 38 mg tin/day (averaging 3–4 mg), mostly in inorganic form, the amount depending largely on intake of canned fruits and juices (the tin from the cans). Inorganic tin is very poorly absorbed from the diet, while organic forms are rapidly internalized. Absorption also depends on the dose, being as high as 50% for a 0.12 mg intake and 3% at 50 mg (Greger et al., 1981). What is absorbed is excreted partly in the bile and only a little in the urine (Table 7.1) (Greger, 1988; Venugopal and Luckey, 1978). At normal intake levels, there is no body accumulation of the element with age. Moreover, average intake values may be meaningless, as diets of fresh and frozen foods contain very little tin (typically 0.12 mg; Greger et al., 1981), whereas those with significant amounts of canned fruits and juices may contain as much as 50 mg. This is because fruit and fruit juices (pineapple, orange), and tomato sauce are usually placed in unlacquered tin cans (Greger et al., 1981), whereas other foods are not. At 50-mg intake levels, Greger has found that zinc balance (retention/absorption) is negatively affected. There are no changes in copper, iron, manganese, or calcium balance, although changes in iron metabolism (decreased hematocrits, hemoglobin, and serum iron) have been observed in rats fed 150 ppm dietary tin (corresponding to about 170 mg intake/person/day). Overall, the oral toxicity of inorganic tin would appear to be quite low, due to its poor absorption at high doses and the relative ease of its excretion. Many organo-tin compounds are much more toxic (Greger, 1988), perhaps because they are more easily absorbed; however, they are not normally prevalent in foods. In man, inhalation may cause a mild benign pneumoconiosis (a lung condition caused by dust), but reports of other forms of toxicity have been negligible.

Nickel

Nickel (Ni) is another element considered essential for mammals (Anke et al., 1990), although its functions are far from understood at this time. About 10 mg are present in the body of the average American (Venugopal and Luckey, 1978), with the largest proportions in skin (18%) and bone marrow (marrow and mineral matrix) (Nomoto, 1974) where concentrations range from 0.1–0.3 μg/g (Nielsen, 1987*b*). Liver and muscle concentrations (in the range of 0.08–0.1 μg/g) appear to be most responsive to levels of dietary intake (Moiseeva, 1973). Certain tissues (lymph nodes, testes) and hair have much higher concentrations (>0.5 μg/g), and nickel concentrates in sweat (⩾0.05 μg/ml) (Nielsen, 1987*b*). In the plasma, nickel concentrations are very low (Table 7.1), and the element is associated with albumin; with the low molecular weight (amino acid) fraction; and with a protein synthesized in the liver and named "nickeloplasmin" by Sunderman et al. (1972) (see below). Serum nickel concentrations rise in response to trauma—as, for example, after myocardial infarction (heart attack) (McNeely et al., 1971), in stroke, and even during labor. The significance of this response is not understood at this time.

During fetal development in rats, nickel is present in high concentrations in amniotic fluid (Kirchgessner et al., 1981) and is also high in fetal liver (Nielsen, 1987*b*). In contrast to other trace elements, the milk concentration *increases* during the suckling period.

Ni^{2+} is probably the main biologic form, and the ion coordinates with four to six ligands, as is common with neighboring transition elements of the periodic table (Figure 7.19). In vitro, it has shown an affinity for thiamin pyrophosphate, pyridoxal phosphate (vitamin B_6), porphyrins, proteins, and peptides (Venugopal and Luckey, 1978), and binding to RNA and DNA has also been demonstrated. It also binds to some of the same sites as Cu^{2+}, notably to the same high affinity, N-terminal-binding site on albumin (Glennon and Sarkar, 1982) and to free histidine (through the imidazole) (Asato et al., 1975). These associations may be clues to its in vivo effects on metabolism and more specifically to its involvement with specific enzymes. Kirchgessner and colleagues (Schnegg and Kirchgessner, 1978) have reported decreased levels of six liver dehydrogenases (DH) in nickel deficiency, including glucose-6-phosphate DH (involved in the production of NADPH via the pentose phosphate shunt), lactate DH (necessary for anaerobic glycolysis, especially in muscle), isocitrate and malate DH (part of the Krebs cycle), and glutamate DH (necessary for net release of nitrogen from amino acids). Most of these are mitochondrial enzymes. In this connection, nickel deficiency has been shown to alter hepatocyte and mitochondrial structure (Nielsen, 1980), especially the endoplasmic reticulum, which appears "unstacked" and disorganized, and mitochondrial respiration (with a re-

Figure 7.19. Periodic table of elements showing the relative position of essential and nonessential elements. (The lanthanoid and actinoid series have been omitted.) The symbols for essential elements present in greater than trace quantities are in large letters; those for trace elements currently recognized as essential are in medium-sized letters followed by asterisks and with the years in which they were first reported to be essential. Symbols for trace elements not currently known to be essential are shown in the smallest letters. Quantities (mg) of the trace elements found in the average 70-kg human are given in parentheses. [*Sources:* Modified from Linder (1978).]

H																H	He
(2.2) Li	(36) Be											(48) B	C	N	O	(3300) Fe* 1972	Ne
Na	Mg											(100) Al	(1100) Si* 1972	P	S	Cl	Ar
K	Ca	Sc	(9) Ti	(10) V* 1971	(3) Cr* 1959	(14) Mn* 1931	(4000) Fe* 17thC	(1.3) Co* 1935	(8) Ni* 1973	(110) Cu* 1928	(2000) Zn* 1934	Ga	(20) Ge	(14) As* 1975	(21) Se* 1957	(200) Br	Kr
(320) Rb	(340) Sr	Y	(340) Zr	(120) Nb	(13) Mo* 1953	Tc	Ru	Rh	Pd	(0.8) Ag	(34) Cd* 1976	In	(42) Sn* 1970	(6) Sb	(7) Te	(15) I* 1850	Xe
(1.4) Cs	(22) Ba	La	Hf	Ta	W	Re	Os	Ir	Pt	Au	(13) Hg	(7) Tl	(122) Pb* 1979	(0.2) Bi	Po	At	Rn
Fr	Ra	Ac															

duced oxidative capacity) and liver lipid content. Kirchgessner et al. (1981) reported decreases in pancreatic amylase. The concept of nickel-dependent enzymes in animal tissues is strengthened by the existence of "nickeloplasmin." This is unlikely to be a carrier protein in the plasma, since it only holds one atom of nickel per 700 kilodalton of protein and this is not exchangeable (Nomoto, 1980). Several actual nickel enzymes (or "cytochromes") have been identified in lower organisms (Nielsen, 1987*b*). The latter include the plant (jack-bean) enzyme, urease, which contains two atoms of tightly bound nickel per molecule (Dixon et al., 1976), as well as several bacterial hydrogenases. The nickel content (if any) of the mammalian enzymes mentioned has not been established. All of these findings suggest a role for nickel in intermediary metabolism. In the kidney (which is initially the most active organ in uptake), nickel associates mainly with a 15 kilodalton glycoprotein (Abdulwajid and Sarkar, 1983), with fragments of glycosaminoglycan, and with a 36-amino acid polypeptide (Templeton and Sarkar, 1985). In urine, some may be lost as a creatine–phosphate complex (Sayato et al., 1981).

The average American probably consumes 0.3–0.6 mg nickel/day, mainly from plant foods, as muscle meats are very low in the element (Table 7.12). This intake is well below the recommended intake of 50 μg/kg body weight proposed by Nielsen (1982) and based on animal studies. Average absorption is about 3%–10% (Nielsen 1987*b*; Venugopal and Luckey, 1978) and is enhanced during pregnancy (Kirchgessner et al., 1981). Absorption increases with dose and may involve the same receptors/mechanism used for uptake of iron and cobalt. The exact interactions between iron and nickel are difficult to interpret at this time, in that nickel deficiency can depress iron absorption and iron deficiency can enhance nickel absorption (Kirchgessner et al., 1981; Nielsen, 1981). Following absorption and distribution, at least 60% of daily nickel losses are normally via the urine. Some is also lost in the bile and considerable amounts can be lost in sweat (Nielsen, 1987*b*). The capacity to vary excretion of the trace element is probably important in maintaining its homeostasis and preventing toxicity.

Nickel is not a toxic trace element, unless inhaled in substantial quantities and in certain forms. (Nickel carbonyl and some other nickel compounds have been shown to cause lung cancer in several animal species.) Based mainly on animal studies, chronic excessive intake or exposure results in degeneration of heart muscle, brain, lung, liver, and kidney (Venugopal and Luckey, 1978).

Table 7.12. Cobalt, Nickel, and Selenium of Some Foods[a]

Food	Cobalt	Nickel	Selenium
Milk	0.03	<0.1	0.07–0.37
Whole wheat	0.75[b]	0.31–0.47	0.04–0.71[b]
Regular flour	0.36[b]	0.18	0.01–0.63[b]
Bran	1.2[b]	—	—
Germ	0.5[b]	—	0.01–0.77[b]
Other grains/ cereals	0.36 (corn)	3[b]	0.15–0.39
Nuts	—	1–5	—
Vegetables	0.2[b]	0.4+	0.01–1.2
Legumes	0.15	0.4–1.6 (3[b])	0.02
Fruits	0.14	0.11–0.2	0.01–1.0
Meats	0.2–0.5	<0.1	1.1
Fish/shellfish	1.6	1.5 (oysters)	0.5–1.5
Egg	0.10	<0.1	1.0
Sugar cane	0.03	—	—
Raw sugar	0.40	—	—
Molasses	0.25	—	—
Spices	0.52		0.24
Cocoa/tea	—	5/8[b]	—
Gelatin	—	5	—

Source: Data from Schroeder (1973), Venugopal and Luckey (1978), and Nielsen (1987*b*).

[a] μg/g, wet weight, unless otherwise indicated.
[b] On a dry basis.

Cobalt

Cobalt (Co) is an intrinsic part of vitamin B_{12}, and as such, is required for two enzymatic reactions central to mammalian metabolism (see Chapter 5): (1) synthesis of methionine from homocysteine to reform tetrahydrofolic acid from methylfolate and thus allow a normal flow of folate metabolism (and thymidine synthesis); and (2) conversion of methylmalonyl to succinyl-CoA, which is necessary for the utilization of odd-numbered carbon fatty acids and some amino acids. It is uncertain whether cobalt has any other essential functions. For one, ruminants, which can be supplied with B_{12} through synthesis by rumenal bacteria, appear to absorb only this form of cobalt (Underwood, 1975; Venugopal and Luckey, 1978). Similarly, cobalt supplied almost exclusively as B_{12} appears to be sufficient for cobalt homeostasis in man. Nevertheless, most of the cobalt normally absorbed is not in the form of B_{12};

likewise, only about 1/10–1/12 of the cobalt in the body is in vitamin form, and it is conceivable that inorganic cobalt may be released from B_{12} during its metabolism to enable other actions. Moreover, a cobalt requirement (other than as B_{12}) has been ascribed to the enzyme, glycylglycine dipeptidase (Venugopal and Luckey, 1978), and perhaps more importantly, inorganic cobalt is known to have important stimulating effects on erythropoiesis. It is noteworthy that this is not an effect of the B_{12} form of cobalt, which in itself is necessary for cell proliferation and erythropoiesis via its effects on folate and thymidine metabolism (see Chapter 5). Large daily doses (usually 20–30 mg, but up to 300 mg) as $CoCl_2$ (not $CoCl_3$) are sometimes used to treat anemias that are refractory to iron, folate, and B_{12} (Gardner, 1953; Venugopal and Luckey, 1978). However, such large repeated doses can also be toxic.

It is generally argued that the action on hematopoiesis is not an essential feature of human cobalt metabolism, but is simply a fortuitous one useful in the treatment of certain anemias. This argument is not "airtight." The mechanism would appear to involve an effect on the kidney that causes it to release erythropoietin, perhaps via stimulation of guanidine cyclase (to form cyclic GMP) and the release of lysosomal enzymes into the plasma (Rodgers et al., 1974). Bradykinin, another kidney hormone (involved in blood pressure reduction), is also released in response to administration of cobalt salts (Smith and Contura, 1974). In line with this, administration of cobalt salts has been shown to cause vasodilation and flushing (LaGoff, 1940), and Schroeder's group (Perry and Schroeder, 1954) was able to lower the blood pressure of eight of nine hypertensive patients by daily treatments with 50-mg oral doses over 10–65 days. (No toxic effects were noted.) This has not been pursued.

Also of interest is the possibility that cobalt has a role in thyroid function (Smith, 1987). An inverse correlation between cobalt availability in food and drink and the incidence of goiter have been reported for certain areas of the Soviet Union; and rat experiments have suggested cobalt may be necessary for synthesis of thyroxine (Blokhima, 1970). Moreover, excess inorganic cobalt intake has resulted in thyroid hyperplasia (Robey et al., 1956) (see below). These phenomenon should be examined further.

The question remains whether inorganic cobalt has a normal role in human metabolism, such as in the release of erythropoietin or thyroid hormone and prevention of hypertension. Although there are no documented cases of what might be considered cobalt deficiency (as seen in animals), even in areas where cobalt deficiency of ruminants occurs, Schroeder (1973) has shown that this element is less concentrated in the tissues of Westerners (with their refined diets, Table 7.2) than in wild animals (0.03 versus 0.05–0.2 ppm). Despite the report of a Scottish infant, living in a cobalt-deficient area, who had a marked geophagia (the urge to eat dirt or clay) that responded to cobalt therapy (Shuttleworth et al., 1961), the possibility of essential, non-B_{12} cobalt actions remains uncertain.

As already mentioned, cobalt salts enhance proliferation not only of bone marrow erythropoietic cells, but also of the cells of the thyroid when given in high doses. This is part of the general toxicity of cobalt that is evident in some people who have received frequent cobalt injections and/or excessive exposure other than through the diet. (Damage to pancreatic cells and heart muscle also occurs.) Injection of cobalt oxides or sulfides has been shown to produce proliferation of otherwise normal cells and to form cancer in animals and humans at the injection site, or in muscle or thyroid (Venugopal and Luckey, 1978). (This does not occur with oral intake.) Sensitivity to cobalt toxicity is much greater in children, where doses of >1 mg/kg body weight must be avoided. Toxicity is increased by ethanol ingestion and deficiencies of thiamin and protein, conditions that are common among heavy drinkers. Indeed, it is thought that the cardiotoxic actions of cobalt contributed to deaths among heavy beer drinkers in the days when cobalt salts were used to promote foaming of this beverage (Venugopal and Luckey, 1978). Intake of sulfur-containing amino acids ameliorated the problem. By reason of such potentially toxic actions, care must be taken in using cobalt salts to enhance erythropoiesis, especially in infants.

The average American probably consumes a very variable 5–20 μg cobalt/day, mainly from vegetables and whole grains (which contain no B_{12}) (Table 7.12). Variations in the levels of cobalt obtained for foodstuffs by different groups suggest that there are problems with the assay methodology. [Many reported values are orders of magnitude higher (Smith, 1987).] (This has not been fully resolved.) In contrast to the other essential transition elements (Figure 7.19), cobalt salts are almost invariably soluble in neutral and alkaline environments and are thus more easily absorbed into the intestinal mucosa, probably by the same transport system used by $Fe^{2+/3+}$. In line with this, iron deficiency enhances cobalt (and iron and lead) absorption. Indeed, at least in rats, iron status appears to be the main regulator of the rate of intestinal uptake of cobalt (and lead), except in acute conditions, such as during hemolysis or blood transfusion (Barton et al., 1981). The cobalt absorbed into the intestinal mucosa is not invariably transferred to blood, but may be lost when intestinal cells are sloughed off, especially with larger doses. Thus, the efficiency of overall absorption is inversely related to dose.

In the plasma, inorganic cobalt is distributed attached to albumin (Figure 7.1). It initially deposits in liver and kidney, and later in bone, spleen, pancreas, intestine, and other tissues. Tissue concentrations are very low (<60 ng/g) and actual values are somewhat uncertain, showing large variations (Iyengar et al., 1978). Nevertheless, liver, heart, kidney, and bone probably have the highest concentrations (Smith, 1987). (This contrasts with the preferential accumulation of B_{12}-cobalt in the liver, where excess is stored.) Excretion of inorganic cobalt is mainly via the urine, the rate of which is thought to be important in the maintenance of cobalt homeostasis (Underwood, 1977).

Boron

The possibility that boron (B) is an essential element for animals and humans was reinvestigated in the early 1980s by Hunt et al. (1983), who reported that chicks exhibited growth retardation (and an elevated serum alkaline phosphatase activity) when given a diet deficient in this element (<0.3? μg/g). Interest was heightened by preliminary studies in postmenopausal women (see below) suggesting that boron might be helpful in alleviating the tendency toward osteoporosis that accompanies decreased secretion of estrogen at this period of life. Nevertheless, an essential (or even helpful) role of the element in animals or man is far from proven at this time. Several rat studies with boron-deficient diets (0.15–0.16 μg/g) in the 1940s failed to demonstrate any pathological symptomology attributable to boron deprivation. As a consequence very little has been done to study the biochemistry, physiology, and nutrition of boron in higher animals and man.

What has been known for some time is that boron is an important and essential trace element for higher (vascular) plants (Aghulon, 1910; Nielsen, 1988; Warrington, 1923) and it is fairly abundant in our diet. In plants, boron is particularly concentrated in the leaves and fruits (Table 7.13), where it is thought to stabilize the cell wall and help to regulate its synthesis (Marschner, 1986). This may or may not explain how it promotes nutrient uptake by roots and its role in plant defense (involving "callose"). The molecular basis of most of its effects is its propensity to form stable complexes with *cis*-di-alcohols (Figure 7.13), such as with hemicellulose, phenolic acids (precursors to lignin), and mannitol (the sugar alcohol of mannose). Boron also forms a stable complex with 6-phosphogluconate. This may divert glucose from the pentose shunt (which in plants goes to production of phenols and lignin) to other fiber-forming pathways (Marschner, 1986).

The boron content of plant parts ranges widely (Table 7.13), but is much higher than that of human and animal tissues (except perhaps the thyroid). Legumes, fruits, and nuts appear to have high concentrations, but (as for other plant parts) will depend on soil content. Recent data on Finnish foods, U.S. diet composites, and other reports (Nielsen, 1988) indicate that daily adult intakes of boron are in the range of 1.7–4.3 mg/day. [Three U.S. reference diet composites (Table 7.13) had concentrations of 3.5–4.6 μg/g dry weight, which (multiplied by an estimated average intake) would calculate to about 1 mg/day, not including drink.]

Studies with boric acid in man, or vegetable boron in animals, indicate that absorption is very efficient, and that most of the boron in the diet (often 90%) is lost in the urine within 3–7 days (Nielsen, 1988). After absorption, boron is carried by the blood plasma to tissues and/or lost by glomerular filtration in the kidneys. Based on studies of human volunteers (Jansen et al., 1984), borate disappears into tissues (and probably urine) at three different rates, with approximate half-lives of a few hours, half a day, and about a day. [It is of interest that amino acid analogs containing boron (specifically borophenylalanine) also disappeared from the blood of hamsters at three different rates (Yoshino et al., 1989)]. Despite an efficient absorption, blood and tissue boron levels of animals and man are quite low, as already mentioned (Table 7.13). Kidney and liver concentrations are higher than those of blood and muscle. Boron also accumulates in bone, although we don't know in what form.

The function(s) of boron, if any, in the human body is (are) far from clear. Indeed, Nielsen (1988) has concluded that the only consistent symptom of boron deprivation seen in experimental animals is growth retardation. Nevertheless, indirect

Table 7.13. Approximate Boron, Lithium, and Aluminum Contents of Tissues and Foodstuffs (μg/g wet weight)

	Boron	Lithium	Aluminum
Human tissues			
Whole blood	0.15	0.005	—
Serum	0.20	0.011	0.005
Liver	0.4	0.007	1.0
Kidney	0.4	—	—
Lung	—	0.060	—
Muscle	0.10	—	0.3
Brain	0.06	—	0.6
Lymph nodes	—	0.20	—
Thyroid of sheep	(7.5)	—	—
Bone per g ash	(6–138)	(0.05?)	1.7
Several endocrine organs (rats)	—	(0.06–0.14)[b]	—
Foods (animal)			
Meats	0.03	Low	0.2
Fish	0.08	0.02–0.1	0.4
Beef liver	0.12	0.04	—
Milk	0.3[c]	0.0014	0.7
Seafoods	2–7	0.05–0.039	—
Foods (plant)[a]			
Vegetables	2	—	2–3
Leaves	7	0.030–0.084	25 (spinach)
Soymeal	28	—	—
Legumes		0.011[d]	—
Fruits			
Apples	70[e]	—	0.1
Pears	106[e]	—	—
Tomatoes	126[e]	—	0.1
Prunes	27	—	—
Raisins	25	—	—
Dates	9	—	—
Nuts/seeds			
Peanuts	18	—	0.2
Almonds	16	—	—
Hazelnuts	11	—	—
Grains	—	0.008–0.053[d]	5.4
Miscellaneous			
Refined flour	0.5	0.003–0.042	2–3
Honey	7	—	—
Brewer's yeast	6[f]	0.68[f]	—
Wines	5[b]	—	—
Herbs	—	—	400–750
US DIET-1	3.6[f]	0.060[f]	—
ARAS-1	4.6[f]	0.102[f]	—
IREA H9	3.5[f]	0.035[f]	—

Source: Nielsen (1986), Clarke et al. (1987*a*), Greger (1988), and Alfrey (1987).

[a] Based on dry weight: 85% or 90% wet weight for vegetables, milk, and fruits; 25% wet weight for grains and nuts; 70%–80% wet weight for meats.

[b] Refractory to dietary deprivation.

[c] Highly variable.

[d] Grown on low lithium soil (Mertz, 1986) (Values may be 1000-fold too high).

[e] Values from one report (may be high).

[f] Diet composites (Clarke et al., 1987*a*); values are per dry weight.

information suggests it may be a factor in bone mineralization: bone is a repository; deficiency increases serum alkaline phosphatase (a symptom of osteoblast/bone replacement activity); several very indirect observations also suggest that boron may ameliorate the actions of hyperparathyroidism induced by other deficiencies (Nielsen, 1988), and there is a hint of some interaction with cholecalciferol (vitamin D) (Hunt and Nielsen, 1981). Also, the boron content of bone and synovial fluid is reduced in rheumatoid arthritis (Ward et al., 1990).

Somewhat more convincing (but still tentative) are preliminary observations in Table 7.14 on the effects of boron supplementation in postmenopausal women. Several women were placed on a low boron (0.25 μg/g) basal diet for four 24-day diet periods (in which magnesium and aluminum intakes were also varied), then supplemented for two periods with 3 mg boron. The higher boron intake significantly reduced loss of calcium in the urine and increased concentrations of circulating estrogen (and testosterone). The two phenomena may be related, as estrogen can inhibit bone demineralization, and this might reduce calcium losses (see Chapter 6). (Resorption of blood calcium filtered through kidney glomeruli could also be involved.) These potentially important prospects could not be confirmed by Beattie and colleagues (Peace et al., 1990) with six volunteers postmenopause, using 21-day periods of a low B diet ±3 mg supplements. All in all, however, it seems possible that boron has a role in human metabolism. It is quite available in food and well absorbed. Moreover, blood levels appear to be quite constant, suggesting homeostatic control (Clarke et al., 1987*b*).

Table 7.14. Influence of Dietary Boron Levels in Parameters of Bone Metabolism in Postmenopausal Women

	Low boron diet (0.25 μg/g)	
	− Supplement	+3 mg B supplement
Urinary excretion of		
Calcium (mg/day)	121	86[a]
Phosphorus (mg/day)	620	600
Magnesium (mg/day)	89	64[b]
Serum levels of		
Estradiol (pg/ml)	17	36[a]
Testosterone (pg/ml)	320	680[a]

Source: Data are mean values for six 24-day diet periods, from Nielsen (1987).

[a] Significant ($p < 0.01$).
[b] Significant ($p < 0.05$).

Lithium

There is recent evidence that lithium (Li) may also be an essential element, or at least useful, for normal animal health and function. Rats (Burt, 1982; Patt et al., 1978) and goats (Anke et al., 1981, 1990) placed on diets very low in the element were less fertile (had fewer offspring) than those receiving amounts normally found in feed. These findings may be related to the observation that lithium tends to be retained by certain endocrine organs (including the ovaries, thyroid, adrenals, and pituitary) in the face of low dietary availability (Mertz, 1986). Growth rates were lower in the goats but not in the rats. Survival was also reduced. Lithium may also be essential for cultured cells (W. Mertz, comment about work of Herbert at TEMA-7).

What is better established is that lithium has useful pharmacologic effects in controlling the swings of manic-depressive psychosis (bipolar disorder), as first discovered by Cade in 1949. The mechanism of the pharmacologic effect is still unknown, but has variously been postulated to involve changes in production or turnover of cAMP or phosphoinositides via effects on G proteins in the brain (Avissar et al., 1988; Worley et al., 1988), and/or effects on cholinergic activity (Jope, 1979; Ortiz and Junge, 1978). What may also be relevant to this disorder is an inhibitory effect of lithium on activation of the glucocorticosteroid-receptor complex (Andreasson, 1982; Junker et al., 1984), an event that precedes migration of this complex to the cell nucleus to initiate transcription of certain genes. (Some of the symptoms of the manic phase of the psychosis can occur in conditions of excess glucocorticosteroid production, and Li^+ would be expected to inhibit the effects of the steroid.) Current recommendations for treatment of this bipolar disorder are to maintain blood lithium concentrations close to 0.8 m*M* (Gelenberg et al., 1989) to optimize psychosis control and minimize kidney toxicity (Gelenberg et al., 1987). This level of serum lithium (translating to 5.5 μg/ml) is about 1000-fold higher than what is normally found in human blood (Table 7.13). The doses needed for this are about 500 mg/day. Other actions of lithium may be related to blood cell function. There is a pump for Li^+/Na^+ exchange in red cells; neutrophil and platelet formation is stimulated by Li^+ (Joffe et al., 1984) (but does not promote leukemia; Gallichio, 1985).

Almost nothing is known about the food and tissue content of lithium (Table 7.13), although it is one of the most abundant elements in nature (Mertz, 1986). Plant and tissue concentrations appear to be low, and a rough calculation of total body content suggests there is less than 1 mg in the human adult (Table 7.1). As Li^+ (like Na^+ and K^+) is probably easily absorbed, this suggests that excretion is equally rapid. (Excretion is via the urine.) Intake is probably also low. Earlier estimates were about 100 μg/day, but it should be highly variable, depending on the region (soil and water), as well as food type. (Lithium is a significant component of "hard water.") Recent determinations on U.S. dietary composites (Table 7.13) giving values of 35–102 ng/g of dry weight, suggest much lower intakes (on the order of 10–25 μg/day), but this would not include the water. [Bottled (mineral) water samples can have 30–80 ng Li/ml (Allen et al., 1989).] The lithium content (or "hardness") of water has been calculated to relate inversely with the incidence of atherosclerosis (Voors, 1970) and even with the rate of homicides (!) in different regions (Dawson et al., 1972).

Lead

It is obvious that lead (Pb) intake is of concern not for its beneficial/essential effects on metabolism, but rather for its toxic actions, which can be especially damaging to children. However, animal experiments by Kirchgessner and Reichlmayr-Lais (1981; Reichlmayr-Lais and Kirchgessner, 1990) support earlier suggestive evidence (Schwarz et al., 1970) that even this trace element is required in small amounts for normal growth and health. A deficiency induced by feeding rats $\leq$50 ppb lead in the diet (versus 1000 ppb in controls) over one or more generations had its most pronounced effects on the hematopoietic system, producing a microcytic, slightly hypochromic anemia, accompanied by decreased iron stores in liver and spleen, as well as decreased growth (Kirchgessner and Reichlmayr-Lais, 1981); however, iron absorption did not appear to be impaired (Reichlmayr-Lais and Kirchgessner, 1985). Further studies are required. Other possible changes observed were decreases in liver catalase (a heme iron enzyme) and in liver concentrations of glucose, triglyceride, and phospholipid (not cholesterol). The biochemical bases for these various changes is unknown. However, there is evidence that lead may be transported on transferrin (the main plasma carrier for iron) and can bind to ferritin (the iron storage protein) intracellularly (Kochen and Greener, 1975*a*, *b*).

Excessive levels of lead in the organism also affect red cell (and overall heme) metabolism, inhibiting two enzymes of heme biosynthesis (δ-aminolevulinate dehydratase and ferrochelatase, which places Fe^{2+} in the porphyrin ring). This also results in anemia. Certain ATPases are also inhibited by excess lead (Vallee and Ulmer, 1972), and at least in vitro, mitochondrial respiration is severely depressed. Red blood cells tend to concentrate the element, and the resulting inhibition of Na^+/K^+ ATPase may result in their increased fragility, further contributing to the anemia of lead toxicity.

Because of its effects on porphyrin and heme production, lead can have widespread effects on energy and drug (or steroid) inactivation: Heme is needed for the cytochromes of mitochondrial electron transport, and mitochondrial respiration is inhibited in lead intoxication (Quarterman, 1986). Similarly, cytochromes are needed for the microsomal mixed function of oxidases (cytochromes P450 and *b*) involved in the metabolism and excretion of steroids and xenobiotics (man-made organic compounds); and the capacity to detoxify CCl_4, for example, is reduced. Reductions in heme synthesis and electron transport may thus account for many or most of the other symptoms of lead toxicity.

There is also a strong connection to calcium (and phosphate) metabolism, involving regulation of absorption (see below) and deposition in bone. More than 90% of total body lead is in the skeleton; and Pb^{2+} binds to intestinal calbindins (Barton et al., 1978), although its deposition and release from bone is not exactly parallel with that of Ca^{2+} (Quarterman, 1986).

Kidney tubule cells also appear to be special targets of lead toxicity, as tubular resorption is impaired, resulting in glycosuria and aminoaciduria. The capacity of the kidney to activate vitamin D (25-OH cholecalciferol $\rightarrow$ 1,25-diOH cholecalciferol) may also be affected (Mahaffey et al., 1982). Kidney damage leading to hypertension may be connected with toxic effects of lead as well, as suggested by studies of the "lead burdens" of hypertensive patients (Batuman et al., 1983). In the cells of kidney tubules, lead may associate with a sulfur-rich protein to form inclusion bodies in the nucleus (see Quarterman, 1986). Similar bodies may form in osteoclasts with excess lead.

There also are actions on the brain, resulting in hyperactivity and other behavioral problems in children, and stunted intellectual development (Harland et al., 1981; Ratcliffe, 1981). Children are more sensitive to toxicity because of their greater capacity for lead absorption. Urban underprivileged children are the most common victims, because they may eat the sweet-tasting white paint on the walls of old buildings, which contains lead. Some of the lead found in the body comes directly or indirectly from lead-containing gasoline, as demonstrated by the correlation between average blood lead concentrations and use of leaded fuels, both of which are declining (Annest et al., 1983). A 63,000-dalton lead-binding protein in brain and kidney may be a clue to the toxic effects of lead in these tissues. Lead displaces calcium from this cytosol protein (and vice versa) and may thus interfere with calcium action.

The average adult absorbs 5%–10% of the lead ingested in the diet, probably by the same mechanism as calcium. Absorption is much more efficient in infants and children (40% or more) and is stimulated by calcium and phosphate deficiency, probably all via increased levels of parathyroid hormone and formation of 1,25-diOH-D_3 (Mahaffey et al., 1982) (see Chapters 5 and 6). Conversely, adequate or high intakes of calcium depress lead uptake. Dietary levels of iron, zinc, copper, and lactose (Spickett and Bell, 1981) may also influence lead absorption (Quarterman, 1986), although the nature of these effects is still not clear. Fasting and food deprivation enhance lead absorption (Quarterman, 1986), as do diets high in fat and/or the direct feeding of bile acids and phospholipids (Tarugi et al., 1982). Absorption is made more efficient by lactose and may also be furthered by the lactoferrin and fat in milk. Phytates tend to suppress absorption.

Once in the body, lead is distributed via the blood, where most is sequestered in the red cells. As with calcium, most of the lead becomes deposited in the bone and the rest in soft tissues, notably liver and kidney. (Muscles retain very little.) With larger doses, bone, hair, liver, and kidney are especially affected. Lead is excreted mainly in the bile, with 10%–20% via urine. Chelating agents, like EDTA and penicillamine remove excess lead from soft tissues, but not from bone, where it must first be mobilized like Ca^{2+}, through the action of parathyroid hormone or glucocorticosteroids (Underwood, 1977). (Pregnancy, trauma, and infection will also mobilize bone lead.)

The average "Westerner" probably consumes 100–300 μg lead/day, although this is highly variable. The lead content of fresh foods is dependent on soil and environmental conditions and closeness to highways and roads (where volatile lead from motor vehicle exhaust is a major factor). Thus, no meaningful average values are available for various fresh food (Table 7.15). It is noteworthy, however, that lead is not concentrated in the germ and bran of whole grains, but is retained during processing of wheat into regular flour. The observation that Westerners accumulate lead slowly and gradually with age implies that the capacity for excretion is not adequate to maintain overall homeostasis. Nevertheless, the average level of intake probably does not represent a major risk to health. Rats, which achieve tissue levels of lead that are similar to humans, have shown no decrease in lifespan (Schroeder and Balassa, 1967).

Estimates of the total lead in the average American adult are in the area of 120 mg (90–400) (Quarterman, 1986; Underwood, 1977). Excessive intake of the element may occur, especially from canned foods and evaporated milk (where lead solder is still the most common sealing method). Repeated studies indicate that such canning increases the lead contents of vegetables, fruits/fruit juices, tuna, and milk manyfold (see Chapter 9, Table 9.12). The increased use of glass jars or seamless aluminum cans, especially for baby foods, is reducing the problem. Another source of extra lead may be calcium supplements made from bonemeal (R. Rucker, personal communication).

Assay of red call δ-amino levulinate dehydratase activity (or urinary δ-amino levulinate excretion) is probably the most sensitive and easiest measure of lead accumulation and toxicity, because of its accessability and the effectiveness of lead inhibition. Whole blood, and especially plasma, concentrations show much less variation with lead status, although levels of 0.4–0.5 μg/ml (whole blood) have been suggested as the upper level of normal for adults (0.25 μg/ml for children). Hair concentrations also show a correlation, but may be determined by outside contamination. (They are normally about 20 μg/g with >40 μg/g in chronic toxicity.)

Table 7.15. Heavy Metal Contents of Some American and English Foods: Lead, Arsenic, and Cadmium

Food	Concentration of metal (μg/g wet weight)			Ratio
	Lead	Arsenic	Cadmium	Zn:Cd
Milk	0.04	0.03–0.06	0.017–0.030	—
Whole wheat	—	0.18	0.05–0.10 (0.26[c])	121
Hard winter	0.50	—	—	—
Common soft	1.00	—	—	—
Regular flour	0.92	—	0.033–0.05 (0.38[c])	17
Bran	—	—	0.88[c]	113
Germ	—	—	1.11[c]	120
Bread				
Whole wheat	—	—	0.15[c]	35
White	0.41	—	0.16–0.19[c]	5
Rice	2[c]	—	3.2[c]	—
Corn	0.2–0.34	—	0.10[b] (0.035–0.15[c])	111
Potatoes	1.6	—	0.046	
Fruits and vegetables	1–12[a]	0.07–0.08[a]	0.016–0.08	13–65[c]
Meats	0.36–0.54[a]	0.10	0.08–0.24 (2–3.5[c])	15
Fish	—	2–8	—	—
Shellfish				
Clams	0.52–0.70[a]	—	0.19–0.27[a]	108
Oysters	0.47–1.11[a]	3–10	0.88–3.1[a]	460
Shrimp	—	42	—	—
Canned				
Fruits/fruit juices	0.02–8.2	—	—	—
Vegetables		—	—	—
Milk	0.20	—	—	—
Cola beverages	—	—	0.015	—

Source: Data from Underwood (1977) and Schroeder (1973).

[a] Range of means.
[b] 0.5 grown with sewage sludge.
[c] Dry weight basis.

Arsenic

The possibility that arsenic (As) is an essential trace element for mammals is suggested by a considerable number of studies in rats, goats, minipigs, and chicks (Anke et al., 1986, 1990). In these studies, diets containing 10–30 ng As/g induced growth retardation and lowered fertility (less conception, more spontaneous abortion, more mortality). In rats and chicks, there were also reports of rough hair, decreased hematocrits, and enhanced erythrocyte osmotic fragility, accompanied by enlarged and engorged spleens that contained abnormally high amounts of iron (Nielsen et al., 1975; Uthus et al., 1983). No differences in red cell metabolism were observed in the goats, and it has been suggested that the high arsenic content of control diets (2–4.5 μg/g) in the rat and chick studies had a pharmacologically favorable effect, producing the difference (Anke, 1986). In the rat, the highest tissue arsenic concentrations are found in red cells (Marafante et al., 1981), where arsenic has a special affinity for the globin portion of hemoglobin (Venugopal and Luckey, 1978). This prominence of blood arsenic is, however, peculiar to the species; in other species, including man, blood levels are no higher than those of other tissues, with hair, nails, and skin showing much greater concentrations.

Other potential effects of arsenic deficiency, seen in goats and minipigs, would include atrophy of heart and skeletal muscle fibers, changes in mitochondrial membranes, a reduction in skeletal mineralization, more tissue manganese, and less plasma uric acid (Anke, 1986). These various observations suggest, but do not prove, that arsenic is truly an essential element for man. As with lead and cadmium, its toxicity is more well known and a much greater threat than its deficiency. [Arsenic is present in our foodstuffs in concentrations much greater than those required to produce deficiency in animals (Table 7.15).]

Little is known about the specifics of arsenic handling and its metabolism by the body, except that it appears to have a special affinity for keratin, the mixture of proteins making up the horny layers of skin, hair, and fingernails. This would account for its accumulation in these parts of the body. In chickens, arsenic (given as inorganic ^{76}As) accumulated in skeletal muscle, liver, lung, kidney, and ovaries in decreasing amounts, as well as in the feathers, but was lost quite rapidly from the body (Anke, 1986). (Rapid turnover is also the rule in other species.) Arsenic has a special affinity for hydroxyl and thiol groups, which allows its interaction with hair and feathers and certain proteins and enzymes (Venugopal and Luckey, 1978). Some competition with selenium, perhaps at the site of absorption, also occurs, as selenium reduces arsenic toxicity, and vice versa, and an excess of one in the body depletes the other.

Despite the notoriety of arsenic as a poison, arsenicals have been important in medicine, and even today, arsenilic acid and nitrophenyl forms of arsenic are used to enhance the growth, health, and feed efficiency of pigs and poultry (Venugopal and Luckey, 1978; Underwood, 1977). (Here, the mode of action may be similar to that of antibiotics, low levels of which are routinely fed to livestock with the same effects.)

Various forms of dietary arsenic are quite readily absorbed from the diet and can also enter the body through the skin or by inhalation. Intake is quite variable and will depend on the proportion and type of seafoods consumed, the natural arsenic content of water, and environmental/work exposure. As shown in Table 7.15, seafoods, especially shellfish and shrimp, tend to accumulate this element in coastal waters. It is noteworthy, however, that Schroeder did not find higher tissue concentrations in the average U.S. adult than in wild animals, suggesting that industrial exposure and food processing are not major factors in determining body burden. Moreover, in Japan, where seafood is more prominent in the diet, intake is no higher than in the United States (0.07–0.17 mg/day), at least as far as the present data show. Estimates of American average daily intakes have varied from 0.06–0.09 mg in the 1960s (Underwood, 1977) to more recent values of 0.010 mg/day as determined by "Market Basket Survey." Frost (1978) has suggested that this may actually be inadequate.

Arsenic is excreted largely through the urine and mostly as methylated derivatives [especially dimethylarsenic (cacodylic) acid]. Because hair, liver, and nails show high concentrations, these should also be considered important excretory routes. Small amounts are lost via intestinal secretion. In general, it is thought that elimination is rapid enough to prevent toxic accumulations of the element, even when there is a high seafood intake or occasional exposure (Underwood, 1977; Venugopal and Luckey, 1978).

Chronic toxicity is characterized by weakness, prostration, aching muscles, gastrointestinal symptoms, peripheral neuropathy [that is, an increased rate of conduction for certain nerves (Valentine et al., 1981)], and changes in the pigmentation of fingernails and skin. Antagonism to thyroid function and stimulation of goiter production may also occur. The intakes required for toxic effects vary with the individual and with the forms of arsenic ingested, so no generalizations can be made. Detection of toxic body burdens or high intake is best achieved by monitoring concentrations in hair and urine, rather than those in blood.

Many animal and epidemiologic (human) studies have implicated arsenic as a carcinogen or cocarcinogen, especially for the skin, lung, and lymphatics. However, other studies have been entirely negative, and moreover, anticarcinogenic actions of arsenic, especially organic forms, have been demonstrated for "spontaneous" and chemically induced tumors in animals (see Chapter 16). Obviously, several other variables must be influencing the ultimate effects of arsenic, if any, on the outcome. [Selenium, too, has anticarcinogenic effects (Chapter 16), and its relative depletion by arsenic might promote carcinogenesis. This would only explain one aspect.]

Aluminum

Aluminum (Al) is one of the most abundant natural elements and is widely used to form pans and foils for food preparation, as an additive in processed foods (notably "American" cheese), and as an ingredient of antiacids and analgesics. It has also been a major contaminant delivered to many patients during kidney dialysis (Altmann et al., 1987). Despite its abundance, aluminum is relatively inert, biologically. Very little is found in plant and animal tissues (and thus in unprocessed foods) (Table 7.13). Even those plants that may be accumulators (certain herbs, like tea leaves, bay leaves, oregano, and thyme; Greger, 1988) do not have much of it in available form. Thus, while intakes are estimated to average about 3–5 mg/day (Alfrey, 1987), urinary excretion is only about 16–85 μg/day, or about 1% (Table 7.1). (Urine accounts for almost all the excretion of parenteral doses, only traces going to the bile.) Nevertheless, tissues do contain significant amounts of aluminum; and with high doses it will tend to accumulate especially in liver, kidney, and bone. (Levels in brain will also increase.)

There is no evidence at present that aluminum is an essential nutrient, although it does have biologic effects. Indeed, bone and brain appear to be the main targets when an excess accumulates. In the case of bone, aluminum appears to inhibit mineralization at the boundary between mineralized and unmineralized hydroxylapatite (Maloney et al., 1982). It also may reduce the proliferation and activity of osteoclasts (involved in promoting mineralization), by depressing release of parathyroid hormone (Dunstan et al., 1984; Greger, 1988) and will acutely depress intestinal phosphate (and fluoride) absorption. (Details of bone mineralization are covered in Chapter 6.) This condition is associated with considerable bone pain.

In the brain, excess aluminum accumulation has been associated with Alzheimer's disease and some other dementias, including that associated with kidney dialysis (dialysis encephalopathy). Although the association has not been consistent, it is clear that for whatever reason (or reasons) high brain aluminum can have dementia as an outcome.

Interest in the connection of aluminum to Alzheimer's disease began with the observations that the element was associated with the "neurofibrillary tangles" and "senile plaques" seen in the forebrains of such individuals (Perl and Brody, 1980; Candy et al., 1986). [The "amyloid" proteins involved have been under intensive study (Sisodia et al., 1990), and a defect in processing of the precursor membrane glycoprotein may be the primary factor in this disease.] At this time, some connection to aluminum intake cannot be entirely ruled out, although genetic factors must also be involved. [A recent survey of the incidence of this disease in various parts of Wales in relation to aluminum in drinking water did show a statistical association, and the authors argue that the form of aluminum in water may be more soluble and available (Martyn et al., 1989).

The molecular actions of Al^{3+} here are not known, although it can bind to brain calmodulin (Seigel and Hang, 1983), which should interfere with the Ca^{2+} activation of numerous enzymes; and it may enhance the activity of cholinesterase (Patocka, 1971), which would increase turnover of acetylcholine, the main neurotransmitter in these cells (also otherwise implicated in memory recall; see Chapter 5 under Choline). It has also been found in association with brain cell chromatin (Crapper et al., 1980). At least some of the excess aluminum binds to ferritin (Joshi, 1989; Fleming and Joshi, 1987), the main repository (and sequestrant) for excess iron (see Iron). Other potential sites of action include phosphate transferring enzymes (involving ATP and Mg^{2+}) (Sorenson et al., 1974).

The connections between aluminum and iron metabolism are not confined to the brain. Aluminum will be sequestered by ferritin also in other tissues; and in blood Al^{3+} is carried by transferrin (Alfrey, 1987), the main carrier for Fe^{3+}. There may also be a relationship at the level of intestinal absorption, in that iron deficiency may enhance aluminum absorption (Fenandez et al., 1990); and excess aluminum induces a microcytic hypochromic anemia (Alfrey, 1987), suggesting an interference with iron transport and/or mobilization (from ferritin). (The anemia can occur in the absence of iron deficiency.)

Cadmium

Evidence that trace amounts of cadmium (Cd) may be essential for normal growth, comes from studies of Schwarz and Spallholtz (1976), who found consistent, small (up to 13%), dose-dependent growth-enhancing effects of 0.05–0.5 ppm cadmium in rats on "ultraclean diets"; and very recent studies in goats by Anke et al. (1990). These observations are consistent with an essential role of the element in the mammalian organism, although at this time, it is not generally accepted that cadmium is essential. From its widespread use in our industries, contamination of our environment, foodstuffs, and bodies with this element is (as with lead) of much greater practical interest. Even if it were essential, cases of deficiency would not be expected to occur in Western society.

Two phenomena would, at least teleologically, suggest cadmium is not essential to the body: (1) it is very poorly transferred to the fetus (across the placental barrier); and (2) it is difficult to shed from the body (suggesting no mechanisms for its excretion). Also, concentrations of cadmium are very low in the tissues of wild animals and Africans versus Americans, especially in comparison with zinc (Schroeder, 1973), a trace element with which cadmium interacts. However, Anke et al. (1990) report that goats on diets containing less than 15 ppm of cadmium exhibited muscle weakness, mitochondrial pathology, and greater mortality than controls on cadmium-supplemented diets. Thus, the issue of "essentialness" remains to be answered unequivocally.

Cadmium enters the diet through most of our foodstuffs, although seafoods and grain products are especially rich sources (Table 7.15). [Part of the latter may be due to contamination of soluble phosphate fertilizers with the metal (Kostial, 1986).] It is estimated that the average American consumes 20–40 μg/day, which is under the maximum 57–71 μg intake limit suggested by the WHO/FAO (Spivey-Fox, 1983). On average, about 5% of dietary cadmium is absorbed, but this varies with iron status, being enhanced in iron deficiency. Absorption efficiency is also influenced by the relative concentrations of zinc and copper in the diet, in a competitive fashion. These ions may share an intestinal absorption mechanism; and induction of metallothionein in the intestinal mucosa occurring with a high intake of Zn^{2+} will trap Cd^{2+} (or Cu^{2+}) in mucosal cells, inhibiting transfer into the blood.

Once in the body, cadmium initially accumulates in the liver, but is ultimately transferred from this and other tissues to the kidney. Cadmium thus occurs mainly in the kidney (and mainly in the cortex), but also in the liver and to a much lesser extent in most other tissues, including bone and teeth. It is noteworthy that the half-life of kidney cadmium is 18–30 years (Spivey-Fox, 1983), underlining the difficulty experienced in getting rid of the element once it has entered the body. Only about 0.01% of the body burden is lost per day, and this is mainly in the urine (Kostial, 1986). Thus, cadmium steadily accumulates with age and accumulates mainly in the kidney, where it also causes most of the damage. Accumulation is in, and damage is to, the proximal kidney tubule, where resorption of small plasma proteins (like β_2-microglobulin and metallothionein) occurs (Friberg, 1984). Cadmium injury to this area eventually results in proteinuria. When concentrations reach 200 μg/g or more, damage appears to be irreversible. It has been estimated that a person consuming 200–300 μg Cd/day (about five to eight times normal intake) will reach such a critical kidney concentration by 50 years of age. Until that stage, metallothionein sequestration may be able to prevent toxicity (Kostial, 1986). Smoking (tobacco use) doubles the average daily cadmium intake and industrial exposure is also a factor. Critical concentrations have been exceeded in certain groups of people and by individuals in various parts of the world, notably Japanese women with "Itai-itai byo" disease, due to contamination of the food supply in certain mining areas. This form of toxicity manifests also in a painful osteomalacia, hence the "itai-itai."

Apart from kidney damage and osteomalacia (in women), excessive cadmium will cause growth retardation, impaired reproduction, hypertension, teratogenesis, and even cancer. Hypertensive symptoms are likely to be connected with kidney damage, as various aspects of kidney function can influence blood volume and pressure. Sodium and water retention are critically important for regulating blood volume (see Chapter 6); bradykinin is a small peptide hormone that reduces blood pressure by causing peripheral vasodilation (see also cobalt, above) and is formed in the plasma from precursor kininogens made in the kidney (and perhaps also some other tissues). Other possible related actions of cadmium are interference with catecholamine metabolism, and injury to cells of the artery wall (Kostial, 1986). These potential connections between kidney toxicity and hypertension prompted Schroeder (1973) to postulate that cadmium toxicity is contributing to the prevalence of hypertension (and atherosclerosis) in our society, today, a postulate borne out by epidemiology and animal studies. In particular, he suggested that the ratio of dietary zinc to cadmium (Table 7.15), and a similar ratio in the kidneys (Table 7.16), might be critical: animals and humans with hypertension have very low ratios relative to normal men, men from less industrialized societies, and

Table 7.16. Zinc to Cadmium Ratios in Kidneys of Animals and Humans

Population	Ratio Zn:Cd (kidneys)
Beef cattle	40
Pork	72
Wild deer	23–70
Coyote	54
Domestic dog	24
Humans	
Africans	6
Americans	1.5
Americans with hypertension	<1.0–1.4
Hypertensive rats (fed high Cd diet)	1.0–1.7

Source: Data from Schroeder (1973).

wild animals. The exact importance of this must be further evaluated.

References

Abbasi AA, Prasad AS, Rabbani P, DuMouchelle E (1980): J Lab Clin Med 96:544.

Abdulla M, Svensson S, Norden A, Ockerman P-A (1981): *In* Howell JMcC, Gawhorne JM, White CL, eds: Trace element metabolism in man and animals (TEMA-4). Canberra: Australian Academy of Science, p 14.

Abdulwajid AW, Sarkar B (1983): Proc Natl Acad Sci USA 80:4509.

Abumrad NN, Schneider AJ, Steel D, Rogers LS (1981): Am J Clin Nutr 34:2551.

Agget PJ, Harries JT (1979): Arch Dis Child 54:909.

Agulhon H (1910): Ann Inst Pasteur 24:321.

Alfrey AC (1987): *In* Mertz W, ed: Trace elements in human and animal nutrition (5th ed). New York: Academic, p 399.

Allen HE, Halley-Henderson MA, Hass CN (1989): Arch Environ Health 44:102.

Altmann P, Al-Salhi F, Butter K, Cutler P, Blair J, Leeming R, Cunningham J, Marsh F (1987): N Engl J Med 317:80.

Anderson BN, Gibson RS, Sabry JH (1981): Am J Clin Nutr 34:1042.

Anderson RA, Polansky MM, Bryden NA, Rogornski EE, Mertz W (1983): Metab Clin Exp 32:894.

Anderson RA (1985*a*): *In* Watson RR, ed: Handbook of nutrition in the aged. Boca Raton, FL: CRC Press, p 137.

Anderson RA (1985*b*): *In* Bostrom H, Ljungstedt, eds: Trace elements in health and disease. Stockholm: Norstedts Tryckeri, p 110.

Anderson RA (1988): *In* Smith KT, ed: Trace minerals in foods. New York: Marcel Dekker, p 231.

Anderson RA, Borel JS, Polansky MM, Bryden NA, Majerus TC, Moser PB (1988): J Trace Elem Exp Med 1:9.

Anderson RA, Polansky MM, Bryden NA, Roginski EE, Mertz W, Glinsmann W (1983): Metabolism 32:894.

Anderson RA, Polansky MM, Bryden NA, Bhathena SJ, Canary JJ (1987): Metabolism 36:351.

Andreassen PA (1982): J Steroid Biochem 17:577.

Anke M (1986): *In* Mertz W, ed: Trace elements in human and animal nutrition, Vol 1. New York: Academic, p 347.

Anke M, Groppel B, Krause U (1990): 7th international symposium on trace elements in man and animals (TEMA-7), Dubrovnik, May.

Anke M, Grun M, Groppel B, Kronemann H (1981): *In* Anke M, Schneider HJ, eds: Mengen-und Spurenelemente. Leipzig: Karl-Marx-Univ, p 217.

Annest JL, Pirkle JL, Makuc D, Neese JW, Bayse DD, Kovar MG (1983): N Engl J Med 308:1373.

Arthur JR, Beckett GJ (1990): 7th international symposium on trace elements in man and animals (TEMA-7), Dubrovnik, May.

Asato N, Van Soestbergen M, Sunderman FW Jr (1975): Clin Chem 21:521.

Avissar S, Schreiber G, Danon A, Belmaker RH (1988): Nature 331:440.

Barrett T (1976): Nature 260:576.

Barton JC, Conrad ME, Holland R (1978): J Lab Clin Med 91:366.

Barton JC, Conrad ME, Holland R (1981): Proc Soc Exp Biol Med 166:64.

Bassett ML, Halliday JW, Powell LW (1980): Dis Mon 26:1.

Batuman V, Landy E, Maesaka JK, Wedeen RP (1983): N Engl J Med 309:17.

Baumann H (1960): Hoppe-Seyler's Z Physiol Chem 320:11.

Becroft DMO, Dix MR, Farmer K (1977): Arch Dis Child 52:778.

Belisle J (1981): Science 212:1509.

Bettger WJ, O'Dell BL (1981): Life Sci 28:1425.

Blokhima RI (1970): *In* Mills CF, ed: Trace element metabolism in animals, vol 1. New York: Academic, p 426.

Bosselut R, Glineur C, Goldberg Y, Begue A, Ghysdael J (1988): Inst Natl Sante Rech Med 165:43.

Bremner I (1990): 7th international symposium on trace element metabolism in man and animals (TEMA-7), Dubrovnik, May.

Bremner I, Beattie JH (1990): Annu Rev Nutr 10:63.

Brewer GJ, Hill GM, Prasad AS, Cossack ZT, Rabbani P (1983): Ann Intern Med 99:314.

Brooks GA, Henderson SA, Dallman PR (1987): Am J Physiol 253:E461.

Bullen JJ, Rogers HJ, Leigh L (1972): Br Med J 1:69.

Burk RF, Gregory PE (1982): Arch Biochem Biophys 213:73.

Burnside J, Darling DS, Chin WW (1990): J Biol Chem 265:2500.

Burt J (1982): Ph.D. dissertation, University of Missouri, Columbia.

Cade JFJ (1949): Med J Austr 2:255.

Campbell CH, Linder MC (1981): Biochim Biophys Acta 678:27.

Candy JM, Oakley AE, Klinowski J, et al. (1986): Lancet 1:354.

Canfield W (1979): *In* Shapcott D, Hubert J, eds: Chromium in nutrition and metabolism. New York: Elsevier, p 145.

Carlisle EM (1974): Fed Proc 33:1758.

Carlisle EM (1982*a*): Fed Proc 41:1115.

Carlisle EM (1982*b*): Nutr Rev 40:193.

Carlisle EM (1986): *In* Mertz W, ed: Trace elements in human and animal nutrition (5th ed). New York: Academic, p 373.

Carpenter G (1981): Biochem Biophys Res Commun 102:81.

Castro-Magana M, Collipp PJ, Chen SY, Cheruvansky T, Maddaiah VT (1981): Am J Dis Child 135:322.

Cavalieri RR (1980): *In* Goodhart RS, Shils ME, eds: Modern nutrition in health and disease (6th ed). Philadelphia: Lea & Febiger, p 395.

Cerkewski FL, Ridlington JW (1988): *In* Hurley LS, Keen CL, Lonnerdal B, Rucker RB, eds: Trace elements in man and animals 6. New York: Plenum, p 273.

Chesters JK, Petrie L, Boyne R, Allen G (1988): J Trace El Exp Med 1:117.

Clarke WB, Webber CE, Koekebakker M, Barr RD (1987*a*): Appl Radiat Isot 38:735.

Clarke WB, Webber CE, Koekebakker M, Barr RD (1987*b*): J Lab Clin Med 109:155.

Cohen D, Ilowsky B, Linder MC (1979): Am J Physiol 236:E309.

Comens P (1960): *In* Seven MJ, Johnson LA, eds: Metal binding in medicine. Philadelphia: JB Lippincott, p 312.

Cook JD (1977): Fed Proc 36:2028.

Crapper DR, Quittkat S, Krishnan SS, Dalton AJ, DeBoni U (1980): Acta Neuropathol 50:19.

Curran GL, Burch RE (1968): *In* Trace substances in environmental health—I (Proceeding of University of Missouri Annual Conference). Columbia: University of Missouri Press, p 69.

Dallman PR (1986): Annu Rev Nutr 6:13.

Danks D (1981): *In* Howell JMcC, Gawthorne JM, White CL, eds: Trace element metabolism in man and animals (TEMA-4). Canberra: Australian Academy of Science, p 479.

Davidson DLW, Ward NI (1988): Epilepsy Res 2:323.

Dawson EB, Moore TD, McGanity WJ (1972): Dis Nerv Syst 33:546.

DeFranciscis P, Oliviero G, Greco AM, Maranelli C, DeMaira E, Monti G (1974): Clin Term 27:61.

Degani H, Gochin M, Karlish SJD, Shechter Y (1981): Biochemistry 20:5795.

Dimond EG, Caravaca J, Benchimol A (1963): Am J Clin Nutr 12:49.

Disler PB, Lynch SR, Torrance JD, Sayers MH, Bothwell TH, Charlton RW (1975): S Afr J Med Sci 40:109.

Dixon NE, Gazzola C, Blakeley RL, Zerner B (1976): Science 191:1144.

Doisy RJ (1972): *In* Hemphill DD, ed: Trace substances in environmental health—IV (Proceedings of University of Missouri Annual Conference). Columbia: University of Missouri Press, p 193.

Douglass JS, Morris VC, Soares JH Jr, Levander OA (1981): J Nutr 111:2180.

Duckworth WC, Solomon SS, Liepnieks J, Hamel FG, Hand S, Peavy DE (1988): Endocrinology 122:2285.

Dunstan CR, Evans RA, Hills E, Wong SYP, Alfrey AC (1984): Calcif Tissue Int 36:133.

Eaton JW, Brandt P, Mahoney JR (1982): Science 215:691.

Eipper BA, Mains RE (1988): Annu Rev Physiol 50:333.

Elwood JC, Nash DT, Streeton DHP (1982): J Am Coll Nutr 1:263.

Evans GW (1980): Nutr Rev 38:137.

Evenson JK, Sunde RA (1988): Proc Soc Exp Biol Med 187:169.

Fernandes G, Nair M, Onoe K, Tanaka T, Floyd R, Good RA (1979): Proc Natl Acad Sci USA 76:457.

Fernandez I, Gomez C, Fernandez MJ, Diaz JB, Cannata JB (1990): 7th international symposium on trace elements in man and animals (TEMA-7), Dubrovnik, May.

Fields M, Lewis CG, Beal T (1989): Metab Clin Exp 38:371.

Fields M, Holbrook J, Scholfield D, Smith JC Jr, Reiser S (1986*a*): J Nutr 116:625.

Fields M, Lewis C, Scholfield DJ, Powell AS, Rose AJ, Reiser S, Smith JC (1986*b*): Proc Soc Exp Biol Med 183:145.

Finch C (1986): Presentation at ISTERH symposium, Palm Springs, CA (December).

Fleming CR, Lie JT, McCall JT, O'Brien JF, Baillie EE, Thistle JL (1982): Gastroenterology 83:689.

Fleming J, Joshi JG (1988): Proc Natl Acad Sci USA 85:3786.

Flynn A, Strain WH, Pories WJ (1972): Biochem Biophys Res Commun 46:1113.

Foster SJ, Kraus RJ, Ganther HE (1986): Arch Biochem Biophys 247:12.

Fraker PK, Zwicki CM, Luecke RW (1982): J Nutr 112:309.

Fraker PJ, Jardieu P, Cook J (1987): Arch Intern Med 147:1699.

Freeland-Graves JH, Han WH, Friedman BJ, Shorey RAL (1980): Nutr Rep Int 22:285.

Friberg I (1984): Environ Health Perspect 54:1.

Frieden E (1971): Advances in chemistry, series 100. Washington, DC: American Chemical Society.

Friedman BJ, Freeland-Graves JH, Bales CW, Behmardi F, Shorey-Kutschke RL, Willis RA, Crosby JB, Trickett PC, Houston SD (1987): J Nutr 117:133.

Frost DV (1978): Adv Exp Med Biol 91:259.

Gallichio VS (1985): Exp Cell Biol 53:287.

Gallop PM, Paz MA, Fluckinger R, Kagan HM (1989): TIBS 14:343.

Ganther HE (1987): *In* Combs GF Jr, Spallholz JE, Levander OA, Oldfield JE, eds: Selenium in biology and medicine, A. New York: Van Nostrand Rheinhold, p 50.

Garcia-Aranda JA, Lifshitz F, Wapnir RA (1984): J Pediatr Gastroenterol Nutr 3:602.

Gardner FH (1953): J Lab Clin Med 41:56.

Gawthorne JM, Howell JMcC, Wyburn RS (1981): *In* Howell JMcC, Gawthorne JM, White CL, eds: Trace element metabolism in man and animals (TEMA-4). Canberra: Australian Academy of Science, p 553.

Geissler U, Gerloff J (1965): Nova Hedwigia 10:565.

Gelenberg AJ, Wojcik JD, Falk WE, et al. (1987): Acta Psychiatr Scand 75:29.

Gelenberg AJ, Kane JM, Keller MB, Lavori P, Rosenbaum JF, Cole K, Lavelle J (1989): N Engl J Med 321:1489.

Gil J, Mirapeix M, Carreras J, Bartrons R (1988): J Biol Chem 263:1868.

Glennon JD, Sarkar B (1982): Biochem J 203:15.

Golberg L, Smith JP (1958): Br J Pathol 39:59.

Goode CA (1991): *In* Linder MC, ed: The biochemistry of copper. New York: Plenum, in press.

Goode CA, Dinh CT, Linder MC (1990): *In* Kies C, ed: Copper bioavailability and metabolism. New York: Plenum, p 131.

Grant ECG, Howard JM, Davies S, Chasty H, Hornsby B, Galbraith J (1988): Br Med J 296:607.

Greger JL (1988): *In* Smith KT, ed: Trace minerals in foods. New York: Marcel Dekker, p 291.

Greger JL, Johnson MA, Baier MJ (1981): *In* Howell JMcC, Gawthorne JM, White CL, eds: Trace element metabolism in man and animals (TEMA-4). Canberra: Australian Academy of Science, p 101.

Grider A, Kao K-J, Klein PA, Cousins RJ (1989*a*): J Lab Clin Med 113:221.

Grider A, Cousins RJ (1989*b*): FASEB J 3:(abstract).

Hafez Y, Kratzer FH (1976): J Nutr 106:249.

Halliday JW, Powell LW (1982): Semin Hematol 19:42.

Hambidge KM, Casey CE, Krebs NF (1986): *In* Mertz W, ed: Trace elements in human and animal nutrition (5th ed), Vol 2. New York: Academic, p 1.

Hamer DH (1986): Annu Rev Biochem 55:913.

Hamilton EI, Minski MJ, Cleary JJ (1972–1973): Sci Total Environ 1:341.

Halsted JA, Ronaghy HA, Abadi P, Haghshenass M, Amirhakemi GH, Barakat RM, Rheinhold JG (1972): Am J Med 53:277.

Harland BF, Harwood JP, Thatcher RW (1981): *In* Howell JMcC, Gawthorne JM, White CL, eds: Trace element metabolism in man and animals (TEMA-4). Canberra: Australian Academy of Science, p 407.

Hawkes WC, Wilhelmsen EC, Tappel AL (1985): J Inorg Biochem 23:77.

Haylock SJ, Buckley PD, Blackwell LF (1983): J Inorg Biochem 19:105.

Henderson SA, Dallman PR, Brooks GA (1986): Am J Physiol 250:E414.

Henkin RI (1984): Biol Trace Elem Res 6:263.

Hetzel BS, Maberly GF (1986): *In* Mertz W, ed: Trace elements in human and animal nutrition, Vol 2. New York: Academic, p 139.

Hodge HC, Smith FA (1954): *In* Shaw JH, ed: Fluoridation as a public health measure. Washington, DC: American Association for the Advancement of Science, p 79.

Holbein BE, Jericho KWF, Likes GC (1979): Infect Immun 24:545.

Hopkins LL Jr, Mohr HE (1974): Fed Proc 33:1773.

Hunt CD, Nielsen FH (1988): *In* Howell JMcC, Gawthorne JM, White CL, eds: Trace element metabolism in man and animals (TEMA-4). Canberra: Australian Academy of Science.

Hunt CD, Shuler TR, Nielsen FH (1983): *In* Anke M, Baumann W, Braunlich HE, Bruckner C, eds: Spurenelement-Symposium. Jena: Friedrich-Schiller-Univ, p 149.

Hurley LC (1968): Fed Proc 27:193.

Hurley LC (1982). *In* Prasad AS, ed: Current topics in nutrition and disease, Vol 6. New York: Alan R Liss, p 369.

Hurley LS, Lonnerdal B (1982): Nutr Rev 40:65.

Hwang DL, Lev-Ran A, Papoian T, Beech WK (1987): J Inorg Biochem 30:219.

Iwata T, Incefy GS, Tanaka T, Fernandes G, Mendez-Bote CJ, Phi K, Good RA (1979): Cell Immunol 47:100.

Iyengar V, Woittiez J (1988): Clin Chem 34:474.

Iyengar GV, Kollmer WE, Bowen HJM (1978): The elemental composition of human tissues and body fluids. Weinham: Verlag-Chemie.

Jacob RA, Skala JH, Omaye ST, Turnlund JR (1987): J Nutr 117:2109.

Janjua KM, Ali S (1986): Pak J Sci Ind Res 29:422.

Jansen JA, Anderson J, Schou JS (1984): Arch Toxicol 55:64.

Jeejeebhoy KN, Chu RC, Marliss EB, Greenberg GR, Bruce-Robertson A (1977): Am J Clin Nutr 30:531.

Joffe RT, Kellner CH, Post RM, Uhde TW (1984): N Engl J Med 311:673.

Jope RS (1979): J Neurochem 33:487.

Joshi JG, Sczekan SR, Fleming JT (1989): Biol Trace Elem Res 21:105.

Junker K, Svenson M, Junker SJ (1984): Steroid Biochem 20:725.

Kelsay JL, Behall KM, Prather ES (1979*a*): Am J Clin Nutr 32:1876.

Kelsay JL, Jacob RA, Prather ES (1979*b*): Am J Clin Nutr 32:2307.

Keshan Disease Group (1979): Chin Med J 92:471, 477.

Kien CL, Ganther HE (1983): Am J Clin Nutr 37:319.

Kies C (1987): Nutritional bioavailability of manganese. Washington, DC: ACS Symposium Series 354, p 46.

Kies C, Aldrich KD, Johnson JM, Creps C, Kowalski C, Wang RH (1987): *In* Kies C, ed: Nutritional bioavailability of manganese. Washington, DC: ACS, p 136.

King JC (1990): 7th international symposium on trace element metabolism in man and animals (TEMA-7), Dubrovnik, May.

Kirchgessner M, Reichlmayer-Lais AM (1981): *In* Howell JMcC, Gawthorne JM, White CL, eds: Trace element metabolism in man and animals (TEMA-4). Canberra: Australian Academy of Science, p 390.

Kirchgessner M, Roth-Maier GA, Schnegg A (1981): *In* Howell JMcC, Gawthorne JM, White CL, eds: Trace element metabolism in man and animals (TEMA-4). Canberra: Australian Academy of Science, p 621.

Klevay LM (1973): Am J Clin Nutr 26:1060.

Klevay LM (1985): Atherosclerosis 54:213.

Klevay LM, Inman L, Johnson LK, Lawler M, Mahalko JR, Milne DB, Lukaski HC, Bolonchuk W, Sandstead HH (1984): Metabolism 33:1112.

Klevay LM, Forbush J (1976): Nutr Rep Int 14:221.

Klug A, Rhodes D (1987): TIBS 12:464.

Kochen J, Greener Y (1975*a*): Pediatr Res 9:323 (abstr no 399).

Kochen J, Greener Y (1975*b*): Pediatr Res 9:323 (abstr no 400).

Koller LD, Mulhern SA, Frankel NC, Steven MG, Williams JR (1987): Am J Clin Nutr 45:997.

Konijn AM, Carmel N, Levy R, Hershko C (1981): Br J Haematol 49:361.

Koslovsky AS, Moser PB, Reiser S, Anderson RA (1986): Metabolism 35:515.

Kostial K (1986): *In* Mertz W, ed: Trace elements in human and animal nutrition, Vol 1. New York: Academic, p 319.

Krishna G, Whitlock W Jr, Feldbruegge DH, Porter JW (1966): Arch Biochem Biophys 114:200.

Krishnamachari KAVR (1987): *In* Mertz W, ed: Trace elements in human and animal nutrition (5th ed). New York: Academic, p 365.

Krishnamachari KAVR (1990): 7th international symposium on trace elements in man and animals (TEMA-7), Dubrovnik, May.

Kumpulainen JT, Wolf WR, Veillon C, Mertz W (1979): J Agri Food Chem 27:490.

Kuvibidila S, Nauss KM, Baliga BS, Suskind RM (1983): Am J Clin Nutr 37:15.

Kuvibidila S, Dardenne M, Savino W, Lepault F (1990): Am J Clin Nutr 51:228.

LaGoff JM (1940): J Qual 38:1.

Lardy HA, Maley GF (1954): Rec Prog Horm Res 10:129.

Lau KHW, Tanimoto H, Baylink DJ (1988): Endocrinology 123:2858.

Layrisse M, Martinez-Torres C (1971): *In* Brown EB, Moore CV (eds): Progress in hematology, vol VII. New York: Grune & Stratton, p 137.

Leach RM Jr (1974): *In* Hoekstra WG, Suttie JW, Ganther HE, Mertz W, eds: Trace element metabolism in animals—2. Baltimore: University Park Press, p 51.

Lee Y-P, Lardy HA (1965): J Biol Chem 240:1427.

Leinfelder W, Zehelein E, Mandraand-Berthelot M-A, Bock A (1988): Nature 331:723.

Leure-duPree AE, McClain CJ (1982): Invest Ophthalmol Vis Sci 23:425.

Levander OA (1986): *In* Mertz W, ed: Trace elements in human and animal nutrition (5th ed). New York: Academic, p 209.

Levin SR (1983): J Biol Inorgan Chem 38:39.

Li ETS, O'Dell BL (1986): J Nutr 116:1448.

Lin IM, Lei KY (1981): J Nutr 111:450.

Linder MC (1978): *In* Stave U, ed: Perinatal physiology (2nd ed). New York: Plenum, p 425.

Linder MC (1983): J Nutr Growth Cancer 1:27.

Linder MC (1990): The biochemistry of copper. New York: Plenum.

Linder MC, Munro HN (1973): Enzyme 115:111.

Linder MC, Munro HN (1977): Fed Proc 36:2017.

Linder MC, Moor JR, Wright K (1981): JNCI 67:263.

Linder MC, Goode CA, Weiss KC, Wirth PL, Vu MH (1989): *In* Abdulla M, Dashtl H, Sarkar B, Al-Sayer H, Al-Naqeeb N, eds: Metabolism of minerals and trace elements in human disease. London: Smith-Gordon, Nishimura, p 219.

Linder MC, Houle PA, Isaacs E, Moor JR, Scott LE (1979): Enzyme 24:23.

Linder MC, Madani N, Campbell CH (1990*a*): 7th international symposium on trace element metabolism in man and animals (TEMA-7), Dubrovnik, May.

Linder MC, Lee SH, Lancey RW, Madani N (1990*b*): 7th international symposium on trace element metabolism in man and animals (TEMA-7), Dubrovnik, May.

Lipschitz DA, Bothwell TH, Seftel HC (1971): Br J Haematol 20:155.

Loeper J, Gay-Loeper J, Rozenzjn L, Fragny M (1979): Atherosclerosis 33:397.

Loeper J, Goy J, Fragny M, Troniou R, Bedu O (1988): Life Sci 42:2105.

Loeper J, Loeper J, Lemair A (1966): Presse Med 74:865.

Lombeck I, Schnippering HG, Ritl F, Feinendegen LE, Bremer HJ (1975): Lancet 1:855.

Lonnerdal B (1988): *In* Hurley LS, Keen CL, Lonnerdal B, Rucker RB, eds: Trace elements in man and animals 6. New York: Plenum Press, p 189.

Lynch SR, Beard JL, Dassenko SA, Cook JD (1984): Am J Clin Nutr 40:42.

Mack U, Cooksley WGE, Feris RA, Powell LW, Haliday JW (1981): Br J Haematol 47:403.

Mahaffey KR, Rosen JF, Chesney RW, Peeler JT, Smith CM, DeLuca HF (1982): Am J Clin Nutr 35:1327.

Maloney NA, Ott S, Alfrey AC, Coburn JW, Sherrard D (1982): Lab Clin Med 99:206.

Mann (1978): Secondary metabolism. Oxford: Clarendon.

Marafante E, Ede-Rade J, Pietra R, Sabbioni E, Bertolero F (1981): *In* Howell JMcC, Gawthorne JM, White CL, eds: Trace element metabolism in man and animals (TEMA-4). Canberra: Australian Academy of Science, p 162.

Marschner H (1986): Mineral nutrition of higher plants. London: Academic.

Marshall LE, Graham DR, Reich KA, Sigman DS (1981): Biochemistry 20:244.

Martyn CN, Barker DJP, Osmond C, Harris EC, Edwardson JA, Lacey RF (1989): Lancet 1:59.

Mason AC (1988): *In* Smith KT, ed: Trace minerals in foods. New York: Marcel Dekker, p 325.

May P, Williams D (1977): FEBS Lett 78:134.

McAuslan BR, Hannan GN, Reilly W, Whittaker RG, Florence M (1980): *In* CSIRO symposium on the importance of copper in biology and medicine. CSIRO: Canberra, Australia.

McConnell KP, Burton RM, Kute T, Higgins PJ (1979): Biochim Biophys Acta 588:113.

McNeely MD, Sunderman FW Jr, Nechay NW, Levine H (1971): Clin Chem 17:1123.

Mertz W (1979): *In* Shapcott D, Hubert J, eds: Chromium in nutrition and metabolism. New York: Elsevier, p 1.

Mertz W (1974): *In* Hoekstra WG, Suttie JW, Ganther HE, Mertz W, eds: Trace element metabolism in animals—2. Baltimore: University Park Press, p 185.

Mertz W (1986): *In* Mertz W, ed: Trace elements in human and animal nutrition, vol 1. New York: Academic, p 391.

Mertz W, Roginski EE (1963): J Biol Chem 238:868.

Messer HH, Armstrong WB, Singer L (1974): *In* Hoekstra WG, Suttie JW, Ganter HE, Mertz W, eds: Trace element metabolism in animals—2. Baltimore: University Park Press, p 425.

Metzler DA (1977): Biochemistry. New York: Academic Press.

Mills CF, Davis GK (1987): *In* Mertz W, ed: Trace elements in human and animal nutrition (5th ed). New York: Academic, p 429.

Milne DB, Nielsen FH, Lykken GI (1990): 7th international symposium on trace elements in man and animals (TEMA-7), Dubrovnik, May.

Mirsky N, Weiss A, Dori Z (1980): J Inorgan Biochem 13:11.

Mitchel WG, Floyd EP (1954): Proc Soc Exp Biol Med 85:206.

Moiseeva SG (1973): Sd Rab Leningrad Get Inst 33:122.

Moore A, Worwood M (1989): Br Med J 298:1248.

Moore JA, Noiva R, Wells IC (1984): Clin Chem 30:1171.

Moynahan EJ (1974): Lancet 2:399.

Mulhern SA, Koller LD (1988): J Nutr 118:1041.

Muller A, Diemann E, Sassenberg P (1988): Naturwissenschaften 75:155.

Munro HN, Linder MC (1978): Physiol Rev 58:317.

Myron DR, Zimmerman TJ, Shuler TR, Klevay LM, Lee DE, Nielsen FH (1978): Am J Clin Nutr 31:527.

Nath R, Sidhu H (1979): *In* Shapcott D, Hubert J, eds: Chromium in nutrition and metabolism. New York: Elsevier, p 241.

Nielsen FH (1975): Fed Proc 34:923.

Nielsen FH (1980): Adv Nutr Res 3:157.

Nielsen FH (1981): *In* Howell JMcC, Gawthorne JM, White CL, eds: Trace element metabolism in man and animals (TEMA-4). Canberra: Australian Academy of Science, p 593.

Nielsen FH (1982): *In* Prasad AS, ed: Clinical, biochemical, and nutritional aspects of trace elements. New York: Alan R Liss, p 379.

Nielsen FH (1987): FASEB J 1:394.

Nielsen FH (1986): *In* Mertz W, ed: Trace elements in human and animal nutrition, Vol 2. New York: Academic, p 245.

Nielsen FH (1988): *In* Smith KT, ed: Trace minerals in foods. New York: Marcel Dekker, p 357.

Nielsen FH, Ollerich DA (1973): Fed Proc 32:329.

Nienhuis AW (1978): N Engl J Med 304:170.

Nomoto S (1974): Shinshu Igathu Zasshi 22:39, 45.

Nomoto S (1980): *In* Brown SS, Sunder FW Jr, eds: Nickel toxicology. New York: Academic, p 89.

Nutr Rev (1981): 39:333.

Nutr Rev (1988): 46:348.

Nuurtamo M, Varo P, Saari E, Koivistoinen P (1980): Acta Agric Scand Suppl 22:57, 77.

O'Dell BL (1981): Phil Trans R Soc London B29:91.

O'Dell BL, Browning JD, Reeves PG (1983): J Nutr 113:760.

O'Dell BL, Browning JD, Reeves PG (1987): J Nutr 117:1883.

Offenbacher EG (1981): Diss Abstr Int B 41:3392.

Offenbacher EG, Pi-Sunyer FX (1988): Annu Rev Nutr 8:543.

Offenbacher EG, Rinko C, Pi-Sunyer FX (1985): Am J Clin Nutr 42:454.

Ohba H, Suketa Y, Okada S (1986): J Inorg Biochem 27:179.

Okada S, Suzuki M, Ohba H (1983): J Inorg Biochem 19:95.

Okada S, Tsukada, H, Ohba H (1984): J Inorg Biochem 21:113.

Oppenheimer JH, Surks MI (1975): *In* Litwack G, ed: Biochemical actions of hormones, Vol III. New York: Academic, p 119.

Oppenheimer SJ, Gibson FD, MacFarlane SB (1986*a*): Trans R Soc Trop Med Hyg 80:603.

Oppenheimer SJ, MacFarlane SB, Moody JB, Bunari O, Hendrickse RG (1986*b*): Trans R Soc Trop Med Hyg 80:596.

Ortiz CL, Junge D (1978): J Exp Biol 75:171.

Osaki S, Johnson DA (1969): J Biol Chem 244:5757.

Patocka J (1971): Acta Biol Med Ger 26:845.

Patt EI, Pickett EE, O'Dell BL (1978): Bioinorg Chem 9:299.

Peace H, Loveridge N, Reid D, Beattie JH (1990): 7th international symposium on trace element metabolism in man and animals (TEMA-7), Dubrovnik, May.

Petering DH (1980): *In* Sigel H, ed: Metal ions in biological systems, Vol II. New York: Marcel Dekker, p 197.

Polansky MM, Anderson RA, Bryden NA, Glinsmann WH (1982): Fed Proc 41:391.

Pond FR, Tripp MJ, Wu ASH, Whanger PD, Oldfield JE (1981): *In* Howell JMcC, Gawthorne JM, White CL, eds: Trace element metabolism in man and animals (TEMA-4). Canberra: Australian Academy of Science, p 365.

Pories WJ, Henzel JH, Rob CG, Strain WH (1967): Lancet 1:121.

Porter KG, McMaster D, Elmes ME, Love AM (1977): Lancet 2:774.

Powell LW, Halliday JW (1978). *In* Powell LW, ed: Metals and the liver. New York: Marcel Dekker, p 145.

Powell LW, Halliday JW (1982): Viewpoint Digest Dis 14:13.

Prasad AS, Brewer GJ, Schoemaker EB, Rabbani P (1978): JAMA 240:2166.

Prohaska JR, Heller L (1982): J Nutr 112:2142.

Prohaska JR, Lukasewycz OA (1981): Science 213:559.

Prohaska JR, Lukasewycz OA (1990): Adv Exp Med Biol (Antioxid Nutr Immune Funct) 262:123.

Quarterman J (1986): *In* Mertz W, ed: Trace elements in human and animal nutrition (5th ed). New York: Academic, p 281.

Rabinowitz MB, Gonick HC, Levin SR, Davidson MB (1983): Diabetes Care 6:319.

Raja KB, Simpson RJ, Peters TJ (1989): Br J Haematol 73:254.

Rajagopalan KV (1988): Annu Rev Nutr 8:401.

Raju KS, Alessandri O, Ziche M, Gullino P (1982): JNCI 69:1183.

Ratcliffe JM (1981): Lead in man and the environment. Chichester, UK: Ellis Harwood.

Reichlmayr-Lais MM, Eder K, Kirchgessner M (1990): 7th international symposium on trace elements in man and animals (TEMA-7), Dubrovnik, May.

Reichlmayr-Lais MM, Kirchgessner M (1985): *In* Hurley LS, Keen CL, Lonnerdal B, Rucker RB, eds: Trace elements in man and animals 6. New York: Plenum.

Reichlmayr-Lais MM, Kirchgessner M (1990): 7th international symposium on trace elements in man and animals (TEMA-7), Dubrovnik, May.

Reiser S, Smith JC, Mertz W, Holbrook JT, Schonfield DJ, Powell AS, Canfield WK, Canary JJ (1985): Am J Clin Nutr 42:242.

Riales R (1979): *In* Shapcott D, Hubert J, eds: Chromium in nutrition and metabolism. New York: Elsevier, p 109.

Richardson T (1976): J Pharm Pharmacol 28:666.

Robey JS, Veazey PM, Crawford JD (1956): N Engl J Med 255:955.

Rodgers GM, Fisher JW, George WJ (1974): Biochem Biophys Res Commun 59:979.

Roeser HP, Lee GR, Nacht S, Cartwright GE (1970): J Clin Invest 49:2408.

Sabbioni E, Marafante E (1981): *In* Howell JMcC, Gawthorne JM, White CL, eds: Trace element metabolism in man and animals (TEMA-4). Canberra: Australian Academy of Science, p 629.

Salin ML, McCord JM (1977): *In* Michelson AM, McCord JM, Fridovich I, eds: Superoxide and superoxide dismutases. New York: Academic, p 257.

Salonen JT (1985): *In* Bostrom H, Ljungstedt N, eds: Trace elements in health and disease. Stockholm: Almqvist and Wiksell International, p 172.

Saner G (1980): Chromium in deficiency and disease. New York: Alan R Liss.

Sass-Kortsak A (1965): Adv Clin Chem 8:1.

Sayato Y, Nakamuro K, Matsui S, Tanimura A (1981): J Pharmacobio-Dyn 4:S-73.

Schiaffonati L, Rappocciolo E, Tacchini L, Bardella L, Arosio P, Cozzi A, Cantu GB, Cairo G (1988): J Exp Mol Pathol 48:174.

Schnegg A, Kirchgessner M (1978): *In* Kirchgessner M, ed: Trace element metabolism in man and animals (TEMA-3). Washington, DC: US Department of Health, Education, and Welfare, p 236.

Schroeder HA (1973): The trace elements and man. Old Greenwich, CT: Devin-Adair.

Schroeder HA, Balassa JJ (1965): Am J Physiol 209:433.

Schroeder HA, Balassa JJ (1967): J Nutr 92:235.

Schwarz K (1974*a*): Fed Proc 33:1748.

Schwarz K (1974*b*): *In* Hoekstra HG, Suttie JW, Ganther HE, Mertz W, eds: Trace element metabolism in animals—2. Baltimore: University Park Press, p 355.

Schwarz K (1977): Lancet 1:454.

Schwarz K, Foltz CM (1958): J Biol Chem 233:245.

Schwarz K, Mertz W (1959): Arch Biochem Biophys 85:292.

Schwarz K, Spallholtz J (1976): Fed Proc 35:255.

Schwarz K, Milne DB, Vineyard E (1970): Biochem Biophys Res Commun 40:22.

Schwarz K, Ricci BA, Punsar S, Karvonen MJ (1977): Lancet 1:538.

Seelig MS (1973): Am J Clin Nutr 26:657.

Shaw JH, Sweeney EA (1980): *In* Goodhart RS, Shils ME, eds: Modern nutrition in health and disease (6th ed). Philadelphia: Lea & Febiger, p 855.

Shuttleworth DS, Cameron RS, Alderman G, Babin HD (1961): Practitioner 186:760.

Sibille JC, Ciriolo M, Kondo H, Crichton RR, Aisen P (1989*a*): Biochem J 262:685.

Sibille JC, Kondo H, Aisen P (1988): Hepatology 8:296.

Sibille JC, Kondo H, Aisen P (1989*b*): Biochim Biophys Acta 1010:204.

Siegel N, Hang A (1983): Biochim Biophys Acta 744:36.

Siimes MA, Dallman PR (1974): Br J Haematol 28:7.

Simon M, MacPhail P, Bothwell T, Lyons G, Baynes R, Torrance J (1987): Br J Haematol 65:239.

Sisodia SS, Koo EH, Beyreuther K, Unterbeck A, Price DL (1990): Science 248;492.

Smith AM, Picciano MF, Milner JA (1982): Am J Clin Nutr 35:521.

Smith RJ, Contura JF (1974): Biochem Pharmacol 23:1095.

Smith RM (1987): *In* Mertz W, ed: Trace elements in human and animal nutrition, Vol 2. New York: Academic, p 143.

Smith CG, Saedi MS, Sunde RA (1989): FASEB J 3:A451.

Solomons NW (1981): Nutrition in the 1980s: Constraints on our knowledge. New York: Alan R Liss, p 97.

Solomons NW (1988): *In* Shils M, Young V, eds: Modern nutrition in health and disease. Philadelphia: Lea & Febiger, p 238.

Solomons NW, Jacob RA, Pineda O (1979): J Lab Clin Med 94:335.

Sonsma T, Hixon T, McWilliams K, Linder MC (1981): *In* Howell JMcC, Gawthorne JM, White CL, eds: Trace element metabolism in man and animals (TEMA-4). Canberra: Australian Academy of Science, p 145.

Soremark R, Ullberg S (1962): *In* Fried M, ed: Use of radioisotopes in animal biology and the medical sciences, Vol 2. New York: Academic.

Sorenson JRJ, ed (1982): Inflammatory disease and copper. Clifton, NJ: Humana Press.

Sorenson JRJ, Campbell IR, Teper LB, Lingg RD (1974): Environ Health Perspect 8:3.

Spickett JT, Bell RR (1981): *In* Howell JMcC, Gawthorne JM, White CL, eds: Trace element metabolism in man and animals (TEMA-4). Canberra: Australian Academy of Science, p 420.

Spivey-Fox MR (1983): Fed Proc 42:1726.

Stanbury JB (1988): *In* Shils M, Young V, eds: Modern nutrition in health and disease. Philadelphia: Lea & Febiger, p 227.

Stemmer KL, Petering HG, Murthy L, Finelli VN, Menden EE (1985): Ann Nutr Metab 29:332.

Stocks P, Davies RI (1964): Br J Cancer 18:14.

Strause LG, Saltman P (1987): *In* ACS Symposium Series 354. Washington, DC: American Chemical Society, p 46.

Strause LG, Hegenauer J, Saltman P, Cone R, Resnick D (1986): J Nutr 116:135.

Sugarman B, Epps LR, Stenbeck WA (1982): Infect Immun 37:1191.

Sun XF, Ting BTG, Janghorbani M (1987): Anal Biochem 6:304.

Sunde RA (1990): Annu Rev Nutr 10:451.

Sunde RA, Sonnenburg WK, Gutzke GE, Hoekstra WG (1981): *In* Howell JMcC, Gawthorne JM, White CL, eds: Trace element metabolism in man and animals (TEMA-4). Canberra: Australian Academy of Science, p 165.

Sunde RA, Evenson JK (1987): J Biol Chem 262:933.

Sunderman FW Jr (1990): 7th international symposium on trace elements in man and animals (TEMA-7), Dubrovnik, May.

Sunderman FW Jr, Decsy MI, McNeely MD (1972): Ann NY Acad Sci 199:300.

Suttle NF (1974*a*): Vet Rec 95:165.

Suttle NF (1974*b*): Proc Nutr Soc 33:299.

Taft LI, Halliday JW, Russo AM, Francis BH (1978): Aust N Z J Obstet Gynaecol 18:226.

Tanner MS (1989): *In* Abdulla M, Dashtl H, Sarkar B, Al-Sayer H, Al-Naqeeb N, eds: Metabolism of minerals and trace elements in human disease. London: Smith-Gordon, Nishimura.

Tanner MS (1990): 7th international symposium on trace elements in man and animals (TEMA-7), Dubrovnik, May.

Tarugi P, Calandra S, Borella P, Vivoli GF (1982): Atherosclerosis 45:221.

Templeton DM, Sarker B (1985): Fed Proc 44:497.

Thomassen PR, Leicester HM (1960): J Dent Res 39:473.

Thompson DB (1988): *In* Smith KT, ed: Trace minerals in foods. New York: Marcel Dekker, p 157.

Thomson CD, Robinson MF, Campbell DR, Rea HM (1982): Am J Clin Nutr 36:24.

Tokuda M, Kashiwagi A, Wakamiya E, Oguni T, Mino M, Kagamiyama H (1987): Biochem Biophys Res Commun 144:1237.

Tolonen M, Halme M, Sarna S (1985): Biol Trace Elem Res 7:161.

Tolonen M, Halme M, Sarna S, Bayer W, Nordberg UR, Westermarck R (1988): TEMA 6:4.

Tolonen M, Sarna S, Westermarck T, Halme M, Nordberg U-R, Keinonen M, Tuominen SEJ, Schrijver J (1987): VitaMinSpur 2:187.

Torrance JD, Gilhooly M, Mills W, Mayet F, Bothwell TH (1982): *In* Saltman P, Hegenauer J, eds: Biochemistry and physiology of iron. New York: Elsevier, p 819.

Turnlund JR, Keyes WR (1990): 7th international symposium on trace elements in man and animals (TEMA-7), Dubrovnik, May.

Tyrala EE, Brodsky EL, Auerbach V (1982): Am J Clin Nutr 35:542.

Underwood EJ (1975): Nutr Rev 36:65.

Underwood EJ (1977): Trace elements in human and animal nutrition (4th ed). New York: Academic.

Urberg M, Zemel MB (1987): Metabolism 36:896.

Uthus EO, Cornatzer WE, Nielsen FH (1983): *In* Lederer WH, Fensterheim RJ, eds: Arsenic: Industrial, biomedical, environmental perspectives. Princeton: Van Nostrand Reinhold, p 173.

Valentine JL, Campion DS, Schluchter MD, Massey FJ (1981): *In* Howell JMcC, Gawthorne JM, White CL, eds: Trace element metabolism in man and animals (TEMA-4). Canberra: Australian Academy of Science, p 409.

Vallee BL, Ulmer DD (1972): Annu Rev Biochem 41:91.

Varma R, Varma RS, Allen WS, Wardi AH (1974): Biochim Biophys Acta 362:584.

Varo P, Lahelma O, Nuurtamo M, Saari E, Koivistoinen P (1980*a*): Acta Agric Scand Suppl 22:89.

Varo P, Nuurtamo M, Saari E, Koivistoinen P (1980*b*): Acta Agric Scand Suppl 22:27, 37, 115, 127, 141.

Varo P, Nuurtamo M, Saari E, Rasanen L, Koivistoinen P (1980*c*): Acta Agric Scand Suppl 22:161.

Venugopal B, Luckey TD (1978): Metal toxicity in mammals, Vol 2. New York: Plenum.

Verch RL, Chu R, Wallach S, Peabody RA, Jain R, Hannan E (1983): Nutr Rep Intl 27:531.

Vinton NE, Dahlstrom KA, Strobel CT, Ament ME (1987): J Pediatr 111:711.

Voors AW (1970): Am J Epidemiol 92:164.

Wacker WC (1978): *In* Hambidge KM, Nichols BL Jr, eds: Zinc and copper in clinical medicine. New York: SP Medical and Scientific Books, p 15.

Wallaeys B, Cornelis R, Sabbioni E (1988): Sci Total Enviorn 71:401.

Wang T, Himoe A (1974): J Biol Chem 249:3895.

Wapnick AA, Lynch SR, Kravitz P, Seftel HC, Charlton RW, Bothwell TH (1968): Br Med J 3:704.

Ward NI, Thompson J, Abou-Shakra FR, Durrant SF, Havercroft JM, Yadegarian L (1990): 7th international symposium on trace elements in man and animals (TEMA-7), Dubrovnik, May.

Warrington K (1923): Ann Bot 40:27.

Waschulewski IH, Sunde RA (1988): J Nutr 118:367.

Webster MH, Waitkins SA, Stott A (1981): J Clin Pathol 34:651.

Weinberg ED (1974): Science 184:952.

Westermarck T, Rahola T, Suomela M, Kallio A-K (1981): *In* Howell JMcC, Gawthorne JM, White CL, eds: Trace element metabolism in man and animals (TEMA-4). Canberra: Australian Academy of Science, p 506.

Westermarck T, Sandholm M (1977): Acta Pharmacol Toxicol 40:70.

Westermarck T, Santavuori P (1984): Med Biol 62:148.

Widdowson EM, Dauncy J, Shaw JCL (1974): Proc Nutr Soc 33:275.

Williams DM (1982): *In* Prasad AS, ed: Clinical, biochemical, and nutritional aspects of trace elements. New York: Alan R Liss, p 277.

Wirth PL, Linder MC (1985): JNCI 75:277.

Wissler JH, Logeman E, Meyer HE, Kautzfeldt B, Hockel M, Heilmeyer LMG Jr (1986): *In* Peeters H, ed: Protides of the biological fluids, Vol 34, p 525.

Wolff HP (1956): Klin Wochschr 15:409.

Worley PF, Heller WA, Snyder SH, Baraban JM (1988): Science 239:1428.

Worwood M, Covell AM, Cragg SJ, Jacobs A (1983): *In* Urushizaki I, Aisen P, Listowsky W, Drysdale JW, eds: Structure and function of iron storage and transport proteins. Amsterdam: Elsevier, p 181.

Yamamoto A, Wada O, Suzuki H (1988): J Nutr 118:39.

Yang GQ (1987): *In* Combs FJ Jr, Spallholz JE, Levander OA, Oldfield JE, eds: Selenium in biology and medicine. Westport: AVI.

Yoshino K, Okamoto M, Kakihana H, Mori Y (1989): Melanoma, p 291.

Zhu L (1981): *In* Howell JMcC, Gawthorne JM, White CL, eds: Trace element metabolism in man and animals (TEMA-4). Canberra: Australian Academy of Science, p 514.

Maria C. Linder, Ph.D.*

8

Energy Metabolism, Intake, and Expenditure

Energy Content of Foods

Direct Calorimetry

The total energy content of foodstuffs is normally defined in terms of kilocalories (kcal) or kilojoules (kJ), as determined by the heat released upon its ignition and total combustion in a bomb calorimeter (direct calorimetry) (Figure 8.1). Specifically, 1 kcal is the amount of heat released that raises the temperature of 1 L of water 1° Celsius. One calorie is the equivalent heat required for 1 ml of water. The popular "Calories" (with a capital "C") are equivalent to the scientist's "kilocalories." Efforts are being made to convert to joules, 1 kcal being equivalent to 4.128 kJ (or about 4.1 kJ; 0.239 kcal/kJ), but the use of "kcal" still very much predominates.

In the total physical combustion of foodstuffs, carbohydrates and fats are completely oxidized to CO_2 and water, and all energy is given off as heat. In the body, exactly the same overall oxidation occurs, in the sense that 1 glucose molecule plus 6 oxygen molecules are converted to 6 CO_2 and 6 H_2O molecules, or that triglyceride (95%–98% of dietary fat) is converted to a specific number of CO_2 and H_2O molecules. Thus, the heat released in a bomb calorimeter is potentially equivalent to the amount of food energy available from its metabolism. In metabolism, however, not all the energy is released as heat, and a certain proportion is trapped in the form of high energy phosphate bonds (~P), which are the driving force for the numerous anabolic processes needed to maintain life and physical activity. For fats and carbohydrates, a maximum of about 40% of the potential energy is retained as high energy phosphate bonds (see below).

With proteins, there is a difference between the energies released in physical/chemical combustion versus metabolism, in that nitrogen-containing residues (mainly urea and ammonia), which are derived from protein and excreted, are not completely oxidized and still contain available caloric energy (as determined by direct calorimetry). This potential energy (which is excreted) must be subtracted from the total to obtain a more accurate figure for potentially available metabolic energy in protein foods.

For carbohydrates and fats as well as proteins, the digestibility of a food and its nutrients is another factor that may lower the actual energy available from metabolism. Digestibility determines absorption, and although this tends to be very high (averaging 95% overall for a mixed diet), it can make a significant difference.

The caloric contents of foods listed in food tables attempt to take both digestibility and efficiency of overall metabolic combustion into account; the values are thus lower than those based on determinations by direct combustion (Table 8.1), as in a bomb calorimeter. Values for individual foods, in food tables from different sources,

* California State University, Fullerton, CA.

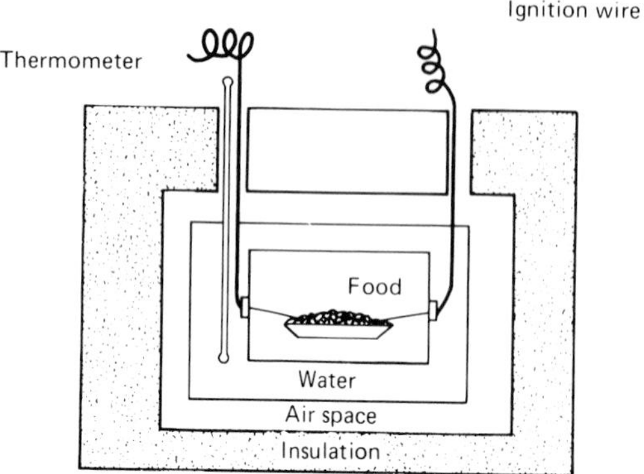

Figure 8.1. Use of a bomb calorimeter to measure the energy content of foods. The food is ignited and burned in a bomb calorimeter, and the heating of the water in the jacket surrounding the chamber is measured. Because the volume of the water in the jacket is known, it is possible to calculate how much heat was released to raise the temperature of 1 L of the water from 14.5°–15.5°C. The total calorimeter is insulated to prevent any heat loss. [*Source:* Based on Reed (1980).]

will show some variation due to (a) differences in the contents of protein, carbohydrate, and fat (and water) among samples of the same foodstuffs; (b) slight differences in the results obtained by direct calorimetry; and/or (c) differences in the assumptions used in calculations (subtraction of digestibility, urea release, etc).

Indirect Calorimetry

During metabolic oxidation, the proportion of oxygen consumed per amount of a specific carbonaceous material oxidized is constant, as is the proportion of carbon dioxide that results. The oxygen consumption per gram for carbohydrates is much less than that for fats (Table 8.1), in that fats are less oxidized to start with; proteins are in between the two, but are closer to carbohydrates. The initial oxidation state also determines the inherent energy content of the nutrient, as determined by direct calorimetry. As a result, the amount of O_2 consumed per kcal of energy produced in metabolic oxidation is quite similar for all three major foodstuffs, varying from 4.5–5.0 kcal/L O_2, from proteins to carbohydrates, respectively (Table 8.1). A common way of determining food energy utilization is thus to measure oxygen consumption. This is the most important form of "indirect calorimetry."

There is also a constant relationship between kcal released and CO_2 production, although values of kcal/L CO_2 are not nearly as similar when fats and carbohydrates are compared (Table 8.1). Consequently, CO_2 production is a less accurate means of determining metabolic energy utilization by indirect calorimetry.

Indirect calorimetric evaluations are aided by measuring the respiratory quotient, or RQ, which indicates the predominant fuels in current use, so that adjustments can be made for the contributions from carbohydrates and fats (and proteins if further information is available; see below). The RQ is the ratio of liters CO_2 produced to O_2 consumed by an individual, which calculates to 1.0 for carbohydrates, about 0.70 for fats, and approximately 0.8 for proteins (Table 8.1). (It is again related to the initial oxidation states of these potential metabolic fuels).

Since the contribution of protein to average caloric intake (in Americans) is only 12%, the RQ is largely determined by the ratio of fat to carbohydrate utilized at any given time or over a 24-hr or longer period. Consequently, the approximate contributions of carbohydrates and fats to energy

Table 8.1. Relationships Among Energy Contents, Oxygen Utilization, and CO_2 Production During Metabolism or Burning of Foodstuffs

	Carbohydrates	Fats	Proteins
Energy content (kcal/g)[a]			
Direct calorimetry	3.7–4.3	9.5	4.0–4.3
Metabolic (av)	4.1	9.3	4.1
O_2 consumed (A) (L/g)	0.75–0.83	2.03	0.97
CO_2 produced (B) (L/g)	0.75–0.83	1.43	0.78
RQ (B/A)	1.00	0.70–0.71	0.80–0.82
kcal produced/L O_2 consumed	5.0	4.7	4.5
kcal produced/L CO_2 produced	5.0	6.6	5.6

Source: Modified from Buskirk and Mendez (1980).

[a] Ethanol contains 7 kcal/g.

expenditures can be determined from any RQ value obtained from 0.70–1.00 (Table 8.2). This is very useful in assessing the effects of various diets, types of physical exercise, and/or degree of exertion as determinants of metabolic fuel utilization.

In order to take the contributions of protein-derived energy into account, values for nitrogen excretion must be available. Most commonly, the nitrogen excreted (in grams) multiplied by 6.25 represents the grams of protein oxidized, multiplied by 0.97 estimates the number of liters oxygen consumed, and multiplied by 0.78 estimates the number of liters CO_2 produced. These liters of O_2 and CO_2 can then be subtracted from the total to obtain amended figures for calculation of an RQ solely dependent on utilization of carbohydrates and fats. From the amended RQ, the proportions of the latter being utilized for fuel may be estimated quite accurately (from Table 8.2). Obviously, this is possible only for periods covering several hours or more, rather than with single or multiple short-term measurements.

For some people, ethanol also becomes a factor in the determination of energy utilization. It contains 7 kcal/g (30 kJ/g) by direct calorimetry. If it were the exclusive fuel, it would result in an RQ closer to that of fats, as it is metabolized via the Krebs cycle and is relatively unoxidized, at the start (see Chapter 3).

Table 8.2. Relationship Between RQ and the Proportions of Carbohydrates and Fats Utilized for Energy

	Percent O_2 consumed in metabolism of		Percent heat produced by oxidation of	
RQ	Carbohydrates	Fats	Carbohydrates	Fats
0.70	0	100	0	100
0.71	1.0	99.0	1.1	98.9
0.72	4.4	95.6	4.8	95.2
0.73	7.85	92.2	8.4	91.6
0.74	11.3	88.7	12.0	88.0
0.75	14.7	85.3	15.6	84.4
0.76	18.1	81.9	19.2	80.8
0.77	21.5	78.5	22.8	77.2
0.78	24.9	75.1	26.3	73.7
0.79	28.3	71.7	29.9	70.1
0.80	31.7	68.3	33.4	66.6
0.81	35.2	64.8	36.9	63.1
0.82	38.6	61.4	40.3	59.7
0.83	42.0	58.0	43.8	56.2
0.84	45.4	54.6	47.2	52.8
0.85	48.8	51.2	50.7	49.3
0.86	52.2	47.8	54.1	45.9
0.87	55.6	44.4	57.5	42.5
0.88	59.0	41.0	60.8	39.2
0.89	62.5	37.5	64.2	35.8
0.90	65.9	34.1	67.5	32.5
0.91	69.3	30.7	70.8	29.2
0.92	72.7	27.3	74.1	25.9
0.93	76.1	23.9	77.4	22.6
0.94	79.5	20.5	80.7	19.3
0.95	82.9	17.1	84.0	16.0
0.96	86.3	13.7	87.2	12.8
0.97	89.8	10.2	90.4	9.6
0.98	93.2	6.8	93.6	6.4
0.99	96.6	3.4	96.8	3.2
1.00	100	0	100	0

Source: Modified from Brody (1945).

Energy Needs of the Human Body

Determinants of Energy Need or Expenditure

The determinants of energy needs may be classified in different ways. Perhaps the most useful is to divide them into the three most basic components defined by (1) basal metabolism, (2) physical activities, and (3) diet induced thermogenesis (DIT), formerly referred to as the specific dynamic action/effect, or heat increment (Table 8.3). To these may be added (in specific circumstances) a component needed for growth, whether it be normal body growth from infancy to adulthood, the growth of the placenta, fetus, and other tissues in pregnancy, muscle growth in body building, etc. The efficiency of energy utilization, as determined by factors such as the digestibility (availability) of foodstuffs, genetic and hormonal factors that affect ~P versus heat production, etc., must also be considered, although they are quantitatively much less important and less well-defined and measurable. Mental activities do not influence energy expenditure.

Basal metabolism. The metabolic activity required for the basic maintenance of body life and function, in as much a steady state as possible, is determined by measuring the oxygen consumption (as well as CO_2 and N excretion) of a person, awake but at complete rest, in a neutral warm environment, after fasting overnight and is called basal metabolism. Such a determination gives a basal metabolic rate, or BMR, usually in kcal (or kJ)/min/kg body weight. Resting metabolic rate (RMR) is the same, except that it includes some energy expended for digestion, absorption, and

Table 8.3. Determinants of Energy Needs/Expenditures

Determinant	Variables
Basal metabolism (staying alive) Maintenance of body tissues and temperature; respiration; heart, kidney, and other basic functions	Age Sex Lean body mass Illness/injury Environmental temperature Hormonal status Stress Pregnancy/lactation
Physical activities (physical exertion)	Degree of exertion Environmental temperature Age/sex/weight
Diet-induced thermogenesis Digestion, absorption, distribution, modification, storage of ingested nutrients Thermogenesis by BAT	Type of diet Genetics
Growth/repair	Normal development Pregnancy/lactation Illness/injury
Efficiency of energy utilization	Diet Genetics Hormonal status

distribution of ingested food and/or other DIT (e.g., determinations are made in a nonfasting state).

In adults, the BMR (or RMR) is most closely related to lean body mass (Keys et al., 1950, 1973). Adipose tissue consists mainly of triglyceride, and this portion of the cell or tissue has little or no metabolic activity. On the basis of nonlean body weight or surface area, there is a significant (10%) average difference in BMR for women versus men (about 0.9 versus 1.0 kcal/kg/hr). This reflects the higher average proportion of body fat in women (about 25% versus 15%). Because of the body fat component, the values of BMR are also lower when based on total versus lean body weight, 0.9–1.0 versus 1.3 kcal/kg/hr, respectively. Body tissues do not contribute equally to BMR; the liver and brain, totaling about 4% of body weight, require more than 40% of the basal oxygen consumption (18%–22% for liver alone); muscle (which may be up to 40% or more of body weight) only accounts for about 25% of basal energy needs.

BMR (per kilogram weight) varies with age, especially in the period of early childhood, when it rises to its highest point (Figure 8.2); it then falls gradually, reaching a more constant level by 20 years of age. With aging, there is gradual shrinkage of metabolically active tissue, and usually an accumulation of more fat, which both contribute to a gradual (slight) decline in BMR. The BMR declines about 10% during sleep. The total RMR (or BMR) of an individual will also be affected by pregnancy, especially in the second and third trimesters when the majority of tissue growth occurs and leads to a greater lean (fat free) body mass. Lactation imposes an additional need to support milk production. This amounts to about 120 kcal/dl of milk produced and might best be considered in the "growth" category (Table 8.3). Illness, fever, burns, and sepsis may also increase BMR (while reducing physical activity). Environmental temperature (and humidity) generally play a negligible role because of the effects of clothing, heating, air conditioning, etc. However, in the extremes of cold or heat, there may be a 2%–5% increase in basal requirements to help regulate body temperature (Buskirk and Mendez, 1980). At extremely cold temperatures, part of the added expenditure is from the hobbling effects of the heavy clothing on muscle action. In extreme heat, enhanced blood flow to the skin for cooling causes an increase of 0.5% in the RMR per degree of temperature rise above 30°C (Buskirk and Mendez, 1980). Normally, it is thought that the body is warmed mainly from the heat released in the pathways of intermediary metabolism (glycolysis, Krebs cycle, etc.), only a portion of the energy of which is reclaimed as ~P (see below). However, the activity of heat-producing brown adipose tissue may at times play a role in this, especially upon cold exposure and in fever (Corbett et al., 1988). The hormonal status of an individual,

Figure 8.2. Changes in basal metabolism from birth to maturity. The values for adult men and women average 33.9 and 28.9 kcal/hr/m², respectively. [*Source:* Redrawn by permission from Brody (1945).]

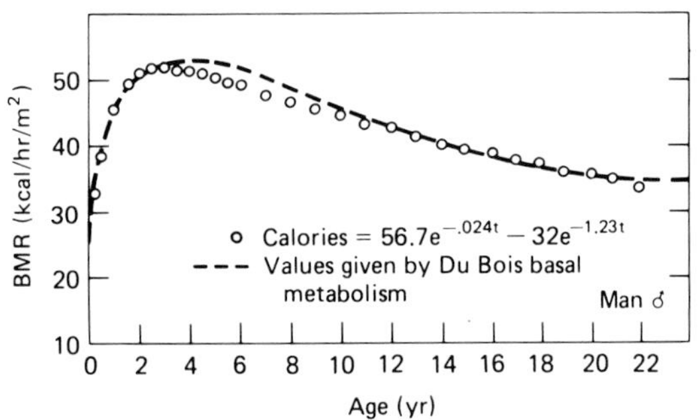

which may be determined by genetics, psychologic stress, and even diet is also a variable determining BMR. Thyroid status is perhaps the most important and can make differences of up to 50% plus (hyperthyroid) or minus (hypothyroid) (Buskirk and Mendez, 1980).

Calculating basal energy expenditure. In practice, many methods have evolved for calculating the energy needs ascribable to basal metabolism (BMR). For the adult person, this is usually based on weight (or surface area), and sometimes also on height and age (see Table 8.4). A simple approach is to use values of 1.0 and 0.90 kcal/hr/kg body weight for men and women, respectively. When figured over 24 hr, this results in values of 1680 and 1173 kcal for an average 70-kg man or 58-kg woman, respectively. More accurate values are obtained with the formulas shown in Table 8.4, or are based on determinations of lean body mass derived from measurements of body density. (Fat has a lower density than lean tissue.) For the average (relatively sedentary) American, BMR is the major determinant of energy needs.

Physical activities. These obviously increase our need for available energy (or ~P) and mobilize the organism to increase fuel utilization and oxygen consumption. By use of portable respirometers, the oxygen consumption (and often CO_2 production) associated with all manner of physical activities has been measured and translated into kcals needed to support these actions. The energy needs associated with various degrees of physical activity and/or occupations are approximated in Table 8.5 and Figure 8.3. Table 8.5 is a composite of the proposed classification of Buskirk and Mendez (1980) and some other information (including that of the Food and Nutrition Board, 1974). Obviously, there is some subjectivity in the designations of degree of physical effort, and categories can be more standardized by relating them to O_2 consumption, as well as to heart and respiratory rate (though the latter two are subject to many other variables).

The values shown for various activities in Table 8.5 and Figure 8.3 include the requirements for basal metabolism (BMR). If the BMR component is subtracted, the contributions of physical activities to energy needs becomes much clearer (Table 8.6). Use of the latter values makes it easier to see the rather small contributions physical activities make to the energy needs of most people (Table 8.7).

Diet-induced thermogenesis (DIT). The third important component in energy calculations is that ascribable to food intake itself, or diet-induced thermogenesis (DIT) (Table 8.3). There are two aspects to the food effect. The first (the major one) is the obligation to expend energy in order to digest, absorb, distribute, and store the nutrients ingested. [This was previously termed the specific dynamic effect/action of food (SDE) or heat "increment."] Second, incoming nutrients can (at least in certain conditions) induce additional heat

Table 8.4. Some Ways of Estimating Basal Metabolic Rate (BMR)[a]

	Equation	Investigators (year)
Men:	BMR[b] $= 66.4730 + 13.751W + 5.0033L - 6.7550A$	Harris and Benedict (1919)
Women:	$BMR = 65.50955 + 9.463W + 1.8496L - 4.6756A$	
Human or animal:	$BMR = 70W^{0.75}$	Brody (1945) and Klieber (1947, 1965)
Men:	$BMR = 71.2W^{0.75}\left[1 + 0.004(30A) + 0.010\left(\frac{L}{W^{0.33}} - 43.4\right)\right]$	Klieber (1965)
Women:	$BMR = 65.8W^{0.75}\left[1 + 0.004(30A) + 0.018\left(\frac{L}{W^{0.33}} - 42.1\right)\right]$	
Men or women:	BMR = 1.3 kcal/hr/kg fat-free body weight (irrespective of sex and age, if 20–60 years)	Grande and Keys (1973, 1978)
Men:	BMR = 1.0 kcal/hr/kg	Useful average for quick estimates
Women:	BMR = 0.9 kcal/hr/kg	

Source: Information from Buskirk and Mendez (1980) and Grande and Keys (1980).

[a] kcal/24 hr.
[b] W, weight; L, height; A, age.

Table 8.5. Relationships Among Respiration, Heart Rate, and Caloric Expenditure for Different Degrees of Physical Activity (in Adults)

Physical effort (with examples)[a]	Respiratory rate (ventilation vol) (L/min)	Oxygen consumption (L/min)	Heart rate (beats/min)	Caloric expenditure[b]	
				kcal/min	kcal/kg/hr[a]
Very light	<10	<0.5	<80	<2.5	
Sleeping, lying, sitting, driving,				1.0–1.1	
sewing, standing, ironing				1.1–1.5	1.3–1.5 av
				1.5–2.5	
Light	10–20	0.5–1.0	80–100	2.5–5.0	
Walking (2.5–3.5 mph), trade work, shopping, table tennis, golf				2.5–3.0	2.6–2.9 av
Moderate	20–35	1.0–1.5	100–120	5.0–7.5	4.1–4.3 av
Walking 3.5–4 mph, dancing, scrubbing floors, weeding, hoeing, cycling, tennis					
Heavy	35–50	1.5–2.0	120–140	7.5–10.0	8.0–8.4 av
Walking uphill with load, pick and shovel work, swimming, basketball					
Very heavy	50–65	2.0–2.5	140–160	10.0–12.5	
Running, climbing					
Unduly heavy	65–85	2.5–3.0	160–180	12.5–15.0	
Exhausting	≧85	≧3.0	≧180	≧15.0	

Source: Modified from Buskirk and Mendez (1980).

[a] Food and Nutrition Board (1974).

[b] Per adult (includes BMR); calculated from O_2 consumption (4.5–5.0 kcal/L O_2 consumed). Does not take into account substantial variations in body size or in physical fitness. The effect of anxiety on heart rate is also not considered.

production by activation of brown adipose tissue. Researchers were alerted to DIT by observing that the RMR increases following ingestion of food, as evidenced by increased oxygen consumption and CO_2 production. The amount of energy required for handling the incoming food is related to the type and quantity of carbohydrates, fats, and proteins eaten (as is the nonobligatory thermic response). Thus, the DIT "expense" is calculated as a percentage of the food calories ingested. (With

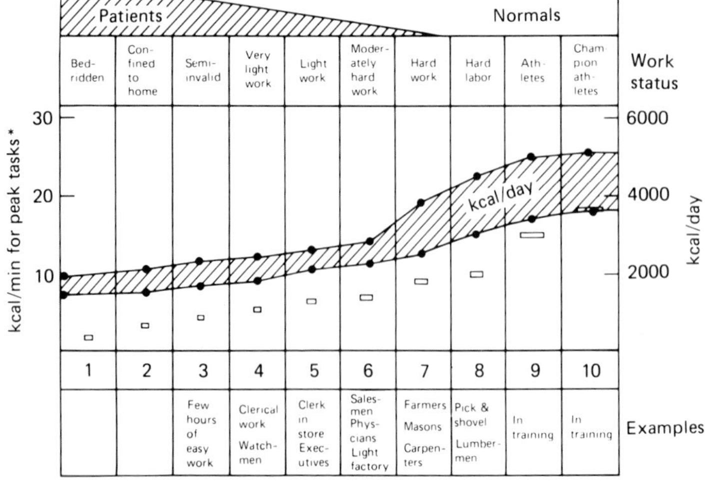

Figure 8.3. Approximate relationship of caloric needs to status of adults. *Bars: Height is determined by energy need during the peak activities performed; width of bar is related to duration of the peak activities. [*Source:* Modified from DuBois (1960).]

Table 8.6. Energy Expenditures Above Basal for Physical Activities

Activity	kcal/kg/hr	Activity	kcal/kg/hr
Bicycling (century run)	7.6	Piano playing (Liszt's "Tarantella")	2.0
Bicycling (moderate speed)	2.5	Reading aloud	0.4
Bookbinding	0.8	Rowing in race	16.0
Boxing	11.8	Running	7.0
Carpentry	2.3	Sawing wood	5.7
Cello playing	1.3	Sewing, hand	0.4
Crocheting	0.4	Sewing, foot-driven machine	0.6
Dancing, foxtrot	3.8	Sewing, motor-driven machine	0.4
Dancing, waltz	3.0	Shoemaking	1.0
Dishwashing	1.0	Singing in loud voice	0.8
Dressing and undressing	0.7	Sitting quietly	0.4
Driving automobile	0.9	Skating	3.5
Eating	0.4	Standing at attention	0.6
Fencing	7.3	Standing relaxed	0.5
Horseback riding, walk	1.4	Stone masonry	4.7
Horseback riding, trot	4.3	Sweeping with broom, bare floor	1.4
Horseback riding, gallop	6.7	Sweeping with carpet sweeper	1.6
Ironing (5-pound iron)	1.0	Sweeping with vacuum sweeper	2.7
Knitting sweater	0.7	Swimming (2 mph)	7.9
Laundry, light	1.3	Tailoring	0.9
Lying still, awake	0.1	Typewriting rapidly	1.0
Organ playing (30%–40% of energy hand work)	1.5	Violin playing	0.6
Painting furniture	1.5	Walking (3 mph)	2.0
Paring potatoes	0.6	Walking rapidly (4 mph)	3.4
Playing ping-pong	4.4	Walking at high speed (5.3 mph)	9.3
Piano playing (Mendelssohn's songs)	0.8	Walking downstairs	[a]
		Walking upstairs	[b]
Piano playing (Beethoven's "Apassionata")	1.4	Washing floors	1.2
		Writing	0.4

Source: Data from Taylor and McLeod (1949).

[a] 0.012 kcal/kg for an ordinary staircase with 15 steps without regard to time.
[b] 0.036 kcal/kg for an ordinary staircase with 15 steps without regard to time.

more intake, more energy is required.) Fat is the least "expensive" in terms of DIT (Table 8.8), requiring relatively little hydrolysis and a fairly direct pathway to storage tissue (see Chapter 3). Carbohydrate is intermediate, requiring considerable metabolism when converted to and stored as triglyceride (Table 8.8), and less when converted to glycogen. Fat, and especially carbohydrate, can also elicit some increased heat production not related to use of energy for nutrient digestion, transport, and storage (see later). Protein is the most "expensive" overall for DIT requiring expenditures of up to 30% of the inherent energy for processing: removal of nitrogen, synthesis of urea, gluconeogenesis, etc. Although there is some controversy, typical mixed diets of Americans probably elicit a thermogenic effect of about 10%. Up to one third of that might be ascribable to "futile cycles" and/or a stimulation of "brown fat" to produce extra heat.

Calculations of Overall Energy Needs

The most common ways of calculating energy needs are summarized in Table 8.7. The amounts of time spent in various activities, per 24 hr, and the quantities of and types of foods consumed must be known, as well as sex, age, body weight, and perhaps even lean body mass. The contributions of basal metabolism and physical exertion are then calculated, either together or separately (as shown), based on known expenditures per weight (and age) for basal and other states. The contribution of diet-induced thermogenesis is added, based on calculations of food energy consumed, times 0.10 depending on the amounts of

Table 8.7. Sample Calculations of Energy Needs

I. Calculations based on BMR, activities, and DIT: 75-kg sedentary adult man

	Individual activity	Total for category
Basal metabolism		= 1800 kcal
1.0 kcal/hr/kg × 24 hr × 75 kg		
Physical activities above basal[a]		
Reading, writing, telephoning, eating, 12.5 hr		
0.4 kcal/hr/g × 12.5 × 75 kg	= 375 kcal	
Walking slowly, 1 hr		
2.0 kcal/hr/kg × 1 × 75 kg	= 150 kcal	
Playing cello, 1 hr		
1.3 kcal/hr/kg × 1 × 75 kg	= 120 kcal	= 645 kcal
Diet-induced thermogenesis		
2500 kcal ingested × 10%		= 250 kcal
Total needs		= 2695 kcal

II. Calculations based on rates that include BMR and DIT: for the "reference" man and woman

Activity	Time (hr)	Man (70 kg)[b]		Woman (58 kg)[b]	
		kcal/min[c]	Total	kcal/min[c]	Total
Sleeping or lying down	8	1.1	528	1.0	480
Sitting	7	1.5	630	1.1	462
Standing	5	2.5	750	1.5	450
Walking	2	3.0	360	2.5	300
Other	2	4.5	540	3.0	360
Total			2808 kcal		2052 kcal

[a] See Table 8.5.
[b] The NRC standard man and woman is 23-years-old, lives and works in a thermally neutral environment, has an office or light industry occupation, and a modest recreational program. From Buskirk and Mendez (1980).
[c] See Table 8.6 (rate includes body size).

Table 8.8. Factors Related to the Energy Available from Ingested Fat, Carbohydrate, and Protein

	Fats	Carbohydrate	Protein	Typical mixed diet[a]
Digestibility (av %)	95	97	91	480
Diet-induced thermogenesis				
(Specific dynamic effect)	(3–4)[b]	10–15	15–20	6–8
% of ingested kcal[f]		31[c]	15–30[d]	10[d]
Energy used for storage only (% kcal)	3	5 (glycogen) 15 (triglyceride) (22)[e]	(<15–20)[b]	(10)[b]
Conversion to ATP (if used directly and not stored)				
~P bonds (mol/100 g nutrient)	50.4	21.1	22.6	34.4
Costs/~P (kcal/bond)	18.6	17.6	22.7	19
Max percent kcal converted to ATP	~40	~40	32–34	39

Source: Based on information from Crist et al. (1980).

[a] 45% of kcal from carbohydrate, 45% from fat, 10% from protein.
[b] Values in parentheses are approximations.
[c] At high glucose infusion rates (mainly converted to fat) (King et al., 1986).
[d] Anderson (1982).
[e] Estimated by Kinney (1988).
[f] Includes storage of 80% of kcal.

protein, carbohydrate, and fat ingested (values closer to 0.06 for a high fat diet, greater than 0.10 for diets high in carbohydrate and protein.) Despite the care invested in these calculations, the values are based on averages that may not apply precisely to a given individual. For example, even when corrected for age, sex, and lean body mass, BMR will still vary up to 30% from one person to another (Pi-Sunyer, 1988). Moreover, the calculations tend to overestimate actual energy expenditures (Anderson, 1982). This is suggested by comparing values of actual energy intakes (from surveys) to recommended values (Table 8.9).

Summary

The fate of food energy is summarized in Figure 8.4 from the viewpoint of metabolism and energy interconversions. Foods eaten begin with a certain value for total inherent energy, as expressed in kcal/g and determined by direct calorimetry. Most, but not all of this potential energy becomes available to the body, because not all is digestible. (Dietary fiber is a notable example, whereas the efficiency of digestion of nutrients is close to, but not as much as, 100%; Table 8.8.) For that portion of foodstuffs digested, the inherent energy largely becomes available to the body, because the digested nutrients can be absorbed. (The undigestible portion is used by intestinal bacteria or is lost in the feces.)

Of the absorbed nutrients, a portion of the inherent energy is lost as components of the urine (like urea) and through various secretions and cell shedding, leaving the majority as net metabolizable energy. The latter is what is estimated and given in common food energy tables. This metabolizable energy is then drawn upon to provide net energy for necessary basal metabolic and physical activities. Also, a percentage is set aside for digestion, absorption, distribution, and storage of "fuels" (Table 8.8). The percentage of inherent food energy actually captured in the form of high energy phosphate bonds (~P) is less than 40% (Table 8.8), and the cost of producing ~P varies somewhat with the nutrient in question, with the cost for production from protein being highest. (This, again, reflects the more complex metabolism involved in converting amino acids to glucose or fat.)

The rest of the inherent metabolizable energy of the ingested nutrients (about 50%) is released as heat, which is largely used to maintain body

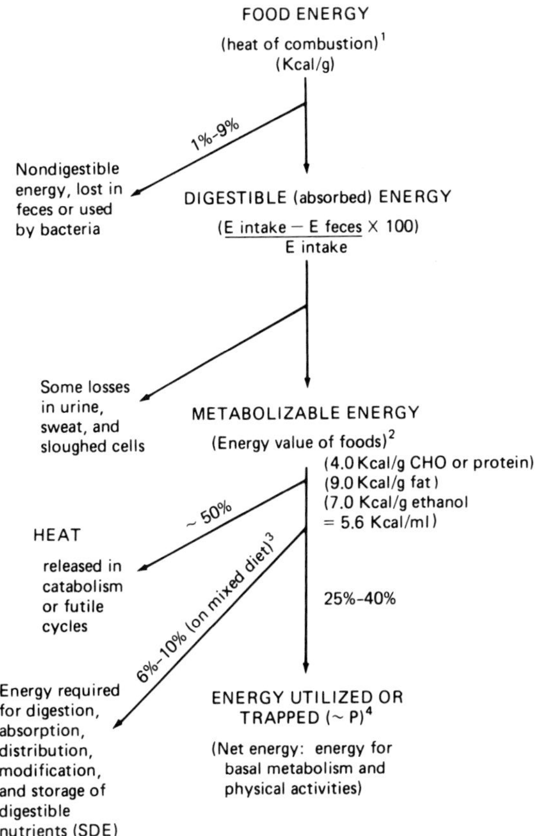

Figure 8.4. The fate of food energy. Footnotes: [1]Heat required to raise the temperature of 1 L of H_2O from 14.5°–15.5°C (determined by direct calorimetry). [2]As found in food composition tables. [3]Most energy required for proteins and carbohydrates (see Table 8.8). [4]High-energy phosphate bond energy, utilizable for anabolic processes.

Table 8.9. Estimated Actual Energy Intakes Versus Recommended Intakes for Average Americans

Age (years)	Actual energy intake (kcal/day)		Recommended energy allowance (kcal/day)	
	Male	Female	Male	Female
20–24	2888	1691	3000	2100
25–34	2739	1638	2700	2000
35–44	2554	1558	2700	2000
45–54	2301	1533	2700	2000
55–64	2076	1382	2400	1800
≥65	1805	1307	2400	1800

Source: Modified from Anderson (1982), based on Health and Nutrition Examination Survey (1977) and Food and Nutrition Board (1981).

temperature. This heat is the product of the well-known, built-in inefficiency of metabolic pathways for catabolism of carbohydrates, fats, and other fuels, plus mechanisms that result in "futile cycles" (Newsholme and Crabtree, 1976): hydrolysis and resynthesis of triglyceride or glycogen; metabolic "shunts" that feed electrons into the coenzyme Q site of electron transport (via $FADH_2$) rather than into the NADH site, resulting in a maximum of 2 rather than 3 ATPs per electron pair (Figure 8.5); and deliberate heat production via "brown fat" and/or direct uncoupling of oxidative phosphorylation in other tissues. Brown fat is a peculiar (often yellowish-brown) form of adipose tissue, generally containing multiple lipid droplets and packed with mitochondria, capable of thermogenesis through uncoupling of oxidative phosphorylation by a 32,000-dalton, specific GDP-binding protein (Heaton et al., 1978; Klingenberg, 1990). Until recently, it was thought that the adult human had only traces of this tissue, although it is difficult to recognize (Himms-Hagen, 1981) and was known to be present in the infant in the scapular region. It is prevalent in animals, especially in those that undergo hibernation. Catecholamines, cold exposure, and high calorie diets can trigger heat production by this tissue, a form of "nonshivering thermogenesis." For other tissues, thyroid hormones may also be important in downregulating the efficiency of ATP versus heat production, perhaps in part, by increasing the shunting of glycolysis electrons (as in Figure 8.5) (Leibel, 1980) and/or increasing membrane ATPase activities (Crist et al., 1980). These factors illustrate that there is some flexibility and/or variability in the production of warmth versus high energy phosphate bonds, which influences the energy needs of individuals and probably allows some adaptation to circumstances.

Figure 8.5. Metabolic sites for loss of glucose energy. Asterisk (*) represents areas where diversionary losses of energy may occur.

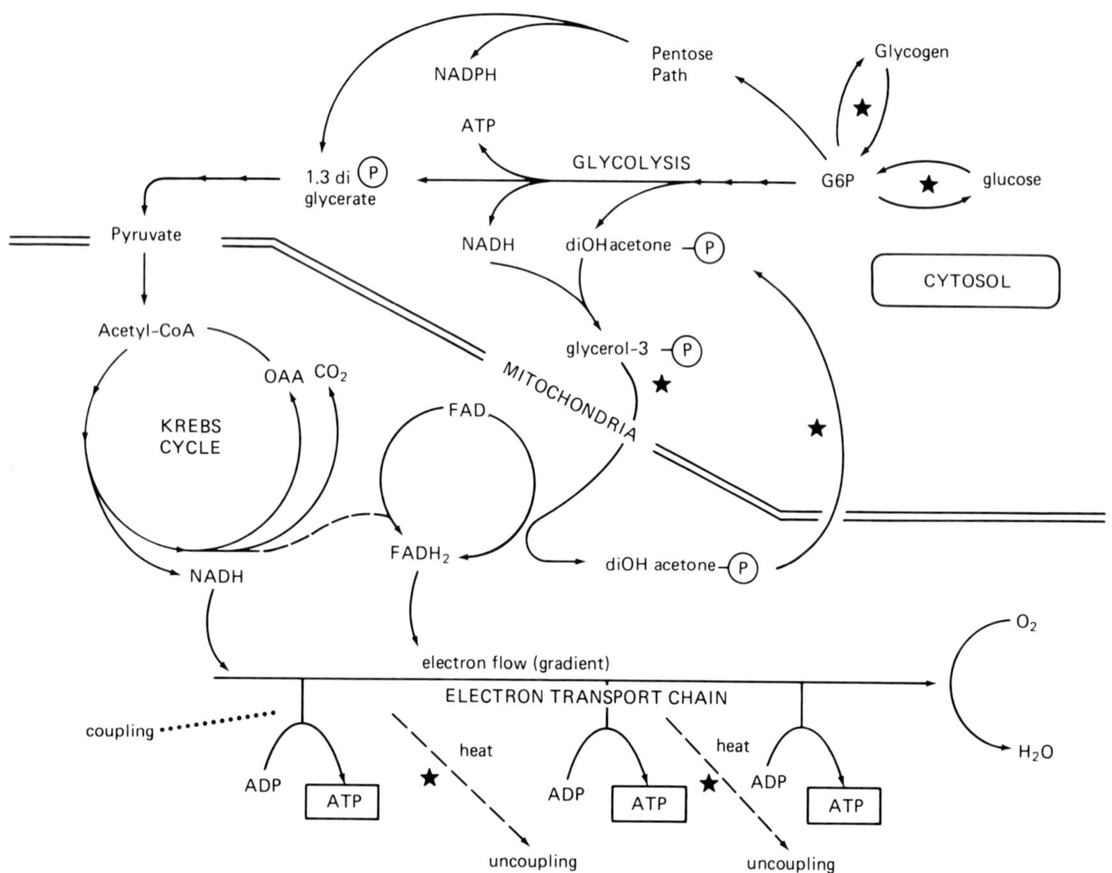

Relation Between Energy Intake and Energy Need

Regulation of Energy Intake

It is clear that there is generally an excellent correspondence between intakes of food energy and energy needs. Individuals of the same height and build, eating as they please, may vary considerably in weight, but each tends to have a constant body weight, which may change, but then only very gradually over time. These observations provide evidence that food energy intake and/or the efficiency of its utilization for fuel is a regulated process. Appetite and thirst mechanisms clearly play a basic role in this, as do psychologic factors. There is also evidence for some homeostatic control of the level of wasteful (heat) versus nonwasteful ($\sim$P) energy utilization to maintain body weight constancy despite variations in caloric intake. At the same time, it is abundantly clear that excesses of caloric intake over expenditures, and vice versa, will result in changes in body weight (see below).

Our understanding of how body weight may be regulated through appetite is still quite limited, although we know that it involves various parts of the hypothalamus, and their effects on the sympathetic and parasympathetic nervous systems, and on the pituitary. A scheme illustrating some of these relationships, and current views on how these may influence food intake (as well as thermogenesis by brown fat), are given in Figure 8.6. Mediated by the cortex, as well as the vagus nerve, signals arrive at the hypothalamus, which are destined to affect its lateral, ventromedial, or paraventricular regions. The ventromedial hypothalamus (VMH) has a particular connection to satiety. When stimulated, it promotes a decreased intake of food and an increased activity of lipolytic enzymes and brown adipose tissue (BAT), via the sympathetic nervous system. The lateral hypothalamus (LH) operates in the opposite direction, stimulating food ingestion (and fat deposition) via the parasympathetic nerves. The paraventricular region (PVN) can influence both of these systems and can (independently) alter the activity of the pituitary to release hormones that will influence metabolism and satiety.

Signals that act on the cortex and hypothalamus to influence these systems include (1) preabsorptive signals from the stomach and intestine, in the form of a variety of hormones (such as cholecystokinin, bombesin, and neurotensin). Cholecystokinin, for example, secreted by the upper small intestine in response to fat and carbohydrate entering from the stomach, stimulates the vagus nerve, which then results in activation of the VMH to induce satiety (possibly via release of oxytocin from the pituitary) (Figure 8.6). Some of the preabsorptive signals increase adipose lipoprotein lipase activity in preparation for uptake and storage of incoming triglycerides (Greenwood et al., 1981). (2) Postabsorptive signals to the hypothalamus come from specific tissues, especially the liver, where the rate of glucose oxidation and/or size of glycogen stores can be translated into a stimulation of the "satiety center" (VMH), also probably via the vagus nerve (Anderson, 1988). (3) Blood levels of nutrients, such as the free fatty acids, glycerol, and ketones associated with fasting, also suppress food intake (Anderson, 1988; Cahill, 1970), presumably via the VMH. (4) The level and turnover of certain metabolites in brain, notably tryptophan and glucose, will also influence satiety. Specifically, a high rate of glucose oxidation is associated with satiety and vice versa (Anderson, 1988); while an influx of tryptophan (as occurs with a high carbohydrate intake and/or intake of tryptophan alone; see Chapter 4) results in more production of 5-OH tryptamine (serotonin), inhibiting food intake (stimulating satiety) and enhancing the preference for protein in future diets (at least in rodents) (Anderson, 1988). Indeed, serotonin has been linked to the regulation of protein intake. Its effects, however, do not appear to involve the hypothalamus (Anderson, 1988).

There are also more cognitive signals that influence appetite and metabolism, such as the taste and smell of food. Drugs (such as opioids), as well as stress (releasing epinephrine from the adrenal medulla), stimulate food intake, probably via the LH and parasympathetic nerves. *Lesions* of the VMH enhance parasympathetic activity and increase total feeding and carbohydrate appetite (Figure 8.6, bottom), at least in rodents. Paraventricular lesions also enhance appetite for carbohydrates. Lesions of the LH enhance sympathetic activity and reduce food intake.

Ideal Body Weight, Obesity, and Body Energy Stores

Standard values for ideal or desirable body weights in the United States are based on data from life insurance files, and are either average values for healthy people of a given height, frame, age, and sex, or are now more commonly based on "body mass index (BMI)," for a given frame

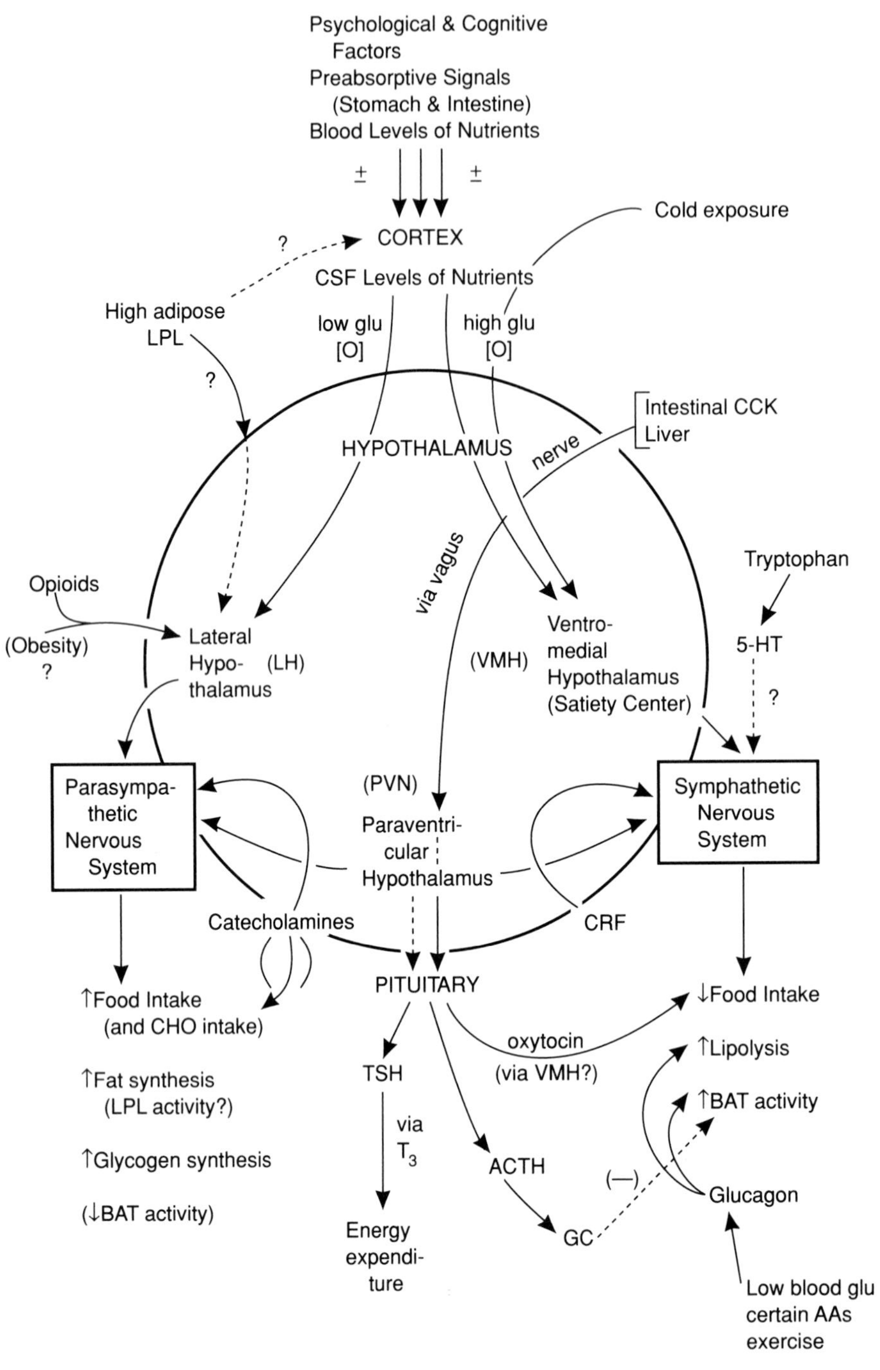

EFFECTS OF LESIONS

LH Lesions
↑Sympathetic activity
↓Food intake
↑BAT activity
↑Core body temperature

PVN Lesions
↑CHO appetite

VMH Lesions
↑parasympathetic activity
↑Total food intake
↑CHO intake
↓BAT activity

(small, medium, large) and sex. BMI (W/H^2), first proposed by Quetelet in 1871 (Pi-Sunyer, 1988), is calculated from weight (kg) and height (meters). It correlates well with the relative size of body fat stores. Desirable and undesirable weights for height are now based largely on the scales proposed by Garrow (1981), in which values of 20–24.9 are considered normal or desirable (see Chapter 13), and larger values represent different grades of overweightedness or obesity (25–29.5, 30–40, >40). Another approach is to define overweight people as more than 20% over their ideal weight. On this basis, and increasingly with age and among women, 15%–38% of the U.S. population is overweight (Pi-Sunyer, 1988). Obesity can be of two types (android and gynoid), with excess fat deposition mainly in the abdominal region or in the hips, respectively. Obesity is associated with a greater morbidity, especially if it is of the android type. [A different type of adipose tissue is involved, with a faster rate of fat turnover (Sims, 1990).]

Obesity often begins in early childhood and already then may be associated with less physical activity (Roberts et al., 1988). Obesity in adolescence generally correlates with obesity in later life. Buskirk and Mendez (1980) have made a distinction between juvenile- and "adult-onset" obesity. Individuals with the former find it more difficult to lose and maintain a lower body weight. As shown in Table 8.10, juvenile-onset obese individuals have about one third more fat cells than individuals who become obese as adults. Of greater interest is that juvenile- and adult-onset obese individuals both have a far greater total fat cell number than normal people with no history of obesity (Table 8.10). The size of fat cells in obese people is also enlarged over that of the normal. Upon drastic weight reduction, the fat cell number is unaltered, but the size of individual adipocytes may become smaller than even in the normal person. It has been suggested that such shrunken cells might make it more difficult for an individual to maintain a leaner body weight. Recent data, showing an increased gene expression and activity of adipose tissue lipoprotein lipase after weight reduction, are consistent with this concept (Kern et al., 1990). (It is noteworthy that obese adults are not just overweight from an excess of fat tissue, but also have a greater lean body mass (Figure 8.7).

Hyperplastic obesity may partly arise from overeating in early childhood (see also Chapter 1). Data from animal studies indicate that caloric intake in early life (before sexual maturation) influences the rate of fat cell proliferation and determines the number of fat cells in the adult (Knittle and Hirsh, 1968). The number is "fixed" before sexual maturity, when the capacity of this tissue for cell proliferation ceases (Chapter 1). (Only changes in cell size occur thereafter.) Nevertheless, the most important factor determining obesity appears to be heredity (Macdonald and Stunkard, 1990; Stunkard et al., 1990). This conclusion comes from recent studies of identical and fraternal twins who were reared apart. The response of pairs of identical twins to deliberate overfeeding (1000 kcal/day for 84 of 100 days) was also much more similar than that of different twin pairs (which was highly variable) (Bouchard et al., 1990). [Among the 12 pairs of male identical twins, the average weight gained (per person) ranged from 4.3–13.3 kg, and there was three times more variance between pairs than within pairs (seven times more if calculations were adjusted for gain in fat mass).] A recent study of

Figure 8.6. Potential mechanisms by which food intake and thermic activity of brown fat are regulated. See text for description of mechanisms involved in appetite/satiety control or BAT thermogenesis, respectively. Arrows indicate stimulation or "results in," unless otherwise indicated. Key: CCK, cholecystokinin; 5HT, 5-OH tryptamine (serotonin); CSF, cerebrospinal fluid; CRF, corticotropin-releasing factor; BAT, brown adipose tissue; CHO, carbohydrate; LPL, lipoprotein lipase; TSH, thyroid-stimulating hormone; ACTH, adrenocorticotropic hormone; GC, glucocorticosteroid; LH, lateral hypothalamus; PVN, paraventricular nucleus of the hypothalamus; VMH, ventromedial hypothalamus; glu [O], glucose oxidation; (−), inhibition. *Source:* Based primarily on Anderson (1988), Billington et al. (1987), Corbett et al. (1988), Grossman (1984), Kern et al. (1990), LeFeuvre et al. (1987), Van Itallie and Kissileff (1985), and Verbalis et al. (1986).

Table 8.10. Number and Size of Fat Cells in Normal and Obese Individuals

	Cell size (μg lipid/cell)	Total cell number ($\times 10^9$)
Normal weight	0.66 ± 0.06	26 ± 6.8
Juvenile-onset obese	0.90 ± 0.05	85 ± 6.9
Adult-onset obese	0.98 ± 0.14	62 ± 4.2
Reduced obese[a]	0.45 ± 0.05	62 ± 5.3

Source: Reprinted by permission from Grinker and Hirsch (1972).

[a] Each subject had lost 50 kg in weight.

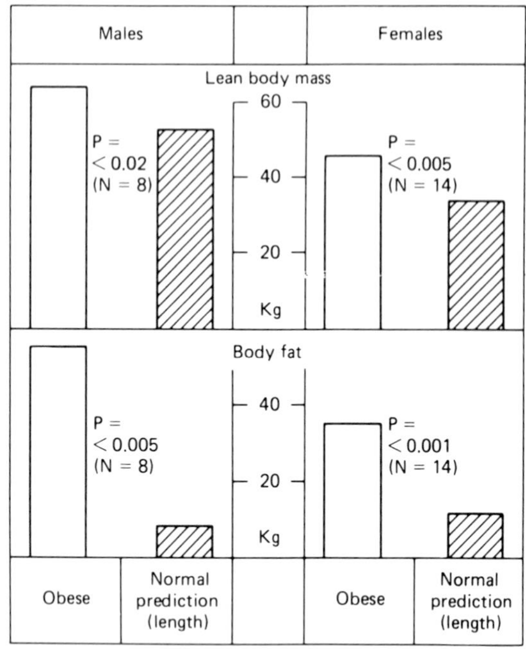

Figure 8.7. Lean body mass of obese individuals. [*Source:* Reprinted by permission from Cheek et al. (1975).]

Native American families indicated that heredity is also the major determinant of basal and resting metabolic rates (Ravussin et al., 1988). Thus, the current overall consensus is that 70% or more of the determination of body weight, obesity, and response to over- (or under-) feeding is heredity.

Normal individuals store the largest proportion of their net metabolizable energy as triglyceride in adipose tissue (Table 8.11), and only a small percentage as glycogen in liver and muscle (if the diet contains a substantial proportion of carbohydrate). The obese person has a much larger amount of triglyceride than the normal individual, but usually has similar amounts of glycogen. Fasting or a low carbohydrate diet will drastically lower carbohydrate stores, while refeeding a high carbohydrate diet will tend to maximize glycogen deposition, especially in muscle after heavy exercise (see below).

When fasting begins, carbohydrate stores are preferentially utilized, but increasingly with time, the body relies on triglyceride stores and prepares for gluconeogenesis from amino acids (especially muscle protein) and other noncarbohydrate precursors (Figure 8.8) (see also Chapter 4, Figure 4.9). As glycogen stores run out, ketones are increasingly produced (Figure 8.8 and Chapter 4, Figure 4.10) and eventually substitute for the majority of the glucose needed by the central nervous system, reducing the breakdown of muscle protein for gluconeogenesis (Chapter 4, Figure 4.9). A similar sequence of steps accompanies the increased utilization of stored fuels during heavy physical activity or exercise (see more below).

Weight Gain and Weight Loss

Substantial and/or long-term differences between the amounts of energy consumed and expended clearly result in changes of body weight, espe-

Table 8.11. Approximate Energy Stores in Normal and Obese Men and Women, Postabsorption, on a Normal Diet

	Tissue	Energy stores g	kcal	%
I. Average 70-kg man[a]				
Triglyceride	Adipose	15,000	100,000	80
Glycogen	Liver	70	280	
	Muscle	120	480	
Glucose	Body fluids	20	80	
Protein	Muscle	6,000	25,000	
Obese 100-kg man[a]				
Triglyceride	Adipose	45,000	300,000	92
II. Average 70-kg person[b]				
Normal diet	Liver	200–350 mmol glu eq/kg[c]		
CHO-free diet[c]	Liver	<75 mmol glu eq/kg		
After high CHO diet[c]	Liver	300–600 mmol glu eq/kg		

[a] Leibel (1980).
[b] Romsos and Clarke (1980).
[c] CHO, carbohydrate; glu, glucose.

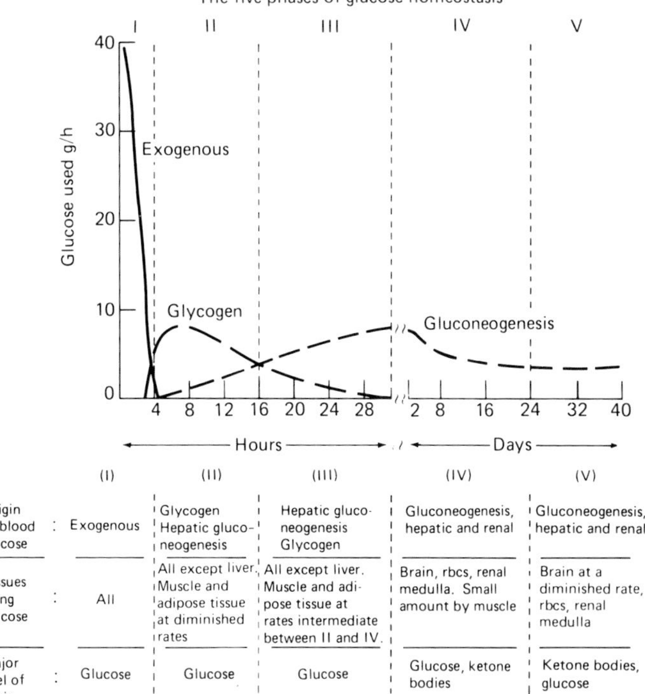

Figure 8.8. Sources of glucose used for energy in various physiologic states. One hundred grams glucose given at 0 time. The five phases of glucose homeostasis are as follows: state I, absorptive; state II, postabsorptive; state III, early fasting; state IV, intermediate starvation; state V, long-term starvation. [*Source:* Reprinted by permission from Ruderman et al. (1976).]

cially (but not exclusively) in terms of body fat. Calculations of energy expenditures as opposed to energy consumed (as described in previous sections) may be used to approximate the net caloric excess, or deficit, occurring for a given individual. This can be used to approximate the rate of weight loss or gain. Some examples are given in Table 8.12. Such calculations must make assumptions about the composition of the tissue lost, and thus, its caloric content. This is far from easy to do. It depends on many factors, including adipose stores, type of diet, length of time on diet, and so on. As shown in Table 8.13 (second column from right), the kcal corresponding to 1 kg of weight loss varies from as little as 2100 to as much as 8200! Knowing that the kcal content of 1 kg triglyceride is 9500, it is clear that the higher values reflect losses largely or exclusively of adipose tissue, while the lower values reflect a much smaller proportion of adipose tissue lost and larger proportions of lean tissue and fluids. It is generally assumed that average adipose tissue (in contrast to triglyceride) has an energy content equivalent of about 7700 kcal/kg, or 3500 kcal/lb (Table 8.12).

From Table 8.13, it is also apparent that weight losses in the early phases of a caloric deficit (in early dieting or starvation) involve less loss of adipose tissue per pound (or kilogram) of weight reduction than after prolonged dieting. This explains the very common high initial weight losses observed when people go on reducing diets, as

Table 8.12. Examples of Estimating Rate of Weight Loss from Deficits in Caloric Intake

Assumptions

Person is a 75-kg sedentary adult man who normally consumes 2600 kcal/day and has an energy need of about 2400 kcal/day (not including energy for DIT).[a] For loss of 1 kg adipose tissue, a deficit of 7700 kcal is required (3500 kcal/lb).

Calculations

(1) If this person reduces his caloric intake 500 kcal/day (a considerable reduction), he will have a deficit of about 500 kcal/day, or 3500 kcal/week, and will lose about 1 lb/week, or 1 kg/2.2 weeks.

(2) On an 800 kcal/day diet, this person will have a daily deficit of about 1600 kcal, and "real" weight loss will be at a rate of about 3 lb or 1.5 kg/week.

(3) On a total fast, the energy requirements of the individual would also probably decrease, and weight loss would probably not exceed 4 lb or 2 kg/week.

[a] See Table 8.7.

Table 8.13. Relationship Between Caloric Deficit and Weight Loss

Status of subjects	Days	Caloric deficit per weight lost kcal/lb[a,b]	kcal/kg	Weight lost per deficit (kg/1000 kcal)
Undernourished	4	1240	2730	0.36
Starved	4	1290	2840	0.35
Starved, working	5	1290	2840	0.35
Semistarved, working[c]	3	1820	2600	0.38
	11–13	3200	7040	0.14
Semistarved, working	12	1950	4300	0.23
Semistarved	24	2420	5320	0.19
Semistarved, prolonged	168	3410	7510	0.13
Overweight, reducing	4	980–1640	2160–3610	0.28–0.46
Overweight, prolonged reducing	63	2800	6170	0.16
Obese, reducing	14+	2730–3730 (Max 3860)	6000–8200 (Max 8500)	0.12–0.17

Source: Summary of many studies; modified from Buskirk and Mendez (1980).

[a] kcal/kg triglyceride = 9300–9500 (4320 kcal/lb).
[b] kcal/kg divided by 2.2 lb/kg.
[c] Brozek et al. (1957).

compared with much slower losses later on. Also, glycogen is preferentially lost in the early phases and is highly hydrated. Thus, 3 g of water (and 0.34 meq of potassium) are lost with every gram of glycogen used (Shils, 1978).

Comparisons of energy intakes and expenditures are also useful in illustrating just how slowly actual fat is lost from the body. As shown in Table 8.12, a net deficit of 500 kcal/day (which is considerable for most people) will result in an adipose tissue weight loss of only 1 lb/week, if the loss is only of adipose tissue. Going on to a more drastic diet or a complete fast will, of course, have much more profound effects, but these will also be likely to interfere with the normal activity, energy, and lifestyle of the individual. In these instances, the body may also institute energy-saving measures, reducing BMR and the urge to perform physical activities, and perhaps even lowering body temperature (Bray and York, 1971).

The composition of the diet, even with equivalent kilocalorie intake, also has profound effects on the type and degree of weight loss observed. As shown in Table 8.14, the proportion of energy from carbohydrate versus fat is especially important as a determinant of fluid (and even protein) losses. Ketogenic (low carbohydrate) diets tend to be associated with greater fluid losses than those that include about half or more of their energy from carbohydrate. Some researchers claim that this can easily be changed by increasing intake of sodium (Bistrian et al., 1976). Moreover, a high protein or amino acid diet (with or without much carbohydrate) is beneficial in minimizing muscle protein losses, while maintaining maximal triglyceride degradation (Baird, 1974; Pi-Sunyer, 1988). Carbohydrate intake will stimulate insulin secretion and reduce glucagon, which will, in turn, reduce the release of free fatty acids and glycerol from adipose tissue (see Chapters 2 and 3; Figures 2.2 and 2.3) (Flatt and Blackburn, 1974; Flatt, 1978). Moreover, the insulin will help minimize muscle protein losses by stimulating muscle protein synthesis (see Chapter 4, Figure 4.2). On the other hand, ingestion of some forms of complex carbohydrate has little effect on insulin release (Chapter 2), and amino acids themselves can cause insulin secretion (see Chapter 4).

Evidence from actual human trials by proponents of exclusively amino acid/protein diets is shown in Table 8.14. However, the results of other studies (also shown) tend to support the use of some carbohydrate (with protein) in reducing diets, especially those that are low (e.g., 800 kcal) or very low (300–400 kcal) in calories. Indeed, within 6 months of their introduction in 1977, very low calorie "liquid protein" diets (containing predigested collagen—a very poor quality protein) were associated with at least 60 sudden deaths among middle-aged women who were, or just had been, on these diets. The majority appeared to have died of cardiac problems. Cardiac arrhythmias, prolonged QT intervals, and epi-

Table 8.14. Effects of Reducing Diets on Weight Loss

Diet	Days on diet	Caloric intake (kcal/day)	Average weight lost (g/day)	Composition of weight lost (g)		
				Water	Fat	Protein
All protein (1.2–1.4 g/kg ideal BW)[a]	300–365	215–345	79–203	ND	ND	3–9
Amino acid (30 g/day)[b]	14	130	286	More	ND	0
Amino acid + CHO (15 g AA + 30 g CHO)[b]	14	195	257	Less	ND	Slight
Ketogenic[c] (70% fat and 5% CHO energy)	10	800	467	286	163	18
Mixed[c] (30% fat and 45% CHO energy)	10	800	278	103	165	10
Ketogenic[d] (all protein)	35	400	286	71	202	13
Mixed[d] (50% CHO, 50% protein)	35	400	228	6	206	16

CHO, carbohydrate; AA, amino acids; BW, body weight; ND, not determined.
[a] Bistrian et al. (1976).
[b] Baird (1974) (patients had been fasting prior to diet).
[c] Yang and Van Itallie (1976) (includes 50 g protein/day).
[d] DeHaven et al. (1980).

sodes of tachycardia (rapid heart beats) were reported for some individuals on such diets (Isner et al., 1979; Lantingua et al., 1980). The exact basis for these phenomena is unclear, although potassium loss has probably been ruled out in many, but not all, cases. A loss of heart muscle protein may be involved (Isner et al., 1979). It should be noted that the most serious adverse responses have arisen with diets containing no carbohydrate or fat, and containing protein equivalents in the form of amino acids (like predigested/hydrolyzed collagen, supplemented with tryptophan). Other very low calorie diets, either based solely on whole (high quality) protein (DeHaven et al., 1980) or on mixtures of whole protein and carbohydrate (with a little fat) (Cambridge diet), have not had these responses, except perhaps long-term (>16 weeks) (Pi-Sunyer, 1988). [NaCl losses and hypotension upon standing have been reported with the exclusively protein, very low calorie diets (DeHaven et al., 1980; Yang and Van Itallie, 1976).] In contrast, less drastic diets (1100–1200 kcal with 60 g protein) appear to be well tolerated and for long periods of time.

The best (safest) means of instituting a weight reduction would thus appear to be to reduce caloric intake in a more balanced way, by cutting back on overall intake of all the foods (especially fatty foods) normally consumed rather than by going on specific diets that drastically alter proportions of protein, carbohydrate, or other food components. Instituting a diet with a lower proportion of fat has additional long-range advantages, as discussed elsewhere (Chapters 3, 15, and 16), as the American diet is top-heavy in fatty foods (related to chronic health problems) and fats are so much more rich in energy, per weight, than carbohydrates.

Similar approaches to diets designed for weight gain are in order, where use of a large proportion of carbohydrates (especially starch) would appear to be the most healthy. Skewing diets to avoid certain classes of foods, especially those containing complex carbohydrate, increases the likelihood of instituting deficiencies in minerals, vitamins, and trace elements (see other chapters).

Body Weight Control Other Than by Adjustment of Caloric Intake

As already described, factors other than the rate of caloric intake influence body weight by varying energy expenditure for physical exercise versus storage and/or heat production. Increasing physical exercise will demand more of the body's available fuel reserves. The weight loss expected from an exercise program can be estimated by comparing intake with expenditure, including that required for increased physical exertion (as previously presented).

The possibility that there is regulation of heat production, and regulation of the efficiency with which available metabolic energy is harnessed to anabolic processes (through formation of ~P) as opposed to heat, has until recently been more controversial. However, there is now a body of suggestive evidence that some homeostatic control of body weight exists in the face of excess or deficient intake, that may function through variations in nonproductive energy losses, including BAT activity. (Relevant studies and observations through 1983 are summarized in Table 8.15.) In the earlier part of this century, "self-studies" by Neumann (1902) and Gulick (1922) indicated that weight changes were minimal, or not as large as expected, when caloric intake was deliberately increased 20%–25%, long-term, and physical activity was held constant. This led to the proposal that there is "luxus consumption," or the enhanced oxidation of excess calories consumed. Since then, other studies have lead to similar findings for groups of people or animals; others have given indications that caloric excesses can increase basal oxygen consumption above what is needed for digestion, absorption, and storage of nutrients and can even increase heat production. In the studies of Kasper et al. (1973, 1975), a few normal individuals were given up to 300–400 g fat/day (2700–3600 kcal) as corn oil or olive oil. With this treatment, some of the subjects experienced sensations of increased warmth and a tendency to sweat, although no heat measurements were made. This study was criticized by Hirsh and Van Itallie (1973) as being insufficiently clear about the degree of heat and water losses involved and for claiming more than the evidence showed. Nevertheless, animal studies have indicated that nonshivering thermogenesis can be induced by cold and/or by excess calories, and that this involves activation of the sympathetic nervous system (catecholamines) and heat generation by BAT (Foster and Frydman, 1978; Himms-Hagen, 1981; Stock and Rothwell, 1981; Sukhatme and Margen, 1982) (Figure 8.6). Moreover, working with humans, Stock and Rothwell (1981) reported the appearance of "hot" areas in the neck and scapular regions of the back (where brown fat is found) in response to sympathomimetic stimulation (ephedrine treatment), as detected by skin thermocouples and infrared thermography (Figure 8.9). It is now quite well-accepted that BAT can occur in human adults, and that in both man and animal its heat-generating activity can be triggered by cold exposure, glucagon, corticotropin-releasing factor (CRF) and even excess calories.

The mechanisms of this regulation have been under intensive study in animals. As with appetite, BAT activity is directly controlled by the sympathetic nervous system (Figure 8.6), presumably via stimuli from the VMH, but also probably via the paraventricular region (through CRF) (LeFeuvre et al., 1987), and more directly even by glucagon (Joel, 1966). Sympathetic stimulation also reduces appetite in the face of satiety (see above) and can thus co-trigger loss of additional calories by heat production.

The effects of treating BAT with glucagon or norepinephrine (as would occur with sympathetic nerve stimulation) are illustrated by data for rats in Table 8.16. Glucagon is released when blood glucose levels fall (as in fasting, exercise, and stress) or in response to cold exposure (see Billington et al., 1987). Treatments with norepinephrine or glucagon increased BAT weight, cell number, and cytochrome oxidase activity (a marker for mitochondria). They also increased BAT lipoprotein lipase activity (which would bring circulating triglyceride and its fatty acids to the tissue at a faster rate) and mitochondrial "GDP-binding," a reflection of the activity of the unique protein of BAT responsible for uncoupling oxidative phosphorylation for heat generation. [The uncoupling protein appears to act by reversing the H^+ gradient generated by the electron transport system, allowing protons to be translocated back into the area of the mitochondrial matrix without generation of ATP. Recent data suggest that H^+ may be carried as part of undissociated fatty acids (Andreyev et al., 1988). The uncoupling protein has been isolated, cloned, and sequenced and bears some homology to other mitochondrial translocator proteins (for phosphate and ADP/ATP) (Klingenberg, 1990).]

BAT activity is increased also by acute cold exposure (which enhances glucagon release, but may also have other effects on the central nervous system and/or hypothalamus and pituitary). Significant increases in activity occur within 20 min of the start of cold exposure (Swick and Swick, 1986) and appear to involve no change in the actual amount of BAT uncoupling protein, determined immunologically (Gribskov et al., 1986). This indicates that the initial effect of cold is to activate or "unmask" existing translocator (uncoupling) protein molecules. However, more long-term, continued treatments (such as with glucagon) appear to result in an enhanced gene expression of the uncoupling protein (Billington

Table 8.15. Summary of Earlier Evidence for Some Homeostatic Control of Body Weight in the Face of Changes in Caloric Intake[a]

	Report result	Reference
Human studies: individuals		
Vary caloric intake, long-term, from 1770–2400 kcal/day	No significant change in body weight	Neumann, 1902
Increase caloric intake, long-term	Weight change not as great as expected from excess calories (assuming 6000 kcal/kg adipose tissue)	Gulick, 1922
Human studies: groups[b]		
Normal people given excess fat calories at 300–400 g fat/day	Weight gain not proportional to excess calories	Kasper et al., 1973
	Sensation of heating: tendency to sweat	Kasper et al., 1975
Normal people given 50% caloric excess	Difficulty in gaining and maintaining excess body weight	Sims, 1976
Normal people given caloric excess of 1500 kcal/day	10.9% increase in basal O_2 consumption	Apfelbaum et al., 1971
Normal people overeating	Associated with increase in exercise-associated metabolic rate	Miller et al., 1967
Normal people greatly reducing their caloric intake	20%+ decrease in basal metabolic rate by 2–3 days	Bray, 1969
Obese versus normal subjects, given 50 g oral glucose	5.2% versus 13% increase in resting metabolic rate; less heat loss	Pittet et al., 1976
Obese versus normal subjects given intravenous epinephrine	9.6% versus 20% increase in resting metabolic rate	Jung et al., 1979
Animal studies		
Dogs fed 30% excess calories for 1 month	No weight gain	Share et al., 1952
Dogs fed 75% excess calories long term	No weight gain	Janowitz and Hollander, 1955
Rats fed 80% excess calories	Gained only 27% of expected extra body weight	Rothwell and Stock, 1979
	Increased resting O_2 consumption	
Genetically obese versus normal mice (same caloric intake)	Greater weight gain	Bray and York, 1971
	Greater proportion of fat	
	Decreased resting O_2 consumption and body temperature	
Monkeys with excess calories (40 kcal/day)	No difference in body weight	Samonds and Fleagle, 1973
Miscellaneous points		
Body weight normally remains quite constant in the adult		Pond, 1983
Species vary greatly in their capacities to convert food energy into available body energy (kcal/kcal): lamb 3%, beef 8%, poultry 13%, pork 23%		

[a] Summarized from Crist et al. (1980); Romsos and Clarke (1980); Leibel (1980).
[b] Additional review in Garrow (1978).

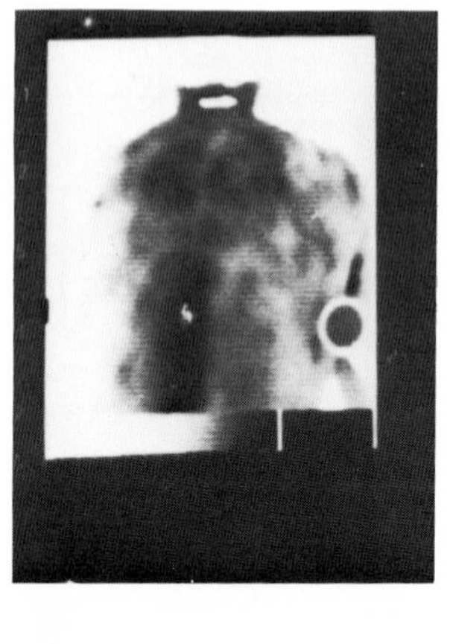
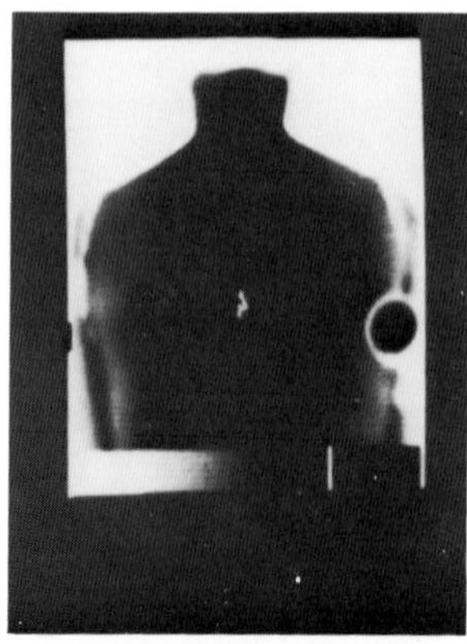
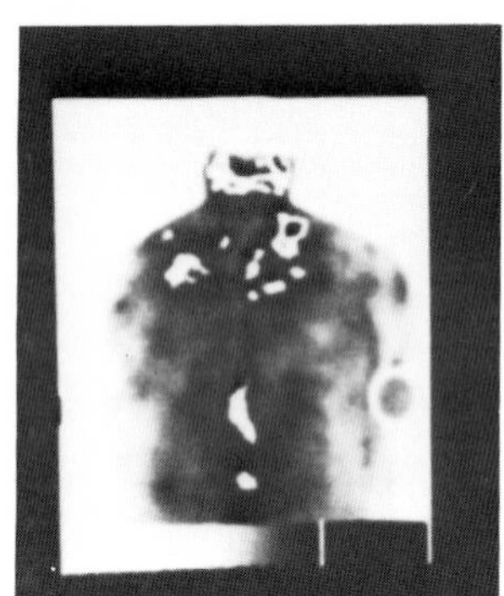
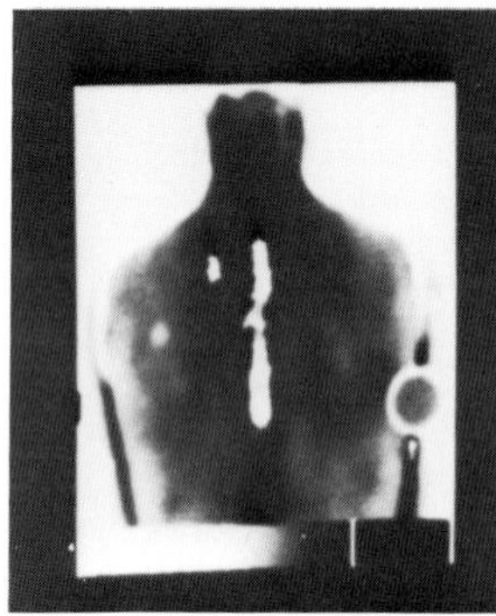

Figure 8.9. Effect of ephedrine on heat production in scapular regions of the body. Infrared thermograms of the back of subjects (left, male; right, female) before (upper thermograms) and 60 min after (lower thermograms) ephedrine administration (1 mg/kg). The white areas increase after ephedrine but are confined to the neck and supra- and interscapular regions. [*Source:* Reprinted by permission from Stock and Rothwell (1981).]

et al., 1989), as shown by cDNA–mRNA hybridization.

Heat production by BAT also appears to be regulated by CRF secreted by the pituitary hypophysis (again, most probably causing activation and/or increased gene expression of the BAT uncoupling protein). This is thought to be mediated by the paraventricular hypothalamus and sympathetic nerves (LeFeuvre et al., 1987) (Figure 8.6). [Adrenalectomy and hypophysectomy enhance CRF release and BAT activity; corticosterone (another end result of CRF release) or mor-

Table 8.16. Effects of Norepinephrine and Glucagon on Brown Adipose Tissue (BAT) in Rats[a]

	Rats		
Parameters	Controls	+Norepinephrine	+Glucagon
Food consumption (kcals/8 days)	1300	1248[b]	1418
Weight gain (g)	56	25[c]	41[c]
BAT			
Final weight (mg/pad)	295	575[c]	405[c]
Protein (mg/pad)	14	73[c]	27[c]
DNA (mg/pad)	305	670[c]	790[c]
Cytochrome oxidase activity (U/pad)	5.5	18.5[c]	9.5[c]
Lipoprotein lipase activity (U/pad)[d]	4.2	—	8.8[c]
GDP-binding activity (U/pad)[d]	5.7	—	11.5[c]

[a] Rats were injected daily with norepinephrine, glucagon, or vehicle (controls) for 18 days. Results are mean values from Billington et al. (1987).
[b] Significant difference from controls ($p < 0.05$).
[c] Significant difference from controls ($p < 0.01$).
[d] After only 5–8 days of treatment.

phine both reduce BAT activity, by decreasing the balance between sympathetic and parasympathetic nervous function (LeFeuvre et al., 1987; Figure 8.6).] CRF treatment has been found to reduce food intake (and enhance BAT) activity in genetically obese, but not in normal rodents, suggesting that a lack of CRF secretion may contribute to some forms of obesity (Rohner-Jeanrenaud et al., 1989). However, obese subjects may also exhibit a reduced thermic response to CRF and other stimuli, as reported in many studies (e.g., James and Trayhurn, 1981; Pitt et al., 1976; Schwarz et al., 1983) but this may be an artifact due to a change in the kinetics of the response. Ravussin et al. (1985) found that differences in the thermic response to intravenous glucose in obese versus normal human subjects could be completely obliterated by equalizing their rates of cell glucose uptake. This was accomplished by infusing more insulin (an average of 6.6 versus 3.0 mU/kg/min), to overcome the well-known phenomenon of "insulin resistance" in such subjects. (Insulin resistance in obesity is thought to reflect a lower density of insulin receptors on the surface of hypertrophied adipocytes.] This resistance is simply a function of enlarged fat stores and is lost upon weight reduction. A reduction in the rate of glucose uptake would mean that uptake of incoming glucose (by tissues from the blood) would also be prolonged, thus changing the kinetics of uptake and presumably also of the thermic response (Ravussin et al., 1985). Indeed, using whole body calorimetry over 24 hr, Blaza and Garrow (1983) were unable to detect differences in overall thermic responses to food, lower temperature, or exercise of obese versus normal individuals. [The obese subjects had a much higher RMR and total energy expenditure, commensurate with their greater total (and lean) body weight.] Similarly, Welle and Campbell (1983) found no differences in the total release of norepinephrine (reflecting activity of the sympathetic nervous system), and in this group of obese, insulin release was greater than in the lean subjects. The overall impression, currently, is thus that obesity in humans is not usually due to a defect in thermic response (relating to BAT or otherwise). Whether this is also true for genetically obese rodents is still not clear.

Apart from BAT, animal studies support the concept that overfeeding may also generate additional heat losses by increasing production of triiodo- from tetraiodothyronine (thyroxine), increasing the numbers and size of cell mitochondria and enhancing ATP breakdown (Crist et al., 1980; Leibel, 1980). Growth hormone (somatotrophin) or epinephrine may also be involved. These hormones may cause heat production indirectly by stimulating the futile release of free fatty acid from adipose tissue (Crist et al., 1980).

There has been some interest in the possibility that *decreases* in BAT activity (or other mechanisms reducing the efficiency of energy metabolism) might contribute to the apparent decreases in BMR observed when caloric intake is restricted (as in dieting and fasting). This would provide a means of conserving energy in the face of caloric deprivation, and thus help in the maintenance of normal body weight. [Weight losses observed with caloric restriction usually are not as great as would be predicted from the deficit in calories involved (Table 8.15).] We do not as yet have sufficient information to fully judge what happens in these cases. However, recent information we do have, suggests that any apparent decreases in BMR either are fully explained by the loss of lean body mass (that accompanies loss of fat) or are only temporary during long-term dieting (James, 1989). Caloric restriction tends to promote a reduction in physical activity which also could lead to energy conservation. Deliberate exercise may also prevent any fall in RMR.

Clearly, BAT and its role in the thermic response to food (DIT) and cold adaptation (via the sympathetic nervous system) are established phenomena in humans. However, the involvement of BAT in decreasing the BMR (or RMR) during calorie restriction is still questionable. The response to cold adaptation indicates BAT can play a role in maintenance or control of body temperature, and animal studies with pyrogens indicate this may also be the case when body temperature is set to a higher level, as in fever (Blatteis, 1976; Corbett et al., 1988). What is still to be clarified is the *degree* of importance of BAT activity in various conditions; many steps in the mechanisms leading to BAT response; and whether some of the individual differences among subjects, even in BMR, might not be ascribable to some aspect of BAT amount or activity.

Energy Needs and Physical Exercise

As already indicated and discussed elsewhere (Chapters 2 and 3), physical exercise requires the organism to draw on its stores of muscle glycogen and adipose triglyceride at a more rapid rate than otherwise. At levels of activity in the moderate to heavy exercise range (oxygen uptake at >40% of the maximum rate), the same sequence of changes with time occur as in fasting (Figure 8.8). However, it should be remembered that muscle glycogen, rather than liver glycogen, is most important for muscle activity, especially when the activity runs into the limitations imposed by the rate of oxygen transport. Indeed, the major fuel (or source of high energy phosphate bonds; ~P) used to form ATP by muscle, will vary depending upon the intensity of the activity and its duration (Table 8.17). Immediately, upon institution of the highest rate of exercise, usually measured as a percentage of maximum oxygen consumption ($VO_{2\,max}$), ~P from creatine-phosphate is the most rapidly available, but is also the most limited in terms of amount. Under intense exercise conditions, the next most important (and the most important while it lasts) is muscle glycogen breakdown and glycolysis. At lower rates of exercise (but above 35%–40% of $VO_{2\,max}$), muscle glycogen is the most important initial fuel, through glycolysis plus oxidative phosphorylation (to the extent the latter can keep up). Glycolysis (to lactate) provides a means of forming ATP without the limitations of oxygen availability. At any rate of exercise, fatty acids become increasingly important with time, in the face of dwindling muscle glycogen stores. [Large-scale mobilization of muscle glycogen stores is triggered when exercise rates are greater than 35%–40% of $VO_{2\,max}$ (Hultman et al., 1988). There is little mobilization at low rates of exercise.] Liver glycogen is also mobilized during exercise, but never becomes a major source of high energy phosphate because of its slow availability (Table 8.17). At rest and low exercise intensity, fatty acids are the major fuel (except during the absorptive phase after a carbohydrate-containing meal, when glucose will be used) (see Chapters 2 and 4). Adaptation to exercise (i.e., training) will tend to increase oxygen transport and thus reduce the RQ of trained versus untrained individuals for the same rate of effort, indicating less reliance on carbohydrate and more in fat.

Table 8.18 summarizes the observations that have been made on changes in energy metabolism and body composition during the act of exercising and the effects of some, or extensive, physical training. In the average person on a mixed diet (who has glycogen stores), the RQ will initially increase when exercise begins (Table 8.18 and Figure 8.10), reflecting an increase in the rate of utilization of muscle (and also liver) glycogen stores (Figure 8.11). For all individuals who have glycogen stores, the RQ will fall progressively with time, reflecting a progressive shift to utilization of energy from fat. For example, an athlete with high glycogen stores will initially derive 90% or more of energy from carbohydrates, while after many hours of exercise, 70%–80% of energy will come from fat (Gollnick, 1984). The rate of glycogen loss, especially from muscle, will depend on the degree of physical effort. Regulating these changes are alterations in hormone secretions, especially insulin and glucagon, with decreased secretion of insulin at the start, followed by increased glucagon release, to lay the groundwork for gluconeogenesis. (Also catecholamine

Table 8.17. Sources and Rates of Mobilization of Energy Stores for Muscle Work

Sources of high energy phosphate	Availability of high energy phosphate equivalents (~P): Maximum rate of mobilization (mol/in)	Availability of high energy phosphate equivalents (~P): Total available (mol/28 kg muscle)	Conditions when primary energy source
Phosphocreatine and other phosphogens	4.4	0.67	Immediate, maximum effort work or exercise
Muscle glycogen to lactate (Glycolysis)	2.35	6.7	Shorter term, maximum effort work or exercise
Muscle glycogen to $CO_2 + H_2O$ (Glycolysis + Krebs cycle)	0.85–1.14	84	Longer term, lower $VO_{2\,max}$ work or exercise
Mobilized liver glycogen (via blood to muscle)[a]	0.16	18	(Never primary source)
Fatty acids (from blood)	0.4	4000[b]	Rest; longer-term or endurance exercise

Source: Estimates of Hultman et al. (1988) for a 70-kg man with muscle at 40% of body weight (28 kg).

[a] Assuming a typical postprandial liver glycogen store.
[b] Per typical adipose tissue stores.

Table 8.18. Effects of Exercise and Training on Body Composition and Metabolism

Changes during exercise
- Overall ↓ in RQ with duration of exercise
- Change from glycogen as main energy source to fat as main energy source
- ↓ Muscle (and liver) glycogen
- ↑ Fat mobilization, with time
- ↑ Gluconeogenesis, with duration of exercise
  - (↑ glucagon secretion)
  - (↑ key gluconeogenic enzymes in liver)
- ↓ Protein synthesis (liver, muscle)
- ↓ Protein content (muscle,[a] liver, plasma)

Changes with training
- ↓ RQ of exercise (more utilization of fat)
- Slight ↑ O_2 consumption/rate of exercise and aerobic capacity ($VO_{2\,max}$)
- ↑ Rate of maximal O_2 consumption ($VO_{2\,max}$)
- Slight ↑ blood flow with exercise
- ↑ Lean body mass/height (local muscle hypertrophy)
- ↓ Percent body fat
- ↑ Glucose tolerance and insulin sensitivity
- ↓ Long-term lactate release by muscle
- ↓ Fasting plasma triglyceride levels
- No change in total cholesterol, though ↓ LDL, ↑ HDL, depending on degree of training

Source: Information from Symposium on Metabolic and Nutritional Aspects of Physical Exercise, FASEB, Chicago, April 1983.

[a] Controversial for determinations made in humans (see text).

release from sympathetic nerves). Gluconeogenesis is needed progressively more as exercise proceeds and glycogen is lost. Mobilization of fat (increased serum levels of free fatty acids) is also increasingly promoted (by glucagon and epinephrine). These events proceed much in the same sequence as in the case of fasting, except in a narrower time frame (Figure 8.12).

With this in mind, it is not surprising that diets high in carbohydrate are preferable for individuals performing physical exercise and for athletes—both those that exercise briefly at maximum O_2 capacity (maximum work) and those involved in endurance efforts. In the first instance, muscle glycogen stores are important for the extra "push" provided by glycolysis (independent of increased oxygen availability). For the endurance athlete, endurance capacity will be prolonged if initial glycogen stores are greater. By the same token, ingestion of carbohydrate (including sugars) too soon before exercise begins will interfere with the normal glycogen (and fat) mobilization processes necessary to support the exercise, because it elicits insulin secretion, which in turn inhibits glycogenolysis and lipolysis. When exercise begins, digestion and absorption of nutrients are also reduced through a marked decrease in stomach emptying (Costill, 1984). Thus, unabsorbed sugar in the stomach will not only be unavailable, but may have osmotic effects on body fluid balance that are unfavorable to exercise. Periodically providing some glucose in sufficient dilution to trained athletes in prolonged exercise (such as bicycling) can spare some of the loss in muscle glycogen and prolong exercise capacity (Costill, 1984). In the long-term, the type of carbohydrate eaten to bolster glycogen stores makes little difference; short-term, glucose tends to go to the muscle and fructose to the liver, so that near exhaustion, the ingestion of some glucose in dilute form may allow prolongation of physical effort for a short time.

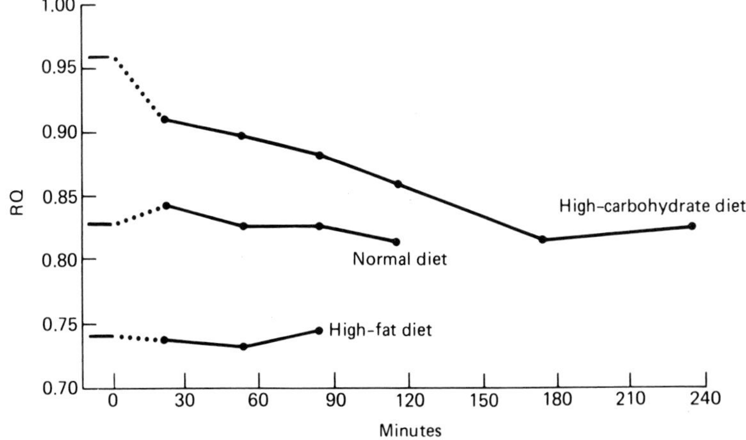

Figure 8.10. Changes in RQ during exercise and while on different diets. Response of a single subject, working at the same rate, while on three different diets. Subject worked to exhaustion in all three cases. [*Source:* Reprinted by permission from Åstrand and Rodahl (1970); data from Christensen and Hansen (1939).]

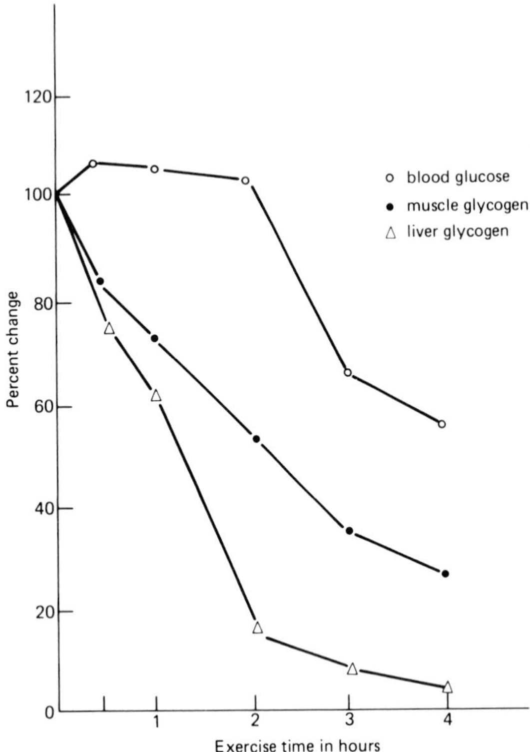

Figure 8.11. Depletion of glycogen in muscle and liver during exercise; studies in rats during 4 hr of swimming. [*Source:* Reprinted by permission from Armstrong et al. (1975).]

Physical exercise, especially when prolonged, puts the organism into glycogenolytic, lipolytic, and ultimately gluconeogenic and ketogenic modes. In line with this, physical exercise reduces protein synthesis and eventually may decrease the protein content of muscle, liver, and plasma. This has been demonstrated in rats subjected to swimming or running (Dohm, 1984) and is supported by some human studies on whole body protein synthesis and the release of 3-methylhistidine, a marker of muscle protein catabolism (Millward et al., 1982; see Chapter 4). An increase in plasma urea and urinary nitrogen excretion (during and after endurance exercise, respectively) has also been observed (Hultman et al., 1988; Rennie et al., 1981), and leucine catabolism to CO_2 (initiated mainly in muscle) can also be accelerated, especially when glycogen stores are low (Lemon and Mullin, 1980). However, not all human studies support an acceleration of muscle protein loss and 3-methylhistidine excretion (Dohm, 1984; Hultman et al., 1988).

The reduction in protein synthesis, with or without the increased catabolism of liver, plasma, and muscle protein, frees up amino acids for gluconeogenic oxidation (Dohm, 1984). Moreover, increases in the key gluconeogenic enzymes of liver (PEP carboxykinase, pyruvate, carboxylase, and others) are observed (see also Chapters 2–4). This allows the flow of amino acid carbon into glucose (and ketone) production, as the glucose available from glycogen stores is used up.

Protein must thus also be considered a daily fuel for physical exercise and other energy-dependent body functions. The high intake of protein in Western countries and Japan provides 12%–15% of calories, average intakes being more than twice U.S. and worldwide RDAs (see Chapter 4). Even with intake restricted to 0.75–0.8 g/kg/day (the RDA), most data suggest there is a sufficient supply of essential amino acids to offset any increase in their catabolism induced by exercise, if normal levels of carbohydrate calories are consumed (Hultman et al., 1988). [An increase of 10% in protein consumption above the RDA would offset any lack induced by a low carbohydrate diet (Hultman et al., 1988).] Similarly, during body building the RDA is thought to supply enough essential amino acids to build the maximum amount of extra tissue that could be expected to accrue (Hultman et al., 1988; Tarnopolsky et al., 1988). [The *timing* of amino acid intake (to coincide with maximal stimulation of muscle protein synthesis, as after insulin secretion) may influence the degree of body building induced by exercise; increasing the *amounts* of protein/amino acid ingested will not.] Nevertheless, some studies suggest that heavy endurance athletes may have a larger requirement for protein. In a study by Tarnopolsky et al. (1988), N-balance was only maintained at an intake rate that was 1.7 times the U.S. RDA. (In the same study, body builders had normal requirements.)

When physical training is instituted, a variety of changes occur that tend to support and ease exercise performance. These are summarized in the second half of Table 8.18. There are increases in aerobic capacity (and oxygen transport), allowing more extensive reliance on fatty acids for fuel and a greater rate of oxygen consumption—thus, a lower RQ for the same degree of effort and less buildup of lactic acid. There is also a decrease in the percentage of body fat, and lean body mass is increased by muscle hypertrophy. Of some interest for long-term health is the observation that the ratio of low-density to high-density lipoproteins in plasma tends to change in favor of a greater

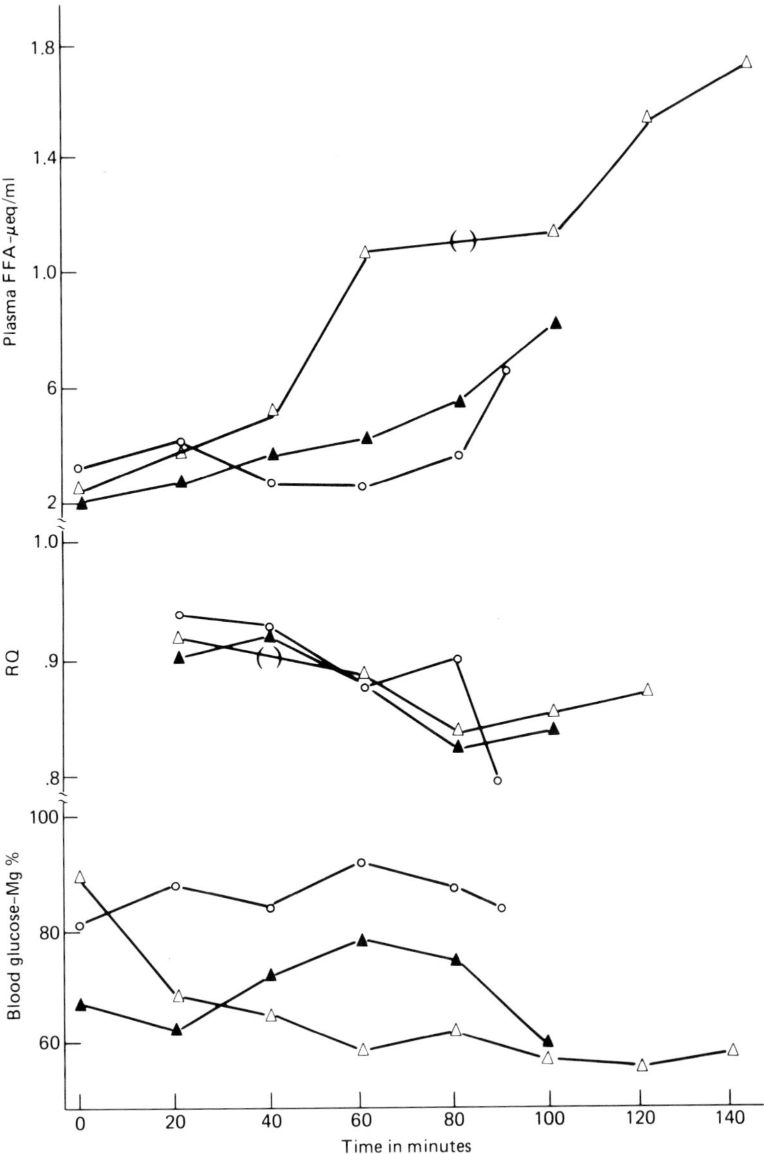

Figure 8.12. Changes in plasma free fatty acids, glucose, and RQ during heavy exercise; 75%–80% of maximum O_2 consumption (bicycle pedaling on an ergometer). Responses of three individuals are presented. [*Source:* Reprinted by permission from Gollnick et al. (1969).]

proportion of high-density lipoproteins (see Chapter 3). [This relates to a reduced atherosclerosis risk (see Chapter 15).] The changes seen in athletic training do occur at least to some degree even in sedentary middle-aged working people, who embark on a limited program of walking, jogging, and running (averaging 8.6 miles a week) for a year or more, as demonstrated by the initial findings of the Stanford Exercise Study (Wood, 1984, 1990).

After very heavy physical exertion (such as a strenuous athletic performance), when glycogen stores have been drained, it takes some time to replenish glycogen reserves. Even when consuming a high carbohydrate diet, maximum levels are likely to be achieved only after 2 days (Figure 8.13). Carbohydrate loading after heavy exercise (and exhaustion of glycogen stores) is nevertheless also the way to maximize subsequent muscle

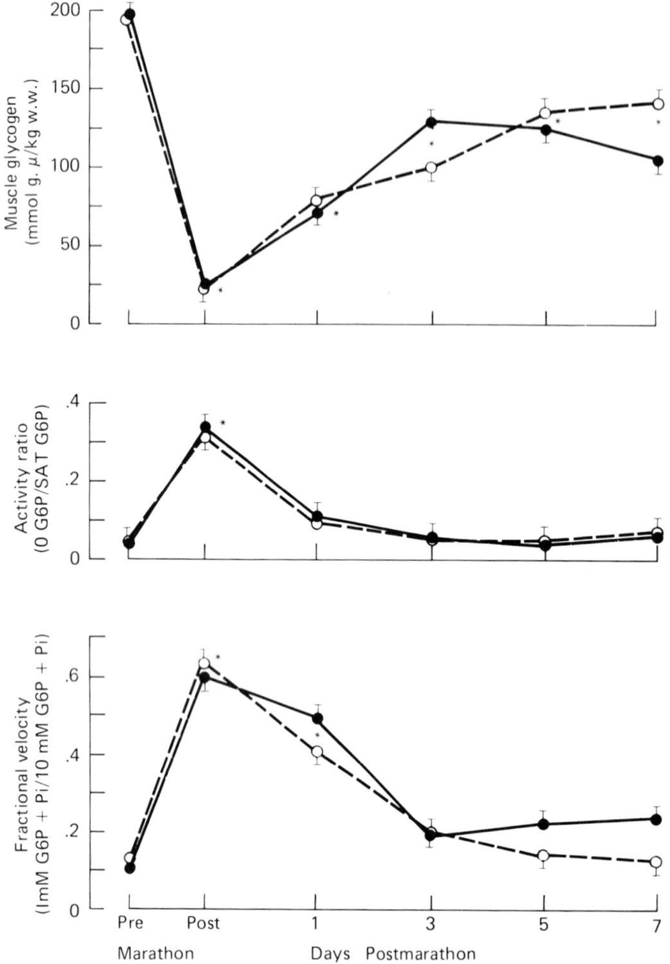

Figure 8.13. Changes in muscle glycogen and glycogen synthetase activity during and after heavy exercise (marathon running). Fractional velocity and activity ratios refer to various forms of glycogen synthetase activity. [*Source:* Reprinted by permission from Sherman et al. (1983).]

glycogen storage (as in preparation for competition) (Hultman et al., 1988).

A decrease in red blood cells and hemoglobin (indicative of anemia) occurs more frequently in athletes, and especially in runners, than in the rest of the population. The data of Hallberg and colleagues (Magnussen et al., 1984*a*, *b*) suggests that this is due to a physiological adjustment of blood volume (increased in training) and usually not to iron deficiency. Nevertheless, athletes may have a higher frequency of low iron stores (Hultman et al., 1988; Par et al., 1984; Wishnitzer et al., 1984). If so, this could be due to a combination of decreased intestinal absorption (in response to iron depletion) and increased losses of iron through the sweat. With excessive exercise, some muscle damage may also occur, leading to loss of myoglobin and hemoglobin in the urine.

References

Anderson GH (1988): *In* Shils M, Young VR, eds: Modern nutrition in health and disease. Philadelphia: Lea & Febiger, p 557.

Anderson JJB (1982): Applied nutrition for health professions: Basic nutrition. Chapel Hill: University of North Carolina.

Andreyev AY, Bondareva TO, Dedukhova VI, Mokhova EN, Skulachev VP, Volkov NI (1988): FEBS Lett 226:265.

Apfelbaum M, Bostarron J, Lacatis D (1971): Am J Clin Nutr 24:1405.

Armstrong RB, Saubert CW IV, Sembrowich WL, Shepherd RE, Gollnick PD (1975): *In* Howald H, Portmans JR, eds: Metabolic adaptation to prolonged physical exercise. Basel: Birkhauser Verlag, p 397.

Åstrand PO, Rodahl K (1970): Textbook of work physiology (1st ed). New York: McGraw-Hill, p 459.

Baird IM (1974): Metabolism 23:645.

Billington CJ, Bartness TJ, Briggs J, Levine AS, Morley JE (1987): Am J Physiol 252:R160.

Billington CJ, Ricquier D, Bouillaud F, Levine AS (1989): Clin Res 37:446A.

Bistrian BR, Blackburn GL, Flatt K-P, Sizer J, Scrimshaw NS, Sherman M (1976): Diabetes 25:494.

Blatteis CM (1976): J Appl Physiol 40:29.

Blaza S, Garrow JS (1983): Br J Nutr 49:171.

Bouchard C, Tremblay A, Despres J-P, Nadeau A, Lupien PJ, Theriault G, Dussault J, Moorjani S, Pinault S, Fournier G (1990): N Engl J Med 322:1477.

Bray GA (1969): Lancet 2:397.

Bray GA, York DA (1971): Physiol Rev 51:598.

Brody GA (1945): Bioenergetics and growth. New York: Hafner.

Brozek J, Grande F, Taylor HL, Anderson JT, Buskirk ER, Keys A (1957): Appl Physiol 10:412.

Buskirk ER, Mendez J (1980): *In* Alfin-Slater RB, Krichevsky D, eds: Human nutrition, a comprehensive treatise, Vol 3A. New York: Plenum, p 49.

Cahill GF Jr (1970): N Engl J Med 128:668.

Cheek DB, Parra A, White J (1975): *In* Clark DB, ed: Fetal and postnatal cellular growth. New York: Wiley, p 453.

Christensen SE, Hansen O (1939): Arch Physiol Scand 81:160.

Corbett SW, Kaufman LN, Keesey RE (1988): Am J Physiol 255:E708.

Costill D (1984): Fed Proc 43.

Crist DA, Baldwin RL, Stern JS (1980): *In* Alfin-Slater RB, Krichevsky D, eds: Human nutrition, a comprehensive treatise, Vol 3A. New York: Plenum, p 159.

DeHaven J, Sherwin R, Hendler R, Felig P (1980): N Engl J Med 302:477.

Dohm GL (1984): Fed Proc 43.

DuBois EF (1960): Proc Am Phil Soc 104:111.

Flatt J-P (1978): *In* Bray GA, ed: Recent advances in obesity research. London: Newman, p 211.

Flatt J-P, Blackburn GL (1974): Am J Clin Nutr 27:175.

Food and Nutrition Board, National Research Council (1974): Recommended dietary allowances (8th ed). Washington, DC: National Academy of Sciences.

Foster DO, Frydman ML (1978): Can J Physiol Pharmacol 56:110.

Garrow JS (1978): *In* Bray GA, ed: Recent advances in obesity research, Vol 2. London: Newman, p 200.

Garrow JS (1981): Treat obesity seriously. Edinburgh: Livingstone.

Gollnick PD, Ianuzzo CD, Williams C, Hill TR (1969): Int Z Angew Physiol 27:257.

Grande F, Keys A (1980): *In* Goodhart RS, Shils ME, eds: Modern nutrition in health and disease (6th ed). Philadelphia: Lea & Febiger, p 3.

Greenwood MRC, Cleary M, Sterngrimsdotter L (1981). *In* Bjorntop P, Cairella M, Howard AN, eds: Recent advances in obesity research III. London: Libby.

Gribskov CL, Henningfield MF, Swick AG, Swick RW (1986): Biochem J 233:743.

Grinker J, Hirsch J (1972): *In* Metabolic and behavioral correlates of obesity. Ciba Foundation Symposium no 8, p 350.

Gulick A (1922): Am J Physiol 60:371.

Heaton GHM, Wagenvoord RJ, Kemp A, Nicholls DG (1978): Eur J Biochem 82:515.

Himms-Hagen J (1981): *In* Beers RF Jr, Basset EG, eds: Nutritional factors: Modulating effects on metabolic processes. New York: Raven, p 85.

Hirsh J, Van Itallie DB (1973): Am J Clin Nutr 26:1039.

Hultman E, Thomson JA, Harris RC (1988): *In* Shils M, Young VR, eds: Modern nutrition in health and disease. Philadelphia: Lea & Febiger, p 1001.

Isner JM, Sours HE, Paris AL, Ferrans VJ, Roberts WC (1979): Circulation 60:1401.

James WPT (1989): Presentation, FASEB.

James WPT, Trayhurn P (1981): *In* Beers RF Jr, Basset EG, eds: Nutritional factors: Modulating effects on metabolic processes. New York: Raven, p 123.

Janowitz HD, Hollander F (1955): Ann NY Acad Sci 63:56.

Joel CD (1966): J Biol Chem 241:814.

Jung RT, Shetty PS, James WPT, Barrand MA, Callingham BA (1979): Nature 279:322.

Kasper H, Schonborn J, Rabast U (1975): Am J Clin Nutr 28:800.

Kasper H, Thiel H, Ehl M (1973): Am J Clin Nutr 26:197.

Kern PA, Ong JM, Saffari B, Carty J (1990): N Engl J Med 322:1053.

Keys A, Brozek J, Henschel A, Mickelsen O, Taylor HL (1950): The biology of human starvation. Minneapolis: University of Minnesota Press.

Keys A, Taylor HL, Grande F (1973): Metabolism 22:579.

King RFGJ, McMahon MJ, Almond DJ (1986): Clin Sci 71:31.

Kinney JM (1988): *In* Shils M, Young VR, eds: Modern nutrition in health and disease. Philadelphia: Lea & Febiger, p 517.

Klingenberg M (1990): TIBS 15:108.

Knittle JL, Hirsch J (1968): J Clin Invest 47:2091.

Lantingua RA, Amatruda JM, Biddle TL, Forbes GB, Lockwood DH (1980): N Engl J Med 303:735.

LeFeuvre RA, Rothwell NJ, Stock MJ (1987): Neuropharmacology 26:1217.

Leibel RL (1980): *In* Bray PD, Marcum VS, eds: Human nutrition, clinical and biomedical aspects. Washington, DC: American Association for Clinical Chemistry, p 239.

LeMagnen J, Devos M (1970): Physiol Behav 5:805.

Lemon PWR, Mullin JP (1980): J Appl Physiol 48:624.

Macdonald A, Stunkard A (1990): N Engl J Med 322:1530.

Magnussen B, Hallberg L, Rossander L (1984*a*): Acta Med Scand 216:149.

Magnussen B, Hallberg L, Rossander L (1984b): Acta Med Scand 216:157.

Miller BS, Munford P, Stock MJ (1967): Am J Clin Nutr 20:1223.

Millward DJ, Davies CTM, Halliday D, Wolman SL, Mathews D, Rennie M (1982): Fed Proc 41:2686.

Neumann RO (1902): Arch Hyg 45:1 [cited by Bray GA (1976): The obese patient. Philadelphia: WB Saunders, p 143].

Newsholme EA, Crabtree B (1976): Biochem Soc Symp 41:61.

Par RB, Bachman LA, Moss RA (1984): Phys Sportsmed 12:81.

Pi-Sunyer FX (1988): *In* Shils M, Young VR, eds: Modern nutrition in health and disease. Philadelphia: Lea & Febiger, p 795.

Pittet P, Chappui P, Acheson K, Techtermann F, Jequier E (1976): Br J Nutr 35:281.

Pond WG (1983): Sci Am 248:96.

Ravussin E, Acheson KJ, Vernet O, Danforth E, Jequier E (1985): J Clin Invest 76:1268.

Ravussin E, et al. (1988): N Engl J Med 318:467.

Reed PB (1980): Nutrition, an applied science. Los Angeles: West Publishing.

Rennie MJ, Edwards RHT, Krywawych SS (1981): Clin Sci 61:627.

Roberts SB, Savage J, Coward WA, Chew B, Lucas A (1988): N Engl J Med 318:461.

Rohner-Jeanrenaud F, Walker C-D, Greco-Perotto R, Jeanrenaud B (1989): Endocrinology 124:733.

Romsos DR, Clarke SD (1980): *In* Alfin-Slater RB, Krichevsky D, eds: Human nutrition, a comprehensive treatise, Vol 3A. New York: Plenum, p 141.

Rothwell NJ, Stock MJ (1979): Nature 281:31.

Ruderman NB, Aoki TT, Cahill GF Jr (1976): *In* Hansen R, Mehlman MA, eds: Gluconeogenesis. New York: Wiley, p 515.

Samonds KW, Fleagle J (1973): Fed Proc 32:901 (abstract).

Schwartz RS, Halter JB, Bierman EL (1983): Metab Clin Exp 32:114.

Share I, Martiniak E, Grossman MI (1952): Am J Physiol 168:229.

Sherman WM, Costill DL, Fink WK, Hagerman FC, Armstrong LE, Murray TF (1983): J Appl Physiol 55:1219.

Shils ME (1980): *In* Goodhart RS, Shils ME, eds: Modern nutrition in health and disease (6th ed). Philadelphia: Lea & Febiger, p 814.

Sims EAH (1976): Clin Endocrinol Metab 5:377.

Sims EAH (1990): N Engl J Med 322:1522.

Stock MJ, Rothwell NJ (1981): *In* Beers RF Jr, Bassett EG, eds: Nutritional factors: Modulating effects on metabolic processes. New York: Raven, p 101.

Stunkard AJ, Harris JR, Pederson NL, McClearn GE (1990): N Engl J Med 322:1483.

Sukhatme PV, Margen S (1982): Am J Clin Nutr 35:355.

Swick AG, Swick RW (1986): Am J Physiol 251:E192.

Tarnopolsky MA, MacDougall JD, Atkinson SA (1988): J Appl Physiol 64:187.

Taylor CM, McLeod G (1949): Rose's laboratory handbook for diabetics (5th ed). New York: Macmillan, p 18.

Van Itallie TB, Kissileff HR (1985): Am J Clin Nutr 42:914.

Verbalis JG, McCann MJ, McHale CM (1986): Science 232:1417.

Welle SL, Campbell RG (1983): Am J Clin Nutr 37:87.

Wishnitzer R, Vorst E, Berrebi A (1984): Int J Sports Med 4:27.

Yang MU, Van Itallie TB (1976): J Clin Invest 58:722.

Maria C. Linder, Ph.D.*

9

Nonnutritive Components of Foodstuffs: Endogenous or Added (Food Additives and Labeling)

Food Additives

A food additive is defined as anything that is not an inherent part of the prepared food. At present, the additives allowed in foodstuffs number about 3900 and cover a broad range of functions, from nutrient supplementation or sweetening to preservatives, stabilizers, and sequestrants (Figure 9.1). About 950 of these additives are on the GRAS List (list of substances "generally recognized as safe"), which was instituted for traditional food additives in 1958 when the Delaney Amendment was passed. The Delaney Amendment forbids the addition of substances to foods that can cause cancer in animals or man, at any dose. This amendment has been under fire as too restrictive, largely due to the case of saccharin, which, without special suspension of the law by Congress, would be banned from foodstuffs (see below). Some of the additives on the GRAS List continue to be under review at this time, stemming from questions that have arisen concerning their chronic safety (see more under caffeine, nitrate/nitrite, and some others, below). Of the several hundred reviewed substances, 14% (Table 9.2) were categorized as not adequately tested. Many of the substances have been approved unconditionally or at current levels of use (Kessler, 1989; Lewis, 1989; Roberts, 1981).

* California State University, Fullerton, CA.

If an additive is not on the GRAS List, it must undergo extensive testing, evaluation, and public hearings before it can be used. The results of acute and long-term toxicity studies in at least two animal species (one of which must not be a rodent or rabbit) must be submitted to the FDA, along with a review of existing information on chemistry, use, function, and safety. If the initial decision of the FDA is favorable, there is a chance for written objections to be submitted, and public hearings are held before the final approval or denial of a request. Additional testing, also by the FDA, may be required. The time and costliness of such studies discourages the addition of substances to the allowable additives list, but makes the U.S. processed food supply among the safest in the world.

In terms of quantity, sucrose, high fructose corn syrup, salt, and other high-calorie sweetening agents comprise the bulk of the substances added to processed foods (Table 9.3). It is estimated that the *average* adult American annually consumes more than 120 lb of sucrose and corn syrup sweeteners, as well as large quantities of salt added to processed foods, including that added in the home. Because individuals consume vastly different proportions of processed foods (from breads and cheeses to ice creams and soft drinks), some people are indeed ingesting enormous amounts of sucrose and other high calorie sweeteners. The remaining average 9 lb/year of food additives consumed per capita consists pri-

Table 9.1. Key Legislation Regulating Food Safety and Additives

1938	Revision of 1906 Pure Food and Drug Act: Cosmetics were included. The FDA was given authority to set standards for recipes, such as for mayonnaise, and for quality. A list of ingredients in order of prevalence was required on labels, including coloring and flavoring agents and chemical preservatives. Sale of food that was harmful to health was forbidden; the burden of proof of harm rested on the government.
1941	Federal Food, Drug, and Cosmetic Act (FD & C Act) required for any food represented for special dietary uses to be labeled with information about vitamin and mineral content. Any food to be used for weight reduction must be labeled with the percent by weight of protein, fat, and carbohydrates and must show the kilocalorie content of a specified serving. Nonnutritive ingredients, such as saccharin, must be indicated on the label.
1946	Agricultural Marketing Act: the USDA was given inspection, certification, and grading authority over meats, poultry, dairy products, eggs, fruits, and vegetables. Some procedures were voluntary; some were in conjunction with state and local governments.
1954	Pesticide Chemical Amendment to FD & C Act: Chemicals added to foods must be proven safe before use. The burden of proof rests on the manufacturer. The FDA was given authority to approve both the use and maximum amounts used.
1958	Food Additive Amendments to FD & C Act: chemicals added to foods must be proven safe before use. The burden of proof rests on the manufacturer. The FDA was given authority to approve both the use and maximum amounts used.
	Delaney Clause: no additive can be regarded as safe for human consumption if it causes cancer in either humans or animals.
	GRAS (Generally Regarded as Safe) List: a list of chemicals approved as safe for human consumption. Chemicals already being used were reviewed by members of the Federation of American Societies of Experimental Biology, and acceptable ones were placed on GRAS List. Future additions must be approved by FDA.
1960	Color Additives Amendment to FD & C Act: all chemical coloring agents added to foods were placed under the Delaney Clause.
1966	Fair Packaging Labeling Act: label information was required in a prominent place. Ambiguous terms for sizes were prohibited.
1976	Toxic Substances Control Act: to regulate interstate commerce on substances which may be carcinogenic; excludes pesticides, drugs, cosmetics, and foods.[a]

Source: Modified from Reed (1980).

[a] Maltoni and Selikoff (1988).

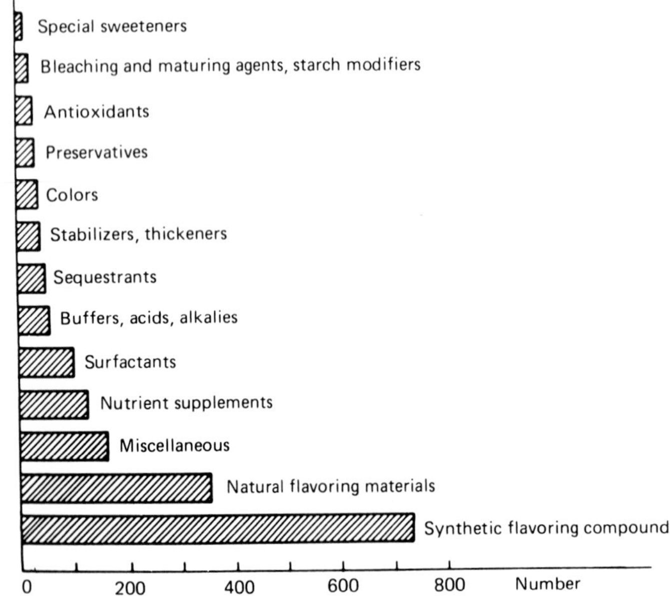

Figure 9.1. Types of food additives used commercially in the United States. [*Source:* Reprinted by permission from Select Committee for Evaluation of GRAS Substances (1977a).]

Table 9.2. GRAS Food Additives Reviewed but Requiring Further Evaluation of Their Safety (as of 1979)[a]

REAFFIRMATION OF SAFETY BUT ADDITIONAL RESEARCH REQUIRED	
BHT, BHA	Some protein hydrolysates
Carrageenan	Caffeine
Oil of nutmeg	Starter distillates
Oxystearin	Soy protein isolate
Monosodium glutamate	Certain modified starches
INFORMATION INSUFFICIENT TO REAFFIRM SAFETY	
Glutamates (glutamic acid, certain salts)	
Protein hydrolysates (soy sauces, enzyme/acid hydrolysates, yeast, and autolysates)	
Sodium chloride	
Certain modified starches	
D- and DL-lactates (given to infants)	
INFORMATION INSUFFICIENT TO JUDGE	
Mono/diglycerides of sulfoacetate, $NaHPO_4$ and citrate	
Japan wax (used in packaging)	
Carnauba wax (used in waxing vegetables/fruits)	
Corn silk	
Methyl and ethyl acrylates (used in packaging)	
Certain iron salts	
Na/NaZn metasilicates; methyl polysilicones	
Manganous oxide	
Starch gelatinized with NaOH	

Source: Roberts (1981).

[a] The substances listed are 14% of the total reviewed; 86% of those tested so far were reaffirmed as safe.

Table 9.3. Relative Quantities of Intentional Food Additives Consumed per Person per Year in the United States

Sweeteners	
Sucrose	63 lb[a]
Corn sweeteners[b]	58 lb[a]
Dextrose	4.2 lb
Salt (NaCl)	6.6 lb[a]
Natural flavoring agents	
MSG	1.9 lb
Others (mustard, pepper)	0.9 lb
Acidity control (acids and bases)	
Citric and propionic acids, NaOH, etc.	1.6 lb
Emulsifiers	
Lecithin, monodiglycerides	1.0 lb
Leavening	
Yeasts, phosphates, carbonates	0.9 lb
Thickeners	
Modified starches	0.8 lb
Leavening control	
Carbonate, phosphates	0.4 lb
Stabilizers	
Carbonates, acacia	0.4 lb
Miscellaneous	
Preservatives, colors, supplements, etc.	1.3 lb

Source: Based on data from Hall (1973).

[a] Data for 1985 (National Research Council, 1989).
[b] 40+ lb/year high fructose corn syrup (HFCS).

marily of monosodium glutamate (flavor enhancer), mustard, pepper, emulsifiers, and starches (used for thickening) (Table 9.3); the hundreds of additives remaining (Figure 9.1) account for only a tiny fraction of the total weight of food additives consumed.

Food Labeling

All processed foods sold across interstate boundaries must carry the following information: ingredients, in decreasing order of abundance (including all additives). If fortified with vitamins, minerals, and/or protein (or if making any nutritional value claims), foods must also carry: nutrition information on energy, protein, carbohydrate, and fat (in calories, or grams, per serving), as well as the content of protein, vitamins A and C, thiamin, riboflavin and niacin, calcium, and iron as a percentage of the U.S. adult RDA. Exceptions to these labeling rules involve those foods with a "standard of identity" (such as mayonnaise, ice cream, or ketchup). The latter must meet certain compositional standards to qualify as a given food type. Special claims made by a manufacturer for a given food are also regulated, such as "sodium-free," "low calorie," or "sugar-free" (Kessler, 1989). More recently, and for the first time, the FDA has begun to allow some health benefit claims, having been encouraged to consider this by the FTC (which regulates interstate commerce and advertising claims). Regulations expected to emerge from the FDA are likely to limit claims to five areas: calcium and osteoporosis; sodium and hypertension; fat and heart disease; fat and cancer; and fiber and cancer (Kessler, 1989). Such regulations would circumvent the traditional ruling by which health claims can only be legally made for items such as drugs.

Specific Food Additives

Preservatives

The preservatives used in processed foods fall into two categories: (1) those designed to prevent oxidation, and (2) those directed at inhibiting microbial growth. Both of these functions are important for the preservation, transport, storage, and nutrient stability of our food supply. Antioxidants are most commonly used to prevent oxidation of lipids, especially the more vulnerable polyunsaturated glycerides. The tocopherols (vitamin E) normally come with triglycerides, especially in plant-derived foods, but a substantial portion of these antioxidants are removed during purification of vegetable oils.

The most common lipid antioxidants added to foods are butylated hydroxytoluene and butylated hydroxyanisole (BHT and BHA) (Figure 9.2 and Table 9.4). Early on, there was some concern that BHT might cause cancer (Brown et al., 1959), but later studies did not confirm this effect. Work in mice indicates that, although BHT may not itself be a carcinogen, it may be a cancer "promoter" (Witschi and Lock, 1978), and it may cause liver enlargement and microsomal enzyme induction (King and McCay, 1981). It may also be a mutagen. On the other hand, BHA (and BHT) may protect against certain kinds of carcinogenesis (King et al., 1979; Lowenfels and Anderson, 1977).

At least one study has shown that long-term feeding of BHA prolongs the life of rodents (Furia, 1972). This study has been criticized on the basis that the controls were deficient in natural antioxi-

Figure 9.2. Structure of specific preservatives. Footnotes: *Butyl group may also occur in this position. †Methyl, propyl, ethyl, or butyl group may be present on ring C.

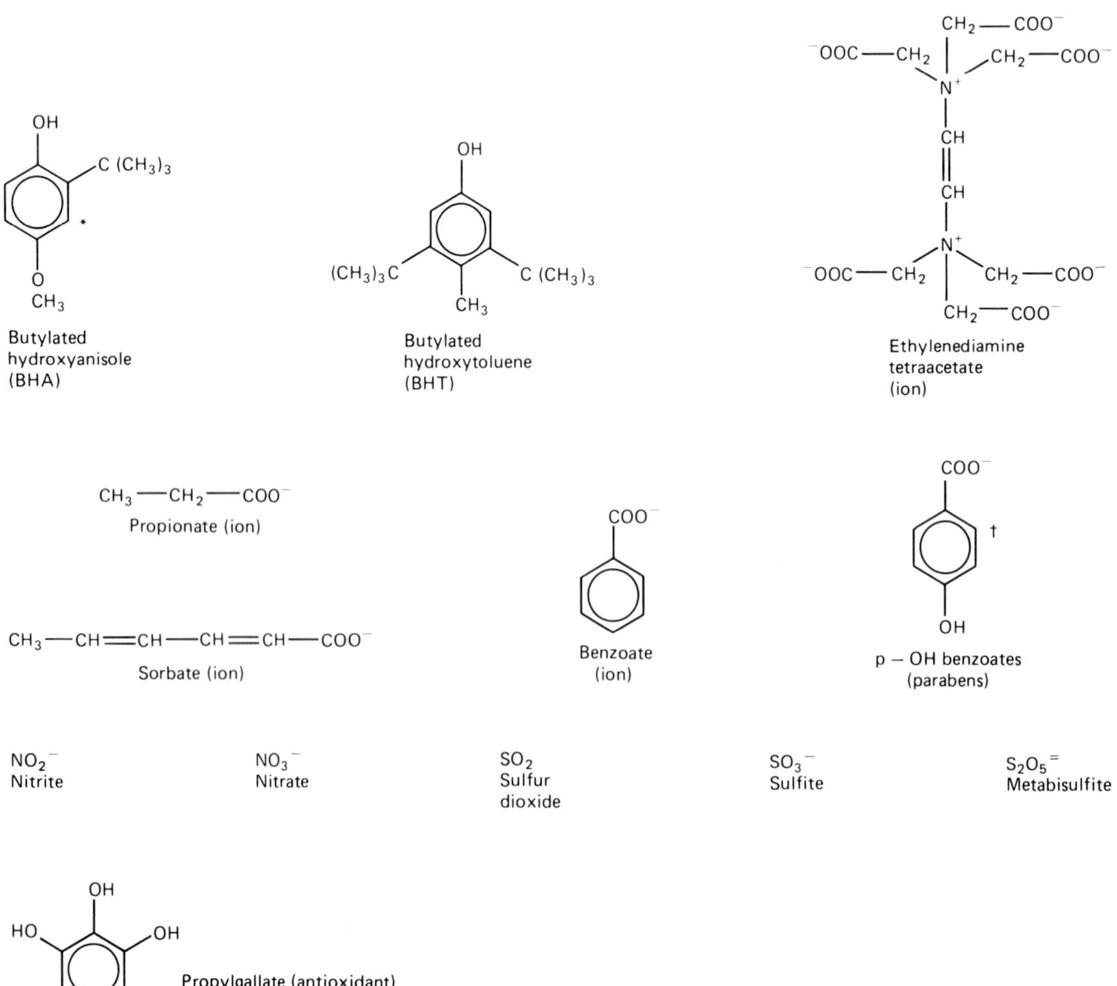

dant intake (vitamin E), but the results have fueled speculation that lipid antioxidants may function to retard the aging process (Harman, 1968).

Use of sequestering agents, such as EDTA (Figure 9.2), represent another approach in the prevention of food oxidation. Here, the chelating agents are inhibiting the capacities of metal ions, like Cu^{2+} and Fe^{3+}, to catalyze oxidative reactions.

The other category of preservatives includes antimould (antifungal) agents like *sorbic* and *propionic acid* derivatives, and antiyeast or antibacterial agents like the *benzoates*, and *sulfur* and *nitrogen oxides* (sulfites, nitrites, etc.) (Figure 9.2 and Table 9.4). Very little is understood about the mechanisms by which these agents inhibit microbial growth (Furia, 1972). The status and toxicities of all of these various substances are summarized in Table 9.4. The benzoates and sorbates (like BHA and BHT) are not normally found in human and animal metabolism. Nevertheless, most are currently on the GRAS List and are, or have recently been, under review (Select Committee for Evaluation of GRAS Substances, 1977*b*).

As of 1986, *sulfites* (bisulfite, HSO_3; metabisulfite, S_2O_3) were withdrawn from the GRAS List (Lewis, 1989) because of the acute reactions exhibited by some asthmatics to foods treated with these agents. These reactions include wheezing, chest "tightness," flushing, and weakness. (Several people died.) The mechanism of the effect is unclear, but does not appear to involve antibisulfite antibodies or the direct stimulation by bisulfites of histamine release from basophils (Stevenson and Simon, 1981). Various sulfites were broadly used in the food industry and in restaurants as sanitizing agents for food containers and equipment; in wine and beer to stop fermentation; on seafoods, vegetables, and fruits (fresh or dried) to prevent spoilage or discoloration; and in green salads, potato chips/fries, guacamole, and seafoods served by restaurants, again to prevent spoilage and discoloration. It is estimated that the average American consumes 2–3 mg of these additives per day, but could have consumed 25–30 mg in one restaurant meal (Stevenson and Simon, 1981). Clearly, very few people react adversely to these intakes, and sulfites can play a useful role in food preservation and manipulation. However, in one study of 61 patients, five (or 8%) were found to react to metabisulfite (R.A. Simon, personal communication). Sulfites are still allowed, but have been banned from use on fresh, raw vegetables, and fruits (as well as from foods considered major sources of thiamin).

Nitrites and *nitrates* bear further mention. These substances have been used primarily in processed meats as potent antibacterial agents, especially to prevent the proliferation of *Clostridium botulinum*. This has been very important in the prevention of spoilage. In fact, it would be difficult to do without these preservatives and still have normal storage, transport, and distribution of processed meat products. Use of nitrites has nevertheless been of concern, as it reacts with secondary amines (such as proline or polyamine derivatives found in foodstuffs) under stomach pH conditions to produce nitrosamines (Figure 9.3). Nitrosamines are potent carcinogens, capable of producing a variety of different kinds of tumors in animal systems. The report by Fine et al. (1977) that ingestion of a spinach and bacon sandwich produces a rapid rise in blood levels of some nitrosamines emphasized the need for continued concern, although the technical difficulty of assaying nitrosamines put these and other results in question (Saul et al., 1981).

Several important discoveries about nitrate/nitrite ingestion and metabolism have been made that indicate that cured and processed meats actually supply only a small fraction of the nitrogen oxides in our bodies. (a) Vegetables are actually a much more important exogenous source than meats (Table 9.5), due at least partly to the extensive use of nitrate fertilizers (see Chapter 10). (b) Balance studies have revealed that 80%–90% of NO_3^- circulating in the body comes from endogenous production (Table 9.6). (c) This endogenous production cannot be ascribed to the work of gut bacteria, as shown in germ-free rats (Green et al., 1981; Witter et al., 1981). Thus, the circulation of nitrite in body fluids is part of the status quo. The pathway by which this ion is produced by animal cells and its purpose [e.g., nutritional or metabolic value (if any)] is unknown at this time. However, the production and circulation of nitrosamines produced from nitrite may be avoidable to some extent and may depend on intake of vitamins C and E.

A less benign aspect of *nitrite* ingestion, when high doses are involved, is the oxidation of circulating hemoglobin to methemoglobin in red cells. The oxidized Fe^{3+} in the heme group can then no longer bind oxygen. A few cases of methemoglobinemia have been reported in infants consuming baby food made with vegetables (like spinach and beets) that tend to accumulate high concentrations of nitrate during their growth (when fertil-

Table 9.4. Uses, Toxicity, and Current Status of Some Food Additives[a]

Additive	Allowed concentration	Use	Toxicity	Current status in U.S.
BHA/BHT	Up to 0.01%–0.02% of fat, in most foods	Antioxidant preservative	0.01% diet, dogs, 1 year, no obvious effect[b]; 2% diet, rats, 6 months, no obvious effects[c]; oral LD_{50}, rats: 2200 (BHA)/80 (BHT) mg/kg; IARC cancer review: animal carcinogen (BHA); NCI carcinogenesis assay negative (NHT)	GRAS, some genetic toxicity (EPA)
Propionates	No limit[d] (other than exceeding what is needed)	Antimicrobial agent (fungal), flavoring agent	Oral LD_{50}, rats: 3.5 g/kg; 1–3 g/day, rats, lifespan, no effects[i] (natural in some cheeses, up to 1%)	GRAS
Sorbates	Limit 0.1%–0.2% (not allowed in cooked sausage)	Preservatives	8% diet, rats, 90 days, no obvious effects; oral LD_{50}, rats: 7.4 g/kg. Potential reproductive effects at high doses	GRAS
Parabens	0.1% maximum	Preservatives	Experimental teratogen/mutagen; 0.05%–0.1% diet, dogs, 1 year, no obvious effects; oral LD_{50}, mice 2–3.7 g/kg body weight	GRAS
Benzoates	Limit 0.1%	Antimicrobial agents, flavoring agents	Skin irritant; lowest lethal dose reported, humans: 500 mg/kg; 80% diet, rats, reduced weight gain, enlarged kidneys and livers, early death[i]; oral LD_{50}, rats: 2.5 g/kg	GRAS, some genetic toxicity (EPA)
Monosodium glutamate	No limit[d]	Flavor enhancer	Experimental teratogen at high doses; CNS effects at high doses; oral LD_{50}, rats: 17 g/kg	GRAS
Caffeine	Limit 0.02%[d]	Stimulant, flavoring agent	Experimental and human teratogen at high doses; lowest dose reported to have reproductive effects in humans: 3.3–6.0 mg/kg; oral LD_{50}, rats: 192 mg/kg	GRAS, some genetic toxicity (EPA)
Carrageenan	No limit[d] [except in restricted meat products: 1.5%	Binder, extender, thickener, (sulfated polygalactose from seaweed)	Probable carcinogen if given i.v. or subcutaneously (IARC): rats (s.c.) minimum dose 525 mg/kg	GRAS
Carnauba wax	No limit[d]	Glaze and anticaking agent (extract of leaves of Brazilian palm)	No data	GRAS
Oil of nutmeg	No limit[d]	Flavoring agent	Potential male reproductive toxicity: lowest dose, mice: 2.4–4 g/kg	GRAS

SO_2/sulfites	Limit 0.05%; not allowed in meats, foods that are recognized as sources of thiamin, or on fresh, raw vegetables, or fruit (except potatoes); allowed in many other foods, including dried fruits and soups, and wine and fresh shrimp	Preservative, bleaching agent	Allergic reactions/pulmonary distress in some humans in oral doses as low as 3 mg or inhaled at levels of 3–4 ppm; 0.05–1.0 g/day, dogs, 1–12 months, no gross microscopic changes[e]; >0.1% rats, thiamin destruction[f]; 11 g/day, humans, decreased protein and fat utilization; 4–5 g: vomiting	Removed from GRAS list, 1986; limited use allowed; on Extremely Hazardous Substance List; genetic effects (EPA)
Brominated vegetable oil	Limit 15 ppm in beverages	Beverage stabilizer (clouding agent)	Reproductive effects at high oral doses in rats: 9–27 g/kg; other studies pending	Allowed additive (limited used)
Aspartame (Nutrasweet)	No limit[d] (except in foods with standard of identity and in baked or cooked foods)	Sugar substitute, sweetener, flavor enhancer	May cause allergic dermatitis in some people at doses of 3.7 mg/kg or more[g]; reproductive toxicity at 4 g/kg in mice[h]	Approved additive
Saccharin	Limit 12 mg/fluid oz in beverages, 30 mg per serving in processed foods	Nonnutritive sweetener	Carcinogen (bladder) at oral doses of 112–224 g/kg (rats); suspected human carcinogen; male reproductive effects (mice) at 2 g/kg; LD_{50}, rats: 14.2 g/kg	Allowed additive (by action of Congress)
Cyclamates	Prohibited in foods	Nonnutritive sweetener	Carcinogen, rats, in oral doses of 63 g/kg; suspected human carcinogen; teratogen, mice, at oral doses of 0.2–5 mg/kg	Prohibited (Delaney Amendment); some genetic toxicity (EPA)
Polysorbate 80	Limit 0.1% in most foods	Adjuvant[b] dispensing agent, solubilizer, stabilizer	Reproductive effects at high oral doses in rats: 635–1270 g/kg; DNA synthesis inhibitor (humans and mice); oral LD_{50}, mice: 8.2 g/kg	Allowed additive
Nitrate/nitrite	Limit 200 ppm (as nitrite)	Curing agent, preservative (meats)	Can form carcinogens; acute toxicity due to methemoglobin formation; oral MLD, rats: 200 mg/kg; oral MLD, dogs: 330 mg/kg	Allowed additive

Source: Data from Furia (1972) and Lewis (1989).

[a] LD_{50}, lethal dose for 50% of animals; MLD, minimum lethal dose; IARC, UN International Agency for Research on Cancer; NCI, National Cancer Institute.
[b] Hodge et al. (1964).
[c] Wilder and Kraybill (1948).
[d] "When used at a level not in excess of the amount reasonably required to accomplish the intended effect."
[e] Rust and Franz (1913): Teratology 28:309 (1983).
[f] Fitzhugh et al. (1946).
[g] Ann Intern Med 104:207 (1986).
[h] Res Comm Psych Psychiat Behav 9:385 (1985).
[i] Harshbarger (1942).
[j] Deuel et al. (1954).

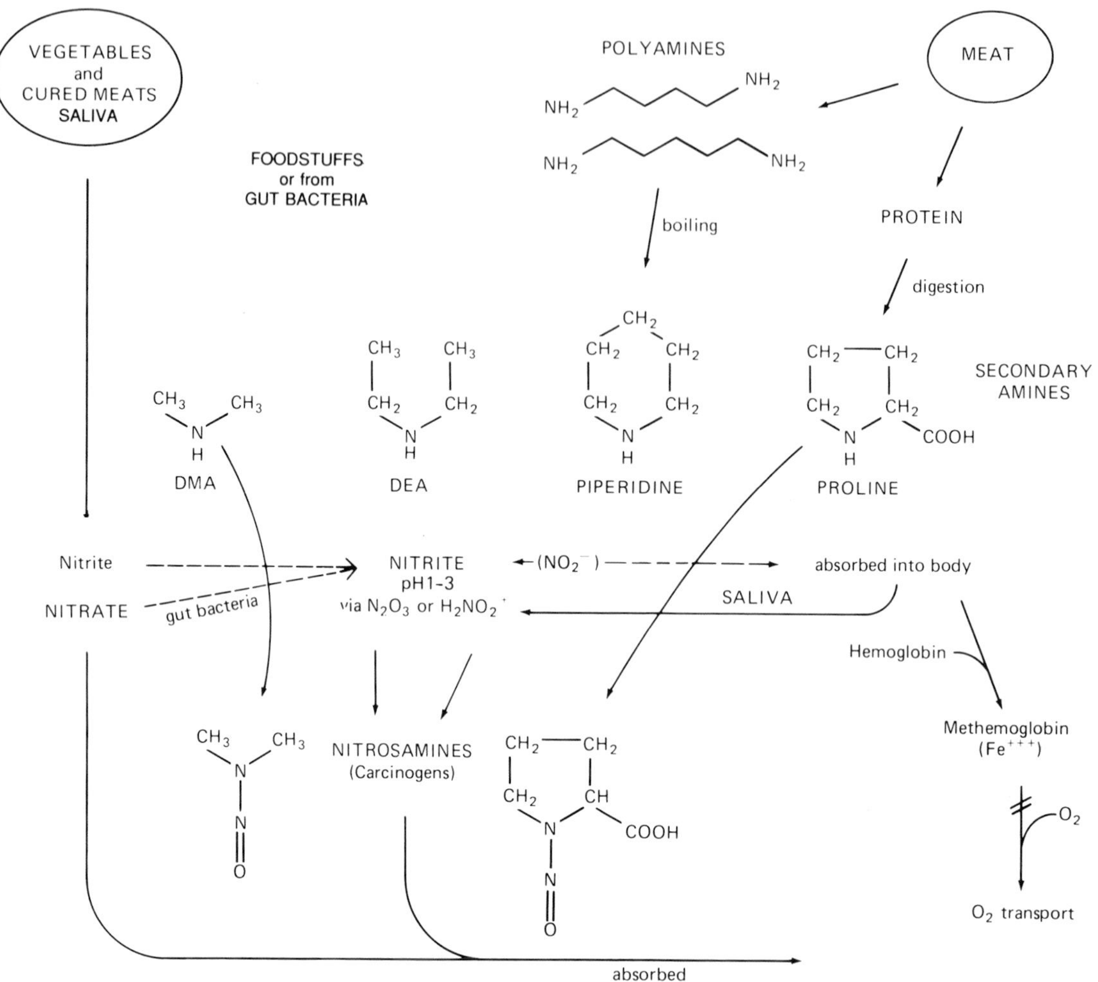

Figure 9.3. Nitrosation of dietary substituents in the stomach: Formation of nitrosamines.

Table 9.5. Estimated Average Daily Nitrate and Nitrite Ingestion by U.S. Residents Based on Per Capita Consumption of Meats, Vegetables, etc.

Source	Nitrate		Nitrite	
	mg	%	mg	%
Vegetables	86.1	81.2	0.20	1.6
Fruit, juices	1.4	1.3	0.00	0.0
Milk and milk products	0.2	0.2	0.00	0.0
Bread	2.0	1.9	0.02	0.2
Water	0.7	0.7	0.00	0.0
Cured meats	15.6	14.7	3.92	30.7
(Saliva)	(30.0)[a]		8.62	67.5
Total	106.0	100	12.76	100

Source: Reprinted by permission from White (1975).

[a] Not included in total.

Table 9.6. Nitrate Balance in Six Human Subjects on Low and High Protein Diets

Subject	Diet	Intake (μmol) $NaNO_3$	Excretion (μmol)
1	Protein-free	72	884
	0.8 g/kg protein	140	551
2	Protein-free	54	1660
	0.8 g/kg protein	86	1300
3	Protein-free	72	1800
	0.8 g/kg protein	155	1830
4	Protein-free	61	1360
	0.8 g/kg protein	117	1350
5	Protein-free	85	655
	0.8 g/kg protein	140	1230
6	Protein-free	60	1230
	0.8 g/kg protein	117	814

Source: Data from Tannenbaum et al. (1978).

ized with nitrates) (Achtzehn and Hawat, 1979). Some poisoning of cattle from intake of high nitrate well water has also been recorded. Nevertheless, these occurrences appear to be quite rare.

Sweeteners

Another category of food additives of special interest is that of low-calorie, or no-calorie, sweeteners. The *cyclamates* (Figure 9.4), which were widely used especially in diet soft drinks, were banned in 1969 under the Delaney Amendment (Table 9.4) when studies in rats showed that intakes of 0.25% of body weight per day, or implantation as waxy pellets in the bladder, produced bladder tumors (Bryan and Erturk, 1970). The results of animal studies (in terms of dosages, especially) cannot be quantitatively extrapolated to the human. Thus, it cannot be said that there is a safe dosage of this carcinogen for humans, hence the Delaney Amendment.

The publication some years later of a report that saccharin (at 5% of the diet) also produces cancer in rats (21 of 200 rats versus 1 of 100 controls) (Munro et al., 1975), in vitro work, and the results of Canadian epidemiologic studies linking a high consumption of "tabletop" artificial sweeteners to an increased likelihood of bladder cancer in men (Canada, NHWM, 1977; Howe et al., 1977), lead to the conclusion that saccharin is indeed also a carcinogen (National Academy of Sciences, 1978) and prompted the FDA to propose the banning of this synthetic sweetener in 1977. Public outcry resulted in special congressional legislation to permit continued use of saccharin, but with labels warning of its potential hazard to health. Pure saccharin was found to be mutagenic by the chromatid exchange test (Wolff and Rodin, 1978), but not by the Ames test (Batzinger et al., 1977). More recent retrospective studies on 9000 and 592 individuals, respectively (Hoover and Strasser, 1980; Morrison and Buring, 1980) indicated that there was relatively little risk associated with then current intakes of saccharin in soft drinks or as a "tabletop" sweetener. Nevertheless, there is some excess risk associated with larger intakes (six or more daily servings and two or more diet drinks), for both men and women (Hoover and Strasser, 1980).

Meanwhile, another sweetener (aspartame), this one a nutritive but low-calorie one, 180 times

Figure 9.4. Structure of sweeteners and methylxanthines.

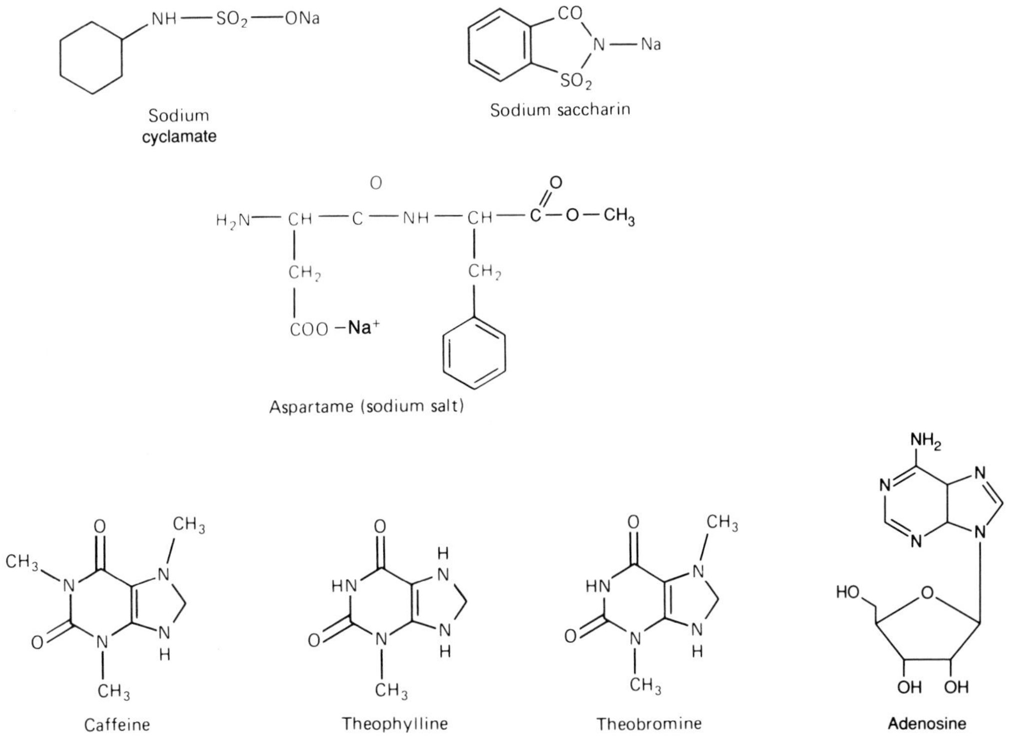

Sodium cyclamate

Sodium saccharin

Aspartame (sodium salt)

Caffeine

Theophylline

Theobromine

Adenosine

as sweet as sucrose, has supplanted most saccharin in soft drinks, after extensive testing and FDA approval (Table 9.4). *Aspartame* (or Nutrasweet) is a methyl ester of the dipeptide, aspartylphenylanine (Figure 9.4). It is deesterified in the small intestine (releasing minute amounts of methanol), and hydrolyzed to its substituent amino acids either in the gut lumen or within intestinal mucosal cells (Stegink, 1987). Initial concerns that this dipeptide might cause brain tumors in rats and other laboratory animals were not confirmed by further studies. The FDA has estimated that this sweetener also should not greatly increase the risk of mental retardation in undiagnosed phenylketonurics, despite an increased intake of up to 3 mg of phenylalanine/kg/day. Anecdotal reports of increased migraine or other headaches associated with aspartame have not been confirmed in double-blind studies involving people making such a claim (Schiffman et al., 1987); but some evidence for increased production of brain norepinephrine (and dopa) was obtained in rats with high doses (Maher, 1988; Tam et al., 1987; Yokogoshi and Wurtman, 1986). As a dipeptide comprised of amino acids normally ingested in much larger quantities (as protein), it would not have been expected that this sweetener would prove harmful to human and animal systems. As a substitute for saccharin, aspartame has one shortcoming; it loses its sweetness (is hydrolyzed) upon prolonged exposure to water and/or heat and thus cannot be used as readily in prepared food products. It is also more expensive, but it can be used in soft drinks, and it substitutes well for saccharin at the table and as a sugar replacement in dry food products.

Some other proteinaceous products are also very sweet, notably thaumatin (a 207 amino acid protein from the katemfe plant), and monellin (an α,β-protein of 94 amino acids from the serendipity berry) (Kim et al., 1988). [Both are African plants.] These proteins are 100,000 times sweeter than sucrose, mole per mole, and several thousand times sweeter on a weight basis. This has not yet been exploited.

Stimulants: Caffeine and Other Methylxanthines

In recent years, there has been some concern about the safety of caffeine as a food additive on the GRAS List. There have been studies to confirm or refute that there are connections between consumption of caffeine or other methylxanthines (Figure 9.4) (present in cocoa and coffee beans) and the incidence of fibrocystic breast disease, birth defects, or pancreatic cancer.

Caffeine belongs to a family of substances that includes theophylline and acts at least partly by inhibiting the phosphodiesterases. The latter degrade cyclic nucleotides, like cAMP. [cAMP is the "second messenger" involved in the effects of many peptide and other nonsteroid hormones, including the catecholamines (see example in Chapter 2, Figure 2.4).] In the presence of methylxanthines, cyclic nucleotide levels are increased, and this is thought to account for some of the actions these compounds have on the central nervous, muscle, and cardiovascular systems, the enhanced breakdown of glycogen and triglyceride, and increased oxygen consumption (Stephenson, 1977). Caffeine, theophylline, and theobromine appear to have differential effects on these systems (Table 9.7), with caffeine being most effective on the central nervous system (alertness, decreases fatigue, etc.) and theophylline on the heart (stimulating heart rate and cardiac output but also decreasing heart rate by vagal stimulation). (As a result, very high doses can cause tachycardia or bradycardia.) Part of the effects of caffeine on the central nervous system probably can also be ascribed to competition with adenosine for binding to receptors in certain neurons (Hunter et al., 1990). [Caffeine, and the methylxanthines as a group, have the same "core base" structure as the purines (Figure 9.4).] Adenosine inhibits neuronal activity, possibly by enhancing the flux of Cl^- through specific channels in the cell membrane/axon, and/or by diminishing adenosine-stimulated phosphoinositide hydrolysis (see Chapter 5, Inositol, or Chapter 6, Calcium) (Narang et al., 1990). High doses of caffeine may reduce hyperactivity in children (Schechter and Timmons, 1985), but its potential side effects would be of concern. [There has also been concern about caffeine transmission to nursing infants from their mothers (Ryu, 1985; Stavchansky et al., 1988).] The caffeine and methylxanthine contents of various foods and beverages are given in Table 9.8.

The possibility of a link between methylxanthine consumption and fibrocystic breast disease was first suggested by Minton (1979), based on observations that abstention from these substances appeared to lead to a regression of signs and symptoms. In a similar study, Brooks et al. (1981) noted improvement in 88% of women abstaining from all sources of methylxanthines, although the effect took some months to be evident. Minton's reports have been criticized for their

Table 9.7. Relative Effects of Methylxanthines on Physiologic Processes

	CNS and respiratory stimulation	Smooth muscle relaxant	Diuresis	Cardiac stimulation	Skeletal muscle stimulation
Caffeine	+++	+	+	+	+++
Theobromine	+	++	++	++	+
Theophylline	++	+++	+++	+++	++

Source: Data from Burger and Mitchell (1978).

Table 9.8. Sources of Caffeine and Other Methylxanthines in the Diet

Source	Theophylline	Theobromine	Caffeine
Coffee			
(% weight)	—	—	0.8–1.8
(mg/cup)			
Bean coffee			85[a]
Instant			60[a]
Decaffeinated			3
(10^6 lb in U.S. per year)[b]			35.1
Tea			
(% weight)	—	—	2.7–4.1
(mg/cup)			
Regular	1	2	50[a]
Instant	1	2	30[a]
(10^6 lb in U.S. per year)[b]	6.0?	3.0	6.0
Cocoa			
(% weight)	—	7.5[a]	0.07–1.7
(mg/cup)	—	232–272	6–42
(10^6 lb in U.S. per year)[b]	—	4.7	0.19
Cola beverages[c] (mg/cup)			
Sugar-free Mr. Pibb			60
Mountain Dew			54
Mello Yellow			52
Tab			46
Coca Cola			45
Shasta Cola			44
Sunkist Orange			40
Mr. Pibb			40
Dr. Pepper			40
Pepsi Cola			38
Diet Pepsi			36
Pepsi Light			36
RC Cola			36
Diet Rite			36
Tablets (mg/tablet)			
Cold (Bromquinine)			15
Allergy (Sinarest, Dristan)			30
Headache (Cope, Excedrin, Anacin)			32–60
Stay-A-Wake (No-Doz, Vivarin)			100–200
Pharmacologic uses	Coronary dilation	Diuresis	Cerebral stimulation Respiratory stimulation (newborns)

Source: Data largely from Graham (1978).

[a] Variable.
[b] Data for 1972.
[c] The *Christian Science Monitor,* August 26, 1981, p 6. Fresca, 7-Up, Canada Dry Ginger Ale, RC 100, Hire's Root Beer—0 mg.

generalizing and even evangelical tone, as well as for a lack of adequate information on changes in the diet, follow-up, and methods of disease assessment (Love et al., 1982; National Coffee Association, 1981). More fundamentally, there is evidence that the majority of women with lumpy breasts show periodic regression even without a change in diet, a factor not controlled for in these studies. The interpretation of existing and future data is complicated by a lack of consensus within the profession on the definition of fibrocystic disease (National Coffee Association, 1981). Case control reports have been contradictory (Boyle et al., 1984; Ernster et al., 1982; Lubin et al., 1985; Parazzini et al., 1986), but suggestive that nonfibroadenomatous processes were promoted. It may be of interest that the results of several double-blind studies of women with premenstrual breast lumps indicate that a significant number respond favorably to daily intakes of 600 IU vitamin E (20 times the RDA) (London et al., 1980, 1985; Sundaram et al., 1965).

Several studies, mainly with animals, have indicated that immoderate caffeine consumption can cause birth defects, reduced fertility, and other reproductive problems (Collins, 1980; Sayka, 1979). Reports on humans (see Jacobson et al., 1981) support the concept of teratogenicity. In three cases described by Jacobson and colleagues, women gave birth to infants with missing fingers or toes and did not appear to have ingested other drugs or agents that might have had such a teratogenic effect. These women consumed between 15 and 25 cups of coffee daily. Others (Linn et al., 1982) have reported no connections between low birth weight or short gestation and intakes of four or more cups of coffee per day, when corrected for smoking. Although the data are scanty, it would seem wise to discourage high levels of caffeine consumption during pregnancy.

The possibility of a connection between methylxanthine consumption and pancreatic cancer is based on a retrospective study of 369 patients with histologically proven cancer of the pancreas and a large group of control subjects with other diagnoses, all interviewed concerning their earlier coffee, tea, tobacco, and alcohol indulgence (McMahon et al., 1981). The authors concluded that there was a statistically significant relationship between the extent of coffee (but not tea) consumption and pancreatic cancer incidence, even when the smoking contribution was eliminated. The results are not very convincing, in that the control subjects showed only a slight shift downward in coffee consumption and, indeed, cover the range from 0 to 5 or more cups a day. The conclusions were not confirmed in another more recent study of 184 patients with pancreatic versus breast or prostatic cancer (Goldstein, 1982), which had a similar distribution of coffee drinkers. The conclusions of the McMahon study have also been questioned because of methodological limitations (Feinstein et al., 1981). It should be mentioned that coffee is only one of many sources of caffeine (Table 9.8) and that others (except tea) were not considered.

As concerns caffeine and blood pressure, long-term health data, collected by IBM since 1968, showed no relationship between chronic patterns of coffee consumption among individuals and systolic or diastolic blood pressure (Bertrand et al., 1978), despite limited data that acute consumption of caffeine (250 mg) by noncoffee-drinkers can cause an increased release of catecholamines and a modest rise in blood pressure (Robertson et al., 1978). Along the same lines, caffeine has been exonerated as a factor in coronary heart disease (Bertrand, 1979). Nevertheless, it can cause heart palpitations. Excessive caffeine intake can also induce tremors, nervousness, and insomnia. Withdrawal can result in headaches. Gastrointestinal effects and diarrhea may also occur with excessive intake. [Recent reports of boiled (but not filtered) coffee inducing hypercholesterolemia probably have nothing to do with caffeine (see Chapter 15, p. 464).] Overall, caffeine is a relatively benign substance in the amounts usually ingested, but intake may be precluded in certain conditions.

Food Colorings

Food colorings are endemic to the typical American diet, and studies indicate that the average young child ingests about 35 mg/day (Table 9.9). The most important sources are soft drinks, ice

Table 9.9. Average Dose of Food Colorings Consumed Daily by Young American Children

Color	Dose (mg/day)
Yellow 5	9.07
Yellow 6	10.70
Red 40	13.80
Red 3	0.57
Blue 1	0.80
Blue 2	0.15
Green 3	0.11
Total	35.26

Source: Data from Weiss et al. (1980).

cream, and candy, although vitamin tablets and child medications can also make a significant contribution. Several of the coloring agents originally allowed in the food supply have been removed from the GRAS List (Figure 9.5). Since 1974, three reds, two blues, two yellows, one green, one violet, and one black (mostly coal tar dyes) have been withdrawn, including FDC Reds 2 and 4 (Figure 9.5). Reasons for their withdrawal or the lowering of allowable contents have been the demonstration in animals that these substances can cause early fetal death, cancer, or have other kinds of toxicity. For example, violet no. 1 was prohibited in 1973 because Japanese studies revealed it could cause cancer in rats at a level of 5% in the diet (Kraybill, 1976). Reds no. 1 and 4 were withdrawn because of damage to liver and other tissues (Maltoni and Selikoff, 1988). Yellow and red no. 1 have been removed because of pharmacologic effects. Amaranth (red no. 2) was shown in FDA and Russian studies to have fetotoxicity in rats when fed at levels of 30 mg/kg body weight or more. However, no mutagenicity was shown in the Ames test or by other similar screening procedures. Controversy remains about the degree of danger to man posed by some of these colorings. Further testing of other food colorings continues.

Food coloring agents have also been implicated as responsible for hyperactivity in some children. Childhood hyperactivity is a very complex, multifactorial problem, the origins of which

Figure 9.5. Structure of present and previously used food colorings. [*Source:* Information from Kermode (1972).]

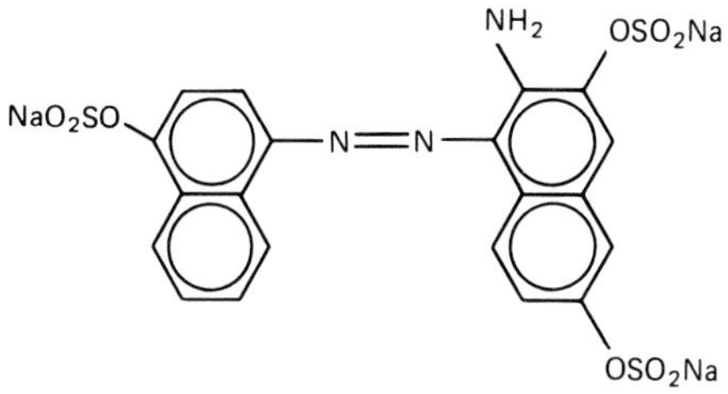

Red 2, amaranth

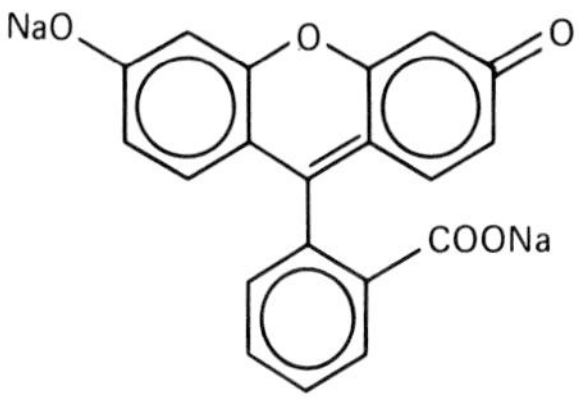

Red 3, erythrosine

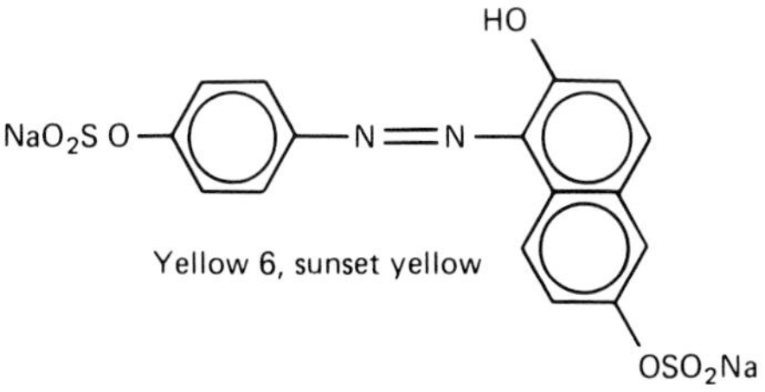

Yellow 6, sunset yellow

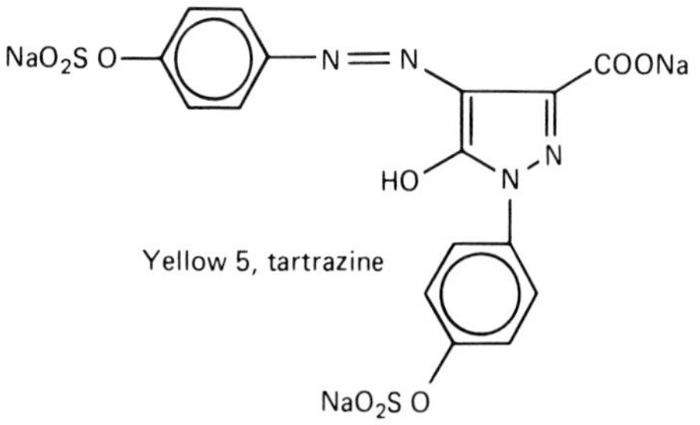

Yellow 5, tartrazine

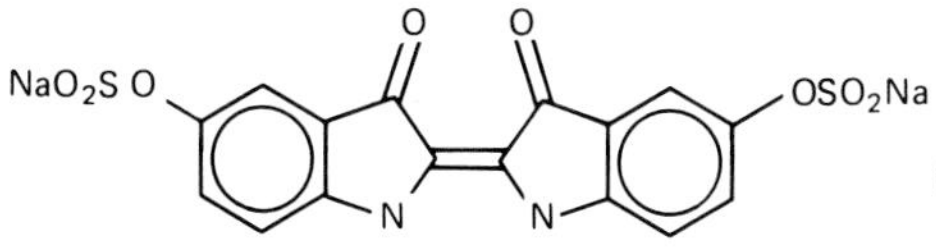

Blue 2, indigotine

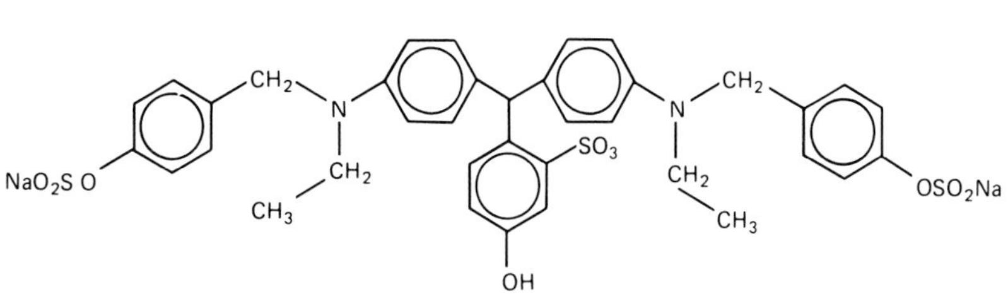

Green 3, fast green

are poorly understood. Nevertheless, the few controlled studies on food colorants that have been carried out suggest that they may be a factor for a small proportion of hyperactive youngsters. Interest in the possibility that food colorants cause hyperactivity originated with Benjamin Feingold's popular book on a diet that he claimed could eliminate or reduce hyperactivity in 50% of children with this problem. Several studies, most recently that of Weiss et al. (1980), indicated a relationship only in a very small proportion of cases when given at doses typical for those found in the general population. In this double-blind study, the behavior of two of 22 children showed a highly significant relation to food color intake versus placebo, as determined by a variety of criteria and the Conners test (Weiss et al., 1980) (Figure 9.6). In other studies, higher doses of colorings may have evoked a much higher incidence of response (Swanson and Kinsbourne, 1980). It should be noted, however, that the Feingold diet excludes not only artificial food colorings, but also preservatives (BHA/BHT), certain spices, aspirin, and various fruits and vegetables high in natural salicylates (notably, citrus and tomatoes). Also, a large percentage of hyperactive children have allergies. The relative importance of allergic reactions and dietary factors other than coloring agents to hyperactivity remains to be evaluated.

Figure 9.6. Behavioral responses of one 3-year-old girl to intake of food colorings versus placebo. Mean total day ratings ± SE, for placebo (open bars) and color intake (hatched bars). Color intake was mixture and amount shown in Table 9.9. [*Source:* Reprinted by permission from Weiss B et al., 1980.]

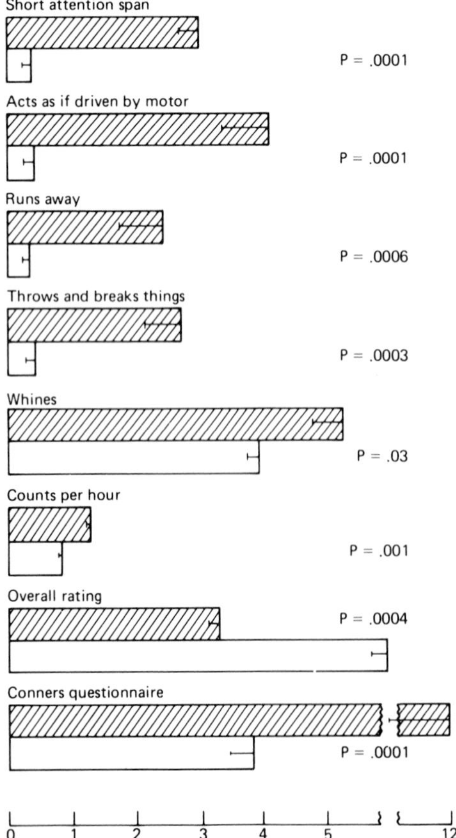

Other Additives

Carrageenan

This red seaweed fiber (see Chapter 2) is widely used as an emulsifier, thickener, and stabilizer in ice cream, puddings, evaporated milk, low calorie diet beverages, and even baby foods. It was temporarily removed from the GRAS List in 1973 because of FDA findings that it produced birth defects in rodents (FDA News, 1982) and may interfere with the immune responses (Bice et al., 1972). Further studies did not confirm teratogenicity (Collins et al., 1979, 1981), but more studies were recommended by the FDA (Roberts, 1981). Directly instilled into the body (other than orally) it may be a carcinogen (Table 9.4). It is still in use.

Inadvertent/Indirect Food Additives

A large number and variety of substances enter the food supply because they are used (a) in producing the foodstuff (hormones and antibiotics in cattle; pesticides and herbicides on vegetable crops), (b) in packaging and preserving (glues, waxes, and lacquers in cans and packages; anti-sprouting agents on roots and tubers; residues of ethylene oxide or dibromide used as a sterilant); or (c) because they become contaminants through industrial or natural pollution (dirt, PCBs, TGEs, etc.) (Table 9.10).

In the cattle, hog, and poultry industries, use of hormonal *growth promoters,* such as mixtures of progesterone and estradiol, is widespread, as is the routine feeding of antibiotics (aureomycin, neooxytetracycline, terramycin, etc.) (Figure 9.7) and the administration of internal antipest agents (phenathiazine). These procedures change the texture and tenderness of meat (estrogen analogs) and ensure faster growth (antibiotics, etc.). The ingestion of antibiotic residues by humans can

Table 9.10. Sources of Common Contaminants of Food, of Industrial and Geologic Origins

Chemical	Source	Food contaminated	Concentrations
Polychlorinated biphenyls (PCB)	Electrical industry	Fish; human milk	12 ppb (milk) (intake 1.8)[a]
Dioxins	Impurities in PCP and other chlorophenols	Fish[b]; cow's milk; beef fat	0.02–0.07 ppt (milk)
Pentachlorophenols (PCP)	Wood preservative	Various foods	
Dibenzofurans	Impurities in PCP/PCB	Fish	
Hexachlorobenzene	Fungicide; industrial byproducts	Animal fat; dairy products; human milk	
Mirex	Pesticide	Fish; edible mammals; human milk	
DDT and related hydrocarbons	Pesticide	Fish; human milk	1–44 ppb (milk) (0.3–6.6 intake)[a]
Alkyl mercury compounds	Manufacture of Cl, sodium lye, acetaldehyde, seed dressing	Fish; grain	
Elemental mercury and salts	Geologic	Fish	
Lead	Auto exhaust; coal combustion; lead industry; solder in can seams; lead-glazed pottery	Vegetables; canned milk; canned fish; acidic foods	
Cadmium	Sewage sludge; smelter operations	Grains; vegetables meat products;	
	Geologic	Fishery products	
Arsenic	Smelter operations	Milk; vegetables; fruits	0.06 ppm (meat, poultry) 0.02 ppm (fruits)
	Geologic	Soft drinks; fish; health food supplements	0.2–0.4 ppm (freshwater fish); 3–18 ppm (marine fish); 11 ppm (shrimp)
Tin	Canning industry	Canned foods	
	Geologic	Fish	
Selenium	Seleniferous soils	Grains	

Source: Modified from Munro and Charbonneau (1982).

[a] Mean daily intake by infants (in μg).
[b] Fish consumption in some areas (like the Baltic) is directly related to plasma levels of dioxins in man (Svensson et al., 1990).

contribute to the development of allergies to these agents (Zanussi, 1978). Residues of most of the substances used are not allowed in the food supply above specific levels; the impossible task of enforcing these rules lies with the USDA, FDA, and state and local officials.

Injection or feeding of diethylstilbesterol (DES) (Figure 9.7) to promote growth in steers has been banned from use under the Delaney Amendment. However, the use of this carcinogenic agent continues largely unchecked in the farming areas of the United States. DES is a potent carcinogen in rodents (McLachlan et al., 1980; Shubik and Rustra, 1979), and there are numerous cases in which uterine and other cancers in women have been traced to the use of this drug in averting miscarriages (Robboy et al., 1982).

In cattle and hogs, bacteriocidal agents or drugs are often used because they enhance feed efficiency and/or prevent infections. One such agent, sulfamethazine, is permitted in hogs until 15 days before slaughter, but several recent studies have found residues in 38%–75% of samples of cow's milk (Ingersoll, 1989; Lewis, 1989) (its

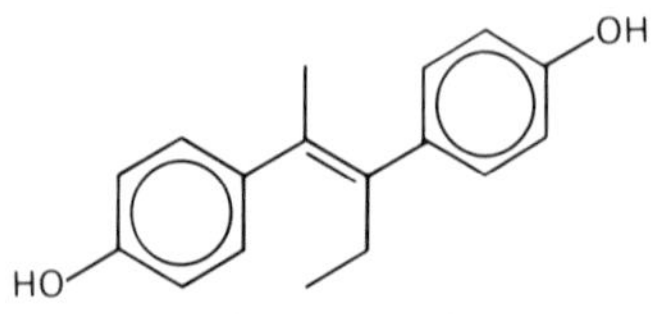

Diethylstilbesterol
(Des)

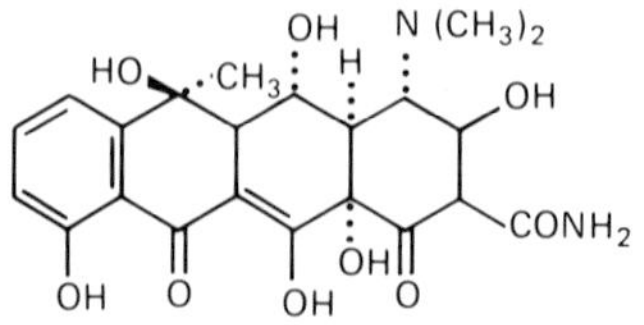

Oxytetracycline (Terramycin)

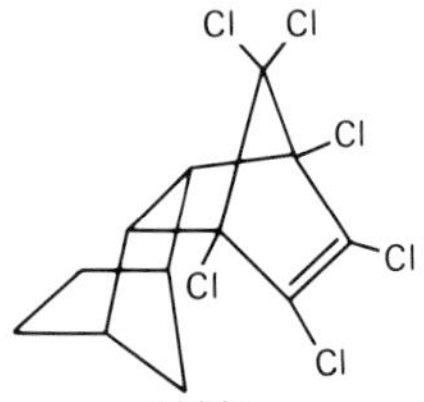

Aldrin
(pesticide)

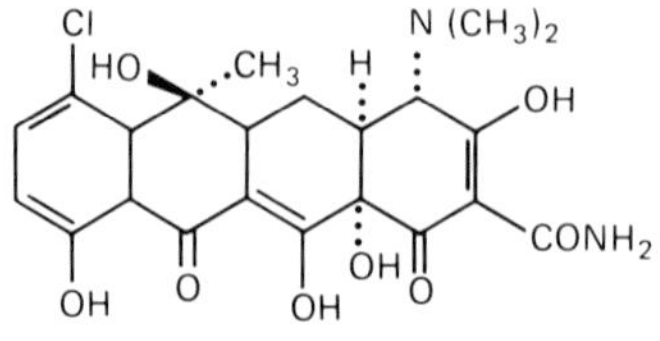

Chlortetracycline
(Aureomycin)

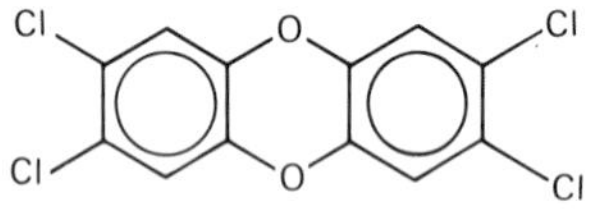

2, 3, 6, 7 tetrachloro-
dibenzodioxin
(potent contaminant
of phenoxyalkanoic
herbicides)

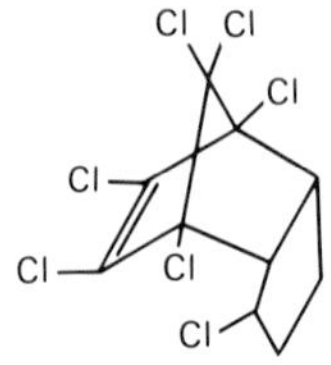

Heptachlor
(pesticide for pineapple fields)
carcinogen
found increasingly in
Hawaiian milk

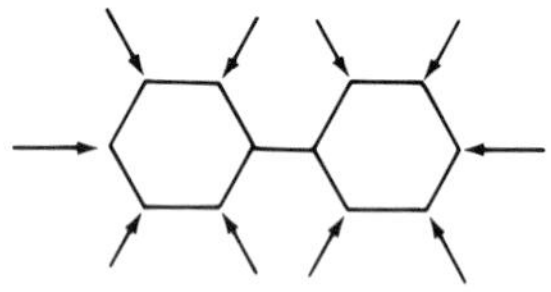

21 — 60% Cl
Polychlorinated biphenyls
(PCBs) (↑) indicate possible
chlorination sites
Concn in fish 0.4-10 μg/g (av. 1.9)
Also high in milk, cheese, and eggs
Human fat has 0-100 μglg

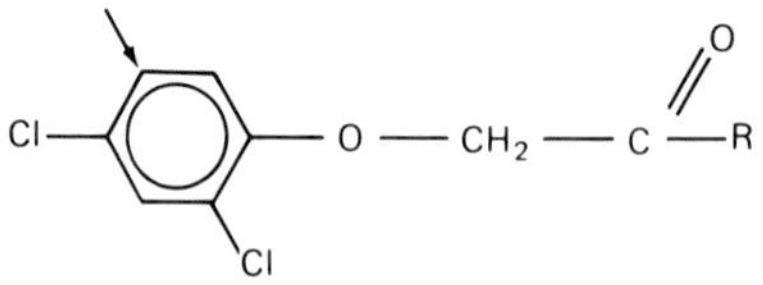

2, 4 – D (or 2, 4, 5) – T
Phenoxyalkanoic
herbicides
(↑) indicates third
chlorination site
(2, 4, 5 — T)

$Cl-CH_2-CH(Br)-CH_2-Br$

DBCP (dibromochloro propane)
pesticide; soil fumigant
mutagen and carcinogen

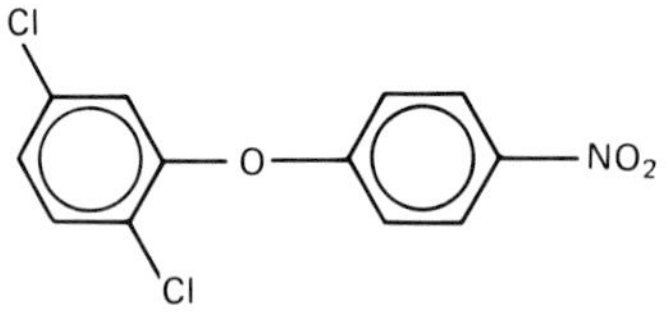

2, 5 dichlorophenyl-p-nitrophenyl ether
(herbicide)

Figure 9.7. Structures of some growth promoters, antibiotics, and food pollutants.

use is prohibited in cows); and for pork there is an average noncompliance of 4%. [Sulfathiazine is a teratogen and probable carcinogen (see Chapter 10, Table 10.17).]

A large variety of pesticides, herbicides, and fungicides are used as agrichemicals on crops and fields (Tables 9.10–9.12), and the EPA has set standards for their allowable levels in produce, usually less than 0.1 ppm. There appears to be a considerable amount of noncompliance with these limits, as illustrated by information in Table 9.12 and reports from the GAO (General Accounting Office of the U.S. Government, 1988). Table 9.12 lists the number of substances registered for use per crop, along with the degree of noncompliance reported; the residues most commonly encountered (the likelihood of produce contamination); evidence on long-term toxicity and on the likelihood that washing with water (and detergent) will reduce contamination. It is noteworthy that imported crops are more often in violation.

The extent of contamination of the food and environment is also still unclear. This is because testing laboratories generally set the lower limits of their assays at the EPA "cutoff." Consequently, most test results come back indicating a residue content of "less than 0.1 ppm" (or less than the particular EPA cutoff); they do not indicate how much contamination there might be at a lower level. (Highly sensitive tests, which are no more expensive to use, are often available, but not generally applied.) For a large proportion of the substances used in agriculture, sensitive and specific tests have not even been developed; nor for most have most of the prescribed toxicity tests been carried out (Bingham, 1988). The data that do exist suggest that there is a "basic" level of contamination with many of these substances, in the range of 5–10 ppb. Together, if not also individually, these residues might have significant health effects.

The large-scale use of *phenoxyherbicides* (and PCBs) contaminated with dioxins on farms, in forestry, and in other industries has also led to a widespread growing contamination of foodstuffs and environment (Table 9.10). These carcinogens accumulate in fat tissue and pancreas and increase the risk of soft tissue sarcoma as well as cancer of the oral and nasal passages (Hardell, 1982).

Numerous *antimycotics*, *slimicides*, and *glues* are used in packaging materials for added food preservation (Table 9.11). Many of these same substances are also used directly in processed foods, and leaching or absorption into the food from packaging is monitored and regulated. The slow release of tin, lead, and some other metals into canned goods also occurs, especially when

Table 9.11. Indirect Additives to the Food Supply

I. Intentional
  Antimycotics employed in the manufacture of food-packaging materials
    Propionates, parabens, sodium benzoate, sorbic acid
  Slimicides used in the manufacture of paper and paperboard that contact food
    Acrolein, alkenyl ($C_{16}C_{18}$) dimethylethylammonium bromide, 4-bromoacetoxymethyl-m-dioxolane, 2-bromo-4′-hydroxyacetophenone, chlorinated levulinic acids, chloroethylene bisthiocyanate, cupric nitrate, disodium cyanodithioimidocarbonate, potassium 2-mercaptobenzothiazole, potassium pentachlorophenate, silver fluoride, silver nitrate, 1,3,6,8-tetraazotricyclo (6,2,1,1,3,6) dodecane, 2(thiocyanomethylthio)-benzothiazole, vinylene bisthiocyanate, etc.
  Preservatives for adhesives in food packaging
    Ammonium benzoate, ρ-benzoxyphenol, 1(3-chloroallyl) 3,5,7-triaza-1-azoadamanthane chloride, 4-chloro-3,5,-dimethylphenol, coconut fatty acid amine salt of tetrachlorophenol, copper 8-quinolinolate, 2-mercaptobenzothiazole sodium or zinc salt, pentachlorophenol, phenol, o-phenylphenol, salicylic acid, sodium dehydroacetate, sodium pentachlorophenate, thymol, etc.

II. Unintentional
  Pesticides and herbicides
    Dieldrin, aldrin, endrin, DDT, 2,4,5-T, etc.
  Hormones and other growth promoters
    Diethylstilbesterol, etc.
  Antibiotics
    Puromycin, tetracycline, etc.
  Antisprouting agents
    Maleic hydrazide, etc.
  Pollutants
    PCBs, TCEs, nitrates, dirt (filth), etc.

Table 9.12. Pesticide/Fungicide/Herbicide Residues Commonly Encountered in Produce at Levels Above Those Sanctioned by the EPA

Produce	Pesticides/fungicides/herbicides				
	No. registered for use on crop	Residues detected at above acceptable levels[a] (no. of pesticides found)	Most common residues (decreasing order)[b]	Potential toxicity[c]	Level reduction by washing?
Apples	>110	1/3 of apples tested	Diphenylamine (DPA)	Teratogen USDA CES: B-4	No
			Captan (Merpan, Orthocide)	Carcinogen, teratogen	Probably not
			Endosulfan (Thiodan, Benzoepin)	Carcinogen; EPA-EHS	Yes
		(43)	Phosmet (Imidan)	EPA-EHS; teratogen, reproductive effects	Yes
			Azinphos-methyl (Guthion)	Teratogen, reproductive effects	Yes
Broccoli	>50	13%	DCPA (Dacthal, Chlorthal dimethyl)	Potential teratogen	Probably not
			Methamidophos (Monitor)	Acute toxic effects at high doses[d,e]	No
		(23)			
			Dimethoate (Cygon, Rogor)	EPA-EHS; teratogen, reproductive effects	?
			Demeton (Systox)	Acute toxicity at high doses	No
			Parathion (Phoskil)	Acute toxicity at high doses[d,e]	Probably
Lettuce	>60	19% (Mevinphos alone)	Mevinphos (Phosdrin)	Possible mutagen[d]	No
			Endosulfan (see apples)	EPA-EHS; carcinogen	Probably not
			Permethrin (Ambush, Pounce)	Reproductive effects, possible mutagen	Yes
		(43)			
			Dimethoate (see broccoli)	EPA-EHS; teratogen, toxic	Partly
			Methomyl (Lannate)	EPA-EHS	No

Potatoes	~90	20%	DDT[f]	Carcinogen	Probably not
			Chloropropham (CIPC)	Possible mutagen[d]	No
		(38)	Dieldrin[f]	Carcinogen	Probably not
			Aldicarb (Temik)	EPA-EHS	No
			Chlordane (Ostachlor, Velsicol 1066)	Carcinogen; EPA-EHS, teratogen	Probably not
Strawberries	>70	>60%	Captan (see apples)	Carcinogen, teratogen	Yes
			Vinclozolin (Ronilan)	Potential mutagen	Probably
		(39)	Endosulfan (see apples)	EPA-EHS; carcinogen	Probably not
		(1/3 had Captan)	Methamidophos (see broccoli)	Acute at high doses[d,e]	No
			Methylparathion (Folidol M, Metacide)	Acute at high doses[d,e]	Probably partly
Tomatoes	>100	~50%[g]	Methamidophos (see broccoli)	Acute at high doses[d,e]	No
			Chlorpyrifos (Dursban)	Teratogen	Probably partly
		(43)	Chlorothalonil (Bravo)	Carcinogen	Yes
		(2% had	Permethrin (see lettuce)	Reproductive effects	Yes
		methamidophos; 19% chlorpyridofos)	Dimethoate (see broccoli)	EPA-EHS; teratogen, reproductive effects	Partly

Source: Based mainly on Lewis (1989), Mott and Snyder (1989), and The Agrichemicals Handbook (1989).

[a] Above cut-off levels set by EPA.
[b] Most commonly found contaminants, in decreasing order of frequency.
[c] Evidence that it can cause cancer or other effects in animals or humans; USDA CES classifications: A-1 (high health hazard) to D-4 (negligible hazard); EPA-EHS = Extremely Hazardous Substances List.
[d] Not much tested.
[e] Long-term feeding (rats); no obvious effects.
[f] Disallowed for use.
[g] Higher levels in imported products.

Table 9.13. Effects of Canned Storage on Lead in Foodstuffs

Food	Lead content (ppm)			pH	Lacquering
	Fresh	Upon opening	After storage[a]		(L/NL)[b]
Grapefruit	0.06	0.14–0.36	0.7	2.9–3.2	NL
Lemon juice	>0.01	0.24	1.0	2.4	L
Orange juice	>0.01	0.18	0.4	3.1	L/NL
Pineapple juice	>0.01	0.12	0.4	3.3	NL
Tomato juice	>0.01	0.23	0.23	4.1	L
		0.15	0.15		NL
Vegetable juice	>0.01	0.1–0.8	0.1–1.1	4.4	L
Evaporated milk[c]	0.04	0.20	—	—	

Source: Data from Bielig et al. (1977).

[a] Open cans, 4 days, 4–20°C.
[b] L, lacquered can; NL, nonlacquered can.
[c] Underwood (1977).

cans remain unlacquered (Greger et al., 1981) and/or the food is acid. Thus, significant amounts of lead may be found in canned pineapple and citrus juices (Table 9.13).

Endogenous Nonnutritive Substances in Food

Apart from "fiber" and pollutants (including pesticides) there are some "natural" substances in food that affect nutritional status and/or are toxins. The ingestion of some of these can be avoided and this is to be desired.

The *aflatoxins* (Figure 9.8) represent a family of potent carcinogens produced by various moulds that grow on cereal grain and nut products. For example (Wogan, 1973), aflatoxin B1, fed at a rate of 400 ppm, in the diet, produced tumors in 83% of rats within 6 months [as compared with a 7% incidence in 24 months with the insecticide, DDT, fed at about the same level (Deichmann et al., 1967)]. The presence of aflatoxins in human food is monitored, especially in imported products such as peanuts. However, the feeding of mouldy grain or corn to animals and fowl is quite common and may account for some of the cancer and necrotic liver disease in these species.

Another source of carcinogens is the *pyrolysis* or *browning* of fat and proteinaceous foods during their preparation. In charcoal broiling, some of the fat dripped on hot coals is transformed into polycyclic hydrocarbons, notably pyrene, fluoranthene, and benz(o)pyrene (Figure 9.8) (the latter is a weak-to-moderate carcinogen in rodents). Oven baking and pan or deep fat frying (except with high heat or repeated heating of the oils) do not have this effect (Lijinsky and Ross, 1967). The production of various pyridine, carboline, and quinoline derivatives (Figure 9.8) during the roasting/pyrolysis of amino acid mixtures/protein or sardines has been implicated in the high incidence of stomach cancer among Japanese (Matsushima, 1982; Yamaizumi et al., 1980) and these are potent mutagens in the Ames assay (see

Figure 9.8. Structures of aflatoxin and some other common toxins that may be in foods.

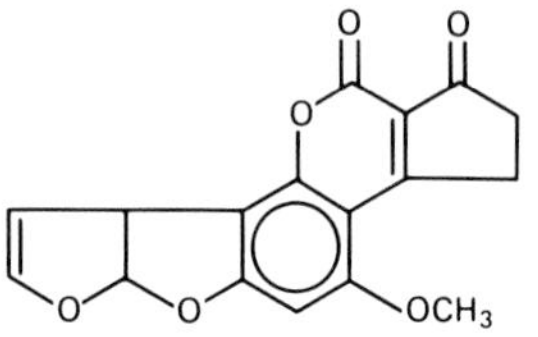

O O O OCH_3

Aflatoxin B_1
(mycotoxin)
aspergillus flavus and parasiticus

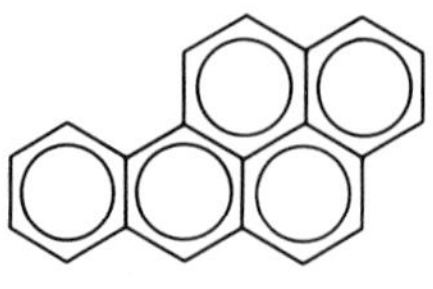

Benzo (o) pyrene
(fat pyrolysis
product)
charcoal grilling
prolonged fat heating

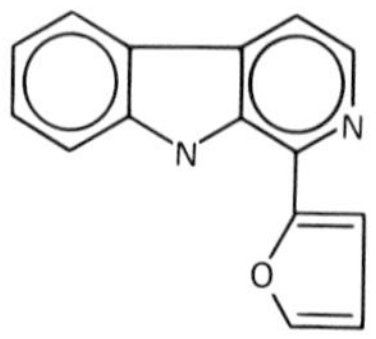

N N O

Trp-P-1
(mutagen from
pyrolysis of
protein)
broiled meats/fish

above). Mutagens may also be formed during cooking (Commoner et al., 1978; Spingarn et al., 1980), although evidence of their harmfulness in humans or animals has not as yet emerged.

Some nitrosation reactions also occur during food preparation (see nitrites/nitrates, above, and Chapter 16). Nitrosamines were discovered to be present in beers produced by a scheme that involved a heat step. Procedures were altered to eliminate this hazard. Formation of oxidized products of cholesterol may also occur during food processing and preparation. Oxycholesterols have been shown to be highly atherogenic in animal systems and may have the same effect in humans (see Chapter 15).

Tannins, phytates, and *oxalates* are natural products found in varying degrees in many plant foodstuffs, often together. Tannins (Chapter 7, Figure 7.3) are a class of polycyclic substances, especially prevalent in tea leaves, spinach, and rhubarb, which are extractable with water and alkaline solutions. Yellow-to-brown in color, they are traditionally used in leather tanning. The presence of high concentrations of these substances inhibits absorption of iron (Torrance et al., 1982) probably through formation of water-insoluble iron–tannin complexes unavailable to the absorptive cells (see Chapter 7).

Oxalic acid salts are often found in the same kinds of plants as the tannins, and are present in high concentrations in all parts of plants of the aroid family (aracae), from which subspecies (colocacia, xanthosoma, and monestera) many Africans and South Americans obtain most of their dietary carbohydrate (see Chapter 6). Oxalates also form insoluble iron (and calcium) salts, thus reducing the dietary availability of these nutrients to the absorptive cells of the small intestine. The presence of oxalate and tannins in spinach renders the otherwise high iron content of this vegetable of little consequence (see Chapter 7). Phytic acid salts (see Chapter 7, Figure 7.3), found mainly in grains, can also form insoluble iron and calcium precipitates and thus influence the dietary availability of these nutrients.

Food Irradiation

Irradiation of food, as it is done for food preservation, is considered a food additive (Lewis, 1989). The FDA currently allows irradiation of foods in certain instances (summarized in Table 9.14). Irradiation may be by γ-rays (from sealed vessels containing ^{60}Co or ^{137}Cs), and x-rays or electrons (generated mechanically). Of the food irradiated (mainly pork, poultry meat, dried herbs, and some fruits), only the pork or its products must be labeled with a special symbol (upper part of Figure 9.9). Highly emotional arguments have been made for and against these practices, but relatively little research has been done to evaluate long-term safety of such products.

What cannot be denied is that irradiation causes chemical changes (which is, of course, why it is used). These changes occur through formation of free radicals, as for example, when fatty acid is irradiated (Merritt et al., 1983). The types of changes that have been documented include alterations in, and cross-linking of, nucleotides in

Table 9.14. Permitted Use of Irradiation in U.S. Foods (1989)

Use	Limitations
For control of *Trichinella spiralis* in pork carcasses or fresh, nonheat-processed cuts of pork carcasses	Minimum dose 0.3 kGy (30 krad); maximum dose not to exceed 1 kGy (100 krad)
For control of *salmonella* and other bacteria in poultry meat	
For growth and maturation inhibition of fresh foods	Not to exceed 1 kGy (100 krad)
For disinfestation of arthropod pests in food	Not to exceed 1 kGy (100 krad)
For microbial disinfestation of dry or dehydrated enzyme preparations (including immobilized enzymes)	Not to exceed 10 kGy (1 Mrad).
For microbial disinfestation of the following dry or dehydrated aromatic vegetable substances: culinary herbs, seeds, spices, teas, vegetable seasonings, and blends of these aromatic vegetable substances. Tumeric and paprika may also be irradiated when they are to be used as color additives [Blends may contain sodium chloride and minor amounts of food ingredients ordinarily used in such blends.]	Not to exceed 30 kGy (3 Mrad).

Source: Modified from Lewis (1989).

A

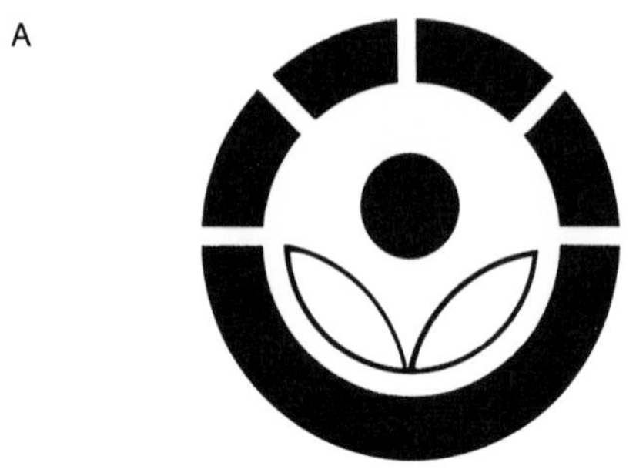

B

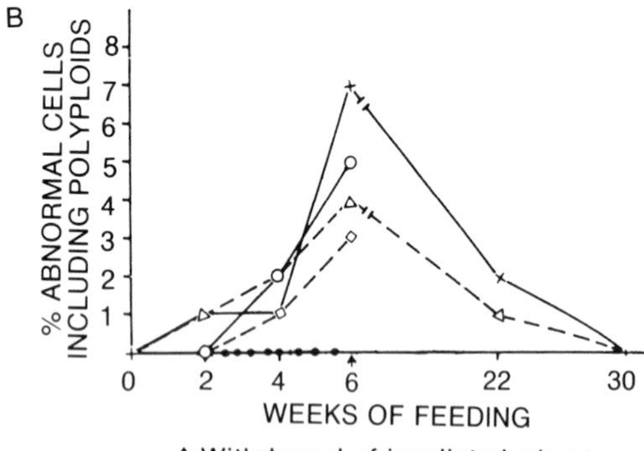

Figure 9.9. Symbol for irradiated meat and poultry products **A.** and effects of eating irradiated wheat on chromosomal changes in malnourished Indian children **B.** (incidence of polyploidy). [*Source:* Reprinted by permission from Bhaskaram and Sadasivan, 1975.]

DNA and RNA; enhancement of lipid peroxidation and formation of benzpyrene quinone (Gower and Wills, 1986); formation of formaldehyde and formic acid from sucrose (Shaw and Hayes, 1966; Steward et al., 1967) and the conversion of nitrate to nitrite (Taub, 1981). (Both formaldehyde and nitrate are mutagenic and/or can form carcinogens.) [Tritsch (1987) pointed out that 6 of 10^7 million bonds will be broken by an exposure to 100 krad. Translated into 100 ml of water, this means 10^{18} of the bonds in that liquid. The OH· radicals formed are extremely reactive, chemically.]

Preliminary human and animal studies also do not look encouraging with regard to the effects of eating irradiated foods (Tritsch, 1987). Five Indian children fed irradiated wheat showed no abnormalities in serum albumin or blood hemoglobin levels, but developed extra chromosomes in their white blood cells, which returned to normal after switching to nonirradiated wheat (Bhaskaram and Sadasivan, 1975) (Figure 9.9B). Similar responses were observed with rats and monkeys (Vijayalaxmi, 1975, 1978). Earlier studies in animals fed irradiated pork or bacon demonstrated some decreased growth, decreased survival of progeny, and increased apparent carcinogenicity, although there were deficiencies in some of the experimental designs (FDA Papers, 1968). Clearly, more work is needed to evaluate whether food irradiation is a harmless process.

References

The Agrichemicals Handbook (1989): Cambridge, UK: The Royal Society of Chemistry.

Achtzehn MK, Hawat H (1979): Z Gesamte Hyg Ihre Grenzgeb 25:242.

Batzinger KP, Ou S-YL, Bueding E (1977): Science 198:944.

Bertrand CA (1979): Exec Health 15:1.

Bertrand CA, Pomper I, Hillman G, Duffy JC, Michell I (1978): N Engl J Med 299:315.

Bhaskaram C, Sadasivan G (1975): Am J Clin Nutr 28:130.

Bice DE, Gruwell DG, Salvaggio JE, Hoffman ED (1972): Immun Commun 1:615.

Bielig HJ, Askar A, Treptow H (1977): Lebensm-Wiss Technol 10:282.

Bingham E (1988): Ann NY Acad Sci 534:1038.

Boyle CA, Berkovitz GS, LiVolsi VA, Ort S, Merino MJ, White C, Kelsey JL (1984): J Nat Cancer Inst 72:1015.

Brooks PG, Gart S, Heldfond AK, Margolin ML, Allen AS (1981): J Reprod Med 26:279.

Brown WD, Johnson AR, O'Halloran MW (1959): Aust J Exp Biol Med Sci 37:533.

Bryan GT, Erturk E (1970): Science 167:997.

Burger ASV, Mitchell JF, eds (1978): Gaddum's pharmacology (8th ed). London: Oxford University Press, p 60.

Canada, Ottawa. National Health and Welfare Ministry (1977): Regulatory affairs—Restriction on saccharin in drug products recommended. Bulletin no 100/77.

Collins TFX (1980): *In* Report on caffeine. Washington, DC: FDA.

Collins TFX, Welsh J, Black TN, Collins EV (1981): Regul Toxicol Pharmacol 1:355.

Collins TFX, Black J, Prew JH (1979): Food Cosmet Toxicol 17:443.

Commoner B, Vithayathil AJ, Dolora P, Nair S, Madyastha P, Cuca GC (1978): Science 201:913.

Deichmann WB, Keplinger M, Sala F, Glass E (1967): Toxicol Appl Pharmacol 11:88.

Duel HJ Jr, Alfin-Slater R, Weil CS, Smyth HF (1954): Food Res 19:1.

Ernster VL, Mason L, Goodson WH, Sickles EA, Sacks ST, Selvin S, Dupuy ME, Hawkinson J, Hunt TK (1982): Surgery 91:263.

FDA News: June 6, 1972.

Feinstein AR, Horowitz RI, Spitzer WO, Battision RN (1981): JAMA 246:957.

Fine DH, Rounbehler DP, Silvergleid A, Song L (1977): Nature 265:73.

Fitzhugh DG, Knudsen L, Nelson A (1946): J Pharmacol Exp Ther 86:37.

Furia TE, ed (1972): Handbook of food additives (2nd ed). Cleveland: CRC Press.

GAO (1988): Report on pesticides in the environment.

Goldstein HR (1982): N Engl J Med 306:997.

Gower JD, Wills ED (1986): Int J Radiat Biol 49:471.

Graham DM (1978): Nutr Rev 36:4.

Green LC, Tannenbaum SR, Goldman P (1981): Science 212:56.

Greger JL, Johnson MA, Baier MJ (1981): *In* Howell JMcC, Gawthorne JM, White CL, eds: Trace element metabolism in man and animals (TEMA-4). Canberra: Australian Academy of Science, p 101.

Hall RL (1973): Nutr Today 8:20.

Hardell LC (1981): Prog Clin Biol Res 32E:357 (Proceedings of the 13th International Cancer Congress, Seattle, September 15, 1982, part E).

Harman D (1968): J Gerontol 23:476.

Harshbarger KE (1942): J Dairy Sci 25:169.

Hodge HC, Fussett DW, Maynard FW, Downs WT, Cove RD Jr (1964): Toxicol Appl Pharmacol 6:572.

Hoover R, Strasser PH (1980): Progress report to the FDA from the NCI concerning the national bladder cancer study. Bethesda: NIH.

Howe GR, Burch JD, Miller AB (1977): Lancet 2:578.

Hunter RE, Barrera CM, Dohanich GP, Dunlap WP (1990): Pharmacol Biochem Behav 35:791.

Ingersoll B (1989): Wall Street Journal, Vol CXXI, no 126, Friday, December 19, p A1.

Jacobson MF, Goldman AS, Syme RH (1981): Lancet 1:1415.

Kermode GO (1972): Sci Am 226:15.

Kessler DA (1989): N Engl J Med 321:717.

Kim S-H, de Vos A, Ogata C (1988): TIBS 13:13.

King MM, McCay PB (1981): Food Cosmet Toxicol 190:13.

King MM, Bailey DM, Gibson DD, Pitha JV, McCay PB (1979): JNCI 63:657.

Kraybill HF (1976): *In* Newberne PM, ed: Trace substances in health, a handbook, part I. New York: Marcel Dekker, p 245.

Lewis RJ Sr (1989): Food additives handbook. New York: Van Nostrand Reinhold.

Lijinsky W, Ross AE (1967): Food Cosmet Toxicol 5:343.

Linn S, Schoenbaum SC, Monson RR, Rosner B, Stubblefield PG, Ryan KJ (1982): N Engl J Med 306:141.

London RS (1980): JAMA 13:1077.

London RS, Sundaram GS, Schultz M, Goldstein PJ (1980): Cancer Res 41:3811.

London RS, Sundaram GS, Murphy L, Manimekalai S, Reynolds M, Goldstein PJ (1985): Obstet Gyn 65:104.

Love SM, Gelman RS, Silen W (1982): N Engl J Med 307:1010.

Lowenfels AB, Anderson ME (1977): Cancer 39:1089.

Lubin F, Ron E, Wax Y, Black M, Furano M, Shitrit A (1985): JAMA 253:2388.

Maher TJ (1988): *In* Belmaker RH, Sandler M, Dahlstrom A (eds): Progress in catecholamine research, part C: Clinical aspects. New York: Alan R Liss, p 55.

Maltoni C, Selikoff IJ, eds (1988): Ann NY Acad Sci Vol 534.

Matsushima T (1982): *In* Molecular interrelations of nutrition and cancer. (MD Anderson Hospital and Tumor Institute, March 4–6, 1981). Houston: MD Anderson Institute.

McLachlan JA, Newbold RR, Bulloc BC (1980): Cancer Res 40:3988.

McMahon B, Yen S, Trichopoulos D, Warren K, Nardi G (1981): N Engl J Med 304:630.

Merritt C Jr, Vajdi M, Bazinet ML, Angelini P (1983): J Am Oil Chem Soc 60:1509.

Minton JP (1979): Am J Obstet Gynecol 135:157.

Morrisoin AS, Buring JE (1980): N Engl J Med 302:537.

Mott L, Snyder K (1989): Pesticide alert. Washington, DC: Natural Resources Defense Council.

Munro IC, Charbonneau SM (1982): *In* Roberts HR, ed. Food safety. New York: Wiley (Interscience), p 141.

Munro IC, Moodie CA, Krewshi D, Grice HC (1975): Toxicol Appl Pharmacol 32:513.

Narang N, Garg LC, Crews FT (1990): Pharmacology 40:90.

National Academy of Sciences (1978): Saccharin: Technical assessment of risks and benefits, report no 1 (November). Washington, DC: National Academy of Science.

National Coffee Association of USA, Inc (1981): Report of the expert panel on methylxanthine consumption and "fibrocystic breast disease," cosponsored by the International Life Sciences Institute. Washington, DC: National Coffee Association of USA, Inc.

National Research Council (1989): Diet and health: Implications for reducing chronic disease risk. Washington, DC: National Academy Press.

Reed PB (1980): Nutrition, an applied science. Los Angeles: West Publishing, p 467.

Robboy SJ, Takaguchi O, Cunha GR (1982): Hum Pathol 13:190.

Roberts HR (1981): *In* Roberts HR, ed: Food safety. New York: Wiley (Interscience), p 239.

Robertson D, Frolich JC, Carr RK (1978): N Engl J Med 298:181.

Rust E, Franz F (1913): Arb Kais-Gesundh 43:187.

Ryu JE (1985): Dev Pharmacol Ther 8:355.

Saul RL, Kabir SH, Cohen Z, Bruce WR, Archer MC (1981): Cancer Res 41:2280.

Sayka PLF (1979): Clin Perinatol 6:37.

Schechter MD, Timmons GD (1985): J Clin Pharmacol 25:276.

Schiffman SS, Buckley CE, Sampson HA, Massey EW, Baraniuk JN, Follett JV, Warwick ZS (1987): N Engl J Med 317:1181.

Select Committee for Evaluation of GRAS Substances (1977*a*): Fed Proc 36:2527.

Select Committee for Evaluation of GRAS Substances (1977*b*). Fed Proc 36:2557.

Shaw MW, Hayes E (1966): Nature 211:1254.

Shubik P, Rustra M (1979): Cancer Res 39:4636.

Spingarn NE, Slocum LA, Weisburger JH (1980): Cancer Lett 9:7.

Stavchansky S, Combs A, Sagraves R, Delgado M, Joshi A (1988): Biopharm Drug Dispos 9:285.

Stegink CD (1987): Am J Clin Nutr 46:204.

Stephenson PE (1977): J Am Dietet Assoc 71:240.

Stevenson DD, Simon RA (1981): J Allergy Clin Immunol 68:26.

Steward FC, Holstein RD, Sugil M (1967): Nature 213:178.

Svensson B-G, Nilsson A, Hansson M, Rappe C, Akesson B, Skerfving S (1990): New Engl J Med 324:8.

Swanson JM, Kinsbourne M (1980): Science 207:1485.

Tam S-Y, Ono N, Roth RH (1987): *In* Kaufman S (ed): Amino acids in health and disease: New perspectives. New York: Alan R Liss, p 421.

Tannenbaum SR, Fett D, Young VR, Land PD, Bruce WR (1978): Science 200:1487.

Taub IA (1981): J Chem Educ 58:162.

Torrance JD, Gilhooly M, Mills W, Mayer F, Bothwell TH (1982): *In* Saltman P, Hegenauer J, eds: The biochemistry and physiology of iron. New York: Elsevier, p 819.

Tritsch G (1987): Food irradiation: Hearing before the subcommittee on health and the environment. Serial no 100-81. Washington, DC: U.S. Government Printing Office.

Underwood EJ (1977): Trace elements in human and animal nutrition. New York: Academic.

Vijayalaxmi (1975): Int J Radiat Biol 27:283.

Vijayalaxmi (1978): Toxicology 9:181.

Weiss B, Williams JH, Margen S, Abrams B, Caan B, Citron LK, Cox C, McKibben J, Ogar D, Schultz S (1980): Science 207:1487.

White JE Jr (1975): J Agri Food Chem 23:886.

Wilder OHM, Kraybill HR (1948): Summary of toxicity studies on BHA (American Meat Institute Foundation). Chicago: University of Chicago.

Witschi H, Lock S (1978): Toxicology 9:137.

Witter JP, Gatley SJ, Balish E (1981): Science 213: 449.

Wogan GN (1973): *In* Busch H, ed: Methods in Cancer Research, Vol III. New York: Academic, p 309.

Wolff S, Rodin B (1978): Science 200:543.

Yamaizumi Z, Shioni T, Kasal H, Nishimura S, Takahashi Y, Nagao M, Sugimura T (1980): Cancer Lett 9:75.

Yokogoshi H, Wurtman RJ (1986): J Nutr 116:356.

Zanussi (1978): *In* Galli CI, Paoletti R, Vettorazzi G, eds: Chemical toxicology of food. Amsterdam: Elsevier, p 271.

Maria C. Linder, Ph.D.*

10

Food Quality and Its Determinants, from Field to Table:
Growing Food, Its Storage, and Preparation

The Central Roles of the Plant and Sun

The plant is central to the nutrition of man and animal, and indeed, to that of almost all creatures. In this sense, it is basic to life on earth as we know it. The plant is the original source of our complex foodstuffs—from starches and sugars to amino acids, fats, and vitamins—and it is responsible for the regeneration of the vital nutrient, oxygen, from the CO_2 waste of our own metabolism (and fuel utilization).

Animals and humans, as well as our industry and transport systems (which burn fossil fuels), do the very opposite. Rather than building nutrients, they break them down into gases and inorganic (or smaller organic) components. The anti-entropy functions of the plant are designed to balance the entropy generated by other living creatures, and one must consider how this balance is to be maintained and how the plants might best be nurtured in support of this task.

The erosion of our forests (such as the Amazon) by the encroachments of civilization is thus of concern, as is the ever-increasing rate of CO_2 production from the burning of fossil fuels. The amounts of CO_2 produced are now so large that they can no longer be fully removed by the oceans or be brought back into the natural cycle of carbon by the dwindling areas of closed forests. Hence, the atmospheric concentration of CO_2 has increased almost exponentially from an estimated 277 ppm in 1740 to 295 ppm in 1900, 316 ppm in 1959, 345 ppm in 1985 and to 351 in 1989 (C.D. Keeling, personal communication; Post et al., 1990). Methane is another heat-trapping gas, the concentration of which has also been increasing. It is released from oxygen-deficient soils (rice paddies), garbage dumps and landfills, and the digestive tract of ruminants. Nitrous oxide, one of the NO_x compounds released from power plants and automobiles, also belongs to the group of factors that trap heat from the sun; and the traces of fluorocarbons accumulating (spray cans, refrigerants), while only present in tiny amounts, are intensely more potent in trapping heat than the gases already mentioned (Ramanathan, 1988). A rise in global temperature, and concomitant weather changes, thus seems inevitable and has begun (Jones and Wigley, 1990).

To perform its enormous, life-supporting tasks, the plant relies on the sun for warmth and energy. Just as life on earth is impossible without the plant, so it is without the sun. The forces of the sun are captured by the plant in the form of complex substances, which we imbibe, releasing the energy needed for our physical and mental actions. The sun enables the plants to build carbohydrates, fats, proteins, and vitamins out of much smaller, less energized substances (like gases and inorganic matter) and to regenerate O_2 from CO_2. Thus, in a sense, the plant is the mediator between living creatures and the forces of the

* California State University, Fullerton, CA.

sun, which, in turn, allow us to exist and develop as physically palpable beings. Our own existence is inexorably tied to plant and sun—a fact that we often forget.

Soil, water, air, and other environmental factors also influence how well plants perform their tasks of producing complex nutrients needed by humans and other forms of life. These factors affect the vitamin, trace element, protein, fat, and carbohydrate contents of fresh plant produce. In some areas the existence and quality of agricultural plants is threatened by effects of human activity on soil, because of acid rain, or heavy metal, and agrochemical contamination. Between the harvest of food crops and their consumption, additional factors come into play that may have major or minor effects on nutrient content. It is the object of this chapter to summarize our present knowledge of the various factors that combine to determine the final nutritive value, or quality, of the food we eat.

Agricultural Determinants of Food Quality

Plant Nutrition and Nurture

Plant nutrition is not nearly so well understood as that of man or animal, although many aspects are clear. The nutrition of the plant involves all phases of matter, or in the ancient Greek sense, all four elements: solid, inorganic mineral matter in the soil (earth), liquid (water), gas (air), and light or warmth (fire) (Figure 10.1). The air gives the plant its most important source of carbon (CO_2) and some oxygen. Together, water and air provide almost all of the substances of plants. Water contributes the main source of hydrogen and oxygen. It also carries soluble nutrients from the soil, like nitrate, phosphate, potash (K_2O), and chelated trace elements. Apart from carbon, hydrogen, and oxygen, the major plant nutrients are nitrate, phosphate, and potassium (Figure 10.1). This accounts for the standard "NPK" analyses of fertilizers applied to fields and crops. The soil provides all of these nutrients, as well as most of the other micronutrients needed by the plant (and ultimately the animal or person eating that plant). Most of the nitrogen for plants is in the form of nitrogenous salts or organic materials like humus. These materials are normally (in Nature) produced by soil microorganisms from organic wastes or through fixation of N_2 from the air. Legumes also have symbiotic N-fixing bacteria in their root nodules, which make this gaseous N_2 much of the nitrogen is added to the soil in the agricultural practices in industrialized countries, much of the nitrogen is added to the soil in the form of soluble nitrates and ammoniates. This circumvents, and in fact reduces, the activity of N-fixing organisms in the soil (McLaren and Skujins, 1971). [It also seriously contributes to the pollution of surface and groundwater in many parts of the United States (National Research Council, 1989) and the world.]

The role of *microorganisms* in the soil and their importance as contributors to, and mediators of, plant nutrition is not adequately recognized or fostered by most current methods of agriculture. Soils are often fumigated to kill microlife and not "fed" with the organic waste materials necessary to promote soil microlife. Consequently, minerals (like phosphate) and trace elements (like zinc and iron) may become increasingly "locked in," that is, unavailable to the plant that has access to them only in soluble form. Microorganisms are capable of dissolving and/or chelating these elements, thereby increasing their availability to plants.

Another important, but neglected, aspect of plant nutrition, which is also influenced by soil microorganisms, is soil structure. Apart from the mix of sand, clay, and rock, the organic matter content, or humus, profoundly influences the texture and nutritional quality of the soil. The organic matter content of the average soil used for commercial growing in this country has declined appreciably from what it was in its virgin state (Oelhaf, 1978), and it is certainly much lower than that of soils which are fertilized with manures and crop residues (see Table 10.1).

With regard to soil structure, the most important functions of organic matter are:

1. To provide a friable texture that allows adequate aeration of plant roots with oxygen—a factor important to root nutrient uptake.
2. To hold moisture, as the organic matter, and especially the humic acids, serve as sponges for water, helping to tideover the soil and plant between periods of rain or irrigation. This is also important for the flow of soluble (available) nutrients to plant roots.
3. To provide a medium for chelating (and holding in available form) inorganic soil nutrients needed by plants.
4. To provide nutrition to soil microorganisms so they can proliferate and make the inorganic portion of the soil more available to plants. (Soil bacteria are capable of slowly digesting even inorganic materials, such as sand, granite, and clay.)

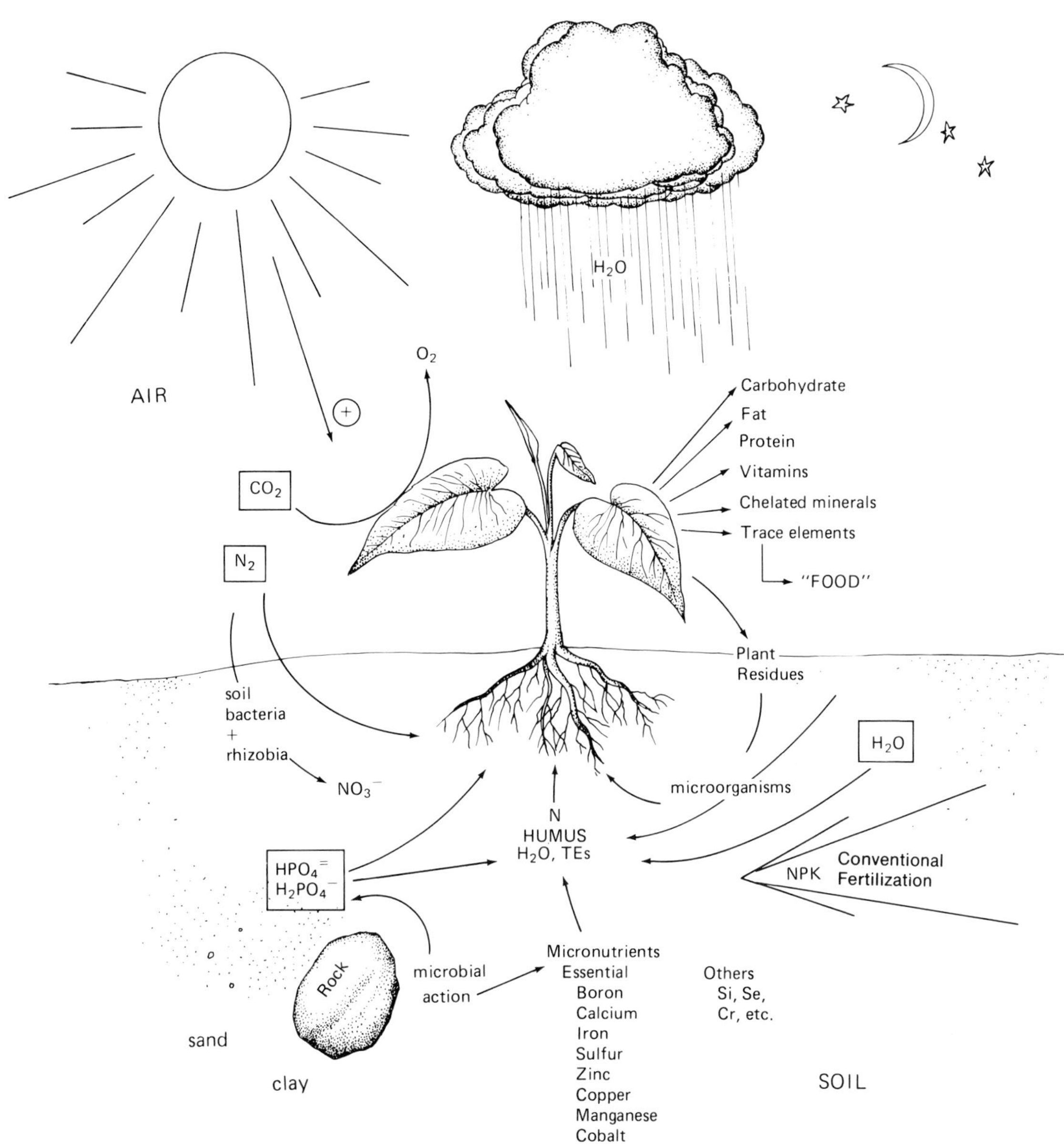

Figure 10.1. Plant nutrition. Key: TEs, trace elements.

5. To buffer changes in soil pH (Table 10.1).
6. In addition, certain forms of organic matter, specifically high nitrogen-containing humic acids, can substitute for inorganic nitrogen in plant nutrition (Schnitzer and Khan, 1972).

Other aspects of soil composition and activity affected by the method of fertilization and especially dependent on soil organic matter are summarized in Table 10.1. Soil organic matter thus influences plant nutrition not only indirectly via soil structure, but also directly as a plant nutrient.

Soil organic matter is composed of a range of materials (and organisms) characterized by various chemical and morphological criteria (Russell, 1973). At least two broader subfractions, sometimes designated "effective" and "stable" humus, can be recognized: the former turns over within months (or a few years), the latter much more slowly (with a half-life of decades). These have somewhat different actions (Table 10.2). The level of soil organic matter depends on climatic and site conditions, the cropping program, and

Table 10.1. Effects of Fertilization Methods on Soil Properties[a]

Soil parameter	Method of fertilization: None	Normal NPK treatment	Humus/compost treatment (one form)[b]
Study A (4 years; $n = 20$)[e]			
pH	5.8 (fallow)	$6.0 \rightarrow 4.7$[c]	$6.8 \rightarrow 7.2$[d]
Study B (18 years; $n = 18$)[f]			
Humus (% dry wt)			
Topsoil 0–4″	2.3	2.8	2.4
Subsoil 10–12″	1.6 (fallow)	1.0	1.7[d]
Subsoil density	1.50	1.53	1.36[d]
Phosphorus (ppm)			
Topsoil	70	130	120
Subsoil	50	40	70[d]
Biologic activity (CO_2 production)	85	81	112[d]
Earthworm holes (no/m^2)	25	25	92[d]
Study C (3 years; $n = 32$)[g]			
Nitrate runoff from fields (ppm)	—	40–59	7–11[d]

[a] Application of compost/humus increases the organic matter and phosphorus content of the lower layer of the soil, reduces nitrate runoff, reduces soil density (increases aeration), and enhances biologic activity.
[b] A sophisticated form of "organic" agriculture known as "biodynamics," practiced especially in Europe and Australia.
[c] Significant change ($p < 0.01$).
[d] Significant difference from NPK treatment ($p < 0.01$).
[e] Recalculated from Pfeiffer (1952) (Linder, 1973); n = number of samples/field plots tested.
[f] Pettersson and von Wistinghausen (1977).
[g] Koepf (1973).

the extent to which animal and vegetable matter is recycled. Crop residues and animal manures restore organic matter and maintain microbial life and fauna. They return nutrients to the soil that were removed during cropping and enhance the capacity for nitrogen fixation. Animal manures can be particularly useful in this regard, a single 500-kg cow (producing 10 tons of manure per year) can supply a large percentage of the nutrients needed for the growth of an "average" crop on 1 hectare (2.5 acres) (Table 10.3). These "nutrients" come from a range of plants and forages "harvested" by the cow, which might otherwise go unused (Baker and Raun, 1989), making farm animals important mediators of recycling and fertility of the land.

The substitution of *humus*, in the form of compost or other "raw" forms of organic materials and wastes, for inorganic chemical fertilizers is termed "organic" or "sustainable" agriculture (Reganold et al., 1990). The kind of organic material used may, or may not, be an adequate source of nutrients for the plants, depending on what it is, how it was produced, and its nitrogen content. Raw manures will initially "overprovide" ammonia-nitrogen, leading to overfertilization (see below), some volatilization, and leaching of the inherent nutrients; later (after nitrification), they will lose a lot to leaching, in comparison to "compost," where the nitrogen has become stabilized. Raw manures contain appreciable amounts of nitrogen in a form not directly available to the plant without microbial intervention and conversion. (Urea or proteins cannot be used directly by the plant.) They may also contain organic acids and other factors harmful to plants. Addition of raw, low nitrogen materials (like straw or clippings) to the soil may temporarily cause a nitrogen deficiency (as microbes will use it to help proliferate and decompose the raw material). It is thus generally preferable to compost raw materials before applying them. Composts made through controlled fermentation by soil bacteria and actinomycetes from high N-containing waste materials may contain forms of humic acid and micronutrients optimal for plant growth and development

Table 10.2. Composition and Functions of Soil Organic Matter

Composition	Plant residues, animal excretions, microorganisms (and other forms of soil life) "effective" humus ($t_{1/2}$, months to a few years) (is decomposed and nourishes the microbial population) "stable" humus ($t_{1/2}$, many years/decades) (lasts much longer; binds soil minerals and water)
Influence on soil structure	The effective humus fraction: creates humic substances that stabilize structure The stable humus fraction: makes light soils more cohesive and increases their water retention; makes heavy soils more porous, improving warming and aeration
Influence on plant nutrition	The effective humus fraction: gives N, P, S, and other nutrients; mobilizes soil minerals/trace elements; air–nitrogen fixed The stable humus fraction: nutrient storage/trapping; slow release
Influence on plant physiology	Both humus fractions: stimulate plant growth and resistance against pathological microorganisms; supplies growth factors and some antibiotics

Source: H.H. Koepf (personal communication).

Table 10.3. Nutrients in the Manure of One 500-kg Cow Excreted in 1 Year

	Average content in 10 tons (g)		Approximate average uptake by crop on 1 hectare (g)
Nutrient	Average	Range	
N	55,000	50–60,000	20,000
P	17,000	15–18,000	6,000
K	55,000	50–60,000	24,000
Mn	500	180–1370	500
Zn	240	100–520	200
Cu	40	20–100	80
B	50	10–130	180
Mo	5	2–10.5	10
Co	2.5	0.5–12	1

Source: Modified from Koepf (1989).

(Table 10.2). (Some of the benefits for food crops are illustrated by data in Tables 10.4 and 10.7.) Thus, plants grown with organic fertilizers may be of the same, better, or poorer quality as those grown by standard means (see below); however, all forms of "organic" agriculture do have an advantage in that they return many (or most) of the elements that were removed from the soils when the crop was harvested.

The details of trace element nutrition in plants are not as well understood as they are for humans and animals. Many fewer elements are currently recognized as essential for the growth, development, and maintenance of plants (Figure 10.1) than are recognized for animals (see Chapter 7). This is partly because of less research and also because it is more difficult to recognize symptoms of deficiency and disease in this phylum. Only about 25 elements are known to be essential for the plant. These include boron, for which we may just be beginning to recognize a human need.

Although it may be that the plant can survive on fewer elements than animals or humans, this is irrelevant when considering food plants that will be used to feed humans and animals. Man depends on the plant for most of the trace elements, and the plant must incorporate them during its growth. It can only do so if these elements are present in the soil or water in available form. As already described, the availability of soil nutrients depends on soil composition, pH, and/or the presence of microorganisms. Promotion of soil microlife will enhance availability if the elements are present (Table 10.1; subsoil phosphate). However, with our present agricultural methods, it is to be expected that soil will increasingly become deficient in various elements, as they are removed and not returned. We have been removing most elements from the soil when we harvest our crops, but we have returned only the most important by quantity: largely N, P, and K. Only when gross deficiencies are recognized are other elements also added. A case can thus be made that our food plants are receiving a refined diet, lacking in micronutrients, just as our own diets have become refined.

A soil may continue to produce large crops despite elemental deficiencies, but the plants may be weakened, and more susceptible to pests and disease (Albrecht, 1970). A partial solution to this problem is to recycle our wastes (including animal and human wastes; Table 10.3), which contain these elements, and to return them to the soil and plants in a palatable and/or tolerable form, such as humus-containing composts. A major fac-

Table 10.4. Effects of Fertilization Methods on Dry Weight, Protein, and Vitamin Contents of Food Plants

	Methods of fertilization			
Vegetable	Regular NPK	Stable manure	Manure and NPK	Composted manure
Spinach				
Dry weight (%)	6.9	9.4[a]	6.5	9.2[a]
Protein (% of control)	100	103	99	101
Nitrate-N (μg/g)	270	20[a]	280	10[a]
Ascorbate (μg/g)	340	560[a]	320	490[a]
β-carotene (μg/g)	28	25	27	25
Sugar (% weight)	0.9	1.0	0.7	1.3[a]
Savoy cabbage				
Dry weight (%)	8.3	13.2[a]	8.7	14.2[a]
Protein (% of control)	100	133[a]	121[a]	135[a]
Ascorbate (μg/g)	440	800[a]	430	780[a]
Celery				
Dry weight (%)	15.0	16.4[a]	15.3	15.9[a]
Protein (% of control)	100	142[a]	118	131[a]
Sugar (% of weight)	2.1	2.3	2.3	2.2

Source: Data from Schuphan (1974). Crops were grown side by side in experimental pots containing a base of sand or "fen" soil plus the fertilizer indicated, all at the same level of nitrogen. Values shown are means for 4–6 average values (2 types of pots planted 2 or 3 times = years). Protein values are given relative to the NPK-fertilized pots (controls).

[a] Indicates values significantly different from control (NPK-fertilized) ($p < 0.01$). (1) Fertilization has significant effects on plant dry weight (water content) as well as protein; mineral fertilizers tend to increase moisture content and decrease protein and dry matter. Differences in sugar and vitamin contents in favor of organic treatment may also occur. (2) Results vary with the particular food crop. (3) Spinach tends to absorb and accumulate nitrate when fertilized with inorganic nitrates.

tor barring this as a total approach is the presence of toxic heavy metals in sewage waste products. This has already become a factor in some areas, where industrial contamination with some metals has exceeded what is tolerated by plants for growth (Table 10.5) (apart from making them toxic to humans and animals). In general, heavy metal contamination is less of an immediate problem for soils with a high pH. The admittedly limited existing data on composted livestock manures suggest that these fertilizers produce food crops of similar quantity but superior quality to those grown (side-by-side) with conventional NPK fertilizers (Tables 10.4, 10.6, and 10.7). Recycling of organic wastes also offers the possibility of reducing nitrate runoff (Table 10.1, bottom) and other forms of pollution of our lakes, streams, and oceans (Singer, 1969) and of reducing the need for nitrate and phosphate fertilizers, which in themselves contribute to water pollution (Spalding et al., 1978; Stout and Buran, 1968; Verduin, 1968).

Table 10.5. Contents of Some Heavy Metals in Normal and Contaminated Arable Land, and Levels Tolerated by Plants[a]

	Heavy metal content (ppm)		
Metal	Commonly found	Heavily contaminated areas	Limit of plant tolerance (ppm)
Zinc	3–50	up to 20,000	300
Copper	1–20	up to 22,000	100
Chromium	2–50	up to 20,000	100
Lead	0.1–20	up to 4000	100
Nickel	2–50	up to 10,000	50
Cadmium	0.1–1	up to 200	3
Mercury	0.1–1	up to 500	2

[a] Data for West Germany (Sauerbeck et al., 1986).

The excessive use of soluble nitrogen fertilizers may have detrimental effects on the nutritional and keeping quality of crops (Goldstein, 1981), as illustrated by the data for potatoes in Table 10.7 (see also below). Of further concern are preliminary data indicating that fertility may be reduced when animals are fed foodstuffs from fields heavily treated with soluble nitrogenous (or other) fertilizers (Hahn and Aehnelt, 1973).

The ultimate nutrient content or composition of a food plant thus depends on a complex set of physical, meteorological, chemical, and biologi-

Table 10.6. Crop Yields on Organic and Conventional Farms Are Similar

Crop	1960[a] Conventional (bushels/acre)	1960[a] Organic (BD)[d]	1972[b] Conventional (tons/acre)	1972[b] Organic (BD)[d]	1974–1976[c] Conventional (bushels/acre)	1974–1976[c] Organic (non-BD)
Wheat	58	73	3.9	4.5	29–38	26–29
Oats	65	70	4.1	4.8	57–62	56–61
Barley	78	89	3.6	2.7	—	—
Peas/beans	65	57	2.5	2.7	—	—
Corn	—	—	—	—	71–94	74–78
Soybeans	—	—	—	—	28–38	30–34
Hay	—	—	—	—	3.5	5

[a] Data from Pfeiffer (1961).
[b] Data from Koepf (1974).
[c] Data from USDA Study Team on Organic Farming (1980).
[d] One form of organic agriculture, termed "biodynamics."

cal factors in the environment during growth. The tendencies fostered by some of these variables can be grouped as indicated in Table 10.8: the coupling of light and heat enhance early ripening, dryness, starch formation, shelf-life, and other factors; while water, humus, and a high nitrogen content foster vegetative processes and leaf formation, along with less amino acid and sugar polymerization and a shorter shelf-life. As a result, the nutrient content of the same plant foods grown in different regions and in different ways will vary enormously. This is not generally appreciated and certainly not taken into account by "Food Tables," in which only average values will be found. The extent of the variation is illustrated by USDA data for just a few crops, from which 95% confidence limits for "normal" values were calculated (Table 10.9). While these data also reflect variabilities inherent in the analytical tests, the range of variability in nutrient content is astounding even if cut in half! Thus, one apple is not going to be like another apple, one potato like another; and, in order to identify effects of environment and growth conditions on food quality, valid comparisons can only be made when studies are carried out under well-controlled conditions, side-by-side.

Plant Breeding and Genetic Engineering

Since World War II, the yields of most major U.S. crops have been enormously increased (Table 10.10). This is largely attributable to the development of plant breeds that inherently produce

Table 10.7. Effects of Fertilization on Yields and Keeping Quality of Potatoes

Fertilization	Nitrogen applied (kg/ha)[a]	Crop yields: Tons/ha	Crop yields: Protein (% wt)	Keeping quality: Tissue darkening[b]	Keeping quality: Pathology (mm)[c]	Keeping quality: Taste points[d] (6 months)
Soluble NPK						
1	62	36	58	30	513	2.4
2	124	35	53[e]	34[e]	489[e]	2.4
Composted manure	108	35	59	27[f]	422[f]	3.0[f]
Fresh manure	123	32[f]	57	29	422[f]	2.8[f]

Source: Data from Goldstein (1981).

[a] Phosphorus applications were similar throughout and potassium applications 20%–50% greater with the manures.
[b] Relative rate of tissue darkening after slicing (oxidation); measured by refractometer.
[c] Potatoes injected with a suspension of potato blight fungus (*Phylophthora infestans*) and the spread of the infection (in mm diameter) measured after 14 days of 18°C.
[d] Mean taste scores for potatoes prepared after 6 months of storage under identical conditions, tested blindly by a panel.
[e] Significantly different from NPK-1 ($p < 0.05$).
[f] Significantly different from both NPK controls ($p < 0.05$).

Table 10.8. Tendencies in Plants Grown Under Two Kinds of Environmental Conditions[a]

Parameter	Tendencies promoted by: Light and warmth (less N, water)	Water, humus, nitrogen
Plant development	Premature ripening	Delayed ripening
	Reproductive processes enhanced	Vegetative processes enhanced
	Leaf metamorphosis enhanced	Delayed leaf metamorphosis
Plant form	Deep, less divided root	Shallow, strongly branching root
	Short internodes	Long internodes
	Leaves small, thick short petioles	Leaves large, thin, long petioles
	Pointed solid structure	Rounded, uniform, soft contour
Pest control	Mainly attacked by insect pests	Mainly attacked by pathogenic fungi
Keeping quality	Long shelf-life	Short shelf-life
Plant composition	High dry matter content	Low dry matter content
	Rel. low crude protein content	Rel. high crude protein content
	High true protein as % of crude protein, nitrate content	Low true protein as % of crude protein, nitrate content
	Low amides, free amino acids (EAA index)	High amides, free amino acids (EAA index)
	Rel. high disaccharides	Rel. low disaccharides
	Rel. low monosaccharides	Rel. high monosaccharides
	High vitamin C	Much pro-vitamin A
	Low enzyme activity in the harvested product	High enzyme activity in the harvested product
	Rich fragrance and taste	Poor fragrance and taste

[a] Modified (mostly re-arranged) from Koepf (1989). Rel, relatively.

Table 10.9. Nutrients of Fruits: Variability in Composition

Nutrient	Content (95% confidence limits)[a]: Apples	Bananas	Oranges
Water (g)	80–88 (126)	66–82 (116)	84–89 (17)
Protein (mg)	124–256 (119)	484–1576 (111)	750–1330 (16)
Fat	0–820 (35)	0–1490 (11)	—
Ash	152–1180 (116)	464–1136 (110)	—
Ca	1–13 (34)	4–8 (5)	—
P	2–12 (114)	—	14–20 (18)
Mg	3–7 (114)	3–54 (103)	2–18 (94)
K	71–159 (74)	301–490 (55)	137–220 (86)
Fe	0.00–0.59 (119)	0.00–0.62 (108)	0.05–0.13 (16)
Zn (μg)	0–94 (15)	102–218 (13)	—
Mn	0–81 (119)	0–456 (103)	7–39 (16)
Cu	0–85 (119)	0–292 (109)	0–77 (16)
Ascorbate (mg)	0–13 (25)	6.6–11.6 (14)	26–71 (75)
Niacin (μg)	0–211 (6)	—	0–886 (75)
Pantothenate	42–80 (6)	276–804 (5)	—
Thiamine	17 (6)	—	69–105 (78)
Riboflavin	9–19 (6)	—	—
Pyridoxine	27–69 (6)	—	34–92 (54)
Folic acid	0–9 (23)	—	—
Retinol equivalents	0–11 (6)	3.5–12.4 (5)	7.4–3.8 (78)

[a] Calculated from data for 100 g samples in USDA Agricultural Handbook No. 8 (means ± 2 SD); number of samples tested in parentheses.

Table 10.10. Escalation of Annual U.S. Crop Yields Largely Attributable to Conventional Plant Breeding

Crop	Cultivated area (per 10^3 ha)	Yield (ton/ha/year)	Total annual production (tons × 10^{-3})
1939–1940			
Maize	36,014	1.80	64,104
Wheat	23,635	0.96	22,453
15 other crops[a]	69,271	—	165,476
1958–1960			
Maize	29,714	3.36	99,891
Wheat	21,419	1.67	35,883
15 major crops[a]	76,303	—	255,614
1978–1980			
Maize	29,338	6.32	185,208
Wheat	25,614	2.22	57,016
15 major crops[a]	77,592	—	368,069

Source: Data from Borlaug (1983).

[a] Rice, barley, sorghum, oats, rye, cotton, soybeans, peanuts, beans, flaxseed, potatoes, sugar beets, hay, corn silage, tobacco.

larger crops and/or may have a greater resistance to disease and insect infestation. The use of controlled plant hybridization has been a major factor in cross-pollinating crops, such as corn and sorghum. In this approach, inbred lines (which have lost their "vigor" through their inbreeding) are crossed, and an explosive recovery of vigor, called heterosis, occurs in the next generation (Borlaug, 1983). This is the generation planted for superior crop yields. Although the nutritional quality of many modern high yielding cultivars has not been carefully assessed, with the notable exception of cases where "high protein" varieties of grain have been bred (International Atomic Energy Agency, 1982), the availability of more food has greatly enhanced the world's capacity to reduce hunger and famine.

The current interest in applying modern principles of genetic engineering to crop plants to increase inherent/symbiotic nitrogen fixation (reducing fertilizer needs), to enhance the efficiency of photosynthesis, and to increase disease and pest resistance may provide for continued high yields in food crops (Abelson, 1983). However, such manipulations alone will not ensure the continued high nutritive quality of plant foods, especially with regard to the micronutrients, unless proper nourishment of the plants (and soils) is also fostered.

Factors Affecting Food Quality After Harvest

Time of Harvest

The maturation and state of ripeness of a fruit or vegetable will clearly influence its content of specific vitamins, proteins, starches, and other nutrients. The handling of fruits and vegetables is dictated by what is most economical, in view of long-range transportation and storage requirements, maintenance of acceptable appearance, flavor, and other hallmarks of quality. Some foods, the so-called "climacteric" fruits, are characterized by a sharp increase in oxygen consumption (and ethylene gas production) at the start of the ripening phase (Figure 10.2); they also can ripen after picking. This makes it possible to harvest some fruits in the unripe state (Tables 10.11 and 10.12) and to control their rate of ripening, which allows for more extensive transportation and longer storage. Other (nonclimacteric) fruits and most vegetables cannot ripen off the vine and cannot be treated in the same way (Table 10.11).

As concerns the nutritional quality of climacteric fruits harvested in the unripe versus ripe state, most studies have focused on potential deficiencies of vitamin C and β-carotene, as these are among the vitamins most vulnerable to food processing or storage destruction (see more below). Numerous studies on many varieties of tomatoes indicate that the ascorbate and carotene contents will be somewhat less if the fruit is picked unripe and allowed to ripen after harvest (on the way to the supermarket), as compared with fruit ripened on the vine; however, the difference is small (J.M. Krochta and B. Feinberg, unpublished review). Surprisingly, avocadoes and bananas actually have a significantly higher final ascorbate content when ripened after picking (Table 10.12) (J.M. Krochta and B. Feinberg, unpublished review). (Indeed, avocadoes only really ripen off the tree.) For nonclimacteric fruits and vegetables, harvest must occur at least in the early "ripe" stage to make them acceptable to the consumer. Here, although changes in various vitamins (and ratios of sugar to starch) occur, it is impossible to generalize about what is best from a nutritional standpoint (Harris and Karmas, 1975). Some vitamins tend to increase (Table 10.12) and others to decrease with increasing maturation, and short of the "senescence" phase (where physiologic or other degeneration begins), various stages are acceptable. Especially for vegetables, the ratio of sugar to starch is important to the consumer; peas

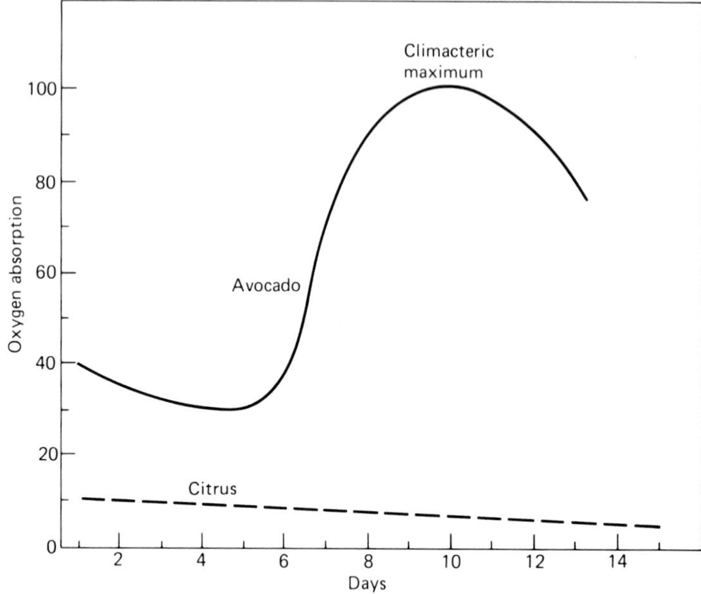

Figure 10.2. Oxygen uptake of a climacteric fruit during ripening. [*Source:* Reprinted by permission from Biale (1975) and the Division of Agriculture and Natural Resources, University of California.]

and corn are harvested on the early side and treated to retard glucose to starch conversion, which occurs with increasing maturity. For easier storage and less sugar accumulation, potatoes are harvested on the late side of maturity (J.M. Krochta and B. Feinberg, unpublished review), which provides potatoes with a better texture and flavor, and there is less of a "browning reaction."

In some cases, mechanics influence procedure. Tomatoes for canning and processing, though belonging to the climacteric fruits, are harvested when the majority are ripe on the vine and by use of mechanical pickers. Special, smaller varieties (which bruise less easily and are retained longer by the vines) are grown for this purpose. These varieties have levels of ascorbate comparable to those of other ripe tomatoes (J.M. Krochta and B. Feinberg, unpublished review). Other foodstuffs harvested mechanically are cherries, carrots, potatoes, corn, and peas, which are destined for processing (including freezing). In contrast, fruits and vegetables sold fresh on the market are harvested by hand to prevent bruising and other damage. Foods harvested mechanically are processed very rapidly (within 10 hr) to prevent spoilage. This also minimizes loss of their nutrients.

Table 10.11. Climacteric and Nonclimacteric Fruits[a]

Climacteric fruits	Nonclimacteric fruits
Tomatoes	Citrus
Avocados	Strawberries
Apples	Other berries
Pears	Pineapples
Peaches	Melons
Apricots	
Bananas	

Source: Table modified from Krochta and Feinberg (1975).

[a] Fruits capable of ripening off the vine, and consuming oxygen during this process (see text).

Table 10.12. Vitamin Contents of Fruits at Different Stages of Maturation[a]

Fruit and vitamin	Vitamin content (μg/g) Unripe	Medium ripe	Ripe	Overripe
Bananas				
Ascorbate	53–58	68–88	91–111	32
Tomatoes				
Ascorbate	142–266	—	137–318	—
β-carotene	3.2–4.3	—	4.0–5.7	—

Source: Data from Krochta and Feinberg (unpublished observations).

[a] 1. The concentration of vitamins in fruits can be very variable, even at the same stage of maturation. 2. The concentration also will change with the state of fruit maturation. 3. Vitamin content tends to be higher in the ripe (but not overripe) versus unripe state.

Crop Fertilization and Treatment

Evidence is accumulating that the method of fertilization can also significantly affect the "shelf-life" of a crop. As indicated by the data in Table 10.13, extensive studies by Samaras (1977) and others in Germany showed a consistent improvement in keeping quality of crops fertilized with composted manures versus soluble nitrogenous (NPK) fertilizers (see also Table 10.7). These data are not widely known, but they clearly illustrate the point that soil treatment affects not only the nutrient content of crops but also their capacity for storage.

Use of insecticides, herbicides, and nematocides and soil fumigants prior to or during growth (see Table 10.17), or fungicides, fumigants, antisprouting agents (and the like) after harvest, may also affect the ultimate quality of the food brought to the table, as residues frequently remain on or in the produce (see also Chapter 9). Some common examples are given in Table 10.17, along with what is known (or not known) about their potential toxicity.

Table 10.13. Method of Nitrogen Fertilization and Its Effects on Storage of Carrots and Other Vegetables[a]

	Mineral fertilizer[b] (Increasing nitrogen)			Organic fertilizer[b]
	1	2	3	
Carrots				
Storage losses (164 days)				
Total weight (%)	26	27	30	29 ± 5
Dry weight (%)	50	58	59	40 ± 14[f]
Rotting (%)	24	31	59	22 ± 5
Peroxidase activity[c] (U/g)	13.9	17.6	19.2	11.4 ± 3.6[f]
SUMMARY—MULTIPLE STUDIES				
Storage losses (% total weight)[d]				
Carrots			30–60[e]	20–50[f]
Red beets			46,74	29,32[f]
Turnips			49,53	34,36[f]
Potatoes			25,35	12,19[f]

Source: Data from Samaras (1977).

[a] Decreased storability of produce is evident with increasing application of mineral fertilizer and in comparison with the organically fertilized foodstuffs, grown in parallel, as evidenced by loss of total weight, dry weight, and percent rotting.

[b] Fertilization during plant growth was with increasing amounts of mineral NPK fertilizer (25,50 and 75 kg/ha) or rotted cow manure (four separate plots with about 150 kg N/ha). Results for the latter are mean ± SD.

[c] Peroxidase activity was measured in juice from the carrots immediately after harvest.

[d] Storage losses over 5–6 months.

[e] Range of mean values for four studies; other values are means for two studies.

[f] Significant difference from NPK-fertilized samples ($p < 0.05$).

Storage, Processing, and Preparation

Following harvest, fruits and vegetables undergo handling and various treatments that will alter (and largely reduce) their nutrient content. Apart from food refining (see Chapters 5 and 7), six factors are mainly responsible for the ultimate degree of nutrient loss and may play a role at any stage of handling, storage, and food preparation. These are temperature, light, oxygen and CO_2, pH, moisture, and microorganisms. Table 10.14 summarizes the effects of most of these factors on the fruit and vegetable contents of vitamins and some other nutrients, as modified from Harris and Karmas (1975). It is clear that most vitamins are quite unstable under some of the conditions that occur in storage or food preparation. Ascorbic acid is especially sensitive to heat, oxygen and alkaline pH, but quite stable in acid (which makes it remarkably stable in unpasteurized citrus juices). Thiamin is extremely unstable in heat; the toasting of bread for as little as 60 sec will lower its thiamin content considerably (Table 10.15). Vitamin A and riboflavin are especially susceptible to light destruction. (The storage of milk in glass bottles may thus reduce its usefulness as a rich source of riboflavin.) Unsaturated fatty acids, and even amino acids, are susceptible to chemical alterations and oxidations upon exposure to heat, air, and light, which lower food quality (see Figure 10.3). The state of moisture is critical not only to the maintenance of vitamin content (through prevention of wilting) but also to determining whether microorganisms that cause rotting or poisoning of the food can proliferate. Wilting not only makes fruit and vegetables unacceptable to the consumer, but results in a general physiologic breakdown of the plant product (J.M. Krochta and B. Feinberg, unpublished review). The minimization of heat exposure and introduction of cooling and refrigeration are most important to minimize nutrient losses during storage and transport. They should also be considered in relation to food preparation (such as canning, blanching for freezing, and cooking or reheating). Further details follow.

Table 10.14. Factors Rendering Nutrients Unstable (U) in Foods or Having Little Effect (S, Stable)

	Factors							
				pH				
Nutrients	Heat	Oxygen or air	Light	Acid	Neutral	Alkaline	Moisture[a]	Microorganisms[b]
Vitamins								
Vitamin A or carotenes	U	U	U	U	S	S	U	U
Ascorbate (C)	U	U	U	S	U	U	U	U
Biotin	U	S	S	S	S	S		U
Choline	S	U	S	S	S	S		U
Cobalamin (B_{12})	S	U	U	S	S	S		U
Vitamin D	U	U	U	S	S	U		U
Folic acid	U	U	U	U	U	S	U	U
Inositol	U	S	S	S	S	S		U
Vitamin K	S	S	U	U	S	U		U
Niacin	S	S	S	S	S	S		U
Pantothenate	U	S	S	S	S	U		U
Pyridoxine (B_6)	U	S	U	S	S	S		U
Riboflavin	U	S	U	S	S	U	U	U
Thiamin	U	U	S	S	U	U	U	U
Tocopherols (E)	U	U	U	S	S	S	U	U
Amino acids								
Isoleucine	S	S	S	S	S	S		U
Leucine	S	S	S	S	S	S		U
Lysine	U	S	S	S	S	S		U
Methionine	S	S	S	S	S	S		U
Phenylalanine	S	S	S	S	S	S		U
Threonine	U	S	S	U	S	U		U
Tryptophan	S	S	U	U	S	S		U
Valine	S	S	S	S	S	S		U
Fatty acids								
Polyunsaturated	S[c]	U	U	S	S	U		U

Source: Modified from Harris and Karmas (1975).

[a] Moist processed foods are always less stable than dry because of greater risk of oxidation, heat effects, and possibilities for microbial growth. In fresh produce, however, adequate moisture to prevent wilting is important in nutrient stability.

[b] Most microorganisms would tend to render the food unpalatable, not so much because of vitamin destruction, but because of toxin production.

[c] If not excessive, such as when dripped on hot coals.

Table 10.15. Thiamin Losses in Bread During Toasting

	Type of bread		
Toasting time (sec)	Whole wheat	Enriched white	Unenriched white
0	0[a]	0	0
30	4	5	9
40	8	7	22
50	12	13	20
60	15	15	27
70	21	17	31

Source: Modified from Harris and Karmas (1975).

[a] Percent lost.

Storage. The least time lost getting vegetables or most fruits from field or garden to table will optimize nutritional quality. Similarly, if time is involved, cooling of the food and maintenance of some humidity are especially important. The institution of a "controlled atmosphere," as in the storage of apples, will also have a profound effect, especially if ripening is to be retarded so marketing can occur weeks and months later on. In some cases, specific chemicals may also be used to reduce microbial or insect attack or to retard sprouting.

Apples (and pears) are best stored either at low oxygen (0.5%–3%) (1%–8% CO_2), 30–40°F ("controlled atmosphere") or under a partial vacuum

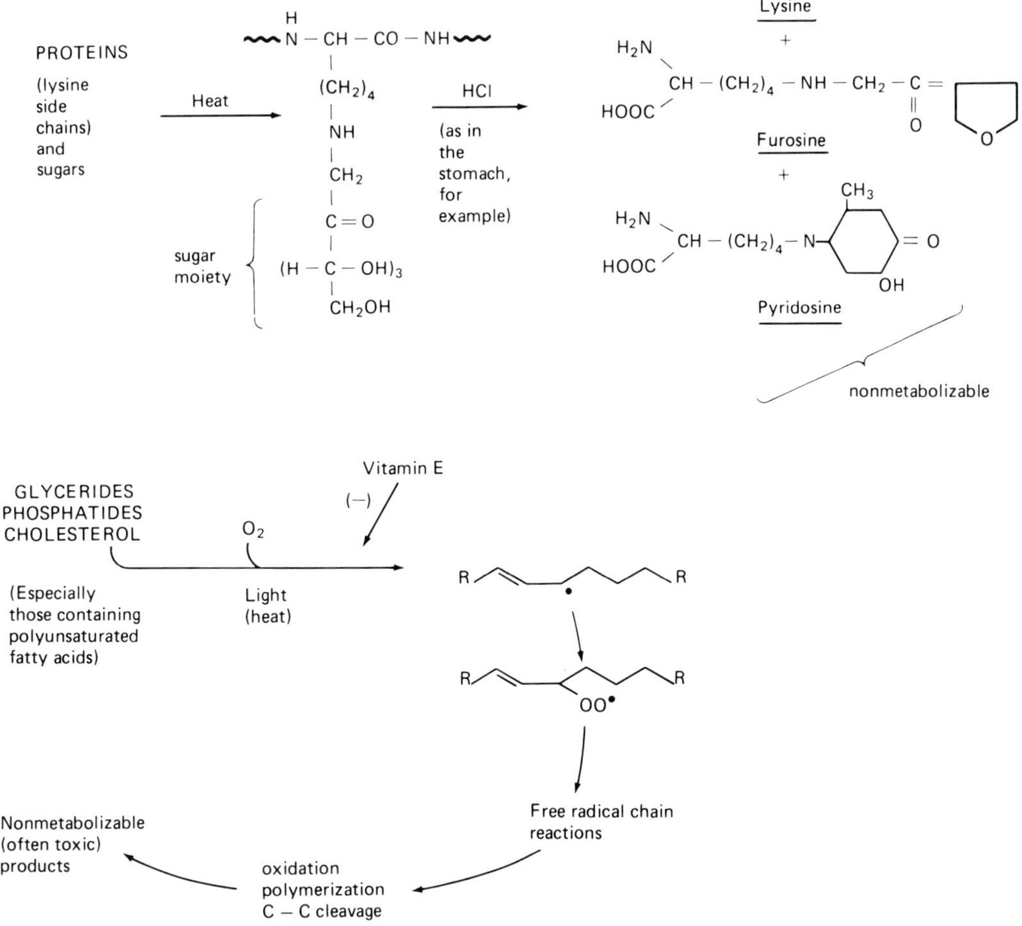

Figure 10.3. Chemical modifications of nutrients that commonly occur in food processing.

(75 torr) at 3°C with humidity near the dew point. The latter procedure is best for firmness and chlorophyll and ascorbate status, but, for some reason, leaves less flavor. The partial vacuum procedure is also sometimes used for currants, cress, peppers, and tomatoes.

Oranges and other citrus tend to be stored at slightly higher temperatures (42°F) for optimal nutrient retention, and their ascorbate content is remarkably stable over 5 months, with fruits generally losing less than 10% to the time of their marketing.

Potatoes are the biggest U.S. food crop, other than the grains (J.M. Krochta and B. Feinberg, unpublished review). Because of their slow respiratory rate, they are stored for up to 12 months, usually under conditions of 45°F, 95% humidity (Table 10.16), and with the application of antisprouting agents, such as isopropyl-N-chlorocarbamylate (CPC) (Table 10.17). Despite the lowered temperature and maintenance of humidity (to prevent wilting), about half the ascorbic acid is lost by 3–5 months (J.M. Krochta and B. Feinberg, unpublished review). As with other crops, the loss is exponential, and thus, most rapid in the early stages of storage. The antisprouting agents remain as a residue that should be washed off. (This may require soap or detergent.) [Some such agents (like maleic hydrazide) have proven to be potent carcinogens.] In Europe, radiation treatment is used as a means of preventing sprouting (or greening) of potatoes, and this procedure has now also been approved for U.S. use (see Chapter 9). The green portion of the potato is associated with the development of some semipoisonous alkaloids that should not be consumed. Antisprouting agents are also commonly used on onions.

Table 10.16. Effects of Various Storage Procedures on Vitamin Retention of Foods[a]

Vegetable and treatment	Vitamin (% lost)			
	Ascorbate	Thiamine	Riboflavin	Carotene
Spinach[b]				
Stored 24 hr, 66–78°F	29	2	5	8
Stored 1 week, 32–40°F	35	15	17	5
Frozen	63	51	40	13
Asparagus[b]				
Stored 24 hr, 66–78°F	40	3	22	9
Stored 1 week, 32–40°F	57	18	27	14
Frozen	24	28	42	24
Potatoes[c]				
Stored 3 months, 45°F, 95% humidity	50–59	0	0–11	0–3
Stored 6 months	40–48	0	0–5	0
Stored 8 months	35–44	0	0–7	0–10
Lettuce[b]				
Stored 48 hr, room temperature	30	—	—	—
Stored 48 hr, refrigerator	40	—	—	—
Stored 48 hr (hydrator)	30	—	—	—
Broccoli[b]				
Stored 48 hr, room temperature	65	—	—	—
Stored 48 hr, refrigerator	10	—	—	—
Stored 48 hr (hydrator)	30	—	—	—
Green beans[b]				
Stored 48 hr, room temperature	25	—	—	—
Stored 48 hr, refrigerator	10	—	—	—
Stored 48 hr (hydrator)	10	—	—	—

[a] 1. Some vegetables store much better than others. 2. Ascorbate losses tend to be greater than for other vitamins. 3. Storage at room temperature is especially detrimental (wilting more likely). 4. Frozen storage detrimental to leafy vegetables.

[b] Data of Gleim and Tressler (1944) from Krochta and Feinberg (unpublished review) compared with the fresh state.

[c] Data of Augustin (1975) from Krochta and Feinberg (1975). Losses computed versus 10-day-old potatoes (data for two varieties).

Sweet potatoes are stored for months at an optimal temperature of 60°F and 85% humidity. During this time, carotene levels may actually increase and then gradually decrease, while ascorbate levels decrease to 50%–60% of harvest levels by 2–3 months. Carrots may also initially increase their β-carotene with long-term cold storage (32–44°F, 85% humidity up to 30 weeks) or short-term storage at room temperature (5–28 days) (J.M. Krochta and B. Feinberg, unpublished review).

Especially for tropical and subtropical fruits, storage cannot occur at temperatures *below* a critical level without causing discoloration, physical breakdown, abnormal ripening, and/or increased susceptibility to growth of pathogenic fungi (J.M. Krochta and B. Feinberg, unpublished review). This is well known for bananas, but also pertains to cucumbers and tomatoes. For these fruits, the "critical" temperature is thought to be about 12–13°C (59–61°F).

Storage of vinefera grapes or papaw fruit from Hawaii begins with a fumigation step, involving SO_2 and ethylene dibromide to control mold rot or insect attack, respectively. Fumigation of dried fruits with SO_2 is also very common, as is treatment of raisins, dates, and other such products with ethylene dibromide (EDB; 1,2-dibromoethane). With EDB, there has been great concern about residues in grains and other products that may be unhealthy to the consumer. [Studies in animals indicate that it is a carcinogen (Table 10.17) (Olson et al., 1973).] Sulfur dioxide is destructive to the vitamin, thiamin (see Chapter 9). Metabisulfites are no longer allowed in fresh fruits and vegetables and must be indicated on the labels of other foods if present in levels at or above 10 ppm. [They can enhance allergic responses and cause acute distress to asthmatic subjects (Stevenson and Simon, 1981).]

Cucumbers, citrus, and almost all fruits and vegetables on the market are "waxed" (Kaplan, 1983; H. Kaplan, personal communication). [Exceptions are strawberries, mushrooms, carrots

Table 10.17. A Sampling of Control Substances Used in Agricultural Production and Storage

Substance	Use on crop or in food	Purpose	Toxicity[a]
Alar (dimethylaminosuccinamic acid)	Animal feed, apples, cherries, grapes, nectarines, peaches, peanut meal, peanuts, pears, tomato products	Plant growth regulator	Carcinogen, teratogen
Aldicarb (2-methyl-2-(methylthio) propionaldehyde-o-methylcarbamoyloxime)	Animal feeds, bananas, beans, citrus, coffee, peanuts, pecans, potatoes, sorghum, soybeans, sugar beets/cane, sweet potatoes	Insecticide Nematocide	EPA-EHS
Bravo (tetrachloro isophthalonitrile)	Broccoli, cabbage, cantalope, carrots, cauliflower, celery, cucumber, lettuce, onions, potatoes, tomatoes	Fungicide	Carcinogen
Captan (1,2,3,6-tetrahydro-*N*-(trichloromethylthio)phthalimide)	Almonds, apples, apricots, beans, cherries, dewberries, grapes, lettuce, nectarines, peaches, peas, plums, raspberries, spinach, strawberries	Fungicide	Carcinogen, teratogen
CPC (isopropyl-*N*-chlorocarbamylate)	Potatoes, onions, carrots	Antisprouting agent	?
DCPA (dimethylchloroterephthalate)	Animal feeds	Herbicide	Potential teratogen[b]
Ethylene dibromide (1,2-dibromoethane)	Cereal grains, corn grits, cracked rice, fermented malt beverages, raisins	Fumigant	Carcinogen, teratogen, reproductive effects
Malathion (diethylmercaptosuccinate-S-ester with o,o-dimethylphosphorothioate)	Animal feed, citrus pulp, grapes, safflower oil	Insecticide	Teratogen, reproductive effects, (probably not a carcinogen)
O-phenylphenol (2-biphenylol)	For packaging (glue)	Fungicide	Experimental carcinogen, teratogen
Sulfamethazine (2-*p*-aminobenzene sulfonamido)-4,6-dimethylpyrimidine)	Animal drug[c] (not permitted in lactating cows)	Antibacterial	Teratogen, probable carcinogen
Tween 60	Vegetables (raw), processed foods (baked goods), oils, drinks, poultry	Wetting agents in "waxing," emulsifier, stabilizer, poultry scalding agent	Experimental tumorigen, reproductive effects

Source: Lewis (1989). (For additional information, see Chapter 9.)

[a] Established experimentally, EPA-EHS (on Extremely Hazardous Substance List).
[b] Not much tested.
[c] Common milk contaminant.

(which are chlorinated), broccoli, and cauliflower.] Waxing is performed for various reasons: to make fruits shiny (apples); to reduce brown spotting (pineapples); to inhibit gas exchange (and inhibit ripening processes or greening of potatoes); as a carrier for fungicides (like *o*-phenylphenol; Table 10.17) (see Chapter 9, Direct Food Additives); and, perhaps most importantly, to prevent loss of moisture (wilting). As already mentioned, wilting is a hallmark not only of physical degeneration, but also of nutritional deterioration.

There are three main components to the "wax": the film former, the emulsifier or other surfactant ("wetting" agent), and the solvent or carrier. As shown in Table 10.18, *film formers* range from hard, natural, or synthetic waxes to mineral and vegetable oils, the latter used especially on vegetables. Apples, citrus, pomegranates, etc. are "shellacked" with a material obtained from the lac bug (native to Sri Lanka and India). (The same material is used in some chocolates and other candies.) The surfactants used are usually in the Tween, Triton, or Span families. The solvent or carrier used is either water or petroleum based and largely evaporates from the produce after application of the wax. Sometimes, preservatives (like the parabens; Chapter 9) or silicon antifoam agents are also added. This process raises the question of whether waxing has altered the quality and quantity of nutrients present, especially in the skin. The substances used have been approved by the Food and Drug Administration and are thought to be nontoxic. However, the waxed cucumber (or apple) has a harder skin, which might increase the likelihood of skin removal. Peeling removes many vitamins and trace elements from most fruits, as these nutrients tend to be more abundant in, and right under, the skin (see Table 5.8, Chapter 5).

Processing. In terms of nutrient retention, various common processing procedures are destructive to vitamins and some other nutrients to various degrees. Freezing and freeze-drying are the best, whereas canning, salting, and sundrying are among the worst. If a food is especially important as a source of protein, fat, carbohydrate, or minerals, a procedure destructive mainly to vitamins may not matter. On the other hand, fruits and vegetables, which are our main sources of vitamins and most trace elements, are best handled to preserve these nutrients for the consumer.

Freeze-drying is probably the best way of preparing a food for long-term storage, with little, if any, loss of inherent nutrients. During the procedure the food is kept frozen, and exposure to light and oxygen is prevented, as drying proceeds under vacuum. pH changes are minimized in the solid or drying state, and microorganisms are killed. The resulting dry material, if kept dry and with little or no oxygen, will last a very long time. Texture will of course be altered and the cost is high.

Freezing processing, as in the preparation of frozen foods for marketing or the home freezer, is a means of rapidly slowing or preventing degenerative reactions in the foodstuff. For optimal freezing storage, minimization of light, and especially oxygen exposure, must be instituted. Oxygen exposure is responsible for "freezer burn," which oxidizes the proteinaceous and other components of the food and renders them impalatable. Some loss of nutrients (especially vitamins) usually occurs prior to freezing, as the fruits or vegetables are chopped and peeled, and this leads to oxidation and/or direct nutrient removal (as in peeling). Also, blanching (the transient dipping in boiling water), to inactivate endogenous enzymes that might otherwise allow ripening and browning type reactions to slowly proceed (even

Table 10.18. Substituents of Preparations Used to "Wax" Fruits and Vegetables for Market

Film Formers	Emulsifiers/surfactants/wetting agents
Waxes	Detergents[a]
Beeswax	Tweens
Carnauba wax (from palms)	Spans
Candalea wax (euphorbia plants)	Triton
Paraffins	Solvents/carriers
Polyethylenes	Water
Oils	Petroleum derivatives
Mineral oils	
Vegetable oils	

[a] As per FDA Code CFR #21 for Direct Food Additives.

in the frozen state), results in some loss of vitamins (and perhaps other nutrients). This results through heat and oxygen exposure and through leaching of some water-soluble nutrients into the blanching water (Fennema, 1975). In freezing, the integrity of the cell walls of the plants is lost, resulting in a change of texture. This allows a slow mixing of juices within the plant and may cause pH changes that alter vitamin stability. This, plus the inherent variability of pH and other factors among fruits or vegetables, has the result that the stability of a given vitamin will vary greatly from one frozen food to another (Tables 10.16 and 10.19).

In contrast to freezing, the *canning* of vegetables or fruits results in an initial destruction of a significant portion of the vitamins present through the thorough boiling required for sterilization. Moreover, after the food has been canned, storage will usually occur at room temperature; in home canning, long-term exposure to light may be a problem when glass containers are employed. Table 10.19 shows that one cannot expect to retain much of the original thiamin and ascorbate content of foods under these circumstances, although once canned, continued destruction may be slow. The loss of ascorbate from canned pineapple juice, for example, is slow because of high acidity and because there is little or no further oxygen exposure.

Various drying methods are popular, especially for fruits in the United States, and for vegetables as well in Europe and elsewhere. Depending on the procedure employed, significant vitamin losses will occur from oxygen, heat, and light exposure and through chopping, peeling, sundrying, or heating. Salting is another preservation procedure that uses the principle of drying, by drawing the water out of the food with externally applied NaCl. The dehydration also kills off microorganisms that would otherwise proliferate. Water-soluble nutrients may be lost from the food as the water migrates to the salt, but as this procedure is usually applied to meats and fish, it may not be as important. Some destruction by heat and oxygen may also occur.

Smoking is another time-honored method of preserving meats and game. It imparts an agreeable flavor from the woodsmoke, while preparing the food for longer storage. Smoking preserves by depositing an external layer of soot on the food. This layer has at least two useful properties (Harris and Karmas, 1975): (1) it contains antimicrobial substances that kill existing microbes and seal the food from further microbial destruction; and (2) it contains antioxidants that also seal off the food and prevent interior and exterior oxidation. One problem is that the smoke usually also contains some mutagenic or carcinogenic substances, like benz(o)pyrene (see Chapter 9). Consequently, commercial "smoked" meats or fish tend to be made by applying "liquid smoke" flavor at lower temperatures than occur in traditional smoking. Storage of the smoked food under refrigeration will obviously enhance the lifespan of its more labile nutrients, and some will be lost in the traditional smoking process from warmth exposure.

Food preparation. The effects of cooking, steaming, broiling, baking, or reheating on the ultimate concentrations of labile nutrients present are obvious from the previous discussions (see Tables 10.20, 10.22, and 10.23). Excess boiling, especially with rapid bubbling, is the worst procedure not only because the length of heat exposure is critical, but also because of the leaching of soluble nutrients into the cooking water, water that may not be ingested. Tables 10.20, 10.21, and 10.23 show the degree of leaching that commonly

Table 10.19. Loss of Vitamins During Freezing/Canning[a,b]

Storage method prior to cooking	Vitamin (% loss as compared with fresh cooked)[b]				
	Carotene	Thiamin	Riboflavin	Niacin	Ascorbate
Frozen, 18°C	12	20	24	24	26
	(0–50)	(0–61)	(0–45)	(0–56)	(0–78)
Canned	10	67	42	49	51
	(0–32)	(56–83)	(14–50)	(31–65)	(28–67)

Source: Data from Fennema (1975).

[a] Mean values for 7–10 vegetables, and range.
[b] All samples were also boiled until done and drained, before analysis. Comparison is with fresh cooked produce.

Table 10.20. Loss of Vitamins During Cooking by Boiling[a]

Vegetable	Vitamin (% lost)[b]			
	Thiamin	Riboflavin	Niacin	Carotene
Green Beans				
Boiling 5–20 min	0–45[c]	25	30	30[c]
(% in water)[d]	(31)	(30)	(8–41)	
Broccoli				
Boiling 13–30 min	5–50[c]	5–50[c]	12[c]	0[c]
(% in water)	(7–46)	(11–54)	(6–13)	
Carrots				
Boiling 5–20 min	0	0	25	1–19[c]
(% in water)	(20)	(55–90)[e]	(42–58)[e]	
Potatoes				
Boiling 20–30 min	0	26	29	
(% in water)	(2–45)	(2–48)	(2–19)	
Spinach				
Boiling 6–10 min	30	20–60	40	3–15[c]
(% in water)	(14–43)	(10–39)		

Source: Data from Lachance (1975) and Lachance and Erdman (1975).

[a] 1. Loss of vitamins through heating. 2. Considerable leaching of vitamins into cooking water. 3. Degree of loss depends on vegetable. 4. Institutional (large-scale) preparation results in greater losses than small-scale home preparation.

[b] From vegetables plus cooking water.

[c] Value given (or greatest loss) is for institutional (large-scale) food preparation.

[d] Percentage of original vitamin recovered in cooking water.

[e] Dehydrated carrots cooked.

occurs and that more leaching occurs with a greater proportion of water to vegetable. [It should be noted that minerals are also lost (Table 10.21).] Oxidation is enhanced by bubbling and there is nothing to be gained by it in terms of cooking speed. (The boiling temperature of water and the temperature of the food in it will be 100°C whether bubbling or not.) There is also nothing to be gained by using more water than needed for evaporation during the cooking process. Thus, nutrient destruction is minimized (1) by cooking at low heat, once boiling has begun, and (2) by using very little water. (Turning the heat down once boiling temperature is attained will also reduce water evaporation.) Overcooking or pre-preparation of meals (which require reheating or "keeping them warm") clearly also allows continued heat (and oxidative) destruction of vitamins and other nutrients prior to ingestion of the food (Tables 10.20 and 10.22).

Steaming (where there is no direct contact with water except as steam), pressure cooking, or microwave cooking (with little or no water) are clearly superior to ordinary boiling (Table 10.23), unless the above-mentioned precautions are instituted, as little or no leaching occurs. (Microwave

Table 10.21. Loss of Food Minerals During Boiling

Vegetables	Mineral (% lost)[a]					
	Calcium	Iron	Phosphorus	Magnesium	Potassium	Sodium
Asparagus	10	13	5	17	8	0
Green beans (cut)	6	18	2	10	3	11
Broccoli	4	38	8	9	14	25
Corn (cut)	6	12	37	9	10	12
Peas (green)	6	21	0	8	10	13
Spinach (leaf)	0	12	0	5	3	6

Source: Modified from Fennema (1975).

[a] Most recovered in cooking water.

Table 10.22. Loss of Vitamins from Meats and Grains During Food Preparation

Foodstuff	Vitamin (% lost) Thiamin	Vitamin B_6
Beef		
Fresh cooked	7	44–58
Cooked, frozen, reheated	10	
Chicken		
Fresh cooked	12	
Cooked, frozen, reheated	25	
Ham		
Freshly prepared	28	43
Cooked, frozen, reheated	28	
Cracked wheat		
Cooked 60 min	18	
Oatmeal		
Cooked 30 min	5	
Bread		
Baked	20	

Source: Data from tables in Lachance and Erdman (1975), except for bread (Matz, 1975).

cooking with larger amounts of water reinstitutes the leaching phenomenon.) However, for the same degree of "doneness," the destruction of vitamins (versus their leaching) will be comparable for all three techniques. This is also the case where baking is concerned.

Broiling, with the heating source above the food, is an acceptable way of "cooking," which probably results in about a comparable degree of nutrient destruction in the interior of the food to that occurring in other forms of food preparing (again, if the same degree of "doneness" is considered). However, the charring of the exterior of the food during broiling will result in the formation of some mutagenic and perhaps carcinogenic substances (see Chapters 9 and 16). Broiling over charcoal, or with the heating element below the food, has the additional problem of promoting carcinogen formation from pyrolysis of fat (which drips down on the coals or heating elements). Benz(o)pyrene, a moderate carcinogen, is the best studied product (Chapter 9).

Table 10.23. Effects of Various Food Preparation Methods on Ascorbate and Thiamin Retention in Foods[a]

Preparation method	Broccoli: Cooking time (min)	Broccoli: H_2O:veg ratio	Broccoli: Percent retention	Green beans: Cooking time (min)	Green beans: H_2O:veg ratio	Green beans: Percent retention
A. Ascorbate						
Boil, covered	20[b]	0.5	74	20	0.5	76
Boil, uncovered	15	4.0	45	20	4.0	60
Microwave	11	—	57	10	—	59
Stir fry	10	—	77	15	—	58
	Broccoli		*Peas*	*Potatoes*		*Spinach*
B. Ascorbate						
Boiling	45–75[d]		68–73	80[d]		49–61
Steaming	59–87		65–68	88–95		—
Pressure cooking	81		88	89–100		—
Microwave	79		62–74	76		56–67
Frying	—		—	78–82		—
	Broccoli		*Cabbage*	*Carrots*		*Potatoes*
C. Thiamine						
Boiling	75(5.5)[c,d]		53(15)	88(9)[d]		83(18)
Pressure cooking	90(0.8)		88(1.3)	85(1)		92(9)
Microwave	76(5.5)		62(6)	91(2.3)		91(6)

Source: Data in A and B are from tables in Lachance and Erdman (1975); C is from Thomas et al. (1949).

[a] Percent retained by food. Note the following: 1. The ratio of water to food influences vitamin losses during boiling (due to leaching). 2. Boiling in a covered container is better than uncovered. 3. Microwave cooking and stir frying (or frying) results in about the same losses as for boiling. 4. Pressure cooking is somewhat superior.

[b] Values are means or range of means (for multiple studies).

[c] Cooking time to same degree of "doneness," in minutes (parentheses).

[d] Percent retention.

In summary, methods of growing, handling, storing, and finally preparing our foods have profound effects on their ultimate nutritional value. An awareness by physicians and consumers of the major procedures that cause destruction, spoilage, or poisoning, and means of circumventing them where possible, is thus important.

References

Abelson PH (1983): Science 219:611.

Albrecht WA (1970): J Appl Nutr 22:23.

Augustin J (1975): J Food Sci 40:1295.

Baker FH, Raun NS (1989): Am J Altern Agric 4:121.

Biale JB (1975): *In* Sinclair WB, ed: The orange. Davis: University of California Press, Division of Agricultural Science.

Borlaug NE (1983): Science 219:689.

Fennema O (1975): *In* Harris RS, Karmas E, eds: Nutritional evaluation of food processing (2nd ed). Westport, CT: AVI, p 244.

Gleim EG, Tressler DK (1944): Food Res 9:471.

Goldstein W (1981): Biodynamics 140:3.

Hahn J, Aehnelt E (1973): Veroeff Landwirtsch Chem Bundesversuchanst Linx 10:277.

Harris RS, Karmas E, eds (1975): Nutritional evaluation of food processing (2nd ed). Westport, CT: AVI.

International Atomic Agency (1982): Induced mutants for cereal grain protein improvement. Technical document no 259, Vienna.

Jones PD, Wigley TML (1990): Scientific Am 264:84.

Kaplan H (1983): *In* Warnowski W, Nagy S, eds: Fresh citrus fruit. Westport, CT: AVI, p. 345.

Koepf HH (1973): Biodynamics 108:20.

Koepf HH (1974): Biodynamics 109:7.

Koepf H (1989): The biodynamic farm. Hudson, NY: Anthroposophic Press.

Krochta JM, Feinberg B (1975): *In* Harris RS, Karmas E, eds: Nutritional evaluation of food processing. Westport, CT: AVI, p 98.

Lachance PA (1975): *In* Harris RS, Karmas E, eds: Nutritional evaluation of food processing. Westport, CT: AVI, p 463.

Lachance PA, Erdman JW Jr (1975): *In* Harris RS, Karmas E, eds: Nutritional evaluation of food processing. Westport, CT, p 529.

Lewis RJ Sr (1989): Food additives handbook. New York: Van Nostrand Reinhold.

Linder MC (1973): Biodynamics 107:1.

Matz SA (1975): *In* Harris RS, Karmas E, eds: Nutritional evaluation of food processing. Westport, CT: AVI, p 244.

McLaren AD, Skujins J (1971): Soil biochemistry. New York: Marcel Dekker.

National Research Council (1988): Alternative agriculture. Washington, DC: National Academy Press.

Oelhaf RC (1978): Organic agriculture. New York: Wiley.

Olson WA, Habermann RT, Weisburger EK, Ward JM, Weisburger JH (1973): JNCI 51:1993.

Pettersson BD, von Wistinghausen E (1977): Bodenuntersuchungen zu einem Langjaerigen Feldversuch in Jaerna, Schweden, Darmstadt. W Germany. Forschungsring zu Biologisch-Dynamischer Wirtschaftsweise (March).

Pfeiffer EE (1952): Biodynamics 10:2.

Pfeiffer EE (1961): Biodynamics 59:1.

Post WM, Peng T-S, Emanuel WR, King AW, Dale VH, DeAngelis DL (1990): Am Scientist 78:310.

Raganold JP, Papendick RI, Parr JF (1990): Sci Am 263:112.

Ramanathan V (1988): Science 240:293.

Russell EW (1973): Soil conditions and plant growth: New York, John Wiley.

Samaras I (1977): Nachernteverhalten unterschiedlich gedungter Gemusearten, mit besonderer Beruchsichtigung physiologischer und microbiogischer Parameter (dissertation). Giessen, Germany: Justus Liebig University.

Sauerbeck D (1986): Vorkommen, Verhalten und Bedeutung von anorganischen Schadstoffen in Boeden. Hohenheimer Arbeiten, Tagung uber Umweltforschung, Februar.

Schnitzer M, Khan SU (1972): Humic substances in the environment. New York: Marcel Dekker.

Schuphan W (1974): Qual Plant Pl Foods Hum Nutr 23:333.

Singer SF, ed (1969): Global effects of environmental pollution. Washington, DC: American Association for the Advancement of Science.

Spalding RF, Gormly JR, Curtiss BH, Exner ME (1978): Groundwater 16:86.

Stevenson DD, Simon RA (1981): J Allergy Clin Immunol 68:26.

Stout PR, Buran RG (1968): *In* Isotopes and radiation in soil organic matter studies. Vienna: International Atomic Energy Agency, p 283.

Thomas MH, Brenner S, Eaton A, Craig V (1949): J Am Dietet Assoc 25:39.

Verduin J (1968): *In* Brady NC, ed: Agriculture and the quality of our environment. Washington, DC: American Association for the Advancement of Science, p 163.

USDA Study Team on Organic Farming (1980): Report and recommendations on organic farming. Washington, DC: US Department of Agriculture.

Stanley H. Zlotkin, M.D., Ph.D., F.R.C.P.(C)*

11

Neonatal Nutrition

Postnatal Growth

The neonatal period includes the period immediately following birth. In this chapter, dealing with nutrition of the healthy full-term infant, it is most appropriate to begin with a comment on growth and the growth process, since growth is more rapid during the first 6 months of life compared to any other time period during the growth cycle. The need for nutrients to support this rapid growth, therefore, is also vital.

Somatic growth during infancy follows a simple curvilinear path often defined as the "S" shaped curve of growth (Hurley, 1980). Although the rate of growth is different among species, the shape of the growth curve is a feature common to all species. When one plots the weight of the organism against time, an S-shaped curve with three distinct stages can be observed (Figure 11.1A). The first stage takes place immediately after birth. In this stage, which is very short, there is a redistribution and loss of body fluids with little or no growth. In the human, 5%–7% of the infant's weight at birth may be lost during the first week of life. It takes time after birth for enough nutrients to be provided and assimilated by the newborn for growth to start. Also, the hormonal milieu (high in catecholamines, glucagon, and cortisol) is not conducive to growth. Birth weight is often not regained until 7–10 days after birth. In the next stage, which is the exponential stage, growth occurs most rapidly. Finally, the third and last stage is the stationary phase. During this stage, growth slows and eventually stops at adulthood.

The next curve (Figure 11.1B) is the "rate of growth" curve (dW/dt). It depicts the change in weight over time. The growth rate is highest at the point of inflection of the curve. In the human neonate, this occurs between 16–24 weeks of age, declining after that age.

As illustrated by the two parts of Figure 11.1, growth is most rapid during the early stages of life (i.e., from birth to 24 weeks of age). In a study on Finnish boys, length velocities fell from 45.8 cm/year between birth and 3 months of age to 14.4 cm/year in the 9- to 12-month interval (Kantero and Tiisala, 1971). During this same period, weight velocities dropped from 10.3–3.4 kg/year. The velocity of length growth is about 15% less for girls compared to boys during the early months of life. In the 9- to 12-month interval, however, no sex difference is apparent.

Genetic Control of Postnatal Growth

The primary determinants of growth rate are genetic (Mueller, 1986). However, the genetic control of growth can be considerably altered by en-

* Division of Clinical Nutrition, Research Institute, The Hospital for Sick Children, and the Departments of Paediatrics and Nutrition, Faculty of Medicine, University of Toronto, Toronto, Ontario, Canada.

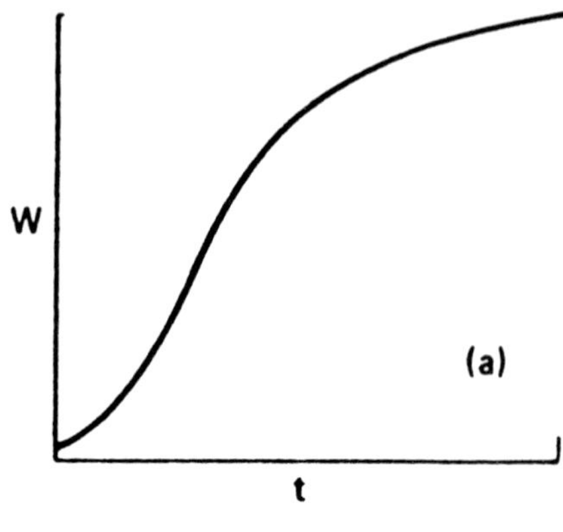

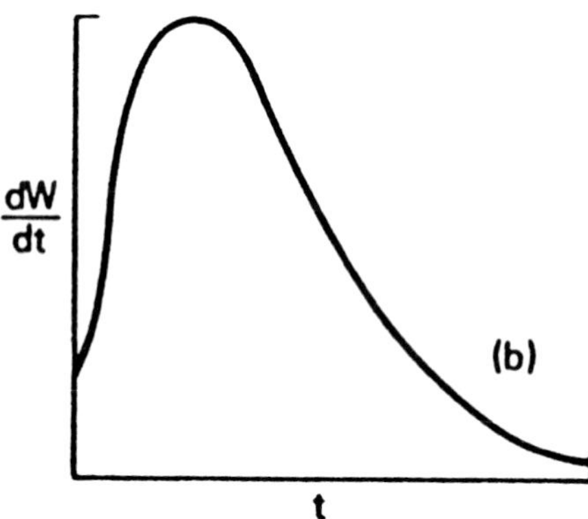

Figure 11.1. Growth of human infants during the first year of life. **(a)** Curve of change in weight per unit of time. An "S"-shaped curve; three distinct stages can be observed. **(b)** Curve of growth rate (dW/dt) per unit of time. [*Source:* Modified from Hurley (1980).]

vironmental factors. Nutrition is one of the major environmental factors that can influence the ability of an individual to meet his/her genetic potential for growth. It is generally true that tall parents have children who tend to grow up to be tall adults, and short parents have children who grow up to be short adults. However, at birth, the correlation between the length of the infant and later adult length is weak (r = 0.3). Similarly, it has been estimated that only 38% of the variation in birth weight can be attributed to heredity. At birth, the major determinant of the size of the infant is the height of the mother and probably the constitution of her bony pelvic structures. Thus, the contribution on the fetus' own genes to size at birth is relatively small. The predominance of maternal factors may be a selective effect to increase the chances of small mothers surviving the birth of infants from large fathers.

After birth, the influence of those powerful, nonhereditary factors that determine birth weight and length diminish, and the individual's own genetic makeup begins to manifest its influence. Postnatal growth is principally genetypically determined; and, by age 2 years, there is a strong correlation (r = 0.8) between the young child's height and final adult height. The rapid change, from dominance of maternal factors controlling growth prior to birth, to endogenous hereditary factors at age 2 years, implies that changes in the rate of linear growth must occur during infancy. "Catch-up" and "catch-down" growth occurs as normal phenomena in infancy (Tanner, 1986). Infants who are short at birth but genetically destined to be "average" or tall will demonstrate accelerated linear growth during the first year of life to achieve their genetic "growth channel" (Figure 11.2); whereas the opposite will be true for those who are long at birth, but genetically destined to

Figure 11.2. This is a graph of length in cm versus age in months. Infants who are short at birth, but who are genetically destined to be "average" length, or tall, will demonstrate accelerated linear growth during the first year of life to achieve their genetic "growth channel." The solid line depicts "catch-up" growth of a short baby on the 10th percentile becoming a "tall" infant on the 75th percentile. [*Source:* Reprinted by permission from Tanner (1986).]

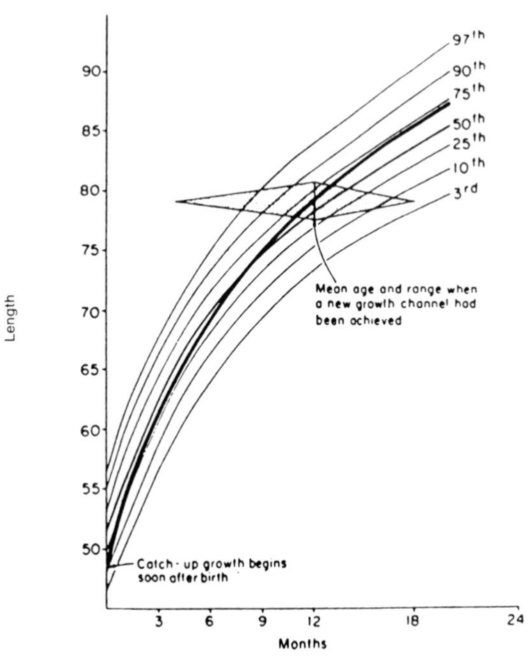

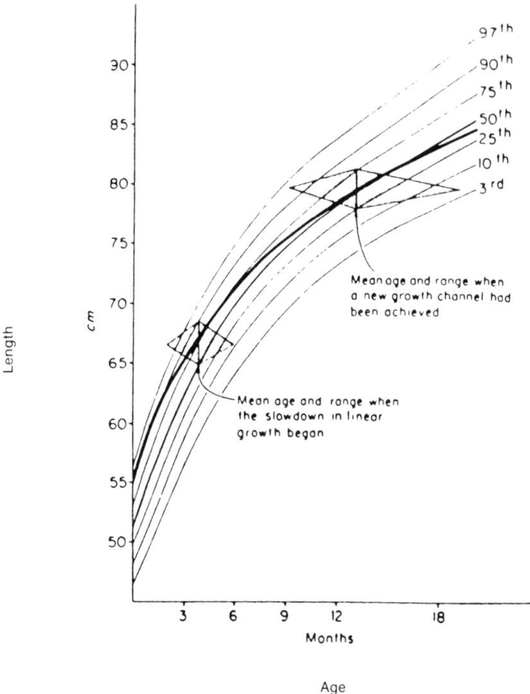

Figure 11.3. This is a graph of length in cm versus age in months. Infants who are long at birth, but who are genetically destined to be "average" length, or short, will demonstrate decelerated linear growth during the first year of life to achieve their genetic "growth channel." The solid line depicts "catch-down" growth of a long baby on the 90th percentile becoming an average length infant between the 50th and 25th percentile. [*Source:* Reprinted by permission from Tanner (1986).]

be "average" in length or short (Figure 11.3) (Smith et al., 1976). Though not necessarily meaningful, the average rate of growth of full-term infants after birth is about 10–12 g/kg/day (Moya, 1991).

Cellular Basis of Growth

Enesco and Leblond made an important contribution to our understanding of growth at the cellular level when they showed that most tissues go through three growth stages (Enesco and Leblond, 1962). The first is known as the hyperplastic stage, and consists of cell division resulting in an increase in cell number. The second stage is one that combines cell hyperplasia with an increase in cell size (hypertrophy). Finally, the third stage, which is normally associated with maturation of a given organ or tissue, is one in which the cells differentiate and increase in size but there is no further increase in cell number. Research, which has established the time sequence of these three stages, has allowed us to predict the effects of under- or overnutrition on growth, depending on the specific timing of the nutritional insult (Widdowson, 1981) (see also Chapter 1).

It is evident that a significant nutritional disturbance occurring during the first phase of cell hyperplasia may thus result in a permanent change in cell number (Brar and Rutherford, 1988). Undernutrition may result in a deficit, while overnutrition may result in an excess number of cells. Different tissues in the same organ, and different organs in the body go through the three phases of cellular growth at different times (see also Figure 1.3). Individuals who are undernourished early in life tend to have decreased skeletal musculature, appropriately proportioned hearts and kidneys, and relatively large brains and skeletons. While retardation in somatic growth may be undesirable, permanent effects on brain growth are clearly of much greater importance.

Neuronal cell division appears to be maximal some time during the second trimester of human gestation, when the fetus is relatively immune to adverse nutritional factors (Hurley, 1980). Nevertheless, cell division in the brain continues through the third trimester and first year of life, with brain DNA content peaking between 12 and 15 months after birth (Figure 1.4). Thus, for the brain, the combined effects of undernutrition occurring during fetal and early postnatal life can be particularly severe. The earlier and longer the period of deprivation, the more severe and long-lasting will be the results. Nonetheless, the human brain appears to have considerable reserves, and infants who have undergone combined fetal and neonatal nutritional insults still may develop normally if placed in a stimulating environment (Grantham-McGregor et al., 1987).

Body Composition and Growth

The major constituent of the body is water. During growth, the proportion of body weight that is water diminishes (Figures 11.4 and 1.5). The percentage of the body that is protein increases steadily during fetal life and continues to increase during the first 1–2 years of life until it reaches levels close to those seen in the adult (Table 1.5; Widdowson, 1981). Apart from calcium, phosphorus, and magnesium (which increase rapidly

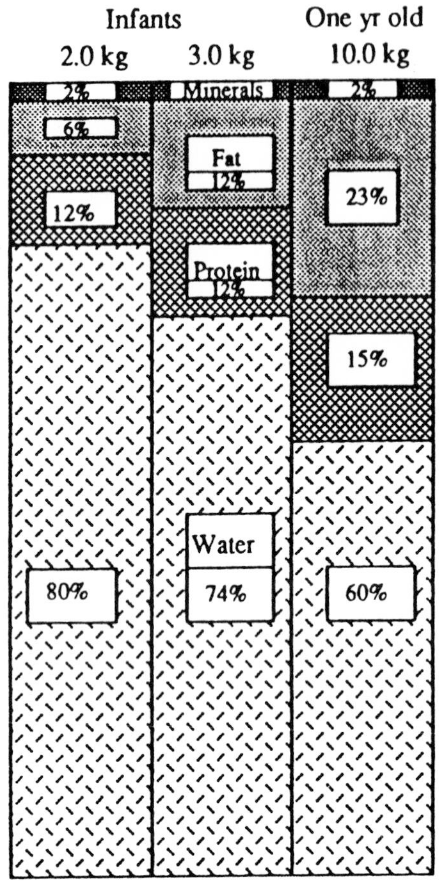

Figure 11.4. Body composition of preterm (2 kg), full-term (3 kg), and 1-year-old infants (10 kg). The figure compares mineral, fat, protein, and water content, each expressed as percentage of total weight. [*Source:* Modified from Widdowson (1981).]

during gestation), the mineral content of the body (as a percentage of body weight) remains fairly constant during fetal life, infancy, and childhood but increases during adolescence. Adipose tissue, on the other hand, increases steadily during the third trimester and the first few months of infancy, peaking somewhere around the fourth or fifth month of life. The proportion of body weight that is adipose tissue then diminishes during the remainder of infancy and early childhood and remains at a relatively low level until puberty is reached.

Growth Patterns

Each part of the body grows at a different rate (Figure 1.2). Differential skeletal growth, for example, results in changes of the shape of the body (Figure 11.5) (Hurley, 1980). At birth, the infant has a large head and short limbs compared with the adult. The head reaches 90% of its final size by 2 years of age, after which only small changes occur. The brain, like the skull, grows most rapidly early in life, reaching its mature weight long before growth as a whole has ceased. It is not until 12 or 13 years of age that adult proportions between body and legs are reached. Skeletal muscle grows slowly during infancy, increasing its rate of growth at puberty. At birth, skeletal muscle accounts for 25% of the total weight of the infant; while at maturity, its contribution rises to 40% of mature body weight in females and 50% in males. The brain, on the other hand, accounts for 10% of body weight at birth, falling to 2% at maturity. These two examples illustrate the differential rate of growth of various components of the body. The timing and duration of nutritional deprivation will determine the extent and significance of the insult to the various organs.

Having established that growth is most rapid during the early months of life in man, it is clear that an adequate supply of nutrients as substrate to support this rapid growth is therefore vital. Let us now consider nutrient needs during the neonatal period.

Nutrient Needs During the Neonatal Period

Energy

The energy requirement has been defined as the amount needed to maintain health, growth, and an "appropriate" level of physical activity (WHO, 1985a). The energy requirements of young infants are widely variable because of varying rates of growth and the variations in the composition of the tissue laid down. For example, as shown in the previous pages, rates of postnatal growth are primarily genetically predetermined and very different among individuals. Similarly, "appropriate" levels of activity for young infants are difficult, if not impossible, to define. Although, in principle, it would be desirable to determine the energy requirements of infants from direct measurements of energy expenditure, this is difficult in practice and has only been accomplished in a limited number of cases. Instead, the energy requirement of infants is most often estimated from the observed nutrient intakes of healthy children growing normally.

A large collection of information on energy intakes (over 4000 data points) has been compiled

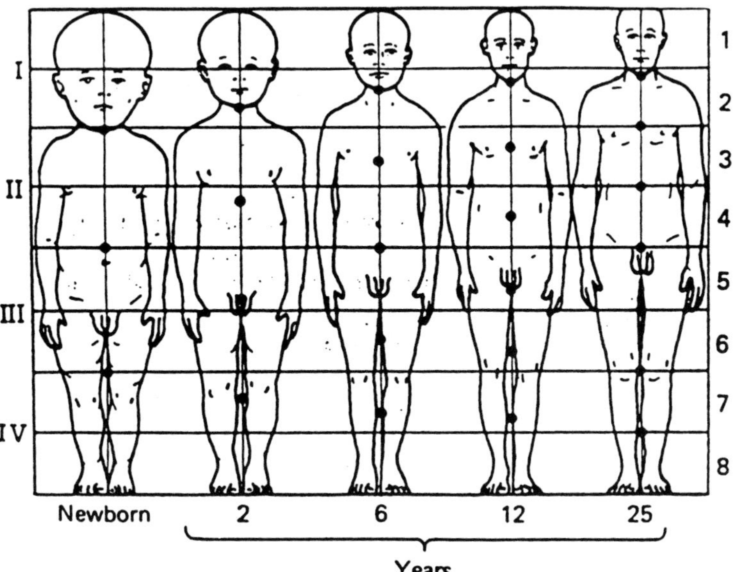

Figure 11.5. The effect of increasing age on the proportion of body parts. This picture illustrates the differential rate of growth of various components of the body. At birth, the infant has a large head and short limbs, compared to the adult. The head reaches 90% of its final size by 2 years of age. At age 12 years, adult proportions between body and legs are reached. [*Source:* Reprinted by permission from Hurley (1980).]

from studies of healthy infants from developed countries (Canada, United States, Sweden, and the United Kingdom) (Whitehead et al., 1981). These average intakes are thus representative for groups of children growing along the 50th centile of the WHO reference standard. In the studies mentioned above, the estimation of intakes of breast milk were made using the "test-weighing" method. Infants were weighed before and after breast-feeding. The difference in weight of the infants before and after feeds represented the volume of milk (and/or other foods) consumed. Using an alternative and more accurate method of estimating milk consumption (the deuterium oxide method), it has recently been determined that test-weighing underestimates milk consumption by about 5% (Coward et al., 1982). Mean values for measured energy intakes during and following the perinatal period (increased by 5%) are shown in Table 11.1. The data demonstrate that (per unit body weight) the highest energy intakes are in the first 3 months. Between 3 and 9 months, intakes decline, only to rise again thereafter. The fall in rate of energy intake in the mid months of the first year of life is considered to be a real phenomenon, representing a period when the very high growth rates (characteristic of the first 3 months of life) have declined, yet full physical activity (walking) has not yet begun to any degree. The combination of slower growth and limited energy expenditure (for activity) results in a lower energy need and, therefore, a lower energy intake. With the increase in physical activity associated with the initiation of crawling and walking, energy intake increases between 9 and 12 months. It is interesting to note that the most recent estimates (WHO, 1985b) of energy needs during the first year of life are 10%–15% lower than those published in 1973 (FAO, 1973), primarily due to more accurate methods of estimating energy intake and expenditure.

Total energy expenditure is, of course, a composite of the utilization of fat, protein, and carbohydrates as sources of energy. Following birth, the average minimum (or resting) energy expenditure varies from 40–60 kcal/kg/day (or 1.67 to 2.5 kcal/kg/hr). The measurement of "minimum energy expenditure" is not identical to "true basal metabolic rate," which is very difficult to assess in the young infant because of frequent feeding. The determination of "minimum energy expenditure" approximates (actually overestimates) basal expenditure, because the measurements are taken

Table 11.1. Estimates of Average Energy Requirements of Infants in the First Year of Life: Past and Present

Age (months)	1985	1971
	(kcal/kg/day)	
0–3	116	120
3–6	99	115
6–9	95	110
9–12	101	105
Average	103	112

Source: WHO, 1985b; FAO, 1973.

after a feed (newborn infants cannot be safely fasted), while the infant is sleeping instead of when the subject has been fasted for 8 hours (Bruck, 1978) (Chapter 8). Thus, it includes energy needed in the digestion, absorption, distribution, and storage of the incoming food (see Chapter 8). About 65% of the energy consumed in the resting metabolic state is needed to support the functioning of liver, heart, kidneys, and especially the brain (Moya, 1991).

During the first 24 hours of life, there is a "minimal energy expenditure" of approximately 50 kcal/kg/day. This is 10 kcal/kg/day higher than the 40 kcal/kg average for the first month, and is probably related to the initiation of feeding. By 1 month of age, "minimal energy expenditure" has increased to approximately 60 kcal/kg/day (Bruck 1978; Karlberg, 1952; Scopes, 1966), and this is maintained throughout the first year of life. Alterations in clothing, environmental temperature, crying, increased heart rate, and fever all influence energy expenditure. For example, an increase in heart rate from 150–200 beats per minute is associated with a net rise in energy expenditure equivalent to 22 kcal/kg/day (Chessex et al., 1981). The estimated contributions of various functions to the total energy needs of the infant at birth and 6 months of age are described in Figure 11.6. They show that resting metabolism accounts for about half of total needs, and that early after birth much of the remainder is needed for growth, while physical activity becomes more important later on. [As in adults, energy to deal with food intake (thermic effect of feeding; "TEF") probably averages 10% of the calories consumed.] It is interesting to note that compared to the adult, where expenditure for physical activity is a major component of the total energy expenditure (Chapter 8), physical activity of the infant only accounts for 10%–15% of the total (Moya, 1991).

As discussed in Chapter 8, the respiratory quotient (RQ) is the ratio between liters of oxygen consumed and CO_2 produced. The ratio for carbohydrate oxidation is 1.0, for fats 0.7, and for proteins 0.9. Measurement of CO_2 production is required to make a precise determination of caloric expenditure from values for oxygen consumption. To differentiate between a reduction in RQ because of lipid or protein oxidation, urinary nitrogen is also measured. Based on the determination that 1 g of urinary nitrogen is equivalent to the expenditure of 26.5 kcal, the protein contribution to overall energy expenditure can be calculated and subtracted. In practice, it is common to assume that 15% of the minimal or basal oxygen consumption is derived from protein, and that the energy expenditure corresponding to a liter of oxygen consumed is 4.8 kcal (Karlberg, 1952).

The infant is born with energy reserves in the form of fat 75% and glycogen 1% averaging about 6800 kcals (Uauy et al., 1990a). (At term, liver glycogen is as much as 10% of liver weight, at least in animals.) With birth, and disconnection from the maternal blood supply of glucose, glycogen stores are immediately mobilized (with

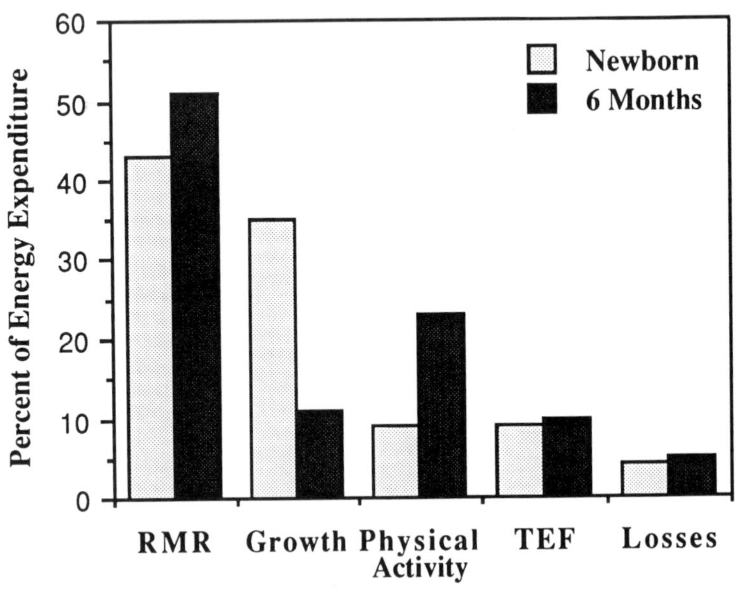

Figure 11.6. Estimated components of energy expenditure in infants. Data are given as percent of energy expenditure. [*Source:* Recalculated from Moya (1991).]

the help of glucagon). Thus, before, and for a significant number of hours after birth, glucose is the primary fuel, and the infant's RQ is about 1.0.

After birth, the RQ gradually falls to 0.8, reflecting a gradual switching to fat as an energy source. During the first 3 days of life, it further declines to a mean value of 0.7. The RQ then rises progressively over the next 3 weeks of life, reflecting the change in fuels available in the infant's diet, particularly lactose (see more below).

Protein

The importance of protein in the diet is that it is a source of amino acids. Amino acids, the end products of protein digestion, have multiple, vital functions in the body (see Chapter 4). Most amino acids are used as substrates for the production of new proteins, synthesized most abundantly (but by no means exclusively) by the liver and muscles. Amino acids are also essential for the synthesis of nonprotein nitrogenous products, such as certain hormones and neurotransmitters. Unlike some nutrients that are stored in the body (i.e., vitamin B_{12} and iron), protein is not stored and must be continually replenished to avoid the adverse effects of protein deficiency.

Although one might expect that the process of protein digestion and absorption are not fully developed during the perinatal period, this is not the case in the infant born at full term (40 weeks after conception). As is the case with older children and adults, orally ingested proteins (usually from milk) are well-digested in the stomach and small intestine to amino acids, small peptides, and dipeptides, despite a lower gastric acidity and less protease availability. The process of protein digestion involves the denaturing actions of acid produced by the stomach; hormones that influence gut motility (as well as pancreatic and gallbladder contractility) (Chapter 1); and the release of protein hydrolyzing enzymes by the pancreas (see Chapters 1 and 4). The products of protein digestion (amino acids and peptides) are actively transported into mucosal cells of the gut by carrier systems which are specific for groups of amino acids and dipeptides. Unlike in the adult, peptides are better absorbed than single amino acids (Moya, 1991). Having passed through the intestinal mucosal cells, the free amino acids are then transported to the liver via the portal vein.

The body has the ability to convert endogenous substrates (i.e., carbonaceous and nitrogenous compounds) to nonessential amino acids. This may be particularly important for the breast-fed neonate, who receives a significant portion of its nitrogen in the form of nonprotein substituents like urea. [Thirty-five percent to 40% of breast milk N is nonprotein in nature (mainly urea, free amino acids, small peptides, and nucleotides).] Although this conversion is possible for more than half of the amino acids, an absence of certain enzymes (needed for specific biochemical conversions) determines that some amino acids cannot be synthesized, de novo, in the body. These amino acids must therefore come from the diet and are classified as "nutritionally essential." In adults, only eight amino acids have generally been considered in that category (Chapter 4; Rose, 1957). In infants and children, nine amino acids cannot be synthesized within the body, histidine being the additional amino acid needed in the diet. The milk content of these amino acids is given in Table 11.2. With age and biochemical maturation, histidine can eventually be synthesized from available substrates within the body, and is thus no longer classified as "nutritionally essential." Conversely, in the infant born prematurely (gestational period <37 weeks), some other amino acids also become essential because of the lower biochemical immaturity, resulting in decreased enzyme activity of specific pathways, including those for synthesis of cysteine from methionine (Gaul et al., 1972; Zlotkin and Anderson, 1982) and tyrosine from phenylalanine (Raiha, 1974); for example, cysteine and tyrosine become "semi-essential" amino acids. As the premature infant gets older and becomes metabolically more mature, cysteine and tyrosine change their status from "semi-essential" to "nonessen-

Table 11.2. Average Essential Amino Acid Composition of Human Milk Protein Compared to Cow's Milk Protein (mg/g crude protein)

Amino acid	Human milk	Cow's milk
Histidine	26	27
Isoleucine	46	47
Leucine	93	95
Lysine	66	78
Methionine + cystine	42[a]	33
Phenylalanine + tyrosine	72	102
Threonine	43	44
Tryptophan	17	14
Valine	55	64
Total	460	504

Source: Modified from WHO (1985c).

[a] Range = 29–60.

tial" amino acids. There may also be a taurine requirement, an amino acid formed from cysteine that is abundant in human milk (Rassin et al., 1990; Tyson et al., 1989).

Estimates of protein requirements during infancy have been derived using a variety of direct and indirect approaches. Direct estimates include: (i) measurement of the content of protein in human milk, taking into consideration the volume of milk consumed by the infant (Macy et al., 1953; Whitehead and Paul, 1981); (ii) observations relating protein nutritional status to intakes of protein by infants living under varied conditions of care and feeding (Viteri et al., 1979); and (iii) direct clinical investigation in which protein intakes are accurately determined and measurements of growth and protein nutritional status are carried out (Fomon et al., 1982). Alternately, an indirect approach to estimating requirements using a factorial approach has been used (WHO, 1985d). For the latter, an amount of protein needed for growth is added to that needed for replacement of obligatory (inevitable) losses.

Of the various estimates of protein requirements outlined above, the intakes of protein by infants breast-fed by healthy women are of particular interest because these intakes are likely to be near the optimal requirement. Since infants fed human milk do not suffer from protein malnutrition, it is safe to assume that the ingestion of protein from human milk meets the requirements for maintenance, growth, and metabolic functions. The average protein content of human milk is 1.15 g/100 ml, except during the first month when the value is 1.3 g/100 ml (Schofield et al., 1985; WHO, 1985b). The protein intakes of healthy infants between birth and age 4 months (Whitehead and Paul, 1981) during the first 4 months are shown in Table 11.3, based on the average volume of milk consumed. The data indicate that average intakes per kilogram drop considerably from the first to the fourth month of age (from 2.5–1.5 g/kg/day).

Information on protein intakes from breast milk for the infant older than 4 months is limited. In developing countries, breast milk is no longer the only source of protein for the infant diet after 4 months of age, and infants depend on some supplementary foods to meet protein requirements. Based on a modified factorial procedure, estimated average protein requirements for infants 6–9 months (combined sexes) have been estimated as being 1.25 g protein/kg/day; and 1.15 g/kg/day for infants at 9–12 months (WHO, 1985d).

Although the majority of proteins are in a form that would be available for digestion and absorption, some of the protein and perhaps 17% of the total nitrogen-containing components of human milk are not bioavailable (Lonnerdal, 1976). Significant amounts of undigested lactoferrin and secretory IgA have been detected in the stool of infants receiving human milk. Excretion of these proteins indicates that the use of values for total protein content of human milk (as in Table 11.3) has led to an overestimation of the protein actually utilized (or needed) by the infant. As already mentioned, not all of the nitrogen in milk is due to protein and amino acids (see Chapter 4), and it is still unclear just how bioavailable milk protein tends to be for the healthy, mature newborn infant.

It is interesting to note that estimates of protein needs derived from the intakes of human milk and factorial analysis are very similar. Yet clearly,

Table 11.3. Average Intake of Protein by Breast-Fed Infants Aged 0–4 Months

Age (months)	Breast milk consumed (ml/day)	Protein intake (g/day)	Weight (kg)	Average intake per day (g/kg/day)
Boys				
0–1	719	9.35	3.8	2.46
1–2	795	9.15	4.75	1.93
2–3	848	9.75	5.6	1.74
3–4	822	9.45	6.35	1.49
Girls				
0–1	661	8.6	3.6	2.39
1–2	731	8.4	4.35	1.93
2–3	780	9.0	5.05	1.78
3–4	756	8.7	5.7	1.53

Source: Modified from WHO (1985e).

calculations based on human milk remain the "gold standard" for determining the protein requirements of the full-term infant, since human milk provides an adequate source of protein until at least 4 months of age.

Since human milk is the "gold standard" source of protein, the essential amino acid content of human milk protein is the reference standard for the amino acid requirements in the perinatal period (Table 11.2). Protein quality refers to the relative nutritional adequacy of the protein source in the infant's diet compared to human milk (see Chapter 4). Infants who are not fed human milk receive an alternate formula containing protein usually derived from cow's milk or soy protein. In the United States, approximately 75% of infants receive cow's milk formula, and 25% receive soy protein-based formula. The amino acid contents of soy and cow's milk-based formulas currently manufactured compare favorably to those of the human milk standard. Thus, if the ingested volume of cow's milk-based or soy protein-based formulas is adequate, amino acid requirements will be achieved. The concentration of protein in formula is, however, invariably higher than in breast milk, a factor that may put an added stress on the kidneys (which must release extra urea) and may also lead to an abnormally high accumulation of amino acids in blood and tissues. [These potential problems are under current debate (Beaton and Chery, 1988; George and DeFrancesca, 1989; Raiha et al., 1986; Young and Pelletier, 1989).] The form of protein in breast milk versus formulas is also different (Table 11.4), formula protein being less abundant in whey and often higher in the (less digestible) casein which is so abundant in cow's milk. Formulas also fail to contain much functional lactoferrin and immunoglobulin A, which are valuable assets in the struggle of the infant to achieve a symbiotic relationship and balance with the bacteria settling its digestive tract (see Chapter 7, under Iron). Certain growth factors and other hormones in breast milk (Table 11.4) may also be important for normal development and for the efficiency of breast milk to support normal growth with a relatively low protein intake (Janas et al., 1987; Koldovsky, 1989).

Lipids, Including Essential Fatty Acids

The full-term infant is born with an abundant fat store that has accumulated during the third trimester (Moya, 1991). Most of this is as triglyceride in white adipocytes, but a small proportion is in brown fat (Chapter 8), which can become a crucial source of warmth to maintain body temperature after birth. Fat is transferred to the fetus across the placenta in the form of fatty acids and ketones, and is also formed from glucose. After

Table 11.4. Differences in the Composition of Human Milk and Formulas

Component	Human milk	Formulas[a]
Total protein concentration (g/dl)	0.85–1.3	1.5–1.6
Type of protein		
Casein : whey	20–30 : 80–70	40–80 : 60–20
Lactalbumin	Alpha form	Beta form or absent[b]
IgA, lactoferrin, lysozyme, lipase	Present	Absent or inactive
Albumin	Present	?
Nonprotein nitrogen concentration (gN/dl)	0.045–0.050	Lower or absent
Taurine	Present	Absent or present[b]
Carnitine	Present	0–?[b]
Nucleotide concentration (mg/dl)	0.15–1.5	0–?[b]
Growth factors, hormones (PTH)	Present	Mostly absent
Oligosaccharides (polyglucose)	Present	Sometimes added
Cholesterol concentration (mg/dl)	10–15	1–6
Phospholipids (mg/dl)	15–20	0–30
Fatty acids (% of fat)		
Linoleic	16	13–33
Linolenic	1	1–5
Docosahexaenoic (DHA)	0.4–0.6	0

Source: Data from Moya (1991).

[a] As of October, 1990.
[b] May be present if formula is based on cow's milk.

birth, lipid becomes a major energy source, first during the initial fast before feeding begins, and from then on, as it is 40%–50% of the total calories in breast milk and formula.

Lipid intake during the perinatal period is important as a concentrated source of energy. In contrast to the infant's limited storage capacity for carbohydrates and protein, energy-rich lipids can be stored in nearly unlimited amounts. In addition to their role as an energy source, lipids are a source of certain fatty acids, including the "nutritionally essential" fatty acids (see Chapter 3). As part of phospholipids and triacylglycerol, these fatty acids are necessary for brain development, are an essential component of all cell membranes, and are the unique carriers of fat-soluble vitamins and hormones in milk. Long-chain polyunsaturated fatty acids (PUFAs) function both as precursors of biologically potent mediators (e.g., prostaglandins, thromboxanes, and leukotrienes) and as vital structural components of membrane systems in all tissues.

it has been known for some time that the fatty acid composition of the triglyceride of adipose tissue can change rapidly to reflect the fatty acid composition of the diet. It has only recently been determined, however, that (at least in primates) the fatty acid composition of the diet also influences the fatty acid composition of the brain (Connor et al., 1985). Although this observation has added to our understanding of the link between diet and body composition, its functional significance remains unknown.

As detailed in Chapter 3, the major lipid classes are the phospholipids, sterols, and glycerides, including fatty acids. A summary of their functions is given in Table 11.5. Two fatty acids,

Table 11.5. Major Functions of Lipids

Lipid class	Function
Glycerides	Storage of fatty acids; source of energy
Phospholipids	Membrane structure; surfactant (lung); source of eicosanoid fatty acids
Sterols	
Cholesterol	Lipoprotein and membrane structure; steroid hormone and bile salt precursor; component of bile
Cholesterol ester	Fat transport and storage
Fatty acids	Energy source; prostanoid precursor

linoleic acid (18:2 n-6) and a-linolenic acid (18:3 n-3), are "nutritionally essential" in humans. These play a role in brain development, cell proliferation, myelination, and function of the retina (Crawford et al., 1978). Within the human body, the biosynthesis of long-chain polyunsaturated fatty acids occurs by a series of chain desaturation and elongation reactions occurring at the carboxy terminus (see Chapter 3, Figure 3.6). There is no direct crossover between unsaturated metabolites from one family to another [i.e., omega-3 (n-3) fatty acids cannot be converted to omega-6 (n-6) fatty acids]. Fatty acids with double bonds at positions n-1 through n-8 cannot be synthesized by vertebrates. Vertebrates (including man) are, therefore, dependent upon dietary sources of these fatty acids; insertion of double bonds in these positions occurs only in plant chloroplasts. Vegetable oils are thus the most important dietary source of the essential fatty acids. Once ingested, man has the ability to further desaturate and elongate the essential (or other) fatty acids.

The metabolism of linoleic acid yields both eicosatrienoic acid (20:3 n-6) and arachidonic acid s(20:4 n-6) (Chapter 3, Figure 3.6). Both of these fatty acids are precursors for the synthesis of prostaglandins (Figure 3.5). The elongation and further desaturation of α-linolenic acid, (18:3 n-3) produces eicosapentaenoic acid (20:5 n-3), a precursor for the prostaglandin-3 series, and docosahexaenoic acid (DHA; 22:6 n-3) (Figure 3.6), a component of brain and retinal phospholipids. Both n-3 and n-6 PUFAs accumulate in the fetus before birth (Clandinin et al., 1980; Uauy et al., 1989), mainly in white fat but also in the brain and retina. Continued availability of these long-chain n-3 and n-6 fatty acids after birth is important for normal development (Carroll, 1989; Uauy et al., 1990a). Premature infants fed breast milk (or formula supplemented with DHA) also have been shown to achieve a better visual acuity when this n-3 fatty acid is administered (Carlson et al., 1989; Moya, 1991). Recommendations are thus that unsaturated fatty acids (mostly linoleic and linolenic acids) should be present at no less than 4% and no more than 12% of total calories (Moya, 1991).

Although essential fatty acid (EFA) deficiency has been described in animals as early as 1929 (Burr and Burr, 1929), such a deficiency was not thought to be of importance in man until the late 1960s. At this time, the first cases of EFA deficiency were described in infants fed formulas based on skim milk (thus, containing little or no fat), and in infants and children who were given intravenous nutrition without a fat source (Caldwell et al., 1972; Collins et al., 1971). Today, deficiencies of linoleic and α-linolenic acids are rare; but if present, deficiencies would be found most often among infants that are very premature (<32 weeks gestation) (Holman et al., 1982). This is because such infants are born with extremely small adipose tissue stores and often receive no essential fatty acids in the first weeks of life. Essential fatty acid deficiency is prevented by providing $\geq$3% of the total energy intake as essential fatty acids (American Academy of Pediatrics, 1985).

Long-chain fatty acids can cross mitochondrial membranes only in the form of acyl-carnitine. Carnitine is thus an essential cofactor for fatty acid oxidation. It has been shown that newborns have a limited capacity for endogenous carnitine synthesis (Borum, 1983). Because fatty acid oxidation and ketogenesis are critical to the survival of newborn infants, an adequate dietary supply of carnitine is also necessary. Plasma and tissue levels of carnitine are low in the newborn. Both human milk (60 nmol/ml) and cow's milk-based formulas, however, are excellent sources of carnitine (Borum, 1983). Thus, despite the newborn's limited capacity for endogenous synthesis, carnitine deficiency is not a problem in the neonatal period.

Fat represents about half of the total energy in human milk. The total fat content of human milk increases from colostrum (with the lowest content), to transitional milk, to mature milk (with the highest content) (Table 11.6). In addition to the changing fat content associated with the length of lactation, there are also diurnal, within-feed, and interindividual differences in milk fat concentrations (Bitman et al., 1983, Hamosh et al., 1985). For example, the fat content rises throughout the day, early morning milk having the lowest amount. The quality of fat in human milk (i.e., the fatty acid pattern) is only partly determined by the pattern of fatty acids in the maternal diet (Harris et al., 1984). However, essential fatty acids and their derived, long-chain PUFAs (C20:4–C22:6), which are important to brain development, are proportionally higher in colostrum and transitional milk than in mature milk, and this phenomenon is independent of the maternal diet.

The fatty acid composition of mature human milk is shown in Table 11.7 (Bitman et al., 1983). The concentration of several classes of fatty acids differ in human and cow's milk. For example, long-chain polyunsaturated fatty acids are present in human, but not cow's milk. As already mentioned, these are important in brain development, cell proliferation, myelination (Crawford et al., 1978), and for the function of the retina (Neuringer et al., 1984). Saturated fats in the C14:0–C18:0 range are found in higher concentrations in human milk; medium chain fatty acids (C8:0–C12:0) are present in higher concentrations in cow's milk. One omega-3 long-chain fatty

Table 11.6. Changes in Human Milk Lipid Composition During Lactation

Lipid class	Lactation day				
	3	7	21	42	84
Total fat (g/L)	20.4	28.9	34.5	31.9	48.7
Triglycerides (%)[a]	97.6	98.5	98.7	98.9	99.0
Cholesterol (%)	1.3	0.7	0.5	0.5	0.4
Phospholipid (%)	1.1	0.8	0.8	0.6	0.6

Source: Adapted from Bitman et al. (1983).

[a] Lipid class as percentage of total lipid by weight. Data are means of 8–41 milk specimens at the different lactation times.

Table 11.7. Fatty Acid Composition of Mature Human Milk[a]

Fatty acid	Chain length and unsaturation	% of total fat
Decanoic	10:0	0.97 ± 0.28
Lauric	12:0	4.46 ± 1.17
Myristic	14:0	5.68 ± 1.36
	15:0	0.31 ± 0.07
Palmitic	16:0	22.20 ± 2.28
Palmitoleic	16:1	3.38 ± 0.39
	17:0	0.49 ± 0.36
Stearic	18:0	7.68 ± 1.85
Oleic	18:1	35.10 ± 2.73
Linoleic	18:2	15.58 ± 1.99
Linolenic	18:3	1.03 ± 0.21
EPA	20:0	0.32 ± 0.11
	20:2	0.18 ± 0.20
	20:3	0.53 ± 0.15
Arachidonic	20:4	0.60 ± 0.29
	20:5	0
	21:0	0.17 ± 0.12
	22:4	0.07 ± 0.16
	22:5 n-6	0.03 ± 0.08
	22:5 n-3	0.11 ± 0.15
DHA?	22:6 n-3	0.23 ± 0.14

Source: Bitman et al. (1983).

[a] Values are means ± SEM of fatty acids in mature milk of mothers of term infants.

acid, docosahexaenoic acid (DHA; 22:6 n-3), an important component of cell membranes, is not found in cow's milk. The concentration of this particular fatty acid in human milk is also low, but increases with maternal ingestion of fish oils high in DHA.

The digestion of fat requires adequate lipase activity and bile salt levels, the former for the breakdown of triglyceride and the latter for emulsification of fat prior to and during lipolysis (Patton, 1981). In the newborn, both pancreatic lipase and bile acid levels are low (Hamosh, 1979). Nevertheless, the fat of human milk is very well-absorbed (90%–95% absorption). This efficient fat absorption depends on alternate mechanisms for the digestion of dietary fat by the breast-fed infant. Two mechanisms aid in the digestion of fat. These are intragastric lipolysis, in which lingual and gastric lipases compensate for low levels of pancreatic lipase; and a bile-salt stimulated lipase present in the *milk*, which aids in the hydrolysis of as much as 30%–40% of milk fat (DeNigris et al., 1985; Hamosh, 1982). This human milk lipase is acid-resistant (i.e., is not inactivated in the stomach), remains active in the intestine for at least 2 hours, and is activated by a lower concentration of bile acids than pancreatic lipase (Hamosh et al., 1975); therefore, it hydrolyzes triglycerides at the low bile acid concentrations present in the intestine of the newborn.

Intragastric lipolysis is catalyzed by lingual lipase, an enzyme secreted from lingual serous glands in the mouth, and by gastric lipase secreted from glands within the gastric mucosa (DeNigris et al., 1985; Patton et al., 1982). Salivary lipase acts primarily on short- and medium-chain fatty acids. Initial hydrolysis of the fat within the core of the milk fat globule by lingual lipase facilitates the subsequent action of pancreatic lipase (and of the bile-salt-stimulated milk lipase) to enhance absorption.

The assisted absorption of fat from human milk is of functional significance, since full-term newborns have low lipase activity of pancreatic origin for at least the first 3 weeks after birth (Fredrikzon and Olivecrona, 1978; Signer et al., 1974). Although the butter fat of cow's milk is relatively poorly absorbed by the newborn infant, cow's milk-based formulas contain no butter fat. Currently, the fat of cow's milk and soy protein-based formulas is a mixture of vegetable fats which are absorbed efficiently, even by the young infant. This still leaves differences between the fatty acid (and other lipid) composition of formulas and breast milk, although their significance (if any) remains unclear. [Another difference is in the cholesterol content (Table 11.4), which is higher in breast milk. Breast-fed infants also have a higher plasma level of cholesterol.]

Carbohydrate

Carbohydrate generally provides between 25% and 50% of the infant's energy needs during the perinatal period, and constitutes about 40% of the calories in breast milk. Although glucose is the major carbohydrate source of energy at the cellular level, infants receiving human milk or cow's milk-based formulas receive mainly disaccharides in the form of lactose. Human milk and most cow's milk-based infant formulas contain 7% lactose; whereas cow's milk contains 5% lactose. Oligosaccharides (of glucose) in human milk provide additional carbohydrate (1.3 g/dl), but only trace quantities of such α-1,4-linked glucose oligosaccharides are present in cow's milk (Blanc, 1981).

The digestion of lactose is the rate-limiting step in its absorption. Lactose is hydrolyzed by lactase, an intestinal villus brush border enzyme (see Chapter 2). Lactase is found in greatest concentration in the proximal jejunum, with decreasing concentrations distally in the small bowel. Lactase activity has been demonstrated in fetuses as young as 24 weeks of gestation; thus, even the infant born prematurely probably has a good capacity for lactose digestion (Figure 11.7) (Antonowicz et al., 1974).

The only other carbohydrate commonly consumed in significant quantities in the first months of life is polyglucose in the form of starch or small (5–10 U) oligosaccharides. Starch, a complex carbohydrate, is a component of infant cereal. Cereal is usually eaten when the infant is older than 4 months of age, although infants as young as 1 month have been given this food. Starch in cereal is almost entirely made up of amylose (Table 2.1; molecular weight >100,000) and the more complex amylopectin (molecular weight 1,000,000). The hydrolysis of starch begins in the mouth, with the action of salivary amylase (which can be detected in the fetus at 20–22 weeks gestation) and continues in the duodenum with maltase, isomaltase, and pancreatic amylase (Figure 11.7), which also develop early in gestation (Auricchio et al., 1965). Breakdown of the interior bonds of amylose results in two smaller saccharides—maltose and malto-triose. These, in turn, are hydrolyzed by the brush border enzyme, maltase.

As already stated, the glucose oligosaccharides

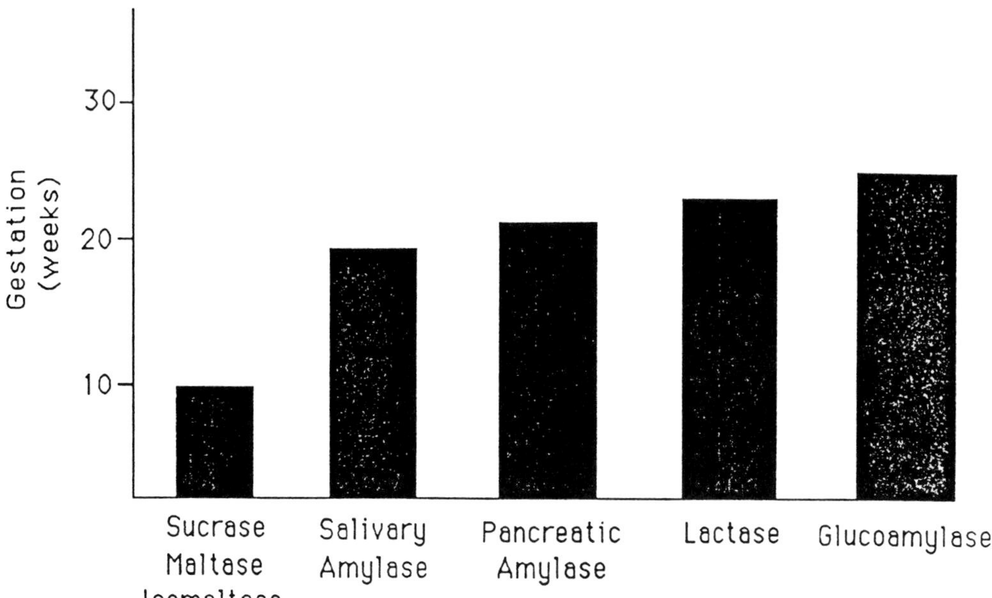

Figure 11.7. The appearance in the fetus of intestinal carbohydrate digestive enzymes. By 23–24 weeks gestation, the digestion of various carbohydrates is not rate-limiting to their absorption. [*Source:* Antonwicz et al. (1974).]

of human milk are present at a concentration of about 1.3% (13 g/L), as already stated. (Cow's milk contains only trace amounts.) Oligosaccharides of 5–10 glucose units are now added to some formulas. These oligosaccharides are also digested by maltase and other brush border enzymes in the small intestine of the newborn infant. In addition to their role as a source of calories, the breast milk oligosaccharides act as a host defense mechanism (with other components of human milk) to protect the newborn from infection. This is because their structure mimics that of bacterial receptors on intestinal cells. The oligosaccharides bind to bacteria, thus blocking bacterial attachment to intestinal cell membranes (Goldman et al., 1986). More specifically, for example, pneumococci can bind to the oligosaccharide portion of pharyngeal cell "receptors"; but human milk contains an oligosaccharide-pharyngeal cell-receptor analogue which binds the pneumococci, thus preventing them from attaching to (and invading) pharyngeal cells (Goldman et al., 1986). Oligosaccharides also influence the growth of intestinal flora by providing substrates for (and thus promoting the growth of) the beneficial bacterium, *Lactobacillus bifidus*, while limiting the growth of other potentially pathogenic bacteria (Blanc, 1981; Carlson, 1985).

Congenital primary disorders of carbohydrate absorption are very rare. Lactose intolerance (Chapter 2) due to a decreased intestinal brush border lactase activity is, however, prevalent in a large proportion of adults, and in children from specific regions of the world during early to mid childhood (Huang and Bayless, 1967; Lebenthal et al., 1975) (i.e., after 11 months of age). Lactose intolerance is common in Southern Asians (Orientals) and Black Africans (Table 11.8). Lactose tolerance and intestinal lactase activity is preserved in Scandinavians and those of Anglo-Saxon background. In white American children, normal lactase activity (and tolerance to lactose) is expected until at least 5 years of age, and in Black children until only 3 years of age (Lebenthal et al., 1975; Welsh et al., 1978).

Vitamins and Minerals

Vitamin D. The results of clinical and epidemiologic investigations have led to a general acceptance of the concept that the amount of minerals and vitamins found in human milk, when fed at a volume to satisfy the energy needs of the healthy growing full-term infant, defines the requirement for the infant during the perinatal period. This estimate of requirement has been accepted by national advisory groups and formula

Table 11.8. Prevalence of Lactase Deficiency Among Adults of Various Ethnic and Racial Groups

Group	Prevalence of lactose malabsorption (%)
Orientals in U.S.	100
Bantu	95
American Indians of Oklahoma	95
Alaskan Inuit	94
Black Americans	81
Children in Ghana	73
Indians in Bombay	64
Mexican Americans	56
White Americans	24
White "Anglo-Americans"	15
Danes	2

Source: Data from Mobassaleh et al. (1985).

manufacturers, so that the quantity of minerals and vitamins found in human milk substitutes (formulas) is at least equivalent to that found in human milk (Table 11.9). The only exceptions to this general rule are with respect to vitamin D (which is very low in human milk), and possibly iron and fluoride. The trace mineral content of human milk is also used to define the requirement for older growing infants, although there are a few exceptions to this general rule, which will be subsequently discussed. The concentration of the water-soluble vitamins is kept universally higher in formulas than in human milk because of the losses associated with sterilization.

Vitamin D is found in especially small amounts in human milk (Hollis et al., 1981). In fact, significant amounts of vitamin D are not present in most foods except certain livers and liver oils (as from cold-water fish). Vitamin D, however, can be synthesized endogenously in the epidermis of the skin upon exposure to sunlight (see Chapter 5). Vitamin D undergoes 25-hydroxylation to 25-hydroxyvitamin D (25-OHD) in the liver, and 1a-hydroxylation in the kidney, to 1,25-dihydroxyvitamin D [1,25-$(OH)_2D$; Figure 5.30]. The latter is an essential hormone whose primary role is to stimulate the absorption of calcium and phosphorus from the small intestine; together with parathyroid hormone (PTH), it also promotes reabsorption of calcium and phosphorus in the kidney, and the mobilization of calcium and phosphorus from bone. In the absence of sufficient vitamin D, children will develop rickets. The clinical signs of rickets, and typical x-ray findings associated with rickets, are shown in Figures 11.8 and 11.9 (Salter, 1970).

For the human infant during the perinatal period, there are three potential sources of vitamin D and its metabolites: placental transfer, endogenous synthesis from the skin, and the diet. Fetal liver stores of vitamin D depend on maternal vitamin D blood levels during pregnancy, which in turn are related to maternal vitamin D nutrition and sunlight exposure (Brooke et al., 1981; Delvin et al., 1982). The placenta can hydroxylate 25-OH D to the active hormone form (Moya, 1991). At birth, infants have plasma 25-OH-vitamin D levels that are related to maternal levels, but are generally lower than those found in their mothers, possibly because of the low concentration of vitamin D binding protein (Bouillon et al., 1981; Tsang et al., 1981). Congenital rickets may develop in neonates from mothers with vitamin D deficiency; however, rickets usually occur beyond the neonatal period, after vitamin D deficiency has been present for some time.

Like adults, newborn infants have the capacity to synthesize vitamin D from 7-dehydrocholesterol in the presence of sunlight. From studies conducted in temperate climates in the United States (Cincinnati, Ohio) and China (Beijing), it was concluded that 2 hours of sunshine exposure

Table 11.9. Vitamin Content of Human Milk and Human Milk Substitutes (Formulas) Expressed as Units per 100 ml of Fluid

	Vitamin											
	A	D	E	K	C	Folate	B_1	B_2	B_6	B_{12}	Niacin	Pantothenate
Food source		(IU)		(μg)	(mg)				(μg)			
Human milk	190	2.2	0.2	1.5	4.3	0.5	16	36	10	0.03	1.47	200
Formula	225	41	1.7	5.7	5.6	8.6	63	105	41	0.14	0.7	277

Source: The vitamin content of formulas is the mean content from Enfamil (Mead Johnson), Similac (Ross Laboratories), and SMA (Wyeth), as per the product monographs.

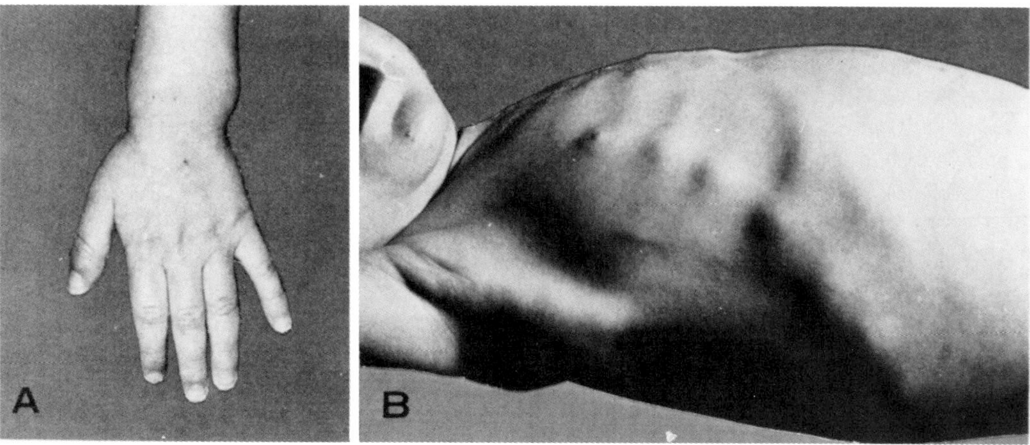

Figure 11.8. Clinical enlargement at the sites of epiphyseal plates. **(A)** Enlargement of the sites of the distal radial and distal ulnar epiphyseal plates in a 1-year-old boy with vitamin D-refractory rickets. **(B)** Enlargement at the sites of the epiphyseal plates at the costochondral junctions in the same child. Because of the beaded appearance, this is known as "richitic rosary." [*Source:* Reprinted by permission from Salter (1970).]

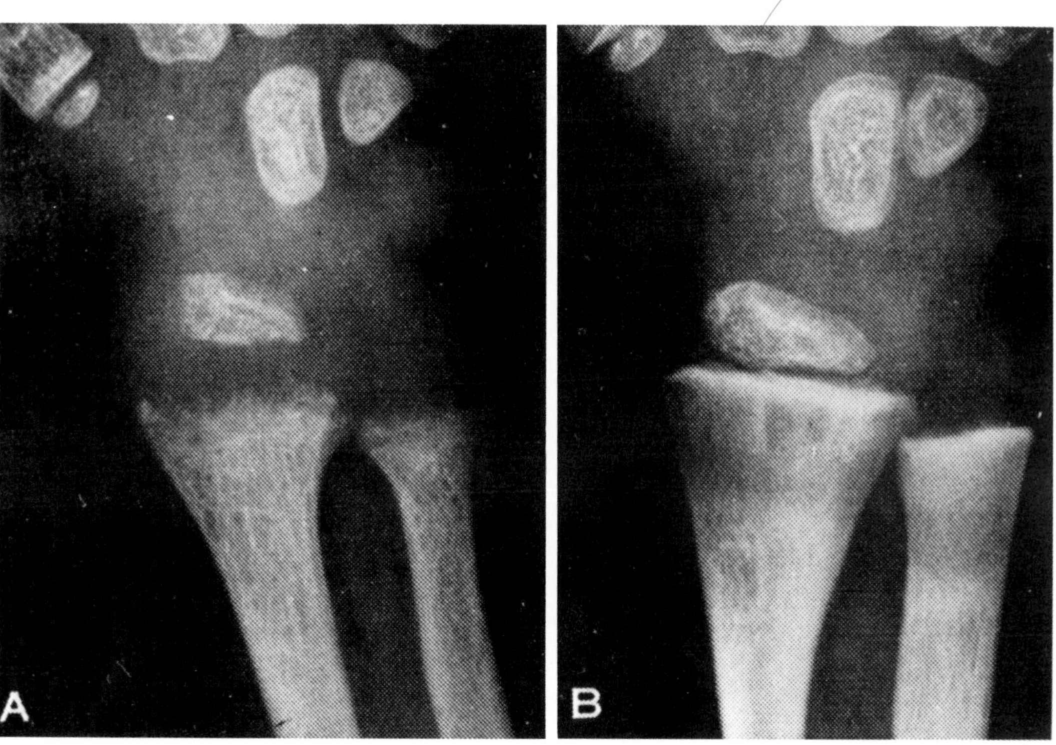

Figure 11.9. **(A)** An x-ray of the wrist of a 3-year-old child with rickets. There is a widened radiolucent zone in the epiphyseal plate (due to uncalcified pre-osseous cartilage and osteoid), generalized rarefaction of the bones, and a coarse trabecular pattern of cancellous bone. **(B)** The same patient following treatment with vitamin D. Now there is normal ossification in the metaphyseal regions and normal generalized density of the bones. [*Source:* Reprinted by permission from Salter (1970).]

per week of fully clothed (hands and head exposed) white, breast-fed infants will maintain serum 25-OH-D concentrations above 11 ng/ml (the lower limit of the normal range) (Ho et al., 1985; Specker et al., 1985).

Dietary intake of vitamin D is the third source for the infant. As mentioned previously, the vitamin D content of human milk is very low but not zero (Hollis et al., 1981). Almost all of the vitamin D activity of human milk can be accounted for by a combination of the parent compound (vitamin D_3) and 25-OH-D_3 (Reeve et al., 1982). The concentration of 1,25-$(OH)_2D_3$ in human milk is negligible. Claims of the discovery of a water-soluble metabolite of vitamin D (vitamin D sulfate) in human milk (Sahashi et al., 1969) have not been verified in subsequent studies (Greer et al., 1982; Lakdawaia and Widdowson, 1977). In North America, today, vitamin D deficiency rickets is rare, but not totally unknown. When diagnosed, it is most often in exclusively breast-fed infants living in the more Northern climactic zones (Bachrach et al., 1979; Edidin et al., 1980). These infants are usually born in the late summer and receive little exposure to sunshine during the fall and winter months. Black-skinned infants are more susceptible than those with fair skin (Clemens et al., 1982; Specker et al., 1985). To prevent rickets, it is currently recommended that exclusively breast-fed infants not exposed to sunlight should receive a vitamin D supplement of 200–300 IU/day (National Research Council, 1989). In addition, commercial infant formulas are fortified with 400 IU of vitamin D/L, specifically to prevent rickets.

Iron. Iron deficiency anemia, although not a problem during the perinatal period, remains the most widespread nutritional problem during the first year of life (Dallman et al., 1984). In recent years, however, several reports have described a declining prevalence of anemia among low-income children, and have provided evidence that iron nutrition in infancy and early childhood has improved, at least in many parts of the world (Miller et al., 1985; Vazquez-Seoane et al., 1985; Yip et al., 1987a, b) (Figure 11.10). This improved iron nutritional status is believed to be due to enrollment of this high-risk group in the Special Supplemented Food Program for Women, Infants and Children (WIC), which was instituted by WHO in the mid-1970s (Yip et al., 1987b).

In full-term infants, iron deficiency anemia rarely develops before 4–6 months of life, because the normal infant accumulates an iron store before birth (Smith and Rios, 1974) (Figure 7.5). Infants at risk for iron deficiency include the following: those born prematurely; those with perinatal bleeding; those with a low hemoglobin concentration at birth or frequent infections; those that have experienced an early and prolonged intake of cow's milk; those with a low vitamin C and/or meat intake; and those exclusively fed breast milk longer than 6 months without the use of supplemental iron.

Although an increased morbidity associated with low hemoglobin concentrations secondary to iron deficiency has been described in the past (Cook and Lynch, 1986), it is now believed that the cognitive and psychomotor behavior of infants may also be influenced by iron deficiency

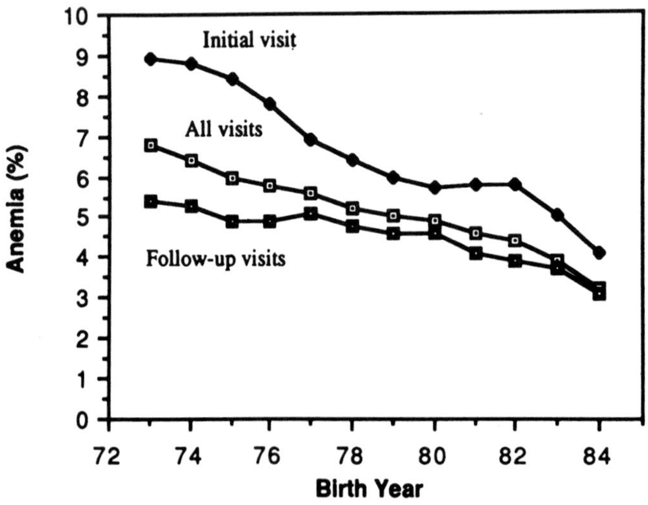

Figure 11.10. Prevalence of anemia in children aged 6–59 months in six selected states (CDC Pediatric Nutrition Surveillance System, 1976–1985). The upper line represents children seen at the initial visit for enrollment into WIC programs ("non-WIC" children). The lower line represents children in the WIC program seen at follow-up visits ("WIC" children). The middle line (all visits) represents the median values. Overall, the prevalence of anemia declined by 54%, from 6.8% in the initial year to 3.1% in the last birth cohort. The "WIC" children consistently had a lower prevalence of anemia than the "non-WIC" children, although the decline of prevalence of anemia was also significant among "non-WIC" children. [*Source:* Reprinted by permission from Yip et al. (1987a).]

anemia (Lozoff, 1990; Oski et al., 1983; Walter, 1990). The neurophysiologic mechanisms mediating the effects of iron deficiency are still largely speculative. It is known, however, that iron is required for the activity of enzymes, such as tyrosine hydroxylase, tryptophan hydroxylase, and monoamine oxidase, which are important in neurotransmitter metabolism (Cook and Lynch, 1986; Hercberg and Galan, 1989).

Postnatal iron requirements can be gauged by the infant's gestational maturity (or birth weight), hemoglobin concentration at birth, rate of growth, rate of blood volume expansion, magnitude of erythropoiesis, and iron losses or iron gains, including transfusions during this period. In the first 1–3 months of life, there is a marked decrease in erythropoiesis, which is normal and results in an actual decrease in red blood cell mass. Hemoglobin concentrations normally decline by 30% from about 170–110 g/L during the 6–8 weeks after birth. Iron released from red cell breakdown enters body stores, so that the iron stores of solid tissues temporarily increase during this phase. During the same time period, obligatory iron losses amount to about 0.24 mg/day (0.04 mg/kg/day) (Smith and Rios, 1974). Since the average iron content of human milk is 0.35 mg/L, and average milk intake is 750 ml/day, the iron intake would be 0.26 mg/day (Fransson and Lonnerdal, 1984). Assuming 50% absorption of iron from human milk, it is quite clear that intake will not meet obligatory iron losses. As more active erythropoiesis resumes, iron stores will eventually be used up if no additional iron is provided. At this point, iron deficiency anemia will occur, if gestational stores are insufficient or an additional iron source is not introduced.

To prevent depletion of iron stores and iron deficiency anemia, it is recommended that breastfed infants receive iron-containing, weaning foods (like infant cereals and/or meat), beginning at or around 6 months of age. Infants receiving formula should receive similar iron-containing, weaning foods somewhat earlier, if the formula is not already iron-fortified. There is no evidence to support the contention that colic is more frequently seen in the infant fed iron-fortified (versus unfortified) formula (Nelson et al., 1988).

Full-term infants rarely develop iron deficiency anemia before 4–6 months of age because of the aforementioned limited early erythropoiesis and the existence of an iron store. When iron-deficient anemia is seen during this time period, the most common cause is diffuse intestinal blood loss associated with the ingestion of fresh (but pasteurized) whole cow's milk. There is evidence that occult blood loss may result from the use of regular cow's milk throughout the first year of life; thus, it may be an unsuitable food for some infants in this period (Fomon et al., 1981; American Academy of Pediatrics, 1983a). [Cow's milk-based (or soy-based) *formulas* do not have this problem and would be preferred.]

Fluoride. In temperate areas where the natural fluoride level is low, the fluoridation of drinking water to 1 ppm reduces the incidence of dental caries in children by 40%–60%, while minimizing the risk of enamel fluorosis. This protection continues into adulthood (WHO, 1985a; Richmond, 1985). The major source of fluoride in the diet is water; thus, intake will depend on exposure of the infant to the local water supply. Plasma fluoride concentrations reflect the level in the diet. Absorption is about 80% from foods and fluids and as high as 97% from supplements, such as the sodium fluoride found in toothpastes (Subba, 1984). Ingested fluoride is rapidly incorporated into the bones and teeth of the growing infant. Excess fluoride is excreted in urine (Krishnamachari, 1987).

Fluoride is incorporated into tooth enamel during the mineralization stage of tooth formation and also by surface adsorption after the tooth has erupted. It strengthens dental enamel by substituting for hydroxyl ions in the hydroxyapatite crystalline mineral matrix of the enamel (see Chapter 7). The resulting fluorapatite is less porous, and thus more resistant to chemical and physical damage.

To avoid confusion, commercial formulas (both cow's milk-based and soy-based) are now manufactured using defluorinated water; thus, they contain very low amounts of fluoride. Any infant, therefore, receiving ready-to-feed formula (premixed with fluoride-free water) should be given supplemental fluoride unless the level in the local water supply is high. It is recommended that infants receive the fluoride supplement for the first 2 years of life, starting in the first 2 weeks of life (American Academy of Pediatrics, 1986). The recommended schedule for fluoride supplementation of infants in communities with varying levels of fluoridation is shown in Table 11.10.

Human milk is very low in fluoride (4–8 ng/ml). Despite maximum intakes by fully breast-fed infants of only about 15 μg/day, a need for fluoride supplementation of this group has not been proven. Nevertheless, the current recommendation for breast-fed infants is no supplementation if the local water supply is adequate in fluoride; otherwise, they should receive the same supplementation as formula-fed infants (American Academy of Pediatrics, 1986).

Zinc. Human milk contains zinc at 2.6 mg/L at 1 month after birth (Vuori and Kuitunen, 1979). If the average milk intake is 700 ml/day when the infant is 1 month of age (Neville et al., 1988), then the zinc intake would be 1.82 mg/day. The zinc concentration of human milk decreases with time, postpartum, while the volume of milk ingested slowly increases. Thus, at age 3 months, with a milk Zn concentration of 1.1 mg/L and an average intake of 750 ml/day, the zinc intake would be 0.83 mg/day. If we assume for an individual infant that there is an appropriate match between the content of zinc ingested from his/her own mother's milk and his/her specific requirement (obligatory losses + needs for storage and growth), then the zinc intake from human milk would equal the dietary requirement for zinc of the human milk-fed infant.

To test whether zinc intake from human milk is adequate, one must look at the zinc status of infants receiving human milk. Until recently, the answer would have been that infants receiving an adequate volume of human milk were indeed invariably receiving an adequate intake of zinc (i.e., that their physiologic requirement was being met). Recently, however, at least five cases of exogenous zinc deficiency have been described in full-term infants (Bye et al., 1985; Kuramoto et al., 1986; Roberts et al., 1987) (Table 11.11). All of the infants were well at birth and were totally breast-fed. An "acrodermatitis-like" skin rash developed between 10–20 weeks after birth, accompanied by low levels of serum zinc. In all cases, the zinc content in the infants' mother's milk was lower than expected, and the zinc ingested by the infants was thus not sufficient to meet their requirements. An inadequate secretion of zinc from the mammary gland, due to a severe deficiency in the mother or to some defect in mammary gland function, is a likely cause of this deficiency disorder. Other than in these rare cases, it is generally believed that for the human milk-fed infant, the amount of zinc in human milk defines the dietary requirement and meets the physiologic requirement, at least until the infant is weaned from milk, even if the mother is deficient.

Table 11.10. Recommended Fluoride Supplementation for Infants

Fluoride in local water supply (mg/l)	<0.3	0.3–0.7	>0.7
Supplement dose (mg F/day)	0.25	0	0

Source: American Academy of Pediatrics (1986).

Table 11.11. Case Characteristics of Full-Term Infants with Zinc Deficiency Due to an Inadequate Human Milk Zinc Content

Birth weight (kg)	Sex	Age at onset (months)	Zn content of milk (mg/L)	Reference values[a,b] (mg/L)
3.7[c]	M	3.5	0.27	0.44 ± 0.2
3.7[d]	F	4	0.03	0.75 ± 0.3
3.0[d]	M	2	0.27	0.75 ± 0.3
—[e]	M	2.5	0.18	1.30 ± 0.3
—[e]	F	2.5	0.14	1.30 ± 0.4

[a] This value corresponds to the postnatal date at which the milk sample was taken.
[b] Vuori and Kuitunen (1979).
[c] Roberts et al. (1987).
[d] Bye et al. (1985).
[e] Kuramoto et al. (1986).

Nucleotides

Human milk also contains small quantities of nucleic acids (RNA and DNA) and nucleotides (cytosine, uridine, adenosine, guanosine, and inosine), the latter mostly as monophosphates, as part of the nonprotein nitrogen fraction (Table 11.4). These are now thought to have beneficial effects on the infant and are even being considered as possible semi-essential or conditionally essential constituents for the diet of the newborn (Moya, 1991; Uauy, 1989, 1990b). Quantities of nucleotides vary from 1.5–15 mg/L (e.g., in the range for certain trace elements) but the quantities of nucleic acids are higher (Sanguansermsri et al., 1974). Among the beneficial effects for which there is evidence from animals and also human studies are: (a) the stimulation of cellular immunity, including natural killer cell activity (Carver et al., 1989); (b) a reduction in the intestinal population of bifidobacteria (Gil et al., 1986); (c) a possibly higher level of n-3 and n-6 polyunsaturated fatty acids in cell membranes; and (d) an enhancement of iron absorption (Moya, 1991). There may also be an influence on the levels of LDL and HDL (a higher ratio of HDL to LDL). These are interesting observations that may soon lead to the general addition of nucleotides to formulas.

Infant Feeding Practices

There is general agreement that human milk is the optimal nutritional choice for healthy newborns. In the United States, the use of breast-feeding from birth has increased from around 29% in 1971 to 61% in 1984 (Figure 11.11) (Martinez and Krieger, 1985; Nichols, 1988). Yet, from 2 months of age onward, formula feeding (primarily cow's milk-based formula) predominates (Martinez and Krieger, 1985). This trend continues until after 6 months of age, when regular cow's milk gradually replaces breast and formula feeding. Although these increases in the incidence and duration of breast-feeding are impressive, it is interesting to note that the greatest increase in breast-feeding has occurred among older, well-educated, more affluent women (Grossman et al., 1990; Martinez and Krieger, 1985). The literature suggests the same trend is not true for younger, poorly educated, and less affluent groups (Grossman et al., 1990).

In addition to its nutritional superiority, human milk is more digestible than cow's milk, has a lower potential renal solute load, is less allergic, and contains anti-infective properties, including lactoferrin, immunoglobulins, complement, and leukocytes (Ogra and Greene, 1982) (See also Table 11.4). In developing countries, it is clear that breast milk protects infants from infections, while formulas that may be mixed with contaminated water do not (Jason et al., 1984). In developed urban centers, however, the protective effects of breast-feeding have not been clearly demonstrated. Conflicting results have been published from observational studies that have used either case-control or cohort designs. Some studies have demonstrated a protective effect from breast-feeding against gastrointestinal and respiratory illnesses and illnesses requiring hospitalizations (Cunningham, 1977, 1979; Downham et al., 1976; Fallot et al., 1980; Larson and Homer, 1978; Watkins et al., 1979). Others have shown little or no protection of breast-feeding against infections (Adebonjo, 1972; Cushing and Anderson, 1982; Leventhal et al., 1986; Pullan et al., 1980; Taylor et al., 1982; Weinberg et al., 1984). A recent prospective study of 500 middle-class urban Danish infants failed to detect any protective effects of breast-feeding against the already low occurrence of infectious illnesses in this population in the first year of life (Rubin et al., 1990). There is no information on rural or poor urban populations from developed countries. However, one may

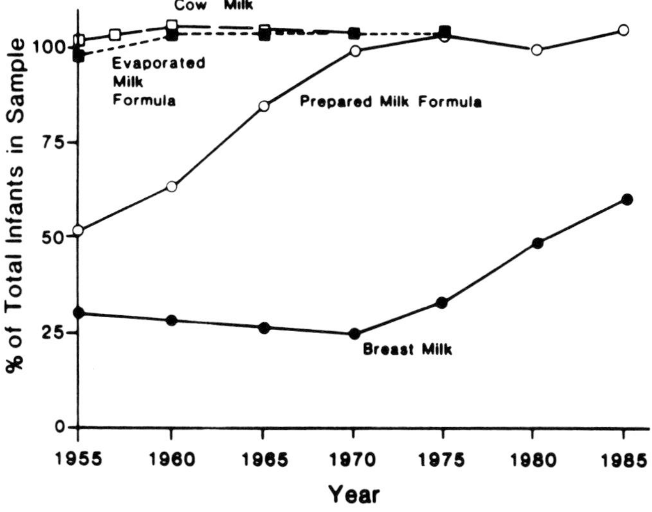

Figure 11.11. Distribution of types of milk feedings during the past 30 years. Infants were 1 week of age at the time of this survey. Prepared milk formulas were commercially available. Cow's milk and evaporated milk formulas were prepared in the home. The use of breast-feeding has increased from around 29% in 1971 to 61% in 1984. [*Source:* Reprinted by permission from Nichols (1988); data from Martinez and Krieger (1985).]

speculate that the protective effects might be similar to those seen in countries with limited sanitation facilities.

Although the manufacturers of infant formulas have done an excellent job in producing safe, nutritionally complete, human milk substitutes, they have, as yet, been unable to duplicate the immunologic properties of human milk. Thus, cow's milk-based formulas still remain the second choice for feeding during the first year of life. Formulas manufactured from soy-protein isolates have been in use since the early 1930s. Since then, the use of these products has expanded appreciably, and they are used for an estimated 10%–15% of all formula-fed infants (American Academy of Pediatrics, 1983b). The indications for the use of soy-based formulas include: (a) vegetarianism, in which animal protein formulas are not desired; (b) the management of galactosemia, primary lactase deficiency, or the recovery phase of secondary lactose intolerance (these formulas contain no lactose); and (c) potentially allergic infants (with a family history of atopy), who have not shown clinical manifestations or allergy (American Academy of Pediatrics, 1983b). It should be noted, however, that recent studies have not found soy-based formulas to be effective in the prophylaxis or treatment of adverse reactions to cow's milk proteins (American Academy of Pediatrics, 1989b). In addition, soy-based formulas are not intended for the routine feeding of premature infants, because of associated hypophosphatemic rickets (Callenbach et al., 1981; Kulkarni et al., 1980).

Weaning is not a single event, but a process that takes place throughout a number of months, beginning optimally between 4 and 6 months of age (Finberg, 1985). The nutritional objective is to achieve a varied diet, with approximately 35%–50% of energy coming from sources other than human milk or formula (American Academy of Pediatrics, 1989a). Variety remains the key to the diet, particularly for infants older than 6 months of age. Solid food must provide an added source of iron, trace minerals, and vitamins to replace and supplement those in that portion of breast milk or formula removed from the diet. Human milk and fortified infant formula continue to be optimal for the milk segment of the diet during the second 6 months of life. The Committee on Nutrition has indicated that cow's milk could be substituted in the second 6 months of age, provided that the amount of energy (calories) from milk does not exceed 65% of total energy, and that the solid food portion of the diet replaces the iron and vitamins deficient in cow's milk (American Academy of Pediatrics, 1983a, 1986).

Overview

This chapter has reviewed the nutrient needs of the neonate in the context of its rapid growth and changing metabolism. It is important to remember that not all nutrients were reviewed, since when human milk is fed at a volume to satisfy the energy needs of the healthy growing infant, by definition, the requirement for the infant has been met. The only exceptions to this general rule are with respect to the human milk content of vitamin D, iron, and fluoride. It is also important to emphasize that growth during the first 6 months of life is faster than at any other time. Provision of an adequate supply of nutrients is necessary to maintain this rapid rate.

Formulas that mimic human milk nutrient composition will also meet the growth requirements of the infant. Such formulas are increasingly available commercially and are being refined as new information on human milk becomes available.

References

Adebonjo FO (1972): Clin Pediatr 11:25.

American Academy of Pediatrics, Committee on Nutrition (1983a): Pediatrics 72:253.

American Academy of Pediatrics, Committee on Nutrition (1983b): Pediatrics 72:359.

American Academy of Pediatrics, Committee on Nutrition (1985): Pediatrics 75:976.

American Academy of Pediatrics, Committee on Nutrition (1986): Pediatrics 78:521.

American Academy of Pediatrics, Committee on Nutrition (1989a): Pediatrics 83:1067.

American Academy of Pediatrics, Committee on Nutrition (1989b): Pediatrics 83:1068.

Antonowicz I, Chang SK, Grand RJ (1974): Gastroenterol 67:51.

Auricchio S, Rubino A, Murset G (1965): Pediatrics 35:944.

Bachrach S, Fisher J, Parks JS (1979): Pediatrics 64:871.

Beaton GH, Chery A (1988): Am J Clin Nutr 48:1403.

Bitman J, Wood DL, Hamosh M (1983): Am J Clin Nutr 38:300.

Blanc B (1981): World Rev Nutr Diet 36:1.

Borum P (1983): Ann Rev Nutr 3:233.

Bouillon R, Van Assche F, Van Baelen H, et al. (1981): J Clin Invest 67:589.

Brar HS, Rutherford SE (1988): Semin Perinatol 12:2.

Brooke OG, Brown IRF, Vleeve HJW (1981): Br J Obstet Gynecol 88:18.

Bruck K (1978): *In* Save U, ed: Perinatal physiology. New York: Plenum, p 455.

Burr GO, Burr MM (1929): J Biol Chem 82:345.

Bye AME, Goodfellow A, Atherton DJ (1985): Pediatr Dermatol 2:308.

Caldwell MD, Jonsson HT, Olmerson HB (1972): J Pediatr 81:894.

Callenbach JC, Sheehan MB, Abranson SJ, et al. (1981): J Pediatr 98:800.

Carlson SE (1985): *In* Barnes LA, ed: Advances in pediatrics, Vol 32. Chicago: Year Book Medical, p 43.

Carlson SE, Cooke RJ, Peeples JM, Werkman SH, Tolley EA (1989): Pediatr Res 25:285A.

Carroll KK (1989): J Nutr 119:1810.

Carver JD, Pimentel B, Barness LA (1989): Pediatr Res 5:286A.

Chessex P, Reichman BL, Verellen JE, Putet G, Smith JM, Heim T, Swyer PR (1981): Pediatr Res 15:1077.

Clandinin MT, Chappell JE, Leong S, et al. (1980): Early Hum Dev 4:121.

Clemens TL, Henderson SL, Adams JS, Holick MF (1982): Lancet 1:74.

Collins FD, Sinclair AJ, Royle JP, Coats DA, Maaynard AT, Leonard RF (1971): Nutr Metab 13:150.

Connor WE, Neuringer M, Lin D, Neuwelt R (1985): XIII Internatl Cong Nutr Abstracts, 104.

Cook JD and Lynch SR (1986): Blood 68:803.

Coward WA, et al. (1982): Hum Nutr Clin Nutr 36:141.

Crawford MA, Hassam AG, Rivers JPW (1978): Am J Clin Nutr 31:2181.

Cunningham AS (1977): J Pediatr 90:726.

Cunningham AS (1979): J Pediatr 95:685.

Cushing AH, Anderson L (1982): Pediatr 70:921.

Dallman PR, Yip R, Johnson C (1984): Am J Clin Nutr 39:437.

Delvin E, Gioleux F, Salle B, et al. (1982): Arch Dis Child 57:754.

DeNigris SJ, Hamosh M, Kasbekar DK, et al. (1985): Biochim Biophys Acta 836:67.

Downham MA, Scott R, Sims DG, Webb JKG, Gardner RS (1976): Br Med J 2:274.

Edidin D, Levitsky LL, Schey W, et al. (1980): Pediatr 65:232.

Enesco M, Leblond CP (1962): J Embryol Exp Morph 10:530.

Fallot ME, Boyd JL, Oski FA (1980): Pediatr 65:1121.

FAO (1973): WHO Technical Report Series, No 522, Geneva, p 33.

Finberg L (1985): Pediatr 75(Suppl):214.

Fomon SJ, Ziegler EE, Nelson SE, et al. (1981): J Pediatr 98:540.

Fomon SJ, et al. (1982): Am J Clin Nutr 35(Suppl 5):1169.

Fransson GB, Lonnerdal B (1984): Am J Clin Nutr 39:185.

Fraser DR (1980): Physiol Rev 60:551.

Fredrikzon B, Olivecrona T (1978): Pediatr Res 12:6321.

Freiburghaus AU, Schmitz J, Schindler M, et al. (1976): N Eng J Med 294:1030.

Gaul G, Sturman JA, Raiha NCR (1972): Pediatr Res 6:538.

George DE, DeFrancesca BA (1989): *In* Lebenthal E, ed: Textbook of gastroenterology and nutrition in infancy. New York: Raven Press, p 239.

Gil A, Corral E, Martinez A, Molina JA (1986): J Clin Nutr Gastroent 1:34.

Goldman AS, Sharpe LW, Goldblum RM, et al. (1986): Acta Paed Scand 75:689.

Grantham-McGregor S, Schofield W, Powell C (1987): Pediatr 79:247.

Greer FR, Ho M, Dodson D, et al. (1982): Pediatrics 69:238.

Grossman LK, Harter C, Sachs L, Kay A (1990): Am J Dis Child 144:471.

Hamosh M (1979): Pediatr Res 13:615.

Hamosh M (1982): Adv Pediatr 29:33.

Hamosh M, Bitman J, Wood DL, et al. (1985): Pediatr 75(Suppl):146.

Hamosh M, Klaeveman HL, Wolf RO, Scow RO (1975): J Clin Invest 55:908.

Harris WD, Conner WE, Lindsey S (1984): Am J Clin Nutr 40:780.

Harvey MAS (1976): J Pediatr 89:225.

Hayward I, Stein MT, Gibson MI (1987): Am J Dis Child 141:1060.

Hercberg S, Galan P (1989): Acta Paediatr Scand Suppl 361:63.

Ho ML, Yen HC, Tsang RC, et al. (1985): J Pediatr 107:928.

Holick MF, MacLaughlin JA, Dopplelt SH (1981): Science 211:590.

Hollis BW, Roos BA, Draper HH, et al. (1981): J Nutr 111:1240.

Holman RT, Johnson RT, Hatch TF (1982): Am J Clin Nutr 35:617.

Huang MH, Bayless TT (1967): New Engl J Med 276:1283.

Hurley L (1980): *In* Developmental nutrition. Englewood Cliffs, NJ: Prentice-Hall, p 5.

Janas LM, Picciano MF, Hatch TF (1987): J Pediatr 110:838.

Jason JM, Nieburg P, Marks JS (1984): Pediatr 73(Suppl):702.

Kantero R-L, Tiisala R (1971): Acta Paediatr Scand 220(Suppl):27.

Karlberg P (1952): Acta Paediatr 41(Suppl 89):13.

Koldovsky O (1989): *In* Lebenthal E, ed: Textbook of gastroenterology and nutrition in infancy. New York: Raven Press, p 97.

Krishnamachari KAVR (1987): In Mertz W, ed: Trace elements in animal and human nutrition. New York: Academic Press, p 365.

Kulkarni PB, Hall RT, Rhodes PG, et al. (1980): J Pediatr 96:249.

Kuramoto Y, Igarashi Y, Kato S, et al. (1986): Acta Dermatol Venerol (Stockholm) 66:359.

Lakdawaia DR, Widdowson EM (1977): Lancet 1:167.

Larson SA, Homer DR (1978): J Pediatr 92:417.

Lebenthal E, Antonowicz I, Shwachman H (1975): Am J Clin Nutr 28:595.

Leventhal JM, Shapiro ED, Aten CB, Berhg AT, Egerter AA (1986): Pediatr 78:896.

Lonnerdal B, et al. (1976): Am J Clin Nutr 29:1127.

Lozoff B (1990): *In* Dobbing J, ed: Brain, behaviour, and iron in the infant diet. New York: Springer-Verlag, p 107.

Macy IG, et al. (1953): National Research Council Publication No 254, Washington, DC: National Academy of Sciences.

Martinez GA, Krieger FW (1985): Pediatr 76:1004.

Miller V, Swaney S, Deinard AS (1985): Pediatr 75:100.

Mobassaleh M, Montgomery RK, Biller JA, et al. (1985): Pediatrics 75(Suppl):160.

Moya FR (1991): *In* Suskind R, Suskind L, eds: Textbook in neonatal nutrition. New York: Raven, in press.

Mueller WH (1986): *In* Falkner F, Tanner JM, eds: Human growth. New York: Plenum Press, Vol 3, p 145.

National Research Council, Commission on Life Sciences (1989): Recommended dietary allowances (10th ed). Washington, DC: National Research Council.

Nelson SE, Ziegler EE, Copeland AM, Edwars BE, Foman SJ (1988): Pediatr 81:360.

Neuringer M, Conner WE, Van Petten C, et al. (1984): J Clin Invest 72:272.

Neville MC, Keller R, Seacat J, et al. (1988): Am J Clin Nutr 48:375.

Nichols BL (1988): *In* Tsang RC, Nichols BL, eds: Nutrition during infancy. Philadelphia: Hanley and Belfus, p 367.

Ogra PL, Greene HL (1982): Pediatr Res 16:266.

Oski FA, Honig AS, Helu B, et al. (1983): Pediatrics 71:877.

Patton JS (1981): *In* Johnson LR, ed: Physiology of the gastrointestinal tract. New York: Raven Press, p 1123.

Pullan CR, Toms GL, Martin AG, Webb JKG, Appleton DR (1980): Br Med J 281:1034.

Raiha NCR (1974): Acta Paediatr Scand 53:147.

Raiha N, Minoli I, Moro G, Bremer HJ (1986): Acta Paediatr Scand 75:887.

Rassin DK, Raiha NCR, Minoli I, Moro G (1990): J Parent Ent Nutr 14:392.

Reeve LE, Chesney RW, DeLuca HF (1982): Am J Clin Nutr 36:122.

Richmond VL (1985): Am J Clin Nutr 41:129.

Roberts LJ, Shadwick CF, Bergstresser PR (1987): J Am Acad Dermatol 6:301.

Rose WC (1957): Nutr Abstr Rev 27:631.

Rubin DH, Leventhal JM, Krasilnikoff PA, Kuo HS, Jekel JF, Weile B, Levee A, Kurzon M, Berget A (1990): Pediatr 85:464.

Sahashi Y, Suzuki T, Higaki M, et al. (1969): J Vitaminol 15:78.

Salter RB (1970): Disorders and injuries of the musculoskeletal system. Baltimore: Williams & Wilkins, p 132.

Sanguansermsri J, Gyorgy P, Zilliken F (1974): Am J Clin Nutr 7:859.

Schofield WN, et al. (1985): Hum Nutr Clin Nutr 39(Suppl).

Scopes JW (1966): Br Med Bull 22:88.

Signer E, Murphy GM, Edkins S, et al. (1974): Arch Dis Child 49:174.

Smith NJ, Rios E (1974): Adv Pediatr 21:239.

Smith DW, Truog W, Rogers JE, Greitzer LJ, Skinner AL, McCann JJ (1976): J Pediatr 89:225.

Specker BL, Valanis B, Hertzberg V, et al. (1985): J Pediatr 107:372.

Subba RG (1984): Annu Rev Nutr 4:115.

Tanner JM (1986): *In* Falkner F, Tanner JM, eds: Human growth. New York: Plenum Press, Vol 1, p 167.

Taylor B, Wadsworth J, Golding J, Butler N (1982): Lancet 1:1227.

Tsang RC, Greer F, Steichen JJ (1981): Clin Perinatol 8:287.

Tyson JE, Laskey R, Flood D, et al. (1989): Pediatr 83:406.

Uauy R (1989): *In* Lebenthal E, ed: Textbook of gastroenterology and nutrition in infancy. New York: Raven, p 265.

Uauy R, Mayfield SR, Warshaw JB (1990a): *In* Oski IF, DeAngelis C, Feigin R, Warshaw J, eds: Principles and practice of pediatrics. Philadelphia: Lippincott, p 261.

Uauy R, Stringel G, Thomas R, et al. (1990b): J Pediatr Gastrcent Nutr 10:497.

Uauy R, Treen M, Hoffman DR (1989): Sem Perinatol 13:118.

Vazquez-Seoane S, Windom R, Pearson HA (1985): N Engl J Med 313:1239.

Viteri FE, et al., eds (1979): Food and Nutrition Bulletin, Suppl 1, Tokyo: United Nations University.

Vuori E, Kuitunen J (1979): Acta Paed Scand 68:33.

Walter T (1990): *In* Dobbing J, ed: Brain, behaviour and iron in the infant diet. New York: Springer-Verlag, p 133.

Watkins CJ, Leeder SR, Corkhill RT (1979): J Epidemiol Commun Health 33:180.

Webb AR, Holick MF (1988): Ann Rev Nutr 8:375.

Weinberg RJ, Tipton G, Klish WJ, et al. (1984): Pediatr 74:250.

Welsh JD, Poley JR, Bhatia M, et al. (1978): Gastroenterology 75:847.

Whitehead RG, Paul AA (1981): Lancet 2:161.

Whitehead RG, et al. (1981): J Hum Nutr 35:339.

WHO (1985a): Energy and protein requirements, report of a joint FAO/WHO/UNU expert consultation, Technical Series Report 724, p 12.

WHO (1985b): Ibid, p 92.

WHO (1985c): Ibid, p 121.

WHO (1985d): Ibid, p 103.

WHO (1985e): Ibid, p 99.

Widdowson EM (1981a): *In* Ritzen M, et al., eds: The biology of normal human growth. New York: Raven, p 253.

Widdowson EM (1981b): *In* Davis JA, Dobbing J, eds: Scientific foundation of pediatrics. London: Heinemann, p 330.

Yip R (1990): *In* Dobbing J, ed: Brain, behaviour and iron in the infant diet. New York: Springer-Verlag, p 27.

Yip R, Binkin NJ, Flashood L, Trowbridge FL (1987a): J Am Med Assoc 258:1619.

Yip R, Walsh KM, Goldfarb MG, Binkin NJ (1987b): Pediatr 80:330.

Young VR, Pelletier VA (1989): J Nutr 119:1799.

Zlotkin SH, Anderson GH (1982): Pediatr Res 16:65.

Lynne M. Ausman* and
Robert M. Russell*

12

Nutrition and the Elderly

Introduction

The increasing numbers of elderly and aged, especially in Western societies, presents new challenges to those concerned with their physical and emotional well-being. Little attention was paid to the role of nutrition and the aging process until about 10 years ago. This topic is of importance, however, for four major reasons:

1. Physiological function decreases with age and there is evidence that eventual physical deterioration in some organs may be associated with diet earlier in life (e.g., the putative role of diet in bone demineralization).
2. There are indications (drawn from epidemiologic studies and laboratory animal experimental studies) that early nutrition may influence the subsequent development of chronic age-related diseases, such as heart disease.
3. While there is good evidence that total energy needs diminish with age, it is not known whether other nutrient needs similarly decrease, remain the same, or increase with aging.
4. Many of the elderly *already* have a variety of conditions necessitating daily pharmaceutical treatment; the interaction of drugs and nutrients may play a major role in the nutrient needs of some elderly persons.

* U.S. Department of Agriculture, Human Nutrition Research Center on Aging, Tufts University, Boston, MA and School of Nutrition, Tufts University, Medford, MA.

Animal Models

Animal studies have yielded the strongest evidence yet that diet plays a major role in longevity and the aging process (see reviews by Guigoz and Munro, 1985; Masoro, 1985, 1989; Walford et al., 1987; and books by the National Research Council, 1981; Snyder, 1989; Weindruch and Walford, 1988).

The most consistent finding from experimental animal studies is that moderate dietary restriction markedly extends the lifespan of the experimental animals studied as compared to control animals fed ad libitum. This is true for nearly all species tested including invertebrates, fish, and homeothermic vertebrates such as mammals (Weindruch and Walford, 1988). The majority of the evidence, however, comes from studies with rodents. The earliest studies by McCay et al. (1935, 1939, 1943) in rats demonstrated that a restriction of total energy intake was associated with a longer lifespan. These findings were subsequently confirmed by other workers (Berg, 1960; Berg and Simms, 1960, 1961; Berg et al., 1962), who also noted a decrease in incidence of glomerulonephritis, cardiovascular changes, and tumors in animals fed the restricted diets.

Dietary restriction by selective removal of individual dietary nutrients (fat, carbohydrate, or protein) has also been accomplished. However, without a concomitant decrease in energy intake, little extension of lifespan is found. Specific restriction of dietary protein was first studied by

McCay et al. (1941) and more extensively by several other laboratories (Bras and Ross, 1964; Davis et al., 1983; Ross, 1959, 1961, 1972, 1976; Ross and Bras, 1971, 1973; Ross et al., 1970; Yu et al., 1984). Moderate protein restriction is often associated with a lower incidence of tumors (Ross, 1971; Ross and Bras, 1973; Weindruch and Walford, 1982) and certain types of kidney disease. Recent studies in mice (Gajjar et al., 1987), however, showed that moderate protein restriction with or without caloric restriction was not related to lifespan or the appearance of renal disease. Clearly, many factors including the species and/or strain of laboratory animal used are important variables in determining the outcome of these experiments.

Ad libitum fed diets adequate in protein but high in fat resulted in lifespans comparable or slightly shorter than those occurring when diets had carbohydrate as the primary energy source (Kubo et al., 1987). When energy restriction was imposed, however, lifespans of animals fed the carbohydrate diet were prolonged over those fed predominantly fat (threefold versus twofold with respect to animals fed ad libitum, respectively).

The effect of high fat diets fed either ad libitum or in restricted amounts has been exhaustively studied. High fat diets per se are associated with obesity, shortened lifespan (French et al., 1953), earlier appearance of tumors (Reddy et al., 1976), decreased cell-mediated immunity (Fernandes et al., 1973), and accelerated aging of collagen (Everitt et al., 1981). The composition of the fat and the amount of dietary antioxidants influence lifespan and tumor development; according to the free radical hypothesis, these variables may also play a role in aging (for review, see Harman, 1981, 1986).

The severity, age of initiation, and duration of the dietary perturbation play an important role in determining the eventual response to the dietary restriction (Weindruch et al., 1986). Most often, energy restriction implemented after weaning and continued through adulthood has prolonged life more than restriction begun in adulthood or imposed only for a short period during weaning (Barrows and Roeder, 1965; Friend et al., 1978; Nolen, 1972; Ross, 1972; Ross and Bras, 1971; Stuchlikova et al., 1975; Weindruch and Walford, 1982). However, a recent study (Yu et al., 1985) in Fischer 344 rats showed similar prolongation of life whether chronic calorie restriction was begun at 6 weeks or at 6 months of age.

By the end of the 1980s, dietary restriction research had extended to a search for mechanisms of action (e.g., how does dietary restriction prolong lifespan). The most common theories of aging are concerned with immunology, cellular proliferation, rate-of-living, rate of DNA repair, free radical damage, and rate of protein synthesis and catabolism. These theories as well as how dietary restriction affects aging and modulates each of the above mechanisms of aging are covered in detail in Weindruch and Walford (1988). Briefly, the restriction of total energy improves immune function, decreases rate of cellular proliferation, decreases basal metabolic rate (rate-of-living), prolongs capacity of cells to repair DNA, generates less free radicals (due to a lower rate-of-living), and increases protein synthesis and degradation rates (aging is associated with decreases in these functions). These are all changes that appear to correlate with a longer lifespan. As indicated above, individual nutrients also have effects on lifespan and may modulate the mechanisms of aging, at least to some extent. For example, increased levels of dietary antioxidants (ascorbic acid, α-tocopherol, retinol) may partially decrease cellular free radical concentrations. It is unclear whether any of these changes are related to the mechanism of aging and subsequent prolongation of life. It is also unclear whether mechanisms of aging operative for invertebrates or small mammals are relevant to aging in large animals and man that have a relatively long lifespan (Weindruch and Walford, 1988). For some organs and biologic systems, such as for sexual organs or the immune system, the dietary restriction not only delays the initial maturation of the system but also delays the decline in function at later ages.

Table 12.1 summarizes selected effects of dietary restriction on various tissue functions.

Nutritional Status of the Elderly

Dietary Intake and Biochemical Measures

The elderly are a diverse population and there are many special factors that may influence their dietary intake (Russell and Sahyoun, 1988). First, the elderly are a very heterogenous group of people with widely varying capabilities and levels of functioning. On the whole, the elderly are more likely to be in marginal nutritional health, and thus at higher risk for frank nutritional deficiency in time of stress or when beset by other healthcare problems. Physical, social, and emotional

Table 12.1. Effect of Dietary Restriction on Selected Biological Parameters

Slows the diminution of kidney function	Hayashida et al., 1986; Maeda et al., 1985; Tucker et al., 1976
Decreases obesity; retains adipocyte responsiveness to hormonal stimulation	Berg, 1960; Bertrand et al., 1980*a*, *b*; Cooper et al., 1977; Nolen, 1972; Voss et al., 1982; Yu et al., 1980
Delays age-associated increase in cholesterol and triglyceride	Liepa et al., 1980; Masoro et al., 1980
Delays age-related changes in connective tissue and muscle	Everitt and Porter, 1976; Herlihy and Yu, 1980; McCarter and McGee, 1987; Yu et al., 1982
Retains normal pancreatic function	Reaven and Reaven, 1981*a*, *b*
Decreases pituitary hormone secretion, possibly due to decreased hypothalamic function	Everitt and Porter, 1976
Delays decay in learning and motor function	Ingram et al., 1987
Delays decline in immune function as judged by T cell mediated immunity and thymus involution	Gerbase-Delima et al., 1975; Makinodan, 1977; Mann, 1978; Walford et al., 1974, 1975; Watson and Safranski, 1981; Weindruch et al., 1980; Weindruch and Suffin, 1980
Delays disease onset in autoimmune disease-prone mice	Dubois and Strain, 1973; Fernandes et al., 1976*a*, *b*, 1977, 1978; Friend et al., 1978; Gardner et al., 1977; Mann, 1978; Nandy, 1982; Weindruch et al., 1979, 1982

problems may interfere with appetite or may affect their ability to purchase, prepare, and consume an adequate diet. These factors are summarized in Table 12.2.

Several studies to determine dietary intakes and nutritional status of the elderly have been carried out over the last 20 years. These range from the nationwide NHANES I (1971–1974) and NHANES II (1976–1980), to several smaller studies of specific populations of free-living and institutionalized elderly (Attwood et al., 1978; Barr et al., 1983; Kohrs et al., 1978; McGandy et al., 1966; Prothro et al., 1976; Sahyoun et al., 1988; Stiedemann et al., 1978). Results obtained with dietary surveys are influenced by the sample population studied, the type of dietary instrument used, and the standards used for interpretation of the actual intake data.

Table 12.2. Factors That Influence Dietary Intake of the Elderly

Whether or not the person lives alone
How many daily meals are eaten
Who does the cooking and shopping
The presence of any physical impediments which would make cooking and shopping difficult
Problems in chewing and denture use
Alcohol and medication use
Whether there is adequate income to purchase the appropriate foods

Methodology of Diet History

Three instruments are currently in use: those involving dietary food records and those involving recall and food frequency questionnaires. The food record requires that an individual records current intake, either in household measures, or more accurately (and expensively) by weighing. Records are usually kept for 3–7 days. The food-recall technique seeks information on consumption for the previous 24-hr period but is particularly inappropriate for older persons with short-term memory problems. The food-frequency approach covers usual food consumption patterns for a whole year, including seasonal variations. All of these approaches should incorporate questions on the use of dietary supplements and alcohol. The various advantages and disadvantages of each method have been reviewed by Marr (1971), Campbell and Dodds (1967) and Block (1982). As demonstrated by Sahyoun and Rasmussen (1988), many variations of these methods tend to underestimate food intake. This is confounded by the fact that the actual food content of some nutrients (especially vitamin B_6, folate, zinc, and chromium) is not well-established.

Dietary Intake Standards

Standards used for interpretation of dietary data in the elderly range from the Recommended Dietary Allowances (RDAs, published by the National Research Council, 1989) in use at the time of the survey (or a percentage of the RDA) to special standards set up especially for a particular study. Since 1974, there have been separate RDAs for individuals 51 years of age or older.

Nutritional Status Surveys

O'Hanlon and Kohrs (1978) reviewed the design and results of 28 dietary surveys, which included data from the elderly. The mean calorie intake in each study was most often found to be below the standard utilized for each particular survey. The results of several large surveys available since that time (Lowenstein, 1982; National Center for Health Statistics, 1983; McGandy et al., 1986; Sahyoun et al., 1988; Garry et al., 1982*a*, *b*) indicate that mean energy intakes (kcal/kg/day) averaged 1792–2171 for males and 1168–1770 for females. These intakes are generally lower than the 1989 RDA of 2300 for males and 1900 kcal/day for females (presuming body weights of 77 kg for males and 65 kg for females). The low intakes may be attributable to the tendency of many methods to underestimate food intake or could reflect the fact that calorie intakes of sedentary individuals may indeed be lower than current estimates.

With respect to the macro- and micronutrients, the nutritional status of elderly people has been estimated by dietary intake and accompanying biochemical parameters. The average protein intakes in NHANES I and II (National Center for Health Statistics, 1982), as well as in other surveys of institutional and free-living elderly, were above the Tenth Edition RDA. Thus, protein nutriture, in the absence of chronic disease, appears to be adequate. In many studies, some serum proteins (albumin, transferrin, retinol-binding protein) appeared to decline with age (Yearick et al., 1980; Jansen and Harrill, 1977; Sahyoun et al., 1988). Often these changes did not correlate with protein intake and may represent normal decreases for the elderly (Munro et al., 1987*a*).

Among the water-soluble vitamins, assessment of vitamin B_6 nutriture and status is quite complex. On the one hand, several studies (McGandy et al., 1986; Sahyoun et al., 1988; Smith et al., 1984) show that vitamin B_6 intakes appear to be well below the RDA and that a fair proportion (6%–28%) of individuals exceeded what would be considered normal for erythrocyte aspartate aminotransferase stimulation tests (see Chapter 13). On the other hand, it is generally accepted that the reported low vitamin B_6 intake values would be somewhat higher if the food table values for vitamin B_6 (as well as for zinc, folate, and vitamin B_{12}) were more complete. Furthermore, as for any nutrient, it may be that current standards for biochemical tests of nutrient status are inappropriate for the elderly. Finally, inferences of deficiency based on biochemical tests should be tempered by the fact that the intraindividual variance in biochemical measures is large enough to account for a portion of the "deficiency" (Garry et al., 1989).

Based on both dietary intake and/or biochemical measures in the NHANES I and II studies as well as other studies (McGandy et al., 1986; Sahyoun et al., 1988; Webb et al., 1990), the evidence for low intakes of calcium and vitamin D appears to be the most substantial; these low intakes are attributable to the low intake of dairy products among certain groups of this population.

Average intakes of most other vitamins and minerals (with an adequate database) appear adequate, although in a few studies, biochemical tests indicate that levels may be low for thiamin, riboflavin, iron, and folate in 5%–20% of the people.

Supplement Use by the Elderly

In a study of elderly receiving "Meals-on-Wheels," 14 of 33 were considered at risk for protein-energy malnutrition (Lipschitz et al., 1985). Supplementation with a liquid polymeric supplement (containing protein and calories) (Ensure Plus) three times daily for 16 weeks increased weight in a majority of subjects. This weight gain was associated with increases in serum albumin, total iron binding capacity, folate, vitamin C, and vitamin B_{12}, thus providing evidence of a generally improved nutritional status.

Vitamin and mineral supplement use was examined as part of the nutritional status survey of free-living elderly in Boston (Hartz et al., 1988). Daily supplement use was reported by 45% of the males and 55% of the females; vitamins C and E were most common. Intakes of micronutrients from dietary sources alone were similar for those who used or did not use supplements. Use of the supplements markedly increased the proportion of individuals whose total daily intake (diet + supplement) was greater than two thirds of the RDA, in the case of vitamins B_6, B_{12}, and D, and folate and calcium. Some of the men and women, however, were observed to consume excessive

(≥10 × RDA) amounts of vitamin A, vitamin E, and thiamin. At least in the case of vitamin A, this could be harmful (see Chapter 5).

These results are consistent with those of other studies. In a study of 3192 elderly (Hale et al., 1982), vitamin supplement use was observed in 45.5% and 34% of the women and men, respectively. Mineral supplement use occurred about half as much. An even greater percent of vitamin-mineral supplementation (72%) was observed in the survey of an affluent community of "health conscious" residents (Gray et al., 1983). Interestingly, consumption of supplements was not related to intake of vitamins and minerals through diet alone.

The effect of supplements on vitamins A and E status was studied in detail in a group of free-living elderly (Krazinski et al., 1989). Serum levels of retinyl esters (storage form of vitamin A), but not retinol, were related to supplementary vitamin A intake. Supplementation with 1–2 times the 1989 RDA led to a 2.5-fold increase in retinyl esters as well as to increased plasma levels of hepatic aspartate aminotransferase, suggesting possible liver damage and vitamin A overload among supplement users. This observation underscores the importance of understanding not only minimal nutritional requirements but toxicities and safety margins for the elderly, since tolerances are not necessarily the same as for young to middle-aged adults.

Anthropometric Measures

Body weight. The association of obesity, as estimated by body weight (and a variety of other techniques) with increased morbidity and mortality is well-known (Build Study, 1979; Garrison et al., 1983; Manson et al., 1987; Metropolitan Insurance Company, 1983; Simopoulos and Van Itallie, 1984). The pattern of distribution of body fat (higher risk with increased waist to hip girth) may also be a factor in the excess morbidity and mortality (Kissebah et al., 1982; Krotkiewski et al., 1983; Lapidus et al., 1984; Larsson et al., 1984). However, since few body weight standards specific for the elderly are currently in use (Russell et al., 1984), determination of their "true" degree of obesity has been problematic. One of the earliest standards developed was based on the accumulated body weight data of 5600 men and women, aged 65 through 94 years, who lived in the community and reported on an ambulatory basis to their doctors (Master and Lasser, 1960). More recent data are available on elderly up through age 74 (from the NHANES I and II studies). From these, Frisancho (1984) has established body weight standards for persons aged 25–54 years and 55–74 years, for sex, age, height, and frame size using elbow breadth as an estimate of frame size (Frisancho and Flegel, 1983). The latter standards are consistent with data based on the Baltimore Longitudinal Aging Study (Andres, 1985; Andres et al., 1985). Since body mass index (kg/m^2) was found to be about 22.5 for both sexes (in NHANES I and II and in several other studies), the summary tables of Frisancho (1984) have been prepared in weight ranges according to height and age but not by gender.

The Metropolitan Life Tables (Metropolitan Insurance Company, 1983), based on people aged 25–59, do not account for possible changes in body weight and height with age, and are thus probably not useful for the elderly. Moreover, they are based on a biased sample of the general population since they represent the experience of the insurance industry. Furthermore, the conclusion of the Build study (1979), that there was less mortality in those elderly with a body mass index greater than that calculated from the Metropolitan Life Tables, indicates that these standards are not accurate or desirable to use after the age of 59. Therefore, we recommend that the Metropolitan Life Tables be used up to age 59 and the NHANES medians thereafter. Some groups (e.g., black women) show a high frequency of obesity.

The degree of obesity or malnutrition in an individual or population has also been calculated from relationships of weight to height. Body mass index (kg/m^2) was used in the institutionalized study in Boston (Sahyoun et al., 1988) to identify obesity. Using the 85th percentile of Body Mass Index in the NHANES I study, a total of 38 of 250 individuals (15.2%) were found to be obese. Both male and female elderly 80+ years of age had a lower body weight than those between 60 and 79 years of age.

Other anthropometric standards. Anthropometric data other than body weight or height (e.g., triceps skinfold) have been used in other surveys to assess the nutritional status of populations (Chumlea et al., 1989; National Center for Health Statistics, 1987; Vir and Love, 1980) and to predict prognosis in the hospital and monitor responses to treatment (Blackburn and Thornton, 1979).

It is accepted that lean body mass declines and body fat stores increase with aging (Forbes, 1976;

see Chapter 1). Body fat is stored subcutaneously in the young but may be deposited intraabdominally and intramuscularly in the elderly (Cohn et al., 1981). Other studies have shown a 40% loss of lean body mass for those over 70 years of age in comparison with young adults (Korenchevsky, 1961).

These changes in body composition should theoretically be reflected in changes of various anthropometric measurements (such as triceps skinfold, midarm circumference, midarm muscle area, and arm muscle circumference), which have been utilized in several investigations of the elderly (Chumlea et al., 1986; Frisancho, 1981; Heymsfield et al., 1982*a*, *b*; Kemm and Allcock, 1984; Mitchell and Lipschitz, 1982). (See Chapter 13 for descriptions of these measures). The standard for obesity of the elderly in the NHANES I and II studies was a triceps skinfold of ≥85% of the median measure in the 20- to 29-year-old groups. By this standard, elderly men were less likely to be obese (at 5%–11%) than elderly women (19%–36%). However, extensive studies by Cohn et al. (1981) demonstrated that body fat contents calculated from triceps skinfold measurements only agreed well with other (better) measures of body fat in the case of young adults (age 20–29), and that there was a discrepancy of 15%–20% in estimates of body fat (based on such measurements) in men and women more than 70 years of age. McEvoy and James (1982) found changes in such correlations in females, but not males, with age. Thus, triceps skinfold thickness cannot accurately be used in the elderly to predict body fat content, and midarm muscle circumference (which is derived from it) is probably also not useful.

Biological Changes in Organ Function During Aging

A decline in organ function normally accompanies the aging process, especially in older individuals. As much as possible, it is important to distinguish between changes in function attributable to age and those that are due to disease. Many changes occurring "normally" with age would be expected to influence nutrient needs, especially when associated with the digestive tract (Rosenberg et al., 1982; Thompson and Keelan, 1986). Table 12.3 reviews documented

Table 12.3. Changes in Organ Function with Aging That May Influence Nutrient Status[a]

Organ function	Physical change	Importance to nutrition
Taste and smell	Decreased taste buds; decreased papilla on tongue; decrease in taste and olfactory nerve endings; change in taste and smell threshold	Loss of ability to detect salt and sweet; decreased palatability causing poor food intake
Saliva secretion	Saliva flow may be reduced	Doubtful clinical significance
Esophageal function and swallowing	Minor changes including disordered contractions and spontaneous gastroesophageal reflux	Doubtful clinical significance
Gastric function and emptying	Decreased secretion of HCL, IF, and pepsin in 20% of healthy population >60 years of age (atrophic gastritis); rapid rate of emptying of liquids, increased proximal small bowel pH, bacterial overgrowth in bowel	Decreased bioavailability of mineral, vitamins, and proteins; decreased absorption of protein bound vitamin B_{12} and folate; increase in bacterial folate synthesis to counteract malabsorption
Liver and biliary function	Minor structural and biochemical changes; activity and drug metabolizing enzymes reduced	Rate of albumin synthesis may be decreased; drug dosages may need to be lower
Pancreatic secretion	Slightly lower bicarbonate and enzyme outputs	Doubtful clinical significance
Intestinal morphology and function	Insignificant or no changes in small bowel morphology	Doubtful clinical significance
Intestinal microflora	Bacterial overgrowth in proximal small bowel	Functional significance unknown; influences supply of water-soluble vitamins and vitamin K

[a] Taken from Rosenberg et al. (1989).

changes in the digestive tract, as well as changes in other organs that may reasonably be expected to affect nutrient requirements.

Nutrient Requirements in Aging

Munro et al. (1987*a*) and Munro (1989) recently summarized our knowledge of nutritional requirements of the elderly. It is widely expected that these may differ from those of young adults, because of changes in organ function (see above), diminished energy needs, and changes in dietary patterns. For example, in one study of healthy Bostonians over the age of 60, 20% were found to have decreased hydrochloric acid secretion in their stomachs (atrophic gastritis) (Krasinski et al., 1986). This resulted in a more rapid rate of emptying of liquids, an increase in proximal small bowel pH (Russell et al., 1986), and an overgrowth of bacteria in the small bowel. These changes could be expected to affect the bioavailability of certain vitamins (folate and vitamin B_{12}), several minerals (iron, calcium, copper, zinc), and protein.

Macronutrients

Energy. Several studies have documented a decreased need for energy by the elderly (James et al., 1989). In a sample of males, the Baltimore Longitudinal Study of Aging found that energy needs decreased from 2700 kcal/day at age 30 years to 2100 kcal/day for those around 80. Two thirds of this reduction was attributable to a decrease in physical activity and, to a lesser extent, to a decrease in basal metabolism (McGandy et al., 1966). These findings have generally been supported by other studies. In NHANES II, young men, aged 24–34, were shown to consume 2700 kcal/day, whereas older men, aged 65–74, consumed 1800 kcal/day. Energy consumption of women fell from 1600–1300 kcal over this age span. Thus, the recommended energy intake from the Tenth Recommended Dietary Allowances is 2300 kcal for the reference 77 kg elderly male and 1900 kcal for the reference 65 kg female 51+ years of age; in both cases, the new RDA for energy is 30 kcal/kg/day, reduced from an earlier RDA of 33–34 kcal/kg/day. After age 75, averages for both sexes are somewhat further reduced. Much of the variation in estimation of energy needs is due to the variability of measuring techniques. A new laboratory method using excretion of administered ${}^{2}H_2{}^{18}O$ may be instrumental in allowing calculation of actual energy consumption of the healthy elderly (Prentice et al., 1985).

Fat. On diets containing average fat levels ($\approx$100 g), the efficiency of fat absorption by the elderly is equivalent to that of young adults (Arora et al., 1989); at higher dietary levels, the elderly showed slightly more fecal fat than the young adults. Other studies have confirmed that the elderly have only a minimally decreased capacity for fat digestion (94.7% versus 96.4%) (Southgate and Durnin, 1970). However, the institutionalized elderly occasionally have fecal fat levels of up to 20% of fecal dry weight (Pelz et al., 1968). One of the most common causes of fat malabsorption in the elderly is bacterial overgrowth of the small intestine, which interferes with the deconjugation of bile salts and thus their detergent function and reabsorption. The presence of increased dietary fiber in many elderly diets could also be a confounding factor. Chylomicron appearance in blood, after a 100 g fat meal, was slower in the elderly than in young adults. However, a slower gastric emptying time (with subsequent slower lipid hydrolysis) may have produced this result (Webster et al., 1977).

There are no recommended dietary allowances for daily fat. However, it is widely felt that a prudent diet, with 30% or less of calories as fat (10% saturated, 10% monounsaturated, and 10% polyunsaturated fatty acids), is just as important in the elderly as in young adults for prevention of chronic diseases, such as heart disease, and for provision of adequate amounts of essential fatty acids.

Protein. As judged by an increased fecal nitrogen content in response to load (Werner and Hambraeus, 1972), high protein diets may be less well-digested and absorbed in the elderly. However, little quantitative information is available.

The Recommended Dietary Allowances recommends 0.8 g protein/kg body weight per day, an amount which is adequate for the elderly when excessive energy intakes are fed (i.e., $\geq$40 kcal/kg/day) (Cheng et al., 1978). However, when the energy intake is decreased to 30 kcal/kg/day, an amount more usual for the elderly, nitrogen balance may not be obtained in more than half the elderly subjects tested (Gersovitz et al., 1982; Uauy et al., 1978). The degree of adaptation of the individual to the lower energy or lower protein intake before an actual experimental trial begins (Munro et al., 1987b) may account for many of the discrepancies in apparent nitrogen needs (or balance) reported in the literature. The most recent studies in physically active young (26.8 ± 1.2 years of age) and middle-aged (52.0 ± 1.9 years) men estimates a mean protein requirement at 0.94 g/kg for both groups, suggesting an RDA greater than the current standard of 0.8 g/kg/day (Meredith et al., 1989). Thus, the current RDA may not be sufficient for elderly who are very active. The age-related erosion of lean muscle mass occurs at such a slow rate that it is difficult, if not impossible, to determine experimentally whether or not any special dietary treatments might influence this process in the short term. The average protein consumption among the free-living elderly in Boston was 1.05 g/kg/day with no evidence that lower intakes were correlated with protein-energy malnutrition (Munro et al., 1987a). Therefore, a daily intake of 1 g/kg (and probably less) will probably meet the needs of this population. A thorough review of protein needs during aging is found in Munro (1989).

Carbohydrate. Most studies indicate that carbohydrate absorption (measured with mannitol, xylose, or 3-O-methyl glucose) is slightly impaired with advancing age. However, decreased renal function is also thought to be involved (Arora et al., 1989; Beaumont et al., 1987; Guth, 1968), as many of these diagnostic tests depend on efficient urinary excretion of the test carbohydrate. Using another approach, Feibusch and Holt (1982) measured breath hydrogen in response to a 100–200 g carbohydrate challenge to estimate carbohydrate malabsorption in subjects 65–89 years of age and found it was increased. However, increased H_2 excretion could result from increased bacterial enzyme activity in the small bowel (as in atrophic gastritis) as well as from increased activity of the colonic microflora (in the presence of unabsorbed carbohydrate). Therefore, the increased breadth hydrogen found in the elderly is not necessarily due to malabsorption of carbohydrate. Lactase activity decreases with age, especially in early life, but other brush border hydrolase activities appear to remain fairly constant (Welsh et al., 1974, 1978). Many elderly tend to avoid the consumption of milk products (which are an excellent source of riboflavin, vitamin D, and calcium) because of the bloating and discomfort of lactose intolerance.

No RDA has been set for dietary carbohydrate. However, the USDA, American Heart Association, and American Cancer Society, among others, are recommending that for all adults (including the elderly) dietary carbohydrate be 55%–60% of calories, with a high proportion of complex over simple sugars.

Minerals

Calcium. The lifelong pattern of calcium intake is widely thought to influence the degree of osteoporosis in the elderly (Becker and Heaney, 1989). Intestinal calcium absorption in both men and women decreases with age (Bullamore et al., 1970; Gallagher et al., 1979). Moreover, the achlorhydria observed in some elderly would be expected to decrease calcium absorption by keeping it less available. Gallagher et al. (1979) studied 94 normal volunteers (aged 30–90) and 52 untreated women with postmenopausal osteoporosis. Fractional calcium absorption decreased with age in these subjects, and did not correlate with calcium intake. In another study, Ireland and Fordtran (1973) showed that the elderly were less able to adapt to a low calcium diet (by enhancing absorption or decreasing urinary excretion) than were the young adults studied. Decreased vitamin D intake and activation in the elderly are widely thought to be partially responsible for the decreased calcium absorption that has been observed (see section on Vitamin D below).

Average calcium intakes for women were about 500 mg/day in the NHANES I and II studies, well below the current RDA of 800 mg/day. In Yugoslavia, Matkovic et al. (1979) showed that metacarpal cortical thickness was greater in a population which routinely consumed 1100 mg calcium/day as compared to a population with a typically low calcium intake (500 mg/day). Although bone loss progressed with age in both groups, the rate of hip fracture was higher in the population with the low calcium intake, suggesting a relationship to impaired bone strength. In a recent study, spinal bone loss in healthy postmenopausal elderly was less in women consuming more than 777 mg calcium/day as compared to those consuming less than 405 mg/day (Dawson-Hughes et al., 1987). One consensus conference on osteoporosis (Spencer and Kramer, 1986) has recommended an intake of 1500 mg/day to ensure adequate calcium absorption. However, a recent study (Dawson-Hughes et al., 1990) showed that calcium supplementation in excess of a total daily intake of 800 mg/day provided no additional benefit. (See also Osteoporosis, Chapter 6).

Iron. Most evidence indicates that, in general, iron absorption does not decline significantly with age (Bunker et al., 1984), although in one study, red cell incorporation of absorbed intestinal iron was reduced by about one third (Marx, 1979). Some individuals do, nevertheless, develop iron deficiency. Inadequate iron intake, blood loss due to chronic disease, and reduced nonheme iron absorption secondary to the hypo- or achlorhydria (from atrophic gastritis) are thought to be responsible (Lynch et al., 1982). The average iron intakes of the elderly men and women in the NHANES I and II studies were 14 and 10 mg/day, respectively (Pilch and Senti, 1984*b*), thus being at or above the 10 mg/day RDA. A 4% prevalence of anemia in men was attributable to chronic disease; iron-deficiency anemia without complicating factors was rare for women. The current RDA for the elderly, therefore, seems adequate.

Zinc. Isotopic studies suggest that zinc absorption decreases with age (Turnlund et al., 1986). Since data from several studies (Garry et al., 1982*a*; Pilch and Senti, 1984*a*) also indicate that the elderly are consuming much less than is recommended (10 mg for men and 7 mg for women, as compared with a 15 mg RDA), a decreased absorptive capacity is likely to make things even worse. There are conflicting data in the literature indicating normal or decreased plasma zinc concentrations in the elderly (Jacob et al., 1985; Sandstead et al., 1982). However, the significance of any decrease in plasma zinc levels is difficult to ascertain since serum zinc decreases in inflammatory (and other) conditions, and diagnosis of zinc deficiency is problematic. Zinc enzyme levels or tissue concentrations available for sampling in humans (blood, urine, feces, hair) respond very little to marginal or zinc deficiency. (See Chapters 7 and 13).

Copper. Copper absorption in the elderly is similar to that of young adults (Turnlund et al., 1982), as determined by isotope studies. As for other minerals, the absorption of copper can be affected by the presence of an excess of some other trace minerals and factors in the diet (see Chapter 7). One recent study suggests that only 1.1 mg of copper may be necessary for copper balance (Gibson et al., 1985), an amount below the usual intake of 2–3 mg (also the RDA) observed in the elderly.

Other trace minerals. Information on the nutritional status and requirement of the elderly with respect to a variety of ultra-trace minerals has been summarized by Yunice and Hsu (1984) and Mertz et al. (1989). Although fragmentary, there is some evidence to suggest that intakes of some of these (e.g., selenium, chromium, and silicon) may be suboptimal.

Vitamins

In recent reviews of vitamin requirements of the elderly, Suter and Russell (1987, 1989) indicate that low to inadequate dietary intakes may account for much of the poor vitamin nutriture observed. Physiological changes associated with the aging gut may, in addition, alter vitamin absorption, thereby influencing (positively or negatively) total dietary vitamin requirements. Table 12.4 lists the major water- and fat-soluble vitamins, the current RDA or Safe and Adequate Daily Dietary Intake, along with an assessment of whether or not the current recommendation is adequate, or may be too high or too low for the elderly. A discussion of certain individual vitamins follows in the paragraphs below; for some vitamins there were insufficient or conflicting data to make this assessment.

Thiamin. Thiamin requirements are linked to overall caloric intake. The current U.S. RDA for the elderly for thiamin is 1.2 mg/day for males and 1.0 mg/day for females, and, when corrected for caloric consumption, should not decrease below 0.5 mg/1000 kcal. The NHANES I and II data indicated that the mean intake was above this amount, although some 3%–8% of women and men were ingesting less than 0.5 mg/1000 kcal. Aging appears to be associated with an increased erythrocyte transketolase-activation coefficient in 3%–25% of normal, free-living elderly (Iber et al., 1982). It is unclear whether such an increase is a normal event in aging or represents nutritional inadequacy. Data on changes in absorption of thiamin with age are not consistent (Thomson, 1966; Breen et al., 1985). Probably the major cause of thiamin deficiency in the elderly is alcoholism accompanied by a too low thiamin intake; for most well elderly, however, the RDA for thiamin appears to be covering their needs.

Riboflavin. The current RDA for riboflavin for the elderly is 1.4 mg/day for males and 1.2 mg/day for females. Deficiency of riboflavin, as diag-

Table 12.4. Estimate of Adequacy of 1989 RDA for Vitamins for the Elderly[a]

Vitamin	Current RDA for age 51+[b]	Adequacy of RDA for elderly	Physiological reason for change
Thiamin	1–1.2 mg	Adequate	—
Riboflavin	1.2–1.4 mg	Adequate	—
Niacin	13–15 mg	I/C data[c]	—
Vitamin B_6	1.6–2.0 mg	May be too low	Nonresponse to B_6 supplements in normal range suggests altered absorption or metabolism
Folate	180–200 μg	Adequate	—
Vitamin B_{12}	2.0 μg	May be too low	Atrophic gastritis and competition from bacterial overgrowth reduce B_{12} availability
Ascorbate	60 mg	Adequate	—
Biotin	30–100 μg[d]	I/C data	—
Pantothenic	4–7 mg[d]	I/C data	—
Vitamin A	800–1000 μg RE	May be too high	Thinner or change in unstirred water layer may lead to increased absorption in elderly; decreased uptake by the liver of newly absorbed vitamin A
Vitamin D	5 μg	May be too low	Lack of sun exposure, reduced vitamin D synthesis in skin and impaired renal 1-α-hydroxylation suggest that dietary requirement might be higher
Vitamin E	8–10 mg	I/C data	—
Vitamin K	65–80 μg[d]	I/C data	—

[a] Taken from Suter and Russell (1987).
[b] RDA for female–male elderly 51+ years of age.
[c] Insufficient or conflicting data.
[d] Safe and adequate daily dietary intake.

nosed by an increase in the erythrocyte glutathione reductase activity coefficient (Chen and Fan Chiang, 1981; Harrill and Cervone, 1977) or decrease in urinary riboflavin excretion (Suter and Russell, 1987), was most often associated with low dietary intakes of riboflavin. There is little evidence for altered absorption of the vitamin (Said and Hollander, 1985), or of altered tissue concentrations with age (Schaus and Kirk, 1957), so that current dietary recommendations should cover the elderly.

Ascorbic acid. Ascorbic acid (vitamin C) is considered one of the chief dietary antioxidants and may play a role in preventing aging. The current RDA for vitamin C for the elderly is 60 mg/day for both men and women. Although vitamin C is widely abundant in many foods, levels of intake in the elderly vary widely. Vitamin C nutriture is adversely affected by factors such as smoking, medications, and emotional and environmental stress (Pelletier, 1975; Sahud and Cohen, 1971). The functional significance of age-related declines in leukocyte and plasma vitamin C levels observed is unclear (Kirk and Chieffi, 1953a; Loh, 1972). Maintenance of the plasma level at 1.0 mg/dl would require, by extrapolation, 75 mg/day for females and 150 mg/day for males (Garry et al., 1982), although there is no evidence that a saturation of the body pool is optimal or desirable in this age group. There is little evidence that vitamin C absorption changes with aging, and reports of changes in tissue concentration with age have not been consistent (Kirk and Chieffi, 1953b; Cheng et al., 1985). Therefore, there is no evidence that vitamin C requirements per se increase with aging.

Niacin. The current RDA for the elderly for this vitamin is 15 mg/day for males and 13 for females, the same as for young adults. A low excretion of urinary N-methyl nicotinamide is most often associated with poor niacin intakes, or with extreme illness or old age. Otherwise, there is little (if any) evidence that niacin requirements change with age (Suter and Russell, 1987).

Vitamin B_6. Since the B_6 content of many foods is not known, reported dietary intakes vary widely and may be underestimates. Nevertheless, serum and plasma B_6 levels in the elderly show a decreasing trend with age. Studies, indicating poor B_6 nutriture based on activity coefficient tests, show that with moderate oral supplementation, some activity coefficients still do not return to normal (Vir and Love, 1977). The current RDA for vitamin B_6 in the elderly is 2.0 mg/day for men and 1.6 for women. However, a study investigating vitamin B_6 requirements of the elderly has just been completed in this laboratory (Ribaya-Mercado et al., 1991). Based on plasma pyridoxal phosphate concentrations, 24-hr urinary xanthurenic acid excretion after a tryptophan load test, and urinary pyridoxic acid excretion, average requirements in both males and females were about 2.0 mg/day. Therefore, recommendations for intakes of vitamin B_6 by the elderly may have to be revised upward by at least 15%.

Folate. Despite a low intake of folate, only 3%–7% of persons in NHANES I (Senti and Pilch, 1984) or among the free-living elderly (Rosenberg et al., 1982) had low serum folate concentrations (i.e., <3.0 ng/ml). In a Swedish study of 35 elderly subjects (Jagerstad and Westesson, 1979), an intake of only 100–200 μg/day brought whole-blood folate concentrations back to normal. Furthermore, although atrophic gastritis can cause folate malabsorption by increasing the pH of the upper small intestine, this is more than offset by the production, availability, and absorption of folate from bacteria overgrowing the small intestine. The current RDA for the elderly is 200 μg/day for men and 180 μg/day for women. Since it is believed that most current methodology to measure the total folate content of food underestimates actual content, real intakes and requirements may prove to be somewhat greater (as suggested in the Ninth Edition of the RDA in 1980).

Vitamin B_{12}. Serum or plasma vitamin B_{12} levels in the elderly are often found to be low (Bailey et al., 1980; Elwood et al., 1971; Garry et al., 1984; Magnus et al., 1982). Low intake of vitamin B_{12}, especially among the poor elderly, and impaired absorption of dietary B_{12} may be responsible. Although atrophic gastritis partially reduces the secretion of intrinsic factor, thereby decreasing B_{12} absorption, this mechanism does not seem to account for the low serum levels. Instead, decreased digestive release of vitamin B_{12} from food, and bacterial overgrowth in the small bowel leading to competition with intestinal cells for B_{12}, are the factors most responsible (Russell, 1986). It may be concluded that the current RDA of 2.0 μg/day is sufficient for most elderly but may be too low for those with atrophic gastritis.

Vitamin A. Although vitamin A is not distributed widely in foods, excess daily intake is stored in the liver (see Chapter 5). Thus, individuals obtain what they need by consuming rich food sources only occasionally. It follows that data obtained from 24-hr recalls cannot give valid estimates. Vitamin A tolerance curves show higher serum retinyl ester levels in the elderly as compared to young adults (Krasinski et al., 1989). More recently, this was shown to be due to reduced clearance (57 versus 31 min) in the elderly of the lipid-rich lipoproteins carrying the retinyl esters (Krasinzki et al., 1990). Carotenes, the vitamin A precursors derived from plant pigments, are an important source of vitamin A and, in addition, may have a beneficial effect in terms of cancer prevention. Thus, although the RDA for the elderly for preformed vitamin A may be lower, it would be prudent to continue to ingest adequate amounts of carotene-containing fruits and vegetables.

Vitamin D. Since vitamin D is found only in a few foods (which include sea food and fortified milk products), it is not surprising that over three quarters of the elderly have vitamin D intakes that are less than two thirds of the RDA. The contribution of sunlight to the vitamin D status of the elderly is also reduced since the elderly receive less sun exposure and have a decreased efficiency of vitamin D synthesis in the skin (MacLaughlin and Holick, 1985). In institutionalized subjects with little access to sunlight exposure, the diet tends not to provide sufficient vitamin D. Supplements of an additional 10 μg (400 IU/day) maintain serum 25-OH-D levels in the normal range (>37.5 nmol/L) (Webb et al., 1990).

In a study of 146 normal and osteoporotic women (Gallagher et al., 1979), calcium absorption decreased with age. Although serum 25-OH-D levels were not decreased in the elderly subjects, those of the active vitamin (1,25-$(OH)_2$-D) were significantly lower, suggesting a reduced conversion of 25-OH-D (see Chapter 5). As in younger people, there was also a significant correlation between serum levels of 1,25-$(OH)_2$-D and intestinal calcium absorption. Elderly patients with osteoporosis had less circulating 1,25-$(OH)_2$-D and decreased calcium absorption compared to normal elderly subjects. Since in some of the elderly the renal 1-α-hydroxylase enzyme appears to be impaired with aging, there may be an argument for including higher amounts of vitamin D in the diet. [By providing additional 25-OH-D substrate, there is evidence this can increase production of the 1,25-$(OH)_2$-D form]. Currently, low-dose supplementation with 10 μg vitamin D/day (twice the RDA) is recommended, to assure at least an adequate availability of the vitamin to the elderly that are homebound or in nursing homes.

Vitamin E. As for vitamin C, the antioxidative properties of vitamin E (tocopherol) may play a role in retarding the aging process. The 1989 RDA for the elderly for vitamin E (expressed as mg of α-tocopherol equivalents) is 10 mg/day for males and 8 for females. Intakes in most populations are reported to be adequate although 40% of the dietary intakes of the free-living population of Garry et al. (1982*a*) were receiving less than <75% of the RDA. (One third of this population took vitamin E supplements.) Since the plasma α-tocopherol is carried passively by the lipid-rich lipoproteins (VLDL and LDL), changes in plasma lipid concentrations with age could influence apparent vitamin E status (Horwitt et al., 1972; Kelleher and Losowsky, 1978). Therefore, it is probably most accurate to express the vitamin E concentration in relation to blood lipid content (Davies et al., 1969). On this basis, there was no relation between the plasma vitamin E–lipid ratio and age in a study by Vatassery et al. (1983). Data examining tissue concentrations (platelets, liver, adrenal glands, heart) of vitamin E with age have been inconsistent, and there is no evidence of an increased need for vitamin E with age based on the erythrocyte hemolysis test (Suter and Russell, 1987). Finally, there is no evidence for an altered vitamin E absorption with aging (Kelleher and Losowsky, 1978). However, due to its antioxidative properties, further studies investigating the role of this vitamin in relation to aging retardation, and the amount which should be recommended for the elderly, are of the utmost importance.

Vitamin K. Little information is available on the vitamin K status of the healthy elderly. Only within the last 10 years has the biochemical methodology been available to measure vitamin K metabolites in the plasma (for a recent example, see Haroon et al., 1987).

With this methodology, it has been possible to show that serum phylloquinone levels vary as a function of gender, age, and serum lipid levels. When expressed per mmol of triglyceride, plasma phylloquinone concentrations in young subjects were 0.82×10^{-6} mmol and those in the elderly 0.62×10^{-6} mmol (Sadowski et al., 1989). The nutritional significance of this decrease in the elderly, if any, is not yet understood. The 1989 RDA for vitamin K for the elderly is 80 μg/day for men and 65 for women.

Drug–Nutrient Interactions

The general subject of drug–nutrient interactions is covered in the last chapter of this book and has been reviewed elsewhere (Roe, 1989). Some considerations and examples particularly relevant to the elderly are briefly covered here.

Various components of the diet are known to influence (accentuate or attenuate) a drug's actions. Nutrients can affect drug action by altering the digestion, absorption, distribution, metabolism, and/or excretion of the drug. A common example of this is the avoidance of milk-product consumption concurrently with tetracycline therapy (see Chapter 19). Less often recognized is that drugs may influence nutritional status. This is particularly important to consider in the elderly who often have multiple chronic diseases and are taking several medications or drugs concurrently. The risk of adverse side effects increases with the number of drugs taken simultaneously and with the duration of drug exposure. Drugs may exhibit their effects on nutritional status through several avenues: effects on food intake, alteration of nutrient absorption, alteration of nutrient metabolism, and alteration in nutrient excretion (Blumberg, 1986).

Mechanisms of Drug–Nutrient Interaction

Food intake. Drugs are known to affect food intake through changes in appetite, taste, smell, and/or fear of adverse clinical symptoms.

Alteration of nutrient absorption. Drugs most commonly impair the absorption of the nutrient from the intestinal lumen by altering either the intestinal milieu (e.g., antacid use decreases the acidity of the small bowel) or by affecting the mucosal cell responsible for the absorption (e.g., laxative abuse may damage the intestinal mucosa and destroy the structure of the microvilli). A variety of other mechanisms have also been elucidated (Blumberg, 1985; Chapter 19). The resultant adverse effect on nutrient absorption may be specific for one or two nutrients or may be a generalized failure of absorption for a whole class of nutrients. However, few studies have been performed in which this has been examined in the elderly.

In a study of 682 free-living elderly, individuals were classified with respect to use of antacid during the preceding year (41% of the males and 36% of the females) (Otradovec et al., 1986). About 10% of the users were classified as heavy users (4–7 times per week during the last week). Calcium containing antacids were associated with significantly decreased levels of serum phosphorus and chloride, magnesium-containing antacids with decreased serum chloride and increased serum magnesium, and aluminum-containing antacids with decreased serum zinc and chloride but increased magnesium. Magnesium- and aluminum-containing antacids also were significantly correlated with decreased HDL cholesterol and increased VLDL cholesterol. These responses suggest an impact of antacids on the nutrient status of the major minerals.

Alteration of nutrient metabolism. Several drugs are known to interfere with the metabolism of specific nutrients. Often, the drugs are known to inhibit an enzyme key to the proper function or use of the nutrient. As an example, Trimethoprim inhibits dihydrofolate reductase activity; thus, persons using this drug can develop megaloblastic anemia through induced folic acid deficiency.

Alteration of nutrient excretion. Tetracycline is known to increase the urinary excretion of vitamin C. Thus, prolonged and/or excessive use of this drug may increase the individual's requirement for the vitamin. Examples of potential nutrient deficiencies (or toxicities) which may develop secondary to drug usage or treatment are listed in Chapter 19.

Alcohol and Nutritional Status in the Elderly

Alcohol is one of the most common drugs used by the population at large. In moderate to large amounts, it is known to adversely affect nutritional status at all levels, including reducing appetite, and impairing nutrient absorption, metabolism, and excretion. It is also associated with the serious problems of hepatic cirrhosis, adenocarcinoma of the mouth, esophagus, gastrointestinal tract and liver, and driving to endanger. However, most elderly individuals consume alcohol in only small amounts. In a survey of 554 nonalcoholic elderly in the Boston area, alcohol use was classified as <5 g/day, 5–14 g/day or 15+ g/day (Jacques et al., 1988). The relation of alcohol intake to nutritional, biochemical, and physical parameters was then assessed. Plasma retinol, ferritin, and HDL cholesterol concentrations were significantly increased and serum copper, zinc, and potassium were significantly decreased in the high versus low alcohol-intake groups. The (statistically significant) effects were small, however, and, therefore, of questionable biological significance; the effects of alcohol on potassium and copper were observed only in patients using diuretics. In conclusion, small to moderate alcohol use would appear to have no major effects on the nutritional status of a nonalcoholic population.

Summary

In advanced age, fewer calories (i.e., less food) are eaten due to the acquisition of a more sedentary lifestyle. With less intake of food, the amounts of certain nutrients consumed may fall below critical levels and, thus, may place the older person at risk of specific nutrient deficiencies. However, in the United States and Western Europe, food supplies are varied enough so that the nutritional status of free-living older people is generally satisfactory. Nevertheless, there are specific groups of elderly people (e.g., the ill, homebound, institutionalized) that show a high prevalence of malnutrition. It should be recognized that malnutrition in aging is not so much related to age or institutionalization per se as it is to chronic illness, depression, dementia, and lack of mobility. The micronutrients that seem to be most problematic for the elderly person living in the United States are calcium, vitamin D, vitamin B_6, and vitamin B_{12}, in that higher intakes of these nutrients may be required by the elderly person to satisfactorily meet his or her metabolic needs. It is possible that the intake of certain nutrients (e.g., antioxidants such as vitamin E, vitamin C, and beta carotene) play a role in "slowing" the aging process by preventing lipid peroxidation and membrane damage. However, whether these effects can be seen when physiologic levels of these vitamins are eaten or only when they are ingested at pharmacologic levels (e.g., in massive doses) is in need of study. Also, in need of study is the area of drug–nutrient interactions, where relatively little detailed work has been carried out in the human. The entire area of nutrition and aging is rapidly evolving and should be followed carefully by the reader, since the recommendations and predictions made in this chapter will likely change quickly over the ensuing years as new information becomes available.

References

Andres R (1985): *In* Andres R, Bierman E, Hazzard W, eds: Principles of geriatric medicine. New York: McGraw-Hill, p 311.

Andres R, Elahi D, Tobin JD, Muller DC, Brant L (1985): Ann Int Med 103:1030.

Arora S, Kassarjian Z, Krasinski SD, Croffey B, Kaplan MM, Russell RM (1989): Gastroenterology 96:1560.

Attwood EC, Robey E, Kramer JJ, Ovenden N, Snape S, Ross J, Bradley F (1978): Age Ageing 7:46.

Bailey LB, Wagner PA, Christakis GJ, Araujo PE, Appledorf H, Davis CG, Dorsey E, Dinning JS (1980): J Amer Geriatric Society 28:276.

Barr SI, Chrysomilides SA, Willis EJ, Beattie BL (1983): Nutr Res 3:417.

Barrows CH, Roeder IM (1965): J Gerontol 20:69.

Baum BJ (1981): J Dental Res 60:1292.

Beaumont DM, Cobden I, Sheldon WL, Laker MF, James OFW (1987): Age Ageing 16:294.

Becker RR, Heaney RP (1989): *In* Munro HM, Danford DE, eds: Nutrition, aging and the elderly. New York: Plenum Press.

Berg BN (1960): J Nutr 71:242.

Berg BN, Simms HS (1960): J Nutr 71:255.

Berg BN, Simms HS (1961): J Nutr 74:23.

Berg BN, Wolf A, Simms HS (1962): J Nutr 77:439.

Bertrand HA, Lynd FT, Masoro EJ, Yu BD (1980*a*): J Gerontol 35:827.

Bertrand HA, Masoro EJ, Yu BP (1980*b*): Endocrinol 107:591.

Blackburn GL, Thornton PA (1979): Med Clin North Am 63:1103.

Block G (1982): Am J Epidemiol 115:492.

Blumberg JB (1985): Drug-Nutrient Interactions 4:99.

Blumberg JB (1986): Transactions, Pharmacol Science 7:33.

Bras G, Ross MH (1964): Toxicol Applied Pharmacol 6:247.

Breen KJ, Buttigier R, Iossifidis S, Lourensz C, Wood B (1985): Am J Clin Nutr 42:121.

Build Study (1979): Chicago: Society of Actuaries and Association of Life Insurance Medical Directors of America, 1980.

Bullamore JR, Wilkinson R, Gallagher JC, Nordin BEC (1970): Lancet 2:535.

Bunker VW, Lawson MS, Clayton BE (1984): J Clin Pathol 37:1353.

Campbell VA, Dodds ML (1967): J Am Dietetic Association 51:29.

Chen LH, Fan Chiang WL (1981): Int J Vitamin Nutr Res 51:232.

Cheng L, Cohen M, Bhagavan HN (1985): *In* Watson RR, ed: Handbook of nutrition in the aged. Boca Raton, FL: CRC Press, p 157.

Cheng AHR, Gomez A, Gergan JG, Lee TC, Monckeberg F, Chichester CO (1978): Am J Clin Nutr 31:12.

Chumlea WC, Roche AF, Mukherjee D (1986): J Gerontol 41:36.

Chumlea WC, Roche AF, Steinbaugh ML (1989): *In* Munro HM, Danford DE, eds: Nutrition, aging and the elderly. New York: Plenum Press.

Cohn SH, Ellis KJ, Sawitsky A, Gartenhaus W, Yasumura S, Vaswani AN (1981): Am J Clin Nutr 34: 2839.

Cooper B, Weinblatt F, Gregerman RI (1977): J Clin Investigation 39:467.

Davies E, Kelleher J, Losowhy MS (1969): Clin Chim Acta 24:431.

Davis TA, Bales CW, Beauchenne RE (1983): Exp Gerontol 18:427.

Dawson-Hughes B, Jacques P, Shipp C (1987): Am J Clin Nutr 46:685.

Dawson-Hughes B, Dallal GE, Krall EA, Sadowski L, Sahyoun N, Tannenbaum S (1990): N Engl J Med 323:878.

Dubois EL, Strain L (1973): Biochemical Med 7:336.

Elwood PC, Shinton NK, Wilson CID, Sweetnam P, Frazer AC (1971): Br J Haematol 21:557.

Everitt AV, Porter B (1976): *In* Everitt AV, Burgess JA, eds: Hypothalamus, pituitary and aging. Springfield, IL: Thomas, p 570.

Everitt AV, Porter BD, Steele M (1981): Gerontology 27:37.

Feibusch JM, Holt PR (1982): Dig Dis Sci 27:1095.

Fernandes G, Friend P, Yunis EJ (1977): Fed Proc 36:1313.

Fernandes G, Friend P, Yunis EJ, Good RA (1978): Proc Natl Acad Sci USA 75:1500.

Fernandes G, Yunis EJ, Good RA (1976*a*): J Immunol 116:782.

Fernandes G, Yunis EJ, Good RA (1976*b*): Proc Natl Acad Sci USA 73:1279.

Fernandes G, Yunis EJ, Jose DG, Good RA (1973): Int J Allergy 44:770.

Forbes GB (1976): Human Biol 48:161.

French CE, Ingram RH, Unram JA, Barron GP, Swift RW (1953): J Nutr 51:329.

Friend PS, Fernandes G, Good RA, Michael AF, Yunis EJ (1978): Lab Invest 38:629.

Frisancho AR (1981): Am J Clin Nutr 34:2540.

Frisancho AR (1984): Am J Clin Nutr 84:808.

Frisancho AR, Flegel PN (1983): Am J Clin Nutr 37:311.

Gajjar A, Kubo C, Johnson BC, Good RA (1987): J Nutr 117:1136.

Gallagher JC, Riggs BL, Eisman J, Hamstra A, Arnaud SB, DeLuca HF (1979): J Clin Invest 64:729.

Gardner MB, Ihle JN, Pillarisetty RJ, Talal N, Dubois EL, Levy JA (1977): Nature 268:341.

Garrison RJ, Feinleib M, Castelli WP, McNamara PM (1983): JAMA 249:2199.

Garry PJ, Goodwin JS, Hunt WC (1982*b*): Am J Clin Nutr 36:902.

Garry PJ, Goodwin JS, Hunt WC (1984): J Am Geriatric Soc 32:719.

Garry PJ, Goodwin JS, Hunt WC, Gilbert BA (1982*c*): Am J Clin Nutr 36:332.

Garry PJ, Goodwin JS, Hunt WC, Hooper EM, Leonard AG (1982*a*): Am J Clin Nutr 36:319.

Garry PJ, Hunt WC, VanderJagt D, Rhyne RL (1989): Am J Clin Nutr 50:1219.

Gerbase-Delima M, Liu RK, Cheney KE, Mickey MR, Walford RL (1975): Gerontologia 21:184.

Gersovitz M, Motil D, Munro HN, Scrimshaw NS, Young VR (1982): Am J Clin Nutr 35:6.

Gersovitz M, Munro HN, Udall J, Young VR (1980): Metabolism 29:1075.

Gibson RS, Martinez OB, MacDonald C (1985): J Gerontol 40:296.

Gray GE, Paganini-Hill A, Ross RK (1983): Am J Clin Nutr 38:122.

Guigoz Y, Munro HN (1985): *In* Finch CE, Schneider EL, eds: Handbook of the biology of aging. New York: Van Nostrand Reinhold, p 878.

Guth PH (1968): Am J Dig Dis 13:565.

Hale WE, Stewart RB, Cerda JJ, Marks RG, May FE (1982): J Am Geriatric Soc 30:401.

Harman D (1981): Proc Natl Acad Sci USA 78:7124.

Harman D (1986): *In* Johnson JE, Walford RL, Harman D, Miguel J, eds: Free radicals, aging, and degenerative diseases. New York: Liss, p 3.

Haroon Y, Bacon DS, Sadowski JA (1987): J Chromatography 384:383.

Harrill I, Cervone N (1977): Am J Clin Nutr 30:431.

Hartz SC, Otradovec CL, McGandy RB, Russell RM, Jacob RA, Sahyoun N, Peters H, Abrams D, Scura LA, Whinston-Perry RA (1988): J Am College Nutr 7:119.

Hayashida M, Yu BP, Masoro EJ, Iwasaki K, Ikeda T (1986): Exp Gerontol 21:535.

Herlihy JT, Yu BP (1980): Am J Physiology 238:H652.

Heymsfield SB, McManus C, Smith J, Stevens V, Nixon DW (1982*a*): Am J Clin Nutr 36:680.

Heymsfield SB, Stevens V, Nail R, McManus C, Smith J, Nixon D (1982*b*): Am J Clin Nutr 36:131.

Horwitt MK, Harvey CC, Dahm CJ Jr, Searey MT (1972): NY Acad Sci 203:223.

Iber FL, Blass JP, Brin M, Leevy CM (1982): Am J Clin Nutr 36:1067.

Ingram DK, Weindruch R, Spangler EL, Freeman JR, Walford RL (1987): J Gerontol 42:78.

Ireland P, Fordtran JS (1973): J Clin Invest 52:2672.

Jacob RA, Russell RM, Sandstead HH (1985): Watson R, ed: Handbook of nutrition in the aged. Boca Raton, FL: CRC, p 77.

Jacques PF, Hartz SC, Russell RM (1988): FASEB Journal 2:A1613.

Jagerstad M, Westesson AK (1979): Scand J Gastroenterol 14(Suppl 52):196.

James WPT, Ralpha A, Ferro-Luzzi A (1989): *In* Munro HM, Danford DE, eds: Nutrition, aging and the elderly. New York: Plenum Press.

Jansen C, Harrill I (1977): Am J Clin Nutr 30:1414.

Kelleher J, Losowsky MS (1978): *In* DeDuve C, Hayaishi O, eds: Tocopherol, oxygen and biomembranes. Amsterdam: Elsevier, p 311.

Kemm JR, Allcock J (1984): Age Aging 13:21.

Kirk JE, Chieffi M (1953*a*): J Gerontol 8:301.

Kirk JE, Chieffi M (1953*b*): J Gerontol 8:305.

Kissebah AH, Vydelingum N, Murray R, Evans DJ, Hartz AJ, Kalkhoff RK, Adams PW (1982): J Clin Endocrinol Metab 54:254.

Kohrs MB, O'Neal R, Preston A, Eklund D, Abrahams O (1978): Am J Clin Nutr 31:2186.

Korenchevsky V (1961): Physiological and pathological aging. New York: Hafner.

Krasinski SD, Cohn JS, Schaefer EJ, Russell RB (1990): J Clin Invest 85:883.

Krasinski SD, Russell RM, Samloff IM, Jacob RA, Dallal GE, McGandy RB, Hartz SC (1986): JAGS 34:800.

Krasinski S, Russell RM, Otradovec CL, Sadowski JA, Hartz SC, Jacob RA, McGandy RB (1989): Am J Clin Nutr 49:112.

Krotkiewski M, Björntorp P, Sjöström L, Smith U (1983): J Clin Invest 72:1150.

Kubo C, Johnson B, Gajjar A, Good RA (1987): J Nutr 17:1129.

Lapidus L, Bengtsson C, Larsson B, Pennert K, Rybo E, Sjöström L (1984): Br Med J 289:1257.

Larsson B, Svärdsudd K, Welin L, Wilhelmsen L, Björntorp P, Tibblin G (1984): Br Med J 288:1401.

Liepa GU, Masoro EJ, Bertrand HA, Yu BP (1980): Am J Physiol 238:E253.

Lipschitz DA, Mitchell CO, Steele RW, Milton KY (1985): J Parenteral Enteral Nutr 9:343.

Loh HS (1972): Int J Vitamin Nutr Res 42:80.

Lowenstein FW (1982): J Am College Nutr 1:165.

Lynch SR, Finch CA, Monsen ER, Cook JD (1982): Am J Clin Nutr 36:1032.

MacLaughlin J, Holick MF (1985): J Clin Invest 76:1536.

McCarter R, McGee J (1987): J Gerontol 42:432.

McCay CM, Crowell MF, Maynard LA (1935): J Nutr 10:63.

McCay CM, Maynard LA, Sperling G, Barnes LL (1939): J Nutr 18:1.

McCay CM, Maynard LA, Sperling G, Osgood HS (1941): J Nutr 21:45.

McCay CM, Sperling G, Barnes LL (1943): Arch Biochem 2:469.

McGandy RB, Barrows CH, Spanias A, Meredith A, Stone JL, Norris AH (1966): J Gerontol 21:581.

McGandy RB, Russell RM, Hartz SC, Jacob RA, Tannenbaum S, Peters H, Sahyoun N, Otradovec CL (1986): Nutr Res 6:785.

McEvoy AW, James OFW (1982): Age Ageing 11:97.

Maeda H, Gleiser CA, Masoro EJ, Murata I, McMahan CA, Yu BP (1985): J Gerontol 40:671.

Magnus EM, Bache-Wiig JE, Aanderson TR, Melbostad E (1982): Scand J Haematol 28:360.

Makinodan T (1977): *In* Finch CE, Hayflick L, eds: Handbook of the biology of aging. New York: Van Nostrand Reinhold, p 379.

Mann PL (1978): Growth 42:87.

Manson JE, Stampfer MJ, Hennekens CH, Willett WC (1987): JAMA 257:353.

Marr JW (1971): World Rev Nutr Diet 13:105.

Marx JJM (1979): Blood 53:204.

Masoro EJ (1985): J Nutr 115:842.

Masoro EJ (1989): *In* Munro HM, Danford DE, eds: Nutrition, aging and the elderly. New York: Plenum Press.

Masoro EJ, Yu BP, Bertrand HA, Lynd FT (1980): Fed Proc 39:3178.

Master AM, Lasser RP (1960): J Am Med Assoc 172:658.

Matkovic V, Kostial K, Simonovic I, Buzina R, Brodarec A, Nordin BEC (1979): Am J Clin Nutr 32:540.

Meredith CN, Zackin MJ, Frontera WR, Evans WJ (1989): J Appl Physiol 66:2850.

Mertz W, Morris ER, Smith JC, Udomkesmalee E, Fields M, Levander OA, Anderson RA (1989): *In* Munro HM, Danford DE, eds: Nutrition, aging and the elderly. New York: Plenum Press.

Metropolitan Insurance Company (1983): Metropolitan height and weight tables. New York: Metropolitan Insurance Company.

Mitchell CO, Lipschitz DA (1982): Am J Clin Nutr 35:398.

Munro HN (1989): *In* Munro HM, Danford DE, eds: Nutrition, aging and the elderly. New York: Plenum Press.

Munro HN, McGandy RB, Hartz SC, Russell RM, Jacob RA, Otradovec CL (1987*a*): Am J Clin Nutr 46:586.

Munro HN, Suter PM, Russell RM (1987*b*): Annu Rev Nutr 7:23.

Nandy K (1982): Mechanisms Aging Development 18:97.

National Center for Health Statistics (1982): *In* Fulwood R, Johnson CL, Bryner JD, Gunter EW, McGrath CR, eds: Vital and health statistics. Series 11-No. 232. DHHS Pub. No. (PHS) 83-1682. Public Health Service. Washington, DC: US Government Printing Office.

National Center for Health Statistics (1983): *In* Carroll MD, Abraham S, Dresser CM, eds: Vital and health statistics. Series 11-No. 231. DHHS Pub. No. (PHS) 83-1681. Public Health Service. Washington, DC: US Government Printing Office.

National Center for Health Statistics (1987): *In* Najjar MF, Rowland M, eds: Vital and health statistics. Series 11, No. 238. DHHS Pub. No. (PHS) 87-1688. Public Health Service. Washington, DC: US Government Printing Office.

National Research Council (1981): Mammalian models for research on aging. Washington, DC: National Academy Press.

National Research Council (1989): Recommended dietary allowances. Washington, DC: National Academy Press.

Nolen GA (1972): J Nutr 102:1477.

O'Hanlon P, Kohrs MB (1978): Am J Clin Nutr 31:1257.

Otradovec CL, Russell RM, Hartz SC, McGandy RB, Jacob RA, Beaton DA (1986): Fed Proc 45:838a.

Pelletier O (1975): NY Acad Sci 258:156.

Pelz KS, Goffried SP, Sooes E (1968): Geriatrics 23:149.

Pilch SM, Senti FR, eds (June 1984*a*): Bethesda, MD: FASEB.

Pilch SM, Senti FR, eds (August 1984*b*): Bethesda, MD: FASEB.

Prentice AM, Coward WA, Davies HL, Murgatroyd PR, Black AE, Goldberg GR, Ashford J, Sawyer M, Whitehead RG (1985): Lancet 1:1419.

Prothro J, Mickles M, Tolbert B (1976): Am J Clin Nutr 29:94.

Reaven EP, Reaven GM (1981*a*): J Clin Invest 68:75.

Reaven GM, Reaven EP (1981*b*): Metabolism 30:982.

Reddy BS, Marisawa T, Vakusich D, Weisburger JH, Wynder E (1976): Proc Soc Exp Biol Med 151:237.

Ribaya-Mercado JD, Russell RM, Sahyoun N, Morrow FD, Gershoff SN (1991): J Nutr 121: In press.

Roe DA (1989): *In* Munro HM, Danford DE, eds: Nutrition, aging and the elderly. New York: Plenum Press.

Rosenberg IH, Bowman BB, Cooper BA, Halstead CH, Lindenbaum J (1982): Am J Clin Nutr 36:1060.

Ross MH (1959): Fed Proc 18:1190.

Ross MH (1961): J Nutr 75:197.

Ross MH (1972): Am J Clin Nutr 25:834.

Ross MH (1976): *In* Winick M, ed: Nutrition and aging. New York: John Wiley & Sons, p 23.

Ross MH, Bras G (1971): J Nat Cancer Inst 47:1095.

Ross MH, Bras G (1973): J Nutr 103:944.

Ross MH, Bras G, Ragbeer MS (1970): J Nutr 100:177.

Russell RM (1986): *In* Hutchinson ML, Munro HN, eds: Nutrition and aging. New York: Academic Press, p 59.

Russell RM, McGandy RB, Jelliffe D (1984): Am J Med 76:767.

Russell RM, Sahyoun NR (1988): *In* Paige DM, ed: Clin Nutr (2nd ed). Washington, DC: CV Mosby, p 110.

Sadowski JA, Hood SJ, Dallal GE, Garry PJ (1989): Am J Clin Nutr 50:100.

Sahud MA, Cohen RJ (1971): Lancet 1:937.

Sahyoun NR, Otradovec CL, Hartz SC, Jacob RA, Peters H, Russell RM, McGandy RB (1988): Am J Clin Nutr 47:524.

Sahyoun NR, Rasmussen NM (1988): Annual meeting of the American Dietetic Association, p 58.

Said HM, Hollander D (1985): Life Sci 36:69.

Sandstead HD, Henriksen LK, Gerger JL, Prasad AD, Good RA (1982): Am J Clin Nutr 36:1046.

Schaus R, Kirk JE (1957): J Gerontol 11:147.

Senti FR, Pilch SM (October 1984): Bethesda, MD: FASEB.

Simopoulos AP, Van Itallie TB (1984): Ann Internal Med 100:285.

Smith JL, Wickiser AA, Korth LL, Grandjean AC, Schaefer AE (1984): J Am College Nutr 3:13.

Snyder DL, ed (1989): Prog Clin Biol Res 298.

Southgate DAT, Durnin JVGA (1970): Br J Nutr 24:517.

Spencer H, Kramer L (1986): J Nutr 116:316.

Stiedemann M, Jansen C, Harrill I (1978): J Am Diet Assoc 73:132.

Stuchlikova E, Juricova-Horakova M, Deyl Z (1975): Exper Gerontol 10:141.

Suter PM, Russell RM (1987): Am J Clin Nutr 45:501.

Suter PM, Russell RM (1989): *In* Munro HM, Danford DE, eds: Nutrition, aging and the elderly. New York: Plenum Press.

Thompson ABR, Keelan M (1986): Canadian J Physiol Pharmacol 64:30.

Thomson AD (1966): Gerontol Clin 8:345.

Tucker SM, Mason RL, Beauchenne RE (1976): J Gerontol 31:264.

Turnlund JR, Durkin N, Costa F, Margen S (1986): J Nutr 116:1239.

Turnlund JR, Michel MC, Keyes WR, Schutz Y, Margen S (1982): Am J Clin Nutr 36:587.

Uauy R, Scrimshaw NS, Rand WM, Young VR (1978): Am J Clin Nutr 31:779.

Vatassery GT, Johnson GJ, Johnson GJ, Krezowski AM (1983): J Am Coll Nutr 4:369.

Vir SC, Love AHG (1977): Int J Vitam Nutr Res 47:364.

Vir SC, Love AHG (1979): Am J Clin Nutr 32:1934.

Vir SC, Love AHG (1980): Gerontology 26:1.

Voss KH, Masoro EJ, Anderson W (1982): Mech Ageing Devel 18:135.

Walford RL, Harris SB, Weindruch R (1987): J Nutr 117:1650.

Walford RL, Liu RK, Gerbase-Delima M, Mathies M, Smith GS (1974): Mech Ageing Devel 2:447.

Walford RL, Liu RK, Mathies M, Lipps L, Konen T (1975): Proc Ninth Intern Congress Nutr 1:374.

Warren PM, Pepperman MA, Montgomery RD (1978): Lancet 2:849.

Watson RR, Safranski DV (1981): *In* Kay MMB, Makinodan T. eds: CRC handbook of immunology in aging. Boca Raton, FL: CRC press, p 125.

Webb AR, Pilbeam C, Hanafin N, Holick MF (1990): Am J Clin Nutr 51:1075.

Webster SGP, Wilkinson EM, Gowland E (1977): Age Ageing 6:113.

Weindruch RH, Suffin SC (1980): J Gerontol 35:525.

Weindruch R, Walford RL (1982): Science 215:1415.

Weindruch RH, Walford RL (1988): The retardation of aging and disease by dietary restriction. Springfield, IL: Charles C Thomas.

Weindruch RH, Cheung ML, Verity MA, Walford RL (1980): Mech Age Dev 12:375.

Weindruch R, Gottesman SR, Walford RL (1982): Proc Nat Acad Sci 79:898.

Weindruch RH, Kristie JA, Cheney KE, Walford RL (1979): Fed Proc 38:2007.

Weindruch R, Walford RL, Fligiel S, Guthrie D (1986): J Nutr 116:641.

Welsh JD, Poley JR, Bhatia M, Stevenson DE (1978): Gastroenterology 75:847.

Welsh JD, Russell LC, Walker AW Jr (1974): Gerontology 66:993.

Werner I, Hambraeus L (1972): *In* Carlson LA, ed: Nutrition in old age. Uppsala: Almquist and Wiksell, p 55.

Yearick ES, Wang M-SL, Pisias SJ (1980): J Gerontol 35:663.

Yu BP, Bertrand HA, Masoro EJ (1980): Metabolism 29:438.

Yu BP, Maeda H, Murata I, Masoro EJ (1984): Fed Proc 43:858A.

Yu BP, Masoro EJ, Murata I, Bertrand HA, Lynd FT (1982): J Gerontol 37:130.

Yu BP, Masoro EJ, McMahan A (1985): J Gerontol 40:657.

Yunice AA, Hsu JM (1984): *In* Rennert OM, Chan NY, eds: Metabolism of trace metals in man. Boca Raton, FL: CRC Press, p 99.

Frank D. Morrow, Ph.D.,
Nadine Sahyoun, R.D.,
Robert A. Jacob, Ph.D.,
and Robert M. Russell, M.D.

13

Clinical Assessment of the Nutritional Status of Adults

Introduction

In recent years, there has been a growing awareness among health care professionals that the nutritional status of hospitalized patients can affect morbidity, mortality, and length of hospital stay (Mullen et al., 1979; Walesby et al., 1978). Because it is readily diagnosed using anthropometric and laboratory tests, protein-calorie malnutrition has been the most frequently reported nutritional disorder (Bistrian et al., 1974; Bushman et al., 1980; Wiensier et al., 1979). Evidence has emerged during the last decade which suggests that the prevalence of micronutrient deficiencies (e.g., vitamins and minerals) is also high among some age groups (Morrow, 1986). Moreover, regardless of their nature, one is reminded that nutritional deficits are not limited to hospitalized subjects and, in fact, are frequently encountered among ambulatory subjects suffering either acute or chronic illness.

As nutritional maladies contribute to both morbidity and mortality, and also respond quickly to appropriate therapy, it is prudent for the clinician to view assessment of patient nutritional status in the same light as the many diagnostic tests currently available. Regrettably, the selection of *which* procedure(s) will provide the best assessment of nutritional status for a *particular* patient has become increasingly difficult. Anthropometric standards are constantly changing (or are unavailable for some age groups) and a plethora of laboratory tests has emerged, many of which are unfamiliar to the physician. Typically, no one or two measurements can provide adequate clinical nutritional assessment of a given patient. Thus, the clinician must carefully choose among those tests or procedures which, when interpreted as a whole, provide components of a comprehensive nutritional workup and assists the physician in undertaking a detailed nutritional assessment. Sections are included below which discuss: (1) medical, social, and dietary history; (2) anthropometric indices of nutritional status; (3) physical examination; and (4) biochemical testing.

Medical, Social, and Dietary History

A detailed medical and social history can alert the health care provider to an existing nutritional problem or the risks of a future nutritional problem. For example, complaints of weight loss, diarrhea, anorexia (lack of appetite), or dysphagia (difficulty swallowing) are symptoms that can adversely affect the nutritional status of the patient. If the patient has increased metabolic needs resulting from infection or fever, increased nutrient losses resulting from open wounds or burns, recent major surgery, or evidence of malabsorption or pancreatic insufficiency, the likelihood of malnutrition is greater, especially if the condition is not recognized early and appropriate nutritional therapy is not initiated.

Table 13.1. List of Key Questions to Be Asked as Part of the Nutritional Assessment of the Adult

1. Is there recent weight gain or weight loss?
2. Are there changes in appetite?
3. Are there changes in sense of smell or taste?
4. Are there problems with chewing or swallowing?
5. Does the individual have poor dentition or poorly fitting dentures?
6. Are there symptoms of gastrointestinal disorders: diarrhea, constipation, nausea, vomiting?
7. Does the individual live alone? If not, who prepares meals? Does he/she know how to cook?
8. Are there adequate cooking facilities and refrigeration in person's home?
9. Is the individual financially able to buy an adequate variety of food?
10. Are one or more meals eaten outside of home?
11. Is the person handicapped? Does this prevent the individual from shopping, cooking, or feeding herself/himself?
12. Does the person take any dietary supplements (e.g., vitamins)?
13. How much alcohol does the individual consume?
14. Does the person use nonprescription drugs?
15. Are there any religious beliefs, food allergies, or ethnic beliefs that prevent adequate food intake?
16. Does the person follow a dietary restriction? Is it doctor-prescribed or self-imposed?
17. Is the individual depressed?

The patient's social and economic situation is a major contributor to an inadequate dietary regimen, and the result may be malnutrition. This is particularly true for the elderly population. In addition, a patient's lifestyle and work schedule may be such that he/she does not allow time to consume regular adequate meals. A subject may skip meals, eat on the run or from a vending machine. To quickly identify those factors that may affect nutritional status, a list of key questions is presented in Table 13.1.

A dietary history obtained by a dietitian can identify those patients who follow fad or monotonous diets or who are noncompliant to dietary instructions. Patients are asked to assess their typical daily intake, or frequency of intake, of specific food items. Self-imposed dietary restrictions due to ethnic or religious reasons or belief in fad diets can seriously affect nutritional status. The Recommended Dietary Allowances (RDAs) are frequently used to determine nutritional adequacy of dietary intakes (Table 13.2). However, these population standards are not individual requirements. They are set to exceed the needs of most healthy individuals (Food and Nutrition Board, 1989), but do not meet the increased metabolic needs of ill patients.

Table 13.2. U.S. Recommended Dietary Allowances for Adults (Ages 25–50)

	Males	Females
Calories	2700	2000
Protein (g)	63	50
Vitamin A (μg, retinol equivalent)	1000	800
Vitamin D (μg)	5	5
Vitamin E (mg, α tocopherol equivalent)	10	8
Vitamin K (μg)	80	65
Vitamin C (mg)	60	60
Thiamin (mg)	1.5	1.1
Riboflavin (mg)	1.7	1.3
Niacin (mg, niacin equivalent)	19	15
Vitamin B_6 (mg)	2.0	1.6
Folate (μg)	200	180
Vitamin B_{12} (μg)	2	2
Calcium (mg)	800	800
Phosphorus (mg)	800	800
Magnesium (mg)	350	280
Iron (mg)	10	15
Zinc (mg)	15	12
Iodine (μg)	150	150
Selenium (μg)	70	55

Anthropometric Evaluation

Anthropometric measurements are valuable because they provide an estimate of the patient's protein and fat reserves. As single measurements they are useful to use along with biochemical, dietary, and clinical parameters to assess the nutritional status of a patient. Anthropometric measures are also useful when they are performed periodically over time to detect changes that indicate a need for intervention or when taken during treatment as an indicator of the efficacy of therapy. These measurements include height in centimeters, weight in kilograms, triceps skinfold thickness in millimeters, and midarm circumference in centimeters. Anthropometric measurements are noninvasive and can be performed easily, quickly, and at little cost to the health care provider. Using these values and the formulas provided below, the following indices may be derived: weight as percentage of usual weight, actual weight, body mass index, triceps skinfold thickness (TSF), and bone-free, upperarm muscle area as percentages of reference standards. The following pieces of equipment are needed: a beam or lever balance scale, a measuring stick or a nonstretchable tape attached to a flat vertical surface, a right-angle headboard, a constant tension skinfold caliper, and an insertion tape measure.

Height and Weight

The subject's height should be measured without shoes. The individual stands up straight, with heels close together touching the wall, arms at the side, and shoulders relaxed. The person looks straight ahead so that the line of vision is perpendicular to the body. The headboard is lowered until it makes contact with the scalp, and height is read in centimeters. The subject should be asked his/her usual body weight and then weighed. The patient's weight for height may then be compared to a reference weight table. The Metropolitan Insurance Company (MET) weight table is derived from actuarial data from people 25–59 years old, and is thought best to represent the desirable weights for heights of a young to middle-aged population. It is suggested that the midpoint of the middle frame for each height be used as the reference standard for the assessment of this age group. These values are provided in Table 13.3. For a quick and approximate estimate of the patient's reference weight, the following formulas may be used:

Male reference body weight
= 127 lb for first 5 ft + 3 lb for every in. over 5 ft

Female reference body weight
= 119 lb for first 5 ft + 3 lb for every in. over 5 ft

Another reference weight table contains the normative values obtained from the Health and Nutrition Examination Surveys (NHANES) I and II data sets (Frisancho, 1984). These normative values are presently the most representative values of the noninstitutionalized adult population in the United States (Table 13.4). All races were included in the NHANES I and II subsample of 21,752. These values are higher than the MET reference weights, which indicates that the general

Table 13.3. Actuarial Reference Data: 1983 Weight-for-Height Table Derived from Life Insurance Data

Height		Weight[a]			
		Male		Female	
in	cm	lb	kg	lb	kg
58	147.3	—	—	114	51.7
59	149.9	—	—	116.5	52.8
60	152.4	—	—	119	53.9
61	154.9	—	—	122	55.3
62	157.5	133	60.3	125	56.7
63	160.0	135	61.2	128	58.0
64	162.6	137.5	62.4	131	59.4
65	165.1	140	63.5	134	60.8
66	167.6	143	64.9	137	62.1
67	170.2	146	66.2	140	63.5
68	172.7	149	67.6	143	64.9
69	175.3	152	68.9	146	66.2
70	177.8	155	70.3	149	67.6
71	180.3	158.5	71.9	152	69.0
72	182.9	162	73.9	—	—
73	185.4	166	75.3	—	—
74	188.0	169.5	76.9	—	—
75	190.5	174	78.9	—	—

[a] Weights represent the midpoint of the middle frame. These values correct the 1983 Metropolitan Tables to nude weights and heights.

Table 13.4. Average Weight for Height for Ages 25–54 from NHANES I and II Data Sets

Height		Weight				Weight/Height	
		Male		Female		Male	Female
in.	cm	kg	lb	kg	lb	(lb/in.)	
58	147	—	—	63	138.6	—	2.39
59	150	—	—	66	145.2	—	2.46
60	152	—	—	60	132.0	—	2.20
61	155	—	—	61	134.2	—	2.16
62	157	68	149.6	61	134.2	2.41	2.16
63	160	71	156.2	62	136.4	2.48	2.17
64	163	71	156.2	62	136.4	2.44	2.13
65	165	74	162.8	63	138.6	2.50	2.13
66	168	75	165.0	63	138.6	2.50	2.09
67	170	77	169.4	65	143.0	2.52	2.13
68	173	78	171.6	67	147.4	2.52	2.16
69	175	78	171.6	68	149.6	2.49	2.17
70	178	81	178.2	70	154.0	2.55	2.20
71	180	81	178.2	—	—	2.51	—
72	183	84	184.8	—	—	2.57	—
73	185	85	187.0	—	—	2.56	—
74	188	88	193.6	—	—	2.62	—

population may be heavier than recommended according to the MET table. NHANES tables may, therefore, be used to indicate where a person's weight for height fits in comparison to the general U.S. population. After consulting the reference weight tables, the following calculations are made:

$$\% \text{ usual weight} = \frac{\text{actual weight}}{\text{usual weight}} \times 100$$

$$\% \text{ reference body weight} = \frac{\text{actual weight}}{\text{reference body weight}} \times 100$$

$$\% \text{ weight change} = \frac{\text{usual weight} - \text{actual weight}}{\text{usual weight}} \times 100$$

Changes in weight over time provide important information on the nutritional assessment of a patient. The rate of weight loss, as well as the amount lost, can reflect the individual's nutritional status. The health provider should be aware that a person who has lost over 10% of his body weight during the previous 6 months may need nutritional support. Often, an overweight person's nutritional status is ignored; however, a rapid weight loss (within 6 months) of 6% of body weight or greater may indicate the loss of somatic muscle protein (Wilmore, 1977). Height and weight can serve as useful screening tools, but at times may be misleading. Edema, ascites, and obesity can mask muscle tissue loss and malnutrition.

Another measure that has gained wide use as a simple index of relative weight is the Quetelet body mass index (BMI). BMI, which is obtained by dividing weight (kg) by height (m) squared (i.e., wt/ht^2) minimizes the contribution of the individual's height. This measure may be determined without performing calculations, by using the nomograph for BMI (Figure 13.1; Burton et al., 1985).

Triceps Skinfold (TSF)

Triceps Skinfold (TSF), an estimate of the patient's fat stores, measures a double layer of skin and subcutaneous fat with a skinfold caliper. Although subscapular, lower thoracic, iliac, or abdominal sites can be used to perform this measurement, the deltoid triceps is most commonly used because of its easy accessibility and the usual absence of edema at this site. The measurement is taken on the right arm, unless edema or paralysis is present, as the standards are based on right-arm measurements. When possible, the subject should be standing with the bare right arm hanging relaxed at the side. An alternate method is to have the subject sit on the edge of a bed or chair, without the arm resting on any surface.

Because the amount of fat overlying the triceps muscle varies, the measurement is taken at the midpoint between the acromial process of the

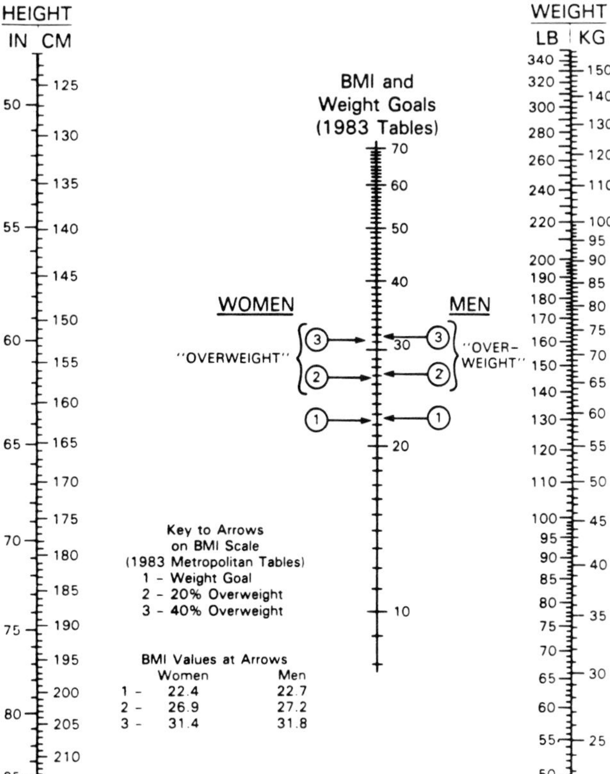

Figure 13.1. Nomograph for body mass index (BMI) (kg/m^2). The ratio weight/height^2 (metric units) is read from the central scale after a straight edge is placed between height and body weight. [*Source:* Burton et al. (1985).]

scapula (shoulder blade) and the olecranon process of the ulna (tip of the elbow). To find this midpoint, the subject bends the arm 90° and a tape measure is placed between these two points. The midpoint is marked on the back of the arm with a pen (Figure 13.2). With the subject's arm hanging relaxed at the side, the marked midpoint is grasped posteriorly between the thumb and forefinger of the examiner's left hand. The fold is raised, allowing the underlying muscle to fall back to the bone. If uncertain, the examiner should have the subject contract and relax the arm muscle to make sure no muscle is included in the fold. The examiner places the calipers on the fold below the fingers, releases the calipers (but not the grasp), and takes a reading to the nearest 0.5 mm (Figure 13.3). For accuracy, it is recommended that the examiner release the fold and repeat the measurement three times. An average of the three measurements should be used to compute the mean thickness.

Arm Muscle Area

Midarm muscle circumference, a widely used measure for estimating the amount of skeletal muscle, was popularized by Jeliffe (1966). Using computerized axial tomography, Heymsfield and coworkers (1982) observed that the equation used to obtain midarm muscle circumference resulted in a 20%–25% overestimate of arm muscle area. The authors, therefore, developed a revised equation which improved the accuracy of the measurement and calculated bone-free arm muscle area. To perform this calculation, the midarm circumference must first be measured. With the subject's right arm relaxed at the side and not resting on any surface, the examiner places the tape measure around the subject's arm at the marked midpoint. This should be done firmly, but without compressing the fat tissue (Figure 13.4). Using midarm circumference and TSF measurements, it is possible to calculate bone-free upper arm muscle area circumference by using the following formula:

Males, bone-free upper arm muscle area (cm^2) = $[(\text{arm circumference (cm)} - 3.14 \times \text{TSF(cm)})^2 \div 4\pi] - 10$

Females, bone-free upper arm muscle area (cm^2) = $[(\text{arm circumference (cm)} - 3.14 \times \text{TSF(cm)})^2 \div 4\pi] - 6.5$

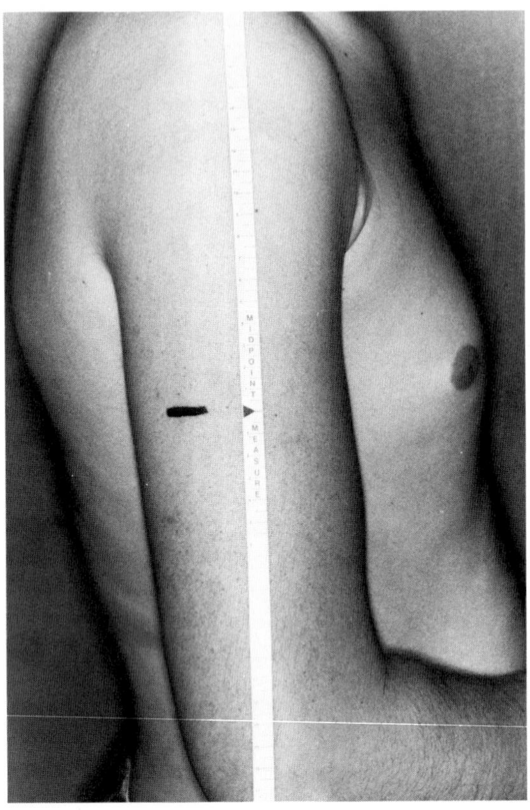

Figure 13.2. Determining midpoint of the upper arm for measurement of midarm muscle circumference (MAMC). Midpoint is halfway between the acromonial process of the scapula and the olecranon process of the ulna.

Interpretation of Standards

Reference standards for some of the anthropometric measurements, such as skinfold thickness and bone-free upper arm muscle area, have been suggested based on normative values obtained from the National Health and Nutrition Examination Survey (NHANES). NHANES was designed to assess the nutritional status of a sample of people representative of noninstitutionalized civilians living in the United States by monitoring changes in nutritional status over time. Population subgroups were defined according to socioeconomic status, sex, age, and race. The first survey (NHANES I), which included dietary data, anthropometric measurements, and biochemical evaluation, was conducted between 1971–1974; and the second survey (NHANES II) between 1976–1980. This survey is expected to be conducted every 5–6 years. Until more information is available to indicate the ideal measurements recommended, the normative values obtained from these surveys are used as reference standards. Table 13.5 summarizes the reference standards suggested for use in assessing anthropometric measurements discussed in this chapter and described in the text.

Height and Weight

The Metropolitan Life Insurance (MET) values have been criticized as a reference standard because they are based on actuarial tables from a

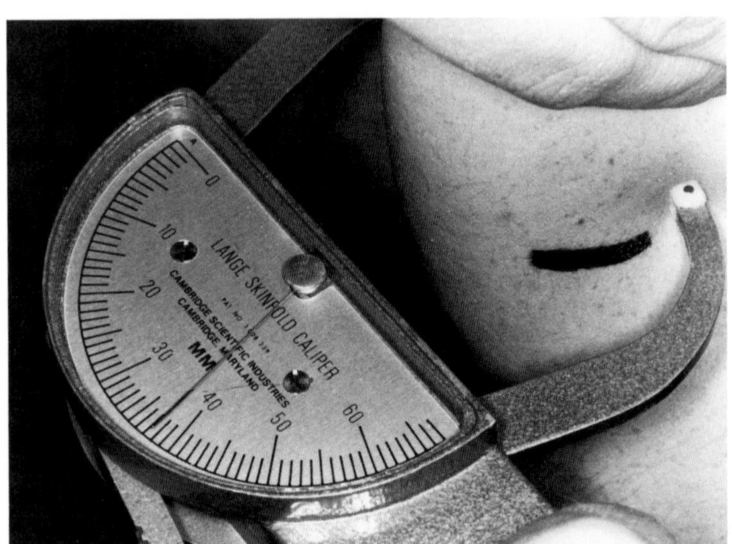

Figure 13.3. Measurement of triceps skinfold thickness (TSF). Large skinfold calipers are used for the measurement. The evaluator maintains a light pinching pressure on the skinfold throughout the measurement.

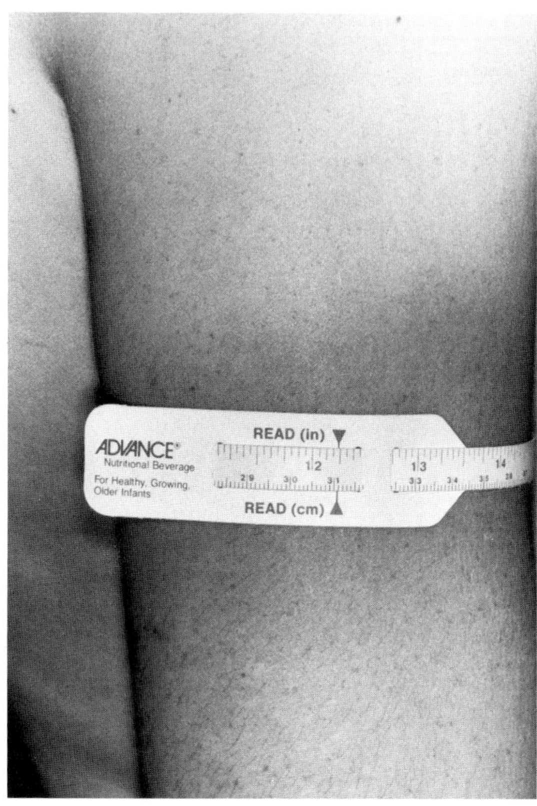

Figure 13.4. Measurement of midarm muscle circumference (MAMC). Midarm circumference is measured with Ross Laboratories insertion tape measure. The evaluator must be careful not to constrict the patient's arm.

young population of healthy, insured individuals. The values are not age-specific, and do not account for the diverse socioeconomic and ethnic differences that characterize the U.S. population. The values derived from the NHANES survey, in contrast, are normative values; however, the weight-for-height measures are high as compared to MET values. Since mortality and morbidity are associated with increased weight, NHANES tables should only be used to compare how a person's weight for height compares to that of the general population. Therefore, until a more appropriate weight-for-height reference table is available, the MET reference table (Table 13.3) is recommended for use for adults up to age 59.

The suggested reference standard for Body Mass Index (BMI) is 22.7 kg/m^2 for males and females. This value is calculated from the MET weight-for-height table. The National Center for Health Statistics set criteria for defining overweight. The criteria adopted by the Consensus Conference on Obesity (Van Itallie, 1985) are BMI values of 27.8 kg/m^2 and 27.3 kg/m^2 for males and females, respectively. These values are the 85th percentiles from NHANES II for age group 20–29 years. This age group was chosen for setting the criteria because young adults are considered relatively lean. The criteria are about 20% over those calculated from the MET values. To assess underweightness, it is suggested to take as cutoff values 20% below those calculated from the midpoint of the MET tables. This corresponds to less than the 5th percentile from NHANES II for ages 20–29 years.

Skinfold Thickness and Arm Muscle Area

The reference standards suggested for triceps skinfold thickness and bone-free upper arm muscle area are derived from the 50th percentile of NHANES I and II data sets for age group 25–54 years. For assessing risks of malnutrition and obesity, the 5th and 85th percentiles of the combined NHANES I and II data sets, respectively, are suggested.

Table 13.5. Suggested Criteria to Judge Risk of Undernutrition and Overnutrition in Adults

Anthropometric parameter	Reference standard Male/female	Risk of undernutrition (% of standard)		Risk of overnutrition (% of standard)	
		Males	Females	Males	Females
Weight for height	—[a]	<80	<80	>130	>130
Body mass index (kg/m^2)	22.7/22.6	<80	<80	>120	>120
Triceps skinfold (mm)	12/23	<40	<50	>170	>145
Arm muscle area (cm)^2	55/31	<70	<70	NA[b]	NA[b]

Source: Data on triceps skinfold and arm muscle area are from Frisancho (1981).

[a] Table 13.3 is used as reference.
[b] NA, Not applicable.

To simplify the assessment of malnutrition in a clinical setting, the percent standard for each actual value may be obtained by using the following formula:

$$\% \text{ standard} = \frac{\text{actual measurement}}{\text{median standard}} \times 100$$

This value is then compared to the percentages suggested in Table 13.5.

Using one parameter to diagnose malnutrition can overestimate the prevalence. Therefore, it is suggested that a combination of dietary, anthropometric, biochemical, and clinical assessments be used to judge the severity of the nutritional problem.

Clinical Assessment

Most clinical signs and symptoms of malnutrition are nonspecific in that they are not related to a single nutrient deficit. Nevertheless, they are useful for recognizing the severely malnourished individual and are presented in Table 13.6. Early clinical signs of malnutrition are lacking or are so nonspecific as to be diagnostically useless (e.g., lassitude, irritability). In our experience, on clinical grounds only, physicians recognize only about one fourth of moderately or severely malnourished patients (as diagnosed by anthropometric and/or biochemical data) (Bushman et al., 1980). Functional tests (e.g., dark adaptation for vitamin A) or target organ tests (e.g., bone density for vitamin D) can lead to the recognition of subclinical deficiencies of a particular nutrient (Posner et al., 1978; Russell et al., 1973). However, functional tests for specific nutrients are mostly lacking or can be affected by factors other than nutrition. For example, taste abnormalities may be due to zinc deficiency, but taste also declines with age and can be affected by drugs or smoking (Greger and Geissler, 1978; Nutrition Reviews, 1979).

There has been recent interest in designing a nutritional index to predict surgical outcome in hospitalized patients. One attempt at this resulted in the derivation of the so-called "prognostic nutritional index" (PNI) (Buzby et al., 1980), which is calculated according to a derived formula into which are plugged values for the patient's serum albumin, triceps skinfold thickness, serum transferrin, and reactivity to recall antigens (mumps, streptokinase-streptodornase, and *Candida*). The higher the PNI value, the worse the outcome. However, other attempts to look at similar predictive indicators have shown that complications of nutritional origin can be just as well predicted by using the serum albumin value alone (i.e., the lower the serum albumin value, the worse the outcome) (Leite et al., 1987). More data are needed before a predictive indicator is generally accepted and used by clinicians for deciding on the need for specific nutritional therapy.

Biochemical Evaluation

Biochemical tests of nutritional status offer several advantages to the clinician over those of (and not overlapping those of) dietary assessment, physical examination, or anthropometry. In general, they are considered to provide greater precision, sensitivity, and specificity than the aforementioned indirect measures of nutritional status and, unlike a dietary history, can even be performed on the patient who is comatose or mentally confused. When prescribed judiciously, laboratory tests can be used to effectively stage or circumscribe a suspected nutritional malady, provide a prognostic index of surgical complications, or monitor adherence to therapeutic interventions. However, with the possible exception of serum albumin, iron binding capacity, and vitamins B_{12} and folate, laboratory measures of nutritional status have not been widely used by the practicing physician. In part, this situation can be attributed to the complexity of the tests themselves, their high cost, and the occasional necessity to provide unusual specimen matrices and handling procedures. As many of the more esoteric nutritional tests are available only through the largest hospital and commercial reference laboratories, the physician is faced with the added burden of locating a facility capable of providing quality nutritional testing.

Recent Advances

With the advent of computerized, robotic analytical instrumentation, the modern clinical chemistry laboratory is, nevertheless, now in a position to provide a comprehensive array of nutritional biochemical testing in a cost-effective manner. For example, the latest generation of centrifugal analyzers can be programmed to provide flexible sample- and reagent-processing steps and to employ one of five different detection modes. Used in combination with robotic liquid-handling systems, these instruments can be used to automate a wide variety of nonchromatographic nutrition-

Table 13.6. Signs and Symptoms of Nutritional Deficiency in Adult Patients

Sign or symptom	Nutrient deficiency
General	
Wasted, skinny	Calorie
Loss of appetite	Protein-calorie
Skin	
Pallor	Folate, iron, vitamin B_{12}
Follicular hyperkeratosis	Vitamin A
Perifollicular petichiae	Vitamin C
Flaking dermatitis	Protein, calorie, niacin, riboflavin, zinc
Bruising	Vitamin C, vitamin K, essential fatty acids
Pigmentation changes	Niacin, protein-calorie
Scrotal dermatosis	Riboflavin
Head	
Temporal muscle wasting	Protein-calorie
Hair	
Sparse and thin	Protein
Easy to pull out	
Eyes	
History of night blindness (especially impaired visual recovery after glare)	Vitamin A
Photophobia, blurring, conjunctival inflammation	Riboflavin, vitamin A
Mouth	
Glossitis	Riboflavin, niacin, folic acid, vitamin B_{12}
Bleeding gums	Vitamin C
Cheilosis	Riboflavin
Angular stomatitis	Riboflavin
Hypogeusia	Zinc
Tongue fissuring	Niacin
Tongue atrophy	Riboflavin, niacin, iron
Neck	
Goiter	Iodine
Parotid enlargement	Protein
Abdomen	
Distention	Protein-calorie
Hepatomegaly	Protein-calorie
Extremities	
Edema	Protein, thiamin
Bone tenderness	Vitamin D
Bone ache, joint pain	Vitamin C
Muscle wasting and weakness	Protein, calorie, vitamin D
Muscle tenderness, muscle pain	Thiamin
Nails	
Spooning	Iron
Transverse lines	Protein
Neurologic	
Tetany	Calcium magnesium
Paresthesias	Thiamin
Loss of reflexes, wrist drop, foot drop	Thiamin
Loss of vibratory and position sense	Vitamin B_{12}
Dementia, disorientation	Niacin

related assays, which heretofore could be performed using only tedious, manual methodologies. High-performance liquid chromatography (HPLC), a methodology previously confined to the domain of the research laboratory, is now commonly found in small- or medium-sized hospital laboratories. Moreover, with recent advances in microprocessor control and data acquisition techniques, HPLCs can now be coupled with the flexibility of a diode array detector, or the specificity of the mass spectrometer. On the horizon, clinicians can look forward to a new generation of nutritional tests involving application of stable isotope technologies. The latest generation of GC-MS and dual isotope ratio spectrophotometers are relatively easy to operate and require only a fraction of the space used by earlier models. Assays developed to date which involve stable isotope applications include a procedure for estimating hepatic reserves of vitamin A (Furr et al., 1989) and a test for estimating vitamin C requirements (Powers, 1987). The result is an ever-expanding array of diagnostically useful nutrition tests from which the physician can choose.

Advances have also occurred in mature laboratory methodologies, such as competitive protein binding and colorimetric techniques. At least two companies have developed convenient kits to quantitate plasma levels of 25-OH vitamin-D, a nutrient which has received heightened interest among clinicians due to the widespread prevalence of osteoporosis among postmenopausal women. Moreover, in response to concerns raised by nutritional biochemists regarding B_{12} analogues, nearly every manufacturer of commercial kits used to quantitate serum levels of B_{12} has developed convenient methodologies based on the highly cobalamin-specific hog stomach intrinsic factor. Finally, at least one company has introduced sensitive, specific colorimetric procedures to quantitate serum levels of zinc and copper. Both methodologies can be readily adapted to a variety of automated chemistry analyzers and, for routine clinical use, may prove to be useful substitutes for the less readily available atomic absorption methodologies.

Categories of Nutritional Tests

Biochemical tests for assessing nutritional status can be categorized into two groups: (1) those that provide a static, unperturbed measure of a nutrient or metabolite in body fluids and tissues; and (2) those that measure a biochemical function dependent upon the nutrient in question or in response to a challenge dose. In the case of vitamin B_6, for example, direct measures include the determination of pyridoxal-5-phosphate (PLP) in plasma, or the 24-hr excretion of 4-pyridoxic acid in urine. Functional measures of B_6 status include the determination of erythrocyte transaminase activity, for which PLP is a cofactor, or the tryptophan-load test in which the relative metabolic flux through a PLP-dependent biochemical pathway is estimated. Functional tests are often regarded to be "time-integrated" measures of nutrient intake (i.e., dependent upon dietary intake over a period of days or weeks). Not all functional tests do, in fact, represent long-term measures of nutrient intake, and many suffer from a lower level of precision than that which can be obtained from direct measures of nutrient levels. The selection of which test(s) is to be used is largely dependent upon the research or clinical application of interest. Table 13.7 represents a compilation of nutritional biochemistries now available to the clinician, including reference ranges and suggested methodologies.

Test Sensitivity and Specificity

Like all laboratory procedures, tests of nutritional status have characteristic sensitivities and specificities. The physician must choose the test (or tests) which can either confirm or deny the evidence obtained from indirect measures of nutritional status (e.g., dietary history or anthropometrics), or provide a differential diagnosis between two possible maladies—of which perhaps only one is nutritionally related. Yet, unlike more commonly performed laboratory procedures, nutritional tests often lack a reference standard by which rigorous determinations of sensitivity and specificity can be made. The situation is exacerbated by the effect that concurrent pathology and drug use may have on the test result itself (see Chapter 19). It is well-known that, in the presence of hepatic disease, normal ferritin levels can be observed even in the face of low body iron stores. Also, plasma levels of retinol and retinol-binding protein are frequently observed to be elevated in the subject with chronic renal tubular disease and, therefore, do not reflect vitamin A adequacy. The validity of even a functional test of vitamin A stores, the relative dose–response test (RDR), has been reported to be jeopardized in the subject who is cirrhotic (Mobarhan et al., 1981).

Finally, one should be aware that reference ranges for some nutritional biochemistry tests should be considered as one-sided. For example, while retinol levels less than 20 μg/dl are indicative of low vitamin A stores in adult subjects, results above the reference range do not necessarily imply hypervitaminosis A. As a general rule, functional tests of nutritional status typically have one-sided reference ranges.

Specimen Collection and Transport

The choice of specimen and the manner in which it is collected and transported to the laboratory are critical considerations for any diagnostic pro-

Table 13.7. List of Recommended Clinical Laboratory Tests for Detection of Micronutrient and Macronutrient Disorders[a]

Nutrient	Analyte	Methodology	Reference range	Remarks
Vitamin A	Retinol	HPLC reverse phase	30–90 μg/dl	Good index for hypovitaminosis; often appears normal during cases of hypervitaminosis A
Vitamin A	Retinyl esters	HPLC normal phase	0–8 μg/dl	Preferred test for cases of suspected vitamin toxicity
Vitamin D	25-hydroxy vitamin D	Ligand-binding assay	8–55 ng/ml	1,25 dihydroxy-vitamin D is not useful for assessing dietary status
Vitamin E	Tocopherol	HPLC reverse phase	500–1800 μg/dl	Values can be falsely elevated in subjects with hypertriglyceridemia
Vitamin K	Prothrombin time	Single-stage functional test	11–15 sec	Not specific for vitamin K status
Vitamin K	Vitamin K_1	Reverse-phase HPLC	0.30–2.64 nmol/L	More specific than hemostasis assay for detection of low vitamin K status
Carotenes	Total carotenoids	Spectrophotometry	40–240 μg/dl	Not specific for beta-carotene
Carotenes	Beta-carotene	HPLC reverse phase	10–85 μg/dl	Will likely become a commonly requested test in research centers due to possible protection against some epithelial cancers
Vitamin B_1	RBC transketolase activity coefficient	Spectrophotometric/ kinetic	0.90–1.29	Suitable for detection of advanced deficiency only
Vitamin B_2	RBC glutathione reductase activity coefficient	Spectrophotometric/ kinetic	0.90–1.34	Good index for long term B_2 status. Can be elevated secondary to hypothyroidism.
Vitamin B_6	RBC aspartate aminotransferase activity coefficient	Spectrophotometric/ kinetic	0.90–2.20	Good index for long term B_6 status
Vitamin B_6	Pyridoxal-5-phosphate	Radioenzymatic	>20 ng/ml	Difficult procedure; choose laboratory with extensive experience with this analyte
Vitamin B_6	4-pyridoxic acid	HPLC reverse phase	>0.50 mg/day	Does not index long-term B_6 status
Folate	Folic acid	Competitive protein binding	3–30 ng/ml	As inappropriate folate therapy can have serious consequences, folate and B_{12} analyses should be performed simultaneously
Vitamin B_{12}	Cobalamin	Competitive protein binding	150–1200 pg/ml	See above regarding folate testing
Vitamin B_{12} or folate	Homocysteine	HPLC-fluorometric	7–22 μmol/L	Total homocysteine can be elevated secondary to either cobalamin or folate deficiency
Vitamin B_{12}	Methylmalonic acid, serum	GC-mass spectroscopy	<900 nmol/L	MMA can be elevated secondary to cobalamin deficiency, but not secondary to folate deficiency
Vitamin C	Ascorbic acid	Colorimetric	0.3–2.0 mg/dl	Recent index of vitamin C intake only; leukocyte levels may better predict tissue stores

(continued)

Table 13.7 *(continued)*

Nutrient	Analyte	Methodology	Reference range	Remarks
Iron	Free RBC porphyrins	Fluorometry	<50 μg/dl	Changes before other measures of iron status; also elevated during plumbism
Iron	Serum iron	Flame AA or colorimetric	50–170 μg/dl	Can be altered due to recent infection or inflammation independent of body iron status; large diurnal variation in serum iron
Iron	Unsaturated iron binding	Colorimetric	130–375 μg/dl	Iron, UIBC, and TIBC are typically performed as a combined profile
Iron	Total iron binding	Colorimetric	245–400 μg/dl	
Iron	Transferrin	Calculation	16–55%	Transferrin saturation = iron ÷ TIBC
Iron	Transferrin	Immunoturbidimetric	200–400 mg/dl	Preferred over iron-binding capacity if available
Iron	Ferritin	Immunoradiometric	12–300 ng/ml	High sensitivity, modest specificity; reflects whole body stores of iron; elevated with infection or inflammation
Zinc	Plasma zinc	Flame atomic absorption	70–130 μg/dl	Relatively low specificity
Zinc	Zinc tolerance test	Flame atomic absorption	100% increase over baseline at 2 hr	
Copper	Serum copper	Flame atomic absorption	55–175 μg/dl	
Copper	Ceruloplasmin	Immunoturbidimetric	15–60 mg/dl	Often elevated in postmenopausal women and subjects with cancers, independent of their copper status
Selenium	Glutathione peroxidase, plasma	Spectrophotometric/ kinetic	455–800 U/L	Sensitive marker of selenium deficiency, but not selenium toxicity
Protein	Prealbumin	Immunoturbidimetric	10–40 mg/dl	Responds to therapeutic parenteral diets more quickly than does albumin due to its shorter half-life in the plasma
Protein	Retinol-binding protein	Immunoturbidimetric	3.0–6.0 mg/dl	Like prealbumin, RBP has short half-life; may be low in zinc deficiency or vitamin A deficiency, regardless of protein status
Anemia	RBC indices	Impedance occlusion	Age/sex stratified	See hematology texts
Niacin	2-Pyridone/ n-methyl-nicotinamide, urine	HPLC cation exchange	>2.4 mg/day	
Niacin	2-Pyridone/ n-methyl-nicotinamide ratio	HPLC cation exchange	Ratio >1.0	Rarely performed
Niacin	RBC NAD/NADP ratio	Reverse-phase HPLC	Ratio >1.0	Newly developed methodology; not fully validated for general use

[a] Some procedures may be available only in specialized laboratories or research centers. Consult the laboratory regarding appropriate specimen matrix and instructions for transport.

cedure. As vitamins serve as cofactors for many biochemical processes, they characteristically possess a plethora of ring structures, conjugated double bonds, and loosely chelated divalent cations. As a result, most vitamins are highly labile, particularly if exposed to significant amounts of UV irradiation or lengthy periods of time at ambient temperatures (see Chapter 10). In practice, it is often necessary to stabilize the nutrient of interest by selecting the proper blood or urine additive and by providing favorable transport and storage conditions. Also, the type of specimen taken is of major importance to both the subject and the analyst. While blood, urine, hair, and saliva are easy to obtain, the sampling of a metabolically important tissue, such as the liver, is very difficult.

Blood as a Test Matrix

Collection of blood specimens for nutritional analysis is most readily accomplished using commercially available evacuated blood collection tubes. Special "trace metal free" tubes (royal blue tops) with or without heparin additive are also available for use in trace element studies. In general, blood tubes should be wrapped in foil to block UV light exposure, placed in crushed ice to stabilize the nutritional analytes, and transported to the laboratory as soon as possible. To allow full clot retraction and avoid hemolysis, serum tubes should be allowed to clot before placing on ice. Transport to distant laboratories can be made in polyfoam packages using blocks of dry ice (4 pounds per 24 hr) and express courier service. Regarding trace metal studies, analysts are advised to avoid rimming the clot with wooden sticks. The latter are rich sources of contaminating metals, especially manganese. Finally, vitamin C, one of the most labile vitamins, requires special preservation using perchloric or metaphosphoric acid within 1 hr of venipuncture. Assays involving erythrocytes or leukocytes require that anticoagulated whole blood be provided. Clinicians are advised to consult the laboratory for specific instructions on the appropriate preservation and transport of the nutrient in question.

Urine as a Test Matrix

In general, urinary tests are not as diagnostically useful as blood tests for several reasons. Of primary concern is the large effect which fluid intake can have on urinary solute concentrations. If unadjusted for volume or some other static measure, the result is usually uninterpretable in terms of a reference range. Second, many nutrients exhibit variable rates of excretion throughout the day, a factor which can be particularly affected by the time elapsed since consumption of the last meal. The rate at which some nutritional analytes are excreted after a loading dose can also be substantially affected by the subject's glomerular filtration rate (GFR). The effect of diminished GFR is not limited to subjects with renal pathologies. GFR is known to fall throughout the life span, and by the eighth decade can reach levels characteristic of modestly advanced kidney disease even in the face of normal levels of serum creatinine and BUN. GFR can be roughly estimated in adult subjects by determination of the endogenous creatinine clearance rate (CRCL), using readily available nomograms (based on body weight and frame size) and a single determination of serum creatinine. A better indication of CRCL involves the collection of a 24-hr urine specimen, two measures of serum creatinine 12 hours apart, and sufficient fluid intake to provide at least 2 ml/min of urine flow. However, as true age- and sex-adjusted CRCL reference ranges are not generally available, it is difficult or impossible to rigorously adjust the excretion of a given nutritional analyte for impaired renal function.

Continuous collection of urine over a timed interval (usually 6–24 hr) is recommended and allows for the expression of the nutrient or metabolite on an excretion basis. Results can then be directly compared to the reference range. Correction for urine osmolality in random urine collections may be achieved by measuring creatinine concentration and reporting the result in terms of analyte per milligram of creatinine excreted. Use of such a "creatinine quotient" is convenient and has often been used where longer urine collection periods are impractical. However, in addition to requiring an extra test for creatinine, the constancy of daily creatinine excretion in free-living subjects may not be as constant as previously reported (Waterlow, 1986) and may vary up to 12%–15% in some individuals. Several comprehensive reviews of this topic are available (Narayanan and Appleton, 1980).

Excretion of creatinine over 6–24 hr has also been used as an index for *completeness* of the urine collection, a concern for the researcher or clinician treating patients who are forgetful or unreliable. Unfortunately, reference ranges for creatinine excretion are quite wide and allow the diagnostician to reliably detect only those subjects who grossly undercollected the timed specimen. A more elegant approach for detection of either incomplete collections or those subjects suffering impaired renal function is the use of nontoxic urinary markers, such as para-aminobenzoic acid (PABA). After an oral administration of a dose on the order of 200–500 mg, both the nutrient of interest and PABA are determined. Recoveries in excess of 91.6% are considered to be complete collections (95% confidence level) and allow for a more reliable interpretation of the nutritional marker (Roberts et al., 1989). The colorimetric assay used to quantitate PABA is not specific for this compound, however, and can result in overestimation of PABA recovery in those subjects consuming certain foods or analgesics, such as acetaminophen.

The following sections provide an overview of current principles and techniques of biochemical tests for assessing body status of specific nutrients in the clinical setting. More detailed information on this subject is available in monographs (Calman, 1981; Labbe, 1981; Sauberlich et al., 1974) and other sources (Sauberlich, 1981*a*, 1984).

Micronutrients: Water-Soluble Vitamins

Vitamin C (Ascorbic Acid)

Effective tests relating a vitamin-C-dependent function to ascorbate status have not been forthcoming. Alternatively, direct quantitation of ascorbate in plasma, leukocytes, erythrocytes, and whole blood has been shown to be a convenient and reliable index of recent dietary intake. Of these, plasma ascorbate determinations are most commonly performed but may not accurately reflect tissue reserves. Ascorbic acid saturation tests have been proposed in which a large oral dose of vitamin C is administered, followed by assessment of changes in serum or urinary ascorbate levels. These tests are tedious, but may serve to better gauge the extent of tissue deficit in an individual subject than that which is provided by plasma levels alone (Neale et al., 1988). Animal studies suggest that leukocyte levels may also better represent whole body stores than does the plasma compartment (Turnbull et al., 1981). Both plasma and leukocyte vitamin C levels have been shown to be reduced in hospitalized subjects (Rose and Nahrwold, 1981).

Studies with humans consuming various levels of dietary ascorbate show that plasma ascorbate levels vary directly with the intake of the vitamin. Plasma levels of 0.4 mg/dl and higher have recently been shown to require an intake of approximately 41 mg/day in young adult males (Jacob et al., 1987). Values less than 0.3 mg/dl are considered deficient, with clinical signs of scurvy appearing at plasma levels below 0.2 mg/dl. As whole blood ascorbate levels do not fall as much upon vitamin C depletion as serum levels do, whole blood levels are considered a less sensitive indicator (Baker et al., 1971; Hodges et al., 1971). Urinary excretion of ascorbate falls to nearly zero in the frankly deficient subject, but, otherwise, is too readily influenced by recent dietary intake to be useful in the assessment of marginal deficiencies. Similarly, levels of salivary ascorbic acid were not found to discriminate well between adequate and deficient intake in adult subjects fed varying levels of the vitamin (Jacob et al., 1987).

Analytical approaches for determining ascorbate in biologic samples include colorimetric, fluorometric, and HPLC methodologies (Sauberlich, 1981*a*, *b*). With the exception of liquid chromatography, all methods depend upon the reducing properties of the vitamin's 1,2-enediol group toward indicator dyes, or the formation of hydrazones and fluorophores. Colorimetric methods are most commonly employed, and include such chromophores as 2,4-dinitrophenylhydrazine (Roe and Keuther, 1943), ferrozine (Butts and Mulvihill, 1975; McGown et al., 1982), and 2,6-dichloroindophenol (Omaye et al., 1979; Sauberlich et al., 1982). The 2,6-dichloroindophenol method is readily automated; however, the DNPH method is generally regarded to be the most sensitive and specific, and remains the most popular. Fluorometric procedures based on o-phenylenediamine are an attractive alternative but require the availability of an automated analyzer capable of fluorescent measurements. Vuilleumier and Keck (1989) have recently reported an automated fluorescent procedure which uses ascorbate oxidase as an analyte-specific oxidizing agent. Detection and quantitation can be easily performed using an automated centrifugal analyzer in fluorescence mode. Any of the above methods can be used for plasma, whole blood, leukocyte, or urinary matrices. Leukocyte measurements, however, require significantly greater amounts of blood and require the additional step of harvesting the white cell fraction. Special leukocyte separation tubes have been recently introduced (Becton-Dickinson), which should expedite this task. Two practical reviews of ascorbate methodologies applicable to either the clinical laboratory (Brewster and Turley, 1987) or the research laboratory (Pachla et al., 1985) have been recently published.

HPLC methodologies using C_{18} reverse-phase separation followed by electrochemical detection are gaining widespread use in the clinical laboratory (Sauberlich et al., 1981*a*, *b*). The method is both sensitive and specific, but detects only the reduced form of ascorbate. Dehydroascorbate (DHA), a component found in plasma and which represents the first oxidative breakdown product of ascorbic acid, is not detected by this methodology. As the conversion of ascorbate to oxidative breakdown products is rapid, some investigators have utilized iso-ascorbate as an internal standard by which losses may be corrected. Other groups, in an effort to estimate total vitamin C using electrochemical detection, have attempted to convert the DHA to reduced ascorbate prior to quantitation by HPLC. The clinician is advised that unless a total vitamin C result is provided by the HPLC procedure, a modified (lower) reference range must be used to interpret patient results.

Certain precautions regarding ascorbate determinations should be mentioned. Vitamin C is among the most labile of the vitamins, and steps must be taken to stabilize the vitamin in plasma, body tissues, or fluids (Olliver, 1967). Minimally, samples should be refrigerated immediately after venipuncture and processed further within 4 hr. EDTA plasma (lavender top blood tube) is preferred over serum since hemoglobin released during the clotting process accelerates destruction of the vitamin. The EDTA anticoagulant also serves to bind iron, copper, and other divalent cations which participate in oxidation-reduction reactions involving vitamin C. A protein-free extract of the plasma should be prepared using an equal volume of 8% (vol/vol) metaphosphoric or perchloric acid containing 0.1% EDTA. Vortex the sample and centrifuge for 5 min. The clear, protein-free extract should be frozen at −20°C until analysis. If the DNPH procedure is to be used, incubation temperatures above 37°C should be avoided, as the generation of ascorbate-2-sulfate will produce spuriously high results (Baker et al., 1973).

Thiamin (Vitamin B_1)

Various approaches have been described for the laboratory evaluation of thiamin status in humans. Urinary excretion of thiamin (Pearson, 1967; Sauberlich, 1967) in a timed collection has, until recently, been the most popular approach. Historically, animal, microbiologic, and chemical assays have been employed. The thiochrome procedure, in which thiamin is reacted with ferricyanide, has been the most widely used, and a recent modification of this method which substantially increases the sensitivity and specificity has been reported (Waldenlind, 1979). HPLC procedures have also gained some support in recent years but, for levels generally encountered in the blood, lack sufficient sensitivity.

As illustrated in Figure 13.5, urinary thiamin excretion varies directly with the dietary intake of thiamin. However, under conditions of low or marginal intake, urinary excretion does not provide information concerning the degree of body thiamin depletion. As a result, while urinary thiamin excretions based on creatinine-corrected random urine samples are useful for population studies, they are not diagnostically useful on an individual basis. Measurements based on 24-hr urine collections are marginally more useful than random collections for the diagnosis of deficiency in individual patients.

Thiamin retention tests (Dewhurst and Morgan, 1970; Lossy et al., 1951; Pearson, 1962*a*), and determination of thiamin-dependent enzyme activity have emerged as reliable functional tests of thiamin status. Thiamin retention tests are performed by administering a load of thiamin (usually 5 mg) parenterally and measuring thiamin

Figure 13.5. Influence of thiamin intake on urinary thiamin excretion and erythrocyte transketolase activity in adult men. [*Source:* Sauberlich et al. (1974).]

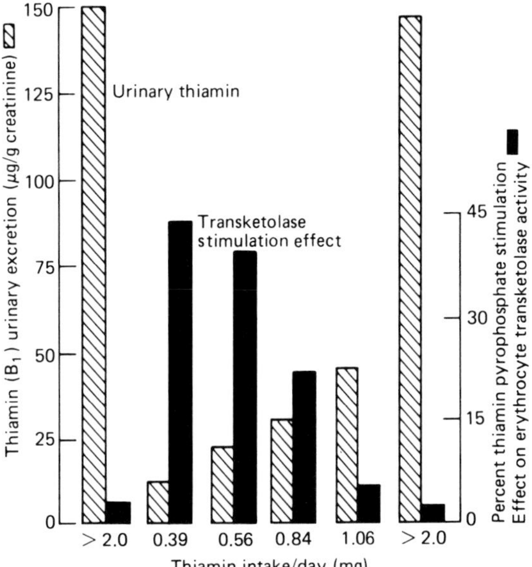

urinary excretion over the following 4-hr period. Deficient subjects excrete less than 20 μg of thiamin over the 4-hr period. The procedure is not practical for population survey use, but is diagnostically useful for estimating the extent of tissue thiamin depletion.

A functional test that is particularly useful in the clinical setting is the erythrocyte transketolase test (Smeets et al., 1971). The procedure measures the activity of transketolase (EC 2.2.1.1), a thiamin-dependent enzyme. The reaction sequence involves monitoring the formation of a glycoaldehyde intermediate from the ketol group of ribulose-5-phosphate. Transfer of the ketol group to a suitable acceptor aldehyde is followed by monitoring the disappearance of NADH at 340 nm. Transketolase activity is assessed in a red cell hemolysate with and without the presence of exogenously added thiamin pyrophosphate (TPP). Hemolysates from subjects who are thiamin-deficient demonstrate a relatively greater stimulation from the added TPP than do subjects who are adequate in thiamin stores. An activity coefficient (AC) is calculated as the ratio of the change in absorbance over time (Δ absorbance) of the stimulated to the nonstimulated hemolysate:

$$\text{Activity coefficient} = \frac{\Delta \text{ Absorbance (stimulated)}}{\Delta \text{ Absorbance (nonstimulated)}}$$

An activity coefficient in excess of 1.3 is generally regarded as deficient. Activity coefficients less than 1.0, while theoretically impossible, are observed and are interpreted as normal. The clinician is advised that some variants of the procedure calculate the "percent stimulation" or "percent activation," values which can be readily converted to an activity coefficient using the above ratio. The erythrocyte transketolase measure has proven to be a relatively simple, yet reliable, functional test of thiamin status. As the split hemolysate provides each subject with its own control, the test is independent of the usual confounding factors, such as age and sex. One precaution involves the lability of the transketolase enzyme. Erythrocyte or whole blood specimens must be kept on ice and analyzed as soon as possible to avoid loss of enzyme activity. Samples can be frozen before analysis, but only for a period of weeks rather than months.

Riboflavin (Vitamin B_2)

Laboratory approaches for assessing riboflavin status are essentially identical to those described for thiamin and include both direct and functional measures of B_2 status. Unlike some other water-soluble vitamins, the body does not metabolize substantial amounts of riboflavin, and urinary excretion appears to correlate well with intake and tissue reserves (Kraut et al., 1961; Morley et al., 1959). Accordingly, the most widely used tests for assessing riboflavin nutriture are those involving direct measures of urinary riboflavin excretion (Horwitt, 1966). Quantitation of whole blood, erythrocyte, or plasma levels of flavin compounds has also been reported, but appear to be of less value than urinary measures. An excellent functional test of B_2 status, erythrocyte glutathione reductase (EGR) activity, is available for use in the clinical setting and does not require the collection of a timed specimen (Nichoalds, 1974).

Determination of urinary riboflavin, expressed per gram of creatinine, has been successfully used for urine collections of less than 24-hr duration. For reasons of diagnostic reliability, however, the 24-hr urine collection is preferred. Reference intervals provided by the ICNND (Manual for Nutrition Surveys, 1963) suggest that values less than 27 μg/g of creatinine are indicative of deficiency in adult subjects. Reference values for children are substantially higher. While dietary intake and tissue reserves are the predominant factors affecting the daily excretion of riboflavin, the reader is advised that urinary riboflavin excretion can be spuriously elevated by physiological conditions frequently encountered in a clinical setting, including negative nitrogen balance, fasting, heat stress, and bed rest. A variation of the urinary excretion test involves the per oral administration of a riboflavin loading dose (5 mg), followed by a timed 4-hr collection period. Tentative guidelines released by the ICNND suggest that adults excreting less than 1000 μg of the load can be considered to be deficient. Reference ranges have not been developed for the B_2 loading test in pediatric subjects.

Riboflavin status has also been evaluated by determining blood, plasma, and erythrocytes concentrations of the two predominant flavin compounds—flavin mononucleotide (FMN) and flavin adenine dinucleotide (FAD) (Pearson, 1962*b*). However, direct blood measurements do not relate well to the degree of tissue riboflavin depletion and are not as responsive to changes in riboflavin nutriture as are urine or EGR tests. While not useful in the clinical setting, direct determination of flavins in tissues (other than blood) have been found to be an ideal index of body riboflavin reserves.

Analytical methods for direct determination of

flavins in blood and tissues include fluorometric (Nichoalds, 1981; Sauberlich, 1981*a*), microbiologic, and solid-phase enzyme-linked competitive binding (Cha and Meyerhoff, 1988). Fluorometric procedures generally provide more consistent results than the microbiologic assays and do not suffer from the problems frequently encountered with biologically based assays. The solid-phase assay is not yet practical for the clinical setting. Quantitation of urinary flavin compounds is readily accomplished using the new HPLC procedure of Chastain and McCormick (1987).

An excellent functional test of riboflavin status, which does not require the collection of a urine specimen, is the erythrocyte glutathione reductase (EGR) test already mentioned. The principle and technique of the functional EGR test is similar to that described previously for the erythrocyte transketolase test of thiamin status. Glutathione reductase (GR) serves to reduce oxidized glutathione (GSSG) in a reaction in which FAD serves as a cofactor:

$$\text{NADPH} + \text{H}+ + \text{GSSG} \xrightarrow{\text{FAD}} \text{NADP}+ + 2\ \text{GSH}$$

The GR activity of unstimulated and flavin-stimulated red cell hemolysates is measured, and an activity coefficient is calculated. Activity coefficient values above 1.3 are generally indicative of deficiency. As for thiamin, some investigators calculate percent stimulation or activation from the same data.

The EGR has all the advantages previously mentioned for the transketolase thiamin test. The GR enzyme is also somewhat more stable than the labile transketolase enzyme. The EGR activity coefficient plateaus rapidly in riboflavin deficiency and does not respond to further decreases in riboflavin tissue reserves. In addition, certain diseases, particularly glucose-6-phosphate dehydrogenase deficiency (Thurnham, 1972), and some drugs, including phenothiazines (chlorpromazine) and tricyclic antidepressants (Pinto et al., 1981), interfere with riboflavin metabolism. The EGR test, however, is convenient and reliable and is the current method of choice for assessing riboflavin status in the clinical situation.

Vitamin B_6 (Pyridoxine)

A greater variety of useful tests is available for assessing pyridoxine status than for thiamin and riboflavin. The methods include determination of free pyridoxine vitamers or metabolites in blood or urine and several functional tests based on vitamin B_6-dependent enzyme actions. Of these methods, the recommended tests include measurement of urinary vitamin B_6 excretion, blood pyridoxal-5-phosphate (PLP) levels, the tryptophan load test, and functional measures of erythrocyte transaminase activity.

The level of free urinary vitamin B_6 (principally as pyridoxal) has been shown to closely correlate with dietary pyridoxine intake in controlled studies with adult subjects (Figure 13.6) (Sauberlich et al., 1972). Adult urinary excretions of vitamin B_6 of less than 35 μg/day (or 20 μg/g creatinine) are indicative of marginal or inade-

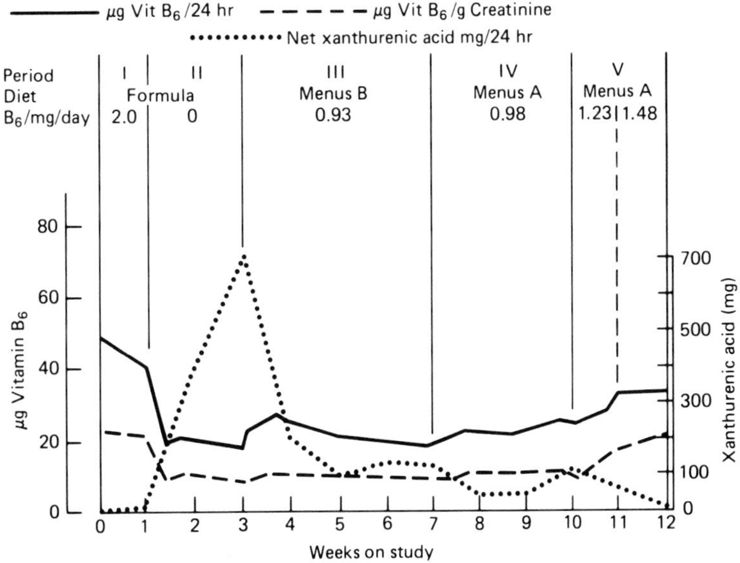

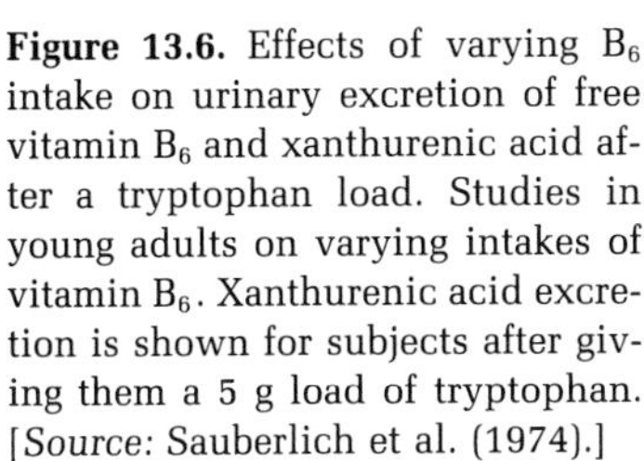

Figure 13.6. Effects of varying B_6 intake on urinary excretion of free vitamin B_6 and xanthurenic acid after a tryptophan load. Studies in young adults on varying intakes of vitamin B_6. Xanthurenic acid excretion is shown for subjects after giving them a 5 g load of tryptophan. [*Source:* Sauberlich et al. (1974).]

quate pyridoxine intakes. Like thiamin, urinary pyridoxine excretions reflect recent dietary intakes rather than the status of tissue reserves. Creatinine-corrected random morning fasting urines are useful for population studies, but 24-hr collections are recommended for diagnostic classification of individuals. From childhood to adulthood, the urinary excretion of pyridoxine, as well as thiamin and riboflavin, per gram of creatinine decreases with age. Therefore, guidelines for interpretation of results depend on the particular age group (Sauberlich et al., 1974). Alternatively, urinary 4-pyridoxic acid (4PA), the principal excretory form of vitamin B_6, can now be readily quantitated using a simple isocratic fluorescent HPLC procedure (Gregory and Kirk, 1979). However, as 4PA reflects only very recent dietary intake, it is suitable only for large nutrition status surveys.

The determination of pyridoxal-5-phosphate, the major coenzyme form of vitamin B_6 in plasma, has been shown to reflect its concentration in muscle, the major storage utilization site for this vitamer (Li and Lumeng, 1981). However, the principal method for determination of plasma PLP levels is technically difficult and requires the purification of B_6-free tyrosine apo-decarboxylase from bacterial cells (Reynolds, 1987). HPLC procedures for the determination of PLP and other B_6 vitamers in plasma have been reported but generally lack sufficient sensitivity for the levels encountered in deficient states, or suffer poor analytical precision (Reynolds, 1983). A new binary gradient HPLC procedure involving postcolumn derivitization has been reported (Sampson and O'Connor, 1989), which appears to provide adequate sensitivity. The latter procedure also provides results for pyridoxal, pyridoxine, and pyridoxic acid. However, the diagnostic utility of these non-PLP vitamers is unknown.

For the routine clinical setting, two functional measures of B_6 status are recommended. The first, the tryptophan load test, involves estimation of metabolite flux through a pathway which includes several B_6-dependent enzymes (see Chapter 5; Figure 5.16). Typically, subjects are provided with a 5- or 10-g tryptophan dose, followed by either a 6-hr or 24-hr urine collection (Brown et al., 1971). Subjects who are marginal or deficient in B_6 excrete significantly larger amounts of a tryptophan metabolite, xanthurenic acid. Excretion in excess of 250 mg per 24 hr is indicative of pyridoxine deficiency (Figure 13.6). Colorimetric procedures for the quantitation of xanthurenic acid are available (Hoes, 1981) and can be readily adapted to an automated chemistry analyzer. Urine specimens for xanthurenic acid can be frozen prior to analysis, but should be analyzed within 1 week of collection to avoid degradative losses. Due to the requirement for a timed urine collection, the tryptophan load test is not suitable for large population studies. Moreover, results must be interpreted with caution due to the interrelation of tryptophan metabolism with diverse metabolic and hormonal factors (Brown et al., 1971; Hattori et al., 1984).

A second functional test that has also been shown to be useful for assessment of body reserves of pyridoxine is the measurement of vitamin B_6-dependent transaminases before and after stimulation with exogenously added PLP. Erythrocyte glutamate-oxaloacetate transaminase (EGOT) and erythrocyte glutamate-pyruvate transaminase (EGPT) are the enzyme systems most typically used, since the red cell matrix is both readily available and may reflect a more time-integrated measure of B_6 intake. These procedures (Bayoumi and Rosalki, 1976; Krishnaswamy, 1971) are similar in approach to those previously described for thiamin and riboflavin, and results are reported as activity coefficients. However, because individual results and normal ranges are more variable than for the thiamin and riboflavin tests, each laboratory must establish its own normal range of results. As the enzymes are important clinical diagnostic tests for liver function, many colorimetric and other techniques are available for determining erythrocyte transaminase activity. However, the reader is advised that commercially available reagents for determination of serum SGPT and SGOT are not suitable due to the presence of PLP in the reaction mixtures. However, the assay is readily automated on discrete chemical analyzers using biochemical reagents which are widely available (Mount et al., 1987).

Folic Acid

As vitamins B_{12} and folic acid are both hematopoietic factors (Chapter 5), deficiencies of either vitamin can result in clinically discernible megaloblastic anemia. It is important, therefore, to distinguish between the two deficiencies prior to undertaking therapeutic interventions. Hence, it is essential that folate assessment methods relate to body folate reserves, independent of vitamin B_{12} status.

The sequence of biochemical and hematologic events in experimental human folate deficiency is shown in Figure 13.7. Serum folate levels are responsive to changes in dietary folate intake and are useful for distinguishing folate from B_{12} deficiency. However, the test is not a good index of overall body folate reserves. Analytical procedures for determination of serum folic acid include microbiological and radiometric competitive protein-binding (CPB) techniques.

The microbiologic assay procedure, which uses a folate-requiring strain of *Lactobacillus casei* (Scott et al., 1974), involves turbidimetric detection after an 18-hr incubation. Although tedious, the *L. casei* assay is considered to be the reference method, especially for tissues or food matrices. The CPB assay is appreciably simpler and faster and, as well, allows for the simultaneous determination of serum B_{12} levels. Two types of commercial folic acid kits are currently available: single-stage (competitive), and two-stage (noncompetitive) involving sequential incubations. Two-stage folate assays provide slightly better sensitivity. It should be noted that matrices other than serum or red cells require pretreatment with hog kidney or chicken pancreas deconjugase prior to quantitation of folates.

Erythrocyte folate content is generally regarded to be less affected by recent changes in folate intake (Mortensen, 1976, 1978) (Figure 13.7) and, therefore, is considered to be the best indicator of depleted tissue folate reserves. Unlike plasma, however, the erythrocyte contains significant amounts of monoglutamate and polyglutamate forms of folic acid, an observation which is of practical significance since the folate-binding proteins used in the commercial kits demonstrate variable affinities for the many forms of folic acid. As a result, dose–response curves for the commercial kits are frequently not as linear for the red cell folates as that observed with the microbiologically based techniques. Moreover, red cell folate levels are not useful for differentiating folate from B_{12} deficiencies, as low red-cell folate levels occur with B_{12} deficiency even in the face of adequate intake (Hoffbrand et al., 1966).

The presence of hypersegmented neutrophils has also been proven to be a reliable index of folate or vitamin B_{12} deficiency. The criteria for defining hypersegmentation in terms of the presence of five- or six-lobed neutrophils has been discussed (Herbert, 1959; Lindenbaum and Nath, 1980; Nath and Lindenbaum, 1979). However, the procedure is time-consuming and somewhat subjective. Other tests for diagnosing folate deficiency include urinary excretion of formiminoglutamic acid (FIGLU) after a histidine load, the deoxyuridine suppression test, the presence of macrocytosis (or macroovalocytosis), and megaloblastic bone marrow. The application of HPLC techniques to the determination of folates in biologic samples has also been reported (Colman, 1981), and a recent technique using affinity media has been shown to provide a profile of all forms of folates present in tissues (Selhub et al., 1988).

The histidine load test and the dU-suppression test are of interest in that they measure the metabolic flux through folate-dependent metabolic pathways and, therefore, are categorized as functional assays. Formiminoglutamate (FIGLU), an intermediate in the folate-dependent conversion of histidine to glutamate, is excreted in excessive amounts in the face of low folate status. A typical

Figure 13.7. Sequential changes that occur when folate deficiency is imposed in man. [*Source:* Herbert (1962, 1967).]

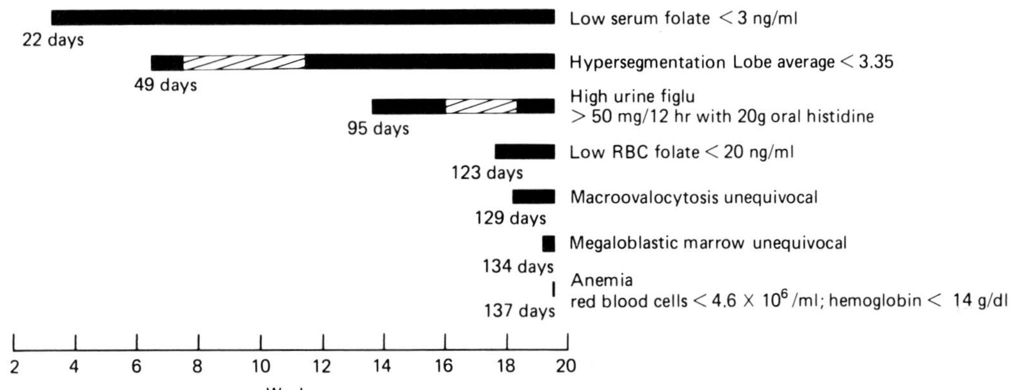

procedure involves oral administration of 15 g of histidine followed by an 8-hr urinary collection. FIGLU is readily measured spectrophotometrically by the method of Chanarin and Bennett (1962). Normal subjects have been reported to excrete less than 17 mg of FIGLU, whereas folate-deficient individuals ranged from 185–2047 mg per 8 hr (Luhby and Cooperman, 1964). However, as elevated excretion of FIGLU has also been observed in a substantial percentage of subjects deficient in vitamin B_{12}, the histidine load has only marginal utility as a test specific for folate deficiency.

The deoxyuridine suppression test (Colman, 1981), a functional assay involving the culture of either lymphocytes or bone marrow aspirates, is unique in that the procedure can directly distinguish between folic acid and cobalamin deficiencies. The test is predicated on well-characterized metabolic pathways involving the folate and B_{12}-dependent conversion of deoxyuridine (dU) to deoxythymidine monophosphate (dTMP) (see Chapter 5, Figures 5.18 and 5.19). The dTMP resulting from these reactions can be subsequently incorporated into genetic material during the de novo synthesis of DNA. The addition of exogenous dU to cultured cells serves to competitively suppress the incorporation of tritiated thymidine into DNA. In the presence of dU (which form nonradioactive dUMP and thus dTMP), incorporation of thymidine tracer in normal cells (i.e., folate and vitamin B_{12} replete) is suppressed by more than 90%. Conversely, the rate of conversion of unlabeled dU to dTMP is impaired in folate- or vitamin B_{12}-deficient cells and, therefore, labeled thymidine incorporation is less effectively suppressed. When performed on bone marrow aspirates, the test is thought to reflect current nutritional status, whereas circulating lymphocytes appear to index past nutritional status (Das and Herbert, 1978). While the dU-suppression test is diagnostically very useful, the procedure is laborious and requires a 3-day incubation. Its use is largely restricted to the research laboratory.

Vitamin B_{12} (Cobalamin)

As discussed previously, the macrocytic anemia caused by either vitamin B_{12} or folic acid deficiency cannot be distinguished by morphological changes alone. However, as the metabolism of folic acid and vitamin B_{12} are closely interrelated, it is essential that the status of these nutrients be evaluated together. Overall, the most useful test for assessing vitamin B_{12} nutriture is the determination of serum vitamin B_{12} levels. Serum vitamin B_{12} levels decrease with lowered total body B_{12} stores. As illustrated in Figure 13.8, serum B_{12} levels of pernicious anemia subjects (the most common form of vitamin B_{12} deficiency) are lower than those of normal subjects and those of patients with folate deficiency. Generally, serum vitamin B_{12} levels below 150 pg/ml are considered to indicate deficiency. As low red cell B_{12} levels are also seen in folate deficiency, erythrocyte determinations of vitamin B_{12} are not as reliable.

Principal techniques for determining serum vitamin B_{12} are, like folate, microbiologic methods using B_{12} requiring strains of *Lactobacillus leichmannii* (Matthews, 1962) and competitive binding (CPB) based assays. For clinical diagnostics, the CPB assay is the overwhelming choice because of its relative simplicity. It has been shown that procedures using impure intrinsic-factor

Figure 13.8. Serum B_{12} concentrations in normal subjects and in patients with pernicious anemia or folate deficiency. [*Source:* Wagstaff and Broughton (1971).]

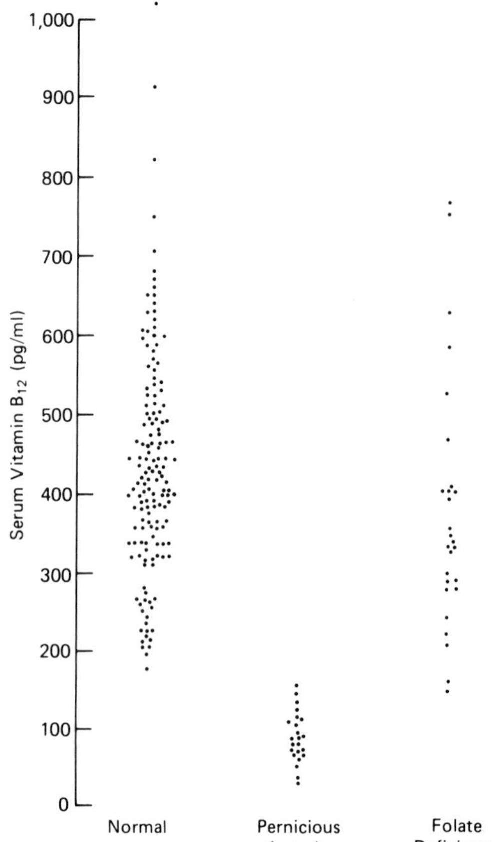

binder can provide spuriously high results in some specimens due to inclusion of cobalamin analogues that have little or no vitamin B_{12} activity (Kolhouse et al., 1978). In response to these concerns, the National Committee for Clinical Laboratory Standards has established guidelines for manufacturers of commercial B_{12} kits, which effectively eliminates this problem (National Committee for Clinical Laboratory Standards, 1980). However, at least one manufacturer provides a kit in which the binding protein is a crude intrinsic factor preparation. True (nonanalogue) B_{12} levels are provided by incubation of the sample with cobinamide to block R-binder protein activity. Assay without the presence of cobinamide may provide a "total" B_{12} level, which includes B_{12} analogues. The clinical significance of "total" B_{12} measures is not clear. As the cobinamide-blocked assay does not provide exactly the same result as a purified intrinsic factor-based assay (Chen, 1987), laboratories planning to use an in-house assay are advised to avoid procedures which are not based on affinity purified hog stomach intrinsic factor.

Generation of blood specimens intended for B_{12} analysis deserves a brief comment. As recent food intake may result in transient increases which are not reflective of tissues stores, all specimens should be from fasting subjects. It is especially important that patients on whom a Schilling test is to be performed have their specimen drawn for B_{12} analysis *prior* to administering either the radioactive cobalamin or receiving the standard 1 mg blocking dose. Serum or plasma are suitable specimens; however, evacuated blood tubes containing heparin or fluoride should be avoided as they promote destruction of cobalamin. Vitamin B_{12} is modestly degraded by exposure to sunlight, but is stable to freezing for several months at −20°C.

Recent reports suggest that two additional measures of B_{12} status, methylmalonic acid (MMA) and homocysteine (THC), may be earlier indicators of marginal B_{12} status than that provided by more traditional indices of B_{12} status. Previous studies had shown drastically elevated urinary excretion of these compounds in cases of overt B_{12} deficiency (Gompertz and Hoffbrand, 1970). However, a study examining levels of MMA and THC in serum reveal that B_{12}-responsive neuropsychiatric disorders have been identified in which traditional indicators of B_{12} status (anemia, mean corpuscular volume, and Schilling test) were either normal or only slightly perturbed (Lindenbaum et al., 1988). In all cases, measures of serum MMA and THC were significantly elevated and responded to treatment with parenteral vitamin B_{12}.

Other urinary B_{12}/folate metabolites have been shown to be excreted in larger amounts also during B_{12} deficiency, and include FIGLU, urocanic acid, and aminoimidazole-carboxamide. None have gained widespread use in the clinical community.

Niacin (Nicotinic Acid)

Measurement of urinary excretion of the major niacin metabolites, N^1-methylnicotinamide (NMN) and 2-pyridone, has been the most popular and reliable method for assessing niacin deficiency. The Interdepartmental Committee on Nutrition for National Defense published criteria for interpreting urinary NMN excretion in adults and pregnant women and suggested 24-hr excretions for adults of less than 0.8 mg/day as representing deficient niacin status and less than 2.4 mg/day as representing low status (Sauberlich et al., 1974). The use of creatinine corrections to allow for assay of random fasting urine samples rather than 24-hr collections is difficult to interpret because of differences in creatinine excretion by age. The ratio of 2-pyridone to NMN has been suggested as a niacin-deficiency marker independent of age and creatinine excretion (Holman and deLange, 1950; deLange and Joubert, 1964; DuPlessis, 1967). Shibata and Matsuo (1988, 1989), however, found that the urinary pyridone/NMN ratio in rats and humans was strongly dependent on the level of protein intake and that the ratio was a measure of protein adequacy rather than niacin status. A recent experimental study of niacin deficiency in adult males found the ratio to be insensitive to a marginal niacin intake of 10 niacin equivalents (NE) per day and not reliable for evaluating an intake of 6 NE/day (Jacob et al., 1989).

Although no tests of niacin derivatives in blood have been in general use as markers of niacin status, results from recent studies suggest that the level of pyridine nucleotides in the erythrocyte, especially NAD, can serve as a measure of niacin intake. Shibata (1987) found that whole blood levels of NAD and NADP reflected niacin intake in free-living women students consuming self-selected diets. In a recent experimental study of human niacin deficiency, erythrocyte NAD levels decreased by approximately 70%, whereas NADP levels remained unchanged when adult male subjects were fed low-niacin diets of either 6 or 10 niacin equivalents per day. The results suggest that the erythrocyte NAD concentration may serve as a sensitive indicator of niacin depletion, and that a ratio of erythrocyte NAD to NADP of <1.0 may identify subjects at risk of developing niacin deficiency (Fu et al., 1989). Concentrations of niacin and niacin metabolites in plasma are normally quite low and, in general, have not been shown to be useful markers of niacin status. As with other water-soluble vitamins, postdose increases in urinary excretion of niacin metabolites (particularly 2-pyridone) after an oral niacin load appear to provide an index of body niacin depletion (Jacob et al., 1989).

Micronutrients: Fat-Soluble Vitamins

Vitamin A

Liver, the major storage organ for vitamin A, contains mostly retinyl esters, with retinyl palmitate as the predominant species. While direct determination of hepatic retinyl esters is the most direct and accurate estimation of vitamin A reserves, the procedure is rarely performed and is limited to those circumstances in which noninvasive biochemical indices have provided inconclusive results. As a result, routine laboratory tests for detection of hypo- or hypervitaminosis A involve quantitation of plasma levels of either the alcohol or the ester form of the vitamin, respectively.

Under normal circumstances, plasma retinol levels are homeostatically regulated by the liver to meet the needs of peripheral tissues. As a result, static (unperturbed) measures of plasma retinol do not generally reflect dietary intake. Once hepatic reserves of vitamin A fall to less than 20 μg/g, a decline in plasma retinol levels is observed. Various guidelines for interpretation of plasma retinol results have been compiled (Food and Agriculture Organization/World Health Organization, 1987; Food and Drug Administration, 1985; International Vitamin A Consultative Group, 1979). In adults, retinol values below 20 μg/dl are usually indicative of inadequate vitamin A intake and lowered tissue stores of the vitamin. Levels between 20 and 30 μg/dl are considered to be indeterminate and warrant further investigation by one or more of the functional measures as described below. Levels above 40 μg/dl are considered adequate to meet the needs of peripheral tissues and are not accompanied by ophthalmic or dermatologic pathologies. Populations which consume diets rich in the preformed vitamin (e.g., North Americans) rather than carotenoids typically have plasma retinol levels in the range of 42–65 μg/dl. Chronic overconsumption of preformed vitamin A can result in vitamin A toxicity with severe clinical consequences (see Chapter 5). The recommended laboratory test for suspected cases of hypervitaminosis A is the quantitative determination of retinyl esters after a 14-hr fast, as described by Bankson et al. (1986). Total retinyl ester levels (mostly as retinyl palmitate) in excess of 11 μg/dl can be considered as indicative of excessive liver stores. Confirmation of vitamin A toxicity requires a liver biopsy. The Bankson et al. procedure is attractive since, it is a normal phase HPLC technique and does not require redissolution of the vitamin A extract into a secondary mobile phase. Moreover, the procedure provides simultaneous quantitation of both retinol and retinyl esters within the same chromatographic run, a feature attractive to the clinical laboratory that must be prepared to confirm putative cases of both hypo- and hypervitaminosis A.

Several functional measures of low vitamin A status have been proposed, including electroretinography and dark adaptation (Hodges and Kolder, 1971; Russell et al., 1973) and the relative dose–response test (RDR). The RDR procedure is based on well-characterized biological mechanisms involving the uptake and release of retinol from the liver after administration of a physiological dose of vitamin A. Specimens are taken both before (A_0) and 5 hours (A_5) after the test dose. The rise in vitamin A levels are calculated as described by Loerch et al. (1979) as:

$$\text{Relative dose–response (RDR) (\%)} = \frac{A_5 - A_0}{A_5} \times 100$$

Subjects with adequate vitamin A stores demonstrate little or no rise in plasma vitamin levels at 5 hr, whereas subjects with low hepatic stores demonstrate an exaggerated increase. Human studies (Flores et al., 1984) suggest that an RDR response $\geq 14\%$ is indicative of hypovitaminosis A. The clinician is advised that under circumstances where the synthesis of apo-RBP may be limiting (e.g., protein-calorie malnutrition or zinc deficiency), a false negative result might be anticipated (Russell et al., 1983). Previous studies have also demonstrated that the RDR also fails to predict vitamin A status in cirrhotic and malabsorptive subjects (Mobarhan et al., 1981).

Under circumstances where little or no preformed vitamin A is consumed in the diet, carotenoids from plant foods are a source of vitamin A.

However, the clinician is advised that plasma levels of carotenoids do not provide a good index of either dietary vitamin A adequacy or of liver vitamin A reserves. Moreover, while HPLC methodologies are now available that can individually quantitate members of the carotenoid family, the most commonly used method for assessment of "carotene" status [hexane extraction of plasma or serum followed by colorimetry at 450 nm] gives an estimate of total carotenoid intake. Absolute levels of beta-carotene, the most active vitamin A precursor, are usually on the order of 20%–30% of the total carotenoid level (Chapter 5, Table 5.8). Subjects consuming large quantities of tomatoes demonstrate an even greater discrepancy as a substantial part of their carotenoid profile is accounted for by lycopene, a carotenoid thought to lack activity as a vitamin A precursor (see Chapter 5, Table 5.7). Low carotenoid levels can be observed even with normal dietary intake if there is fat malabsorption, liver disease, chronic abuse of mineral oil laxatives, and/or a febrile condition. Administration of kanamycin or neomycin can cause transitory decreases in plasma carotenoids due to malabsorption. [They do not interfere with absorption of retinol.]

Three major analytical methods are commonly used for determining retinol levels in plasma: (1) spectrophotometry, (2) fluorometry, and (3) HPLC. An excellent review of these methods, including their limitations, has been authored by Turley and Brewster (1987). The colorimetric Carr–Price technique and its many modifications have been commonly used and depend on the formation of a transient blue complex in the presence of antimony trichloride and trifluoroacetic acid. Both retinol and its esters are detected by the method, as are the carotenoids. The method is sufficiently sensitive and is reproducible when close attention is given to the problems of correction for carotene content and rapid color losses. However, the reagents are hazardous and highly corrosive to laboratory instrumentation. Another spectrophotometric procedure, the method of Bessey et al. (1946), can be used, which does not require the use of corrosive reagents. Retinol is quantitated by its natural absorption at 325 nm after extraction into a suitable solvent, such as petroleum ether. Specificity is imparted to the assay by measuring the absorbance before and after exposure of the sample to UV light to destroy the retinol moieties. Sensitivity is generally poor.

The fluorometric determination of retinol provides a three- to fourfold greater sensitivity than for colorimetric procedures, but can suffer spuriously high results due to the presence of phytofluene, a pigment found in reddish-colored vegetables and fruits. A modification of this procedure corrects for phytofluene interference by its prior removal with silicic acid columns, or by the use of a bichromatic detection mode (Thompson et al., 1971). With the advent of modern, automated fluorometers, the fluorometric technique has become increasingly popular in the clinical setting and now surpasses the Carr–Price approach for routine applications.

A number of HPLC techniques are available for the quantitation of retinol, and all provide good sensitivity and unsurpassed specificity compared to colorimetric or fluorometric methodologies. The reverse-phase HPLC method of Bieri et al. (1979) provides simultaneous determination of both retinol and tocopherol in a single 5-min chromatographic run and is under consideration by the American Association for Clinical Chemistry as a Selected Method. Retinol acetate is used to assess analytical recovery during the initial liquid extraction steps. Within-run and between-run coefficients of variation are approximately 4% and 6%, respectively. As mentioned earlier, the Bankson et al. (1986) normal-phase HPLC method is an attractive alternative when tocopherol levels are not required. Procedures in which retinoids, carotenoids, and tocopherols are simultaneously quantitated in a single chromatographic run are very useful for the research setting, but are generally too demanding for use in the routine clinical laboratory (MacCrehan and Schonberger, 1987; Milne and Botnen, 1986; Thurnham et al., 1988).

The generation of plasma specimens intended for use in the quantitation of retinol or retinyl esters deserves some comments. Retinol is characterized by a ring structure and a series of unconjugated double bonds which make the molecule highly susceptible to degradation by UV light (Chapter 5, Figure 5.25). Specimens should be drawn in the fasting state (especially important for determination of retinyl esters) into EDTA-containing evacuated blood tubes. If immediate processing is not practical, the specimen should be foil-wrapped and placed on ice. Centrifugation and freezing (in the dark) should proceed within 6 hr of venipuncture. Specimens can be analyzed up to 8 months after collection if kept frozen at −70°C in small 2 ml cryovials with minimal air space above the sample. Larger tubes containing small volumes of plasma suffer significant oxidative losses due to trapped air. An excellent study examining the stability of retinol and carotenoids in frozen specimens has been recently reported (Craft et al., 1988).

Vitamin E (Tocopherol)

Clinical interest in determining vitamin E status in humans has been largely restricted to either neonates or adult subjects suffering from a variety of malabsorptive or hepatobiliary conditions. Other instances of either vitamin E deficiency or excess have been virtually unknown. Recent studies have suggested, however, that tocopherols may play an important role in the aging process, immune function, and as an anticancer agent. As a result, clinical laboratories are observing a significant increase in the number of requests related to determination of tocopherol status.

Vitamin E can be measured in a variety of matrices, including serum, erythrocytes, leukocytes, and platelets. Plasma is the most commonly used matrix and its levels are thought to reflect both dietary intake and body tissue reserves. Colorimetric, fluorometric, and liquid chromatographic assays have been developed. The colorimetric procedures are based on the Emmerie–Engel reaction, in which solvent-extracted tocopherols participate in the reduction of ferric iron to ferrous iron. The latter is reacted with α,α_1-dipyridyl to produce a red chromophore absorbing at 510 nm. Correction for contributions from carotene and retinol are accomplished using prior chromatographic removal, hydrogenation to nonreactive species, or by subtraction using assays specific for these compounds. As the corrections required to impart vitamin E specificity are both laborious and inexact, this procedure is no longer in common usage (Turley and Brewster, 1987). A sensitive fluorometric procedure which allows simultaneous quantitation of vitamins A and E has gained some popularity in the clinical setting (Hansen and Warwick, 1969). After precipitation of serum proteins with ethanol, fat-soluble vitamins are extracted into hexane and are quantitated at 340 nm after excitation at 295 nm.

HPLC (liquid chromatographic) techniques involving either fluorometric or spectrophotometric detection are gaining widespread acceptance due to their sensitivity as well as specificity. The normal phase methods allow for the separation and quantitation of vitamin E isomers (α, β, and γ) and do not require drying of the extract and redissolution into mobile phase. However, clinicians do not generally require individual quantitation of tocopherol isomers. Furthermore, since normal phase methods are not readily adapted to provide simultaneous determination of plasma retinol levels, they have not gained the widespread use enjoyed by the reverse-phase methodologies (Bieri et al., 1979). Analysts using HPLC methodologies are advised that tocopherol acetate is not as suitable as retinol acetate for use as an internal standard, since its presence in the plasma from subjects receiving total parenteral nutrition may cause severe underestimation of the true levels of vitamin E (Turley and Catignani, 1985). Alternatively, dl-tocol can be used as an internal standard for vitamin E quantitation (De Leenheer et al., 1979).

Several functional tests of vitamin E status have been used or have been proposed. All are based on the natural antioxidant character which tocopherols impart to lipid moieties, particularly plasma membranes. The most commonly employed functional test of vitamin E status is the erythrocyte fragility test. The test using hydrogen peroxide as the lysing agent is probably the most commonly used (Leonard and Losowksky, 1967) and is technically simple to perform. The amount of hemoglobin released upon hemolysis due to hydrogen peroxide is compared to a distilled-water control specimen. Values in excess of 20% hemolysis are considered to reflect tocopherol deficiency. While not yet commonly employed in the clinical laboratory, the quantitation of erythrocyte malondialdehyde release after in vitro incubation of red cells with hydrogen peroxide (Cynamon et al., 1985) has also been used as a functional measure of in vivo lipid peroxidation secondary to vitamin E deficiency. Finally, measurement of expired pentane and ethane has also been proposed as a reliable test of vitamin E status (Dillard et al., 1977; Lemoyne et al., 1987) and has recently been shown to relate positively to increased lipid peroxidation in patients receiving parenteral nutrition (Lemoyne et al., 1988; Van Gossum et al., 1988).

The clinician is reminded that all indirect (i.e., functional) measures of vitamin E status reflect tissue antioxidant capabilities, of which tocopherol is only one determinant (Chapter 5, Figure 5.33). Thus, while experimental studies of human vitamin E depletion have documented the increased susceptibility of red cells to hemolysis, the results obtained from deficient and nondeficient populations were shown to overlap (Sauberlich et al., 1974). Also, since vitamin E is largely carried within the lipoprotein fractions, expression of total plasma tocopherols per unit of total plasma lipid provides a more accurate index of vitamin E status than that provided by levels expressed on a plasma volume basis. An adequate level is 0.8 mg total tocopherol per gram of total lipid in adults (Horwitt et al., 1972) or 0.6 mg/g in older children (Farrell et al., 1978). However, rapid postnatal changes preclude the use of tocopherol : lipid indices in the newborn and should be expressed on a per volume basis (Gutcher et al., 1984). Levels in excess of 6.4 mg/L can be regarded as adequate in this age group.

Vitamin D (Calciferol)

The increasing use of modern analytical techniques, such as competitive protein-binding (CPB) assays, HPLC, and mass spectrometry, has greatly expanded the number of approaches available for assessing vitamin D nutriture. Tests developed before 1970 were tedious and nonspecific and included a variety of bioassays and the measurement of vitamin D-related analytes, such as alkaline phosphatase, serum calcium, or serum phosphate. More recently developed techniques allow direct quantitation of the biologically important vitamin D metabolites in serum, 25-hydroxyvitamin D (25-OH-D), and 1,25-dihydroxyvitamin D [1,25-$(OH)_2$-D]. Analytical methods for determining the plasma concentrations of 25-OH-D and 1,25-(OH)-2-D must possess extremely high sensitivity and specificity, since the concentration ranges are 8–55 ng/ml and 16–65 pg/ml respectively.

Various methods have been reported that combine two analytical approaches to achieve the required total specificity and sensitivity. Examples include column chromatography (eg, silica, Sephadex-LH gels) and HPLC as separative techniques (specificity) and CPB, RIA, and mass spectrometry as detection techniques (sensitivity). These techniques have been reviewed and critiqued (Duncan and Haddad, 1981). Although they are complex and tedious to set up and run, they provide more direct and reliable information than do the older assessment methods. The first practical assays developed to quantitate 25-OH-D without prior chromatographic purification demonstrated concentrations of the vitamin nearly twice those observed by chromatographically based methods (Belsey et al., 1974; Justova et al., 1976). Bouillon et al. (1984) subsequently reported a direct assay of 25-OH-D based on competitive protein binding (CPB), which produces results similar to those from chromatographic methodologies. Recently, commercial kits for the direct assay of 25-OH-D have been introduced. The kits include all of the materials necessary to perform the required sample preparation steps and provide acceptable correlations with the chromatographically based assays. Most CPB assays of 25-OH-D use dextran-coated charcoal for separation of the bound and free tracer (tritiated) vitamin.

As the major circulating metabolite of vitamin D (Chapter 5, Figure 5.30), 25-OH-D has been shown to be the best index of body vitamin D stores and is clinically useful both as an indicator of vitamin D deficiency and vitamin D toxicity. The 1,25-$(OH)_2$-D metabolite, although the most metabolically active regarding mineral homeostasis, is not regarded as a good measure of vitamin D nutriture. Laboratory measures of 1,25-$(OH)_2$-D are recommended only for patients with hypocalcemic and hypercalcemic disorders. The first assays developed for 1,25-$(OH)_2$-D were, like 25-OH-D, tedious and cumbersome to perform. The analytical requirements for providing accurate and precise quantitation of 1,25-$(OH)_2$-D are exacerbated by the fact that circulating levels are nearly 1000-fold less than the monohydroxylated form of the vitamin. Recently, two methods have been reported which utilize a calf-thymus receptor specific for 1,25-$(OH)_2$-D to provide relatively straightforward quantitation of this vitamin D metabolite (Hollis, 1986; Reinhardt et al., 1984). This laboratory (Morrow) purifies the thymus receptor from freshly slaughtered animals and prepares large batches in lyophilized form for use over a period of several months. Alternatively, commercial kits have been introduced for quantitation of 1,25-$(OH)_2$-D, which are based on the single-extraction (Hollis, 1986) procedure. Another manufacturer provides a commercial kit for quantitation of 1,25-$(OH)_2$-D, which utilizes a dual extraction approach.

Vitamin K

Vitamin K is necessary for the biosynthesis of prothrombin, blood-clotting factors (VII, IX, and X), and for a number of other proteins (not related to hemostasis (Chapter 5). Analogous to laboratory measures of vitamin D metabolites, direct quantitation of vitamin K compounds (K_1, K_2, K_3) has been difficult to achieve in body tissues and fluids because of their molecular similarity and very low concentrations. As a result, routine diagnostic tests to diagnose putative vitamin K deficiency are based on functional measures of the clotting system. The most frequently performed tests include prothrombin time, partial thromboplastin time, and bleeding time. As a number of other factors involved in the clotting cascade may cause abnormal coagulation results, these tests are nonspecific for vitamin K. However, normalization of the functional response after administration of phylloquinone (K_1) is generally regarded as evidence of latent vitamin K deficiency. Alternative explanations for delayed clotting times include hepatic disease, drugs, or genetic abnormalities.

A more sensitive but, nevertheless, indirect test for vitamin K deficiency has been proposed (Blanchard et al., 1981). The test is a radioimmunoassay for abnormal prothrombin, a species which appears in the circulation when vitamin K-dependent γ-carboxylation of glutamic acid residues of prothrombin is diminished due to low vitamin K status (Chapter 5). Direct HPLC assays of serum vitamin K levels have also been reported that involve chromatographic separation of the nonpolar vitamin K species on reverse-phase columns followed by UV detection (LeFevre et al., 1979, 1982). Prior removal of neutral lipids is required in order to eliminate interferences. While highly specific for vitamin K_1, the UV-based methods generally provide only modest sensitivity. Electrochemical reduction of vitamin K followed by fluorescence detection has been reported and provides enhanced sensitivity (Hart et al., 1984; Ikenoya et al., 1979). Of more interest to the clinical laboratory is an elegant procedure that eliminates the need for electrochemical reduction and provides quantitative conversion of the vitamin to its naturally fluorescent form (Haroon et al., 1986). On-line catalytic reduction is accomplished by use of powdered metallic zinc. A recent report by the same laboratory (Sadowski et al., 1989) provides reference values for young and elderly adults consuming a freely selected diet.

Micronutrients: Trace Metals

Iron

Determination of iron status is one of the most frequently requested laboratory procedures related to nutritional assessment, and deficiencies of this trace element are encountered with relatively high prevalence throughout the world (Baker and DeMaeyer, 1979). The need to assess latent or developing iron deficiency is apparent, not only to prevent anemia, but also due to increasing evidence that suggests that marginal iron deficiency in the existing absence of anemia may be detrimental to health (Baker et al., 1977; Cook and Finch, 1979). Indeed, overt anemia is neither a sensitive nor a specific indicator of iron status, and this condition should be viewed as the final stage in a continuous spectrum of iron intakes. The clinical presentation observed in instances of iron deficiency is complicated by the fact that the condition is frequently secondary to more severe maladies (e.g., malignancy or occult bleeding). Therefore, it is necessary for the clinician to choose among those laboratory tests, which are not only sensitive markers of iron status, but which can provide a differential diagnosis between low iron intake and excessive iron losses.

Figure 13.9 illustrates the course of four biochemical indices of status during the development of iron deficiency. The most definitive laboratory procedure for defining iron reserves is cytochemical staining of blood marrow aspirates

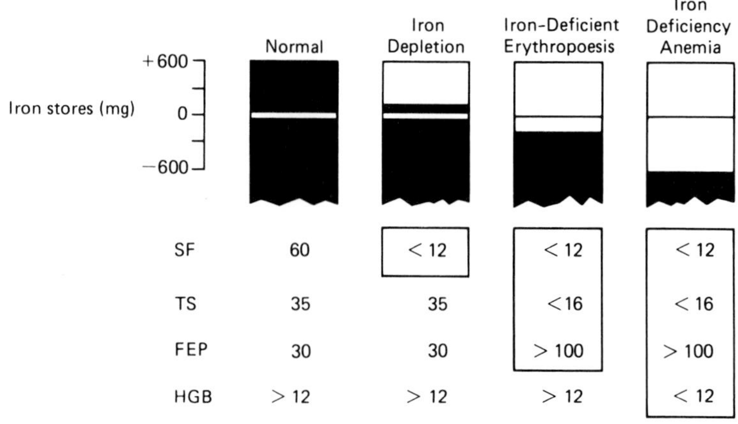

Figure 13.9. Iron status in relation to body iron stores. Various measures of body iron status are shown in relation to body iron stores (shaded areas), SF (serum ferritin), TS (transferrin saturation), FEP (free erythrocyte protoporphyrins), and HGB (hemoglobin). Negative iron stores represent depletion from circulating red cells. [*Source:* Cook and Finch (1979).]

using the Prussian blue reaction. However, the procedure is invasive and is not routinely performed. When iron stores are only modestly diminished, serum ferritin is generally regarded to be the most sensitive laboratory index. Values less than 12 ng/ml represent depleted stores, especially in males. However, serum ferritin levels are substantially affected by chronic inflammatory processes and concurrent liver disease (Chapter 7, Table 7.4). Under such circumstances, one can observe normal levels even in the face of diminished iron reserves. At least one manufacturer now provides a two-site immunoradiometric assay (IRMA) for ferritin which utilizes a solid-phase magnetic separation technique. The method is rapid, provides excellent sensitivity and precision, and is readily adaptable to automation. Clinicians are advised to rerun ferritin analyses on diluted specimens from those subjects suspected of having hemochromatosis. Some ferritin assays can erroneously demonstrate "normal" counts on specimens with extremely high levels of ferritin, a situation somewhat analogous to antigen excess in an immunoturbidimetric assay.

Alternatively, the clinician can request the determination of transferrin saturation (TSAT) [i.e., the ratio of serum iron levels to the serum total iron binding capacity (TIBC)]. During iron deficiency, the major determinant of TIBC (transferrin) is elevated, and serum iron levels fall. TSAT values less than 16% are indicative of jeopardized iron status. TIBC values are decreased with chronic inflammatory disease and malignancy (Fairbanks and Klee, 1986). A number of procedures have been developed for the quantitation of serum iron and iron-binding capacities. Many of the colorimetric assays are based on the formation of the highly colored iron/ferrozine complex first reported by Stookey (1970). These procedures are inexpensive and readily adaptable to discrete analyzers. A similar ferroin compound has been developed which is more specific for ferrous iron and eliminates significant interference from serum copper (Higgins, 1981). Alternatively, serum iron levels can be quantitated by flame atomic absorption spectrophotometry after chelation and extraction with bathophenanthroline, or after protein precipitation with hot trichloroacetic acid. Direct assay of serum samples by atomic absorption spectrophotometry is to be avoided due to the contribution from hemoglobin iron released during the clotting process.

Using a formula, the absolute levels of transferrin can be estimated as:

$$\text{Transferrin (mg/dl)} = 0.70 \times \text{TIBC (mg/dl)}$$

The relationship is not entirely linear since a small portion of serum iron is not bound to transferrin. Moreover, the actual regression equation is somewhat dependent upon the instrumentation and methodology being used and, therefore, should be empirically determined by each laboratory. For laboratories so equipped, transferrin can be determined directly using a variety of immunoturbidimetric or nephelometric procedures available from reagent manufacturers. The clinician is reminded that transferrin is an acute phase-affected protein, and its levels may not be indicative of iron status in the presence of inflammatory conditions.

The determination of free erythrocyte photoporphyrins (FEP) has also been promoted as a test of iron status that identifies impaired erythropoiesis secondary to iron deficiency. It is particularly of value when there is a need to distinguish between bona fide iron deficiency and the genetic condition, thalassemia minor. FEP levels are elevated during iron deficiency but are normal in cases of this thalassemia. FEP levels can also be elevated in plumbism (lead poisoning). In both iron deficiency and plumbism, the first step of heme synthesis is blocked. Both conditions can be readily treated, and FEP assays are frequently included in health-screening programs conducted in the nation's public schools. Subsequent testing is required to distinguish between the two conditions whenever elevated FEP values are observed.

Zinc

Zinc, the second most abundant trace element in the body after iron (Chapter 7, Table 7.1), is involved in a large number of metabolic functions. Over 100 enzymes have been found to be dependent upon zinc as a cofactor (Chapter 7, Figure 7.7), an observation which probably accounts for the diverse effects of zinc deficiency. As with the nutrients discussed previously, laboratory tests for assessing zinc nutriture either involve a direct determination of zinc in a body tissue or fluid, or the assessment of a biochemical function dependent upon zinc. Direct determinations of zinc can be performed on plasma, hair, urine, erythrocytes, and saliva. Functional tests include serum alkaline phosphatase, lactic dehydrogenase, ribonuclease, erythrocyte carbonic anhydrase, and taste and smell acuity. All of the above indices decrease with zinc deficiency, except ribonuclease activity, which increases (Jacob, 1986).

Although the tests described above have been shown to correlate with zinc deficiency in animals and humans, no single procedure has proven to be a definitive indicator of dietary intake or body reserves. Moreover, test results must be interpreted with caution, as they may be confounded by clinical conditions unrelated to the subject's zinc status. Examples of the latter include hypoalbuminemia, hepatic cirrhosis, immediate postsurgical periods, bacterial endotoxin, and therapeutic steroid regimens (Jacob, 1986).

Direct assay of zinc in plasma, red cells, cerebral spinal fluid, and urine can be accomplished by the dithiozone compleximetric method (Helwig et al., 1986; Kagi and Vallee, 1958) by fluorometry (Mahanand and Houck, 1968; Watanabe et al., 1963) or by flame atomic absorption spectrophotometry (Smith et al., 1983). The colorimetric and fluorometric procedures are tedious, offer only modest specificity, and are no longer commonly performed in the clinical laboratory environment. A new zinc-specific colorimetric method, based on the procedure of Homsher and Zak (1985), has been reported and is now available as a commercial kit. The method is both sensitive and specific, and is readily adaptable to automation on most discrete analyzers. Flame atomic absorption spectrophotometry (an AACC Selected Method) is the assay of choice in those laboratories equipped with the necessary instrumentation. Specimens are first diluted fivefold in water and measured against external atomic absorption standards prepared in 5% (vol/vol) glycerol to account for differential viscosity. Analysts are advised that quantitation of zinc by flame atomic absorption should be performed in conjunction with deuterium background correction in order to provide adequate precision. Accuracy can be ensured by use of bilevel serum-based assayed control materials which are available commercially. These materials can be used to monitor accuracy for a number of trace and ultratrace metal analyses.

Specimen collection for zinc should be performed using guidelines previously reported for trace metal analyses (Adeloju and Bond, 1985; Ericson et al., 1986; Katz, 1985). For routine evaluations, plasma is the preferred specimen. Serum values tend to be variably elevated due to the destruction of zinc-rich platelets during the clotting process. Therefore, blood should be collected into commercially available evacuated blood tubes treated to remove trace metal contamination. Moreover, as nearly 80% of blood zinc is contained in the red cell fraction, even microhemolysis is to be avoided. Hemolysis can be minimized by ensuring immediate processing of the specimen and by using low speed (2000 g) centrifugation. Fasting plasma values tend to be higher than postprandial specimens. Values less than 70 μg/dl are regarded as zinc-deficient.

Zinc concentrations in hair have been reported to be an indicator of long-term zinc nutriture. However, hair zinc levels demonstrate a seasonal variation (Strain et al., 1966) and above-normal levels can occasionally be observed in zinc-deficient subjects due to the extremely slow rate at which hair grows under such circumstances. Determination of urinary zinc levels has also been reported (Baer and King, 1984), and values fall rapidly with diminished zinc intake. The presence of catabolic conditions (e.g., fasting, trauma, surgery) can lead to accelerated rates of zinc excretion and can lead to normal values in spite of low zinc status. Urinary zinc analysis should be performed on a 24-hr specimen collected into a plastic container previously washed with mineral acids to remove contaminating metals. A suitable procedure is to fill the container overnight with a solution of 10% hydrochloric and 10% nitric acid, followed by extensive rinsing with deionized water. In order to avoid loss of zinc onto the plastic surface and to avoid precipitates, the container should contain 15–20 ml of 35% (vol/vol) reagent grade hydrochloric acid. For reasons of safety, patients providing their own collections must be advised to avoid contact with the acid additive. Values less than 150 μg/day represent abnormally low excretion and warrant follow-up with other indices of zinc status.

Copper

The occurrence of copper deficiency in human populations is not widespread and is largely limited to cases involving long-term parenteral nutrition, special dietary regimens, or genetic abnormalities. Deficiencies in pediatric subjects are the most commonly reported, especially in those subjects receiving high calorie, low copper rehabilitative diets (Cordano et al., 1966). Deficiency is characterized by anemia, hypoproteinemia, neutropenia, and diarrhea. Instances of copper toxicity are also not that uncommon and can arise from either chronic hemodialysis (Blomfield et al., 1971) or from industrial accidents involving inhalation of copper fumes.

Measurement of serum copper levels is generally regarded as providing the best assessment of copper deficiency. Decreased circulating copper levels have been observed in copper-deficient subjects. Additionally, copper levels increase when copper supplementation is initiated. Like zinc, other factors not related to copper nutriture can affect serum copper levels, including cancer, pregnancy, and inflammation (Chapter 7, Table 7.8). Also, like zinc, plasma copper levels may exhibit slight diurnal variation, with the highest levels in the morning. Hair copper has also been proposed to be a useful index of copper status. However, a progressive increase in human hair copper levels from the proximal to distal end of the shafts has been observed and is attributed to airborne contamination. Therefore, it is suggested that only the most proximal hair segments be analyzed as a test of copper nutriture. Urinary copper and cuproenzymatic activities may also be helpful in some circumstances. Unlike zinc, however, urinary excretion of copper is quite low (less than 60 μg/day) (Chapter 7, Figure 7.8) and is somewhat independent of intake. Nevertheless, an effect of depleted body copper may be lowered urinary copper excretion as observed in some patients undergoing TPN with copper-deficient solutions. The cuproenzymes most suitable for assessing copper status are serum ceruloplasmin, erythrocyte superoxide dismutase (SOD), and leukocyte cytochrome oxidase.

Laboratory methods for assessment of copper status have been reviewed (Jacob, 1981; Solomons, 1979). The most common methods in use today are flame or flameless atomic absorption spectrophotometry, emission spectroscopy, and colorimetry. The colorimetric procedure reported by Peterson and Bollier (1955) and modified by Rice (1960) demonstrates high specificity and molar absorptivity for divalent copper but is quickly being replaced by the bathocuproine reagent, originally introduced by Zak and Ressler (1958). The latter procedure has been adapted for the Cobas centrifugal analyzer (Kossman, 1983) and is now available as a commercial kit. For those laboratories so equipped, the reference method for determination of serum copper is flame atomic absorption spectrophotometry as described by Alcock (1987). Specimens should be collected so as to avoid hemolysis using trace metal free evacuated blood tubes as described previously for zinc. Unlike zinc, serum is the preferred matrix.

Selenium

Selenium has long been recognized as a nutrient essential for human health. However, studies during the last decade, suggesting that selenium may be protective against cardiovascular disease (Shamberger et al., 1978) and some cancers (Jansson et al., 1978; Schrauzer et al., 1977), has led to an increased interest among clinicians in the routine determination of selenium status. Direct measures of selenium status can be provided by quantitation of the element in serum, red cells, or whole blood. Alternatively, determination of glutathione peroxidase, a seleno-enzyme, can be useful as a screening procedure in subjects with possible selenium deficiency.

As selenium is nearly equally distributed between the red cell and plasma compartments, either matrix can adequately serve to index selenium status. Determination of urinary selenium has also been reported, but its clinical utility is largely restricted to instances of suspected selenium toxicity (Glover, 1967). Unlike zinc or iron, contamination of laboratory disposables with selenium is not commonly encountered. Nevertheless, it is good practice to observe precautions similar to those cited previously, particularly with regard to the use of commercially available "trace metal free" evacuated blood tubes. In those instances where either red cell selenium or glutathione peroxidase levels are to be determined, it is essential to collect blood into trace metal free tubes containing heparin anticoagulant. Urinary specimens should be acidified to a pH less than 3.0 with reagent-grade hydrochloric acid in order to avoid selenium losses associated with bacterial generation of hydrogen selenide, a volatile form of the element.

Determination of selenium in any of the matrices listed above can be accomplished using one of three methodologies: fluorometric determination after complexing with decalin; electrothermal atomic absorption spectroscopy (EAA); and hydride generation atomic absorption spectrophotometry (HGAA). The decalin fluorometric procedure is relatively straightforward and is still the most commonly used method for the clinical laboratory. However, while the procedure can be substantially automated, it does require prior digestion of the sample in order to remove all traces of organic material (Brown and Watkinson, 1977; Watkinson, 1979). For laboratories so equipped, serum selenium can be determined without prior digestion using flameless EAA. The specimen must be pretreated with a nickel-based matrix modifier in order to reduce the volatility of the various forms of selenium. Quantitation is provided by the method of standard additions. Although only 20–30 specimens can be analyzed per day, the EAA methods are generally more precise than either the fluorometric or the HGAA procedures (Krumpulainen and Koivistoinen,

1981). Analysts are advised that the HGAA procedure can show a slight negative bias relative to other methods of selenium determination due to the loss of selenium hydride at tubing connectors (Shamberger, 1978).

Determination of plasma or red cell glutathione peroxidase (GPX), the only presently well-established selenoenzyme in humans (Chapter 7), can also be useful in cases of suspected selenium deficiency. GPX (EC 1.11.1.9) has been reported to be markedly reduced in cases involving long-term total parenteral nutrition, in which selenium had been omitted from the formulation. Plasma enzyme levels quickly normalize after sodium selenite replacement therapy is initiated. However, red cell GPX activity may remain low for up to 6 weeks after repletion has commenced (Cohen et al., 1985). While the determination of plasma or red cell GPX cannot replace direct measures of selenium status, the procedure is readily automated on most centrifugal analyzers (Jacobson et al., 1988) and, therefore, can serve as an inexpensive screening test. Analysts are advised that the rate of the enzyme reaction is highly dependent upon hydrogen peroxide or t-butyl peroxide substrate concentration.

Other Essential Trace Metals

Other trace metals essential to humans include manganese, molybdenum, chromium, and cobalt (Chapter 7). With the possible exception of chromium, the prevalence of human clinical pathology resulting from deficiencies of these elements has not been well-studied. Comprehensive sources of information regarding the metabolism and assessment of these metals in humans are available (see Chapter 7; and Prasad, 1978; Prasad and Oberleas, 1976).

Macronutrients: Dietary Protein

Protein-Calorie Malnutrition (PCM)

Various forms of PCM affect muscle (somatic) and nonmuscle (visceral) compartments differently. It is useful to have tests that can differentiate between the types of PCM [e.g., marasmus (the calorically deprived type) versus kwashiorkor (the protein-derived type)]. A variety of biochemical tests is available that offer greater sensitivity than clinical techniques and has some ability to distinguish among the various forms of PCM.

Total serum protein and albumin have commonly been measured; however, albumin is generally recognized as a more reliable and sensitive indicator of protein nutritional status than total protein levels. For example, total protein levels have been shown to be high in tropical and subtropical populations known to be consuming inadequate protein intakes (Pearson, 1966). In the elderly, however, protein synthesis has been reported at a lower setpoint than in younger adults (Mitchell and Lipschitz, 1982). Generally, serum albumin levels below 2.8 g/dl indicate severely deficient protein nutriture. Clinically apparent cases of marasmus, however, may show nearly normal total protein and albumin levels. Certain specific transport proteins, whose hepatic synthesis may be limited by insufficient amino acid supply, have been shown to be indicators of protein deficiency and to aid differentiating various forms of PCM. These include transferrin, retinol-binding protein, prealbumin, and ceruloplasmin—all of which have shorter half-lives than albumin and thus appear to be more sensitive indicators of PCM. Although recent reports suggest that these visceral proteins respond more quickly to therapeutic diets than does serum albumin (Winkler et al., 1989), it is not yet clear whether they are superior to albumin for the detection of inadequate intake of dietary protein.

The ratio of certain nonessential to essential (NE/E) serum amino acids has been shown to be increased in children with primary protein deficiency (Arroyave, 1970). Various amino acid indices have been suggested. One index, by Whitehead (1969), is as follows:

$$\text{Amino acid ratio (NE/E)} = \frac{\text{glycine} + \text{serine} + \text{glutamine} + \text{taurine}}{\text{isoleucine} + \text{leucine} + \text{methionine} + \text{valine}}$$

Values above 3 are considered to represent primary malnutrition. The index is useful for assessing protein malnutrition in children rather than adults, and is responsive to specific protein deficiency rather than general PCM. However, the determination of free serum amino acids is involved and tedious, and the amino acid ratio test is not recommended as a routine test for PCM.

Because creatinine excretion is dependent on lean body mass, which is decreased as a result of protein depletion, the urinary creatinine-to-height ratio is decreased in PCM (Nutrition Reviews, 1971; Viteri, 1972; Viteri and Alvarado, 1970). As the creatinine-height index is calculated as the ratio of creatinine excreted daily in the test subject to that excreted by the normal child of the same height, the test is somewhat age-independent (except in old age due to declining renal function). Simple and reliable methods are available for urinary creatinine determinations. The method has some sensitivity toward detecting subclinical protein deprivation, but it is not well-suited to field use since 24-hr, or at least precisely timed, urine collections are needed for accurate results.

Other urinary products that have been shown to index protein depletion include hydroxyproline and the urea-to-creatinine ratio. In all cases, the tests are more reliable when 24-hr urine collections are obtained; however, the hydroxyproline index has been useful as the creatinine-corrected quotient on random samples from population studies. The hydroxyproline index is age-dependent, and its best use has been found in the assessment of children's protein intakes and growth rates. The test does not distinguish between protein and calorie malnutrition, and certain subjects with kwashiorkor are found with unexpectedly high hydroxyproline excretions. The urea-to-creatinine ratio is useful as a measure of recent protein intake rather than body protein status.

An approximate measure of total body nitrogen balance has been derived to closely follow the course of protein repletion of the malnourished hospital patient. The formula requires a 24-hr urinary urea nitrogen (UUN) measure (Mackenzie et al., 1974):

$$\text{Nitrogen balance} = \frac{\text{dietary protein intake (g/day)}}{6.25} - [\text{UUN (g/day)} + 4]$$

In a patient being protein-repleted, a positive balance of 4 g/day is desirable. The formula cannot be used for patients with renal disease or those patients with enhanced protein loss diseases, such as enteropathy, burns, or skin diseases.

Measures of immunologic status, including decreased total lymphocyte count (<1500/cu mm) and reactivity to skin antigens, have been shown to correlate with both protein and calorie deprivation (Menkins et al., 1977). Although there are no known decreases in lymphocyte count with age, T cell function reportedly decreases with age. This finding questions the utility of skin-sensitivity testing in the elderly.

Other tests that have been proposed as indicators of protein intake or status are the urinary sulfur-to-creatinine ratio, leukocyte pyruvic kinase, and plasma-to-urine RNase activities.

Macrominerals

Assessment of body status of the macrominerals—sodium, potassium, calcium, magnesium, and phosphorus—is routinely performed by determination of serum levels. Flame emission, atomic absorption spectrophotometric, and ion-selective electrode methodologies are commonly used. The methods are detailed in instrument manuals and in clinical chemistry texts, along with guidelines for the interpretation of results (Henry et al., 1979).

References

Adeloju SB, Bond AM (1985): Anal Chem 57:1728.

Alcock NW (1987): *In* Pesce AJ, Kaplan LA, eds: Methods in clinical chemistry. Washington, DC: CV Mosby.

Arroyave G (1970): Am J Clin Nutr 23:703.

Baer MT, King JC (1984): Amer J Clin Nutr 39:556.

Baker EM, Hodges, RE, Hood J, Sauberlich HE, March SC, Canham JE (1971): Am J Clin Nutr 24:444.

Baker SJ, DeMaeyer EM (1979): Am J Clin Nutr 32:368.

Baker SJ, Chichester CO, Cook JD, Darby WJ, DeMaeyer EM, Hallberg L, Kahbn SG, eds (1977): A report of the International Nutritional Anemia Consultative Group. Washington, DC: Nutrition Foundation.

Baker EM, Hammer DC, Kennedy JL, Tolbert BM (1973): Anal Biochem 55:641.

Bankson DD, Russell RM, Sadowski JA (1986): Clin Chem 32:35.

Bayoumi RA, Rosalki S (1976): Clin Chem 22:327.

Belsey R, DeLuca HF, Potts JT (1974): J Clinic Endo Metab 38:1046.

Bessey OA, Lowry OH, Brock MJ, Lopez T (1946): J Biol Chem 166:177.

Bieri JG, Tolliver TJ, Catignani GL (1979): Am J Clin Nutr 32:2143.

Bistrian BR, Blackburn GL, Hallowell E, Heddle R (1974): JAMA 230:858.

Blanchard RA, Furie BC, Jorgensen M, Kruger SF, Furie B (1981): N Engl J Med 305:242.

Blomfield J, Dixon SR, McCredie DA (1971): Arch Intern Med 128:555.

Boddy K, Adams JF (1972): Am J Clin Nutr 25:395.

Bouillon R, Herck EV, Jan I, Tan BK, Baelen HV, DeMoor P (1984): Clin Chem 30:1731.

Brewster MA, Turley CP (1987): *In* Pesce AJ and Kaplan LA, eds: Methods in clinical chemistry. Washington, DC: CV Mosby.

Brown MW, Watkinson JH (1977): Anal Chem Acta 89:29.

Brown RR, Miller ON, Coursin DB, Rose DP (1971): Am J Clin Nutr 24:653.

Burton BT, Foster WR, Hirsch J, Van Itallie TB (1985): Intl J Obesity 9:155.

Bushman L, Russell RM, Warfield L, Curry G, Iber F (1980): J Am Dietet Assoc 77:462.

Butts WC, Mulvihill HJ (1975): Clin Chem 21:1493.

Buzby GP, Mullen JL, Matthews DC, Hobbs CL, Rosato EF (1980): Amer J Surg 139:160.

Calman KC, chairman (1981): Proc Nutr Soc 40:147.

Cha GS, Meyerhoff ME (1988): Anal Biochem 168:216.

Chanarin I, Bennett MC (1962): Br Med J 1:27.

Chastain JL, McCormick DB (1987): Am J Clin Nutr 46:830.

Chen IW (1987): *In* Pesce AJ and Kaplan LA, eds: Methods in clinical chemistry. Washington, DC: CV Mosby.

Cohen HJ, Chovaniec ME, Mistretta D, Baker SS (1985): Am J Clin Nutr 41:735.

Colman N (1981): *In* Labbe RF, ed: Clinics in laboratory medicine. Symposium on laboratory assessment of nutritional status, Vol 1. Philadelphia: WB Saunders.

Cook JD, Finch CA (1979): Am J Clin Nutr 32:2115.

Cordano A, Placko RP, Graham GG (1966): Blood 28:220.

Craft NE, Brown ED, Smith JC (1988): Clin Chem 34:44.

Cynamon HA, Isenberg JN, Nguyen CH (1985): Clin Chim Acta 151:169.

Das KC, Herbert V (1978): Br J Haematol 38:219.

deLange DJ, Joubert CP (1964): Am J Clin Nutr 15:169.

De Leenheer AP, DeBevere V, De Ruyter MGM, Claeys AE (1979): J Chrom 162:408.

Dewhurst WG, Morgan HG (1970): Am J Clin Nutr 23:379.

Dillard CJ, Dumelin EE, Tappel AL (1977): Lipids 12:109.

Duncan WE, Haddad JG (1981): *In* Labbe RF, ed: Clinics in laboratory medicine. Symposium on laboratory assessment of nutritional status, Vol 1. Philadelphia: WB Saunders.

DuPlessis JP (1967): An evaluation of biochemical criteria for use in nutrition status surveys. Council for Scientific and Industrial Research report no 261. Pretoria, South Africa: National Nutritional Research Institute.

Ericson SP, McHalsky ML, Rabinow BE, Kronholm KG, Arceo CS, Weltzer JA, Ayd SW (1986): Clin Chem 32:1350.

Fairbanks VF, Klee GG (1986): *In* Tietz NW, ed: Textbook of clinical chemistry. Philadelphia: WB Saunders, p 1578.

Farrell PM, Levine SL, Murphy MD, Adams AJ (1978): Am J Clin Nutr 31:1720.

Flores H, Campos F, Araujo CRC, Underwood BA (1984): Am J Clin Nutr 40:1281.

Food and Agriculture Organization/World Health Organization. Requirements of vitamin A, iron, folate, and vitamin B_{12} (1987): Report of a joint Food and Agriculture Organization/World Health Organization expert committee. Rome, Italy: Food and Agriculture Organization and Geneva, Switzerland: World Health Organization. FAO Nutrition Meetings report series, WHO technical report series.

Food and Drug Administration (1985): Assessment of the vitamin A nutritional status of the U.S. population based on data collected in the Health and Nutrition Examination Surveys (HANES), Department of Health and Human Services, SM Pilch, ed: Life Sciences Research Office, FASEB, Bethesda, MD.

Food and Nutrition Board, National Research Council (1989): Recommended Dietary Allowances (10th rev ed) Washington, DC: National Academy of Sciences.

Frisancho AR (1981): Am J Clin Nutr 34:2540.

Frisancho AR (1984): Amer J Clin Nutr 40:808.

Fu CS, Swendseid ME, Jacob RE, McKee, RW (1989): J Nutr, in press.

Furr HC, Amedee-Manesme O, Clifford AJ, Bergen HR, Jones AD, Anderson DP, Olson JA (1989): Amer J Clin Nutr 49:713.

Glover JR (1967): Ann Occup Hyg 10:3.

Gompertz D, Hoffbrand AV (1970): Br J Haematol 18:377.

Greger JM, Geissler AH (1978): Am J Clin Nutr 31:633.

Gregory JF, Kirk JR (1979): Amer J Clin Nutr 32:879.

Gutcher GR, Raynor WJ, Farrell PM (1984): Am J Clin Nutr 40:1078.

Hansen LG, Warwick WJ (1969): Amer J Clin Pathol 51:538.

Haroon Y, Bacon DS, Sadowski JA (1986): Clin Chem 32:1925.

Hart JP, Shearer MJ, McCarthy PT, Rahim S (1984): Analyst 109:477.

Hattori M, Kotake Y, Kotake Y (1984): Acta Vitaminol Enzymol 6:221.

Helwig HL, Hoffer EM, Thielen WC (1966): Amer J Clin Pathol 45:160.

Henry JB, Todd-Stanford-Davidson (1979): Clinical diagnosis by laboratory methods (16th ed). Philadelphia: WB Saunders.

Herbert B (1959): The megaloblastic anemias. New York: Grune & Stratton.

Herbert B (1962): Trans Assoc Am Physician Phila 75:307.

Herbert B (1967): Am J Clin Nutr 20:562.

Heymsfield SB, McManus C, Smith J, Stevens V, Nixon DW (1982): Amer J Clin Nutr 36:680.

Higgins T (1981): Clin Chem 27:1619.

Hodges RE, Kolder H (1971): *In* Bieri JG, chairman: Summary of proceedings of workshop on biochemical and clinical criteria for determining human vitamin A nutriture, January 28–29. Washington, DC: Food Nutrition Board, National Academy of Sciences—National Research Council.

Hodges, RE, Hood H, Canham JE, Sauberlich HE, Baker EM (1971): Am J Clin Nutr 24:432.

Hoes MJ (1981): J Clin Chem Clin Biochem 19:259.

Hoffbrand AV, Newcombe NF, Mollin DL (1966): J Clin Pathol 19:17.

Hollis BW (1986): Clin Chem 32:2060.

Holman SIM, deLange DJ (1950): Nature 165:604.

Homsher R, Zak B (1985): Clin Chem 31:1310.

Horwitt MK (1966): Am J Clin Nutr 18:458.

Horwitt MK, Harvey CC, Dahn CH, Searcy MT (1972): Ann NY Acad Sci 203:223.

Ikenoya S, Abe K, Tsuda T (1979): Chem Pharm Bull 27:1237.

International Vitamin A Consultative Group (1979): Guidelines for the eradication of vitamin A deficiency and xerophthalmia. VI Recent advances in the metabolism and function of vitamin A and their relationship to applied nutrition. New York: The Nutrition Foundation.

Jacob RA (1981): *In* Labbe RF, ed: Clinics in laboratory medicine. Symposium on laboratory assessment of nutritional status, Vol 1. Philadelphia: WB Saunders.

Jacob RA (1986): *In* Tietz NW, ed: Textbook of clinical chemistry. Philadelphia: WB Saunders, p 977.

Jacob RA, Skala JH, Omaye ST (1987): Am J Clin Nutr 46:818.

Jacob RA, Swendseid ME, McKee RW, Fu CS, Clemens RA (1989): J Nutr 119:591.

Jacobson B, Quigley G, Lockitch G (1988): Clin Chem 34:2164.

Jansson B, Jacobs MM, Griffin AC (1978): *In* Schrauzer GN, ed: Gastrointestinal cancer—Epidemiology and experimental studies: Inorganic and nutritional aspects of cancer. New York: Plenum Press, p 305.

Jeliffe DB (1966): The assessment of the nutritional status of the community. Geneva: WHO.

Justova V, Starka L, Wilczek H, Pacovsky V (1976): Clin Chim Acta 70:97.

Kagi JHR, Vallee BL (1958): Anal Chem 30:1951.

Katz SA (1985): Amer Clin Prod 4:8.

Kolhouse JF, Kindo J, Allen NC, Podell E, Allen RH (1978): N Engl J Med 299:785.

Kossman KT (1983): Clin Chem 29:578.

Kraut H, Ramaswamy SS, Wildemann L (1961): Int Zeit Vit 32:25.

Krishnaswamy K (1971): Int J Vit Nutr Res 41:240.

Krumpulainen J, Koivistoinen P (1981): Kemia-Kemi 8:372.

Labbe RF, ed (1981): Clinics in laboratory medicine: Symposium on laboratory assessment of nutritional status, Vol 1. Philadelphia: WB Saunders.

Lefevre MF, De Leenheer AP, Claeys AE (1979): J Chrom 186:749.

Lefevre MF, De Leenheer AP, Claeys IV, Stayaert H (1982): J Lipid Res 23:1068.

Leite JFMS, Antunes CF, Monteiro JCMP, Pereira BTV (1987): Br J Surg 75:426.

Lemoyne M, Van Gossum A, Kurian R, Jeejeebhoy KN (1988): Am J Clin Nutr 48:1310.

Lemoyne M, Van Gossum A, Kurian R, Ostro M, Axler J, Jeejeebhoy KN (1987): Am J Clin Nutr 46:267.

Leonard PJ, Losowsky MS (1967): Am J Clin Nutr 20:795.

Li TK, Lumeng L (1981): *In* Leklem JE, Reynolds RD, eds: Methods in vitamin B_6 nutrition: Analysis and status assessment. New York: Plenum Press, p 289.

Lindenbaum J, Nath BJ (1980): Br J Haematol 45:511.

Lindenbaum J, Healton EB, Savage DG, Brust JCM, Garrett TJ, Podell ER, Marcell PD, Stabler SP, Allen RH (1988): N Engl J Med 318:1720.

Loerch JD, Underwood BA, Lewis KC (1979): J Nutr 109:778.

Lossy FT, Goldsmith GA, Sarret HP (1951): J Nutr 45:213.

Luhby AL, Cooperman JM (1964): Adv Metab Disorders 1:263.

MacCrehan WA, Schonberger E (1987): Clin Chem 33:1585.

Mackenzie T, Blackburn GL, Flatt JP (1974): Fed Proc 33:683.

Mahanand D, Houck JC (1968): Clin Chem 14:6.

Manual for Nutrition Surveys (2nd ed) (1963): Interdepartmental Committee on Nutrition for National Defense. Washington, DC: Superintendent of Documents, U.S. Government Printing Office.

Matthews DM (1962): Clin Sci 22:101.

McGown EL, Rusnak MG, Lewis CM, Tilotson JA (1982): Anal Biochem 119:55.

Menkins JL, Pietsch JB, Bubenick O (1977): Ann Surg 186:241.

Metropolitan Insurance (1983): Metropolitan Height and Weight Tables. New York: Metropolitan Insurance Company.

Milne DB, Botnen J (1986): Clin Chem 32:874.

Mitchell CO, Lipschitz DA (1982): Am J Clin Nutr 36:340.

Mobarhan S, Russell RM, Underwood BA, Wallingford J, Mathieson RD, Al-Midani H (1981): Am J Clin Nutr 34:2264.

Morley HH, Edwards MA, Moller II, Woodring MJ, Storvick CA (1959): J Nutr 69:191.

Morrow, FD (1986): Clin Nutr 5:112.

Mortensen E (1976): Clin Chem 22:982.

Mortensen E (1978): Clin Chem 24:663.

Mount JN, Heduan E, Herd C, Jupp R, Kearney E, Marsh A (1987): Ann Clin Biochem 24:41.

Mullen JL, Gertner MH, Buzby GP, Goodhart GL, Rosato EF (1979): Arch Surg 114:121.

Narayanan S, Appleton HD (1980): Clin Chem 26:1119.

Nath BJ, Lindenbaum J (1979): Ann Intern Med 90:757.

National Center for Health Statistics, Division of Health Examination Statistics (1976–1980): Data from the Second National Health and Nutrition Examination Survey, unpublished.

National Committee for Clinical Laboratory Standards (1980): Guidelines for evaluating a B_{12} (cobalamin) assay. Villanova, PA.

Neale RJ, Lim H, Turner J, Freeman C, Kemm JR (1988): Age Ageing 17:35.

Nichoalds GE (1974): Clin Chem 20:624.

Nichoalds GE (1981): *In* Labbe RF, ed: Clinics in laboratory medicine: Symposium on laboratory assessment of nutritional status, Vol 1. Philadelphia: WB Saunders.

Nutr Rev (1971): 29:134.

Nutr Rev (1979): 37:283.

Olliver M (1967): *In* Sebrell WH, Harris RS, eds: The vitamins, Vol I (2nd ed). New York: Academic.

Omaye ST, Turnbull JD, Sauberlich HE (1979): Meth Enzymol 62:3.

Pachla LA, Reynolds DL, Kissinger PT (1985): J Assoc Off Anal Chem 68:1.

Pearson WM (1962*a*): JAMA 180:49.

Pearson WM (1962*b*): Am J Clin Nutr 11:462.

Pearson WM (1966): *In* Beaton GH, McHenry EW, eds: Nutrition: A comprehensive treatis, Vol III. New York: Academic.

Pearson WM (1967): Am J Clin Nutr 20:514.

Peterson RE, Bollier ME (1955): Anal Chem 27:1195.

Pinto J, Yee PH, Rivlin RS (1981): J Clin Invest 67: 1500.

Posner D, Russell RM, Absood S, Connor T, Norris A, David C, Martin L (1978): Gastroenterology 74:866.

Powers, HJ (1987): Int J Vitam Nutr Res 57:455.

Prasad AS, Oberleas D (1976): Trace elements in human health and disease-vol 2. Essential and toxic elements. New York: Academic.

Prasad AS, ed (1978): Trace elements in human metabolism. New York: Plenum.

Reinhardt TA, Horst RL, Orf JW, Hollis BW (1984): J Clin Endo Metab 58:91.

Reynolds RD (1983): Fed Proc 42:665.

Reynolds RD (1987): *In* Pesce AJ and Kaplan LA, eds: Methods in clinical chemistry. Washington, DC: CV Mosby.

Rice EW (1960): J Lab Med 55:325.

Riordan JF, Vallee BL (1976): *In* AS Prasad, ed: Trace elements in human health and disease, Vol 1. New York: Academic, p 227.

Roberts SB, Morrow FD, Evans WJ, Shepard DC, Dallal GE, Meredith CN, Young VR (1989): Am J Clin Nutr 51:485.

Roe JH, Keuther CA (1943): J Biol Chem J 147:399.

Rose RC, Nahrwold DL (1981): Anal Biochem 114:140.

Russell RM, Iber FL, Krasinski SD, Miller P (1983): Hum Nutr Clin Nutr 37C:361.

Russell RM, Multack R, Smith V, Frill A, Rosenberg IH (1973): Lancet 2:1161.

Sadowski JA, Hood ST, Dallal GE, Garry PJ (1989): Amer J Clin Nutr 50:100.

Sampson DA, O'Connor DK (1989): Nutr Res 9:259.

Sauberlich HE (1967): Am J Clin Nutr 20:528.

Sauberlich HE (1981*a*): *In* Nutrition in health and disease and international development (symposium from the XII International Congress of Nutrition). New York: Alan R. Liss.

Sauberlich HE (1981*b*): *In* Labbe RF, ed: Clinics in laboratory medicine: Symposium on laboratory assessment of nutritional status, Vol 1. Philadelphia: WB Saunders.

Sauberlich HE (1984): Present knowledge in nutrition (5th ed). New York: Nutrition Foundation.

Sauberlich HE, Canham JE, Baker EM, Raica N Jr, Herman YF (1972): Am J Clin Nutr 25:629.

Sauberlich HE, Dowdy RP, Skala JH (1974): Laboratory tests for the assessment of nutritional status. Boca Raton, FL: CRC Press.

Sauberlich HE, Green MD, Omaye ST (1982): *In* Seib P, Tolbert B, eds: Ascorbic acid: Chemistry, metabolism, and uses. Advances in chemistry series, No. 200. Washington, DC: American Chemical Society.

Schrauzer GN, White DA, Schneider CJ (1977): Bioorganic Chem 7:23.

Scott JM, Ghanta V, Herbert V (1974): Am J Med Technol 40:1225.

Selhub J, Darcy-Vrillon B, Fell D (1988): Anal Biochem 168:247.

Shamberger RJ, Wills CE, McCormack LJ (1978): *In* Hemphill DD, ed: Trace substances in environmental health, Vol 12. Columbia, MO: University of Missouri Press, p 59.

Shibata K (1987): J Clin Biochem Nutr 3:37.

Shibata K, Matsuo H (1988): Agric Biol Chem 52:2747.

Shibata K, Matsuo H (1989): J Nutr 119:896.

Smeets EHJ, Muller H, Dewael J (1971): Clin Chim Acta 33:379.

Smith JC, Butrimovitz GP, Purdy WC (1983): *In* Cooper GR, ed: Selected method of clinical chemistry, Vol 10. Washington, DC. American Association for Clinical Chemistry, p 75.

Solomons NW (1979): Am J Clin Nutr 32:856.

Stookey LL (1970): Anal Chem 42:779.

Strain WH, Steadman LT, Lankau CA (1966): J Lab Clin Med 68:244.

Thompson JN, Erdody P, Brien R (1971): Biochem Med 5:67.

Thurnham DI (1972): Ann Trop Med Paraisitol 66:505.

Thurnham DI, Smith E, Flora PS (1988): Clin Chem 34:377.

Turley CP, Brewster MA (1987): *In* Pesce AJ, Kaplan LA, eds: Methods in clinical chemistry. Washington, DC: CV Mosby.

Turley CP, Catignani GL (1985): Chem 31:1761.

Turnbull JD, Sudduth JH, Sauberlich HE, Omaye ST (1981): Int Vit Nutr Res 51:47.

Van Gossum A, Sharift R, Lemoyne M, Kurian R, Jeejeebhoy KN (1988): Am J Clin Nutr 48:1394.

Van Itallie TB (1985): Ann Intern Med 103:983.

Viteri FE (1972): Nutr Rev 30:24.

Viteri FE, Alvarado J (1970): Pediatrics 46:696.

Vuilleumier JP, Keck E (1989): J Micro Analysis 5:25.

Wagstaff M, Broughton A (1971): Br J Haematol 21:581.

Waldenlind L (1979): Nutr Metab 23:38.

Walesby RK, Good RW, Bentall HH (1978): Lancet 1:76.

Watanabe S, Frantz W, Trottier D (1963): Anal Biochem 5:345.

Waterlow JC (1986): Human Nutrition: Clinical Nutrition 40C:125.

Watkinson JH (1979): Anal Chem Acta 105:319.

Weinsier RL, Hunker EM, Krumdiech CL, Butterworth CE (1979): Am J Clin Nutr 32:418.

Whitehead RG (1969): Proc Nutr Soc 28:1.

Wilmore DW (1977): The metabolic management of the critically ill. New York: Plenum.

Winkler MF, Gerrior SA, Pomp A, Albina JE (1989): Perspectives in Practice 89:684.

Zak B, Ressler N (1958): Clin Chem 4:43.

Claude Pichard, M.D., Ph.D.† and
Khursheed N. Jeejeebhoy, M.B., B.S.,
Ph.D., F.R.C.P. (C)*

14

Metabolic Consequences of Total Parenteral Nutrition

Introduction

Nutritional support of patients has become of particular importance because improvements in the treatment of sepsis, cardiorespiratory failure, metabolic abnormalities, and surgical techniques have allowed patients to survive to a point where malnutrition becomes a limiting factor in their progress. Nutritional deficiency is especially likely to occur in patients with a prolonged inability to eat, such as those who have undergone surgery and radiochemotherapy or in those with gastrointestinal diseases compromising absorption of an oral diet (Brennan, 1979; Champault and Patel, 1979; Willicuts et al., 1977). The imbalance between intake and requirements results in wasting of muscle and other tissues, a negative nitrogen balance (Waterlow and Jackson, 1981), and multisystem dysfunction which, together, ultimately promote clinical complications, such as infection, poor wound healing, and increased mortality (MacLean et al., 1975; Mullen et al., 1980; Rombeau et al., 1982). Recently, the use of parenteral nutrition has provided the means of preventing or reversing the metabolic consequences of malnutrition in patients with a nonfunctioning bowel unable to take or absorb orally given nutrients.

* Department of Medicine, University of Toronto and St. Michael's Hospital, Toronto, Ontario, Canada.
† Service de Dietetique et de Nutrition, Hopital Cantonal Universitaire de Genève, Genève, Switzerland.

We thank Dr. Alan Bruce-Robertson for his thoughtful comments and untiring editorial efforts. This work was supported by the Fond National Suisse pour la Recherche Scientifique, Berne, Switzerland, and the Société pour l'Encouragement de la Recherche sur la Nutrition en Suisse, Lausanne, Switzerland and the Medical Research Council of Canada with grants MT.3204 and MA.9814.

In addition, patients with permanent injury to the gastrointestinal tract can be fed intravenously on a long-term basis at home. Thus, many patients who would have slowly succumbed to starvation are now able to live relatively normal and productive lives despite having a nonfunctional bowel.

Indications for Total Parenteral Nutrition

Total parenteral nutrition (TPN) is now widely available and technically moderately easy to administer; however, it should not be employed when nutrients can be provided effectively via the enteral route for two main reasons. First, parenteral nutrition is expensive compared with enteral feeding, and second, there is a greater potential for complications, such as infections. When assessing the indications for parenteral nutrition in a given patient, two major questions need to be addressed. First, does the patient need nutritional support, and second, is the parenteral route the preferred way of providing nutrients to the patient? The main indications for nutritional support are listed in Table 14.1. These will now be discussed in detail.

Malnutrition or Potential for Malnutrition

It is obvious that if a patient is malnourished, an attempt must be made to provide adequate nutrition. However, while advanced malnutrition is easy to recognize, early malnutrition is difficult to define clinically, especially with a view to initiating nutritional support before the occurrence of complications. Thus not only malnutrition, but even a strong potential for the development of malnutrition, should be an indication for nutritional support.

Injury and Sepsis

Trauma results in major losses of nitrogen, potassium, and phosphorus which are correlated with muscle cell catabolism (Cuthbertson, 1932). Furthermore, injury and sepsis substantially increase the metabolic rate and need for energy (Kinney, 1987). It is also commonly observed that patients with injury and sepsis develop marked muscle wasting and hypoproteinemia. Thus, the occurrence of injury and sepsis should alert the physician to the fact that nutritional support may be necessary and can be initiated before the occurrence of the adverse effects of malnutrition.

Bowel Rest

In several gastrointestinal diseases, symptoms may become worse with oral feeding. For example, pain related to acute pancreatitis will be increased by oral feeding. In patients with high small bowel fistula, the output will increase and the fistula will remain open if oral feeding is continued. It is believed, but not demonstrated, that TPN may promote fistula closure. It is also thought that bowel "rest," by precluding oral intake, may aid the resolution of Crohn's disease, although controlled trials have resulted in controversial results (Dickenson et al., 1980; Greenberg and Jeejeebhoy, 1981; Greenberg et al., 1988; Holm, 1981). It is difficult to believe that bowel "rest" occurs in fasting patients because of the existence of migratory myoelectric complexes of the gut. Although the efficacy of bowel "rest" in the treatment of these disorders has not been substantiated by controlled trials, there are clinical situations where avoiding oral feeding may reduce discomfort, avoid vomiting, and reduce diarrhea. Obviously prohibiting all oral intake in a patient will soon lead to malnutrition unless parenteral nutrition is provided.

Table 14.1. Indications for Nutritional Support

Malnutrition or potential for malnutrition
Injury and sepsis
Bowel rest
Adjuvant preoperative therapy to improve the nutritional status
Adjuvant therapy to improve the nutritional status of a cancer patient
Massive ileal and/or jejunal resection
Massive small bowel resection
Chronic small bowel obstruction not amenable to surgical alleviation
Growth retardation

Adjuvant Preoperative Therapy for Improving Nutritional Status

Malnutrition is correlated with increased morbidity in patients undergoing major surgery (Champault and Patel, 1979; Muller et al., 1982). Thus, there are theoretical reasons for providing nutritional support to malnourished patients preoperatively. Nutrition for a period shorter than 2 weeks does not change anthropometry or plasma protein levels (Fan et al., 1988) but muscle function has been improved by only 2 days of a glucose and potassium infusion (Chan, 1986). Unfortunately, data showing that preoperative nutrition reduces complications have not been consistently obtained by controlled trials. Therefore, if there is evidence of malnutrition, and surgery can be delayed, preoperative nutrition should be continued for at least 1 week. Because of its potential for infectious complications, preoperative parenteral nutrition should be undertaken with extreme caution in situations where the absence of bacteremia is especially important, as, for example, in orthopedic or intracranial procedures.

Cancer Therapy

Weight loss commonly occurs in patients with cancer. Several studies have shown that important weight loss is associated with a poor prognosis (Lanzotti et al., 1977). Thus, several investigators attempted to determine whether providing nutritional support would improve the prognosis.

Controlled trials have demonstrated neither improvement in survival nor an improved effect of chemotherapy in patients given parenteral nutrition (Brennan, 1981; Evans et al., 1987). Recently, Mullen et al. (1980) and Bozetti et al. (1988) have shown that, in selected patients with cancer and hypoalbuminemia (indicative of protein malnutrition), parenteral nutrition may decrease postoperative morbidity. Further controlled trials are required to assess the role of nutritional support in cancer cachexia (see end of chapter).

Indications for Home TPN

Over the past two decades, parenteral nutrition has become available for long-term use at home for patients who have suffered irreversible bowel injury to a degree that they are unable to derive nourishment from an oral diet. Thus, patients can be provided with a means of receiving adequate nutritional support, while living relatively normal and productive lives. The indications for home parenteral nutrition include the following.

Total Jejunoileal Resection

Efficient oral nutrition is not possible in these patients and death due to starvation ensues if nutrition is not provided parenterally.

Massive Small Bowel Resection

Massive small bowel resection results in severe malnutrition in the patient who is unable to maintain oral nutrition despite careful attention to the use of defined formula diets and other supplements. It should be realized too, that for some of these patients, an oral diet may be feasible through the use of extreme measures, such as eating every 2 hr. However, this would result in the patient defecating approximately as frequently as eating and in becoming a social cripple. Such a patient would obviously benefit from home TPN despite being able to get by nutritionally with an oral diet. In some patients, the remaining bowel may adapt with time, resulting in adequate bowel function so that eventually home TPN can be discontinued.

Chronic Small Bowel Obstruction

When chronic small bowel obstruction is not amenable to surgical alleviation, home TPN should be considered. In these patients, eating will result in abdominal pain and vomiting, which, in turn, will condition the patient to avoid eating and thus result in malnutrition. Chronic obstruction may occur in several clinical situations, such as Crohn's disease (with multiple strictures not amenable to a simple surgical solution), scleroderma, and the pseudoobstruction syndrome. In fact, in the last condition, home TPN has revolutionized the outlook for affected persons.

End-Jejunostomy Syndrome

In this condition, the patient has lost those areas of small and large bowel where intestinal contents are concentrated (fluids reabsorbed). Therefore, there is copious loss of isotonic bowel contents after eating. Nutrients may be absorbed adequately, but severe deficiency of fluid and electrolytes, especially magnesium, ensues. These patients require parenteral fluid and electrolyte supplementation, which can now be provided via home TPN.

Growth Retardation

An unfortunate consequence of Crohn's disease in childhood and adolescence is cessation of growth and maturation. Several studies have demonstrated that this occurs as a result of decreased caloric intake due to anorexia or to provocation of symptoms (such as abdominal pain or diarrhea) rather than to malabsorption of ingested nutrients (Kelts et al., 1979). Growth retardation may even occur in the presence of relatively inactive bowel disease. This may be due to the fact that decreased oral intake will reduce or prevent the occurrence of obstruction or diarrhea. Nutritional support, both enterally and parenterally, has resulted in catch-up growth and the onset of puberty (Prader et al., 1963).

Choice of Nutritional Support System

The rational use of nutritional support depends on the identification of malnutrition or the potential for malnutrition, definition of the risks of malnutrition, and demonstration of the reversal of such risks by nutritional support. Nutritional support in the hospital should be based on the history of the patient's food intake, his/her present nutritional state, and his/her ability to metabolize nutrients. Clinical nutrition consists of a spectrum of approaches which should be in-

Table 14.2. Situations Where TPN Is Preferable to Enteral Nutrition

Severe malabsorption
Short bowel
Small bowel mucosal atrophy
Intestinal mechanical obstruction
Gastric or/and intestinal hypomotility
High risk of intrapulmonary aspiration
Depressed level of consciousness
Tracheoesophageal fistula
Therapeutic "bowel rest"
Crohn's disease
Fistula
Pancreatitis
Pancreatic fistula

tegrated, proceeding from a normal oral diet to parenteral nutrition and vice versa until the patient is discharged. The program should be initiated on arrival of the patient and modified according to the clinical course. A normal or modified oral diet should be used whenever possible and the nutrient intake and tolerance should be monitored. However, if oral intake is consistently poor, enteral feeding should be started. If there is intolerance to enteral feeding or if the gut is not functional, TPN should be given (Table 14.2). The critical role of an on-site dietitian needs to be emphasized in this context.

Nutrient Requirements

Patients who are candidates for TPN have often been subjected to previous starvation. During starvation and malnutrition, energy requirements are met by mobilization of fatty acids from adipose tissue stores (see Chapter 3). However, despite the availability of energy from endogenous fat stores, there is a continuing loss of amino acid nitrogen from muscle as alanine and glutamine (Chapters 4 and 17). This is associated with losses of intracellular ions, such as potassium, magnesium, and phosphorus (Table 14.3). These losses of intracellular electrolytes and nitrogen from muscle and other tissues result in loss of cell function and mass (Russell et al., 1983*a*). Studies have shown that during fasting, obese subjects exhibit changes in muscle function before any significant changes in standard parameters of nutritional assessment (Table 14.4) (Russell et al., 1983*b*). From Figures 14.1–14.3, it will be observed that, before starvation, the muscle exhibits 30% of its maximal force when stimulated at 10 Hz, relaxes quickly, and shows no appreciable loss of force when continuously stimulated for 30 sec. After starvation, the muscle exhibits 49% of its maximal force when stimulated at 10 Hz, relaxes slowly, and loses force when stimulated continuously (i.e., fatigues). All these changes in

Table 14.3. Intracellular Muscle Potassium, Phosphorus, and Magnesium During Malnutrition (mmol/L of intracellular water)

	Potassium	Phosphorus	Magnesium
Well nourished	139.3 ± 4.1[a]	63.7 ± 1.8	12.9 ± 0.7
Malnourished	106.7 ± 4.0[b]	54.7 ± 2.0[b]	10.6 ± 0.3[b]

Source: Unpublished observations of soleus muscle of rats. Controls fed ad libitum and malnourished fed 25% of intake of control rats for 7 days.

[a] Values are means ± SEM.
[b] Significant decrease ($p < 0.005$, t test).

Figure 14.1. The effects of diets on force of stimulated muscle contraction. Values are means ± SEM. $*p < 0.01$ and $**p < 0.02$ for differences indicated. [*Source:* Reprinted by permission from Russell et al. (1983*b*).]

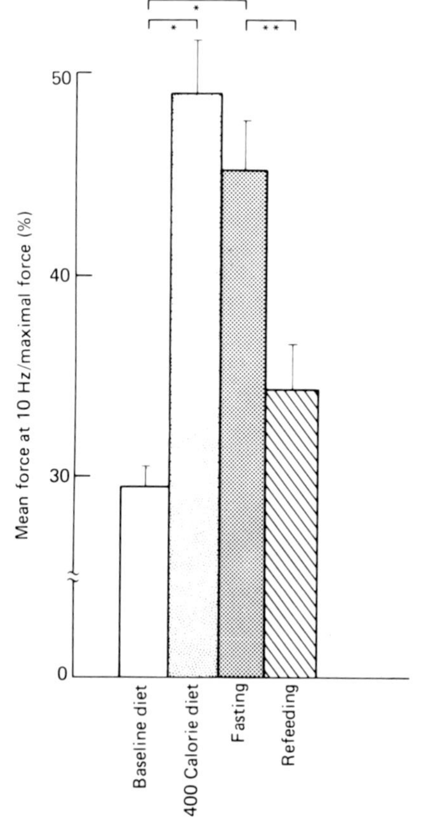

Table 14.4. Values for Standard Parameters Used in Nutritional Assessment of Obese Subjects While Fasting or on a Very Low Calorie Diet[a]

	Albumin (g/dl)	Total iron binding capacity (μg/dl)	Creatinine height index (%)	Lean body weight (kg)	Body fat (%)	Total weight (kg)
Baseline diet	3.9 ± 0.2[b]	268 ± 21	135 ± 7	64 ± 3	45.7 ± 1	120.5 ± 6.0
400-kcal diet	3.7 ± 0.1	263 ± 12	124 ± 8	62 ± 3	45.0 ± 2	114.0 ± 6.0[c]
Fasting	3.9 ± 0.1	245 ± 18	115 ± 8	60 ± 2	46.0 ± 1	109.0 ± 6.0[c]

Source: Reprinted by permission from Russell et al. (1983*b*).

[a] Patients are those of the same group as shown in Figures 14.1–14.3.
[b] Values are means ± SEM.
[c] Significant decrease in total body weight compared with that during baseline diet ($p < 0.05$, *t* test).

function revert to normal with refeeding. Furthermore, Chan (1986) recently reported normalization of the muscle relaxation–contraction characteristics in malnourished patients after a 2-day intravenous infusion of glucose and potassium (K^+). This finding points to the crucial role of K^+ for muscle electrophysiology and the probable need for repletion of intracellular K^+ before the initiation of protein synthesis and the recovery of gross muscle mass.

Complete restoration of cell function and mass can only occur if a variety of nutrients is administered. To restore intracellular protein, and ions such as potassium, magnesium, zinc, and phos-

Figure 14.2. Maximal muscle relaxation rate (MRR) as affected by diet. Values are shown as in Figure 14.1. [*Source:* Reprinted by permission from Russell et al. (1983*b*).]

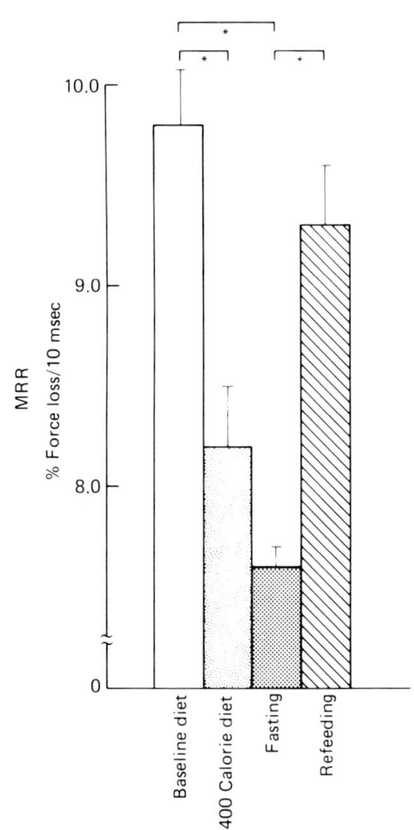

Figure 14.3. Muscle fatiguability in persons on various diets. Values are shown as in Figure 14.1. [*Source:* Reprinted with permission from Russell et al. (1983*b*).]

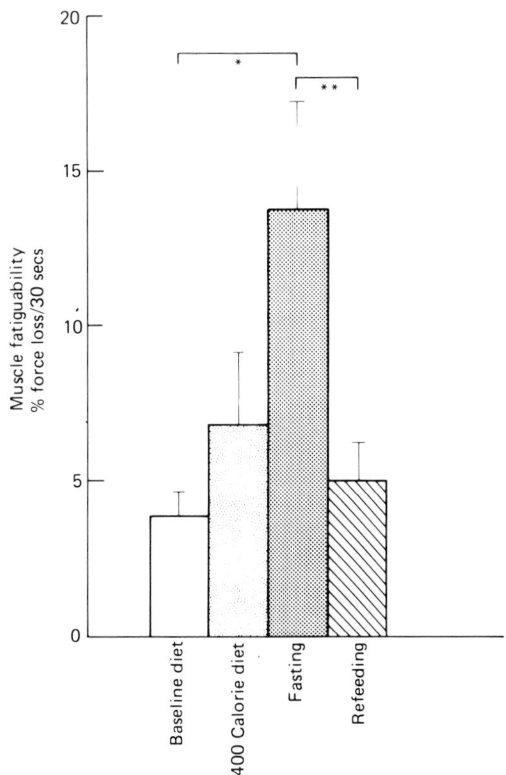

phate, it is necessary to give amino acids and the above-mentioned ions. The need for the concurrent administration of proteins and intracellular ions has been highlighted by the findings of Rudman et al. (1975), who showed that a positive nitrogen balance during TPN only occurred if adequate phosphate and potassium were included in the infusion. Similarly, Wolman et al. (1979) showed that zinc was necessary to optimize nitrogen retention. In addition, energy from fat and glucose is required to optimize nitrogen utilization and also to meet energy requirements. Essential fatty acids (especially linoleic and linolenic acids, see Chapter 3) which cannot be synthesized from carbohydrates must also be supplied. The requirements for each of these specific nutrients will now be discussed systematically.

Lipid

Although fat has long been recognized as an important source of calories and essential fatty acids, it was the last major nutrient to gain approval in the United States for intravenous administration. During the past few decades, more insight has been gained into the metabolic demands of trauma and disease, and with this realization, physicians have begun to augment dextrose solution with amino acids to offset the losses of visceral and somatic protein resulting from prolonged periods of physical stress. The addition of amino acids greatly improved the quality of nutritional therapy, but the hypertonicity of solutions containing sufficient calories to allow anabolism of the administered amino acids proved to be damaging to peripheral veins and introduced the risks of phlebitis and thrombosis. The possible solutions were either to dilute the infusate to reduce its osmolality (which was inadvisable, especially for patients at risk of fluid overload), or to infuse the hypertonic solutions through a large central vein, such as the superior vena cava. (The rapid blood flow through this vessel dilutes the hypertonic infusate and prevents its prolonged contact with venous endothelium.) Due to the risks of central vein TPN (vide infra), investigators turned to isotonic fat as a means of delivering high concentrations of nonprotein calories via peripheral veins.

TPN with fat is now considered a safe, important component of balanced, nutritional support, offering the following advantages over regimens containing dextrose as the sole nonprotein caloric substrate.

1. As mentioned above, TPN admixtures containing fat as a source of nonprotein calories can be infused peripherally, allowing the mildly depleted patient to avoid the risks associated with central venous cannulation.
2. Fat has twice the caloric value of carbohydrate (9 kcal/g versus 4 kcal/g); thus, coinfusing a fat emulsion will increase the caloric density and decrease osmolarity without substantially altering the total fluid volume infused. Coinfusing fat calories will decrease the dextrose requirements and can thereby decrease some of the risks associated with a high dextrose intake (e.g., hyperglycemia, aggravated insulin requirements, and osmotic diuresis).
3. Fat provides essential fatty acids (not present in dextrose) and can thus prevent and/or correct the syndrome of essential fatty acid deficiency.

Composition of lipid emulsions. The physical structure of intravenously administered fat is identical with that of chylomicrons—an hydrophobic triglyceride core surrounded by a thin shell of a highly polar phospholipid. The only difference between fat emulsions and chylomicrons is that the former contain no protein, and the latter are coated with a variety of apoproteins from the moment of synthesis. However, almost immediately upon introduction into the bloodstream, fat emulsion particles acquire free cholesterol, apoproteins, and cholesteryl esters. At this point, they become (with the exception of the absence of the nontransferable apolipoprotein B) physically, compositionally, and metabolically indistinguishable from human chylomicrons. The fatty acid composition of the triglyceride varies according to the source of the oil (i.e., soya bean, safflower) used to prepare the emulsion.

Complications. Problems with the administration of parenteral fat emulsions will occur only if they are infused at rates that exceed the patient's capacity to clear triglycerides from the circulation. Administering fat emulsions in excess of the maximal clearance rate can lead to hypertriglyceridemia. Marked hypertriglyceridemia is believed to have a number of undesirable effects and therefore should be avoided. As with chylomicrons, the maximal rate of clearance is related to the levels of lipoprotein lipase present (Huttenen and Nikkila, 1973); caution is therefore recommended when administering fat emulsions to patients who might have low levels of this enzyme, such as patients with familial hypertriglyceridemia, diabetes mellitus, or hypothyroidism (Bierman, 1972; O'Hara et al., 1966). Insulin and thyroid hormone are essential for lipoprotein lipase synthesis, and therefore, should be replaced in deficiency states prior to infusing lipid emulsions. With the exception of type I hypertriglyceridemia, there is no absolute contraindication for infusing lipids. Acute respiratory distress syndrome is believed to be a contraindication as is the presence of acute pancreatitis. The balance of currently available data is that lipid infusions have not been shown to aggravate pancreatitis nor to have adverse effects on gas exchange.

Protein

In providing protein there are two major considerations, the amino acid composition and the total amount of nitrogen given.

Amino acid composition. As discussed in Chapter 4, studies have demonstrated that the growth of an animal depends not only on the amount of protein fed, but also on the source of protein (Munro, 1964). Some protein, such as egg, induces rapid growth even when fed in small quantities. In contrast, other protein, such as wheat gluten, even in large quantities, does not induce the same rate of growth. In adult humans, amino acid mixtures similar to the composition of egg protein give optimal nitrogen retention. Rose, Holt, and Nagakawa independently, as summarized by Munro (1972) defined the amino acid requirements of normal humans (Table 14.5). Protein in human tissue is made up of 20 different amino acids, of which eight cannot be synthesized by the body and thus are termed essential. Two nonessential amino acids, arginine and histidine, may become essential under certain circumstances, such as during childhood or in patients with renal failure. Three of the essential amino acids, the branched-chain amino acids (leucine, isoleucine, valine), are not oxidized by the liver and are metabolized by muscles. Earlier solutions of amino acids used for TPN were made from casein hydrolysates and were not ideal in terms of their essential amino acid content. Currently, most institutions use solutions made from crystalline amino acids (Table 14.6), which are more effective in promoting nitrogen retention than protein hydrolysates (Anderson et al., 1974). In a controlled study (Patel et al., 1973) (Table 14.7) comparing oral casein with oral casein hydrolysate and intravenous casein hydrolysate, it was shown that oral casein hydrolysate resulted in a nitrogen balance similar to that achieved with intravenous casein hydrolysate. Furthermore, nitrogen balance with oral casein was much better than with oral casein hydrolysate. Thus, hydrolysis resulted in changes that made the product less efficiently utilized orally or intravenously than

Table 14.5. Minimal Essential Amino Acid Requirements (for Normal Subjects) and Relationship to Compositions of Intravenous Amino Acid Infusions

	Minimal requirement[a]			Casein hydrolysate[b] (% weight)	Crystalline amino acid mixture[c] (% weight)
	Children (mg/kg)	Adults mg/kg	Adults % of total		
Isoleucine	28	10	2.4	4.4	7.3
Leucine	49	13	3.1	8.2	9.5
Methionine and cystine	27	13	3.1	2.7	4.0
Phenylanine and tyrosine	27	14	3.3	5.2	5.3
Threonine	34	6	1.4	4.8	5.2
Tryptophan	4	3	0.7	0.9	1.6
Valine	33	13	3.1	5.7	8.1
Lysine	59	10	2.4	7.3	7.3
Total essential AA	261	82	19.3	39.2	47.4
Total nonessential AA	439	343	80.7	60.8	52.6
Daily intake (g/kg)	0.70	0.425		1.7–3.0[d]	1.7–2.1[d]

[a] Data adapted from that assembled by Munro (1972).
[b] Data from Anderson et al. (1974) reported as free essential amino acids. Total nonessential amino acids includes all peptide-bound amino acids, as well as the nonessential amino acids.
[c] Manufacturer's monograph (Aminosyn 7%, Abbott).
[d] Assuming 2–3 L 5%–7% solution infused daily, and body weights of 58–70 kg.

Table 14.6. Amino Acid Composition of Commercially Available Amino Acid Solutions[a]

Composition	Travasol[b] 5.5%	Aminosyn[b] 5%	Vamin[b] 7%	Amigen[c] 5%
Essential amino acids				
Isoleucine	0.263[d]	0.360	0.390	0.26
Leucine	0.340	0.470	0.525	0.41
Lysine	0.318	0.360	0.385	0.31
Methionine	0.318	0.200	0.190	0.13
Phenylalanine	0.340	0.220	0.545	0.20
Threonine	0.230	0.260	0.300	0.19
Tryptophan	0.099	0.080	0.100	0.035
Valine	0.252	0.400	0.425	0.31
Nonessential and semi-essential amino acids				
Alanine	1.149	0.640	0.300	0.15
Arginine	0.570	0.490	0.300	0.18
Histidine	0.241	0.150	0.240	0.13
Proline	0.230	0.430	0.810	0.45
Serine	—	0.210	0.750	0.30
Tyrosine	0.022	0.044	0.050	0.06
Glycine	1.140	0.640	0.210	0.11
Cysteine/Cystine	—	—	0.140	—
Aspartic acid	—	—	0.405	0.35
Glutamic acid	—	—	0.900	1.30

[a] Data from Manufacturers' monographs.
[b] Crystalline amino acid solution.
[c] Casein hydrolysate.
[d] Concentration expressed as percent weight.

the parent protein. Since peptides in oral hydrolysates would be absorbed and utilized, it was concluded that the difference might be due to changes in the amino acid pattern due to loss of cysteine and tyrosine (insoluble amino acid) from the hydrolysate. Subsequently, a crystalline amino acid mixture, designed to have more sulfur-containing and aromatic amino acids than casein, was found to give the same nitrogen balance as first-class oral protein (Anderson et al., 1974) (Table 14.7). It was shown by Rose (1938) that for optimum nitrogen balance, amino acids have to be given in certain proportions and in specified minimal amounts. Mixtures with correct proportions have since been referred to as "balanced."

The optimal composition of crystalline amino acid solutions has yet to be defined. There is a wide variety of commercially available solutions that vary slightly in the ratio of essential to nonessential amino acids. Currently, the majority of nonessential amino acids is given in the form of glycine and alanine rather than glutamate, because the last may cause central nervous system toxicity when given intravenously (Olney et al., 1973). Whether the infusion of excessive glycine and alanine has any deleterious effects on protein synthesis or results in systemic toxicity is unknown, but is currently being investigated. Leucine and its transaminated analogue, α-ketoisocaproic acid, appear to enhance protein synthesis and inhibit proteolysis (Buse and Reid, 1975; Li and Jefferson 1978; Sherwin, 1978). There are conflicting data on whether these actions of leucine can be used to improve nitrogen balance in patients with trauma and sepsis (Hammarqvist et al., 1988; Walser, 1984*b*). At the

Table 14.7. Nitrogen Balances Obtained with (A) Oral and Intravenous Casein Hydrolysate and Oral Casein, and (B) an Intravenous Defined Crystalline Amino Acid Solution and Oral Protein (1 g/kg/day)

	Nitrogen balance (g/day)
A. Oral casein hydrolysate	+ 0.8 ± 0.2[a]
Intravenous casein hydrolysate	+ 0.7 ± 0.3
Oral casein	+ 3.0 ± 0.1
B. Intravenous defined crystalline amino acid solution	+ 2.2 ± 0.3
Oral protein (egg or milk)	+ 2.0 ± 0.6

Source: (A) Data from Patel et al. (1973); (B) data from Anderson et al. (1974).

[a] Values are means ± SEM.

present time, there is no demonstrated role for the branched-chain amino acid-enriched solutions in patients with sepsis or injury (Bonau et al., 1984; Daly et al., 1983; Freund et al., 1988). The efficiency of the branched-chain keto analogues in these patients remains to be demonstrated (Walser 1984*a*, *b*).

Thus, the quantity of protein needed to maintain nitrogen balance is dependent on the nutritional quality of the protein given, and thus upon the amino acid composition. If an amino acid mixture is deficient in an essential amino acid or if there is an imbalance in the essential amino acids, nitrogen balance is not achieved in experimental animals and in patients receiving parenteral nutrition (Patel et al., 1973). It should be noted that amino acid solutions that contain only the essential amino acids are probably not as well utilized as more balanced solutions containing essential and nonessential amino acids (Anderson et al., 1974). Finally, our knowledge of amino acid requirements is based on data derived from normal adults, who need only to maintain their tissue protein. There are no similar data for malnourished patients (who are repleting tissue) or septic and injured patients, and those with specific illnesses (who may have different requirements).

Total nitrogen intake. In normal subjects, net nitrogen retention occurs only when nonprotein calories are given in sufficient amounts to meet estimated metabolic needs (Calloway and Spector, 1954). In the study cited, positive nitrogen balance was achieved only when about 15 g of nitrogen was fed (orally) with about 3000 kcal/day. Hence, for years it was believed that a positive nitrogen balance could occur only in conjunction with a positive energy balance. Recently, Blackburn et al. (1973) have shown that infusing amino acids alone into malnourished patients results in significant protein-sparing. Greenberg et al. (1976) showed that the protein-sparing action was based on the amount of amino acid(s) given and did not depend on the substrate–hormone profile (Table 14.8). The glucose-containing infusions resulted in higher insulin levels and low levels of free fatty acids. In contrast, patients given amino acids alone or with lipid did not have high insulin levels and had higher free fatty acid levels. Despite these differences, there was no difference in nitrogen balance in the groups receiving similar amounts of nitrogen. In later studies, Greenberg and Jeejeebhoy (1979) showed that a positive nitrogen balance was possible even with hypocaloric infusions in malnourished patients if the rate of amino acid infusion was about 2 g/kg of ideal body weight (IBW) per day. This finding confirmed the experience of Bozetti (1976) and was supported by Elwyn (1980). Thus, the most important determinant of a positive nitrogen balance is the amount of amino acids given. This concept is supported by the observation of Collins et al. (1978), who showed that

Table 14.8. Blood Parameters Related to Energy Metabolism and Nitrogen Balance in Patients Receiving Various Intravenous Mixtures[a]

	Composition of infusate			
Parameters	Glucose	Amino acid	Amino acid and lipid	Amino acid and glucose
Plasma glucose (mg/dl)	130 ± 7	90 ± 15	100 ± 13	117 ± 6
Blood lactate (μM)	1.097 ± 0.144	779 ± 29	775 ± 49	975 ± 73
Blood pyruvate (μM)	111 ± 18	71 ± 6	81 ± 7	96 ± 7
Plasma-free fatty acids (μM)	341 ± 38	618 ± 41	759 ± 50	428 ± 42
Blood β-hydroxybutyrate (μM)	122 ± 26	1288 ± 199	1405 ± 296	214 ± 59
Blood acetoacetate (μM)	56 ± 17	574 ± 70	644 ± 118	105 ± 38
Immunoreactive insulin (ng/ml)	1.30 ± 0.27	0.66 ± 0.10	0.71 ± 0.14	1.67 ± 0.35
Immunoreactive glucagon (ng/ml)	203 ± 37	296 ± 32	307 ± 17	208 ± 21
Nitrogen input (g/3 days)	0 ± 7	42 ± 2	39 ± 2	40 ± 3
Nitrogen balance (g/3 days)	−45 ± 5	−20 ± 3	−17 ± 5	−21 ± 4
Significance (p)				
versus glucose		<0.001	<0.001	<0.001
versus other treatments		>0.3	>0.3	>0.3

Source: Data from Greenberg et al. (1976).

[a] Pooled data for days 2 and 3 of treatment: values are means ± SEM.

body nitrogen was maintained equally well with amino acids alone as with amino acids plus glucose (the latter in quantities sufficient to meet or exceed the patient's energy requirements).

Stable adults require only 0.4 g/kg/day of nitrogen to maintain zero balance (Table 14.5). However, malnourished patients need to be in significantly positive nitrogen balance, which is best achieved by giving more amino acids. The gain in nitrogen is linear with nitrogen intake when that intake is in the range of 0.25–2.0 g/kg/day, subject to increased needs for increased metabolic rate and less with decreased energy intake. Above an intake of 2 g/kg/day, there is no increase in nitrogen retention. In malnourished, septic subjects, Roulet et al. (1983) showed that providing about 1.5 g of amino acids/kg body weight resulted in a zero or positive nitrogen balance.

However, the administration of substantial amounts of amino acids must be tempered by the fact that altered renal and/or hepatic function will reduce tolerance to amino acid loads. Considering these factors, it seems desirable generally to prescribe 1.0–1.5 g/kg ideal body weight/day of a balanced amino acid mixture.

Energy

Energy requirements can be predicted from the Harris-Benedict equation (Chapter 8, Table 8.4) (Harris and Benedict, 1919), based on age, sex, and size, or by indirect calorimetry (Chapter 8). Depleted subjects have a lower than normal energy expenditure, but this is appropriate for their reduced body size. About 20 kcal/kg/day will meet their initial requirements, and subsequently 25 kcal/kg/day will result in weight gain and restoration of the lean body mass.

In contrast, injury and sepsis are associated with an increased basal energy expenditure. It had previously been thought that patients with these conditions might require 4000–6000 kcal/day, but it is now recognized that these figures are largely exaggerated. Not only are these values much greater than required by the patient, but such intake can lead to serious complications, due to the increased energy expenditure required for distribution and metabolism of the extra nutrients, and the increased oxygen consumption and carbon dioxide production; it is also associated with hyperglycemia and the development of a fatty liver. Recent studies (Askanazi et al., 1980; Baker et al., 1984; Roulet et al., 1983) have shown that the energy requirements of septic-injured patients are only 13%–14% above the predicted value, derived from the Harris-Benedict equation. Thus, approximately 30–35 kcal/kg IBW/day should be sufficient to maintain and/or restore the lean body mass in these patients.

The major energy sources used in TPN (as in normal nutrition) are carbohydrates and lipids. Jeejeebhoy et al. (1976*a*) showed that nitrogen balance was the same when patients were provided with 1 g/kg amino acids/day and 40 kcal/kg/day of nonprotein calories which are either as glucose alone or as 83% fat and 17% glucose. These findings have been confirmed by several other investigators (Burke et al., 1979; Gazzaniga et al., 1975; Nordenström et al., 1983; Wannamacher et al., 1980) and are in contrast to studies by Long et al. (1974) and Woolfson et al. (1979), who showed that there was better nitrogen retention when glucose was the only source of nonprotein calories. Roulet et al. (1983) showed that ventilated septic patients who received 50% of their calories as fat had a better protein synthesis to catabolism ratio than those who received glucose alone. MacFie et al. (1981) showed that total body nitrogen was gained in postoperative patients only when 60% of their nonprotein calories was given as fat. The need for obligatory fat oxidation was further supported by the studies of Carpentier et al. (1979), who showed that fat oxidation and fatty acid turnover continued even when the patients were receiving parenteral nutrition in which all the caloric requirements were met by infused glucose. Parallel observations by others (Askanazi et al., 1980; Burke et al., 1979; Wolfe et al., 1979) have shown that the injured-septic patient, including the burn patient, has an obligatory need for fat energy. Such patients continue to oxidize significant amounts of fat even when receiving all their nonprotein calories as glucose. Furthermore, they do not utilize all the infused glucose calories for energy, and while some excess is stored, possibly as glycogen, the rest is converted to fat. Glucose calories infused in gross excess of requirements or ability to oxidize glucose is consequently associated with the development of fatty liver in patients whose TPN contains excessive glucose. As observed earlier (Jeejeebhoy et al., 1973), replacing fat isocalorically with glucose has resulted in the development of fatty liver, a phenomenon that was reversed by restoration of the fat intake. This finding has been corroborated by others (Messing et al., 1977, 1979).

Although the depleted patient without trauma and/or sepsis can metabolize glucose, as well as fat, critically ill patients appear to have an obligatory need for fat energy. Wolfe et al. (1979) showed that 4 mg/kg/min is the maximum glucose oxidation rate, and if this infusion rate is exceeded in critically ill, insulin-resistant patients, the excess glucose is retained but not oxidized. The fate of the unoxidized glucose is speculative, but the concurrent development of fatty liver and increased CO_2 production, which is disproportionate to the oxygen consumption seen under these circumstances, suggests that glucose is being used for fat synthesis. In association with the ability to oxidize glucose, the critically ill patient continues to oxidize fat resulting in the respiratory quotient (RQ) remaining below 1.0 (see Chapter 8), despite giving all exogenous calories as glucose. Askanazi et al. (1980) showed that infusing hypercaloric glucose to injured-septic patients resulted in a hypermetabolism, which was characterized by increased catecholamine excretion, oxygen consumption, and CO_2 production. This last effect is of special concern in patients with respiratory failure. Another major drawback to the prolonged use of glucose as the sole nonprotein caloric source is the eventual onset of essential fatty acid deficiency (EFAD), which will be discussed below. The minimal dose of a 10% lipid emulsion necessary to prevent EFAD in adults receiving TPN ranges from 150–350 ml/day, depending on the concentration of linoleic acid present. Finally, Baker et al. (1984) have shown that the need to infuse insulin for maintaining euglycemia during TPN is reduced when a fat–glucose mixture is used as a source of nonprotein energy when compared with a regimen using glucose alone. In summary, by using balanced glucose–lipid TPN, we can prevent the complications associated with the administration of substantial amounts of glucose. These include hepatic steatosis, CO_2 retention and EFAD, hypo- or hyperglycemia, and the need to add insulin to the TPN regimen.

Based on the above information, it would appear prudent to provide about 25–35 kcal/kg/day of an equicaloric mixture of glucose and lipid. Such a regimen results in fewer complications, is well tolerated and utilized by depleted patients, and is advantageous in the seriously ill hypermetabolic ones.

Micronutrients

Micronutrients are essential for the proper utilization of protein, carbohydrate, fat, and electrolytes. Essential fatty acids, trace elements, and vitamins constitute the three major groups of micronutrients. Vitamins and trace elements are essential because they regulate metabolic processes in many different ways, either as coenzymes or as elemental constituents of enzymes complexes, and so are vital for normal cellular activity. Essential fatty acids are required for prostaglandin synthesis and cell membrane integrity.

Essential fatty acids. As described in detail in Chapter 3, linoleic and linolenic acids cannot be synthesized endogenously in humans, and so must be provided from external sources. They are present in many natural foods, but clearly patients receiving TPN without lipid will develop a syndrome of EFAD. The clinical signs of this syndrome are a red, eczematoid, scaly dermatitis on the face, palms, soles, extremities, chest, and trunk; alopecia, brittle nails, intertriginous skin with oozing, thrombocytopenia, poor wound healing, reduced resistance to infection, and fatty infiltration of the liver. This syndrome can be reversed by supplementation with linoleic acid, but not with linolenic acid. Recently, linolenic acid has been claimed to be necessary to avoid neuropathy, and thus, it may be essential for the nervous system in man (Holman et al., 1982).

The main essential fatty acid is linoleic acid. Linoleic acid is a precursor of arachidonic acid which is needed for prostaglandin synthesis (see Chapter 3, Figure 3.4). It has been shown that patients given fat-free TPN develop biochemical evidence of EFAD within 2 weeks (Goodgame and Fischer, 1977) without any change in linoleic acid stores (12% of total fatty acids). Deficiency develops rapidly because of suppressed lipolysis resulting from high insulin levels secondary to high glucose infusion (Wene et al., 1975). Clinical deficiency can be avoided by giving 2%–4% of total calories as linoleic acid.

Trace elements. As described in Chapter 7, there are at least 15 trace elements currently recognized as essential for animals. In humans, the recognition of the value of trace elements has been slower, but with the advent of TPN, several syndromes due to trace element deficiency have become apparent, thus demonstrating the essentiality of supplementation with these nutrients. Among them copper, chromium, iodine, iron, selenium, zinc, and cobalt as vitamin B_{12} are clearly essential. Iron and zinc deficiencies are especially common and may develop more rapidly than for other elements. Clinical situations with increased requirements are frequent (iron in chronic bleeding, zinc in diarrhea, gastrointestinal fistula, surgical drainage, hypermetabolism) and the normal requirements are clearly higher than for other trace elements. Table 14.9 lists the recommended daily intakes for most of these trace elements in TPN. A major difficulty in the determination of requirements of vitamins and trace elements in TPN is the fact that blood, plasma, or serum levels of these nutrients may not necessarily reflect their content in the tissues, their biological activity, or their balance state (see Chapters 7 and 12). Hence, detailed balance studies of trace elements and investigations of the functional effects of intravenously administering these elements should be performed in order to determine their requirements.

IRON. Iron is an essential constituent of porphyrin-based compounds incorporated into proteins, such as hemoglobin, myoglobin, and the cytochromes (see Chapter 7, Figure 7.1). Smaller amounts of tissue iron are associated with other components, including iron–sulfur enzymes, and all of these have important metabolic functions. Iron is found in storage or transport forms bound to ferritin (or hemosiderin) and transferrin proteins, respectively. (For further information, see Chapter 7.)

The prevalence of iron deficiency anemia is high especially among premature infants, young or pregnant women, malnourished patients, and those who have been subject to a surgical procedure or have gastrointestinal disease. In the absence of anemia, there is no proof that iron deficiency results in disability except fatigue. Anemia is considered the first effect of iron deficiency, and occurs when iron stores have been used up. The first biochemical sign of *incipient* deficiency is a reduction in serum ferritin to below 12 μg/L, unless the patient also has an inflammatory process or liver disease (which elevates serum ferritin; see Table 7.4). Total serum iron also decreases, and the iron-binding capacity of transferrin is increased. When less iron than needed is available, hemoglobin synthesis becomes impaired and anemia becomes manifest.

In patients receiving TPN, needs could (theoretically) be enhanced by abnormal losses; but no carefully controlled studies of iron needs have yet been carried out. Peter et al. (1980) found that up to 25 mg of iron given weekly to patients receiving TPN significantly reduced the need for blood transfusions. A dilute solution of iron-dextran can be used to provide 1–2 mg of iron/day, according to the sex and age of patients, to meet physiological losses. Additional needs, related to abnormal losses (such as bleeding) would be met by infusing a calculated amount of iron dextran. In patients receiving home TPN, we give 1–2 mg/day and monitor the bone marrow at intervals of 1–2 years.

ZINC. Zinc is the most abundant of the trace elements, other than iron and fluoride (see Chapter 7, Table 7.1), amounting to between 22 and 35 mmol, of which 99% is intracellular and only 1% is extracellular. Therefore, it is not surprising that plasma zinc is a poor indicator of zinc stores or zinc balance. Zinc is an important element in many metalloenzyme systems (see Chapter 7, Figure 7.7). Because it is important for nucleic acid synthesis (Prasad et al., 1978), cell proliferation requires the presence of zinc. It also has an important role in the maintenance of cellular immunity

Table 14.9. Recommended Daily Dose of Trace Elements for TPN

Trace element	Chemical source	Daily i.v. dose of element
Chromium	Chromic chloride	20 μg
Copper	Cupric chloride	300 μg None with severe liver disease
Iodine	Potassium iodide	120 μg
Iron	Iron dextran	Men: 1 mg Women: premenopausal: 2 mg postmenopausal: 1 mg
Manganese	Manganous chloride	700 μg None with severe liver disease
Selenium	Selenious acid	120 μg
Zinc	Zinc sulphate	2.2 mg 12.2 mg/kg small bowel fluid loss 17.1 mg/kg stool loss

(Prasad et al., 1978) and delayed hypersensitivity, insulin secretion, and nitrogen retention. In studies where parenteral nutrition was given without zinc supplementation, plasma zinc levels dropped at a steady rate, with subnormal levels appearing after 2–7 weeks (Fleming et al., 1977; Solomons et al., 1976). Clinical zinc deficiency during unsupplemented TPN has been observed (Arakawa et al., 1976; Kay and Tasman-Jones, 1975) and consists of a scaly and pustular rash starting around the mouth and over the joints, eventually spreading over the entire body. Also, there may be alopecia, erythema of the palms and soles with desquamation, loss of the senses of taste and smell, eye changes with blepharitis and conjunctivitis, behavioral changes, impaired delayed cutaneous hypersensitivity, and resistant skin infections (Golden et al., 1978). The skin infections are usually due to staphylococci and fungi and will not disappear until zinc is provided. Supplementation with zinc reverses this entire clinical syndrome and also improves nitrogen balance and insulin secretion.

Zinc requirements during TPN are determined by urinary and gastrointestinal losses. The major source of zinc loss is from the gastrointestinal tract in patients with diarrhea and ostomies. In such patients, the losses may vary between 3 and 20 mg zinc/L of diarrhea or ostomy fluid (Wolman et al., 1979). The concentration of zinc in gastrointestinal dejecta is less when the losses are from stomach and upper bowel and higher when the site of loss is the ileum and colon. Urinary losses are increased by increased muscle catabolism, since zinc is an integral part of muscle.

The daily parenteral requirements of zinc have been shown to be about 2.5–3.0 mg in patients without diarrhea compared with an oral Recommended Dietary Allowance (RDA) of 15 mg (absorption 30%–50%; see Chapter 7). Patients with diarrhea and ostomies have greater requirements for zinc because they can lose about 10–12 mg/L of upper intestinal fluid, and 17–20 mg/L of diarrheal stool (Wolman et al., 1979). Because the urinary losses of zinc are relatively modest and are independent of the infusion rate, zinc infusions may be given even in the presence of renal failure. The form of zinc administered in TPN is usually zinc sulphate.

COPPER. Copper deficiency has been noted during TPN, but less frequently than that of zinc. In children it results in a hypochromic, normocytic anemia, leukopenia, and skeletal abnormalities (osteoporosis and metaphyseal irregularity) (Karpel and Peden, 1972). Anemia and leukopenia have also been observed in adults with low plasma copper concentrations (which occur in copper deficiency; see Chapter 7) and the abnormalities have responded to copper supplementation (Bernard et al., 1977; Dunlop et al., 1974; Vilter et al., 1974). As with zinc, the plasma level is nevertheless a poor indicator of copper status (see Chapter 7). Shike et al. (1981*a*) found daily requirements of intravenous copper (usually given as cupric chloride) to be approximately 300 μg in patients without diarrhea and 500 μg in patients with substantial fluid losses from the gastrointestinal tract. This compares with an oral RDA of 2 mg (30%–60% absorption; Chapter 7). The dose must be decreased in patients with obstructive jaundice, for copper is excreted via the biliary tract and might otherwise accumulate to reach toxic levels. In cases of severe liver disease, copper supplementation should be avoided.

CHROMIUM. Chromium is required for the peripheral action of insulin. Deficiency of chromium causes insulin resistance and glucose intolerance—a condition only corrected when chromium is added to the diet (Mertz and Roginski, 1971) (see Chapter 7). Direct evidence of the role of chromium deficiency in humans was first presented by Jeejeebhoy et al. (1977), who described a patient who developed weight loss, peripheral neuropathy, ataxia, and glucose intolerance associated with normal levels of insulin but low levels of chromium in blood and hair after 3.5 years of home TPN. Despite very large amounts of insulin, the neuropathy did not improve, and the glucose intolerance continued. When chromium was infused there was dramatic improvement in the neuropathy, and insulin was no longer required. Freund et al. (1979) have described another patient receiving long-term TPN who developed central nervous system abnormalities and glucose intolerance associated with low levels of serum chromium, all of which were corrected rapidly with chromium supplementation.

Unlike zinc and copper, adequate balance studies have not been performed for chromium. It appears that 20 μg chromium/day in the form of chromic chloride is sufficient to prevent deficiency, but further studies of doses and forms of the trace element are necessary.

IODINE. Although adequate balance studies have not been done for iodine, it appears that about 120 μg/day of iodine supplementation in TPN does not result in hyper- or hypothyroidism in patients on a long- or short-term TPN regimen. However, it should be recognized that patients being treated with povidone-iodine in their dressings will likely absorb sufficient amounts for their needs.

MANGANESE. Manganese is a cofactor for enzymes necessary in the synthesis of glycoproteins and glycolipids (see Chapter 7). Its deficiency has been associated with defective growth, dysfunction of the reproductive system, and central nervous system abnormalities in animals. Many of these effects of manganese deficiency can be explained in terms of its effects on mucopolysaccharide biosynthesis. To date, there have been no direct reports of manganese deficiency in humans.

The recommended daily infusion is about 700 μg/day. This dose should be reduced in patients with cholestatic jaundice, since manganese is excreted via the biliary tract. In the case of severe liver disease, manganese supplementation is avoided because excessive accumulation of this element in the basal ganglia may otherwise occur, leading to a Parkinson-like syndrome.

MOLYBDENUM. Molybdenum is an essential component of xanthine (De Renzo et al., 1953), sulfite (Cohen et al., 1971) and aldehyde (Mahler et al., 1954) oxidases (see Chapter 7). Xanthine oxidase catalyzes the conversion of oxypurines to uric acid, and when it is absent, there will be increased levels of oxypurines and decreased levels of uric acid. Sulfite oxidase influences the conversion of sulfite to sulfate (see Chapter 7, Figure 7.11). The lack of sulfite oxidase has been shown to cause neurological abnormalities (Cohen et al., 1973). Abumrad et al. (1981) have described a patient receiving TPN who was infused with amino acid solutions containing sulfite and who developed a comatose state. This state was reversed by supplementing the TPN with molybdenum at a rate of 300 μg/day. That a molybdenum deficiency was present was supported by the concurrent finding of hyperoxypurinemia, hypouricemia, and low sulfate excretion.

Although molybdenum excretion is mainly in urine, its loss in intestinal secretions is increased markedly in patients with short bowel or Crohn's disease. In addition, there is increased excretion of molybdenum with increased sulfate intake or with endogenous sulfate production, as occurs with increased muscle catabolism. Molybdenum also interacts with copper and increases its excretion (see Chapter 7).

The daily requirements for molybdenum have not been well established. It appears that 20 μg molybdenum/day in the form of molybdenum chloride is sufficient to prevent deficiency. However, it is not clear whether this small amount becomes available as a contaminant in TPN solutions.

SELENIUM. Vitamin E and selenium are interrelated in their actions, and a deficiency of one can be partially corrected by giving the other. Selenium is an essential component of the enzyme glutathione peroxidase (see Chapter 7). This enzyme, together with catalase, superoxide dismutase, and vitamin E provides a line of defense against oxidative damage by peroxides and free radicals (see Chapter 5, Figure 5.33).

Selenium deficiency is known to cause muscular dystrophy, pancreatic necrosis and fibrosis, exudative diathesis, and various other syndromes in different animals (Underwood, 1977). Human selenium deficiency has been implicated in Keshan's disease (Keshan Disease Research Group, 1979*a*, *b*), a congestive cardiomyopathy occurring in certain rural areas in China (where the soil has a low selenium content). It has been associated with a poor selenium status, as evidenced by low whole blood glutathione peroxidase activity and low hair selenium content. Its incidence has been decreased 82% with prophylactic selenium supplementation. In patients receiving long-term TPN, selenium deficiency may develop and result in cardiomyopathy (Fleming et al., 1982; Johnson et al., 1981; Quercia et al., 1984). Also, in 1979, van Rij et al. described a patient receiving long-term TPN who developed incapacitating bilateral muscular pain in her quadriceps and hamstring muscles that was associated with a markedly decreased plasma selenium level. Complete recovery was achieved within 3 weeks of initiating selenium supplementation.

The daily requirements for selenium are not well established at present. The dietary intake of selenium varies from 18–220 μg/day in different parts of Canada (Robinson et al., 1973; Thompson et al., 1975). Balance studies in six patients with no selenium supplementation in their TPN solution showed a negative balance with a mean loss of 10 ± 1.7 μg/day (Fischer, 1979). The need for selenium may be conditioned by other factors, such as the vitamin E status, heavy metal intake, other oxidants, and abnormal losses (see Chapter 7). The role of these factors needs to be studied. The form of selenium administered in TPN is usually selenious acid and we give 120 μg/day.

OTHER TRACE ELEMENTS. A TPN need for other trace elements including fluorine, tin, arsenic, silicon, aluminum, vanadium, cadmium, lead, and mercury, has not yet been demonstrated.

Vitamins. Vitamin requirements during TPN, with the exception of a few, have not been studied in detail. As a result, most current recommendations are based on an extrapolation from oral RDA and studies using commercially prepared multivitamin preparations. Table 14.10 outlines current practices for intravenous vitamin supplementation. Pharmaceutical stability and variability of needs (in terms of hypermetabolism, sepsis, trauma, and carbohydrate loads) have not been adequately evaluated. Thus, the suggested amounts are in excess of the oral RDA, but provide a demonstrably safe intake for the patients. When further information becomes available, these intakes may have to be adjusted. Nichoalds et al. (1977), studying six patients on a regimen of long-term TPN, have demonstrated that regular use of a well-known multivitamin infusion will maintain adequate blood levels of many water-soluble vitamins, including thiamine, riboflavin, pyridoxine, niacin, pantothenic acid, and ascorbic acid. Additionally, Jeejeebhoy et al. (1976*b*) have reported vitamin intakes and levels in six long-term TPN patients, again demonstrating that adequate levels of water-soluble vitamins can be provided by routine multivitamin preparations.

Table 14.10. Dose of Vitamins Recommended for TPN

Vitamin	Supplementation
Water-soluble vitamins	
Thiamine (B_1)	5 mg/day
Riboflavin (B_2)	5 mg/day
Niacinamide	50 mg/day
Pantothenic acid	15 mg/day
Pyridoxine (B_6)	5 mg/day
Folic acid	0.6 mg/day
Vitamin B_{12}	5 μg/day
Biotin	60 μg/day[a]
Ascorbic acid (C)	300 mg/day
Fat-soluble vitamins	
Vitamin A	2500 IU/day
Vitamin D	None added
Vitamin E	50–100 IU/day additional to that in lipid emulsion[b]
Vitamin K	10 mg/week

[a] Recommended by the American Medical Association.
[b] Different fat emulsions contain different amounts of vitamin E (35–50 IU/500 ml).

THIAMINE (B_1). Thiamine is an integral part of the carboxylase enzyme complex that is necessary for the metabolism of α-keto acids, such as pyruvate (see Chapter 5, Figure 5.3). Some cells, such as neurons, depend on glucose for energy unless ketones are available in sufficient concentration to meet their metabolic needs. During TPN, the continuous infusion of insulin suppresses ketogenesis, as does sepsis. Thus, in patients receiving TPN, neurons are exclusively dependent on glucose for energy and are particularly vulnerable to thiamine deficiency. Kishi et al. (1979) found that 5 mg/day of thiamine was sufficient in patients receiving TPN (compared with an oral RDA of 1.54–1.90 mg). Most multivitamin preparations contain at least this amount. The higher requirements for thiamine during TPN may be due to the large carbohydrate loads given during the practice of TPN.

RIBOFLAVIN (B_2). Deficiency of riboflavin can lead to photophobia, cheilosis, glossitis, and pruritus of the skin with inflammation, especially of the anogenital region. A daily infusion of 5 mg in patients receiving TPN has avoided clinical deficiency. The oral RDA is 1.2–1.5 mg (see Chapter 5, Figure 5.4).

NIACIN. Deficiency of niacin can lead to the syndrome of pellagra, which consists of erythema and pigmentation of the skin, glossitis, stomatitis, and diarrhea. Delerium and confusion may also develop. A daily infusion of 50 mg of niacinamide in patients receiving TPN is recommended. This is more than double the oral RDA of 13–19 mg (see Chapter 5, Figure 5.5).

PANTOTHENIC ACID. Disease states due to deficiency of pantothenic acid have not been described in man. The recommended daily infusion in patients receiving TPN is 15 mg, which is similar to recommendations for oral intake (see Chapter 5, Figure 5.6).

PYRIDOXINE (B_6). Deficiency of vitamin B_6 can lead to dermatitis, seborrhea, intertrigo, neuropathy, and changes in mental status (see Chapter 5). A daily infusion of 15 mg in patients receiving TPN has avoided clinical deficiency; the oral RDA is 2–2.2 mg.

B_{12} AND FOLIC ACID. Deficiencies of B_{12} and folate have a combination of hematologic, gastrointestinal, and neurologic manifestations. These substances are not provided in many of the multivitamin preparations. B_{12} has long been used par-

parenterally in patients with pernicious anemia who cannot absorb vitamin B_{12} taken orally. A daily maintenance dose of 5 μg of B_{12} is given to these patients, and the same dose is recommended for patients receiving TPN. Folate deficiency is relatively common in severely malnourished hospitalized patients, and although 5 mg/day is often given, Lowry et al. (1978) have shown that 0.6 mg/day is normally sufficient.

VITAMIN C. Deficiency of vitamin C (ascorbic acid), when extreme, can lead to the syndrome of scurvy, characterized by perifollicular hemorrhages in the skin, gingivitis, and infections. Infusion of 300–500 mg/day (five times or more the oral RDA) is recommended, since for its other roles (e.g., antioxidant) ascorbic acid may be needed as an antioxidant in considerably greater amounts than for its antiscorbutic effect.

BIOTIN. Until recently, biotin deficiency had only been observed in man under two conditions. The first is a genetic syndrome of biotin-responsive carboxylase deficiency (Roth et al., 1976; Sweetman et al., 1977). The second is an acquired biotin deficiency which occurs only in association with substantial raw egg ingestion (Scott, 1958). The white of egg contains avidin, a protein capable of binding biotin intraluminally and preventing its absorption (see Chapter 5). Jeejeebhoy et al. (1976*b*) found low plasma biotin levels in six long-term home TPN patients, but were unable to discover any clinical pathology: adding biotin did not change the clinical picture.

However recently, there have been several reports of biotin deficiency with prolonged TPN (Innis and Allardyce, 1983; Khalidi et al., 1984; Mock et al., 1981) with manifestations including dermatitis, alopecia, paresthesias, delirium, depression, nausea, vomiting, and possibly fever. It is still unclear whether routine biotin supplementation in TPN is necessary. However, patients receiving TPN with biotin-free preparations who develop the above-mentioned symptoms without explanation should be given a trial of biotin therapy. The American Medical Association has recommended administration of 60 μg/day for patients receiving TPN.

VITAMIN A. This vitamin is essential for the integrity of epithelial surfaces and synthesis of retinal pigments and is important in protecting against infection. In patients on a regimen of long-term TPN, 2500 IU/day maintain normal serum levels for periods of several years. When vitamin A was withdrawn from 12 home TPN patients, who had previously been receiving 2500 IU of vitamin A, 11 of the patients still had normal serum vitamin A levels after 6 months (Jeejeebhoy et al., 1976*b*). The other patient who did not receive vitamin A for 12 months had a low serum level. These findings indicate that for most patients, the 2500 IU daily dose was sufficient to build or maintain stores in the liver.

Uncertainties about the dose remain, for it has recently been shown that vitamin A adsorbs to the polyvinylchloride used for the bags and tubing of the TPN administration system. Also, the vitamin is fairly labile, especially in the presence of light and heat (see Chapter 10). Howard et al. (1980) found a 30% decrease in the concentration of vitamin A in the TPN fluid during the first 8 hr of infusion; Hartline and Zachman (1976) found a 50% decrease in 24 hr. Consequently, vitamins should only be added to TPN solutions just prior to infusion.

VITAMIN D. A prospective study of bone biopsies performed prior to the onset of home TPN (containing vitamin D) and repeated after at least 1 year of this treatment, showed that these patients developed histological osteomalacia (Shike et al., 1980). Furthermore, after several years of home TPN, a number of patients were noted to have bone pain and some developed bone fractures. Further studies showed that the osteomalacia was associated with intermittent hypercalcemia, hypercalciuria, and loss of skeletal calcium (Shike et al., 1981*b*) (see Chapters 5 and 6 for definitions). Levels of 25-OH-D were normal, those of 1,25-diOH-D were low, and those of parathyroid hormone were suppressed, suggesting that neither excess vitamin D nor hyperparathyroidism was the cause of the observed metabolic problems. Nevertheless, withdrawal of the vitamin from the TPN on a prospective basis resulted in a return to normal bone structure and an increase of tetracycline uptake by bone (an index of better bone formation). Withdrawal of the vitamin was also associated with clinical remission of the symptoms.

Interestingly, Izsak et al. (1980) described the occurrence of pancreatitis secondary to hypercalcemia in several patients on a TPN regimen. The hypercalcemia was thought to be due to the vitamin D content of the infusion and not to the calcium (then routinely infused), since the hypercalcemia persisted after the calcium was discontinued, and resolved only after vitamin D was withdrawn.

It appears that administering vitamin D intravenously to patients receiving long-term TPN increases their propensity to develop metabolic bone disease. It is thus recommended that all vitamin D supplements be withdrawn from home TPN patients, and that they be encouraged to expose themselves to sunlight to maintain normal vitamin D levels through endogenous production (see Chapter 5). Patients receiving shorter courses of TPN in a hospital may be given once weekly, a multivitamin preparation containing 500 IU of vitamin D.

VITAMIN E. Vitamin E is supplied to patients receiving TPN in part by vitamin preparations and in part by that present in the lipid solutions. Jeejeebhoy et al. (1976*b*) have shown that serum α-tocopherol levels decrease slightly in long-term TPN patients, even with daily lipid infusions. Thurlow and Grant (1980) have described 10 patients receiving TPN who developed increased red blood cell fragility and increased platelet aggregation in conjunction with low serum vitamin E levels. These abnormalities were corrected in seven patients with 50 IU/day, 1-α-tocopherol daily, but not by 25 IU/day. It is current practice to provide about 50–100 IU/day in addition to that in the infused lipid.

VITAMIN K. Vitamin K is required for the synthesis of several coagulation factors (see Chapter 5, Figure 5.35) through carboxylation of glutamate side chains (see Chapter 5). Under normal circumstances, it is derived both from the diet (mainly plants) and from gut bacteria. In patients receiving TPN, the gut bacteria may be a sufficient source of vitamin K, but because there may be changes in the bacterial flora of the nonactive gut (especially if the patient is receiving antibiotics) supplementation with vitamin K is advisable. Ten milligrams of Synkavite (menadiol sodium diphosphate, a synthetic vitamin analogue; Chapter 5, Figure 5.34), given weekly, is sufficient.

In summary, current vitamin recommendations are given in Table 14.10. At the Toronto General, a Division of the Toronto Hospital, it is current practice to supply daily a multivitamin preparation containing all of the vitamins, except for A, D, E, K, and biotin. Vitamin E is supplied by the lipid solutions used in the TPN regimen (50% of the nonprotein calories), but this may not be adequate (see above). Vitamin K is given once weekly to both inpatients and home TPN patients.

Fluid and Electrolytes

Water. The solutions used for TPN should have a caloric density of about 1 kcal/ml. Adult patients generally require about 35 ml water/kg body weight/day and about 30 kcal/kg body weight/day or in other words about 2–3 L of fluid to provide the daily energy requirements. Accordingly, the patient must be able to excrete this water load. The amount of fluid given will have to be altered in situations where water excretion is compromised, such as in renal, hepatic, or cardiac failure, or in case of cerebral edema. When fluid restriction is necessary, 20% lipid emulsions (which contain about 4 kcal/ml), up to 70% dextrose solutions, and up to 10% amino acid solutions can be used to increase the caloric density and the protein intakes. Unfortunately, highly concentrated dextrose is viscous and difficult to infuse. Furthermore, the osmolarity increases with the substrate concentration and only the administration of TPN into a large central vein is then possible. Thus, when severe water restriction is essential, nutritional requirements are unlikely to be met.

Electrolytes. The importance of fluid and electrolytes for promoting tissue perfusion and ionic equilibrium is self-evident. Malnutrition is associated with major changes in electrolyte balance. With malnutrition there is a loss of the intracellular ions, potassium, magnesium, and phosphorus, together with a gain in sodium and water. A positive nitrogen balance upon refeeding is not achieved unless these lost ions are supplied in sufficient amount at least to maintain balance (Freeman, 1981; Rudman et al., 1975). A positive balance of sodium and water may be seen during refeeding with carbohydrate (MacFie et al., 1981). This process is referred to as "refeeding edema" and disappears concomitantly with improvement in the nutritional status. In malnourished patients, particularly elderly subjects and those with cardiopulmonary disease or renal insufficiency, refeeding has to be undertaken very carefully because of the risk of pulmonary edema.

Recommendations for electrolyte supplementation are given in Table 14.11. They have to be altered to meet special needs, such as occur in cardiac, renal and hepatic dysfunction.

Sodium. The average intake of sodium during TPN is about 120 mmol (2.8 g)/day, but this can be reduced to 20–40 mmol (0.5–0.9 g)/day if salt restriction is necessary. In general, severely mal-

Table 14.11. Standard Electrolyte Supplementation for TPN

Sodium	100–120 mmol/day
Potassium	80–120 mmol/day
Calcium	8–10 mmol/day
Phosphorus	14–16 mmol/day
Magnesium	12–15 mmol/day

nourished patients (especially the elderly and those with cardiopulmonary or renal disease) when refed orally or parenterally with a system rich in carbohydrate, quickly develop peripheral edema and may even develop severe pulmonary edema. This may be related to the finding that feeding carbohydrate tends to induce sodium retention (De Fronzo, 1981); this is exaggerated in malnourished patients who already have an excess of total body water. Thus, refeeding should be performed cautiously in such patients, initially restricting the intake of both sodium and fluid.

Potassium. When a malnourished patient is refed, there is a disproportionately greater retention of potassium than nitrogen during the first 2 months (Rudman et al., 1975). Infusing glucose plus amino acids causes a greater increase in total body potassium than infusing amino acids alone (Collins et al., 1978). Therefore, at least 90–120 mmol (3.5–4.7 g) potassium/day should be provided in the TPN solutions to avoid hypokalemia and to assist in achieving positive nitrogen balance. Patients with renal failure should receive less potassium. Additional potassium should be provided for those patients undergoing vigorous nasogastric suctioning, or those with diarrhea or fistula losses.

Magnesium. Like potassium, magnesium is retained during TPN, especially during the phase of positive nitrogen balance. In fact, it has been shown that a positive nitrogen balance cannot be achieved without providing magnesium (Freeman, 1981). Magnesium balance can usually be maintained by providing 12–15 mmol (0.29–0.36 g) of magnesium daily compared to an oral RDA of 0.35 g (see Chapter 6).

Phosphorus. Phosphate deficiency commonly occurred in the early days of TPN prior to the realization of the need for phosphorus supplementation. In fact, positive nitrogen balance will not occur in the absence of added phosphate (Rudman et al., 1975). Thus, potassium, magnesium, and phosphate are the three intracellular cations required for the repletion of cell mass. If inorganic phosphorus (as $H_2PO_4^{2-}$ and HPO_4^{-}) is not supplemented during TPN, hypophosphatemia may result and lead to serious neurological symptoms (Silvis and Paragas, 1972). About 10–20 mmol (0.3–0.6 g) of elemental phosphorus should be provided daily, versus an oral RDA of 0.6 g (see Chapter 6).

Calcium. Hypercalcemia may appear as a complication of TPN and may even result in pancreatitis (Iszak et al., 1980). The mechanism involved is not known, but it is not due to the continued infusion of TPN solution, because it may persist for several weeks even after the TPN has been discontinued (Manson, 1974). The phenomenon tends to occur when vitamin D is added to the TPN solutions (Shike et al., 1980, 1981*b*) and may be associated with metabolic bone disease that is indistinguishable from osteomalacia. Hypercalciuria and a markedly negative calcium balance usually accompany the hypercalcemia (Shike et al., 1980). After withdrawing the vitamin D, the hypercalcemia, hypercalciuria, and bone pain improve (Shike et al., 1981*b*). We currently recommend about 10–12 mmol (0.4–0.48 g) calcium/day, compared with an oral RDA of 0.8 g (10%–40% absorbed) (see Chapter 6).

Acid–Base Disorders Unique to Parenteral Nutrition

Metabolic Acidosis

Because the normal kidney can excrete about 300 mmol of ammonia daily when a chronic acid load is given (Halperin et al., 1985), exceedingly high protein intakes would be required to be the sole cause of metabolic acidosis. These amounts are never infused during TPN, and so, if metabolic acidosis does occur during TPN, one can conclude that it is caused by other factors.

The most common renal cause of metabolic acidosis attributable to TPN is a defect in the excretion of ammonia (Fraley et al., 1978). The cause of this defect is unknown. There is no evidence to suggest hyperkalemia, renal cortical necrosis, or a decrease in circulating glutamine as the cause. Rather, the cause may be an interstitial nephritis, which can compromise ammonium ion delivery to the collecting duct (Sajo et al., 1981). Infusing hypertonic dextrose leads to a modest rise in blood lactate levels, but unless an underlying defect in intermediary metabolism is present, significant clinical acidosis will not occur (Goldman et al., 1961; Merritt et al., 1981). Lactic acidosis has been reported in five pediatric oncology patients who were receiving 4% Freamine amino acid mixture and 25% glucose (wt/vol). In two of these patients, the lactic acidosis resolved after decreasing the amount of glucose infused, whereas in the other three it appeared to be an integral part of the disease (Merritt et al., 1981).

Metabolic acidosis can also occur as a result of the infusion of fructose or sorbitol, both of which can be metabolized to lactate. Fructose infusions may lead to lactic acidosis (Bergstrom et al., 1968; Sahebjami and Scalettar, 1971), especially in patients with inborn errors of metabolism leading to fructose intolerance (Chapter 18). In adults, clinical acidosis has not been observed when only 25% of the nonprotein calories in TPN is given as fructose (Vinay et al., 1981). In contrast, infants receiving TPN solutions with fructose or sorbitol have developed severe acidosis and hyperlactatemia (Aynsley-Green et al., 1974; Harries, 1972). The acidosis with fructose infusions is due to binding of ATP phosphate as fructose-1-phosphate, thus depleting ATP levels in the liver (Bode et al., 1973).

Increased levels of blood free fatty acids and ketones may occur with infusion of hypocaloric amino acid solutions (containing fewer calories than required for metabolic needs) in so-called "protein-sparing" therapy (Greenberg and Jeejeebhoy, 1979; Greenberg et al., 1976). The ketoacidosis that occurs is usually mild and remains so.

All amino acid mixtures have some free ammonia and titratable acid. In practice, this does not appear to produce a significant proton load during TPN (Chan et al., 1972; Greenberg et al., 1976). In fact the titratable acidity of a synthetic amino acid mixture causing acidosis is only 10–15 meq/L. However, some protein and amino acid preparations may have high free ammonia concentrations, which lead to elevated blood ammonia concentrations in vulnerable subjects (Chan et al., 1972; Heird et al., 1972*a*, *b*; Johnson et al., 1972).

The main cause of an increased proton load is the metabolism of basic amino acids (arginine, histidine, and lysine). Currently, amino acid mixtures contain acetate (metabolized to bicarbonate) to buffer the proton load produced by the metabolism of basic amino acids. In contrast to adults, infants receiving hypertonic glucose and protein hydrolysate solutions parenterally may develop metabolic acidosis due to hyperosmolality (Sotos et al., 1962). TPN does not lead to hyperosmolality in adults because of the greater capacity of adults to utilize the infused glucose and amino acids. In contrast, this capacity is limited in immature low-birth-weight infants, who will develop hyperglycemia, hyperammonemia, acidema, and hypertonicity if infused too rapidly.

Metabolic Alkalosis

Depletion of the extracellular fluid volume, chloride, and potassium can lead to metabolic alkalosis during TPN. The kidney will normally excrete bicarbonate in the face of a net base load, and thus, unless renal failure is present, severe metabolic alkalosis should not occur as a result of TPN.

Respiratory Acidosis or Alkalosis

In septic-injured patients and those with markedly impaired pulmonary function, high carbohydrate loads may lead to elevated arterial pCO_2 as a result of increased CO_2 generation (Roulet et al., 1983). This, in turn, may lead to difficulties in attempting to wean the patient off a ventilator. By decreasing the amount of glucose infused, the amount of CO_2 produced will decrease, and it may then become easier to wean the patient.

Controversies in TPN

TPN in Cancer

Cachexia is one of the earliest and most dramatic manifestations of malignancies. The mechanisms involved in the development of malnutrition in cancer are not well defined. In the past, it was believed that the malnutrition was due to inadequate intake of nutrition, secondary to anorexia, taste abnormalities, depression, or the effects of radio- and/or chemotherapy, at a time when the metabolic requirements were increased. Recently, there has been growing evidence that cancer-induced malnutrition may be due to altered metabolism, as well as to decreased availability of nutrients. Abnormalities in carbohydrate metabolism with an increase in Cori cycle (gluconeogenic) activity, decreased glucose tolerance, and peripheral insulin resistance have all been shown to occur. In patients with weight loss, abnormalities of circulating amino acids have been described, but the data are conflicting (Clarke et al., 1978; Kelley and Waisman, 1957; Rudman et al., 1971; Wu and Bauer, 1960; Young et al., 1967). As well, cancer leads to loss of body fat early in the course of the disease (Shike et al., 1984).

It is still unknown whether TPN can reverse the effects of cancer cachexia and modify these alterations in metabolism. In a controlled trial, Shike et al. (1984) have shown that cancer patients, when given TPN, gain weight and retain K^+ but continue to lose body nitrogen. However, in this study, survival did not improve by giving TPN. Indeed there are no well controlled studies showing improved overall survival in cancer patients provided with TPN. The possibility that nutritional support may stimulate tumor growth without any benefit to the host is an obvious concern. Animal and human studies have provided conflicting data on this point. It is likely that improved nutrition will lead to some increased tumor growth, because both tumor and normal host cells are dependent on adequate nutrition. At the same time, this increase in tumor cell growth may be useful therapeutically, since actively dividing cells are those that are most sensitive to the cytotoxic effects of chemotherapeutic agents. In a specific group of cancer patients, malnutrition is caused by dysphagia or bowel obstruction. In such patients, the cause of malnutrition is simply starvation. In this group, nutritional support might be beneficial.

In summary, the benefits of nutritional support in cancer patients remain unclear. Further controlled studies are required before more definite guidelines for its use become available.

TPN in Renal Failure

Renal insufficiency often leads to various metabolic disorders that may be associated with weight loss, inability to eat, and electrolyte disorders (potassium and magnesium). Malnutrition is common in those who undergo dialysis or who are suffering from debilitating intercurrent illnesses that preclude adequate oral nutrition. In addition, the patients often suffer from dyspepsia or anorexia. If the patient cannot be adequately maintained on an enteral regimen due to his/her gastrointestinal symptoms or dysfunction, then intervention with parenteral nutrition is necessary to prevent malnutrition and further deterioration in an already compromised host. The parenteral regimen has to be modified so as to restrict fluid and electrolyte intake. By using a 20% fat emulsion as part of the TPN regimen, the fluid intake can be decreased, thus decreasing the requirement for water removal during dialysis. There is no evidence that fat emulsions interfere with clearance during peritoneal or hemodialysis.

Although carbohydrate and fat utilization are impaired in patients with renal failure, dialysis can restore metabolism to a nearly normal state. Consequently, nutritionally depleted patients who undergo regular dialysis can receive infusions of amino acids and calories sufficient to satisfy their nutritional requirements. It is important to provide an adequate amount of protein and calories and to tailor the requirements for dialysis around this, rather than to restrict the vital nutrients due to limitations imposed by the desire to perform dialysis less frequently. The caloric requirements for these catabolic patients are usually about 30 kcal/kg. An equicaloric mixture of fat and carbohydrate is effective in meeting the needs of these patients.

Solutions providing free L-amino acids are preferable to protein hydrolysates, since there is the possibility that some of the peptide-bound amino acids present in hydrolysates may not be metabolized and could accumulate in renal failure. Furthermore, it has been shown that providing essential amino acids as the sole source of nitrogen will promote protein synthesis and decrease muscle proteolysis. Infusing solutions with a predominance of essential amino acids has reduced azotemia in patients with renal failure. On the basis of this observation, considerable attention has been given to formulating an optimal amino acid solution for patients in acute renal failure in order to minimize the azotemia and avoid dialysis. A mixture containing only essential amino acids has been shown to improve survival by comparison with controls receiving glucose and amino acids, but without reduction of the need for dialysis in such patients (Abel et al., 1973; Giordano, 1963; Saba et al., 1983; Walser, 1984*a*, *b*). However, others have shown no difference between infusing a balanced amino acid mixture and one containing only essential amino acids (Feinstein et al., 1981). Some authorities recommend that the protein intake should not exceed 40 g/day, given as an equal quantity of both essential and nonessential amino acids. Other investigators maintain that protein should not be restricted in hypercatabolic patients with renal failure and recommend as much as 120 g protein/day for some patients who are injured. Despite the possibly increased requirements for dialysis with increased administration of protein, such therapy is sometimes needed to enhance the utilization of nutrients in severely ill patients. Optimal protein intake for patients in renal failure is still unclear and further studies are required. Despite the retention of sodium, potassium, magnesium, and phosphate in patients with renal failure, giving TPN results in the rapid utilization of potassium, magnesium, and phosphate for tissue anabolism, and as a result, there is an increased requirement for these electrolytes. In fact, nitrogen balance and glucose utilization will be impaired in the presence of potassium deficiency. Thus, the need for these electrolytes depends on both the amount excreted by the kidneys and the rate of tissue anabolism. An attempt should be made to measure the losses of electrolytes in diarrheal stools, fistula drainage, and d-tube suction (the latter used to drain the stomach as in gastric or upper intestinal obstruction), and this amount should be added to the infusion mixtures.

Our current practice is first to place the patient on alternate day dialysis (and if needing water removal, ultrafiltration) and second to give a balanced amino acid solution containing 50% of essential amino acids at 1 g/kg body weight/day in a regimen of full TPN. Only Na, K, Mg, and P intakes are restricted, to the extent required to maintain normal electrolyte levels.

TPN in Hepatic Failure

Despite the restraints on the amount of protein that can be given to patients in hepatic failure, without precipitating or aggravating encephalopathy, there is still a definite need for protein in these patients—for restoration of lean body mass and for protein synthesis within the liver to restore its enzymatic function. Patients with hepatic failure have an alteration in their protein metabolism, as evidenced by the distortion of their circulating amino acid pattern, with an increase in aromatic amino acids and methionine, and a decrease in the branched-chain amino acids. This distortion in the amino acid pattern is believed to alter neurotransmitter metabolism in the brain, causing an increase of false neurotransmitters, such as octopamine. These imbalances, as well as many other factors, may contribute to the evolution of hepatic encephalopathy. As a result of these findings, Fischer et al. (1976) advocate the use of a solution rich in branched-chain amino acids and poor in aromatic amino acids and methionine for patients with hepatic failure. However, infusions of branched-chain amino-acid-enriched amino acid mixtures have not resulted in constant clinical and electroencephalographic improvement (Wahren et al., 1983). In addition, when the use of branched-chain amino-acid-enriched solutions has been compared with the use of standard amino acid solutions, there has been no difference in mortality (Aubin et al., 1983). At the present time, branched-chain amino-acid-enriched mixtures cannot be considered to be of proven efficacy in patients with liver failure, so that no recommendations can be given regarding the optimal amino acid balance.

Despite previous fears of using lipids in patients with liver disease, there is no evidence to suggest a detrimental effect of lipids, and in fact, there may be a beneficial effect of providing lipid as a source of calories, thus decreasing the requirements for carbohydrate. Lipid emulsions can be infused safely in jaundiced patients and are cleared normally, as the clearance in the liver of infused fat is quite insignificant. Shortly after the infusion of the fat emulsion, fat particles undergo hydrolysis by lipoprotein lipase, resulting in the release of free fatty acids, which are mostly oxidized in muscle. By contrast, the liver has a much more important role in carbohydrate metabolism, since the liver is the primary site for the conversion of carbohydrate to fat. Thus, high carbohydrate loads may be detrimental to hepatic function and may precipitate the formation of a fatty liver. By providing fat as a source of nonprotein calories, the requirements for carbohydrate will decrease, and thus the risk of developing a fatty liver will decrease.

Sodium and water restriction is indicated in patients with severe liver insufficiency who have an expanded extracellular space. Vitamins and trace elements can be given in the usual quantities, with the exceptions of copper and manganese which should be withheld in severe liver disease. Patients with alcoholic cirrhosis may benefit from increased vitamin intakes, notably thiamine (50–100 mg/daily), which must be administered prior to the infusion of a carbohydrate load.

Summary

TPN is an effective and often life-saving means of providing adequate nutrition, fluid, electrolytes, trace elements, and vitamins for various conditions. In the proper hands, it is a valuable tool for the clinician, but in inexperienced hands, its use can result in serious consequences.

References

Abel RM, Beck CH Jr, Abott WM, Ryan JA Jr, Octo Barnett G, Fischer JE (1973): N Engl J Med 288:695.

Abumrad NN, Schneider AJ, Steel D, Rogers LS (1981): Am J Clin Nutr 34:2551.

Anderson GH, Patel DG, Jeejeebhoy KN (1974): J Clin Invest 53:904.

Arakawa T, Tamura T, Igarashi Y, Suzuki H, Sandstead HH (1976): Am J Clin Nutr 29:197.

Askanazi J, Carpentier YA, Elwyn DH, Nordenstrom J, Jeevanandam M, Rosenbaum SH, Gump FE, Kinney JM (1980): Ann Surg 191:40.

Aubin J-P, Pomier-Layrargues G, Bories P, Mirouze D, Bellet-Herman H, Michel H (1983): Gastroenterol Clin Biol 7:209 (abstract).

Aynsley-Green A, Baum JD, Alberti KGMM, Woods HF (1974): Arch Dis Child 49:647.

Baker JP, Detsky AS, Stewart S, Whitwell J, Marliss EB, Jeejeebhoy KN (1984): Gastroenterology 87:53.

Bergstrom J, Hultman E, Roch-Norlund AE (1968): Acta Med Scand 184:359.

Bernard LZ, Shadduck RK, Zeigler Z (1977): Am J Hematol 3:177.

Bierman EL (1972): Isr J Med Sci 8:303.

Blackburn GL, Flatt J-P, Clowes GHA, O'Donnel TF (1973): Am J Surg 125:447.

Bode JC, Zelder O, Rumpelt HJ, Wittkamt U (1973): Eur J Clin Invest 3:436.

Bonau RA, Ang SD, Jeevanandam M, Daly JM (1984): J Parenter Enteral Nutr 8:622.

Bozetti F (1976): Surg Gynecol Obstet 142:16.

Bozetti F, Agradi E, Ravera E (1988): Clin Nutr 8:35.

Brennan MF (1979): Cancer 43:2053.

Breenan MF (1981): N Engl J Med 305:375.

Burke JF, Wolfe RR, Mullany CJ, Matthews DE, Bier DM (1979): Ann Surg 190:274.

Buse MG, Reid SS (1975): J Clin Invest 56:1250.

Calloway DH, Spector H (1954): Am J Clin Nutr 2:405.

Carpentier YA, Askanazi J, Elwyn DH, Jeevanandam M, Gump FE, Hyman AI, Burr R, Kinney JM (1979): J Trauma 19:649.

Champault G, Patel JC (1979): Chirurgie 105:751.

Chan JCM, Malekzadeh M, Hurley J (1972): JAMA 220:1119.

Chan STF (1986) Br Med J 293:1055.

Clarke EF, Lewis AM, Waterhouse C (1978): Cancer 42:2909.

Cohen HJ, Drew RT, Johnson J, Rajagopalan KV (1973): Proc Natl Acad Sci USA 70:3655.

Cohen HJ, Fridovich T, Rajagopalan KV (1971): J Biol Chem 246:374.

Collins JP, Oxby CB, Hill GL (1978): Lancet 1:778.

Cuthbertson DP (1932): Q J Med 25:233.

Daly JM, Mihranin MH, Kehoe JE, Brennan MF (1983): Surgery 94:151.

De Fronzo RA (1981): Can J Surg 19:505.

De Renzo EC, Kaleita E, Heytler P, Oleson JJ, Hutchings RL, Williams JH (1953): Arch Biochem Biophys 45:247.

Dickenson RJ, Ashton MG, Axon ATR, Smith RC, Yeung CK, Hill GL (1980): Gastroenterology 79:1199.

Dunlop WM, James GW III, Hume DM (1974): Ann Intern Med 80:470.

Elwyn DH (1980): Crit Care Med 8:9.

Evans WK, Nixon DW, Daly JM, Ellenberg SS, Gardner L, Wolfe E, Shepherd FA, Feld R, Gralla R, Fine S, Kemeny M, Jeejeebhoy KN, Heymsfield S, Hoffman FA (1987): J Clin Oncol 5:113.

Fan ST, Lau WY, Wong KK, Chan YPM (1988): Clin Nutr 8:23.

Feinstein EI, Blumenkrantz MJ, Healy M, Koffler A, Silberman H, Massry SG, Kopple JD (1981): Medicine 60:124.

Fischer JE (1979): JAMA 241:496.

Fischer JE, Rosen HM, Ebeid AM, James JH, Keane JM, Soeters PB (1976): Surgery 80:77.

Fleming CR, Lee JT, McCall JT, O'Brien JF, Baillie EE, Thistle JL (1982): Gastroenterology 83:689.

Fleming CR, McGill DB, Berkner S (1977): Gastroenterology 73:1077.

Fraley DS, Adler S, Bruns F, Segal D (1978): Ann Intern Med 88:352.

Freeman JB (1981): *In* Hill GL, Jeejeebhoy KN, Kinney JM, eds: Parenteral nutrition Canada. Present status and newer developments. Princeton Junction, NJ: Communications Media for Education, p 43.

Freund H, Atamian S, Fischer JE (1979): JAMA 241:496.

Freund HR, Muggia-Sullam M, LaFrance R, Fischer JE (1988): Clin Nutr 7:139.

Gazzaniga AB, Bartlett RH, Shobe JB (1975): Ann Surg 182:163.

Giordano C (1963): J Lab Clin Med 62:231.

Golden MHN, Golden BE, Harland PSEG, Jackson AA (1978): Lancet 1:1226.

Goldman HI, Karelitz S, Seifter E, Acs H, Schelle NB (1961): Pediatrics 27:921.

Goodgame JT, Fischer JE (1977): Ann Surg 186:651.

Greenberg GR, Fleming CR, Jeejeebhoy KN, Rosenberg IH, Sales D, Tremaine WJ (1988): Gut 29:1309.

Greenberg GR, Jeejeebhoy KN (1979): J Parenter Enteral Nutr 3:427.

Greenberg GR, Jeejeebhoy KN (1981): *In* Pean AS, Weterman IT, Booth CC, Strober W, eds: Developments in gastroenterology: Recent advances in Crohn's disease. The Hague: Martinus Nijhoff, p 492.

Greenberg GR, Marliss EB, Anderson GH, Langer B, Spence W, Toveee EB, Jeejeebhoy KN (1976): N Engl J Med 294:1411.

Halperin ML, Goldstein MB, Stinebaugh BJ, Jungas RL (1985): *In* Seldin DW, Giebisch G, eds: Physiology and pathology of electrolyte metabolism. New York: Raven, p 1471.

Hammarqvist F, Wernerman J, Von der Decken K, Vinnars E (1988): Clin Nutr 7:171.

Harries JT (1972): *In* Wilkinson AW, ed: Parenteral nutrition (an international symposium in London. April 30–May 1, 1971). London: Churchill Livingstone, p 266.

Harris JA, Benedict FG (1919): *In* JA Harris, ed: A biometric study of basal metabolism in man. Philadelphia: Carnegie Institution of Washington, publication no 279, JB Lippincott, p 223.

Hartline JV, Zachman RD (1976): Paediatrics 58:448.

Heird WC, Dell RB, Driscoll JM Jr, Grebin B, Winters RW (1972*a*): N Engl J Med 287:943.

Heird WC, Nicholson JF, Driscoll JM Jr, Schillinger JN, Winters RW (1972*b*): J Pediatr 81:162.

Holm I (1981): Acta Chir Scand 147:271.

Holman RT, Johnson SB, Hatch TF (1982): Am J Clin Nutr 35:617.

Howard L, Chu R, Feman S, Mintz I, Ovesen L, Wolf B (1980): Ann Intern Med 93:576.

Huttenen JK, Nikkila EA (1973): Eur J Clin Invest 3:483.

Innis SM, Allardyce DB (1983): Am J Clin Nutr 37:185.

Izsak EM, Shike M, Roulet M, Jeejeebhoy KN (1980): Gastroenterology 79:555.

Jeejeebhoy KN, Anderson GH, Nakhooda AF, Greenberg GR, Sanderson I, Marliss EB (1976*a*): J Clin Invest 57:125.

Jeejeebhoy KN, Chu RC, Marliss EB, Greenberg GR, Bruce-Robertson A (1977): Am J Clin Nutr 30:531.

Jeejeebhoy KN, Langer B, Tsallas G, Chu RC, Kuksis A, Anderson GH (1976*b*): Gastroenterology 71:943.

Jeejeebhoy KN, Zohrab WJ, Langer B, Phillips MJ, Kuksis A, Anderson GH (1973): Gastroenterology 65:811.

Johnson JD, Albritton WL, Sunshine P (1972): J Pediatr 81:154.

Johnson RA, Baker SE, Fallon JT, Maynard EP, Ruskin JN, Wen Z, Ge K, Cohen HJ (1981): N Engl J Med 304:1210.

Karpel JT, Peden VH (1972): J Pediatr 80:32.

Kay RG, Tasman-Jones G (1975): Aust N Z J Surg 45:325.

Kelley JJ, Waisman HA (1957): Blood 12:635.

Kelts DG, Grand RJ, Shen G, Watkins JB, Werlin SL, Boehme C (1979): Gastroenterology 76:720.

Keshan Disease Research Group of the Chinese Academy of Medical Sciences, Beijing (1979*a*): Chin Med J 92:471.

Keshan Disease Research Group of the Chinese Academy of Medical Sciences, Beijing (1979*b*): Chin Med J 92:477.

Khalidi N, Wesley JR, Thoene JG, Whitehouse WM Jr, Baker WL (1984): J Parenter Enteral Nutr 8:311.

Kinney JM (1987): J Parenter Enteral Nutr 11:90.

Kishi H, Nishii S, Ono T, Yamagi A, Kasahara N, Hiraoka E, Okada A, Itakura T, Tagaki Y (1979): Am J Clin Nutr 32:332.

Lanzotti VJ, Thomas DR, Boyle LE, Smith TL, Gehan EA, Samuels ML (1977): Cancer 39:303.

Li J, Jefferson L (1978): Biochim Biophys Acta 544:351.

Long JM, Wilmore DW, Mason AD Jr, Pruitt BA Jr (1974): Surg Forum 25:61.

Lowry SF, Goodgame JT, Maher MM, Brennan MF (1978): Am J Clin Nutr 31:2149.

MacFie J, Smith RC, Hill GL (1981): Gastroenterology 80:103.

Maclean LD, Meakin JL, Taguchi K, Buignan JP, Philton KS, Gordon J (1975): Ann Surg 182:207.

Mahler HR, Mackler B, Green DE, Bock RH (1954): J Biol Chem 310:465.

Manson RR (1974): Arch Surg 108:213.

Merritt RJ, Ennis CE, Thomas DW, Sinatra FR (1981): J Pediatr 99:247.

Mertz W, Roginski EE (1971): *In* Mertz W, Cornatzer WE, eds: Newer trace elements in nutrition. New York: Marcel Dekker, p 123.

Messing B, Bitoun A, Galian A, Mary JV, Goll A, Bernier JJ (1977): Gastroenterol Clin Biol 1:1015.

Messing B, Latrive J-P, Bitoun A, Galian A, Bernier JJ (1979): Gastroenterol Clin Biol 3:719.

Mock DM, deLorimer AA, Liebman WM, Sweetman L, Baker H (1981): N Engl J Med 304:820.

Mullen JL, Buzby GP, Matthews DC, Smale BF, Rosato EF (1980): Ann Surg 192:604.

Muller JM, Dienst C, Brenner V, Pichlmaier H (1982): Lancet 1:68.

Munro HN (1964): *In* Munro HN, Allison JB, eds: Mammalian protein metabolism, vol 1. New York: Academic, p 38.

Munro HN (1972): *In* Wilkinson AW, ed: Parenteral nutrition (an international symposium, London, April 30–May 1, 1971). London: Churchill Livingstone, p 34.

Nichoalds GE, Meng HC, Caldwell MD (1977): Arch Surg 112:1061.

Nordenström J, Askanazi J, Elwyn DH, Martin P, Carpentier YA, Robin AP, Kinney JM (1983): Ann Surg 197:27.

O'Hara DD, Porte D Jr, Williams RH (1966): Metabolism 15:123.

Olney JW, Ho OL, Rhee V (1973): N Engl J Med 289: 301.

Patel DG, Anderson GH, Jeejeebhoy KN (1973): Gastroenterology 65:427.

Peter ML, Maher M, Brennan MF (1980): J Parenter Enteral Nutr 4:601.

Prader A, Tanner JM, von Harnack GA (1963): J Pediatr 62:646.

Prasad AS, Rabbani P, Abbasii A, Bowersox F, Fox MRS (1978): Ann Intern Med 89:483.

Quercia RA, Korn S, O'Neil D, Dougherty JE, Ludwig M, Schweizer R, Sigman R (1984): Clin Pharmacol 3:531.

Robinson MF, McKenzie JM, Thompson CD, van Rij AL (1973): Br J Nutr 30:195.

Rombeau J, Barot LR, Williamson CE, Mullen JL (1982): Am J Surg 143:139.

Rose WC (1938): Physiol Rev 18:109.

Rose WC (1949): Fed Proc 8:546.

Roth K, Cohn R, Yandrasitz J, Preti G, Dodd P, Segal S (1976): J Pediatr 88:229.

Roulet M, Detsky AS, Marliss EB, Todd TRJ, Mahon WA, Anderson GH, Stewart S, Jeejeebhoy KN (1983): Clin Nutr 2:97.

Rudman D, Vogler WR, Howard CH, Gerron CG (1971): Cancer Res 31:1159.

Rudman D, Millikan WJ, Richardson TJ, Bixler TJ II, Stackhouse WJ, McGarrity WC (1975): J Clin Invest 55:94.

Russell DMcR, Prendergast PJ, Darby PL, Garfinkel PE, Whitwell J, Jeejeebhoy KN (1983*a*): Am J Clin Nutr 38:229.

Russell DMcR, Leiter LA, Whitwell J, Marliss EB, Jeejeebhoy KN (1983*b*): Am J Clin Nutr 37:133.

Saba TM, Dillon BC, Lanser ME (1983): J Parenter Enteral Nutr 7:62.

Sahebjami H, Scalettar R (1971): Lancet 1:366.

Sajo IM, Goldstein MB, Sonnenberg H, Stinebaugh HJ, Wilson DR, Halperin ML (1981): Kidney Int 20: 353.

Scott D (1958): Acta Med Scand 162:69.

Sherwin RS (1978): J Clin Invest 61:1471.

Shike M, Harrison JE, Sturtridge WC, Tam CS, Bobechko PE, Jones G, Murray TM, Jeejeebhoy KN (1980): Ann Intern Med 92:343.

Shike M, Roulet M, Kurian R, Whitwell J, Stewart S, Jeejeebhoy KN (1981*a*): Gastroenterology 81:290.

Shike M, Russell DMcR, Detsky AS, Harrison JE, McNeill KG, Shepherd FA, Feld R, Evans WK, Jeejeebhoy KN (1984): Ann Intern Med 101:303.

Shike M, Sturtridge WC, Tam CS, Harrison JE, Jones G, Murray TM, Husdan H, Whitwell J, Wilson DR, Jeejeebhoy KN (1981*b*): Ann Intern Med 95:560.

Silvis SE, Paragas PD (1972): Gastroenterology 62:513.

Solomons NW, Layden TJ, Rosenberg IH, Vo-Khactu K, Sandstead HH (1976): Gastroenterology 70:1022.

Sotos JF, Dodge PR, Talbot NB (1962): Pediatrics 30:180.

Sweetman L, Bates SP, Hull D, Nyhan WL (1977): Pediatr Res 11:1144.

Thompson JN, Erdoby P, Smith DC (1975): J Nutr 105:274.

Thurlow PM, Grant JP (1980): J Parenter Enteral Nutr 4:586.

Underwood EJ (1977): Trace elements in human and animal nutrition (4th ed). New York: Academic, p 314.

van Rij AM, Thomson CD, McKenzie JM, Robinson MF (1979): Am J Clin Nutr 32:2076.

Vilter RW, Bozian RC, Hess EV (1974): N Engl J Med 291:188.

Vinay P, Bourbeau D, Durancea A, Doyle D, Heppel J, Gougoux A, Lemieux G (1981): Clin Invest Med 4:87.

Walser M (1984*a*): J Parenter Enteral Nutr 8:37.

Walser M (1984*b*): Clin Sci 66:1.

Wahren J, Denis J, Desurmont P (1983): Hepatology 3:475.

Wannemacher RW, Kaminski MR, Dinterman RE, Bostian KA, Hadick CL (1980): J Parenter Enteral Nutr 2:507.

Waterlow JC, Jackson AA (1981): Br Med Bull 37:5.

Wene JD, Connor WE, DenBesten L (1975): J Clin Invest 56:127.

Willicuts HD (1977): J Parenter Enteral Nutr 1:25 (abstract).

Wolfe RR, Durkot MJ, Allsop JR, Burke JF (1979): Metabolism 20:1031.

Wolman SL, Anderson GH, Marliss EB, Jeejeebhoy KN (1979): Gastroenterology 73:458.

Woolfson AMJ, Heatley RV, Allison SP (1979): N Engl J Med 300:14.

Wu C, Bauer JM (1960): Cancer Res 20:848.

Young SE, Griffin AC, Milner AN, Stehlin JS (1967): Cancer Res 27:15.

Maria C. Linder, Ph.D.*

15

Nutrition and Atherosclerosis

Introduction

Atherosclerosis is characterized by a thickening of the internal layer of the walls of major blood vessels (see below), especially arteries, resulting in a constriction of the vessel lumen and a restriction of blood flow and vessel elasticity. This promotes the formation of occlusive blood clots and can result in injury to heart, brain, and lung tissue, which may be fatal. Cardiovascular disease, including myocardial infarction (heart attack) and stroke, is the major cause of death in "Western" society, accounting for more than 50% of all deaths in the United States, with 60% of deaths in individuals 65 years and older. This death rate is three times that from all forms of cancer (Naito, 1980). However, there has been a significant 20% decline in death from heart disease in the United States since 1968, a trend that has been ascribed to the increasing effectiveness of hospital care, sophisticated surgery, and a decline in smoking. Dietary factors and life-style may also play a role, as will be evaluated in this chapter.

Along with these changes have been changes in our views on the genesis of atherosclerosis in man and the potential roles of diet in this process. Much of the recent information has not as yet filtered down to the average physician. Controversy continues to reign in many areas, but several trends in knowledge and theory are apparent. Of particular interest is evidence: (1) that the development of atherosclerotic plaques represents an "injury response" on the part of the arterial wall to damage perpetrated on the epithelial cell layer; (2) that dietary (or other) modulation of prostaglandin, thromboxane, and leukotriene production, as by fish oils or aspirin, may be an important determinant of response; and (3) that dietary fiber, magnesium, antioxidants, and some micronutrients (such as chromium, copper, and silicon) may be important in long-term prevention or retardation of the atherosclerotic process. The matter of importance (or lack of importance) of cholesterol and fat intake to the genesis and/or development of atherosclerotic disease is another important aspect that has been fraught with controversy and hotly debated by experts with divergent views, but for which the beginnings of a resolution are apparent. All of these matters are reviewed below.

Atherosclerosis and Its Genesis

Atherosclerosis is a disease of the vasculature in which a large proportion of the inner surface of the major arteries develops raised plaques that consist of mounds of smooth muscle cells, fiber, lipid, and debris, with varying degrees of necrosis, calcification, and hemorrhage (Figure 15.1C). These plaques represent a thickening of the intimal layer of the arterial wall, which projects into

* California State University, Fullerton, CA.

the lumen and causes a decrease in blood flow and vessel elasticity. This promotes the formation of occlusive thrombi (clots) and can lead to myocardial infarction and stroke. Less obtrusive and complex plaques are also found: the "fatty streaks," which consist of proliferated smooth muscle cells with varying quantities of intra- and extracellular lipid (probably including oxidized LDL in macrophages) (Figure 15.1B), and fibrous plaques, where connective tissue fiber forms a cap over deeper deposits of extracellular lipid and cellular debris, and the developing mound begins to encroach upon the lumen (Figure 15.1C). There appears to be a relationship between the average age at which the various plaque forms are found, beginning with the fatty streaks (the only form normally seen in children) and progressing to the fibrous plaques (sometimes seen already in the teens) and then to the raised complex plaques seen in most Westerners by middle age (Figure 15.1D) and increasingly thereafter. Thus, it is tempting to think of these plaque forms as different stages of the same disease process (Wilson, 1976); indeed, this is generally assumed.

Experimental observations in animals lend further support to the idea of successive stages. It has been shown that factors injuring the arterial wall will promote a response progressing through roughly the same stages, depending on the severity of the insult inflicted. Factors promoting this reaction, at least experimentally, include mechanical injury, heat and cold, and a variety of chemical agents, from mutagens and even viruses to homocysteine and oxidized cholesterol and oxidized LDL (Wilson, 1976; Ross, 1986). (Further information on these agents is detailed below.) The sequence of events thought to occur may be summarized as follows:

1. The layer of endothelial cells that covers the connective tissue matrix of the artery wall is injured and disrupted, exposing a portion of the underlying matrix to blood cells and plasma substituents. This may come about either directly, by mechanical means or by the chemical actions of cytotoxic agents circulating in the blood; or indirectly, after formation of fatty streaks.

   In the latter case, it has been postulated (Steinberg et al., 1989) that LDL entering the areas beneath the intact endothelial layer may under certain conditions be oxidized to a cytotoxic (and atherogenic) product. Oxidized LDL attracts monocytes (and any resident macrophages) to this part of the artery wall to engulf the material. The result may initially be a "fatty streak" (with foam cells), and the vascular endothelium may still be intact. However, it may progress to cell necrosis and disruption of the endothelium if LDL oxidation persists, and/or oxidized LDL is released from macrophages that have been killed by it, poisoning the layer of endothelial cells. (Further information on oxidized LDL is given below.)
2. Disruption of the endothelium (as mentioned above) triggers a further series of changes leading toward atherosclerosis. Endothelial cells normally produce PGI_2 (prostacyclin; Figures 3.5 and 3.13), which inhibits platelet aggregation. Activated platelets (e.g., after stimulation by thrombin, involved in clotting or by catecholamines) release TXA_2 (thromboxane A_2), which stimulates their aggregation, and PDGF (platelet-derived growth factor), which stimulates smooth muscle cell proliferation. Similar growth factors are produced by cells of the developing plaque itself (Libby et al., 1988), especially macrophages (Ross et al., 1990), as are LTB_2 (leukotriene B_2), another attractant for blood monocytes and leukocytes (Leaf and Weber, 1988). Injury to the endothelial layer thus promotes platelet aggregation, further cell invasion, and cell proliferation—a complex of effects involving specific prostaglandins, thromboxanes, leukotrienes, and growth factors. [Platelet aggregability is clearly also a factor in the initiation of acute myocardial infarction (MI) (heart attack). The incidence of MI shows a diurnal variation, being highest on rising in the morning, when serum epinephrine and norepinephrine are highest.]

   As a consequence, smooth muscle cells in the connective tissue layer (media) (Figure 15.1) migrate into the intima and proliferate, forming new cells. Monocytes also enter the area. These various cells can also produce triglyceride and cholesterol, which may account for some of the lipid that begins to accumulate (Wilson, 1976). Much of the accumulated lipid, however, is probably from LDL: mainly phospholipid and cholesterol ester (and free cholesterol) (Sassen et al., 1989).
3. The gaps in the endothelial layer also promote adherence of blood platelets to the scarring surface area, and these may provide an additional source of accumulating fat. Some fat (and cholesterol) also continues to enter via

A Normal Arterial Wall

Intima
Media
Adventitia
Endothelial cells
Internal elastic lamina
Smooth muscle cells

B Fatty Streaks

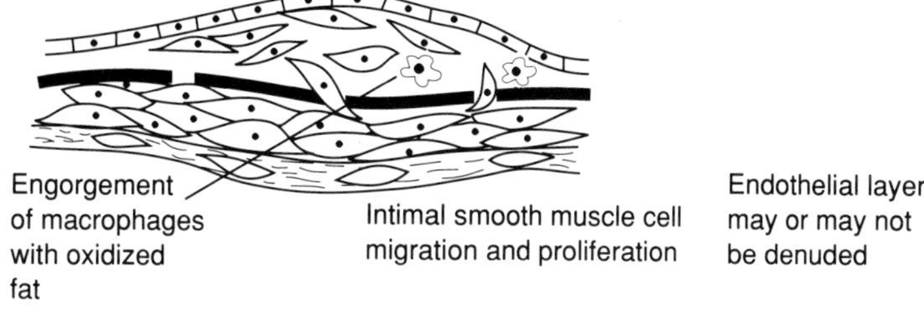

C Fibrous Plaques

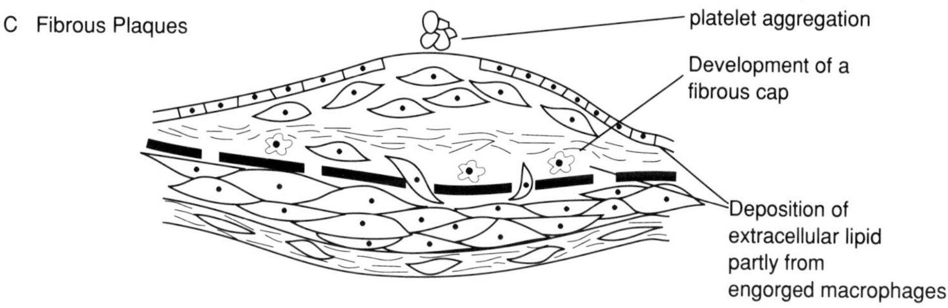

D Complex Raised Plaques

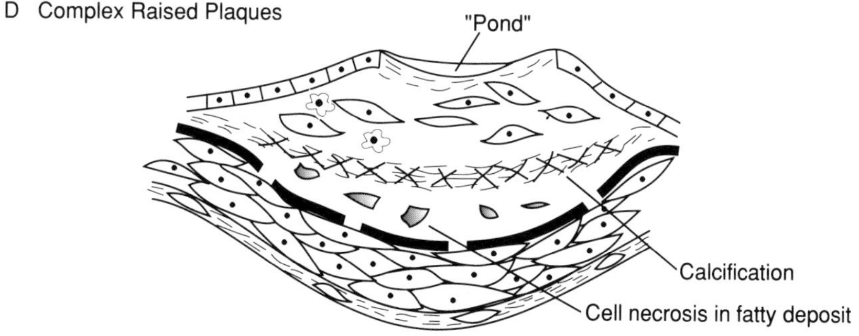

plasma lipoproteins, especially LDL, and some of it leaves the developing plaque (presumably via HDL and apolipoprotein E; see Chapter 3).

4. With severe or continuing damage, cell proliferation and lipid accumulation continue, and a scar tissue layer is laid down, which may trap extracellular lipid and cells below it (versus toward the arterial lumen). (Collagen and elastin are secreted by smooth muscle cells.)

Figure 15.1. Various forms (stages) of atherosclerotic lesions, showing fatty streaks **(B)** and plaques **(C, D)** in comparison with the normal artery wall **(A).** Note the normally intact endothelial cell layer, which may or may not be disrupted at the fatty streak stage, but is clearly disrupted at later stages (promoting platelet aggregation).

Part of the lipid at the base of the plaque appears to be in the form of crystalline cholesterol (or oxidized cholesterol), which may have precipitated after hydrolysis of cholesterol-esters coming from LDL (Small, 1988). Incoming cholesterol (closer to the lumen of the artery) is mostly in the form of fatty acid esters.

5. Trapped cells will die, leading to necrosis and cell debris within the plaque. It is thought that this stage of plaque development may be irreversible (Wolinsky, 1981). Cell death may be promoted by oxidized LDL (Steinberg et al., 1989).
6. Calcification (a laying down of hydroxylapatite) may also begin as part of the process of scarring. From this view, the whole process of plaque development is thus an "injury response" on the part of the wall of the major arteries to various forms of assault, and the plaque itself is a variously developed strengthening or shoring-up of the vessel wall.

The concepts for such a sequence of events have emerged from the observations and thoughts of many investigators over the last 15–20 years. What has more recently been added to the picture are details about the modulation of atherogenesis by various, sometimes opposing prostaglandins, thromboxanes, and leukotrienes (reviewed, e.g., by Leaf and Weber, 1988), and the discovery that oxidized rather than normal LDL may be a factor in the process (as reviewed by Steinberg et al., 1989). The observations on prostaglandins and related products of 20 and 22 carbon polyunsaturated fatty acids stem from an interest in the potentially beneficial effects of fish oils containing docosahexaenoic and eicosapentaenoic acids (DHA/EPA), of which more will be mentioned below. Background information on the metabolism and actions of these fatty acids and their products is given in Chapter 3.

As concerns the observations on oxidized LDL, work by a number of different groups (with a variety of approaches) has shown that oxidatively modified LDL is a potent cytotoxic agent, a potent chemoattractant for macrophages/monocytes, and is rapidly phagocytosed by them via "scavenger" receptors not identical with the LDL receptor (apo B/E) (Brown et al., 1980; Parthasarathy et al., 1986). Moreover, oxidation of LDL can and does occur in the human, as indicated by the presence of specific antibodies. It probably occurs not in the blood, but in tissue beneath the endothelial cell layer (which can still be intact); and it may involve a lipoxygenase and phospholipase A_2 (Steinberg et al., 1989), initiating a free radical chain of events that alters lipoprotein composition and structure. The oxidized product inhibits migration of macrophages out of the area. These phenomena would help to explain observations in animals that binding of blood monocytes to the (intact) layer of endothelial cells can be an early event in atherogenesis and may underlie the development of foam cells and fatty streaks beneath a nondisrupted, nondenuded vascular epithelium. It also may help to explain why in some cases, but not in others, elevations in blood LDL (more traditionally viewed as elevated blood cholesterol, a major risk factor in atherosclerosis) could lead to atherogenesis; and, indeed, how otherwise altered LDL (as by glycation; the chemical binding of glucose or other sugars, as in diabetes; see Chapter 2), and perhaps even chylomicron remnants carrying oxidized cholesterol from the diet, might promote the atherosclerotic process. What is not so clear is what would trigger the oxidation of LDL within the body. A variety of cells are capable of carrying out such an oxidation (as shown in culture), including monocytes, macrophages, smooth muscle, and even endothelial cells (see Steinberg et al., 1989). Inflammatory or immune processes might be initiators; and nutrients capable of oxidation/reduction might play a modulatory role.

An additional twist to this view is that of Stehbens (1989). He sees the phenomenon of lipid accumulation in macrophages as a lipid storage disorder: either artificially inducible in animals by cholesterol feeding (and not causing "conventional" human atherosclerosis) or caused genetically in some humans by the gene for familial hypercholesterolemia.

As will be detailed more thoroughly below, evidence from animal experiments and observations in man indicate that the process of plaque formation may be reversible, especially in the early stages before fibrous infiltration has occurred (Wissler and Vesselinovich, 1977), but even to some extent later on (Blankenhorn, 1981). This also fits with the "injury response" analogy. In this regard, it is noteworthy that plaque formation is a normal process that takes place, to some extent, in all animals and humans with age and occurs especially at bends or other stress points in the arterial system, places that need to be strengthened against rupture and where high pressure or turbulence is found (Meyer Texon; see Altschule, 1974). As reported in animals, new "bends" in the arteries created by surgery result in plaque development, especially at the points of maximum stress. A highly speculative correlary thought would be that high blood pressure might contribute to atherogenesis by "stressing" certain parts of the vasculature.

Benditt (1976) has introduced the additional concept of atherosclerosis as a kind of cancer of the arterial wall, noting the importance of smooth muscle cell proliferation to the process, the eventual necrosis, and, most importantly, the fact that plaques may originate from proliferation triggered in a single cell and its progeny, in analogy to theories of malignant transformation and tumor development. Specifically, he has found that most individual human plaques from black women heterozygous for the X-linked enzyme, glucose-6-phosphate dehydrogenase, contain either the A or B form of the enzyme, but not both, implying that most plaques are of monoclonal origin. The concept of atherosclerosis either as a scarring or neoplastic response to injury of the artery wall thus seems to explain why a variety of agents, from mechanical (blood pressure) to chemical and dietary (CO and other poisons in cigarette smoke; homocysteine; oxidized cholesterol; high LDL or oxidized LDL), might affect the process.

Epidemiology and Risk Factors in Atherosclerosis

Epidemiologic studies comparing the population (or subpopulations) of countries around the world, or subgroups within a single country, have identified a number of factors of life-style and diet associated with a greater risk of serious cardiovascular disease. These "risk factors" have been ranked according to their calculated contributions to the prevalence and severity of atherosclerosis or have been subcategorized as major or minor factors, based on the available statistics. A summary of currently accepted categorizations is given in Table 15.1, along with some of the statistics upon which these are based. It should be noted that the term, "risk factor," has been deliberately used instead of "cause," in that epidemiology cannot identify the nature of the connection between the phenomena and atherosclerosis, and also because the mechanism of cause and effect is not understood (e.g., for smoking) and/or a direct causal (initiating) effect is unlikely (dietary fat).

Smoking, high blood pressure, and elevated levels of plasma/serum cholesterol have been identified as the main risk factors emerging from such data for men (Sytkowski et al., 1990). Recent studies indicate that for women, obesity is also a major factor (Manson et al., 1990), with stress, lack of exercise, elevated plasma triglycerides, and others being secondary. For both sexes, the ratio of HDL to LDL cholesterol is thought to be more specifically and inversely related to incidence and more significant than the relation to total serum cholesterol. Though not extensively studied, the concentration of plasma apolipoprotein B also appears to be a highly significant risk factor in coronary artery disease, which may not be surprising in that it is the main apoprotein associated with LDL, the major carrier of cholesterol (Sniderman et al., 1980). Based on the Framingham Massachusetts Heart Study and others (Pekkanen et al., 1990), a synergistic relationship between risk factors is suggested, resulting in more than an additive effect when multiple risk factors are present together (Figure 15.2). Important and highly significant positive overall correlations have been reported also for the intake of animal protein, or total fat, or cholesterol (even sugar) and the incidence of cardiovascular disease (Table 15.1), with negative correlations to starch, vegetable protein, and fiber.

As part of the background to changes in disease incidence, trends in the consumption of various nutrients in the United States from 1909 to recent times may be illuminating (Table 15.2). Notably, cholesterol intake did not change (it has dropped more recently), while that of animal protein, vegetable oil, and sugar markedly increased, and intake of vegetable protein, starch, and fiber declined. During this period, the contribution of cardiovascular disease to mortality increased, but many other aspects of our life-style also changed, making it difficult to assess the impact of dietary change alone from the data.

Interpretation of the epidemiologic data is problematic also for other reasons. Diet surveys are prone to errors resulting from such differences as those between nutrient availability and actual consumption in a country; variable intake; and poor or inaccurate recall of consumption (Stehbens, 1989). Statistics based on the responses of individuals (rather than groups) often show relatively poor correlations between intakes of specific nutrients and prevalence of atherosclerosis or levels of specific serum factors. Estimates of mortality from atherosclerotic disease are also quite approximate (Stehbens, 1989), as are the accuracy of blood cholesterol determinations (which have a coefficient of variation of 5%–10% for any given sample; Hegsted and Nicolosi,

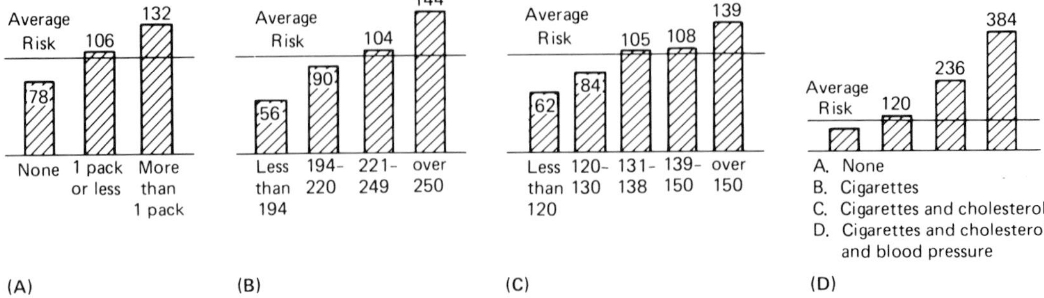

Figure 15.2. Risk factors in heart attack (based on the Framingham, MA, heart study). These graphs demonstrate the extent to which particular risk factors increased the danger of coronary heart disease for 30- to 62-year-old men in Framingham, MA. Columns below the black horizontal line indicate lower-than-average risk. **(A)** Cigarette smoking. A man who smokes more than a pack of cigarettes a day has nearly twice the risk of heart attack of a nonsmoker. **(B)** Cholesterol. A man with a blood cholesterol measurement of 250 or more (mg/dl) has about three times the risk of heart attack of a man with one below 194. **(C)** Blood pressure. A man whose blood pressure at systole (the moment the heart contracts) is over 150 has more than twice the risk of heart attack of a man with blood pressure under 120. **(D)** Number of risk factors increases danger. A combination of three major risk factors can increase the likelihood of coronary heart attack disease in a 45-year-old man with an abnormal blood pressure of 180 systolic and a cholesterol level of 310. [*Source:* Reprinted by permission from *Coronary Heart Disease: Risk Factors and Diet Debate.* Courtesy National Dairy Council (1974).]

1987), further muddying any interpretation. There are also contradictions, as for example, that death from cerebrovascular accidents (strokes) tends to show a negative correlation to fat intake, or serum cholesterol, in the same groups where the reported mortality from coronary heart disease shows a positive relationship (Iso et al., 1989; Yerushalmy and Hilleboe, 1957). [Both of these diseases are thought to be manifestations of atherosclerosis, and yet serum cholesterol is not a risk factor for stroke, while blood pressure and smoking still seem to be (along with maternal history) (Colditz et al., 1988; Welin et al., 1987).] Similarly, there has been a discrepancy between the patterns of change in rates of mortality from heart attack in women versus men over many years (that for women decreased, that for men increased), suggesting no relation to diet (Oliver, 1982). There are data showing no correlation between fat intake and the severity of atherosclerosis (McGill et al., 1968); between serum lipids and cardiovascular disease or disease severity (see McGee et al., 1984; Stehbens, 1989); and between intakes of butterfat (Yudkin, 1957) or dairy products (Kahn, 1970; Olson, 1979) and cardiovascular disease. All of this suggests that existing epidemiologic data must be viewed with caution and that any conclusions derived from them should be considered tentative. Evidence relating indi-

Table 15.1. Risk Factors in Atherosclerosis

Primary risk factors
Smoking (1 or more packs a day)
Blood pressure (diastolic > 90 mm Hg; systolic > 105 mm Hg)
Elevated plasma cholesterol [>240–250 mg/dl (can be hereditary)]
Secondary risk factors
Elevated plasma triglycerides
Obesity
Diabetes
Chronic stress
Birth control pills
Vasectomy
Correlation of mortality with intake of certain nutrients[a]
Positive correlations ($p < 0.05$)
Animal protein (0.782[b])
Cholesterol (0.762)
Meat (0.697)
Total fat (0.676)
Eggs (0.666)
Sugar (0.638)
Total calories (0.633)
Animal fat (0.632)
Negative correlations ($p < 0.05$)
Starch (−0.464)
Vegetable protein (−0.403)
No correlations ($p > 0.05$)
Plant sterols, fish, vegetable fat, vegetables

Source: Information from Naito (1980) and Connor (1980).

[a] Men 55–59 years of age (Connor, 1980).
[b] Correlation coefficient.

Table 15.2. Trends in Dietary Consumption Associated with Increased Cardiovascular and Degenerative Diseases in the United States

	1909	1972	Change
Caloric intake			−4%
Protein intake (g)	102	102	0
Animal protein	53	69	+30%
Vegetable protein	49	32	−35%
Ratio animal/vegetable protein	1.08	2.16	+100%
Fat consumption			+26%
Animal/vegetable fat	4.9	1.6	−67%
Linoleic/saturated fat	0.21	0.40	+90%
Cholesterol (mg)	509	556	+9%
Carbohydrate intake			−21%
Starch/sugar	2.15	0.89	−59%
Sugar (total available)	156	205	+31%
Crude fiber intake			−50%

Source: Data from Krichevsky (1979).

vidual dietary factors and mechanisms to atherosclerosis risk is detailed below.

Cholesterol and Atherosclerosis

Highly significant associations have been demonstrated between daily cholesterol intake and mortality from coronary heart disease when different populations around the world are compared (Figure 15.3). Even industrialized countries like Japan (where average intake is low) have a much lower mortality from coronary heart disease than the United States, Canada, and Australia, where intake is uniformly high. It is noteworthy that cross-national comparisons cover a very broad range of cholesterol intakes (from <5.0 mg/day to >600 mg/day), versus *intra*national comparisons, where intake tends to be more uniform (spanning only about 200–500 mg/day in the United States). In Western populations, fasting plasma/serum cholesterol concentrations increase with age (Figure 15.4), as does the risk of myocardial infarction and the incidence of atherosclerotic disease. (Levels in women tend to be lower than in men until after menopause.) Moreover, numerous dietary studies in rabbits, rodents, monkeys, and many other species have indicated that the addition of substantial amounts of cholesterol and saturated fat to the diet will induce a type of atherosclerosis, sometimes of the type seen in man. [It should be noted, however, that in rabbits (a favorite choice of researchers), the plaques usually are different and consist of "foam cells," with little or no smooth muscle cell proliferation, fibrosis, or calcification (Wilson, 1976), and the same can be true for other animals (Stehbens, 1989).] Other evidence relating cholesterol intake to atherogenesis includes data showing that a drastic lowering of cholesterol intake in monkeys with arterial occlusions will result in a gradual, drastic

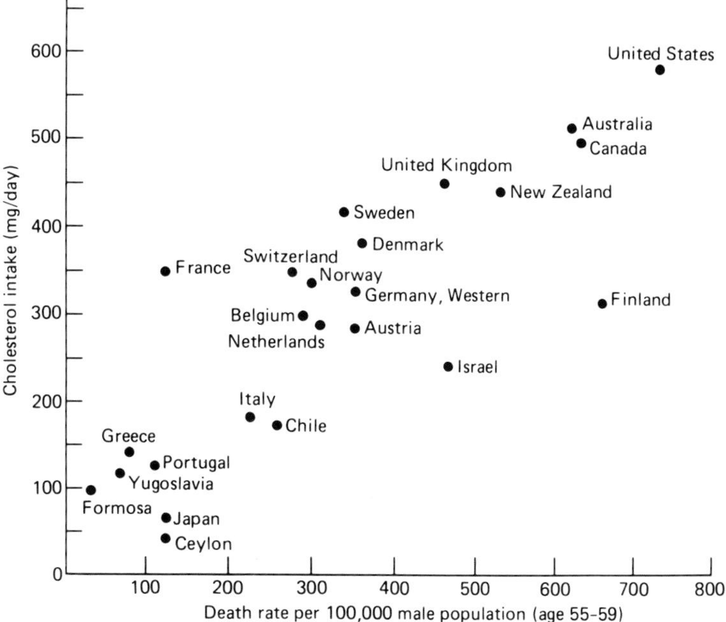

Figure 15.3. Relationship between death rate from coronary heart disease, and average daily cholesterol consumption in 24 countries (1952–1956). A similar relationship may prevail between animal protein intake and heart disease. [*Source:* Reprinted by permission from Conner (1980).]

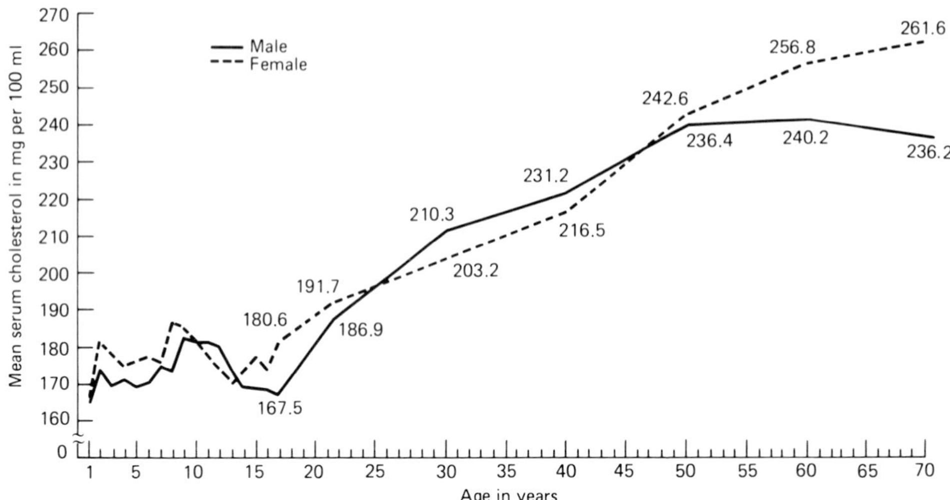

Figure 15.4. Mean serum cholesterol concentrations in the U.S. population throughout life. [*Source:* Reprinted by permission from Abraham et al. (1978).]

lowering of plasma cholesterol concentrations and a regression of atherosclerotic plaques (Armstrong et al., 1970). Also, in humans, a drastic lowering of cholesterol intake may reduce plasma cholesterol 10%–15% (Connor, 1980; Chapter 3), and some special x-ray studies indicate that even more drastic measures to lower plasma cholesterol (through the use of bile acid binding resins) may be accompanied by some plaque regression and a lower risk of cardiovascular disease (see below). These various data are consistent with the concept that cholesterol intake is a causative agent in atherogenesis, and they have served as the basis for the long-popular medical policy of placing patients with atherosclerosis on cholesterol-free or low-cholesterol diets. Nevertheless, the demonstration that cholesterol, per se, is really a causative factor is far from clear, and some researchers would argue that the emphasis on cholesterol has obscured other aspects of the relation between diet and atherosclerosis, which may be of equal importance.

From the other vantage, the association between cholesterol intake (or plasma level) and atherosclerosis may not be what it seems. For one, high cholesterol intake is a consequence of the generous consumption of meats, eggs, and dairy products (and, thus, more animal protein). As will be detailed further on, there is some reason to suppose that excessive consumption of animal protein, in the absence of sufficient micronutrients (especially B_6), might in itself cause atherosclerosis by promoting accumulation of homocystine—a potent smooth muscle cell and arterial endothelial poison derived from incomplete degradation of sulfur-containing amino acids (see Chapter 4). Thus, high cholesterol intake might fortuitously be associated with increased atherosclerosis in Western society. Second, it is well-known that certain subpopulations, such as the Greenland Eskimo (Bang and Dyerberg, 1972) and Masai herdsmen (Ho et al., 1971) and some other tribes (Shaper et al., 1963) in East Africa, who consume moderate or very great quantities of cholesterol, have a low incidence of atherosclerotic disease and do not have increased levels of cholesterol. [Indeed, the Masai have subsisted mainly on milk, blood, and meat, with about 66% of their calories coming from animal fat, and with intakes of cholesterol of up to 2 g/day (Ho et al., 1971). It is also noteworthy that carnivorous wild animals are not much troubled by atherosclerosis (Vastesaeger, 1968).] Thus, dietary cholesterol intake is not invariably associated with atherosclerotic effects or hypercholesterolemia; indeed, this is true also within populations (such as Americans) that have an overall high cholesterol intake (Report of Working Group, 1981).

Nor does diet have a profound influence on plasma cholesterol concentrations in Western populations. It is well-known that altering cholesterol and saturated fat intakes alters plasma cholesterol only 10%–20%. This is not surprising if one recalls the biochemical and physiologic events underlying the presence of cholesterol in the blood in very low density and low density lipoproteins (VLDL and LDL). [Eating several or no eggs per day makes little or no difference

(Flynn et al., 1979; Truswell, 1978), except in "cholesterol-sensitive" individuals (see Chapter 3); and the Framingham Study (Dawber, 1982) found no correlation between serum cholesterol levels and egg consumption.] (For a more thorough review, see Chapter 3.) Plasma cholesterol concentrations are determined by the relative rates of entry and clearance of low density lipoproteins (LDL) (and sometimes also VLDL) from the blood. The majority of cholesterol is synthesized within the body, mainly in liver and intestine, but also in peripheral cells and tissues, and does not come from the diet. In most tissues, endogenous synthesis is "feedback" controlled by cholesterol, so that excessive dietary intake results in reduced endogenous (especially liver) production. Finally, evidence suggests that the main factor in hypercholesterolemia is a reduced capacity for clearing LDL cholesterol from the blood, as, for example, in familial hypercholesterolemia, where there is a relative lack of cellular receptors for LDL (see Chapter 3), or copper deficiency, where hypercholesterolemia may also result from a decreased rate of plasma cholesterol turnover (see Chapter 7). Thus, it would appear that hypercholesterolemia reflects an abnormally reduced capacity of the body to dispose of cholesterol, and/or an incapacity to regulate endogenous production. (The reader is encouraged to review cholesterol metabolism, as described in Chapter 3.)

A 10%–15% reduction in serum cholesterol due to decreased cholesterol intake and increased unsaturated fat intake has also been reported to have little effect on incidence of, and mortality from, cardiovascular disease (Dayton et al., 1968; McMichael, 1977; Oliver, 1982; Paterson et al., 1963). Most recent is the report of the Multiple Risk Factor Intervention Trial Research Group (1982), in which a three-prong intervention program was instituted, with special efforts to reduce blood pressure and smoking, as well as to lower cholesterol and saturated fat intakes to less than 300 mg and 10% of calories, per day, respectively. In this study, there was no significant difference in the mortality of the intervention versus nonintervention groups, although the possibility was raised that toxicity from drug intervention for blood pressure might have obscured beneficial results of diet and smoking. Even assuming that there is a significant correlation between risk of mortality and serum cholesterol (as in the data from the Framingham study; Figure 15.2), calculations suggest that lowering serum cholesterol (by 15%–20%) would only increase the lifespan a few days to a few months (Taylor et al., 1987). As already mentioned, and adding to the confusion, is evidence suggesting that a greater risk of stroke (also ascribed to the atherosclerotic process) accompanies lower serum cholesterol concentrations (Gordon et al., 1981; Kagan et al., 1980; Yerushalamy and Hilleboe, 1957), as well as deaths due to cancer and other noncardiovascular causes (Gordon et al., 1981; Williams et al., 1981). The latter observation has also been discounted (Feinleib, 1983).

Several other points argue against a causal connection between cholesterol intake and atherogenesis. Studies in which macaque monkeys were exposed to an atherogenic high cholesterol diet, with and without one of several anticalcifying drugs, showed a marked difference in the degree of aortal atherosclerosis, as evidenced by composition and appearance of the aorta (Figure 15.5) (Kramsch et al., 1981). Animals receiving the atherogenic diet and anticalcifying drug developed little or no atherosclerosis, despite very high concentrations of cholesterol in the blood (averaging 450–470 mg/dl). This is another instance where hypercholesterolemia and atherosclerosis have been disassociated. (Disassociation is also demonstrated in a reverse way by the fact that mechanical injury, and other insults to the endothelial lining of the arteries, can cause plaques in the *absence* of hypercholesterolemia.)

Another important point is that much of the animal evidence linking a high dietary cholesterol intake to the induction of something like atherosclerosis may perhaps be explained by the presence in these diets of potent atherogenic cholesterol oxidation products (Wilson, 1976). In animal studies, high cholesterol diets are typically made by mixing various amounts of purified or semipure cholesterol with the other dietary components. Cholesterol (in its purified state) is fairly unstable and easily oxidized at room temperature when exposed to air. More than 32 oxidation products have been isolated from such material. Indeed, 26-hydroxycholesterol has especially been found associated with atherosclerotic plaque (NS Bhacca, personal communication). In contrast to cholesterol per se, these oxidation products are highly toxic to smooth muscle cells in vitro and are potent atherogenic agents in vivo (Imai et al., 1976; Taylor et al., 1975). In a normal human diet, oxidation of cholesterol is less likely because cholesterol is part of the food mixture in which antioxidants, like tocopherols (vitamin E), are also present. However, oxidation products similar to those found in USP cholesterol have

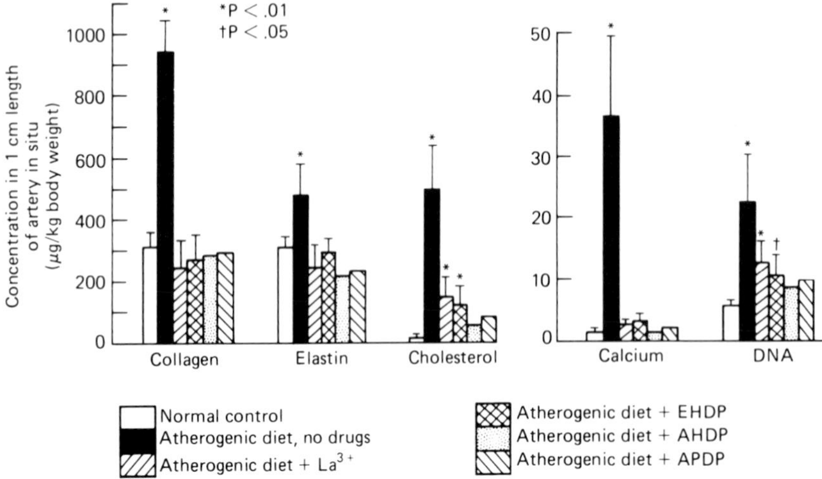

Figure 15.5. Effects of anticalcifying drugs on atherogenesis in monkeys on an atherogenic diet: composition of the intimal and medial layers. [*Source:* Reprinted by permission from Kramsch et al. (1981).]

been detected in powdered eggs and whole milk (Wilson, 1976). Thus, many experiments in which "cholesterol" induced atherosclerosis in animals might be artifacts of oxidized cholesterol action.

Along the same lines, factors that trigger oxidation of LDL (as described in the earlier section on atherogenesis) and perhaps even other alterations in LDL may be much more important than LDL (or dietary) cholesterol per se. [In this connection, serum from patients with cardiovascular disease (but not from normal subjects) was found to enhance accumulation of cholesterol in cells cultured from the aorta (Chasov et al., 1986).] Oxidation may be triggered in the artery wall by immune/inflammatory processes, resulting in accumulation of (abnormal) LDL within macrophages. Glycation of LDL protein (as occurs especially in diabetes) may result in a similar engorgement by intimal/medial macrophages (Lopez-Virella et al., 1988; Steinberg et al., 1989), which would help to explain the greater susceptibility of diabetics to atherosclerosis. [Acetaldehyde adducts of LDL (formed in connection with alcohol abuse) might be handled the same way.] Moreover, antibodies formed against the altered LDL (which have been detected in the circulation) would form antigen-antibody complexes (with the altered LDL), which might contribute to the problem by stimulating platelet aggregation and/or localized inflammation, resulting in endothelial cell injury (Steinberg et al., 1989). This suggests that atherosclerosis could be a kind of autoimmune disease (at least in some cases). Clearly, dietary substances that would work against chemoalteration of LDL and/or cholesterol (e.g., reducing agents such as vitamin E and butylated hydroxytoluene; Steinberg et al., 1989) might also work against the initiation and propagation of atherosclerosis.

Observations on the cytotoxicity and atherogenicity of oxidized cholesterol or LDL imply that the oxidation state (or propensity to oxidation) is what is important, rather than overall levels of serum cholesterol or LDL. Serum cholesterol may even have emerged as a risk factor in atherosclerosis because of cholesterol/LDL oxidation.

As already indicated, the correlation between cardiovascular disease incidence and serum cholesterol is only significant when groups (or populations as a whole) are compared and not on the basis of values for individuals (see earlier, or Stehbens, 1989). The lack of individual correlations indicates that the actual variable involved has not been identified. (It might, of course, be oxidized serum lipid or lipoprotein.) Steinberg et al. (1989) postulate that high serum cholesterol would (presumably by mass action) increase the interstitial fluid concentrations of serum lipoproteins, and that somehow this would result in more oxidation of LDL. It seems more reasonable, however, to suppose that the real determinant must be still another (or other) factor (or factors), such as inflammation or antibody-antigen interactions, that determine(s) an individual's propensity to oxidize these substances (which may then, of course, also be inhibited by antioxidants, etc.). Heredity may also be a factor in this propensity (and is clearly also a major determinant of atherosclerosis) (Austin et al., 1987; Stehbens, 1989).

Although it is far from clear that cholesterol itself is a causative agent in atherosclerosis, it is clear that plasma cholesterol (on LDL) is a source of some of this lipid for the plaque, especially in the more advanced stages of plaque development and/or if plasma concentrations are high. Although rabbits are not a very good model for human atherosclerosis, Figure 15.6 shows that in rabbits, with plaques induced by mechanical injury, uptake of LDL cholesterol increases with plasma LDL cholesterol concentrations. Studies by Bjorkerud and Bondjers (1976) suggest that below 400 mg/dl, the capacity for cholesterol elimination from the aortic wall matches the rate of uptake in regions with intact endothelium (low injury regions), but that the threshold for balance of uptake and elimination is lower in regions where the endothelium has been disrupted and plaque has formed. Thus, a substantial lowering of plasma cholesterol concentrations (as achieved by treatment with clofibrate, niacin, neomycin, cholestyramine, and other drugs and resins) (see below) may be of some preventive help in re-

Figure 15.6. Uptake of cholesterol ester by aortic regions after mechanical injury: relation to serum cholesterol concentration. [*Source:* Reprinted by permission from Björkerud and Bondjers (1976).]

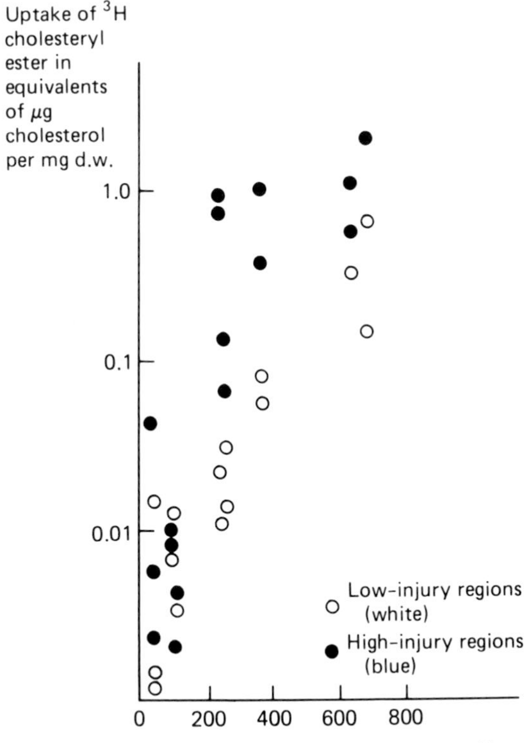

achieving a balance between uptake and elimination and may reduce cholesterol accumulation in the plaque. Evidence is accruing that such treatment may in fact contribute to a very slow regression of atherosclerotic plaques, especially if the "injury-response" inducing factors (like smoking) are removed (see below). These considerations, of course, ignore the matter of LDL (or cholesterol) oxidation and how that might be involved in these events.

Prostaglandins, Fish Oils, Aspirin, and Atherosclerosis

As discussed in Chapter 3, the triacylglycerols found in fish oils (high in eicosapentaenoic and docosahexanenoic acids—EPA/DHA) have been the focus of considerable research because of their potential benefits in fighting atherosclerotic disease (Leaf and Weber, 1988). As detailed in Figure 3.13, ingestion of these fats results in a variety of physiological responses that should be beneficial. These include reductions in synthesis of VLDL and blood pressure (also in essential hypertension; Bonaa et al., 1990), as well as the production of a spectrum of prostaglandins, thromboxanes, and leukotrienes, which reduce the likelihood of platelet aggregation and migration of monocytes and macrophages into areas of arterial injury. As already discussed (Chapter 3), these effects are thought to occur at least partly through the production of fatty acid-derived hormones alternative in structure to those formed from arachidonic acid (Figure 3.5). Evidence that this indeed occurs in man is given in Figure 15.7, and shows a decrease in platelet aggregability (determined in vitro with collagen) and production of thromboxane A_2 (as mirrored by its urinary metabolite TXB_2), with increased production of EPA-derived prostaglandin PGI_3 (that works against platelet aggregation), all at various times after the start of increased and then decreased ingestion of cod liver oil (CLO).

The major enzymes initiating formation of the various prostaglandins and thromboxanes, the cyclooxygenase, is inhibited by aspirin and some other antiinflammatory agents. Aspirin inhibition is irreversible, involving enzyme modification and inactivation (Oates et al., 1988a; Roth et al., 1975). Some recent prospective studies have indicated that a low intake of aspirin may have beneficial effects on the rate of cardiovascular accidents (heart attacks) (Physicians' Health Study, 1988; Steering Committee of the Physicians' Health Study Research Unit, 1989). These results are explained by the interference of aspirin with pros-

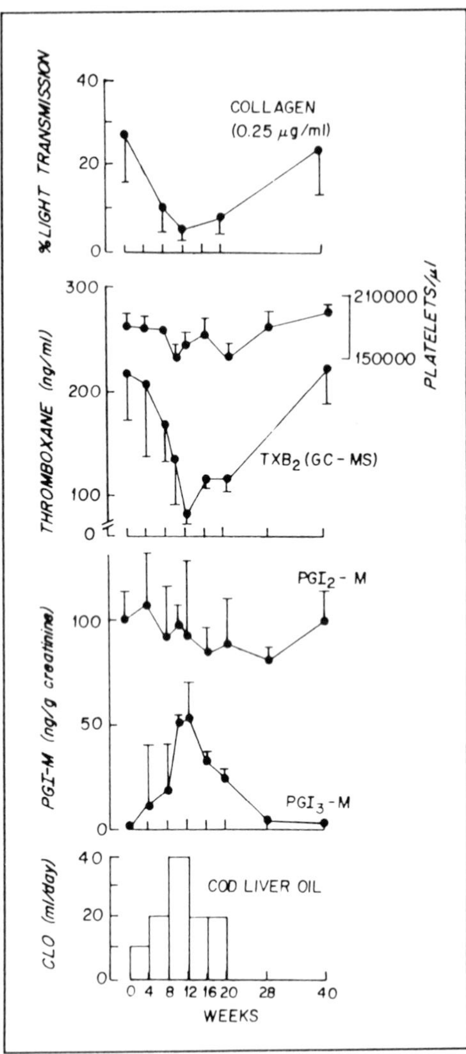

Figure 15.7. Effects of fish oil (cod liver oil; CLO) supplementation at various doses **(bottom),** on platelet aggregability (with collagen) **(top);** platelet number, and urinary metabolites of thromboxane A_2 (data for TXB_2); prostacyclin (data for PGI_2-M) and eicosanoid-derived PGI_3 (PGI_3-M). [*Source:* Reprinted by permission from Leaf and Weber (1988).]

taglandin metabolism. Specifically, inactivation of cyclooxygenase in platelets (in the absence of EPA/DHA) would reduce production of TXA_2, important in stimulating aggregation. Production of prostacyclin (PGI_2) by endothelial cells (a prostaglandin inhibiting platelet aggregation) would not be inhibited as much, in part because platelets will be exposed to higher doses of aspirin (during absorption and initial blood transport) before its extensive hydrolysis to salicylate in the liver (Gambino et al., 1988); and because endothelial cells have nuclei and can replace the cyclooxygenase, while the platelet enzyme would be permanently inactivated and only replaced with new platelets. [Fish oils (EPA/DHA) also reduce the number of platelets formed, but not their mass (Goodnight, 1988).] The overall result would be less TXA_2 relative to PGI_2 and thus less platelet aggregation and activity. This may be an important factor in atherosclerosis progression (see earlier). In the double-blind studies with aspirin cited, the physicians who were subjects (some 22,071 between 40 and 84 years of age) took 325 mg (or a single pill) of aspirin (or placebo) every second day for 5 years. The rate of myocardial infarction (heart attack) was 255 per 100,000 with aspirin, as compared with 440 with placebo, a 44% reduction in risk. Risk was reduced only in individuals over 50 (and especially over 60—more than 50%) and extended to the risk of fatal heart attacks (which was reduced 64%). Aspirin also appeared to be helpful against the restenosis (swelling and constriction) that can follow angioplastic surgery (to remove plaque inside coronary blood vessels) (Schwartz et al., 1988), presumably due to a reduction in the injury response of the artery. However, in another study in which groups of elderly subjects who did or did not use aspirin on a regular basis were compared (Paganini-Hill et al., 1989) over 6.5 years, the risk of heart attack was reduced only in the men and not in the women, and there were significant increases in the risks for ischemic heart disease and kidney cancer. These results must give us pause but may not reflect the effects of aspirin alone, as aspirin intake was not imposed on the subjects (in random fashion), but was by self-selection and could have reflected other physical problems. However, the risk of stroke may also be higher, as suggested by the data from the Physicians' Health Study (1988) (although there were too few cases to establish statistical significance). Thus, more information is needed to fully evaluate the benefits and risks of the treatment. [In some individuals, for example, there would also be a greater risk of ulcers, as prostaglandins also control the overproduction of stomach acid.] There might also be a greater risk of asthmatic/anaphylactoid attack (Oates et al., 1988a).

What is of considerable interest, however, is that ingestion of relatively large doses of fish oil may have the same beneficial effects as aspirin relating to thromboxanes and prostaglandins, and may in addition be helpful, in terms of lowering VLDL synthesis, by enhancing red blood cell deformability, increasing fat "tolerance," and lowering blood pressure (see Chapter 3). Thus, fish oils are likely to provide a broader spectrum of benefits than aspirin. Indeed, animal studies in pigs (Weiner et al., 1986), guinea pigs (Ziemlanski et al., 1987), and monkeys (Davis et al., 1987) have shown a dramatic inhibition of atherogenesis by fish oil supplementation. An example of the difference in plaque formation with and without 30 ml daily doses of cod liver oil in pigs on a 2.3% cholesterol, high fat diet (with balloon abrasion of the descending coronary artery) for 16 months (fish oil given in the last 8 months) is shown in Figure 15.8. It is of interest that in these studies, blood cholesterol concentrations were uniformly elevated (to >560 mg/dl at the end of the study) whether or not the animals received fish oil supplement; whereas in another study, with monkeys (Parks et al., 1989), hypercholesterolemia itself was prevented or decreased by the fish oil supplementation, and the LDL was smaller and had a reduced content of esterified cholesterol. In the case of pigs, switching to a diet with no cholesterol and a high n-3 fatty acid content resulted in complete regression of arterial lesions in the descending aorta but not in the coronary arteries (Sassen et al., 1989). The significance of these findings remains to be evaluated but suggests differential sensitivities of parts of the vasculature with regard to atherosclerotic and anti-atherosclerotic stimuli.

Figure 15.8. Effects of fish oil on development of injury and diet-induced atherosclerotic plaque in pigs. Segments of coronary arteries of pigs on an atherogenic diet (peanut oil + lard = 52% of kcals; + cholesterol at 4.3% weight of diet), without **(A)** and with **(B)** cod liver oil supplementation (30 ml per day, containing 12% EPA). Animals were fed the diets for a total of 8 months, and balloon abrasion of this artery was instituted 3 weeks into the diet. [Hematoxylin and eosin stain; magnification 24-fold.] [*Source:* Reprinted by permission from Weiner et al. (1986).]

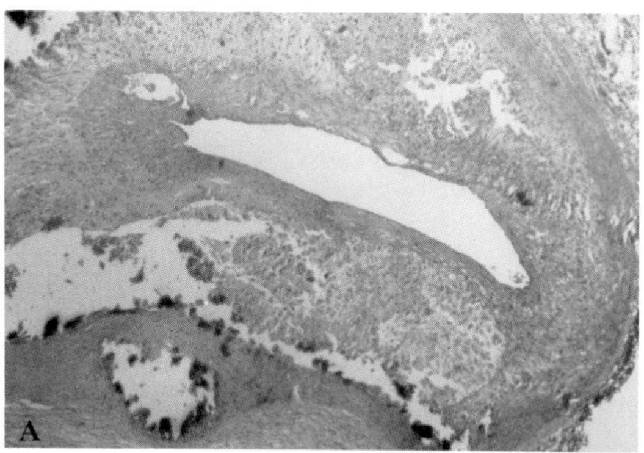

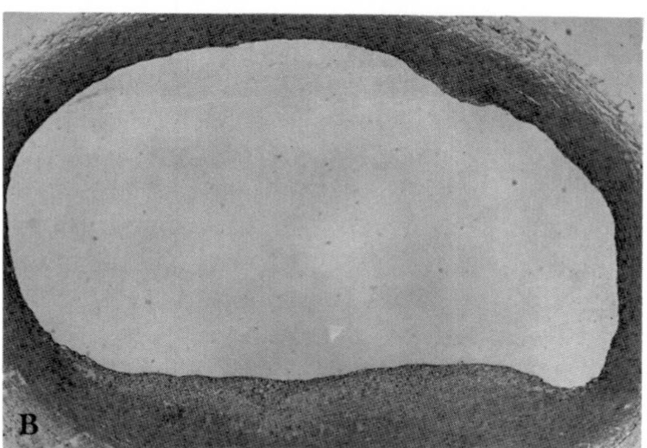

In man, fish oil also tends to lower blood cholesterol (Table 3.5) but is more effective against blood triglycerides. It will also tend to lengthen clotting time (due to inhibition of platelet aggregation). Insulin resistance may be prevented, as suggested by studies with rats on a high fat diet (polyunsaturated or saturated fat) (Storlien et al., 1987). Insulin resistance (glucose intolerance) is another risk factor in atherosclerosis (Zavaroni et al., 1989). Indeed, LDL from diabetics (which is probably glycated) is rapidly removed by macrophages (Slavina et al., 1987), thus resembling oxidized LDL (see earlier discussion). (Perhaps it is also "toxic.") Epidemiologic studies of human populations with different levels of fish and/or marine mammal consumption, particularly those on the Greenland Eskimo as compared with their less fish-eating Danish or North American counterparts (Bang and Dyerberg, 1980; Dyerberg, 1986), are consistent with these concepts. [A good review of the subject is given by Leaf and Weber (1988).] A more recent supporting study is that of Kromhout et al. (1985) on middle-aged men in The Netherlands, where data suggested that consumption of as few as two fish dishes per week (30 g fish per day) lowered the incidence of fatal coronary heart disease about 50% [also see data from the Western Electric Study (Shekelle et al., 1985)]. [Not all such data on fish consumption have been positive, however (Vollset et al., 1985; Curb et al., 1985).] A considerable reduction in restenosis after angioplasty has been documented for subjects given daily doses of 3.2 g EPA + 2.2 g DHA in addition to aspirin (and dipyramidole) (Dehmer et al., 1988); and several studies in animals indicate protective effects against injury to the coronary or cerebral artery or against ventricular arhythmias (see Leaf and Weber, 1988).

EPA and DHA, in fish and marine mammals, derive from the marine phyto- and zooplankton that constitute the bottom of their food chain

(Leaf and Weber, 1988). Apparently, some terrestrial ferns and mosses (and, therefore, some nonruminant game animals) can also be significant sources of EPA and DHA (Tinoco, 1982). Fish high in EPA and DHA and available to Americans include salmon, black cod, mackeral, brook trout, herring, and sardines (see Chapter 3). [Most common fish are low in fat, including EPA and DHA (cod, sole, red snapper, etc.; WH Harris and WE Connor, University of Oregon, personal communication).]

Other experiments with cats and dogs support the concept that these fish oils reduce the likelihood of injury to brain and heart from experimental stroke and myocardial infarction (Black et al., 1979; Culp et al., 1980). On the other hand, potential toxic effects of such fatty acids, causing increased bleeding, "yellow fat disease," cardiac necrosis (Vergroesen et al., 1981), as well as ulcers, platelet and immune malfunction, and changes in the metabolism of kidneys that are already diseased (Leaf and Weber, 1988; Oates et al., 1988*b*) must not be ignored. Further studies will help to place in context the implications of these various findings and their potential importance for reducing the incidence of atherosclerosis in Western society.

Inhibition of Atherogenesis by Components from Milk, Garlic, and Onions

Essential oils of garlic and onion have also been shown to reduce platelet aggregation (Vanderhoek, 1980) and to lower plasma triglyceride concentrations, with smaller effects on cholesterol (Bordia et al., 1975; Sainani et al., 1976). One of the active ingredients in these effects appears to be ajoene (Figure 15.9) formed from alline (the substance responsible for part of the odor of garlic) with the help of a compartmentalized enzyme (allinase) released when the garlic is crushed (Jain and Apitz-Castro, 1987). Ajoene was isolated from ethanol extracts but is not present in most commercial garlic powders or preparations (that are steam distillates). It inhibits the aggregation of platelets at a late stage (that may involve the exposure of fibrinogen receptors for platelet binding) (Apitz-Castro et al., 1986). Its action does not interfere with prostanoid metabolism, is synergistic with that of other agents (like prostacyclin and aspirin), and has no effect on clotting. As already discussed, platelet aggregation (and concomitant activation) is an initiating event for both the atherosclerotic process and the formation of thrombi (clots) that could lead to myocardial (or other) infarctions (heart attack, etc.).

Earlier reports attributed these and other actions of garlic *and* onion to a more generalized version of this compound, plus its precursors (propylallyl disulfide, etc.; Figure 15.9) and suggested that they inhibited the synthesis of thromboxanes that promote platelet aggregation (Vanderhoek, 1980). Fairly large amounts of these oils (such as 50 g) were required for an effect. This is hard to achieve by simple dietary means, as the oils comprise only 0.06%–0.1% of the weight of the garlic and only 0.005% of the weight of the onion. However, Jain and Apitz-Castro (1987) estimate that 3–5 g of garlic per day, crushed to form ajoene, should have a clinically significant effect.

Observations that populations consuming a high milk or yogurt diet have a low incidence of atherosclerosis has led to the isolation of two milk factors capable of markedly reducing endogenous (liver) cholesterol synthesis (Ahmed et al., 1979). One is orotic acid (Figure 15.9), a precursor of pyrimidines, which blocks the cholesterol pathway, probably at HMG CoA reductase (see Chapter 3). The other has a similar, but not yet fully defined, structure and inhibits synthesis further along the pathway. In line with this, sour milk, yogurt, and whole cow's milk are hypocholesterolemic in man and animal (Krichevsky, 1979; Mann, 1977). [This again goes contrary to the prevalent concept that (because of their cholesterol) milk and dairy products contribute to atherogenesis.] These various findings may eventually lead to new dietary approaches to atherosclerosis prevention.

Ethanol and Coffee Consumption in Relation to Atherosclerosis

Several epidemiological studies have linked moderate alcohol consumption (as compared with overindulgence or abstention) to a lower risk of coronary heart disease (see Moore and Pearson, 1986). More recent data suggest the same benefit for middle-aged women consuming 3–9 drinks per week (Stampfer et al., 1988), and a seeming benefit against the risk of ischemic stroke was also calculated. In contrast, low ethanol intake (from abstention to 1 drink a day) had no significant effect on blood pressure, but high intakes caused an increase, suggesting a greater risk of atherosclerosis (Saunders, 1987). The initial explanation for the beneficial ethanol effect has been that it increases levels of HDL, a factor

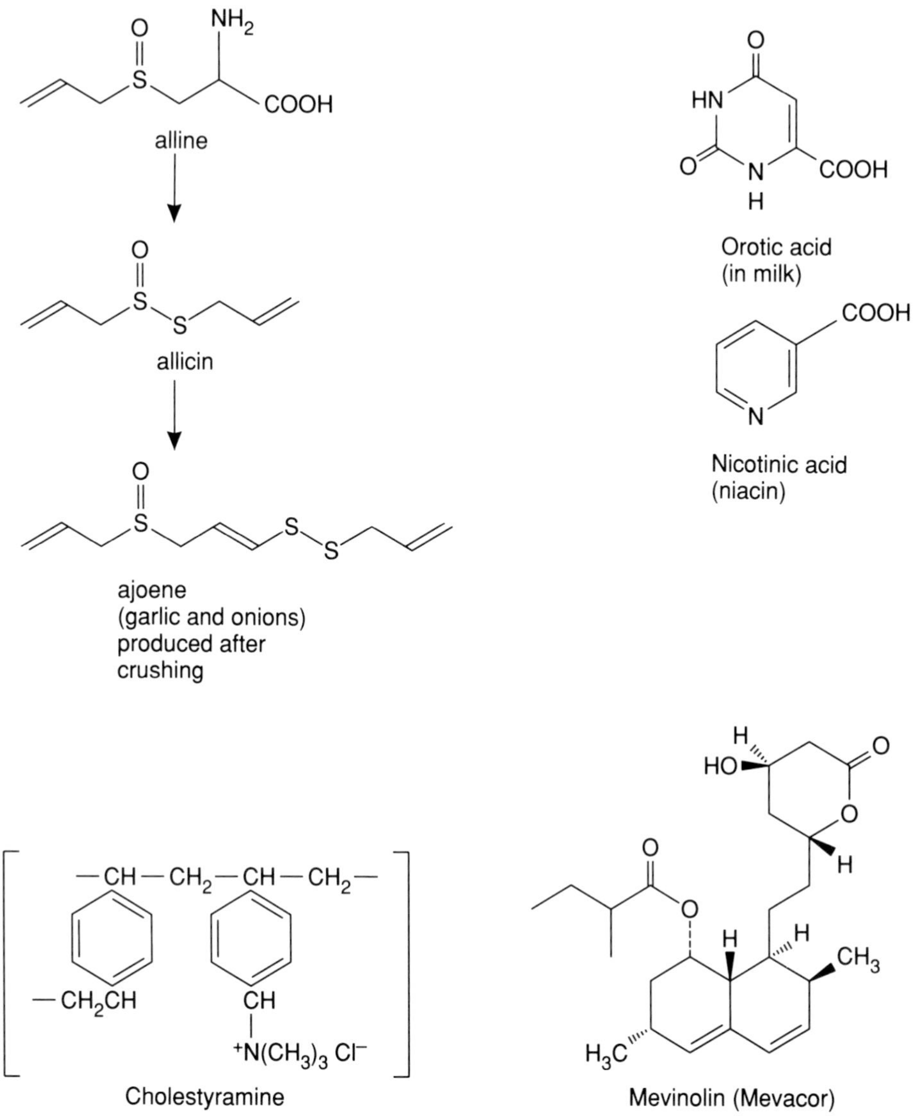

alline

allicin

ajoene
(garlic and onions)
produced after
crushing

Orotic acid
(in milk)

Nicotinic acid
(niacin)

Cholestyramine

Mevinolin (Mevacor)

Figure 15.9. Various antiatherogenic and/or hypocholesterolemic agents.

inversely associated with atherosclerotic risk (Belfrage et al., 1977; Thornton et al., 1983). This now seems less likely, as it has been found that the subfraction of HDL responding positively to ethanol is the one (HDL_3) not epidemiologically favored to reduce atherosclerosis (Haskell et al., 1984). [There was no effect of ethanol on the "good" HDL (HDL_2).] A recent British study questions the conclusions of the original epidemiologic studies, showing first that the inverse relationship of alcohol consumption to cardiovascular mortality was present only in subjects with diagnosed cardiovascular diseases and, second, that there was movement of subjects from one drinking category to another during the period under study (mostly away from more drinking) that may have skewed the results (Shaper et al., 1988). If there is a beneficial effect it might again have to do with the activity and aggregability of platelets. Tabakoff et al. (1988) have shown that platelets from alcoholics are much more resistant to various activating stimuli. [This again should lower their contributions to atherogenesis and clot formation, which occurs through their production of TXA_2 and PDGF (thromboxane A_2 and platelet-derived growth factor).]

As concerns coffee, numerous epidemiologic studies, often contradictory, have suggested overall that coffee consumption (and/or the life-style associated therewith) may be related positively to hypercholesterolemia (a risk factor in atherosclerosis) (see Thelle et al., 1987). Some studies have shown that coffee consumption tends to be associated with smoking and intake of more calories and saturated fat (Aro et al., 1989; Solvoll et al., 1989), which would account for such a relationship. However, a recent 9-week trial of the effects of boiled or filtered coffee, on the serum cholesterol levels of young men, strongly suggests there is a hypercholesterolemic factor in the roasted, ground coffee extracted by 10-min steeping in boiling water (but not with a drip filter method of coffee brewing). [There was a gradual increase in cholesterol, amounting to 10% by the end of 9 weeks) (Bak and Grobbee, 1989).] Boiling/steeping coffee is common in Scandinavia and may explain the results of some of the many Scandinavian epidemiologic studies. Whether this has any clear relation to either atherosclerosis or mortality, however, is another (still unanswered) question.

Protein Intake and Atherosclerosis

As already noted (Table 15.2), changes in the dietary habits of Americans over the last 80 years were accompanied by a threefold increase in mortality from cardiovascular disease, although more recent mortality rates are on the decline. Since 1909, intake of saturated fat, starch, and fiber has been lower, sugar and animal protein consumption has soared, and vegetable protein intake has also been lower. Another interpretation of these data is that Americans reduced their consumption of vegetables and whole grains in favor of more meat and refined sugar and flour. Thus, the ratio of animal to vegetable protein has almost doubled, and there has been a reduction in intake of many micronutrients, especially the trace elements and certain vitamins. As already indicated, epidemiologic studies have found an association between consumption of animal protein and atherosclerosis equally strong to that of animal fat or cholesterol (Table 15.1). Moreover, Krichevsky (1979) has summarized considerable evidence from human and animal studies that, even in purified diets, animal protein tends to be hypercholesterolemic, while vegetable protein is hypocholesterolemic. In several rabbit (and chicken) studies, casein with or without cholesterol has proven more atherogenic than soy protein, and consumption of casein has reduced excretion of sterols and bile acids as well as the turnover of plasma cholesterol (Carroll, 1982). [More recent studies confirm the relatively atherogenic nature of casein over soy protein (Krichevsky et al., 1988c; Vahouny et al., 1985).] The mechanism of the animal protein effect is unclear, especially as the amino acid composition is not all that different (see Table 4.2). The further finding that homocystine, a catabolite of S-amino acids, is a potent atherogenic agent, plus the fact that vitamin B_6 deficiency promotes accumulation of this substance and is likely on our "Western" diets (Fincham et al., 1987), may offer at least a partial explanation for the epidemiologic data and influence of dietary trends. It cannot, however, explain the detrimental casein effect seen in the animal studies. [Here, one might wonder whether alterations induced by processing—or even traces of oxidized cholesterol—might not be involved.]

Returning to the matter of homocystine, methionine catabolism proceeds through a series of steps designed to produce cysteine and divert these and the other carbons to energy metabolism (Chapter 4, Figure 4.11; Chapter 5, Figure 5.16). Sulfur is excreted as sulfate, derived from cysteine. (For further details, see Chapter 5, Vitamin B_6.) A key step in the pathway is production of cystathionine from homocysteine and serine, a reaction dependent on pyridoxal phosphate (an activated form of vitamin B_6). A relative lack of this vitamin has a particular effect on this enzyme pathway and results in accumulation of homocysteine, which is formed during methylation reactions in which methionine is the methyl group donor. [More recently, lack of folate and vitamin B_{12} have also been implicated (see Chapter 4).] (Methionine is an important cosubstrate in many methylation reactions, apart from playing a structural role in most proteins.) The homocysteine that accumulates during a reduction of its catabolism forms dimeric homocystine and is excreted in the urine. Homocystine accumulation and excretion also occurs in the genetic disorder "homocystinuria" (see Chapters 4, 5, and 18). Sulfur amino acids tend to be less prevalent in plant versus animal proteins, especially the legumes (see Chapter 4) (although this is not the case for soybeans); and vegetarians are known to consume less of these amino acids (Chapter 4, Table 4.3). Moreover, unrefined plant-derived foods are much richer in B vitamins and vitamin B_6. Coupled with the tendency of most Americans and Europeans to consume more than twice as much protein as required for normal health, some homocystine accumulation would be expected to occur frequently in many Americans. Therefore, it is possible that this is a factor in the development and prevalence of atherosclerotic disease.

In 1969, McCully first made a connection between homocystinuria and the precocious development of atherosclerosis when he determined that homocystinuric children, 7–13 years of age, displayed evidence of advanced vascular disease and thromboses at autopsy. Following this, McCully and Ragsdale (1970) demonstrated that homocystine could rapidly induce atherosclerosis in rabbits, due to promotion of smooth muscle cell hyperplasia (McCully and Wilson, 1975), accompanied by the laying down of abnormal proteoglycans in the aorta (McCully, 1970, 1972, 1975). These findings were confirmed by John and Thomas (1972). (This normally occurs in the atherosclerotic process.) The potential connection to vitamin B_6 deficiency was obvious from the fact that the enzymatic step involved is dependent on the vitamin and that some homocystinurics even respond to high levels of B_6 intake (Barber and Spaeth, 1969). Of interest, too, are earlier findings that pyridoxine deficiency caused atherosclerosis in baboons (Rinehard and Greenberg, 1949).

All of the facts supporting a connection between B_6 deficiency and atherosclerosis have been reviewed by McCully and Wilson (1975). Certainly, there is considerable evidence of marginal or overt B_6 deficiency in a portion of the American population. (See Chapter 5 for further details.) The availability of folate is also often limiting, and B_{12} is low in people with pernicious anemia (although there appear to be no reports on the incidence of atherosclerosis in this group). Available evidence implicates high protein and low B_6 consumption (as well as low folate and B_{12}) in the promotion of atherogenesis, but the true impact of these factors on the prevalence of atherosclerosis remains to be assessed, especially in relation to other dietary components and risk factors.

Fiber and Atherosclerosis

Since the early 1970s, there has been a great deal of interest in the possibility that those parts of our foodstuffs, especially grains, fruits, and vegetables, not digested by enzymes secreted by man may indirectly be important to our health because they influence the physical state of the gut contents, food and bowel transit time, and have varying capacities for adsorbing or diluting bile acids/salts, sterols, and some nutrients. Burkitt et al. (1974) were the first to suggest a connection between fiber intake and the incidence of colon cancer, later extending this to cardiovascular and other common diseases of "Western" man. Nevertheless, Walker (1974) and others had earlier implicated a lack of dietary fiber in atherosclerotic risk, and it is well-known that vegetarians (who almost by definition consume a high fiber diet) are less likely to develop the disease. [However, they also generally consume less animal protein, more vitamins, and less cholesterol.)

The best definition of dietary fiber and best methods for its assay are still in debate, but chances for a resolution of the confusion look brighter every day (see Chapter 2). Fiber is a heterogeneous category of materials with a range of quite different chemical and physical properties. Different foods contain different relative proportions of these substances, and both variabilities go a long way toward explaining the lack of agreement about the effects of dietary fiber as a whole. (See Chapter 2 for further details on structure, function, and action.)

As concerns cardiovascular disease, epidemiologic associations implicate a relative lack of food fiber intake with a higher risk of cardiovascular disease and hypercholesterolemia. From the evidence at hand, soluble fiber, such as pectin (in fruits) or oat bran, would appear to have the most consistent beneficial effects, both on plasma cholesterol concentrations in humans and in experimental animals, and on the development of atheromas in rabbits (Krichevsky and Tepper, 1977). Krichevsky (1979) has cited 11 studies in humans, all but two of which demonstrated a hypocholesterolemic effect (4%–42%, mean 11%) with various daily doses of pectin (6–50 g). More consistent and dramatic effects have occurred in animals, with pectin as 2.5%–10% of the diet. More recently, oat bran (Anderson et al., 1984) and corn bran (Earll et al., 1988) have become "hot items" with regard to lowering blood cholesterol (Table 15.3), although the scale of effects observed is not all that great and may have reached exaggeration in the minds of the public. Guar gum (at 36 g/day) is probably also hypocholesterolemic (Jenkins et al., 1975). Typical examples of these findings are given in Table 15.3. Studies with various forms of bran and cellulose have not shown these fiber forms to be effective overall, although there are individual reports that some high cereal fiber diets will lower plasma lipids (Munoz et al., 1979). Animal studies (Table 15.4), on the other hand, have not always found pectin to be beneficial or

Table 15.3. Effects of Fiber on Human Plasma Cholesterol Concentrations[a]

	Fiber amount[b]	Plasma cholesterol (fasting) (mg/dl)			Reference
		Total	LDL	HDL	
Control		280	190	31	Anderson et al. (1984)
+ Oat bran	28	226*	149*	29	
Control		298	—	50	Earll et al. (1988)
+ Corn bran	17	248*	—	49	
Control		300	221	32	Anderson et al. (1984)
+ Beans[c]	25	244*	170*	28	
Control		387	—	45	Tuomilehto et al. (1988)
+ Guar gum	20–27	333	—	49	
Control		180	101	55	Abraham and Mehta (1988)
+ Psyllium	21	139*	85*	49*	

[a] Unless otherwise indicated, subjects were their own controls.
[b] g/day supplement. Increase in total fiber consumption.
[c] Pinto and navy beans.
* $p < 0.01$ (or less) for difference from controls.

better than cellulose, either in reducing blood cholesterol (Krichevsky et al., 1988*b*; rats) or the apparent rate of atherogenesis (Krichevsky et al., 1988*a*; monkeys). Clearly, much confusion remains.

The mechanism of action of the pectins and/or other soluble fibers and/or gums would appear to be to bind (and thus enhance excretion from the body of) cholesterol and its bile acid derivatives (see Chapter 3). (Production of bile acids is the main route for catabolism of cholesterol.) In addition, fiber will increase the rate at which foodstuffs as a whole pass through the digestive tract, and this in itself might enhance the daily fecal loss of cholesterol and bile acids. Studies with drugs that reduce or increase transit time have demonstrated that the efficiency of dietary cholesterol absorption (and, thus, probably also cholesterol resorption, after biliary secretion) can be dramatically affected (DeLeon et al., 1982). [In the latter experiments, normal transit time averaged about 7 hr, as judged by excretion of a ^{99}Tc-labeled colloid marker, with a cholesterol absorption efficiency of 35%–43% (with 450–550 mg in the diet), which fell to 21%–27% when transit time was reduced by fiber to 4–5 hr. (It is also noteworthy that increasing the transit time beyond 7 hr did not improve absorption efficiency.)] All kinds of fiber enhance the rate of transit of dietary components through the gut (see Chapter 2). Thus, fiber may act both by directly binding cholesterol and its derivatives and indirectly by

Table 15.4. Effects of Fiber on Cholesterol Metabolism (Rat Studies)

Type of fiber	Effect on total plasma cholesterol	Other effects on cholesterol	Reference
Oat gum	Decreased	—	Jennings et al. (1988)
Oat bran	Decreased	Decreased liver cholesterol	Shinnick et al. (1988)
	Decreased	—	Ney et al. (1988)
Pectin	—	Decreased intestinal absorption	Vahouny et al. (1988)
	—	Increased sterol excretion	Ide and Horii (1989)
	Usually decreased	—	See Krichevsky (1987)
Guar gum	—	Decreased intestinal absorption	Vahouny et al. (1988)
	Decreased	—	See Krichevsky (1987)
Cellulose	No change	—	Jennings et al. (1988); Ney et al. (1988)
	—	Delayed intestinal absorption	Vahouny et al. (1988)
	—	No change in sterol excretion	Ide and Horii (1989)
Alfalfa	—	Decreased intestinal absorption	Vahouny et al. (1988)

reducing small bowel transit time. As a consequence, less cholesterol and bile acid is resorbed, and the liver removes more cholesterol from the circulation to form more bile, thus lowering blood cholesterol concentrations (see Chapter 3).

The relative effectiveness of one form of fiber over another therefore depends on its relative affinity for the various bile acids and sterols (Krichevsky, 1978) (although pectins have not been tested) and its relative capacity to lower gut transit time. Turning to existing studies in which effects on bile acid and sterol excretion have been measured, these are often contradictory. It may be that methodological problems and great individual variability among subjects are responsible. The method of storage of fecal material, for example, and the variability of feces from one time to another in an individual will greatly influence the data obtained (Bell, 1981). The silicon content of the fiber in question may also be a factor (see below). Even if it is eventually proven that pectins, and perhaps some other fibers, are hypocholesterolemic, the question remains as to how important this is to the progression and/or regression of atherosclerosis (see above), especially when cholesterol concentrations are below 250 mg/dl (Reiser, 1978; Figure 15.10).

Atherosclerosis and Micronutrients

The possibility of a connection between the intake of vitamin B_6 and the development of atherosclerosis has already been explained (above). Vitamin E has also been the focus of attention as a possible antiatherogenic agent. The current status of this concept was well-reviewed by Wilson in 1976 and has not changed significantly since that time. Suffice it to say that there is no convincing evidence that
sured by ser
related to th
rotic disease or
less, oxidation pro
terol, and LDL, inclu
ules (see Chapter 7, Vit
detected in atheromatous p
with the severity of the disease. A
cited, oxidized forms of cholesterol an
potent atherogenic agents and might be les
alent in diets containing more vitamin E or ot
antioxidants. The initial long-term studies of Wilson (1976), in which rabbits were given low concentrations of cholesterol (0.05%) relative to vitamin E (1%), do suggest that, under certain conditions, the vitamin has an inhibitory effect on atherogenesis—in this case, accompanied by a lowering of serum cholesterol. However, it seems unlikely that this would be a major factor in disease prevention. It is still possible that occasional benefits to man accrue from other actions of the vitamin, as perhaps the promotion of a collateral blood supply (Puente-Dominguez and Dominguez, 1955) and a decrease in intermittent claudication (see Chapter 7), although studies of Gillilan et al. (1977) with angina patients given 1600 IU/day for 6 months showed no significant reduction in angina attacks or symptoms of functional heart muscle impairment. One of the mechanisms of vitamin E action may be to prevent production of the

Figure 15.10. Relationship between serum cholesterol concentrations and death, from all causes and from coronary heart disease. Data are for U.S. white males, aged 30–59, from the National Cooperative Pooling Project. [*Source:* Reprinted by permission from Reiser (1978).]

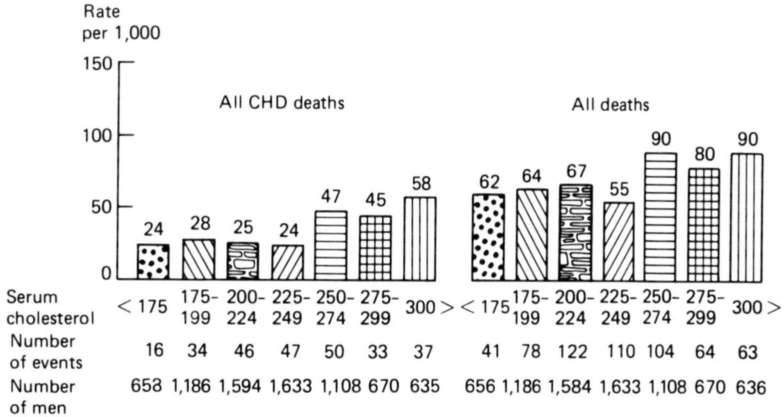

ctor, PDGFc, by aortic endothelial cells, s also inhibited by omega-3 (n-3) fatty ish oils) and BHT (butylated hydroxyto-) (Fox and DiCorleto, 1988). The availability her reducing equivalents (in the form of glu- hione), as well as phospholipase A_2 activity an Kuijk et al., 1987), and trace elements (such as Se and Cu) should be important as well in the inhibition of lipid peroxidative processes that are promotional for atherosclerosis.

The possible actions of several trace elements on the atherogenic process has not been well-studied but should not be ignored. Some of these actions may be via cholesterol. Copper deficiency, which also occurs to varying degrees, may be necessary for the proper turnover, or clearance, of plasma cholesterol (see Chapter 7) and for the antiperoxidative action of superoxide dismutase, also implicating this trace element in hypercholesterolemia. Chromium and vanadium may be inhibitory to endogenous cholesterol synthesis, and there is evidence that a deficiency of the former does occur in Americans and may be common (see Chapter 7). In further support of links between lack of these trace elements and atherosclerosis, Ivanov (1975) showed a drastic preventative effect of vanadium pentoxide in guinea pig atherogenesis, and Punsar et al. (1977) showed an inverse relationship between the concentration of chromium in Finnish drinking water (but not urinary Cr excretion) and the incidence of advanced atherosclerotic disease. [Chromium may also act by inhibiting platelet aggregation (Boyle, 1977).] Deficiencies of these trace elements may thus lead to overproduction of cholesterol, hypercholesterolemia, and/or enhanced platelet aggregation.

Along similar lines, silicon intake in the drinking water and as part of dietary fiber has been associated inversely with a reduced incidence of atherosclerosis, leading to the concept of Schwarz (1977), that a lack of silicon plays a role in the development of atherosclerosis. (For a full discussion of these data, see Silicon, Chapter 7.) Silicon appears to be less prevalent in the diseased aorta, especially where calcification has occurred, and may be an important component in the metabolism and structure of connective tissue (and thus the aortic matrix). This leaves open the possibility of all kinds of effects connected to the "injury response" and plaque formation. In foodstuffs, silicon is especially associated with dietary fiber, providing the possibility of more direct connections between fiber consumption and atherosclerosis. In East versus West Finland (where it has been studied), the silicon content of the water supply is one of the few diet factors that correlates with differences in the incidence of coronary heart disease (see Chapter 7). Chromium is "in the same boat." Also, Bassler (1978) has re-

Table 15.5. List of Studies with Evidence of Regression of Atherosclerotic Lesions in Humans

Principal investigator (year)	Conditions of regression	Evidence of regression
Ashoff (1924)	Post World War I, semistarvation	Aortic atherosclerosis reduced
Wilens (1947)	Wasting disease, 40- to 60-year-olds	Less severe atherosclerosis correlated with weight loss
Vartiainen (1946)	Post World War II, malnutrition	Less atherosclerosis, especially in 30- to 49-year age group
Rivin (1954)	Carcinoma of the prostate and breast, estrogen-treated	Diminution of coronary atherosclerosis
Zelis (1970)	Hyperlipoproteinemias treated with clofibrate and diet	Improvement of peripheral circulation
Buchwald (1974)	Ileal bypass operation for hyperlipoproteinemia	Angiographic evidence of regression of coronary atherosclerosis
Blankenhorn (1975)	Clofibrate, niacin, and diet in postcoronary patients	Angiographic evidence of regression of coronary and femoral arter atherosclerosis
Barth et al. (1987)	Vegetarian diet; 34% cals fat; P/S ratio 2; <100 mg cholesterol/day	Quantitative computer-assisted angiographic evidence of regression or lack of progression in coronary arteries of 14 of 25 subjects (4 years)
Brown et al. (1990)	Cholesterol + niacin or Lovastatin in subjects with coronary disease	Arteriography showed less progression and some regression compared to the control group on conventional therapy

Source: Updated from Wissler and Vesselinovitch (1976).

Table 15.6. Summary of the Effects of Various Drugs and Resins on Hypercholesterolemia and Death from Cardiovascular Disease

Substance	Effect on blood cholesterol		Mechanism (?)	Effects on CHD mortality[a]	Potential side effects	Reference	Study
	LDL	HDL					
Nicotinic acid/niacin	Decreased	Increased	Decreased synthesis of VLDL	Decreased recurrence of MI, decreased mortality	Flushing	Conner et al. (1986)	Coronary Drug Project
Colestipol	Decreased	Variable increase	Binding/excretion of bile acids and cholesterol enhanced	Probably decreased (decreased first time MI); decreased progression (angiography)	May decrease absorption of other drugs; may increase blood TG	Blankenhorn et al. (1987)	Cholesterol Lowering Atherosclerosis Study
Cholestyramine	Decreased		Inhibition of cholesterol synthesis?	?	Possible carcinogen	Gordon et al. (1986); Lipid Research Clinics Program (1984a); Levy et al. (1984)	Clinic Coronary Primary Prevention Trial; NHLBI Type II Intervention Trial
Lovastatin (Mevacor) (Mevinolin)	Decreased	Slight/ variable increase	Inhibition of liver HMG-CoA reductase; LDL receptors increased	?	GI disturbances; painful muscles; liver damage; cataracts	Lovastatin Study Group II (1986); Tobert et al. (1982)	Lovastatin Study Group
Gemfibrozil (Lopid)	Slight decrease (11%)	Increased (11%)	Decrease VLDL and cholesterol synthesis?	Probably decreased (34% decreased first time MI)	Increased risk of gallstones; increased bleeding time	Frick et al. (1987); Manninen et al. (1988)	Helsinki Heart Study
Probucol (Lorelco)	Decreased somewhat	Decreased	Decreased LDL oxidation; enhanced LDL removal/clearance; structure like BHT	? (Lower, in rabbits)	Reduces HDL	Kalevi and Lewis (1987)	
Clofibrate	Decreased		Decreased VLDL and cholesterol synthesis	Probably decreased	Carcinogen	Committee of Principal Investigators (1978)	WHO Trial
Fish oil	Decreased somewhat	Little change	Decreased VLDL synthesis; decreased atherogenesis	? (Inuit)	Slight increase in bleeding time		See Chapter 3

TG = triacylglycerol/triglyceride

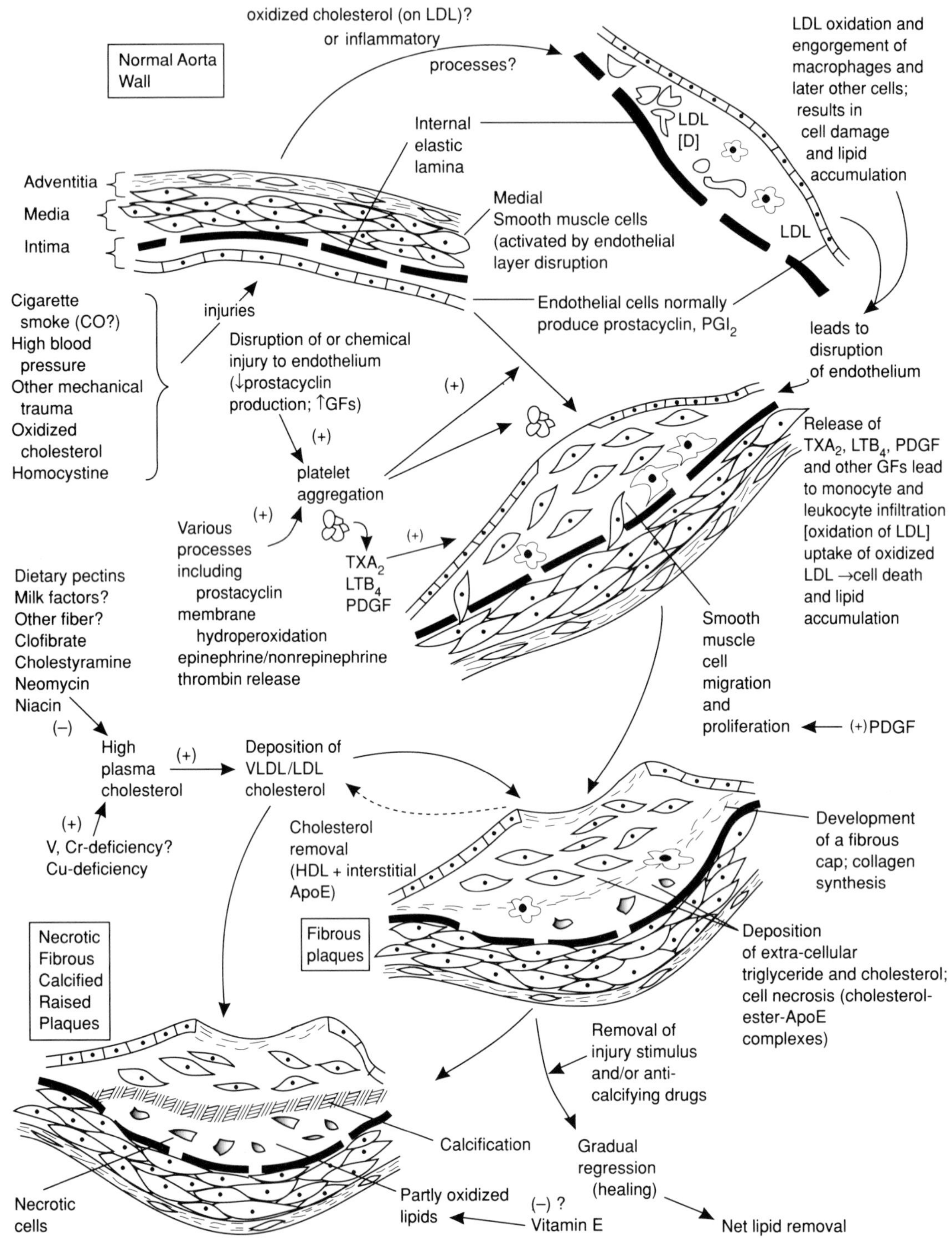

Figure 15.11. Summary of pathways postulated for atherogenesis, and factors that may affect the process: GF, growth factor; VLDL, chylomicron/VLDL remnants with ApoE (with very high fat and cholesterol diets); LTB_4, leukotriene B_4; PDGF, platelet-derived growth factor; PGI_2, prostglandin I_2 (= prostacyclin); TXA_2, thromboxane A_2; (+), stimulation; (−), inhibition. [*Source:* Based on information from Bjorkerud and Bondjers (1976), Ardlie (1981), Wilson (1976), Wissler and Vesselinovitch (1977), Leaf and Weber (1988), and Steinberg et al. (1989).]

ported improvement in cardiac patients who have been given a high silicon diet. Zinc may also be important, by providing for the normal production of glycosaminoglycans in the artery (Philip and Kurup, 1977). The availability of magnesium, a major mineral (Chapter 6), may also be important, as suggested by earlier epidemiologic data on "hard" versus "soft" drinking water (Karppanen, 1981) and more recent reports on beneficial effects of infusing Mg^{2+} during acute myocardial infarction (Morton et al., 1984). Patients with ischemic heart disease appear to have a lower Mg status determined by Mg loading, as shown by a recent Danish study (Rasmussen et al., 1988).

Regression of Atherosclerosis

Evidence is accumulating from various directions that a slow regression of atherosclerotic disease can take place when the factors assaulting the vascular system (perhaps responsible for an "injury response") are removed or reduced, and/or drugs and resins are used to markedly lower plasma cholesterol concentrations. A summary of the types of evidence available is given in Table 15.5. Perhaps most impressive are the data of Blankenhorn (1981) and Crawford and Blankenhorn (1979), who developed a sensitive angiographic technique for following individual lesions in specific arteries (like the femoral) in living individual men and women over several years. The initial results of these studies indicate that regression of raised plaques does occur, but at a very slow rate (visible over years), just as progression of atherosclerotic disease is a slow process in the average American. (Blankenhorn estimates an average increase in artery surface involvement of 2%/year, beginning in the 20s.) Regression does not occur in all individuals. Smoking is a major factor (perhaps even the most important one) in promoting disease progression, and cessation of smoking also evokes the fastest and clearest evidence of disease regression.

The authors believe that a drastic (25%–30%) reduction in plasma cholesterol, achieved by a combination of diet and pharmacologic agents, is important in promoting regression, as is control of hypertension. In the context of theories previously discussed, inhalation of tobacco smoke and hypertension might cause chemical and mechanical injury to the artery endothelium, initiating the atherosclerotic process. Lowering plasma cholesterol might then reduce the accumulation of cholesterol and oxidized LDL in the plaque. Agents that have been used to achieve a drastic lowering of plasma cholesterol (Table 15.6) are clofibrate and lovastatin, inhibitors of HMG CoA reductase and thus endogenous cholesterol synthesis, and 3–6 g niacin, which inhibits VLDL synthesis (see Chapter 3). Other cholesterol-lowering agents are cholestyramine and cholestipol, resins that bind bile acids and thus promote loss of cholesterol derivatives from the body, and neomycin, a non-absorbable aminoglycoside antibiotic that has a similar bile acid binding effect (at doses of 0.5–2 g/day). Use of cholestyramine and especially clofibrate is not always advisable because side effects can occur (*The Medical Letter* 22:65, 1980), and clofibrate is mutagenic in the Ames assay (Ames, 1982). Additional drugs are (a) gemfibrozil (an analog of clofibrate), which raises HDL concentrations with little effect on LDL (Manninen et al., 1988) [blood HDL levels are inversely associated with atherosclerosis risk]; and (b) probucol, a hypocholesterolemic agent (mechanism unknown) (also a reducing agent that travels on LDL; Steinberg et al., 1989). It may interfere with oxidation of LDL and thus work against the atherosclerotic process.

Overview

Figure 15.11 summarizes the postulated pathway of the "injury response" and atherogenesis, and the connections postulated between the various promotional or inhibitory factors mentioned and this process.

References

Abraham S, Johnson CL, Carroll MD (1978): *In* Total serum cholesterol levels of children 4–7 years. Washington, DC: US Department of Health, Education, and Welfare (publication no 78-1655).

Abraham Z, Mehta T (1988): Am J Clin Nutr 47:67.

Ahmed AA, McCarthy RD, Porter CA (1979): Atherosclerosis 32:347.

Altschule MD (1974): Exec Health 10:1.

Ames BN (1982): Progr Clin Biol Res 131D:121 (13th International Cancer Congress, Seattle, September 15, part D).

Anderson JW, Story L, Sieling B, Chen W-JL, Petro MS, Story J (1984): Am J Clin Nutr 40:1146.

Apitz-Castro R, Ledezma, E, Escalante J, Jain MK (1986): Bioch Biophys Res Comm 141:145.

Ardlie NG (1981): *In* Miller NE, Lewis B, eds: Lipoproteins, atherosclerosis, and coronary heart disease. Amsterdam: Elsevier, p 107.

Armstrong ML, Warner ED, Conner WE (1970): Circ Res 27:59.

Aro A, et al. (1989): J Intern Med 226:127.

Austin MA, King M-C, Bawol RD, Hully SB, Friedman GD (1987): Am J Epidiol 125:308.

Bak AAA, Grobbee DE (1989): N Engl J Med 321:1432.

Bang HO, Dyerberg J (1972): Acta Med Scand 192:85.

Bang HO, Dyerberg J (1980): Adv Nutr Res 3:1.

Barber CW, Spaeth BL (1969): Pediatr 75:463.

Barth JD, Jansen H, Kromhout D, Reiber JH, Birkenhager JC, Arntzenius AC (1987): Atherosclerosis 68:51.

Bassler TJ (1978): Br Med J 1:6117.

Belfrage P, Berg B, Hagerstrand I, Nilsson-Ehle P, Tornquist H, Wiebe T (1977): Eur J Clin Invest 7:127.

Bell FC (1981): Am J Clin Nutr 34:1071.

Benditt EP (1976): Ann NY Acad Sci 275:96.

Black KL, Culp B, Madison D, Randall OS, Lands WEM (1979): Prostagland Med 5:247.

Blankenhorn DH (1981): Am J Surg 141:644.

Blankenhorn DH, Nessim SA, Johnson RL, Sanmarco ME, Azen SP, Cashin-Hemphill L (1987): JAMA 257:3233.

Bjorkerud S, Bondjers G (1976): Ann NY Acad Sci 275:180.

Bonaa KH, Bjerve KS, Straume B, Gram IT, Thelle D (1990): N Engl J Med 322:795.

Bordia A, Bansal HC, Arora SK, Singh SV (1975): Atherosclerosis 21:15.

Brown G, Albers JJ, Fisher LD, Schaefer SM, Lin J-T, Kaplan C, Zhao X-Q, Bisson BD, Fitzpatrick VF, Dodge HT (1990): N Engl J Med 323:1289.

Brown MS, Basu SK, Falk JR, Ho YK, Goldstein JL (1980): J Supramol Str 13:67.

Burkitt ET, Walker ART, Painter MS (1974): JAMA 225:526.

Canner PL, Berge KG, Wenger NK, et al. (1986): J Am Coll Cardiol 8:1245.

Carroll KK (1982): Fed Proc 41:2792.

Chazov EL, Tertov VV, Orekhov AN, et al. (1986): Lancet 2:595.

Colditz GA, Bonita R, Stampfer MJ (1988): N Engl J Med 318:937.

Committee of Principal Investigators (1978): Br Heart J 40:1069.

Connor WE (1980): *In* Garry PJ, ed: Human nutrition, clinical and biochemical aspects. Washington, DC: American Association for Clinical Chemistry, p 44.

Consensus Development Conference (1985): JAMA 253:2080.

Crawford DW, Blankenhorn DH (1979): Annu Rev Med 30:289.

Culp BR, Lands WPM, Lucches BR, Pitt R, Romson J (1980): Prostagland Med 20:1021.

Curb JD, Reed DM (1984): N Engl J Med 313:821.

Davis HR, Bridenstine RT, Vesselinovitch D, Wissler RW (1987): Atherosclerosis 7:441.

Dawber TR, Nickerson RJ, Brand FN, Pool J (1982): Am J Clin Nutr 36:617.

Dayton S, Pearce ML, Hashimoto S, Dixon WJ, Tomiyasu U (1968): Circulation 40(Suppl 2):1.

Dehmer GJ, Popma JJ, van den Berg EK, Eichhorn EJ, Prewitt JB, Campbell WB, Jennings L, Willerson JT, Schmitz JM (1988): N Engl J Med 319:733.

DeLeon MP, Iori R, Barbolini G, Pompei G, Zaniol P, Carulli N (1982): N Engl J Med 307:102.

Dyerberg J (1986): Nutr Rev 44:125.

Earll L, Earll JM, Naujokaitis S, Pyle S, McFalls K, Altschul AM (1988): J Am Dietetic Assoc 88:950.

Feinbeib M (1983): Cancer Res 43(Suppl):2503s.

Fincham JE, Faber M, Weight MJ, Labadarios D, Taljaard JJF, Steytler JG, Jacobs P, Kritchevsky D (1987): Atherosclerosis 66:191.

Flaim E, Ferreri LF, Thye FW, Hill JE, Ritchey SJ (1981): Am J Clin Nutr 43:1103.

Flynn MA, Nolph GB, Flynn TC, Kahrs R, Krause G (1979): Am J Clin Nutr 32:1051.

Flynn MA, Nolph GB, Osio Y, Sun GY, Lanning B, Krause G, Dally JC (1986): J Am Dietet Assoc 86:1541.

Fox PL, DiCorleto PE (1988): Science 241:453.

Frick MH, Elo O, Haapa K, et al. (1987): N Engl J Med 317:1237.

Gambino MC, Passaghe S, Chen ZM, Bucchi F, Gori G, Latini R, de Gaetano G, Cerletti C (1988): J Pharmacol Exp Therap 245:287.

Gillilan RE, Mondell B, Warbasse JR (1977): Am Heart J 93:444.

Goldstein JL, Ho YK, Basu SK, Brown MS (1979): Proc Natl Acad Sci USA 76:333.

Goodnight SH, Jr (1988): Sem Thrombosis Hemostasis 14:285.

Goodnight SH Jr, Harris WS, Conner WE (1981): Blood 58:8.

Gordon DJ, Knoke J, Probstfield JL, Superko R, Tyroler HA (1986): Circulation 74:1217.

Gordon T, Kannel WB, Castelli WP, Dauber TR (1981): Arch Inter Med 141:1128.

Harris WS, Connor WE (1980): Trans Assoc Am Physicians 93:148.

Haskell WL, Camargo C Jr, Williams PT, Vranizan KM, Krauss RM, Lindgren FT, Wood D (1984): N Engl J Med 310:805.

Ho K-J, Biss K, Mikkelson B, Lewis LA, Taylor CB (1971): Arch Pathol 91:387.

Ide T, Horii M (1989): Brit J Nutr 61:545.

Imai H, Werhessen NT, Taylor CB, Lee KT (1976): Arch Pathol 100:565.

Iso H, Jacobs DR, Wentworth D, Neaton JD, Cohen JD (1989): N Engl J Med 320:904.

Ivanov VN (1975): Cor Vasa 17:75.

Jain MK, Apitz-Castro R (1987): TIBS 12:252.

Jenkins DJA, Newton C, Leeds AR, Cummings JH (1975): Lancet 1:1116.

Jennings CD, Boleyn K, Bridges SR, Wood PJ, Anderson JW (1988): Proc Soc Exp Biol Med 189:13.

John R, Thomas J (1972): Biochem J 127:251.

Kagan A, Popper JS, Rhoads CG (1980): Stroke 11:14.

Kahn HA (1970): Am J Clin Nutr 23:879.

Kalevi L, Lewis B, eds (1987): *In* Olsson AG, ed: European heart journal, Vol 8 (Suppl E): Atherosclerosis, biology and clinical science. Edinburgh: Churchill Livingstone.

Karppanen H (1981): Artery 9:190.

Kramsch DM, Aspen AJ, Rozler LJ (1981): Science 213:1511.

Krichevsky D (1978): Lipids 13:982.

Krichevsky D (1979): Adv Nutr Res 2:181.

Kritchevsky D (1987): Scan J Gastroenterol 22(Suppl 1986):129.

Krichevsky D, Tepper SA (1977): Atherosclerosis 27:239.

Krichevsky D, Davidson LM, Scott DA, Van der Watt JJ, Mendelsohn D (1988*a*): Lipids 23:164.

Krichevsky D, Tepper SA, Satchithanandam S, Cassidy MM, Vahouny GV (1988*b*): Lipids 23:318.

Krichevsky D, Tepper SA, Weber MM, Klurfeld DM (1988c): Artery 15:163.

Kromhout D, Bosschieter EB, Coulander C deL (1985): N Engl J Med 312:1205.

Leaf A, Weber PC (1988): N Engl J Med 318:549.

Leren (1966): Acta Med Scand Suppl 466:1.

Levy RI, Brenske JF, Epstein SE, et al. (1984): Circulation 69:325.

Libby P, Warner SJC, Salomon RN, Birinyi LK (1988): N Engl J Med 318:1493.

Lipid Research Clinics Program (1984*a*): J Am Med Assoc 251:351.

Lipid Research Clinics Program (1984*b*): J Am Med Assoc 251:365.

Lopez-Virella MF, Klein RL, Lyons TJ, Stevenson HC, Witztum H (1988): Diabetes 37:550.

Lovastatin Study Group II (1986): J Am Med Assoc 256:2829.

Mann GV (1977): Atherosclerosis 26:335.

Manninen V, Elo MO, Frick MH, Haapa K, Heinonen OP, Heinsalmi P, Helo P, Huttunen JK, Kaitaniemi P, Koskinen P, Maenpaa H, Malkonen M, Manttari M, Norola S, Pasternack A, Pikkarainen J, Romo M, Sjoblom T, Nikkila E (1988): J Am Med Assoc 260:641.

Manson JE, Colditz GA, Stampfer MJ, Willett WC, Rosner B, Monson RR, Speizer FE, Hennekens CH (1990): N Engl J Med 32:882.

McCully KS (1969): Am J Pathol 56:111.

McCully KS (1970): Am J Pathol 59:181.

McCully KS (1972): Am J Pathol 66:83.

McCully KS (1975): Ann Clin Lab Sci 5:147.

McCully KS, Ragsdale BD (1970): Am J Pathol 161:1.

McCully KS, Wilson RB (1975): Atherosclerosis 22:215.

McGee DL, Reed DM, Yano K, Kagan A, Tillotson J (1984): Am J Epidem 119:667.

McGill HC Jr, Arias-Stella J, Carbonell LM, Correa P, de Veyra EA Jr, Donoso S, Eggen DA, Galindo L (1968): Lab Invest 18:498.

McMichael J (1977): Eur J Cardiol 5/6:447.

Moore RD, Pearson TA (1986): Medicine 65:242.

Morton BC, Nair RC, Smith FM, McKibbon TG, Poznanski WJ (1984): Magnesium 3:346.

Multiple Risk Factor Intervention Trial Research Group (1982): JAMA 248:1465.

Munoz MJ, Sandstead HH, Jacob RA, Logan GM, Reck SJ, Klevay LM, Dintzis FR, Inglett GE (1979): Am J Clin Nutr 32:580.

Naito HK (1980): *In* Brewster MA, Naito KH, eds: Nutritional elements and clinical biochemistry. New York: Plenum, p 277.

Ney DM, Lasekan JB, Shinnick FL (1988): J Nutr 118:1455.

Oates JA, Fitzgerald GA, Branch RA, Jackson EK, Knapp HR, Roberts LJ (1988*a*): N Engl J Med 319:689.

Oates JA, Fitzgerald GA, Branch RA, Jackson EK, Knapp HR, Roberts LJ (1988*b*): N Engl J Med 319:761.

Oliver MF (1982): Exec Health 29:1.

Oliver MF (1986): Lancet I: 982.

Olson RE (1979): In RI Levy, BM Rifkind, BH Dennis, N Ernst, eds, Nutrition, lipids, and coronary heart disease. New York, Raven, p 349.

Paganini-Hill A, Chao A, Ross RK, Henderson BE (1989): Brit Med J 299:1247.

Parks JS, Wilson MD, Johnson FL, Rudel LL (1989): J Lipid Res 30:1535.

Parthasarathy S, Printz DJ, Boyd D, Joy L, Steinberg D (1986): Arteriosclerosis 6:505.

Paterson JC, Armstrong R, Armstrong EC (1963): Circulation 27:229.

Pekkanen J, Linn S, Heiss G, Suchindran CM, Leon A, Rifkind BM, Tyroler HA (1990): N Engl J Med 322:1700.

Phillip B, Kurup PA (1977): Indian J Biochem Biophys 14:354.

Physicians' Health Study (The DCCT Research Group) (1988): N Engl J Med 318:245.

Puente-Dominguez JL, Dominguez R (1955): Rev Espan Cardiol 9:930.

Punsar S, Wolf W, Mertz W, Karvonen MJ (1977): Ann Clin Res 9:79.

Rasmussen HS, McNair P, Goransson S, Balslov S, Larsen OG, Aurup P (1988): Arch Intern Med 148:329.

Reiser R (1978): Am J Clin Nutr 31:869.

Relman AS (1988): N Engl J Med 318:245.

Rinehardt JF, Greenberg LD (1949): Am J Pathol 25:481.

Ross R (1986): N Engl J Med 314:496.

Ross R, Masuda J, Raines EW, Gown AM, Katsuda S, Sasahara M, Malden LT, Masuko H, Sato H (1990): Science 248:1009.

Roth GJ, Stanford N, Majerus PW (1975): Proc Nat Acad Sci (USA) 72:3073.

Sainani GS, Desai DB, More KN (1976): Lancet 2:575.

Sassen LMA, Koning MMG, Dekkers DHW, Lamers JMJ, Verdouw PD (1989): Eur Heart J 10(Suppl F):173.

Saunders JB (1987): Br Med J 294:1045.

Schwarz K (1977): Lancet 1:454.

Schwartz L, Bourassa MG, Lesperance J, Aldridge HE, Kazim F, Salvatori VA, Henderson M, Bonan R, David PR (1988): N Engl J Med 318:1714.

Shaper AG, Jones KW, Jones M, Kyobe J (1963): Am J Clin Nutr 13:135.

Shaper AG, Wannamethee G, Walker M (1988): Lancet 2:1267.

Shekelle RB, Liu S, Raynor WJ Jr, Lepper M, Maliza C,

Rossof AH, Paul O, Shryock AM, Stamoer J (1981): Lancet 2:1185.

Shekelle RB, Missell LV, Oglesby P, Shryock AM, Stamler J (1985): N Engl J Med 313:820.

Shinnick FL, Longacre MJ, Ink SL, Marlett JA (1988): J Nutr 118:144.

Slavina ES, Madanat AY, Pankov YA, Syrkin AL, Tertov VV, Orekhov AN (1987): N Engl J Med 319:836.

Small DM (1988): Arteriosclerosis 8:103.

Sniderman A, Shapiro S, Marpole D, Skinner B, Teng B, Kwiterovich PO Jr (1980): Proc Natl Acad Sci USA 77:601.

Solvoll K, et al. (1989): Am J Epidemiol 129:1277.

Stampfer MJ, Colditz GA, Willett WC, Speizer FE, Hennekens CH (1988): N Engl J Med 319:267.

Steering Committee of the Physicians' Health Study Research Unit (1989): N Engl J Med 321:129.

Stehbens WE (1987): Lancet I: 606.

Stehbens WE (1989): Nutr Rev 47:1.

Steinberg D, Parthasarathy S, Carew TE, Khoo JC, Witztum JL (1989): N Engl J Med 320:915.

Storlien LH, Kraegen EW, Chisholm DJ, Ford GL, Bruce DG, Pascoe WS (1987): Science 319:885.

Sytkowski PA, Kannel WB, D'Agostino RB (1990): N Engl J Med 322:1635.

Tabakoff B, Hoffman P, Lee JM, Saito TR, Willard B, De Leon-Jones F (1988): N Engl J Med 318:134.

Taylor WC, Pass PM, Shepard DS, Komaroff AL (1987): Ann Intern Med 106:605.

Taylor CB, Peng K, Imai H, Mikkelson B, Lee KT, Werthessen NT (1975): *In* Proceedings of the International Conference and Workshop on Atherosclerosis, London, Ontario, September 1.

Thelle DS, Heyden S, Fodor JG (1987): Atherosclerosis 67:97.

Tinoco J (1982): Prog Lipid Res 21:1.

Tobert JA, Bell GD, Birtwell J, et al. (1982): J Clin Invest 69:913.

Truswell AS (1978): Am J Clin Nutr 31:977.

Tuomilehto J, Silvasti M, Aro A, Koistinen A, Karttunen P, Gref C-G, Ehnholm C, Uusitupa M (1988): Atherosclerosis 72:157.

US Department of Health, Education and Welfare (1978): Vital and health statistics, series 11, no 207. Washington, DC: National Center for Health Statistics (DHEW publication no 78-1655).

Vahouny GV, Adamson I, Chalearz WS, Satchithanandam S, Muesing R, Klurfeld DM, Tepper SA, Sanghvi A, Kritchevsky D (1985): Atherosclerosis 56:127.

Vahouny GV, Chen I, Tepper SA, Kritchevsky D, Lightfoot FG, Cassidy MM (1988): Am J Clin Nutr 47:201.

Vanderhoek JY, Makheja AN, Bailey JM (1980): Biochem Pharmacol 29:3169.

van Kuijk FJGM, Sevanian A, Handelman GJ, Dratz EA (1987): TIBS 12:31.

Vastesaeger MM (1968): J Atherosclerosis Res 8:377.

Vergroesen AJ, ten Hoor F, Hornstra G (1981): *In* Beers RF Jr, Bassett EG, eds: Nutritional factors: Modulating effects on metabolic processes. New York: Raven, p 539.

Vollset SE, Heuch I, Bjelke E (1984): New Engl J Med 313:821.

Walker ARP (1974): Ann Intern Med 80:663.

Weiner BH, Ockene IS, Levine PH, Cuenoud HF, Fisher M, Johnson BF, Daoud AS, Jarmolych JJ, Hosmer D, Johnson MH, Natale A, Vaudreuil C, Hoogasian JJ (1986): N Engl J Med 315:841.

Weinstein R, Stemerman MB, Maciag T (1981): Science 212:818.

Williams RR, Sorlie PD, Feinlab M, McNamara PM, Kannel WB, Dawber TR (1981): JAMA 247:247.

Wilson RB (1976): Br Rev Sci Nutr 8:325.

Wissler RW, Vesselinovitch D (1977): *In* Schettler G, ed: Atherosclerosis, Vol 4. Berlin: Springer-Verlag, p 330.

Wissler RW, Vesselinovitch D (1976): Ann NY Acad Sci 275:363.

Wolinsky H (1981): Science 212:6.

Yerushalmy J, Hilleboe HE (1957): NY State J Med 57:2343.

Yudkin J (1957): Lancet II: 155.

Zavaroni I, Bonora E, Pagliara M, Dall'Aglio E, Luchetti L, Buonanno G, Bonati PA, Bergonzani M, Gnudi L, Passeri M, Reaven G (1989): N Engl J Med 320:702.

Ziemlanski S, Panczenko-Kresowska B, Wielgus-Serafinska E, Zelakliewicz K (1987): Nutr Internat 3:104.

Maria C. Linder, Ph.D.*

16

Nutrition and Cancer Prevention

Cancer Incidence, Origins, and Effects of Diet

Cancer is responsible for about 20% of deaths in the United States and is recognized as the second most important "killer." Heart disease accounts for about 38%, stroke 10%, and others 5% or less. It is well-recognized that the majority of cancer cases are ascribable to environmental factors, and three categories of carcinogens are known (Figure 16.1): chemicals, radiation, and viruses. These may all be found in the environment. However, the most important sources for man would appear to be chemicals in tobacco smoke and the diet. Exposure to radiation is much less important overall. Viruses may play an even smaller role: There are few cases where viruses have been firmly implicated as responsible for cancer in man, except for Burkitt's lymphoma and a few others. Indeed, the ease of inducing viral transformation in tissue culture in the laboratory may have exaggerated the importance of viral carcinogenesis for mammals. The importance of smoking to cancer incidence cannot be overstated, as illustrated by the data in Table 16.1. In human epidemiologic studies, the contribution of smoking must always be subtracted before other factors can be related to disease incidence. The time relation between increased indulgence in smoking and detection of an increased incidence of lung cancer (Figure 16.2) is illustrative of the long lag seen in humans between exposure to carcinogen and tumor development, in this case 25–30 years! This presents a great handicap in assessing "risk factors" in human carcinogenesis.

The mechanism (or mechanisms) by which carcinogenesis proceeds, resulting in the growth of a detectible malignant tumor in a person, is poorly understood, despite impressive progress in the identification of so-called oncogenes implicated in the process. [Hence, the "black box" in Figure 16.1.] Oncogenes generally are normal genes (Nicolson, 1984, 1985) involved in the cell "circuitry" by which proliferation is controlled (Figure 16.3), and include growth factors (Goustin et al., 1987), their receptors (R), G proteins or tyrosine kinase activities initiating second messenger effects (such as on phospholinositides, Ca^{2+} flux, and the activity of protein kinase C); and growth regulatory genes, resulting in DNA replication and cell proliferation (Bishop, 1987; Nowell, 1986).

Carcinogenesis is undoubtedly a multistep, highly complex, even potentially reversible, process, taking place over many years. Two major phases are recognized: initiation, during which a carcinogen triggers a change that may lead to cancer; and promotion, during which noncarcinogenic factors enhance the likelihood of cancer development (Figure 16.1). Details of theories on the mechanism(s) of carcinogenesis are not the

* California State University, Fullerton, CA.

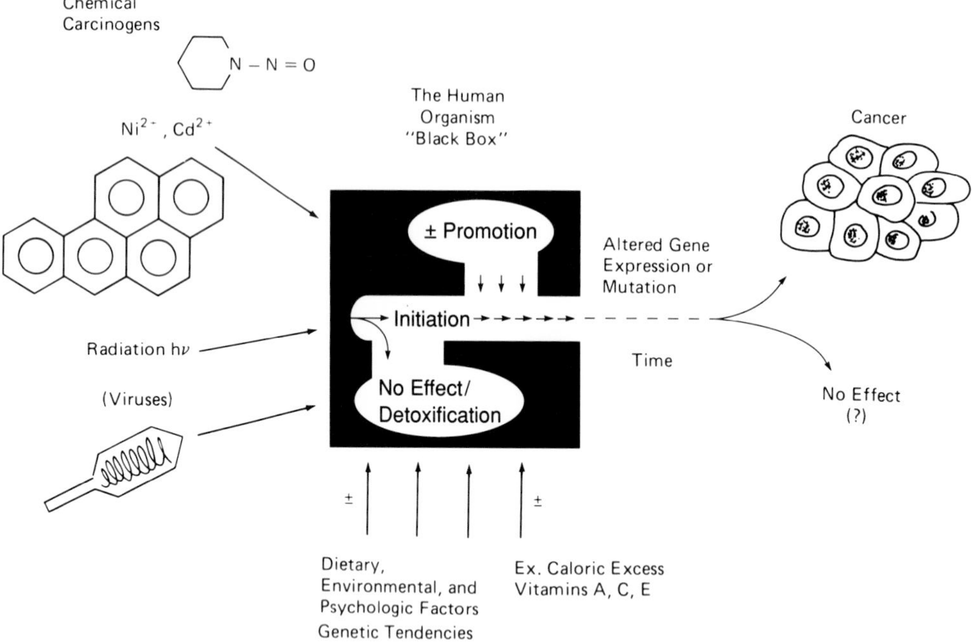

Figure 16.1. Carcinogenesis. The human organism receives exposure to carcinogenic agents **(left of figure)** which results in largely unknown changes, within the "Black Box," changes that involve multiple steps and possibilities, in at least two phases: initiation and promotion. Promotion may or may not succeed initiation of carcinogenesis. Even with promotion, a malignant growth may not result. Changes that occur are over a long time period, and are modulated by many kinds of factors, including diet **(bottom of figure),** the final outcome being (or not being) a change in gene expression and/or mutation that may or may not ultimately result in formation of a malignant tumor.

proper subject of this book, except to say that it is generally thought that tumors develop from genetic changes in individual cells (clones) (Fialkow, 1979); the tumor contains a diversity of cells, only some of which are malignant (Nicolson, 1987); malignancy tends to be associated with chromosomal alterations, especially increases in chromosome number and/or gene translocation, so that cells are genetically "unstable" (again with considerable diversity within a tumor) (Nowell, 1987); oncogene expression in tumor cells tends to be increased over that in nor-

Table 16.1. U.S. Cancer Deaths Attributable to Smoking, as Predicted for 1981

	Males		Females	
Site of cancer	Estimated deaths	% attributed to smoking[a]	Estimated deaths	% attributed to smoking
Lung	77,000	97	28,000	74
Mouth	6300	78	2850	46
Esophagus	5800	83	2300	50
Pancreas	11,500	28	10,500	22
Larynx	3100	99	600	57
Bladder	7300	28	3300	22
Kidney	4900	28	3200	22
All tumors	227,500	41	192,500	14

Source: Reproduced by permission from Reif (1981).

[a] For males, the figures include fatalities attributed to smoking cigars and pipes, as well as cigarettes.

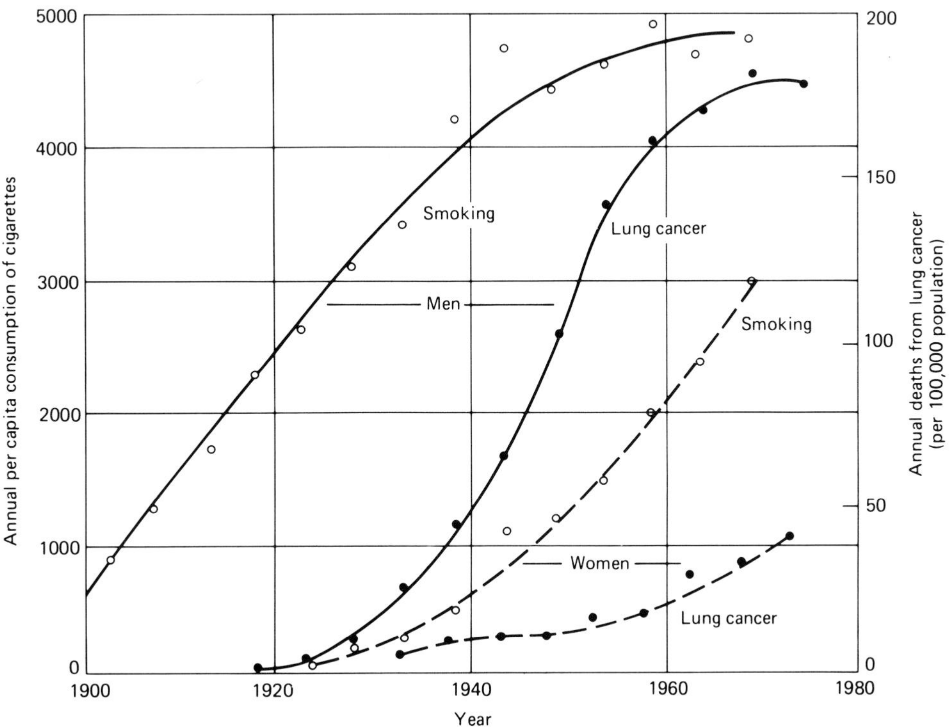

Figure 16.2. Smoking habits and annual death rates from lung cancer in England and Wales. [*Source:* Reprinted by permission from J. Cairn (1975) *Scientific American* 233:64, as quoted in Ames (1979).]

mal tissue (Ohuchi et al., 1986). [At least in human cancer this is ascribable mainly to gene duplication (as with extra chromosomes) or gene translocation, rather than to mutation of "normal" protooncogenes (Nicolson, 1987).] Expression of currently recognized oncogenes is probably not the critical factor in developing metastatic cancer cells (Gallick et al., 1985); and phenotypic expression of the tumor cells (as well as their regression) will be influenced by their microenvironment (Mintz and Illmensee, 1975; Pierce et al., 1979), including tissue architecture and other cells in the tumor (Miner et al., 1982).

Additional points would be that: (1) a large variety of quite different chemical substances (as well as x-rays, etc.) have been shown to induce carcinogenesis; (2) tumors can occur with single or multiple exposure to the carcinogen; (3) the actions of various carcinogens may be synergistic in promoting tumor development; (4) the proportion of exposed people (or animals) developing malignancies will vary greatly, depending, in part, on the degree or dose of exposure (or animal species concerned), but also depending on many other factors, some of which are not well-defined; and (5) evidence increasingly suggests that components of the diet play an important role in modulating the effects of carcinogens on the body (Figure 16.1).

Modulation may be inhibitory to the carcinogenic process, or conversely, it may promote the formation of neoplasms. Apart from diet, psychologic and genetic tendencies also play a modulating role, as may environmental factors. A description of what is currently known of the modulatory effects of the diet is the main purpose of this chapter. The ultimate result of the interactions between carcinogens and modulating factors within the battlefield of the body will, or will not, be the development of a malignant tumor in one or another organ. From what is currently known, it seems likely that specific long-term preventative alterations in dietary habits would significantly affect and reduce the incidence of most major forms of cancer in our society.

Figure 16.4 shows the trends in incidence for the various types of cancer most prevalent in Americans, a finding that is also typical for "Western man" as a whole. The main killers are lung, prostate, and gastrointestinal cancer in men; breast, gastrointestinal, and now, also, lung cancer in women. Of the gastrointestinal forms,

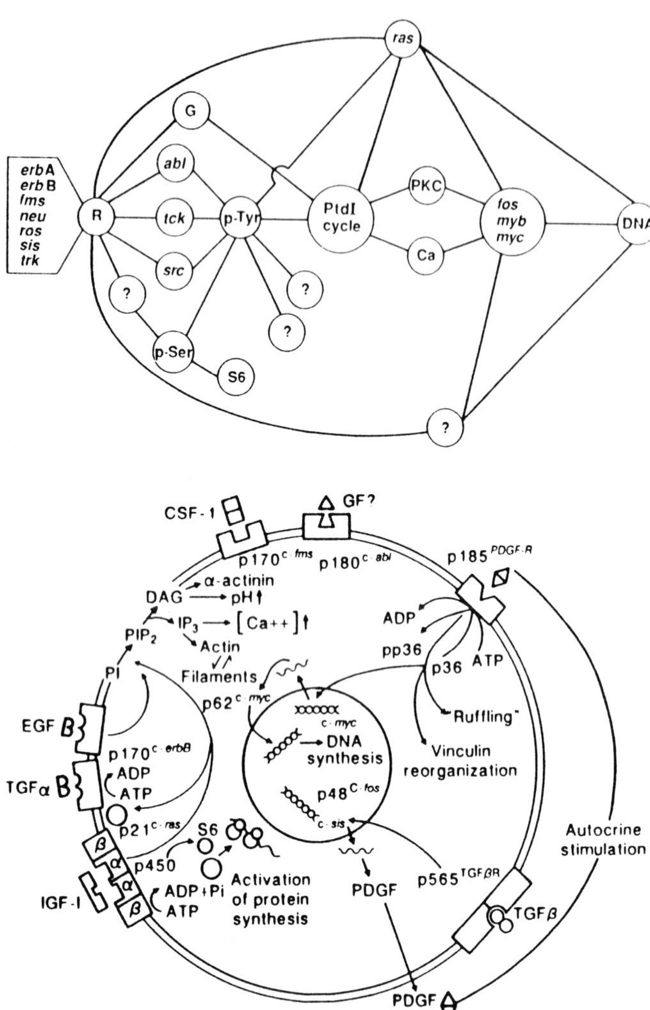

Figure 16.3. Involvement of C-proto-oncogene products in the regulation of cell proliferation. **(A)** Hypothetical scheme placing these proteins in the circuitry for growth regulation, including growth factor receptors (R), tyrosine phosphorylation (tyrosine kinase), G-proteins, protein kinase phosphorylation (phosphoserines), activation of the phosphatidyl inositol cycle (Ptdl cycle), protein kinase C (PKC), changes in cellular Ca^{2+} concentrations (Ca), and stimulation of the expression of growth-involved genes. The positions of oncogene involvement are indicated by their three letter, lowercase codes to the left of (or preceding) where they are active. [*Source:* Reprinted by permission from Bishop (1987).] **(B)** A more detailed view of many of these growth factor-related processes, showing oncogene products as peptides of different apparent molecular weight (Ex., p 21), with c-three letter superscripts, next to receptors or other factors they may encode in different normal and cancerous cells. The designation "pp" refers to a phosphorylated product. [*Source:* Reprinted by permission from Goustin et al. (1986).]

colon or rectal cancers greatly predominate, with a much lower (and falling) incidence of stomach cancer. Until very recently (and with the exception of lung cancer in women), it appeared that cancer rates had stabilized. However, statistical analyses of data from the late 1960s through 1980s (Davis et al., 1990; Pollack and Horn, 1980) indicate that there has been a new upsurge, less than half of which can be ascribed to smoking (Smith, 1980). The upsurge appears to be in breast cancer, malignant melanoma, brain tumors, and multiple myeloma, with a 15% increase in overall cancer death rates from 1968–1987 (Davis et al., 1990). The conjecture is that this represents the impact of increasing exposure to industrial chemicals, the production of which has burgeoned since the early 1950s. Some discussion of the major additives or contaminants of our food supply that may be responsible is found in Chapter 9 (including diethylstilbesterol, aflatoxins, nitrosamines, artificial sweeteners, food colors, pesticides, PCBs, etc.). Another list of chemicals that at times have found their way into our diet is given in Table 16.2, which shows their relative effectiveness in inducing tumors in rats or mice. (The lifespan of rats and mice is somewhere between 1 and 3 years.) The levels of chlorinated hydrocarbons present in human fat (in this case, in Canada) are given in Table 16.3. Almost all of these hydrocarbons are carcinogens (Ames, 1979). There are also, of course, some "natural" carcinogens in the food supply (Ames, 1983b), but it seems less likely that their supply has increased in more recent decades, nor has it been documented that they have contributed to the current incidence of human cancer, except in the

Table 16.2. Incidence of Tumors After Giving Carcinogens to Rats and Mice

Continuous administration	Concentration in diet (ppm)	Time waited (months)	% tumors
Compound			
Aldrin (insecticide)	10	12	100
Aflatoxin B_1 (fungal toxin)	400	6	83
Tween 60 (emulsifier)	600	18	23
Benzpyrene (pyrolysis product)	1000	18	10
	10,000	12	74
Mirj 45 (emulsifier)	250,000	24	15
DDT (insecticide)	200–800	24	7
Sodium cyclamate (sweetener)	50,000	24	3
Single dose	**Dose/mouse (mg)**	**Time waited (months)**	**% tumors**
Compound			
Benzpyrene (pyrolysis product)	0.1	9	65
8-Hydroxyquinoline (preservative)	4–5	13	70
Maleic hydrazide (antisprouting agent)	3	12	18
	55	12	73
Senecio alkaloids (plant products)	4–5	8	25

case of contaminating aflatoxins (in some developing countries).

Of the various forms of cancer, those of the colorectum, breast, and prostate have been related to a high intake of fat, meat, and protein, and usually to low intakes of fiber and selenium; lung and epithelial cancers are related at least partly, to a lack of β-carotene or vitamin A; pancreatic cancer has been related to higher intakes of animal fat and protein, but also to sugar, coffee, and margarine consumption; stomach cancer is related to smoked, salted, or charred meats and fish, and the formation of nitrosamines. Formation of nitrosamines and of fat oxidation products capable of inducing a spectrum of different tumors in animals is inhibited by vitamin C or E in vitro and may be limited in vivo by the same antioxidants, as well as by other antioxidants like glutathione (formed from cysteine). Copper and copper-chelating agents may be protective against hepatoma (liver cancer) and other forms of cancer. Ethanol intake has been implicated in promotion of oral and esophageal cancers; and, in general, vegetables (especially the cruciferi—broccoli, cabbages) have been associated with preventative effects (Graham, 1979).

Based on the data available in 1982, the Committee on Diet, Nutrition and Cancer of the U.S. Academy of Sciences made four recommendations to reduce cancer incidence (Table 16.4). Although not universally accepted by experts on the subject, these recommendations are endorsed by a substantial proportion of investigators and still hold, overall. They represent a first attempt at preventative action against cancer by nutrition. The last part of the table summarizes evidence relating to additional dietary substituents (total calories, protein, selenium), where evidence is less developed. Details of most of these aspects, relating diet to cancer prevention, follow below.

Table 16.3. Chlorinated Hydrocarbons in Human Fat

Compound	Amount[a] (μg/kg wet wt)	% of samples containing residues
PCB	907	100
Hexachlorobenzene	62	100
BHC (lindane)	65	88
Oxychlordane	55	97
Trans-nonachlor	65	99
Heptachlor epoxide	43	100
Dieldrin	69	100
p,p′-DDE	2095	100
o,p′-DDT	31	63
p,p′-TDE	6	26
p,p′-DDT	439	100

Source: Data from Ames (1979).

[a] Mean of 168 Canadian samples.

Table 16.4. Summary of 1982 Dietary Recommendations Related to Cancer

Recommendation 1	Reduce intake of both saturated and unsaturated fat
Summary of evidence	The epidemiologic evidence was judged to be good, although not entirely consistent. The inconsistencies are explained in the report. The laboratory data were found to be supportive of the epidemiologic findings. The evidence concerning the proposed mechanisms for the action of fat was sparse, but indicative of a promotional effect
Type of evidence	Epidemiologic evidence: cancers of the breast, colon, prostate, and other sites Correlations: international and intranational Migrant studies Case control studies Laboratory evidence: tumors of the mammary gland, intestine, pancreas, liver, and other organs Spontaneous tumors Chemically induced: multiple carcinogens Dose–response: dose of carcinogen versus dose of fat Type of fat: saturated and unsaturated Species: mice or rats Measurements: incidence, lifespan, tumor multiplicity Transplantable tumors X-ray-induced tumors
Recommendation 2	Include fruit, vegetables, and whole grain cereal products in daily diet, especially citrus fruits and carotene-rich and cabbage family vegetables
Summary of evidence	The epidemiologic evidence derived from correlation, case control, and cohort studies was judged to be overall consistent with laboratory data from in vitro and in vivo tests designed to examine the effects of selected components of fruits and vegetables on carcinogenesis
Type of evidence	Epidemiologic evidence (1) Index of carotene or vitamin A intake: mostly case control and cohort studies showing inverse association Lung cancer: Norway, Singapore, United States Cancers of larynx, bladder, esophagus, stomach, colon-rectum, and prostate in various countries Serum vitamin A and total cancer incidence: cohort studies in United States and United Kingdom (2) Index of vitamin C intake: case control studies showing inverse association Stomach and esophageal cancer (mainland United States, Iran, Hawaii, Norway, Japan) Limited evidence for laryngeal cancer (3) Raw or cruciferous vegetable intake and inverse association Case control and cohort studies of stomach and colon cancer in different parts of the world, including the United States Laboratory evidence (1) Vitamin A and related compounds Vitamin A deficiency: higher incidence of chemically induced carcinogenesis in lung, bladder, and colon (in rats mostly) Vitamin A excess: lower incidence of chemically induced lung, forestomach, cervix, and skin cancer (in rats, mice, or hamsters); exceedingly high doses enhance incidence in some studies Vitamin A may act via effect on cell differentiation Retinoids: inhibit chemically induced neoplasia of breast, bladder, skin, lung, etc., in most studies; also cause regression of skin papillomas α-Carotene: data limited (2) Vitamin C Inhibits nitrosation in vitro and in vivo: limited, unimpressive data on inhibition of carcinogenesis in rats; regresses and/or prevents malignant transformation of cells in culture (3) Nonnutritive chemicals in fruits and cruciferous vegetables Indoles, phenols, flavones, aromatic isothiocyanates, and β-sitosterol inhibit carcinogenesis in vivo, act as blocking agents, antiinitiators, or antipromoters

(continued)

Table 16.4. *(continued)*

	Vegetables tested in animals and humans induce mixed function oxidase and glutathione S-transferase activity Some flavonoids (e.g., quercetin in onions) are mutagenic, but extracts of most fruits and vegetables are antimutagenic
Recommendation 3	Minimize consumption of cured, pickled, and smoked food
Summary of evidence	The epidemiologic data on esophageal cancer are limited compared to those for stomach cancer. Laboratory experiments to test the carcinogenicity of some components of cured, pickled, or smoked foods support the epidemiologic findings
Type of evidence	Epidemiologic studies: correlation, migrant, case control Esophageal cancer: China Stomach cancer: Japan, USSR, Norway, Iceland, Hungary, United States (Hawaii, high-risk states of Wisconsin, Minnesota, and Michigan) Experimental studies Nitrate and nitrite (cured meats, vegetables): no direct evidence of carcinogenicity; nitrite mutagenic in mammalian systems; both converted to N-nitroso compounds in vitro and in vivo N-nitroso compounds: over 90% of ~300 compounds tested are carcinogenic in multiple species and mutagenic in various systems Polycyclic aromatic hydrocarbons [benzo(a)pyrene, dibenzanthracene, benzathracene] (smoked foods, fatty meats, vegetables, and fruits from contaminated areas) cause cancers of multiple organs in multiple species; strongly mutagenic
Recommendation 4	Drink alcohol only in moderation
Summary of evidence	Higher incidence of colorectal cancer among excessive beer-drinking populations in some parts of the world, including the United States Excessive alcohol consumption, especially if combined with cigarette smoking, linked to increased risk of cancers of the mouth, larynx, esophagus, and respiratory tract Postulated mechanisms: alcohol may act as a carcinogen, cocarcinogen, or promoter; as a solvent facilitating intracellular transport of carcinogens; as an inducer of microsomal enzymes; as a source of putative carcinogens (contaminants); through an effect on nutritional or immunologic status
Lack of recommendations	On intake of total calories, dietary fiber, protein, and selenium

Explanation	Food component	Epidemiologic data	Laboratory data
	Total calories	Epidemiologic evidence indirect and limited	Reduction in total food intake decreases age-specific tumor incidence: effect of calories per se versus macronutrients not clear
	Dietary fiber	International correlations, good; intranational correlations, poor	Different fiber components inhibit or enhance carcinogenesis depending on condition
		Case control data inconsistent for total fiber, limited for fiber components; fat, possible confounding variable	Results inconsistent and difficult to equate with human studies
	Protein	Epidemiologic data limited and weaker compared to fat, especially case control studies	Overall, low-protein diets inhibit and high-protein diets enhance tumorigenesis, but data are inconsistent and limited compared to fat
	Selenium	Epidemiologic data limited to a few geographic correlation studies	Antitumorigenic effect, but frequently at doses that may be toxic in humans

Source: Modified from Palmer (1983). Based on Report by the National Academy of Sciences (U.S.) Committee on Diet, Nutrition, and Cancer, 1982.

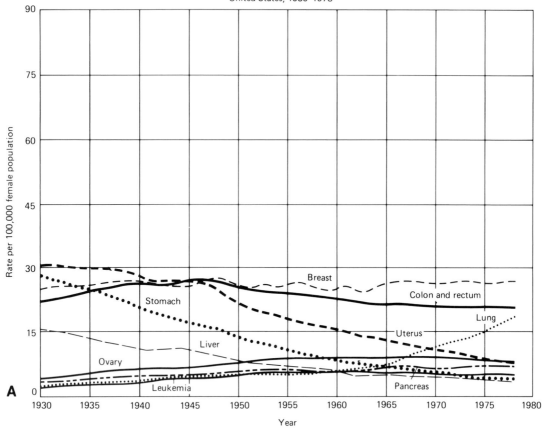

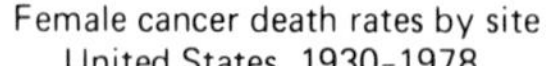
Female cancer death rates by site
United States, 1930-1978
Rate per 100,000 female population
90
75
60
45
30
15
0
Breast
Colon and rectum
Stomach
Lung
Uterus
Liver
Ovary
Leukemia
Pancreas
1930
1935
1940
1945
1950
1955
1960
1965
1970
1975
1980
Year

A

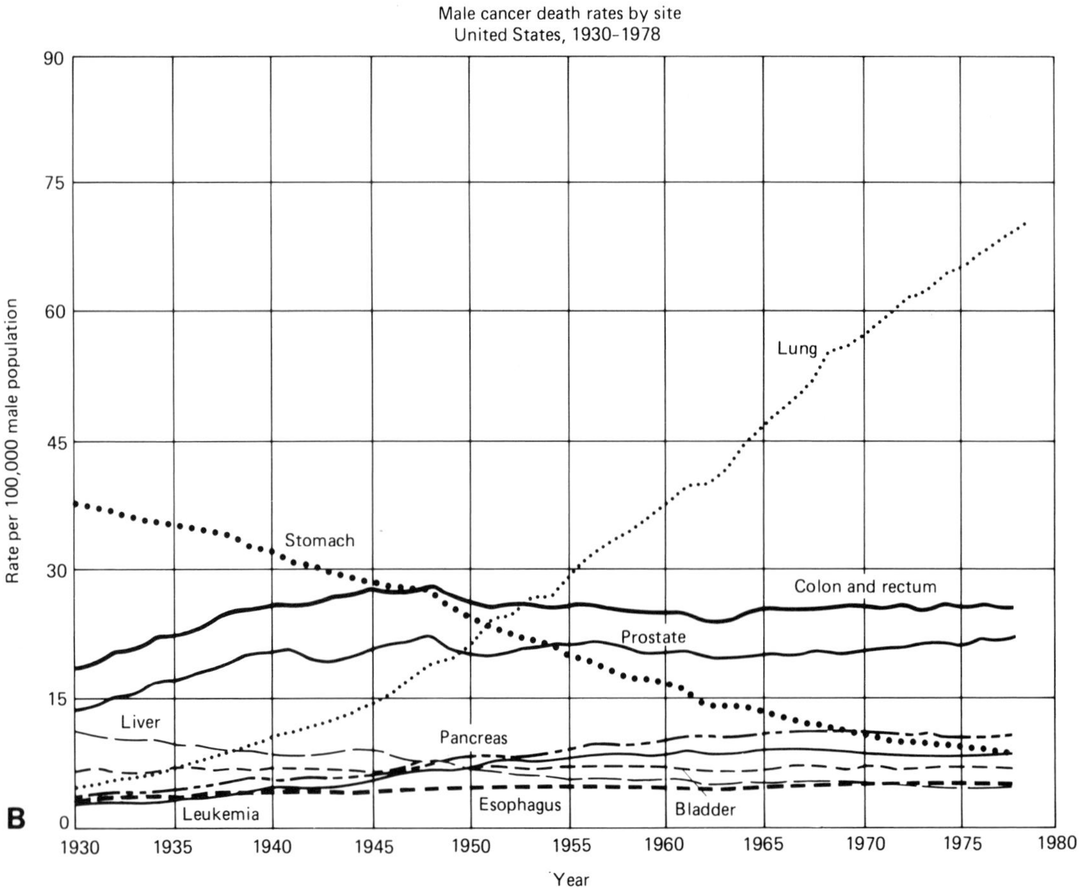

Male cancer death rates by site
United States, 1930-1978
Rate per 100,000 male population
90
75
60
45
30
15
0
Lung
Stomach
Colon and rectum
Prostate
Liver
Pancreas
Leukemia
Esophagus
Bladder
1930
1935
1940
1945
1950
1955
1960
1965
1970
1975
1980
Year

B

Table 16.5. Correlation Coefficients for Connections Between Intake of Various Dietary Components and the Incidence of Some Forms of Cancer and Heart Disease

	Rice	Maize	Beans	Cattle meat	Pork	Eggs	Milk	Animal oil and fat	Beer	Animal calories	Proteins	Fat
Colon	−0.34[a]	−0.67	−0.68	0.54	0.60	0.75	0.48	0.64	0.62	0.84	0.49	0.74
Breast (female)	−0.50	−0.66	−0.70	0.58	0.62	0.75	0.55	0.64	0.56	0.84	0.48	0.75
Prostate	−0.58	−0.53	−0.66	0.47	0.48	0.48	0.52	0.51	0.44	0.76	0.52	0.72
Atherosclerotic heart disease	−0.40			0.48			0.59	0.48		0.74	0.51	0.73

Source: Reprinted by permission from Correa (1981).

[a] Negative correlations denote inverse correlations; positive, positive correlations. The size of the correlation coefficient indicates the strength of the correlation (closer to 1.0 = stronger). All coefficients shown are significant ($p < 0.05$).

Fat, Fiber, and Cancer

Numerous epidemiologic calculations have associated intake of a high fat or low fiber diet with an increased risk of developing specific forms of cancer, especially cancer of the colon and breast, but also prostate (and some other sites). When cancer ascribable to tobacco use is excluded, these forms of cancer, together, account for the majority of American cancer deaths. Typically, data supporting a promotional role of fat (or suppressive role of fiber) in tumor incidence are obtained by comparing the average diets of different countries around the world (Figure 16.5, Table 16.5; Willett et al., 1990), or by comparing vegetarians with those on a typical "Western" high-fat, low-fiber diet. (Vegetarians exhibit a lower incidence of most cancer forms.)

The association between fat intake and cancer development is not new (see studies of A.F. Watson, E. Mellanby, and A. Tannenbaum in the 1930s and 1940s). However, only recently has the nature and importance of this connection begun to be evaluated. The interest in dietary fiber as a modulating component is also recent, dating largely from suggestions of Burkitt et al. (1972, 1974). These stemmed from experience with diet and disease patterns of native Africans. It is clear from the present vantage that both factors are probably important in the development of colon cancer and that examination of only one of these variables without controlling for, or considering, the other may lead to confusion in our interpretation of the results. Consequently, some comparisons of fat intakes and cancer incidence [e.g., for subpopulations within the United States (Enig et al., 1979*a*, *b*); Kolonel et al., 1981)] may show no correlation to colon cancer. (Nevertheless, both studies do show a positive relation to breast cancer.) What renders the epidemiologic findings more meaningful is a considerable wealth of animal work that corroborates the effects of the dietary factors experimentally. In the areas of colon and breast cancer development, mechanisms have been proposed that may ultimately explain (or help to explain) the relationships to diet. For other cancers that may also be affected by fat and fiber, work has not progressed as far.

Figure 16.4. (A) Female cancer death rates by site, United States, 1930–1978. **(B)** Male cancer death rates by site, United States, 1930–1978. Rate of population standardized for age on the 1970 U.S. population. [*Source:* Data from National Vital Statistics Division and Bureau of the Census, United States. American Cancer Society, 1981. Reprinted by their permission.]

Fat

Historically, it is estimated that until the last century the fat content of the average human diet was about 20% of calories or less (Cohen, 1987*a*; Walker, 1988), a phenomenon that still prevails today in some cultures and in underdeveloped countries. Indeed, the major increases in fat intake and cancer incidence have occurred in the Western world over the last 150 years. As already indicated (Figure 16.5), epidemiologic data have generally shown a strong correlation between fat intake and cancer, especially for breast and colon cancer, and when different countries are compared (Howe et al., 1990). [Within countries, correlations have not always been significant (Rosen et al., 1988).]

Animal studies, showing an enhancement of tumor incidence, have greatly strengthened the connection to fat intake, as illustrated by data in Tables 16.6 and 16.7. Moreover, for colon cancer, it has become clear that the effect is on the promo-

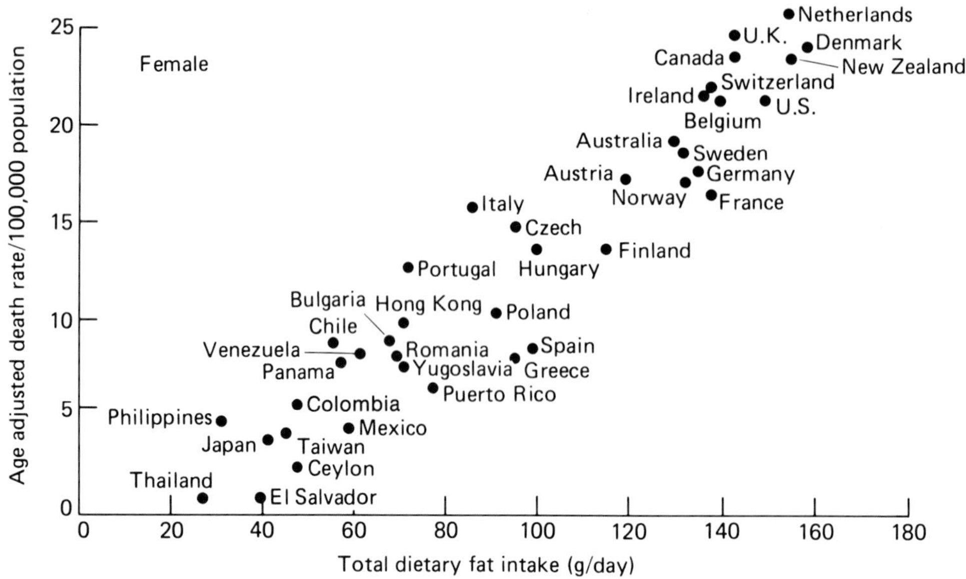

Figure 16.5. Epidemiologic relation between total fat intake and mortality from breast cancer around the world. [*Source:* Data are from the mid-1960s. Reprinted by permission from Carroll (1975).]

tional rather than initiating phase of carcinogenesis (e.g., a high fat diet fed after, rather than during, exposure to carcinogen has the same effect as feeding it throughout). In the case of breast cancer, an effect on initiation may also be present (Table 16.7).

In general, the type of fat does appear to make a difference, as summarized in Table 16.8. At least for experimental colon cancer, plant oils high in linoleic acid (the most important essential fatty acid) appear to enhance tumorigenesis more than those containing more saturated or shorter chain fatty acids (olive and coconut oil) or than animal (beef) fat or fish oil. In general, the same trends are apparent for mammary and other forms of cancer induced in experimental animals. (For particulars on the compositions of these oils and fats, see Chapter 3, Table 3.6.) The mechanisms of the effects of fat are thought to involve changes in bile acids, prostaglandins, and/or other hormones, as will be described.

Table 16.6. Colon Tumor Incidence in Rats Fed Carcinogen Plus Diets High or Low in Fat

Diet fat	Protein	Carcinogen	% rats with colon tumor
5% Lard	25% Casein	DMH[a]	17
20% Lard	25% Casein	DMH[a]	67
5% Corn oil	25% Casein	DMH[a]	36
20% Corn oil	25% Casein	DMH[a]	64
6% Beef fat	19% Beef protein	DMH[a]	35
24% Beef fat	40% Beef protein	DMH[a]	57
6% Corn oil	19% Soybean protein	DMH[a]	35
24% Corn oil	40% Soybean protein	DMH[a]	54
5% Beef fat	22% Casein	MNU[b]	27
20% Beef fat	22% Casein	MNU[b]	34

Source: Data from Reddy (1979).

[a] Female F344 rats, at 7 weeks of age, were given weekly subcutaneous dimethylhydrazine at a dose rate of 10 mg/kg body weight for 20 weeks and autopsied 10 weeks later.

[b] Male F344 rats, at 7 weeks of age, were given intrarectally methylnitrosurea, 2.5 mg/rat twice in 1 week, and autopsied 30 weeks later.

Table 16.7. Effects of Lard and Corn Oil on Carcinogenesis Promotion[a]

Dietary fat		Mammary tumor incidence (%) at the following ages (weeks)			
Type	Content (% wt)	17	20	21	23
Fed fat during DMBA treatment					
Corn oil	5	9	20	26	40
Corn oil	20	17	43	57	66
Lard	5	6	24	45	45
Lard	20	29	51	57	71
Fed fat after DMBA treatment[b]					
Corn oil	20	29	51	63	63
Lard	5	11	17	34	34
Lard	20	11	23	37	37

Source: Data from Rogers and Wetsel (1981).

[a] There were 35 rats per group, fed dimethylbenzanthracene (DMBA). Results are based on gross diagnosis.
[b] All rats in these groups were fed 5% corn oil *during* DMBA treatment.

Fiber

As for fat intake, fiber intake (especially from cereal grains—bread and porridge) declined a great deal in the Western world since the end of the last century, in part with the advent of widespread milling and refining of grains and flour (Cohen, 1987*a*; Walker, 1988). With very few exceptions, epidemiologic studies support a protective effect of dietary fiber for the development of human colon cancer (Jacobs, 1986). Case control studies in man have been less consistently positive, but animal studies suggest that the type of fiber (and type of carcinogen) may be the key to a positive response, the less soluble fibers of wheat bran, cellulose, hemicellulose, and psyllium being more protective, the more soluble ones (oat bran, alfalfa, pectins, and guar gum) less so, or even promotional of colon cancer (Calvert et al., 1987; Jacobs, 1986; Jenkins et al., 1986; Roberts-Anderson et al., 1987). (Examples are given in Table 16.9.) Insoluble fibers provide more bulk and dilution of the contents of the gastrointestinal tract; soluble fibers are more readily digested by colonic bacteria, providing short-chain fatty acids that can be used by intestinal cells (see Chapter 3). This may explain the sometimes tumor-enhancing effects of soluble fiber. [Soluble forms of fiber also bind

Table 16.8. Type of Fat and Carcinogenesis Promotion by Site in Experimental Animals[a]

	Enhancement of chemical carcinogenesis in				
Type of fat	Colon	Breast	Liver	Pancreas	Lung
Corn oil	+++,−	+++	+++	++	+++
Safflower oil	+++				
Sunflower oil	+++	++			++
Linoleate		+++[b]			
Olive oil	−				
Coconut oil	−,+	+,−	+++	−	
Lard/beef tallow	++,−	++	++,−		
Hydrogenated	−,+				
Fish oil (n-3)	−,+				
Effect is on	promotion	promotion and initiation	promotion and initiation	promotion	promotion and initiation

Sources: Cohen (1987*b*), Reddy (1987), Nelson et al. (1988), and Ip et al. (1985).

[a] In general, the influence of feeding a low versus high fat diet on tumor incidence was compared. Increased tumor incidence and degree of enhancement is indicated by (+) = positive and (−) = negative.
[b] Metastases were enhanced in a transplantable tumor model (Hubbard and Erickson, 1987).

Table 16.9. Effect of Different Forms of Dietary Fiber on Incidence of Colon Tumors in Rats

Study and type of fiber	Diet (%)	Animals with tumors (%)	Significance[a]	Tumors/ tumor-bearing rat	Carcinogen[b]
I. Control	0	86	—	3.0	DMH
Wheat bran (± bile salts)	10	64–67	$p < 0.05$	1.6–1.8	
II. Control	0	50	—	1.9	DMH
Cellulose	9.7	30	$p < 0.05$	1.3	
Psyllium	9.7	20	$p < 0.05$	1.8	
III. Control	5	57	—	1.5	AOM
Wheat bran	+15	33	$p < 0.05$	1.2	
Alfalfa	+15	53	NS	1.3	
Pectin	+15	10	$p < 0.05$	1.0	
Control	5	69	—	1.5	MNU
Wheat bran	+15	59	NS	1.7	
Alfalfa	+15	83	NS	2.8	
Pectin	+15	60	NS	1.3	
IV. Control	0	33 (29)[c]	—	1.1	DMH
Cellulose	10	49 (38)	NS (NS)[c]	1.0	
Oat bran	20	57 (22)	NS (NS)	1.2	
Pectin	10	42 (13)	NS ($p < 0.05$)	1.0	
Guar gum	10	63 (8)	$p < 0.05$ ($p < 0.01$)	2.0	

Sources: (I) Calvert et al. (1987), studied 2–6 weeks; (II) Roberts-Anderson et al. (1987), studied 22 weeks; (III) Watanabe et al. (1979), studied 8 weeks; (IV) Jacobs and Lupton (1986), studied 30 weeks.

[a] Compared to controls.
[b] DMH = dimethylhydrazine; AOM = azoxymethane; MNU = methylnitrosurea.
[c] Tumors of the small intestine.

more cholesterol and bile acids, and tend to have a more beneficial (lowering) effect on blood cholesterol.] Only indirectly is fiber implicated in protection against breast and prostate cancer (Table 16.5; rice, maize, and beans), and this has not been studied in animal models.

Mechanisms of Fat and Fiber Effects

Colon Cancer

Both fat and fiber are thought to act indirectly to influence formation of colon cancer by altering the extent of biliary secretion, and especially the colon concentration of bile acids and their derivatives. These substances, in turn, act as "promoters" of the carcinogenic process, a process "initiated" by other chemical substances in the local, colonic epithelium. (Bile acids do not in themselves cause colon cancer in animals.) In support of this concept are observations that: (1) fat intake is positively related to the secretion (and excretion) of bile acids; (2) bile acids and derivatives, especially in the nongermfree gut, "promote" chemical carcinogenesis (Reddy, 1981); (3) specific bile acid derivatives, like lithocholic acid, produced from chenodeoxycholic and cholic acids (the main liver-produced forms) by gut bacteria, are cancer "promoters" even in germfree animals (Reddy, 1981); and (4) the most bulk-producing forms of fiber are the most effective at reducing colon carcinogenesis in experimental animals and are also the most effective at diluting the cancer-promoting (or cocarcinogenic) bile acids and derivatives in the colon. The mechanism by which certain bile acids promote carcinogenesis is thought to involve a stimulation of cell proliferation (Wargovich et al., 1983). At least in the case of wheat bran, there may be an additional or alternative, nonbile acid-involving protective effect: In one study, the inclusion of excess bile acids in the feed of rats treated with chemical carcinogen did not impair the effectiveness of the bran in reducing development of colon tumors (Calvert et al., 1987; Table 16.9).

Of special interest, too, are observations that Western populations with similar intakes of fat (and protein, etc.), but quite different intakes of fiber, will have a quite different incidence of colon cancer and that their feces will contain different proportions of the bile acids and their derivatives. Table 16.10 illustrates data obtained by Reddy and colleagues (Reddy, 1979) for male volunteers in Finnish and U.S. urban areas. The Finns, with a much greater intake of cereal grain in the form of a traditional rye bread, and more of their protein and fat from milk and dairy products, had almost three times the fecal bulk of New Yorkers and an average of about two bowel movements per day. This may explain why, despite a high intake of fat, they had a lower incidence of colon cancer. Concentrations (but not total quantities) of bile acids and the relative proportions of lithocholic and trihydroxycholanic acid were also much lower in the case of the Finns, due to dilution by the dietary fiber. [The importance of the diluting effect is borne out by other studies (Nigro et al., 1987).] Fecal mutagens (as determined by the Ames test in three different bacterial strains) were also much more prevalent in the feces of the typical New Yorkers versus the Finns (or New York vegetarians) (Table 16.10). The results of a Mayo Clinic study of 1600 patients, followed over 20 years, are also relevant. These patients had had their gallbladders removed, resulting in a continuous, uncontrolled secretion of bile acid. As would be predicted from the hypothesis advanced, these patients had twice the normal incidence of colon cancer.

Effects of dietary fiber on the "transit time" of materials taken orally does not appear to be a major factor in colon carcinogenesis, in that women more generally are constipated than men yet have a lower incidence of colon cancer (Eastwood et al., 1976). Also, white versus Japanese-Hawaiians, with similar diets, have the same incidence of colon cancer, but a different gut transit time (Glober et al., 1974). The relative importance of the bacterial metabolism (especially anaerobic metabolism) of bile acids in tumor promotion is still unclear. The group of Reddy, Wynder, and others at the American Health Foundation believes this may be important, whereas others, such as Hill et al. (1981) and Kay (1981), stress they have found few effects of diet on the composition of the bacterial flora. Reddy (1981) has reported elevated bacterial 7α-dehydroxylating activity in feces from colon cancer patients. Similar data of Hill et al. (1981) (see Table 16.11) show a difference in the percentage of individuals with "NDH" clostridia (capable of modifying steroids), comparing colon cancer patients with other groups. But this does not in itself tell you which came first, the clostridia or the cancer. Indeed, considering the long time lag to tumor development, observations—that patients in the first stage of a potentially precancerous large bowel condition (polyps less than 1 cm in diameter) do not have a higher-than-normal prevalence of clostridia (Hill et al., 1981)—suggest, if anything, that clostridial infiltration follows long after initiation and the early events of tumor development.

An apparent protectiveness of calcium intake may also bear on the actions of bile acids in colon carcinogenesis promotion. A number of prospective and retrospective epidemiologic studies (Sorenson et al., 1988), including the Finnish study cited in Table 16.10, and most recently a Swedish study (Rosen et al., 1988), have identified milk, dairy products, and/or calcium per se as factors associated with a decreased risk of colon cancer in man. It is thought that the Ca^{2+} forms less soluble salts of the bile acids which are then not reabsorbed. In support of this concept, mice that were fed extra deoxycholic acid to stimulate proliferation of their colonic epithelium showed little or no such stimulation when calcium lactate was instillated intrarectally (Wargovich et al., 1983) (Fig. 16.6). The overall conclusion is that factors that influence the nature, secretion, solubility, and dilution of bile acids in the gut (notably fat intake, some forms of fiber, and calcium) all work to protect the colon against the promotion of carcinogenesis. An additional variable influenced by fat intake may be the production of prostaglandins (see under Breast Cancer).

Breast Cancer

The current hypothesis of greatest interest, which explains the association between breast cancer and fat intake, is that the latter influences the secretion and metabolism of various hormones that promote or inhibit the growth of tumors, most notably the estrogens and prostaglandins. A substantial percentage of breast cancers is estrogen-dependent for growth, and at least in higher doses, estrogens (notably diethylstilbesterol, DES; Melnick et al., 1987; see Chapter 9) are known to initiate and/or promote carcinogenesis. In further support of this concept are observations that vegetarian women (and men) (who consume less fat) tend to have lower plasma concentrations of estrogens (and androgens) (especially estrone) and excrete 2–3 times more estrogen via the feces compared to nonvegetarian control subjects (Goldin et al., 1981, 1982; Hill, 1981; Howie and Shultz, 1985). Recent studies demonstrate that a low fat diet (20% versus 40% of calories) will substantially lower serum concentrations of nonprotein-bound estradiol (and testosterone) in women before (but not after) menopause (Ingram et al., 1987). (Most cancer initiation and promotion probably occurs before menopause.) A higher crude fiber intake has also been associated with lower serum estrogen (Howie and Shultz, 1985), all of which might help to explain the lower incidence of cancer in vegetarians. Prolactin might also be a factor. Blood levels appear to be lower in vegetarians (Goldin et al., 1981; Hill et al., 1981); and in animals, prolactin promotes breast carcinogenesis and fat promotes prolactin secretion (Cohen, 1981). [Prolactin levels also are higher in nonvegetarian men (Howie and Schultz, 1985), and this might perhaps underlie the connection between fat and prostate cancer.]

Obese individuals have a greater risk of breast cancer (and cancer of the colon or endometrium) (Kirschner et al., 1981). Some studies *have* suggested that obesity may cause an increased retention and decreased turnover of estrogens (Zumoff, 1981), as well as increased plasma concentrations of the hormones. Increased peripheral tissue production of estradiol from androstenedione may also occur. These various views of the connection between fat and breast cancer are still controversial, in that Carroll (1981) found no associations among fat intake, prolactin levels, and tumor incidence in rats, and Gray et al. (1982*a*, *b*) found no differences in plasma hormone levels, either among girls on vegetarian versus regular diets, or girls from the United States, Chile, Japan, and Papua (New Guinea) on different diets—differences that could be statistically related to their intakes of fat, fiber, fish, milk, and other foodstuffs. However, fat may promote the effectiveness of estrogens (and progesterone) on mammary cell growth (Welsch, 1987), and this may occur by other means. Obviously, the estrogen hypotheses require further substantiation.

The other hypothesis of note for mammary cancer is that the effect of dietary fat may be via production of linoleic acid-derived prostaglandins. Linoleic acid is converted to arachidonic acid, which (as an important substituent of membrane phospholipids) is released in response to neutral and hormonal triggers and becomes the substrate for formation of specific eicosanoids (prostaglandins, thromboxanes, leukotrienes) that influence cell metabolic activity, growth, and migration. (See Chapter 3 for details on eicosanoid forms, functions, and the relation to type of dietary fat.) That prostaglandins (or thromboxanes) derived from arachidonic acid are involved in tumor promotion is supported by the following

Table 16.10. Comparisons of Nutrient Intakes, Feces, Fiber, and Bile Acid Excretion Among Middle-aged Men in Kuopio, Finland, and New York City[a]

	Kuopio	New York
Total protein	94.8 ± 3.5	86.7 ± 2.0
Total fat	96.6 ± 2.3	99.6 ± 1.7
Saturated fats	53.7 ± 1.4	47.7 ± 1.3
Other fats	42.9 ± 1.6	51.9 ± 1.7
Carbohydrate	317.6 ± 4.2	283.2 ± 3.7
Total calories (kcal/day)	2521 ± 39	2380 ± 20
Protein calories (% total)	15.0 ± 0.4	14.6 ± 0.3
Fat calories (% total)	34.3 ± 0.5	37.9 ± 0.5
Number of bowel movements/day	1.85	1.00
Fecal dry matter (%)	22.0 ± 1.0	28.7 ± 2.0[b]
Dry feces excreted (g)	60.3 ± 7.6	22.3 ± 1.0[b]
Fecal fiber (g)	24.8 ± 2.2	9.2 ± 0.8[b]
Total bile acids		
(mg/g)	4.59 ± 0.42	11.7 ± 0.54[b]
(mg/day)	277 ± 22	275 ± 14
Lithocholic acid (mg/g)	1.40 ± 0.16	3.27 ± 0.15[b]
3α, 7β, 12α triOH, 5β-cholanic acid	0.04 ± 0.01	9.12 ± 0.01[b]
Other bile acid derivatives	0.93 ± 0.08	3.8 ± 0.26[b]
Mutagenic activity (% of fecal samples)	13	22
(No. of systems in which positive)	1	4

[a] Data obtained from 3-day diet recall (diet histories) and typical foodstuffs consumed by the volunteers; averages ± SEM (Reddy, 1979, 1981).

[b] Significantly different from Kuopio ($p < 0.05$).

[c] In at least 1 of 5 test systems

Table 16.11. Frequency of Steroid Dehydrogenating Clostridia in Patients with Large Bowel Cancer

Patient group	No. studied	% carrying NDH clostridia
Controls (normal healthy persons)	116	38
Large bowel cancer patients	120	83
Dukes A cases	16	88
Large bowel polyp cases	74	42
Adenomatous, >2 cm diameter	18	78
Adenomatous, <1 cm diameter	22	13
Nonadenomatous	16	31
Patients with long-term ulcerative colitis[a]	82	29
Those patients who went on to develop adenocarcinoma or severe dysplasia	9	67

Source: Data from Hill et al. (1981).

[a] Patients with colitis involving the whole of the large bowel for more than 10 years.

findings. (1) Linoleic acid (and plant oils high in this fatty acid) are most effective and may even be essential (Ip et al., 1985) in promoting (or initiating) mammary tumor development and metastases, as shown in animal models (Table 16.8 and 16.12). (2) Indomethacin, an inhibitor of the cyclooxygenase that initiates prostaglandin (and thromboxane) formation, has been shown to inhibit mammary tumor development in rats (McCormick et al., 1985) (and also colon tumors in rats; Narisawa et al., 1981). (3) Fish oils, containing n-3 fatty acids, which produce a different set of eicosanoids (see Chapter 3), tend not to promote (and may in fact inhibit) tumorigenesis. This has been shown for the colon of rats (Nelson et al., 1988; Reddy, 1987) and also for human prostatic tumors, implanted into nude mice (Karmali et al., 1987). (4) The type of fat ingested does influence the type of prostaglandin found in the tumor itself (Table 16.12), and breast cancers produce substantial amounts of prostaglandins (Rosen, 1987*a*). (5) The types of fatty substances found on the surfaces of the tumor would also appear to be related to their degree of malignancy, as suggested by recent NMR data (Smith and Chmurny, 1990). Finally, (6) differences in prostaglandins may help to explain why certain Mediterranean populations (notably Greeks and Spaniards) ingesting mainly olive oil, also have a lower incidence of colon and breast cancer.

Animal studies indicate that the amount of fat eaten is clearly critical, and moreover, initial studies of Cohen (1987*a*, *b*) and others (Ip et al., 1985) suggest that the dose–response to fat is not linear, but involves a "threshold" beyond which all responses are positive. Based on animal studies, Cohen proposes this threshold to be at about 20%–25% of caloric intake, a very low fat diet by Western standards, but one more prevalent in certain cultures and developing nations (Hebert and Wynder, 1987). This would be consistent with findings that only very low intakes of fat reduce levels of serum estrogens and androgens (Boyar et al., 1988; Ingram et al., 1987), and would help to explain failures to correlate breast cancer incidence with fat intakes that were greater than 30% of calories (Mills et al., 1988; Willett et al., 1987*a*).

Table 16.12. Effects of a High Intake of Different Kinds of Fat on Mammary Tumorigenesis in Rats

	Tumor		Serum arachidonic acid	Tumor	
Type of fat	Incidence (%)	Time of first appearance	(% fatty acid)	PGE_2 (ng/g)	PGF_2 (ng/g)
Control[a]					
Low fat intake	60–66	118–146	—	—	—
Experimental (high fat)					
Safflower oil	87	85	82	38	76
Corn oil	87	80	56	23	130
Olive oil	63	148	7	5	64
Coconut oil	47	157	0.8	3	27

Source: Data of Cohen (1987*b*).

[a] Control rats were fed 5% fat, experimentals on high fat (23% by weight). N-nitrosomethylurea was the initiating carcinogen.

Vitamins and Cancer

Vitamin C

Use of megadoses of vitamin C in cancer therapy has been strongly promoted by Linus Pauling and his Scottish physician colleague, Ewan Cameron, based on theoretical and speculative considerations (Cameron et al., 1979), and findings that patients terminally ill with various forms of cancer had a much longer survival when treated with 10 g doses of the vitamin than similar patients without any treatment (Cameron and Pauling, 1976, 1978). For these reports, the "control groups" were obtained from the records of hundreds of similar patients in the same region who had not been treated. The data are difficult to interpret, in that they do not address the problem of a "placebo" effect. Indeed, the double-blind study of Creagan et al. (1979) at the Mayo Clinic found no difference in the response of 123 patients treated daily with similar dosages of vitamin C (4×2.5 g/day) or with a placebo of similar color and taste. In this study, both treatment groups survived twice as long as patients usually do when affected with terminal cancer of various kinds. This indicates strongly that a favorable response to placebo can occur in cancer patients, a finding underscored by evidence that the psychologic orientation of the cancer patient plays a role in his/her survival (Bahnson, 1969). The study of Creagan was criticized for not fully checking on patient compliance, the extent to which the vitamin was absorbed, and whether the placebo group was also treating itself with extra vitamins and/or large amounts of fruits and vegetables. Cameron (1980) and Pauling (1980) also stressed that the difference between Creagan's results and their own could be due to the continued use of chemotherapy and radiation in the patients at Mayo Clinic. However, *all three* factors were addressed in a subsequent study (Moertel et al., 1985) which replicated the earlier Creagan results. Thus, it seems unlikely that high ascorbate treatments would benefit terminal cancer patients beyond offering them hope or extra care. At the same time, treatment of terminal patients with vitamin C is in most cases probably no worse than conventional therapy.

Several studies on cells in tissue culture show no distinction between the cytotoxicity of the vitamin to malignant versus normal cells, with the possible exception of melanoma cells high in copper (Bram et al., 1980). [Here, the thought is that oxidation of ascorbate, enhanced by copper, increases the rate of production of peroxide, leading to cellular damage (Prasad, 1980).] The concentrations of ascorbate required for cytotoxicity are high, usually in the range of 1 mM, but are within range of what can be achieved with intakes of 10 g/day in man (10 g = 50 mmol in a 50–70 kg person ~ 0.8–1 mM, not correcting for efficiency of absorption, rates of excretion, etc.). Such doses might have cytotoxic effects on the patients' normal cells as well. DeClerck and Jones (1980) have observed that the extracellular matrix material, produced by smooth muscle cells in cultures with plenty of vitamin C, is more readily ingested and invaded by tumor cells than matrix produced by a vitamin-C-deficient culture—an observation that tends to argue against a protective action of the vitamin through stimulation of tumor encapsulation or inhibition of tumor cell invasion. There are some reports of protective effects of high doses of C on carcinogenesis in animal models (Birt, 1986); in other cases, carcinogenesis was actually stimulated. Although the possibility of positive actions via stimulation of the immune system (see Chapter 7) have not really been ruled out, the effects of high doses of this antioxidant are clearly complex and would seem to offer little hope to subjects who have cancer.

Vitamins C and E in the Prevention of Nitrosamine Formation

As already described in Chapter 9, nitrosamines are formed by reaction of nitrite (NO_2^-) with amines (or amides) under conditions of low pH (pH 2–4), such as occur in the stomach (see Chapter 9, Figure 9.3). Nitrite can react with primary, secondary, or tertiary amines, but stable nitrosamines are usually the products of the nitrosation of secondary amines—as, for example, pyrrolidine (formed from polyamines present in most meats) or dimethylamine. (Primary amines are usually deaminated; tertiary amines are converted to secondary amines.) (Nitrosamides can be formed by reaction with amide groups, such as those of glutamine and asparagine.) Most nitrosamines (and probably nitrosamides) are carcinogens; nitrosopyrrolidine is a moderate one, and dimethylnitrosamine is a strong one (Mirvish, 1981*a*). The reactivity of a given amine will depend on its basicity and the pH of the environment, which also influences the concentration of nitrous acid (HNO_2) (pK 3.4). Nitrous acid forms N_2O_3 ($2HNO_2 \rightarrow H_2O + N_2O_3$), the reactive species for nitrosation (Mirvish, 1981*a*). Body fluids contain substantial amounts of nitrite, whether a

Table 16.13. Average Daily Nitrosamine Intakes from Various Sources

Source	Form of nitrosamine	Daily intake (μg/person)
Cigarette smoke	Numerous	17
Auto interiors	N-nitrosodimethylamine N-nitrosodiethylamine N-nitrosomorpholine	0.2–0.5
Cosmetics	N-nitrosodiethanolamine	0.4
Beer	N-nitrosodimethylamine	0.3–1.0
Scotch whiskey	N-nitrosodimethylamine	0.03
Cured meats, cooked bacon	N-nitrosohydroxypyrrolidone	0.2

Source: Modified from Scanlan (1983).

person consumes processed meats and vegetables high in this substance or not (see Chapter 9, Nitrate), and the diet contains secondary amines capable of forming carcinogenic nitrosamines. Nitrosamines of many kinds can thus be formed in the bodies of humans or animals under the right conditions (or in foods prior to ingestion), and many of these have been shown to induce cancer in various organs of different animal species. Traces of nitrosamines do occur in the food supply, especially in cured meats and some alcoholic beverages (Scanlan, 1983). (Many beers contained significant quantities until recently, when methods of processing were changed.) From the data available, daily intakes will vary greatly depending on dietary (and smoking) habits. Countries with a high rate of gastric cancer tend to have a high nitrate content in food and drinking water (Gold et al., 1987) (Table 16.13). [The incidence of stomach cancer is relatively low in Western countries.] Hypoacidity in the stomach (as occurs in pernicious anemia) enhances nitrite (and thus presumably nitrosamine) production, and is associated with a higher risk of cancer (Ruddell et al., 1978). Therefore, it is likely that a proportion of the cancer cases in humans may be attributed to the actions of these agents.

Vitamins C and E are both antioxidants and, as such, have been examined for their capacities to inhibit the nitrosation process. The effectiveness of ascorbic acid under test-tube conditions is well-documented, as shown by some data in Table 16.14. It involves the reaction of HNO_2 (as N_2O_3) with either ascorbic acid or its anion (Figure 16.7), thus competing with amine-nitrosation reactions (Mirvish, 1981*a*). This approach has been used by some food processors to lower the possibility of nitrosamine formation in prepared foods. Usually, 500 ppm ascorbate is added to the 120 ppm $NaNO_2$ used as an antibacterial preservative (see Chapter 9). The potential inhibitory effects of tocopherols (vitamin E) have also been investigated (Mergens, 1982; Newmark and Mergens, 1981), and the occurrence of nitrosation by N_2O_3 within a hydrophobic environment (like fat tissue or cell membranes) has been recognized. It is thought that this latter type of nitrosation is most affected by the lipid-soluble tocopherols (Figure 16.8). Thus, both types of antioxidant vitamins may be important in maintaining reduced levels of nitrosamines in the body, as may other antioxidants like glutathione (produced from cysteine and other amino acids). [Phenols (such as tannic acids) found in plant foods also can inhibit nitrosation (Shils, 1988).]

The question is whether this is so in vivo and, if it is, at what levels of dietary (or supplemental) intake will inhibition occur. Several investigators have inhibited the induction of tumors in animals

Table 16.14. Inhibition of Nitrosamine Formation by Vitamin C: Morpholine[a]

pH	Time (min)	Nitrosamine yield without inhibitor (%)	% inhibition by Ascorbate	Urea	Ammonium sulfamate
1	45	7	—	95	100
2	30	20	98	24	100
3	30	65	100	2	99
4	30	34	100	—	71

Source: Reprinted by permission from Mirvish (1981*b*).

[a] Conditions: 25 m*M* morpholine, 50 m*M* nitrite, 100 m*M* inhibitor, 25°C.

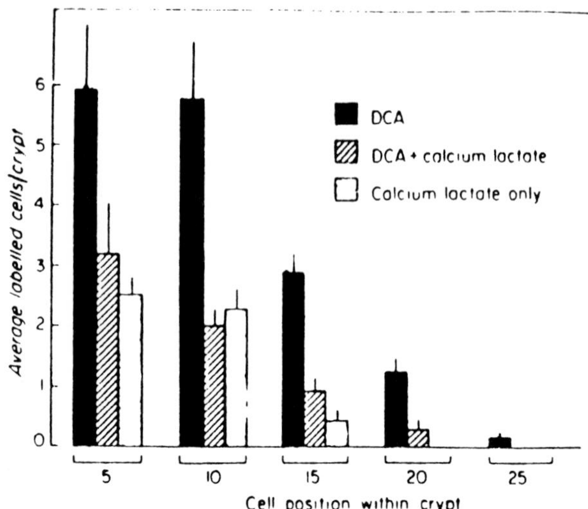

Figure 16.6. Effects of bile acid and calcium on the proliferation of colonic epithelium. Mice received deoxycholic acid (DCA), intrarectally 24 hr before death, and daily oral calcium lactate supplements. (Controls received oral calcium lactate alone.) Cell proliferation was measured at different levels in the intervillus crypts of the colon, by incorporation of ^{3}H-thymidine. [*Source:* Reprinted by permission from Wargowich et al. (1983).]

consuming large amounts of nitrite and amines with very large doses of ascorbic acid (Mirvish, 1981*a*). For example, 37%–91% inhibition was achieved with ascorbate concentrations of 5.8–23 g/kg of food (Mirvish, 1981*a*). Lower doses were not tried, probably because inhibition appeared to fall off quite rapidly at the lower end of the range examined. Of course, in these kinds of studies, concentrations of the nitrosation substrates ingested were also inordinately high. Vitamin E has been used in numerous studies to inhibit carcinogenesis induced by ultraviolet light (Black and Chan, 1975) or polycyclic hydrocarbons (Newmark and Mergens, 1981). Again, doses have been very large, usually 50–200 times normal daily intakes. Very large doses were also found to inhibit the increased synthesis of nitrosamines induced in humans by the administration of nitrate and proline (Wagner et al., 1985); and epidemiologic studies (Bjelke, 1983; Staehelin et al., 1987) suggest a significant inverse relationship between low-adequate versus above-adequate intakes of ascorbate (as well as vitamin E and carotenes) and the incidence/mortality from cancers of the upper gastrointestinal tract (mouth to stomach), which may be encouraging. Also, several prospective studies have found a consistent association between a higher general cancer risk and a low serum level of α-tocopherol (Knekt et al., 1988), and low serum vitamin C concentrations have been associated with a higher risk of cervical cancer or dysplasia (Orr et al., 1985; Romney et al., 1985, 1987). Protection by vitamin C against

Figure 16.7. Mechanism for the inhibition of nitrosation reactions by ascorbate. The ratio of k_2/k_1 is 230 : 1. [*Source:* Reprinted by permission from Mirvish (1981*b*).]

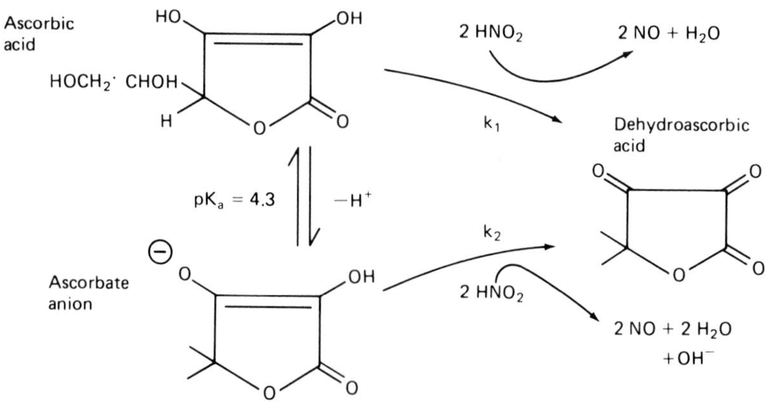

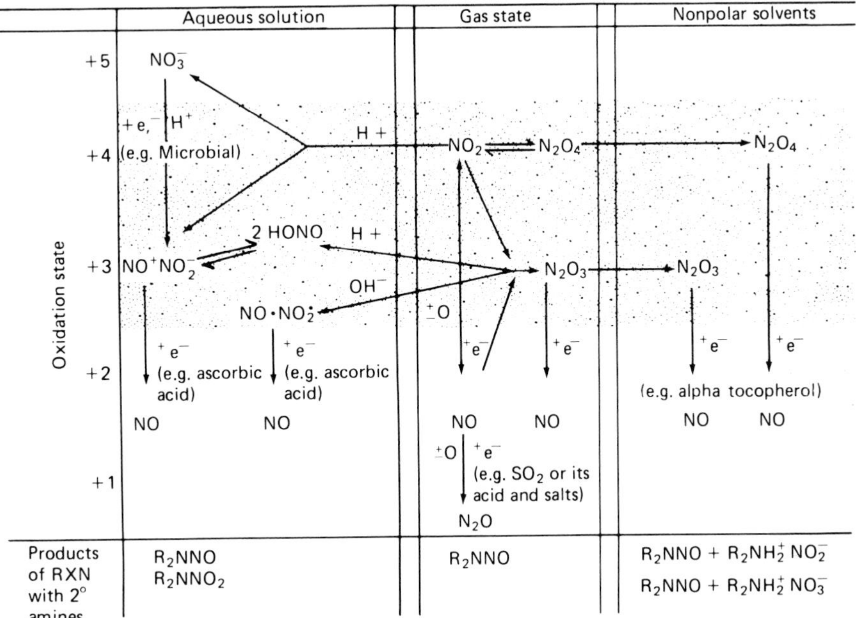

Figure 16.8. Potential nitrogen oxide states and nitrosation reactions in aqueous, gaseous, and lipid environments. Shaded area designates oxides capable of nitrosating secondary amines. [*Source:* Reprinted by permission from Newmark and Mergens (1981).]

carcinogenesis has also been observed in some animal studies, but not in others (Birt, 1986). Most (but not all) of this would be consistent with actions of the antioxidant vitamins on nitrosamine formation.

Antioxidant Vitamins and Fecal Mutagens

Suggestive evidence linking potential anticarcinogenic actions to reasonable doses of both vitamins C and E in humans was obtained by Bruce and colleagues at the University of Toronto, who observed that the content of certain mutagens in human feces appeared to be related to intakes of these vitamins (Bruce, 1983). The original basis for this work was the Ames test (Ames, 1979), in which the reversion to normal of mutant strains of bacteria requiring an amino acid for growth is assessed following their exposure to potential mutagenic agents. As a large proportion of carcinogens are also mutagens, the Ames test (and other similar tests) can be used as a form of screening procedure for potential carcinogens (Tennant et al., 1987). However, certain classes of carcinogens are not mutagenic in these tests, and, conversely, not all mutagens are carcinogenic. Bruce and colleagues showed that organic extracts of human feces often contained mutagens, the concentrations of which varied greatly with the individual. More importantly, groups of individuals on diets containing amounts of vitamins C and E closer to, or above, those recommended by the government tended to carry lower burdens of fecal mutagens than groups on diets low in these vitamins (Bruce, 1983; Dion et al., 1982). Also, individuals with high mutagen levels reduced them dramatically by taking supplements. The main mutagens involved were found to be highly unsaturated mono-fatty acid-glycerol-ethers (termed fecal pentaenes), produced by gut bacteria (Kingston et al., 1981; Van Tassell et al., 1986). However, a recent study, in which patients with polyps that had been resected were placed on supplements of vitamins C and E (or placebo) for 2 years, showed no difference in the recurrence of polyposis (Bruce, 1987). This suggests there is no link of these mutagens to colon cancer, but does not obviate a possible benefit of these vitamins to *gastric* cancer incidence (through nitrosation inhibition).

Retinoids (Vitamin A), Carotenoids, and Cancer

Interest in the possibility that consumption of retinoids is related to the incidence of epithelial cancers in man stems from the demonstration by

Saffiotti and colleagues in the 1960s that lung carcinogenesis, induced by benz(o)pyrene in hamsters, could be inhibited by vitamin A (retinyl palmitate) (Saffiotti et al., 1967); also, epidemiologic data have shown an inverse relationship between intakes of retinoids (or pro-retinoid-containing vegetables) and the incidence of lung and other epithelial cancers: Bjelke (1975) studying 8300 men, and Shekelle et al. (1981) studying 2000 Western Electric employees over 19 years, for intakes versus lung cancer; Staehelin et al. (1987) studying for plasma levels and lung and stomach cancer; and use of isotretinoin (an analog of vitamin A) in the prevention of skin cancer in susceptible subjects (with xeroderma pigmentosa) (Kraemer et al., 1988). The possible relationship of retinoids to epithelial cancers of many kinds (be it skin, lung, gastrointestinal, bladder, or glandular) would have a theoretical base in our present knowledge that retinoids are necessary for differentiation of epidermoid and glandular cells, differentiation being "opposite" to the tendency of cancer cells to lose their differentiated characteristics (become more anaplastic). Thus, retinoids might act to suppress the malignant phenotype even in transformed cells by promoting expression of normal epithelial genes. (See Chapter 5 for details of vitamin A functions.)

Several problems stand in the way of promoting the use of retinoids in the prevention and/or treatment of epithelial cancers: (1) most forms of the vitamin are toxic in the dose ranges that may be required; (2) animal studies indicate that responses of retinoids have not been uniformly positive in terms of cancer prevention or inhibition (Birt, 1986). Indeed, in some systems, carcinogenesis has been enhanced (or promoted) by retinoid treatment (Levij and Polliack, 1968; Levij et al., 1969; Schroder and Black, 1980). (The tumor promoter, croton oil, had the same effect, and very high doses were applied.) (3) Human epidemiologic and prospective studies now tend to support a role for plant carotenoids more than (animal-derived) retinoids in cancer prevention (La Vecchia et al., 1984; Mackerras et al., 1988; Menkes et al., 1986; Wald et al., 1988). Also, despite extensive experimentation to produce retinoid analogs of vitamin A with strongly anticarcinogenic effects (Bollag and Matter, 1981) and minimal toxicity, few analogs have proven better than the naturally occurring "13-*cis*" or "all-*trans*" retinoic acids (Moon, 1989). Certainly, at this stage in our knowledge, it would not be advisable to use doses of *retinoid* vitamin A much above those recommended for daily intake (RDA) for cancer therapy or prevention. Indeed, in one study, the experimental treatment of bladder cancer patients against recurrence had to be halted because of retinoid toxicity (Gunby, 1978). At the same time, it is well-known that a substantial segment of the U.S. population has a low vitamin A/carotene intake, and evidence strongly suggests that some prevention will accrue from adhering to the RDA. Indeed, Lower and Kanarek (1981) have argued that the epidemiologic data showing an inverse connection between retinoid intake and lung cancer (Nettesheim et al., 1979) or bladder cancer (Mettlin and Graham, 1979) only apply in comparing deficiency with normal intake. Animal studies also implicate vitamin A deficiency in epidermoid cancer incidence more consistently than the excess treatment of normal animals implicates the vitamin in cancer suppression (Lower and Kanarek, 1981).

As concerns mechanism, many animal or organ culture studies indicate that retinoids can prevent both the apparent initiation (Chopra and Wilkoff, 1977) and promotion (Levij and Polliack, 1968; Merriman and Bertram, 1979; Verma et al., 1978) of chemical carcinogenesis in many systems (Sporn and Newton, 1981).

Clearly, retinoids do have antitumor cell, differentiation-promoting effects on several epithelial cell systems that may be useful, especially in subjects at high risk, such as those with xeroderma pigmentosa, where the relatively nontoxic retinoid, isotretinoin (13-*cis* retinoic acid), has been used (Kraemer et al., 1988). It may even induce differentiation of leukemic cells (Wathne et al., 1988). Nevertheless, carotenoids may have even more potential, in that they are sources of retinoids but probably also have additional, independent functions (see Chapter 5, Carotenes). Many surveys have implicated intakes of yellow and green vegetables (Colditz et al., 1985) or carotenes with a lower human cancer risk (lung, mouth, esophagus, cervix, larynx, skin, and possibly pancreas; Connett et al., 1989; Gold et al., 1985), even when corrected for the contributions of smoking. This conclusion is supported by recent animal studies in which similar as well as independent effects of carotenoids (versus retinoids) were observed. The examples in Table 16.15 illustrate first, that β-carotene and the nonvitamin A-producing carotenoid, canthaxanthin, usually have very similar inhibitory effects on epithelial cell tumor development or growth (I and II); second, that they can be effective where retinoids are not (II). A human study, however, showed no reduction in skin cancer incidence over 5 years in subjects taking daily 50 mg supplements of β-carotene versus placebo (Greenberg et al., 1990) (more than 40% developed new cancers during the 5-year period). Similarly, antioxidant vitamins C and E, but not β-carotene and canthaxanthin, depressed tumor formation in mice given dimethylhydrazine (Colacchio et al., 1989).

As concerns the mechanism(s) of the nonretinoid action of carotenoids, the supposition is that it may have something to do with their antioxidant capacity. This is consistent with the data in Table 16.15 (IV), in which vitamin E was also tested. Carotenes are very effective scavengers of oxygen radicals at lower oxygen tensions (such as prevail in tissues in vivo) (Burton and Ingold, 1984; Dimitrov, 1986). This might protect precancerous, genetically unstable cells from damage that would lead to further changes in gene expression or chromosome rearrangement. Alternatively or additionally, the carotenoids might enhance the likelihood of an immune response, leading perhaps to increased production of tumor necrosis factor (TNF) by the host, as suggested by the studies of Shklar and Schwartz (1988) in Table 16.15II. TNF, also known as cachectin, has been implicated in the killing of tumor cells, as its name implies. Although those possibilities are just beginning to be studied, they present exciting prospects. Certainly, and in contrast to most retinoids, intake of large amounts of carotenoids is benign, even in excess (Bendich, 1988).

Vitamin B_6 and Cancer

There has been considerable work on the possibility that a deficiency of vitamin B_6 (pyridoxine) might contribute to cancer development (Brown, 1988; Merrill and Henderson, 1987). Many bladder, breast, and lymph cancer patients appear to have elevated urinary levels of tryptophan metabolites, considered symptomatic of B_6 deficiency (see Chapter 5). Those patients with elevated urinary metabolites also had more recurrences of bladder cancer (Yoshida et al., 1970); and many aromatic amines are known to be bladder carcinogens (Brown, 1988). Several intervention trials in animals (Birt et al., 1987) and man (Brown, 1988; Newling et al., 1984) have failed to show a benefit of supplementing with pyridoxine on tumor incidence or recurrence; but Brown (1988) has argued

Table 16.15. Effects of Carotenoids and Retinoids on Tumor Growth and Host Responses in Rodents

Animals and treatments	Tumor size	Tumor incidence (%)	
			Precancerous lesions (%)
I. Rat gastric epithelium			
Controls	—	22	64
β-Carotene or canthaxanthin	—	7.4	66
			TNF-pos. tumor cells[a] (%)
II. Hamster buccal pouch			
Control/sham	1400 (mm^3)	—	1.1–1.3
Retinoic acid (13-*cis*)	1900	—	3.6
β-Carotene	100	—	66
Canthaxanthin	400	—	20
α-Tocopherol	<50	—	55
III. Rat submandibular salivary gland			
Controls	7.0 (g)	71 (39)[b]	—
Retinyl palmitate	4.7	59 (45)	—
β-Carotene	3.2	67 (53)	—
Canthaxanthin	1.8	70 (47)	—

Sources: (I) Santamaria et al. (1987). Rats were given low levels of N-methylnitrosurea in the drinking water at the start of the studies and fed (or not fed) carotenoids. (II) Shklar and Schwartz (1988). Tumors were induced by topical application of dimethylbenzanthracene (DMBA), prior to injection of the vitamins. (III) Alam et al. (1988). Rats were fed different diets during induction and development of tumors initiated by dimethylbenzanthracene.

[a] Tumor cells positive for tumor necrosis factor (TNF) were determined by histochemistry.

[b] The percentage of gastric lesions showing malignant (carcinomatous) changes versus mild to severe dysplasia are indicated.

that this was probably because the animals or subjects studied were not deficient in the vitamin. On the other hand, the long-term survival of some subjects operated for endometrial carcinoma appeared to be enhanced by pyridoxine supplementation (Ladner and Salkeld, 1985).

There may be an alternative reason for the presence of increased tryptophan metabolites in the urine of bladder, breast, and lymphoid cancer patients. Activation of the immune system, and the release of IL-2 or interferon (see Chapter 17), may induce an increase in the capacity of nonhepatic tissues to degrade tryptophan to kynurenine, via a more newly discovered enzyme, indoleamine dioxygenase (Bryne et al., 1986; Takikawa et al., 1986). Thus, the excretion of not fully degraded tryptophan metabolites may reflect the host's response to the tumor, rather than any deficiency of B_6. This will have to be explored more fully.

Minerals, Trace Elements, and Cancer

The only major mineral of current interest in cancer nutrition is calcium, already described under the section on colon cancer. As concerns trace elements, numerous epidemiologic studies have linked intakes of plant foods, especially cereal grains, with a decreased incidence of the most common cancers found in our society. Conversely, a high consumption of fat, sugar, and refined processed foods has been associated with an increased incidence of the same diseases. Apart from changes in the intakes of fat, fiber, and some vitamins, these dietary patterns are consistent with an association between the intake of certain trace elements and cancer incidence. The potential carcinogenic action of some trace elements, notably Ni and Cd, has been recognized and studied for some time (Furst, 1977; Sunderman, 1977). Only recently, the potential anticarcinogenic actions of trace elements have also become the focus of experimental work by researchers in various parts of the world. The status of this work is described below.

Selenium

The possibility that the level of selenium intake might be related to the incidence of certain forms of cancer stemmed from animal studies on skin cancer produced with dimethylbenzanthracene (Shamberger, 1970) and from the epidemiologic work of Shamberger and Willis (1971) on U.S. populations. Such a connection has since been supported by further epidemiologic studies of subpopulations of Americans and populations worldwide (Clark, 1985; Jacobs and Griffin, 1981). More importantly, numerous animal studies have demonstrated that selenium can inhibit both the initiation and growth of spontaneous or chemically induced tumors, making this trace element the one of greatest current interest in the field of cancer prevention.

In evaluating the data, it should be remembered that selenium (like vitamins C and E) plays a role in the oxygen radical scavenging and metabolizing system of the body (see Chapter 5, Figure 5.33), and that many of the symptoms of selenium deficiency in animals can be relieved by vitamin E, and vice versa (see Chapter 7). Selenium is part of the enzyme, glutathione peroxidase (responsible for disposing of harmful peroxides), and also interacts with S-amino acid metabolism. Other selenoproteins of unknown function continue to be discovered. Much of the selenium we ingest is in the form of selenoamino acids in proteins, although inorganic forms, like selenite (S_2O_3), are of equal biologic interest (see Chapter 7). The form of selenium ingested may be very important in defining the biologic effect. Selenium is, nevertheless, also one of the more toxic trace elements and should not be taken in doses much above those consumed by populations on a naturally adequate (or high) selenium diet.

Epidemiologists have linked a lower selenium intake statistically with a higher incidence of cancers of the colon, rectum, prostate, breast, and leukocyte (Schrauzer et al., 1977) by comparing different populations around the world and different areas of the United States where the soil's selenium content varies (Figure 16.9). [Low selenium New Zealand is an exception (Cohen, 1987*a*).] Mean blood selenium concentrations in persons from different states (in the U.S.) are associated inversely with the incidence of breast cancer (Schrauzer et al., 1977). Shamberger et al. (1976) have shown inverse associations between the selenium content of local forage crops in the United States and incidences of cancer of the tongue, esophagus, stomach, intestine, rectum, liver, pancreas, bladder, and lung, as well as Hodgkin's lymphoma (Jacobs and Griffin, 1981). The meaningfulness of such associations, particularly within the United States, where there is a great deal of food transportation, may be questioned, although soil/crop conditions would probably also be reflected in local water and milk selenium concentrations. These latter might

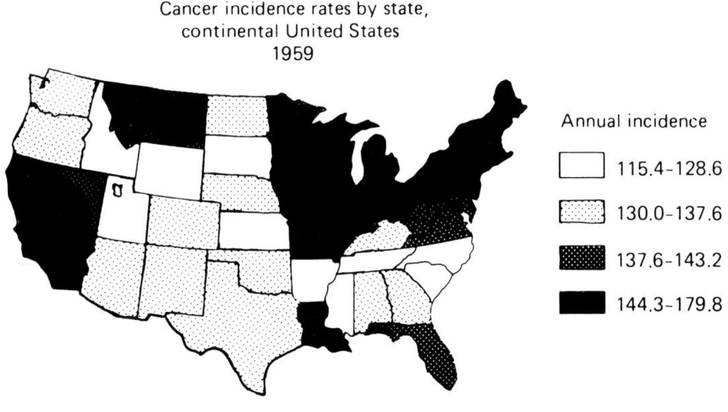

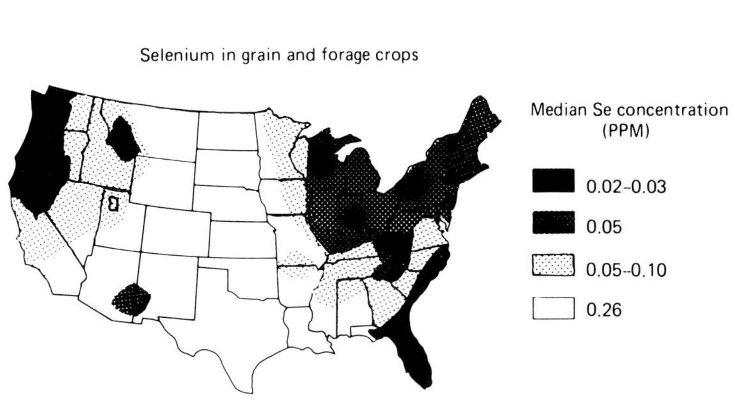

Figure 16.9. Relationship between cancer incidence rates and soil selenium contents, by state. **(Top)** Cancer incidence rates for the continental United States, 1959. **(Bottom)** Median selenium concentrations (ppm) in grains and forage crops in the continental United States. [*Source:* Reprinted by permission from Schrauzer (1978).]

therefore be of greater import. It should be noted that the forms of cancer most consistently associated with a low selenium intake are also those influenced the most by high fat and lower fiber diets (see earlier). Thus, prevention of the oxidation of fats and/or bile acid modification by selenium compounds might be involved.

Numerous animal studies have shown that the induction of tumors that occur spontaneously (breast tumors in C_3H mice) or chemically can be inhibited by supplementation with fairly high levels of selenium (usually as sodium selenite) in diet or drinking water (Table 16.16), given during and/or after the chemical carcinogen (Birt, 1986; Jacobs and Griffin, 1981). Thus, the effects of selenium may be particularly on the promotion phase. Effects on initiation are not ruled out and seem likely where activation of carcinogens by microsomal enzymes may be required (Jacobs and Griffin, 1981). Beneficial effects of selenium on tumor proliferation, once tumor cells have already appeared, have been obtained in mice inoculated with L1210 leukemia cells and given the trace element, as Na_2SeO_3, by injection or in the drinking water (Milner and Hsu, 1981). (The treated animals had a 50%–65% increase in survival time.) However, not all animal studies have found added Se to be beneficial: Birt et al. (1988) have reported that 2.5 ppm of dietary Se failed to prevent N-nitroso-bis(2-oxopropyl)amine-induced pancreatic carcinogenesis, and even enhanced the promotional effect of a high fat diet on the process. The scanty data available on selenite versus organic forms suggest the latter tend to be protective, but are perhaps not as potent, as shown by studies with organic selenium-containing yeast extracts (Greeder and Milner, 1980; Kalin et al., 1980) versus selenite, selenate, and/or selenium dioxide. Trimethylselenonium (a major excretory form), however, may not be effective (Ip and Ganther, 1988). (Arsenite, on the other hand, counters the protective action of selenite, and trimethylselenonium makes arsenite protective, or vice versa.) Schrauzer (1978) has suggested that a doubling of the average selenium intake of Americans would be enough to raise blood concentra-

Table 16.16. Effects of Selenium Feeding on Incidence of Tumors in Mice and Rats

	Control group (regular diet)	Experimental groups	
		Selenium diet	Other diet
Spontaneous breast tumors: mice[a]		(2 ppm)	(As-Se diet)
Number of animals	30	30	30
Tumor onset age (months)	4.5	16	8
Lifespan after onset	1.1	2.0	1.8
Number of tumors, 22 months	12	5	18
Percent tumor incidence	41	17	62
Number multiple tumors	2	0	5
Liver tumors: rats[b]	(0.05% 3′-MeDAB)[c]	(6 ppm)	(Se in water)
Number of animals	15	15	15
Weight at end of study (g)	370	360	365
Survival at end of study (%)	80	100	93
Final tumor incidence (%)	92	46	64

[a] Schrauzer (1978).
[b] Griffin and Jacobs (1977).
[c] 3′-methyldiazoaminobenzene.

tions to the levels found in areas with a lower incidence of cancer. Certainly, a conservative approach such as this is all that can be condoned at this time. Questions remain about (1) the relative effects (including toxicity) of different forms of Se in carcinogenesis and in normal body function, and (2) the distribution of different forms of selenium in different foodstuffs and water (see Chapter 7). Meats, seafood (mainly selenocysteine in proteins), and grains (higher in selenite) remain the major dietary sources, although levels in mushrooms and garlic are also quite high.

Copper

As with selenium, many studies show that simultaneous feeding of copper supplements to rodents given chemical carcinogens inhibits the development of malignant tumors in the liver (Brada et al., 1974; Fare and Howell, 1964; Kamamoto, 1973), kidney (Carlton and Price, 1973), and other tissues (Linder, 1981), and may prolong life in rodents with ovarian and breast cancers (Burki and Okita, 1973). Studies in tissue culture indicate that copper, especially in the form of low molecular weight chelates, is cytotoxic to tumor cells, causing inhibition of DNA synthesis and cell proliferation (Petering, 1978). (It should be noted that "normal" proliferative cells in tissue culture are also adversely affected.) A variety of low molecular weight chelates, including Cu-diisopropylsalicylate, have been used to inhibit tumor development and growth in animal models (Oberley and Oberley, 1988; Sorenson, 1985). The mechanism of action may involve enhanced oxidative fragmentation of the DNA catalyzed by the entering copper or copper chelates (Marshall et al., 1981). Bleomycin, a bacterial or fungal ionophore with high affinity for copper has been used experimentally in human cancer patients to aid in therapy, with favorable results (Carter et al., 1976; Umezawa, 1979). However, almost no other human studies have been carried out in which a connection between copper intake or treatment (supplementation) and cancer incidence has been sought. The one exception is a Welsh study connecting the higher copper (and lower zinc) content of garden soils (used to grow vegetables) to a decreased incidence of cancer of the stomach, a form of cancer more prevalent in that region (Stocks and Davies, 1964). Although all these observations do not as yet make a case for a significant influence of copper intake on cancer development in humans, the additional observations that copper metabolism is thoroughly altered in the host early in tumor growth suggests a more fundamental relationship between alterations of copper metabolism and the cancer process (Linder et al., 1981). Plasma copper concentrations, including those associated with ceruloplasmin and transcuprein, are increased (Wirth and Linder, 1985), and this is an early phenomenon in the growth of the malignancy (Coates et al., 1989; Diez et al., 1989; Linder, 1981; Linder et al., 1981). Liver and kidney copper concentrations decline, and there is increased synthesis and secretion of ceruloplasmin, the major copper transport protein of plasma that also gives extracellular protection against oxygen radicals (see Chapter 7, Copper; Linder, 1991). The specific activity of ceruloplasmin oxidase activity is also enhanced, as is intestinal absorption of copper (Cohen et al., 1979). The purpose of these changes is unknown, but might be: (1) to increase delivery of copper to vital tissues, including immune cells (copper is important for cell-mediated and humoral immunity; Prohaska and Lukasewycz, 1990; Linder, 1991); (2) protect pretumor cells against promotion by oxygen radicals; and/or (3) protect normal cells against such radicals released to induce tumor necrosis. Alternatively, they might provide adequate copper for tumor cell proliferation (cytochrome oxidase and angiogenesis) and/or serve more directly to inhibit tumor growth. [Copper tends to accumulate in tumors (Diez et al., 1989; Linder, 1981).]

Other Trace Elements

Less extensive data on relations of other trace elements to carcinogenesis are available, and in general provide no clear picture of their usefulness in disease prevention. Deficiency of zinc (Pories et al., 1977) or supplementation with excess zinc (Ciapparelli et al., 1972) have both been shown to inhibit chemical tumor induction in a variety of rodents (Jacobs and Griffin, 1981). These kinds of findings may not be surprising in view of the broad range of biologic functions of this trace element in all areas of metabolism, from "zinc fingers" and cell proliferation to protein degradation (see Chapter 7). However, the results imply that only in the lower or upper extremes of intake would zinc have an influence on tumor prevention, and, in the long-term, neither state is compatible with optimal health.

Some trace elements have also been shown to inhibit carcinogenesis induced by other trace elements. Notably, the induction of testicular tumors or sarcomas by cadmium is inhibited by selenium (Griffin, 1979) or zinc (Gunn et al., 1963) and nickel sarcomas by manganese (Sunderman et al., 1974). Isolated experiments implicate various other trace elements as anticarcinogens, from cobalt and aluminum to germanium and vanadium (Jacobs and Griffin, 1981). Arsenite has been implicated both as an anticancer agent, when fed to mice in low concentrations over their lifespan (Kanisawa and Schroeder, 1967), and as a promoter of the growth rate of implanted tumors (Schrauzer and Ishmael, 1974). The significance, if any, of these findings cannot be evaluated at this time.

As concerns iron, one observation may be of some use: High body stores are associated with a slightly higher cancer risk, as demonstrated by data from several epidemiologic and prospective trials (Stevens et al., 1986, 1988; Selby and Friedman, 1988). [Overload was assessed by transferrin levels and iron saturation.] Iron overload is associated with a general increase in tissue damage (and increased risk for heart attack, liver necrosis, and mortality; see Chapter 7), presumably due to its enhancement of oxygen radical formation. Such radical formation might promote carcinogenesis (Cerutti, 1985). Clearly, high body iron stores and overload are to be avoided as much as possible, and not just to reduce the risk of cancer. Cancer is also associated with increases in (iron-poor) serum ferritin (Table 7.4), and cell surface binding of ferritin molecules to lymphocytes has been observed in several forms of cancer (Moroz et al., 1985). The significance of these observations is still unknown.

Other Food Factors and Cancer

Indoles in Cruciferous Vegetables

The ingestion of cruciferous vegetables of the brassica family (brussel sprouts, cabbages, broccoli, etc.) has been associated epidemiologically with a lower general human cancer risk (Graham et al., 1979). In experimental animals, this family of vegetables has been shown to inhibit formation of mammary tumors (Wattenberg, 1983), at the initiation stage [e.g., when fed during exposure of rats to dimethylbenzanthracene (DMBA) (Stoewsand et al., 1988)]. The active ingredients would appear to include benzoyl-isothiocyanate and several indoles (indole-3-acetonitrile, indole-3-carbinol, and 3,3′-di-indolylmethane) (Loub et al., 1975). These substances are known to induce drug metabolizing and conjugating enzymes (microsomal hydroxylases, GSH-S-transferase, and glucuronidating enzymes), in liver, intestine, and lung, both in animals (Wattenberg, 1983) and in man (Pantuck et al., 1984). These inductions will tend to inactivate, and enhance the water solubility and excretion of, drugs as well as potential carcinogens. In some cases, they may enhance tumorigenesis by causing carcinogen activation. Whether other actions may be involved is currently unknown. In general, the data available suggest that ingestion of cruciferous vegetables is beneficial to the long-term health of human beings.

Caffeine

Caffeine intake has been of interest as a possible contributor to the incidence of pancreatic cancer, but the data are not strong (see Chapter 9, Caffeine and Methylxanthines). A recent epidemiologic report, however, suggests that coffee may increase pancreatic cancer risk (with or without caffeine) in smokers only (Graham, 1987). Both coffee and smoking induce secretion of pancreatic proteases, but it is not known if or how this may be relevant. Caffeine has also been implicated in fibrocystic disease of the breast (see Chapter 9), which can lead to breast cancer. Human epidemiologic data as well as animal studies do not support a positive connection between caffeine and breast cancer (Phelps and Phelps, 1988; Rohan and McMichael, 1988). Indeed, caffeine was found to retard mammary carcinogenesis in rats induced with diethylstilbesterol (Petrek et al., 1985). It also showed a negative correlation to colon cancer (Jacobsen and Thelle, 1987). The negative association could be due to effects of caffeine on lipid metabolism, particularly a reduction in biliary secretion that might lead to less fat absorption and/or less promotion of carcinogenesis by bile acids.

Alcohol

Excessive alcohol consumption has been associated with an increased risk of developing cancers of the mouth, esophagus, and larynx (Byers and Graham, 1984). Recently, associations of increased breast cancer risk and moderate alcohol consumption have also been made in many epidemiologic studies (Graham, 1987; Harvey et al., 1987; Hiatt et al., 1988; Schatzkin et al., 1987; Willett et al., 1987). These associations may at least partly be fortuitous. For example, there are positive associations for beer and hard liquor, but not for wine (Willett et al., 1987b), suggesting that something other than ethanol may be involved. There have also been a few studies in which no positive correlation was found to breast cancer (Harris and Wynder, 1988; Lindegard, 1987). Nevertheless, alcohol was found to enhance spontaneous mammary tumor expression in C_3H mice (Schrauzer et al., 1979), and the production of acetaldehyde from ethanol is known to form protein and other adducts (see Chapter 3, Ethanol), and may also cause damage to DNA. This may help to explain the mechanism by which ethanol could initiate or promote changes that lead to cancer. The increase in risk for breast cancer associated with ethanol consumption appears to be quite moderate (on the order of +40% for 1–2 drinks per day), but may well be significant. The risk increases with greater consumption and then also becomes a major factor (with smoking) for cancer of the oral cavity.

Laetrile

The material commonly called "laetrile," which had been the focus of some interest as an anticancer drug among the lay public, is actually "amygdalin," a glycosylated form of laetrile (mandelonitrile) (Figure 16.10). It was isolated earlier in this century from apricot pits, and was first synthesized in 1924 by Hudson. Touted since the late 1940s and early 1950s as an anticancer agent by Howard Beard and Ernst Krebs (of pangamic acid, vitamin B_{15}, fame; see Chapter 5), the theory of its effects on tumor cells has been that intracellular β-glycosidases, presumably higher in tumors than in nonmalignant cells, produce mandelonitrile (laetrile) from amygdalin; amygdalin then, either spontaneously or through intervention of a lyase, dissociates into benzaldehyde and cyanide (Figure 16.10). Cyanide inhibits cell respiration and kills the tumor cells, which, it is theorized, might have much less rhodanese enzyme than normal cells to detoxify the cyanide. Thus, the crux of the theory is that the relative rates of cyanide production versus destruction allow a greater (more toxic/killing) accumulation of cyanide in neoplastic versus normal cells.

Unfortunately, there is almost no evidence to support this contention, except that shown in Figure 16.10 for one particular type of mammary tumor. Moreover, there has been no survey of the cyanide concentrations achieved in normal versus neoplastic animal tissues after injections of amygdalin, although blood concentrations of cyanide have been measured and are elevated. [This has, in fact, led to the accidental death of some healthy people (especially children) (McAnalley et al., 1981).] Oral dosage is much more toxic than injection, because intestinal bacteria hydrolyze the amygdalin to cyanide. By the intravenous route of injection, the material appears to be fairly benign, as shown in animals (Burk et al., 1959) and humans (below).

The report of Moertel et al. (1982) on the National Cancer Institute-supported trials of this "drug" has left the medical community with at

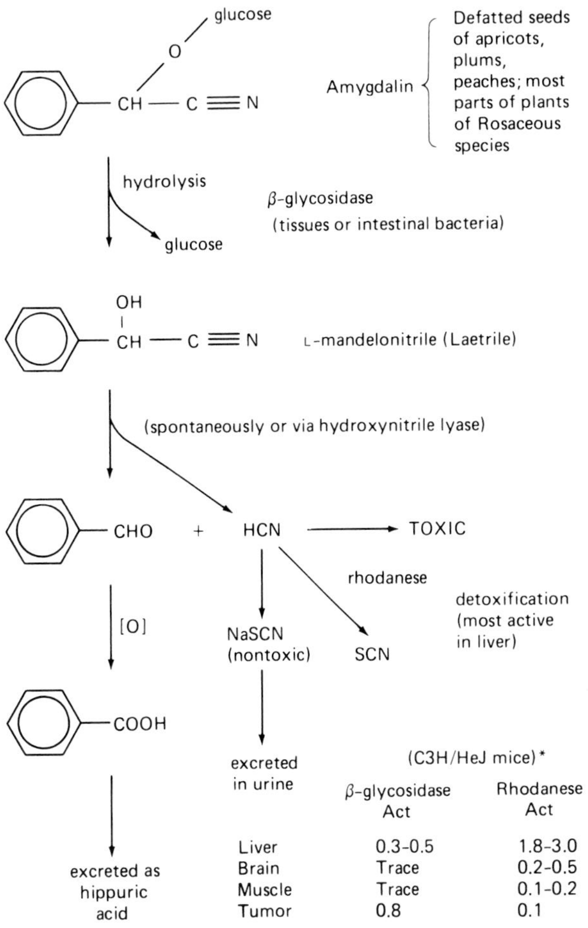

glucose
O
CH — C ≡ N
Amygdalin { Defatted seeds of apricots, plums, peaches; most parts of plants of Rosaceous species
hydrolysis
glucose
β-glycosidase
(tissues or intestinal bacteria)
OH
CH — C ≡ N
L-mandelonitrile (Laetrile)
(spontaneously or via hydroxynitrile lyase)
CHO + HCN → TOXIC
rhodanese
detoxification (most active in liver)
[O]
NaSCN (nontoxic)
SCN
COOH
excreted in urine
excreted as hippuric acid

(C3H/HeJ mice)*

	β-glycosidase Act	Rhodanese Act
Liver	0.3-0.5	1.8-3.0
Brain	Trace	0.2-0.5
Muscle	Trace	0.1-0.2
Tumor	0.8	0.1

Figure 16.10. Sources, forms, and metabolism of laetrile. Data at the bottom are values obtained by Manner et al. (1978) for the levels of two of the principal enzymes involved in laetrile metabolism, as measured in normal tissues and tumors of the rat.

least the temporary feeling that the "laetrile controversy" has been laid to rest once and for all; that this material, even with concomitant changes in diet and additions of vitamin supplements and pancreatic enzymes, is of no benefit to the cancer patient. In the study of 178 terminally ill patients conducted at four U.S. Cancer Centers, no differences were observed in terms of cure rate, disease progression, improvement of symptoms, extension of lifespan, etc., in patients with or without this therapy. (The control group consisted of half of the patients and received no special treatment.) In both cases, 50% of the patients died within 5 months and 80% by 8 months; there was only one case that showed some regression, and this was only transient. Clearly, it indicates that "laetrile" alone, or in combination with certain dietary changes and supplements, has little or no beneficial effect for most cancer patients with very advanced terminal disease. In all fairness, it should be pointed out that no other treatments in current use by the medical profession have been shown to be any better for such patients, and so it is not a test of the potential efficacy of this drug (or treatment regimen) that might be compared with chemotherapeutic and radiation treatments in current use, where these are effective to some degree (Bross, 1982). We have thus gathered little knowledge from the clinical trials and are still faced with the following dilemma. Although we may not, in conscience, feel able to "test the untested" (laetrile) in patients who might benefit from conventional therapy, we know that this is the only way in which it can adequately be tested.

Usually, in such a dilemma, one turns to animal studies. Here, the existing reports give little support to the concept that amygdalin therapy would be useful. Several studies with amygdalin alone, in a variety of animal test systems where tumors were induced spontaneously, by chemical means, or implanted in rodents, failed to show either toxicity or tumor inhibitor effects, or any other obvious benefits to the tumor-bearing animals (Stock et al., 1978*a*, *b*). However, laetrile did not interfere with conventional therapeutic treatments either. Only Manner et al. (1978) have reported some positive effects with amygdalin injected intramuscularly and combined with massive oral doses of vitamin A plus intratumor injections of a mixture of proteolytic and other enzymes. (In these studies, 50% of rats with enzyme alone and with amygdalin or vitamin A had remissions, and 76% of rats with all three treatments had remissions.) Physicians using "laetrile" in other countries also give enormous (500,000 IU) daily doses of vitamin A and oral or intratumoral proteolytic enzymes to patients. (They also change the diet, give large amounts of vitamin C, coffee enemas, etc.) Obviously, intratumoral injections are very risky in humans. Thus, it seems unlikely that amygdalin would be useful in human cancer therapy.

References

Alam BS, Alam SQ, Weir JC Jr (1988): Nutr Cancer 11:233.

Ames BN (1979): Science 204:587.

Ames BN (1983*a*): Progr Clin Biol Res 131 (13th International Cancer Congress, 1982).

Ames BN (1983*b*): Science 221:1256.

Bahnson CB (1969): Ann NY Acad Sci 164:319.

Bendich A (1988): Nutr Cancer 11:207.

Birt DF (1986): Proc Soc Exp Biol Med 183:311.

Birt DF (1987): Adv Exp Med Biol 206:69.

Birt DF, Julius AD, Hasegawa R, St John M, Cohen SM (1987): Cancer Res 47:1244.

Birt DF, Julius AD, Runice CE, White LT, Lawson T, Pour PM (1988): Nutr Cancer 11:21.

Bishop JM (1987): Science 235:305.

Bjelke E (1975): Int J Cancer 15:561.

Bjelke E (1983): Prog Clin Biol Res 131 (13th International Cancer Congress, 1982).

Black HS, Chan JT (1975): J Invest Dermatol 65:412.

Bollag W, Matter A (1981): Ann NY Acad Sci 359:9.

Boyar AP, Rose DP, Loughridge JR, Engle A, Palgi A, Laakso K, Kinne D, Wynder EL (1988): Nutr Cancer 11:93.

Brada Z, Altman NH, Bulba S (1974): Proc Am Assoc Cancer Res 15:145.

Bram S, Froussard P, Guichard M, Jasmin C, Augery Y, Sinoussi-Barre F, Ray W (1980): Nature 284:629.

Bross IJD (1982): N Engl J Med 407:118.

Brown RR (1981): Cancer Res 41:3741.

Brown RR (1988): *In* Leklem JE, Reynolds RD, eds: Clinical and physiological applications of vitamin B_6. New York: Alan R Liss, p 279.

Bruce WR (1983): Progr Clin Biol Res 132D (13th International Cancer Congress, 1982, part D).

Bruce WR (1987): Cancer Res 47:4237.

Bryne CI, Lehmann LK, Kirschbaum JG, Borden EC, Lee CM, Brown RR (1986): J Interferon Res 6:389.

Burk D, McNaughton AR, Von Ardenne M (1959): Minerva Chir 24:1164.

Burki HR, Okita GT (1973): Br J Cancer 23:591.

Burkitt DP, Walker ARP, Painter NS (1972): Lancet 2:1408.

Burkitt DP, Walker ARP, Painter NS (1974): JAMA 229:1068.

Burton GW, Ingold KU (1984): Science 224:569.

Byers GW, Graham S (1984): Adv Cancer Res 41:1.

Calvert RJ, Klurfeld DM, Subramaniam S, Vahouny GV, Kritchevsky D (1987): J Nat Cancer Inst 79:875.

Cameron E (1980): N Engl J Med 302:298.

Cameron E, Pauling L (1976): Proc Natl Acad Sci USA 73:3685.

Cameron E, Pauling L (1978): Proc Natl Acad Sci USA 75:4538.

Cameron E, Pauling L, Leibovitz B (1979): Cancer Res 39:663.

Carlton WW, Price PS (1973): Food Cosmet Toxicol 11:827.

Carroll KK (1975): Cancer Res 35:3374.

Carroll KK (1981): Cancer Res 41:3695.

Carter SK, Ichikawa T, Mathe G, Umezawa H (1976): Gann Monograph on Cancer Research, no 19.

Cerutti PA (1985): Science 227:375.

Chopra DP, Wilkoff LJ (1977): J Natl Cancer Inst 58:923.

Ciapparelli L, Retiel DH, Fatti LP (1972): S Afr J Med Sci 37:85.

Clark LC (1985): Fed Proc 44:2584.

Coates RJ, Weiss NS, Daling JR, Rettmer RL, Warnick GR (1989): Cancer Res 49:4353.

Cohen DI, Illowsky B, Linder MC (1979): Am J Physiol 36:E309.

Cohen LA (1981): Cancer Res 41:3808.

Cohen LA (1987*a*): Scientific Am 257:42.

Cohen LA (1987*b*): Preventive Med 16:468.

Colacchio TA, Memoli VA, Hildebrandt L (1989): Arch Surg 124:217.

Colditz GA, Branch LG, Lipnick RJ, Willett WC, Rosner B, Posner BM, Hennekens H (1985): Am J Clin Nutr 41:32.

Connett JE, Kuller LH, Kjelsberg MO, Polk BF, Collins G, Rider A, Hulley SB (1989): Cancer 64:126.

Correa P (1981): Cancer Res 41:3685.

Creagan ET, Moertel CG, O'Fallon JR, Schutt AJ, O'Connell MJ, Rubin J, Frytak S (1979): N Engl J Med 301:687.

Davis DL, Hoel D, Fox J, Lopez A (1990): Lancet 2:474.

DeClerck YA, Jones PA (1980): Cancer Res 40:3228.

Diez M, Arroyo M, Cerdan FJ, Munoz M, Martin MA, Balibrea JL (1989): Oncol 46:230.

Dimitrov NV (1986): *In* Bland J, ed: A year in nutritional medicine (2nd ed). New Canaan, CN: Keats, p 167.

Dion PW, Bright-See EB, Smith CC, Bruce WR (1982): Mut Res 102:27.

Eastwood MA, Eastwood J, Ward M (1976): *In* Spiller

GA, Amen RJ, eds: Fiber in human nutrition. New York: Plenum, p 207.
Enig MG, Munn RJ, Keeney M (1979*a*): Fed Proc 38:2217.
Enig MG, Munn RJ, Keeney M (1979*b*): Fed Proc 38:2437.
Fare G, Howell JS (1964): Cancer Res 24:1279.
Fialkow PJ (1979): Annu Rev Med 30:135.
Frasca JM (1981): Diss Abstr Internatl B 37:3202.
Furst A (1977): *In* Kraybill HF, Mehlman MA, eds: Advances in modern toxicology, environmental cancer, Vol 3. New York: Wiley.
Gallick GE, Kurzrock R, Kloetzer WS, Arlinghaus RB, Gutterman JU (1985): Proc Natl Acad Sci USA 82:1795.
German J, ed (1983): Chromosome mutation and neoplasia. New York: Alan R Liss.
Glober GA, Klein KL, Morre JO, Abba BC (1974): Lancet 2:80.
Gold EB, Gordis L, Diener MD, Seltser R, Boitnott JK, Bynum TE, Hutcheon DF (1985): Cancer 55:460.
Goldin BR, Adlercreutz H, Dwyer JT, Swenson L, Warram JH, Gorbach SL (1981): Cancer Res 41:3771.
Goldin BR, Adlercreutz H, Gorbach SL, Warram JH, Dwyer JT, Swenson L, Woods MN (1982): N Engl J Med 307:1542.
Goustin AS, Leof EB, Shipley GD, Moses HL (1986): Cancer Res 46:1015.
Graham S (1987): N Engl J Med 316:1211.
Graham S, Haenszel W, Bock FG, Lyon JL (1979): J Natl Cancer Inst 63:879.
Gray GE, Williams P, Gerkins V, Brown JB, Armstrong B, Phillips R, Casagrande JT, Pike MC, Henderson BE (1982*a*): Prevent Med 11:103.
Gray GE, Pike MC, Hirayama T, Tellez J, Gerkins V, Brown JB, Casagrande JT, Henderson BE (1982*b*): Prevent Med 11:108.
Greeder GA, Milner JA (1980): Science 209:825.
Greenberg ER, Baron JA, Stukel TA, Stevens MM, Mandel JS, Spencer SK, Elias PM, Lowe N, Nierneberg DW, Bayrd G, Vance JC, Freeman DH Jr, Clendenning WE, Kwan T, the Skin Cancer Prevention Group (1990): N Engl J Med 323:789.
Griffin AC (1979): Adv Cancer Res 29:419.
Griffin AC, Jacobs MM (1977): Cancer Lett 3:177.
Gunby P (1978): JAMA 240:609.
Gunn SA, Gould TC, Anderson WA (1963): J Natl Cancer Inst 31:745.
Harris RE, Wynder EL (1988): J Am Med Assoc 259:2867.
Harvey EB, et al. (1987): J Natl Cancer Inst 78:657.
Hebert JR, Wynder EL (1987): N Engl J Med 317:165.
Hiatt RA, Klatsky AL, Armstrong MA (1988): Cancer Res 48:2284.
Hill MJ (1981): Cancer Res 41:3778.
Hill T, Garbaczewski L, Helman P, Walker ARP, Garnes H, Wynder EL (1981): Cancer Res 41:3817.
Howe GR, Hirohata T, Hislop TG, Iscovich JM, Yuan J-M, Katsouyanni K, Lubin F, Marubini E, Modan B, Rohan T, Toniolo P, Shunzhang Y (1990): J Natl Cancer Inst 8:561.
Howie BJ, Shultz TD (1985): Am J Clin Nutr 42:127.
Hubbard NE, Erickson KL (1987): Cancer Res 47:6171.
Ingram DM, et al. (1987): J Natl Cancer Inst 79:1225.
Ip C, Ganther H (1988): Carcinogen 9:1481.
Ip C, Carter CA, Ip MM (1985): Cancer Res 45:1997.
Jacobs LR (1986): Proc Soc Exp Biol Med 183:299.
Jacobs MM, Griffin AC (1981): *In* Zedeck MS, Lipkin M, eds: Inhibition of tumor induction and development. New York: Plenum.
Jacobs LR, Lupton JR (1986): Cancer Res 46:1727.
Jacobsen BK, Thelle DS (1987): Brit Med J 294:4.
Jenkins DJA, Jenkins AL, Rao AV, Thompson LU (1986): Am J Gastroent 81:931.
Kalin NH, Risch SC, Poen RM, Insel T, Murphy DL (1980): Science 290:825.
Kamamoto Y, Makiura S, Sugihara S, Hiasa Y, Arai M, Ito N (1973): Cancer Res 33:1129.
Kanisawa M, Schroeder HA (1967): Cancer Res 27:1192.
Karmali RA, Reichel P, Cohen LA, Terano T, Hira A, Tamura Y, Yoshida S (1987): Anticancer Res 7:1173.
Katsouyanni K, Willett W, Trichopoulos D, Boyle P, Trichopoulos A, Vasilaros S, Papadiamantis J, McMahon B (1988): Cancer 61:181.
Kay RM (1981): Cancer Res 41:3774.
Kingston DGI, Wilkins TD, Van Tassell RL, MacFarlane RD, McNeal CJ (1981): Banbury Rep 7:215.
Kirschner MA, Ertel N, Schneider G (1981): Cancer Res 41:3711.
Knekt P, et al. (1988): Am J Epidemiol 127:28.
Kolonel LN, Hankin JH, Nomura AM, Chu FY (1981): Cancer Res 41:3727.
Kraemer KH, DiGiovanna JJ, Moshell AN, Tarone RE, Peck G (1988): N Engl J Med 318:1633.
Krichevsky D (1983): Cancer Res (Suppl) 43:2491s.
Krichevsky D, Tepper SA (1977): Atherosclerosis 27:339.
Ladner HA, Salkeld RM (1985): Strahlensschutz Forsch Prax 26:63.
La Vecchia C, Franceschi S, Decarli A, Gentile A, Fasoli M, Pampallona S, Tognoni G (1984): Int J Cancer 34:319.
Levij JS, Polliack A (1968): Cancer 22:300.
Levij JS, Rwomushana JW, Polliack A (1969): J Invest Dermatol 53:228.
Linder MC (1990): The biochemistry of copper. New York: Plenum.
Linder MC (1981): J Nutr Growth Cancer 1:27.
Linder MC, Moor JR, Wright K (1981): J Nat Cancer Inst 67:263.
Lindegard B (1987): N Engl J Med 317:1285.
Loub WD, Wattenberg LW, Davis DW (1975): J Natl Cancer Inst 54:985.
Lower GM Jr, Kanarek MS (1981): Nutr Cancer 3:109.
Mackerras D, et al. (1988): Am J Epidemiol 128:980.
Manner HW, DiSanti SJ, Maggio MI, Michaelsen TI, Rose V (1978): J Manip Physiol Therapeut 1:246.
Marshall LE, Graham DR, Reich KA, Sigman DS (1981): Biochemistry 20:244.

McAnalley BH, Gardiner TH, Garriott JC (1981): Vet Hum Toxicol 22:400.

McCormick DL, Madigan MJ, Moon RC (1985): Cancer Res 45:1803.

Melnick S, Cole P, Anderson D, Herbst A (1987): N Engl J Med 316:514.

Menkes MS, Comstock GW, Vuilleumier JP, Helsing KJ, Rider AA, Brookmeyer R (1986): N Engl J Med 315:1250.

Mergens WJ (1982): Ann NY Acad Sci 393:61.

Merrill AF, Henderson JM (1987): Ann Rev Nutr 7:137.

Merriman RL, Bertram JS (1979): Cancer Res 39:1661.

Mettlin C, Graham S (1979): Am J Epidemiol 110:225.

Mills PK, Annegers JF, Phillips RL (1988): Am J Epidemiol 127:440.

Milner JA, Hsu CY (1981): Cancer Res 41:1652.

Miner KM, Kawaguchi T, Uba GW, Nicolson GL (1982): Cancer Res 42:4631.

Mintz B, Illmensee K (1975): Proc Natl Acad Sci USA 72:3585.

Mirvish SS (1975): Ann NY Acad Sci 258:175.

Mirvish SS (1981*a*): *In* Burchenal JH, Oettgen HF, eds: Inhibition of tumor induction and development. New York: Plenum, p 101.

Mirvish SS (1981*b*): *In* Burchenal JH, Oettgen HF, eds: Cancer achievements, challenges and prospects for the 1980s. New York: Grune & Stratton, p 557.

Moertel CG, Fleming TR, Creagan ET, Rubin J, O'Connell MJ, Ames MM (1985): N Engl J Med 312:137.

Moertel CG, Fleming TR, Rubin J (1982): N Engl J Med 306:201.

Moon RC (1989): J Nutr 119:127.

Moroz C, Kupfer B, Marcus H, Twig S, Parhami-Seren B (1985): Protides Biol Fluids 3:659.

Morrison DG, Daniel J, Lynd FT, Moyer MP, Esparza RJ, Moyer RC, Rogers W (1981): Nutr Cancer 3:81.

Narisawa T, Sato M, Tani M, Kudo T, Takahashi T, Goto A (1981): Cancer Res 41:1954.

Nelson RL, Tanure JC, Andrianopoulos G, Souza G, Lands WEM (1988): Nutr Cancer 11:215.

Nettesheim P, Snyder C, Kim JCS (1979): Environ Health Perspect 29:89.

Newling DW, Robinson MR, Lockwood R, Stevens I, Byar D, Sylvester R (1984): EORTC Monogr Ser 13:269.

Newmark HL, Mergens WJ (1981): *In* Zedeck MS, Lipkin M, eds: Inhibition of tumor induction and development. New York: Plenum, p 127.

Nicolson GL (1984): Exp Cell Res 150:3.

Nicolson GL (1987): Cancer Res 47:1473.

Nigro ND, Bull AW, Klopfer BA, Pak NS, Campbell RL (1979): J Natl Cancer Inst 62:1097.

Nowell PC (1986): Cancer Res 47:2203.

Oberley LW, Oberley TD (1988): Mol Cell Biochem 84:147.

Ohuchi N, Thor A, Page DL, Hand PH, Halter SA, Schlom J (1980): Cancer Res 46:2511.

Orr JW, Wilson K, Bochford C, Cornwell A, Soong SJ, Honea KL, Hatch KD, Singleton HM (1985): Am J Obstet Gyn 151:632.

Palmer S (1983): Cancer Res (Suppl) 43:2509s.

Pantuck EJ, Pantuck CB, Anderson KE, Wattenberg LW, Conney AH, Kappas A (1984): Clin Pharmacol Therapeutics 35:161.

Pauling L (1980): N Engl J Med 302:694.

Petering DH (1978): *In* Schrauzer GN, ed: Inorganic and nutritional aspects of cancer. New York: Plenum, p 179.

Petrek JA, Sandberg WA, Cole MN, Silberman MS, Collins DC (1985): Cancer 56:1977.

Phelps HM, Phelps CE (1988): Cancer 61:1051.

Pierce GB, Lewis SH, Miller GJ, Mohitz E, Miller P (1979): Proc Natl Acad Sci USA 76:6649.

Pollack ES, Horn JW (1980): J Natl Cancer Inst 64:1091.

Pories WJ, DeWys WD, Flynn A, Mansour EG, Strain WH (1977): Adv Exp Med Biol 91:243.

Prasad KN (1980): Life Sci 27:275.

Prohaska JR, Lukasewycz OA (1990): Adv Exp Med Biol (Antioid Nutr Immune Funct) 262:123.

Reddy BS (1979): Adv Nut Res 2:199.

Reddy BS (1981): Cancer Res 41:3700.

Reddy BS (1987): Preventive Med 16:460.

Reif AE (1981): Scientist 69:437.

Roberts-Anderson J, Mehta T, Wilson RB (1987): Nutr Cancer 10:129.

Rogers AE, Wetsel WC (1981): Cancer Res 41:3735.

Rohan TE, McMichael AJ (1988): Int J Cancer 41:390.

Romney SL, Basu J, Vermund S, Palan PR, DuHagupta C (1987): Ann NY Acad Sci 498:132.

Romney SL, DuHagupta C, Basu J, Palan PR, Karp S, Slagle S, Dwyer A, Wassertheil-Smoller S, Wylie-Rosett J (1985): Am J Obstet Gyn 151:976.

Rosen M, Nystrom L, Wall S (1988): Am J Epidemiol 127:42.

Ruddell WSJ, Bone ES, Hill MJ, Walters CL (1978): Lancet 1:521.

Saffiotti U, Montesano R, Sellakumar AR, Borg SA (1967): Cancer 20:85.

Santamaria L, Bianchi A, Ravetto C, Arnaboldi A, Santagati G, Andreoni L (1987): J Nutr Growth Cancer 4:175.

Scanlan RA (1983): Cancer Res (Suppl) 43:2435s.

Schatzkin A, Jones DY, Hoover RN (1987): N Engl J Med 316:1169.

Schrauzer GN (1978): Adv Exp Med Biol 91:323.

Schrauzer GN, Ishmael D (1974): Ann Clin Lab Sci 4:441.

Schrauzer GN, McGinnes JE, Ishmael D, Bell LJ (1979): J Stud Alcohol 40:240.

Schrauzer GN, White DA, Schneider CJ (1977): Bioinorg Chem 7:23.

Schroder EW, Black PH (1980): J Natl Cancer Inst 65:671.

Selby JV, Friedman GD (1988): Intl J Cancer 41:677.

Shamberger RJ (1970): J Natl Cancer Inst 44:931.

Shamberger RJ, Willis CE (1971): Clin Lab Sci 2:211.

Shamberger RJ, Tytko SA, Willis CE (1976): Arch Environ Health 31:231.

Shekelle RB, Liu S, Raynor WJ Jr, Lepper M, Maliza C, Rossof AH (1981): Lancet 2:1185.

Shils ME (1988): *In* Shils ME, Young YR, eds: Modern nutrition in health and disease. Philadelphia: Lea & Febiger, p 1381.

Shklar G, Schwartz J (1988): Eur J Cancer Clin Oncol 24:839.

Smith RJ (1980): Science 209:998.

Smith ICP, Chmurny GN (1990): Anal Chem 62:853A.

Sorenson AW, Slattery ML, Ford MH (1988): Nutr Cancer 11:135.

Sorenson JRJ (1985): Comp Therapy 11:49.

Sporn MB, Newton DL (1981): *In* Zedeck MS, Lipkin M, eds: Inhibition of tumor induction and development. New York: Plenum, p 71.

Staehelin HB, Gey KF, Brubacher G (1987): Ann NY Acad Sci 498:124.

Stevens RG, Beasley RP, Blumberg BS (1986): J Nat Cancer Inst 76:605.

Stevens RG, Jones DY, Micozzi MS, Taylor PR (1988): N Engl J Med 319:1047.

Stock CC, Martin DS, Kennematsu S, Fugmann RA, Mountain IM, Stockert E, Schmid AF, Tarnowski GS (1978*a*): J Surg Oncol 10:89.

Stock CC, Tarnowski GS, Schmid FA, Hutchison DJ, Teller MN (1978*b*): J Surg Oncol 10:81.

Stocks P, Davies RI (1964): Br J Cancer 18:14.

Stoewsand GS, Anderson JL, Munson L (1988): Cancer Lett 39:199.

Story JA (1980): *In* Brewster MA, Naito HK, eds: Nutritional elements and clinical biochemistry. New York: Plenum, p 383.

Sunderman FW (1977): *In* Goyer RA, Mehlman MA, eds: Advances in modern toxicology, toxicology of trace elements, Vol 2. New York: Wiley, p 257.

Sunderman FW, Lau TJ, Cralley LJ (1974): Cancer Res 34:92.

Takikawa O, Yoshida R, Kido R, Hayaishi O (1986): J Biol Chem 261:3648.

Tennant RW, Margolin BH, Shelby MD, Zeiger E, Haseman JK, Spalding J, Caspary W, Resnick M, Stasiewicz S, Anderson B, Minor R (1987): Science 236:933.

Umezawa H (1979): *In* Hecht SH, ed: Bleomycin: Clinical, biochemical and biological aspects. New York: Springer-Verlag, p 24.

Van Tassell RL, Schram RM, Wilkins TD (1986): *In* Knudson I, ed: Genetic toxicology of the diet. New York: Alan R Liss, p 199.

Verma AK, Royce HM, Shapas BG, Boutwell RK (1978): Cancer Res 38:793.

Wagner DA, Shuker DEG, Bilmazes C, Obiedzinski M, Baker I, Young VR, Tannenbaum SR (1985): Cancer Res 45:6519.

Wald NJ, et al. (1988): Brit J Cancer 57:428.

Walker ARP (1988): Front Gastrointest Res 14:199.

Wargovich MJ, Eng VWS, Newmark HL, Bruce WR (1983): Carcinogen 4:1205.

Watanabe K, Reddy BS, Weisburger JH, Kritchevsky D (1979): J Natl Cancer Inst 63:141.

Wathne K-O, Norum KR, Smeland E, Blomhoff R (1988): J Biol Chem 263:8691.

Wattenberg LW (1983): Cancer Res (Suppl) 43:2448s.

Welsch CW (1987): Preventive Med 16:475.

Wilkins TD (1986): *In* Knudson I, ed: Genetic toxicology of the diet. New York: Alan R Liss, p 199.

Willett WC, Stampfer MJ, Colditz GA, Rosner BA, Hennekens CH, Speizer FE (1987*a*): N Engl J Med 316:22.

Willett WC, Stampfer MJ, Colditz GA, Rosner BA, Hennekens CH, Speizer FE (1987*b*): N Engl J Med 316:1174.

Willett WC, Stampfer MJ, Colditz GA, Rosner BA, Speizer FE (1990): N Engl J Med 323:1664.

Wirth PL, Linder MC (1985): J Nat Cancer Inst 75: 277.

Yoshida O, Brown RR, Bryan GT (1970): Cancer 25:773.

Zumoff B (1981): Cancer Res 41:3805.

William R. Beisel, M.D.*

17

Nutrition and Infection

Introduction

Infectious illnesses constitute the most common form of disease in human beings and other mammalian species. It is typical for a growing child to experience well over 100 discrete episodes of infection before reaching adult life, even in advanced modern societies. Still greater problems with infection occur in underdeveloped areas, where poverty, poor sanitary conditions, and malnutrition are commonplace (see Figure 17.1). Malnutrition often increases the frequency and severity of infectious diseases, especially in infants and children (Brown et al., 1981; Good et al., 1982).

A wide variety of pathogenic microorganisms, including viruses, bacteria, rickettsiae, spirochetes, and parasites, can invade the human host to initiate an infection. The resultant illness may vary in severity from mild to life-threatening, and in duration from brief, self-limited episodes to chronic, persistent infections or infestations. Disease manifestations may emerge as a direct consequence of the organisms per se or because of the toxic products they secrete or release. Less common disease mechanisms may emerge as secondary interactions of a host defensive mechanism with the invading organism or its products. To illustrate this latter point, the deposition of antigen–antibody complexes on the basement membrane of renal glomeruli leads to glomerulonephritis (Bright's disease) after infections by certain streptococcal subtypes.

A complex interactive battle occurs between the invading microorganism and defensive mechanisms of the host. Metabolic and biochemical responses of the host contribute to these defenses, which eventually determine the outcome of each episode of infection. It is the purpose of this chapter to describe and review the biochemical, metabolic, and hormonal responses documented to occur in the host during an infectious illness and to define the nutritional consequences and costs of these underlying fundamental aspects of host defense.

Symptomatic infectious illnesses and even some asymptomatic ones are accompanied by direct or functional losses in the body content of many nutrients and by a redistribution in the body localization of others. The magnitude of these changes is dependent on the severity and duration of an infection. The widespread diverse metabolic responses to acute, generalized febrile infections are generally predictable and relatively stereotyped. They are antigenically nonspecific and occur despite differences in the causative microorganisms (see Figure 17.2) and irrespective of the localized or systemic nature of the inciting disease or its specific etiology. These diverse early reactions to infection are termed, collec-

* Department of Immunology and Infectious Diseases, The Johns Hopkins School of Hygiene and Public Health, Baltimore, MD.

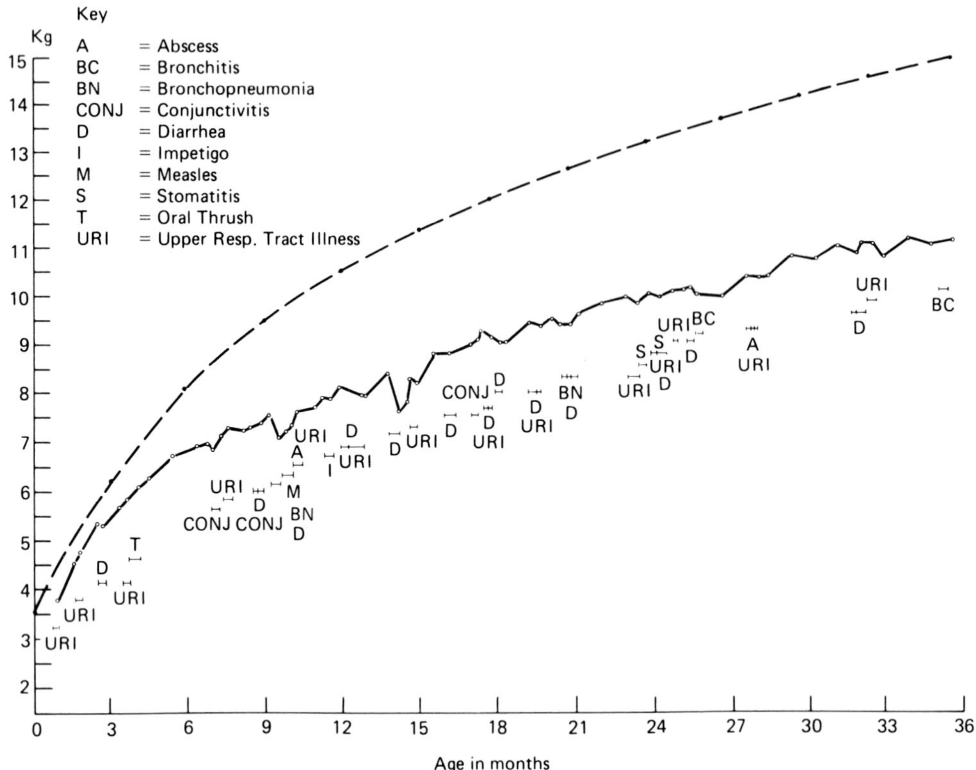

Figure 17.1. Chronological documentation of the infections suffered by a single Guatemalan Indian infant. The cumulative effect of these infections on body weight measurements (open circles) is shown in comparison to the anticipated normal growth curve (dashed line, closed circles). [*Source:* Reprinted by permission from Mata et al. (1977).]

tively, the acute phase response. The resultant consequences of the acute phase response also tend to be predictable. Additional varieties of metabolic, biochemical, and nutritional responses are produced by infections that become localized within a predominant single-organ system, as exemplified by the sizeable losses of fluid and electrolytes in diarrheal infections, the diverse biochemical and metabolic consequences of hepatitis, the anoxia and direct nutrient losses via sputum that occur during pneumonia, or the wasting of bone and muscle that accompanies paralytic forms of infection.

If the infectious process can be cured or eliminated naturally by host defensive mechanisms, lost body nutrients can then be reacquired and body stores reconstituted. This restoration may take a period of weeks to months. If, on the other hand, the infectious process is not eliminated and becomes subacute, chronic, or progressive, body composition becomes markedly altered and a new "relative equilibrium" of body nutrient balances emerges, but at a cachectic, severely wasted level (see Figure 17.3). As documented by Mata et al. (1977), a similar dangerous nutritional status can develop, especially in infants and young children, when a patient suffers a closely spaced series of different infections (see Figure 17.1).

Host Defense Mechanisms

In order to prevent entry of pathogenic microorganisms into the body or to eliminate those that do gain access, the human and animal host possesses a variety of defensive mechanisms. As outlined in Table 17.1, the nonspecific defenses are characterized by both passive and active components that respond to infections of any kind. In addition, the generally more powerful immune defenses are triggered by antigenic components of specific single microorganisms.

Passive defensive components include the anatomical barriers formed by skin, mucous mem-

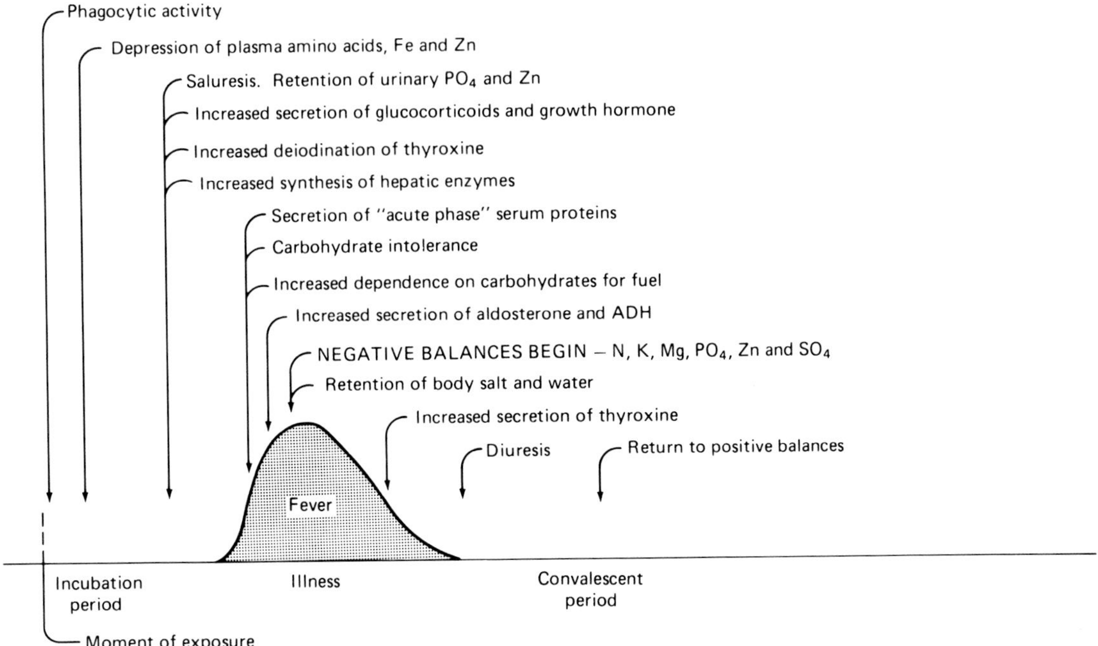

Figure 17.2. Schematic indication of the sequence and relative time of onset of various predictable metabolic, biochemical, and physiologic responses to a brief febrile infectious disease. Note the temporal relationships to the moment of exposure and to the febrile period. [*Source:* Reprinted by permission from Beisel (1977).]

branes, and tissue fascial planes. Normal secretions of the body, including tears, saliva, gastric juice, and mucous, constitute additional barriers. Normal serum contains a number of proteins that serve as antimicrobial factors in host defense. These include substances such as lysozyme, transferrin, complement, and other proteins with opsonic functions. Even proteins of the kinin system and the cascade of blood-clotting factors can become involved in host defensive functions, depending on the nature of the infection being faced.

Active components of host defense can be subdivided into specific and nonspecific defenses. The nonspecific components respond in a relatively similar manner to a large variety of different pathogenic microorganisms. These components include the production of phagocytic cells and the synthesis of proteins such as interferon, lysozyme, and acute-phase reactants. The antigenically specific responses are provided by the immune system and require a capacity for "memory." They include the many interrelated components of the immune system that are able to respond to the unique physiochemical, three-dimensional molecular configuration of specific, antigenic structures of microorganisms, their components, or their products. Specific immunity is generated by an interplay of both the humoral and cell-mediated arms of the immune system.

It is important to note that the function of all active host defensive mechanisms and many of the passive ones require an ongoing capacity of body cells to synthesize new proteins. For this reason, any nutritional deficit or imbalance that influences protein synthetic functions can lead, in turn, to functional impairment of some defensive mechanism and, thus, generally, to a weakening of host resistance. It would be an oversimplification, however, to conclude that malnutrition always leads to an increased incidence of infectious diseases and to disease processes of increased severity. In some instances, the malnourished state of the host makes it difficult for an invading microorganism to acquire certain nutrients from host tissues that the organism needs for its own growth and replication. In such a situation, the infectious process would be less severe than expected (Beisel, 1982*b*; Keusch and Scrim-

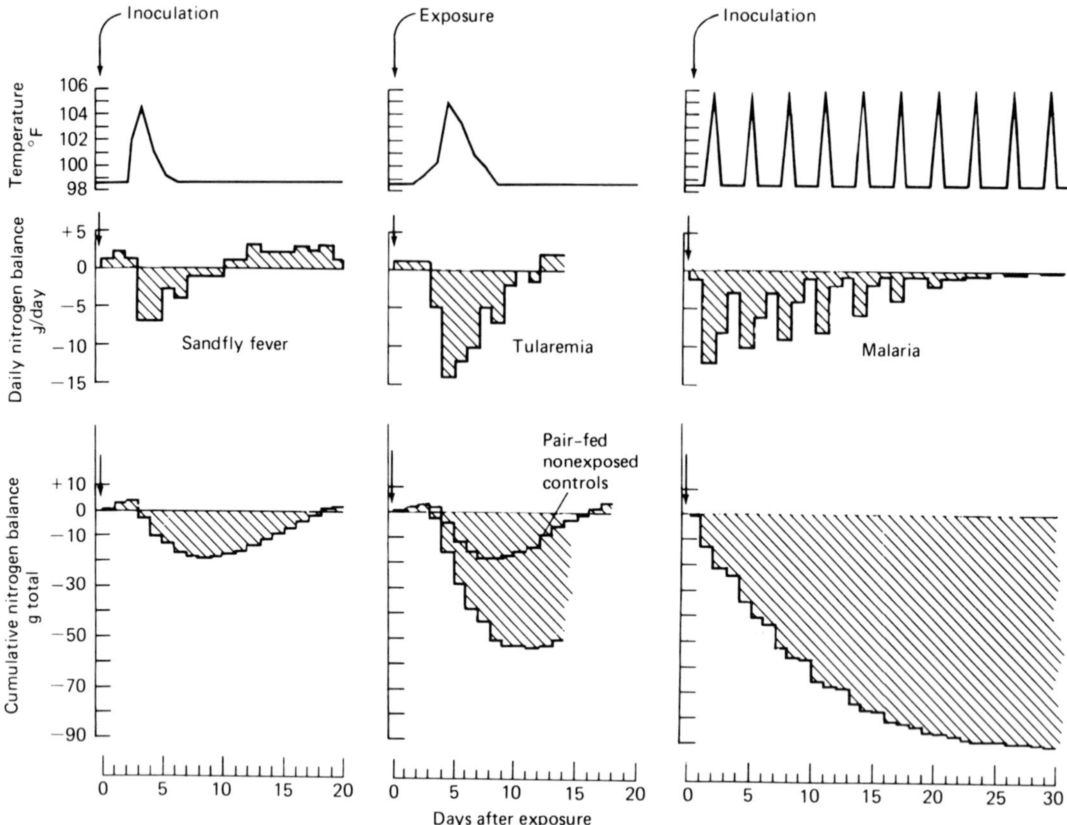

Figure 17.3. Effects of experimentally induced infections in man. Averaged data from volunteers with experimentally induced sandfly fever or tularemia (Beisel et al., 1967) or luetic patients with therapeutically induced malaria (Howard et al., 1946). Daily nitrogen balance data (middle) and cumulative balance (bottom) are shown in relationship to the febrile response (top). Note the difference in cumulative balance in tularemia in comparison to that of pair-fed healthy control subjects. Note also the magnitude and duration of cumulative losses. [*Source:* Reprinted by permission from Beisel (1977).]

shaw, 1986; Scrimshaw et al., 1968). This phenomenon is seen most often in viral or parasitic diseases.

Malnutrition does not have a uniform, across-the-board effect on all aspects of host defense. Rather, some components of the host's defensive mechanisms are more resistant to malnutrition than are other components (Beisel, 1982*a*, *b*). While generalized protein-energy malnutrition is the most common and important cause of immunologic dysfunction, a growing body of evidence indicates that isolated deficiencies of many single nutrients can also impair some aspect of host immunity (see Table 17.2). In addition, excesses of some single nutrients, such as iron, zinc, or vitamin E, or imbalances among some nutrients, such as the essential amino acids, can also cause a functional disruption of immune system components (Beisel, 1982*a*).

The nonspecific active components of host defense represent a relatively primitive system that responds in a common or generally uniform manner to an invasion by many different forms of infectious microorganisms or to tissue injury due to other causes. As shown in Figure 17.4, this system possesses an endocrine-like signal mechanism that serves to activate the widely dispersed, physiologically separate components of the system. Phagocytic cells, predominantly neutrophils and macrophages, are generally the first kind of host cell to interact with invading microorganisms or damaged host tissues. When these cells become activated by an inciting stimulus (see Figure 17.4), they release endogenous mediator substances that circulate as messengers to distant sites; other products of phagocytizing neutrophils and macrophages help to initiate a local inflam-

Table 17.1. Nonspecific (i.e., Nonimmunological) Factors that Influence Host Defenses

- Passive factors that may alter host susceptibility or resistance
  - Normal microbiologic flora
    - Skin, EENT, GI, and GU tracts
  - Anatomic barriers and pathways
    - Surfaces (dermal, mucosal, and endothelial)
    - Fascial planes
    - Body spaces
    - Tubular structures (ureters, vessels, ducts, etc.)
  - Exogenous body secretions
    - Mucin, HCl, lysozyme
  - Physiochemical environment within normal tissues
  - Nutritional factors
  - Normal physiologic factors
    - Age, sex, and race
    - Circadian rhythm
  - Disease-related factors
    - Specific illnesses, i.e., diabetes, leukemia
    - Hodgkin's disease, alcoholism, etc.
    - Injury and trauma
  - Iatrogenic factors
    - Drugs, i.e., corticosteroids, antimetabolites, antimicrobials, etc.
    - Radiation
    - Foreign bodies, i.e., vascular prostheses, catheters, implanted drains, etc.
  - Miscellaneous
    - Fatigue
    - Occupational and environmental factors

- Active factors that respond to the presence of most infectious diseases
  - Inflammatory reactions
    - Rapidly active local factors
      - Amines (histamine, 5-OH-tryptamine, serotonin)
      - Polypeptides (leukotaxine, kinin, complement, and clotting factors)
      - Enzymes (proteases, lysozyme, etc.)
      - Prostaglandins
    - Vasodilatation, heightened vascular permeability
    - Chemotactic substances
    - Localized hypoxia, acidosis, necrosis
    - Fibrin deposition
  - Febrile response
  - Phagocytic functions
  - Metabolic responses
    - Protein catabolism and anabolism
    - Carbohydrate formation and utilization
    - Lipid formation and utilization
    - Mineral, electrolyte, and trace element metabolism
    - Vitamin utilization
  - Endocrine responses
  - Hormone-like factors
    - Interleukins (IL-1, IL-2, IL-6, etc.)
    - Tumor necrosis factor (cachectin)
    - Colony-stimulating factors (CSF)
    - Thymosin
  - Nonspecific antimicrobial factors in plasma
    - Interferon
    - Lysozyme
    - Complement and properdin
    - Nonspecific opsonins
  - Plasma proteins
    - Clotting factors
    - Complement system components
    - Kinin system components
    - Acute phase reactant proteins
    - Carrier proteins for nutrients, hormones, etc.

matory reaction (Wright, 1981). These endogenous mediators are now termed cytokines. They include lymphokines (produced by lymphocytes) and monokines (produced by monocytes and macrophages). Cytokines function as hormones, stimulating responses in nearby or distant cells and tissues (see Figure 17.4). The monokine, Interleukin-1 (IL-1), is the principal stimulus and coordinator of the acute phase response (Dinarello, 1985, 1987; Kluger et al., 1985; Powanda and Beisel, 1982), although some influence may be exerted by other cytokines such as IL-2, IL-6, Tumor Necrosis Factor (TNF) (Dinarello et al., 1986), and the Interferons (INF). IL-1 stimulates hypothalamic centers to initiate fever, anorexia, somnolence, and the pituitary secretion of hormones. Fever can also be produced by IL-2, IL-6, TNF, and INF (see Figure 17.5). IL-1, and perhaps IL-6 as well, cause the liver to take up amino acids, zinc, and iron and to initiate the synthesis of various enzymes, acute-phase reactant proteins, and lipoprotein–triglyceride complexes for release into the plasma. Cytokines also stimulate the bone marrow to manufacture and release additional phagocytic cells; they initiate or modulate, by as yet undefined mechanisms, various endocrine gland responses to infection; and they serve to help activate immunological lymphoid responses of an antigen-specific variety (Powanda and Beisel, 1982).

Table 17.2. Effects of Malnutrition on the Immune System and on Nonspecific Host Defense Mechanisms

	Host resistance to infection	Lymphoid tissues	Lymphocyte changes in: Cell numbers	Lymphocyte changes in: Mitogenic responses in vitro
Generalized malnutrition				
Marasmus/kwashiorkor	Markedly decreased	Atrophic	T cells low, but null cells increased	Depressed if assayed in patient's own serum
Cachexia due to trauma, disease, or malignancy	Markedly decreased	Atrophic	Depressed slightly	Depressed
Uncomplicated starvation	Unchanged for long periods	Eventual atrophy		May eventually decline
Mineral deficiencies				
Iron	Decreased	Lymphocyte depletion	Low T cell counts	Variable declines
Zinc	Markedly decreased	Generalized atrophy Lymphocyte depletion	T_{4+} and NK cell counts low	Poor
Copper	Decreased	Generalized atrophy Cell membrane alterations	Splenic T cells and NK cells decreased	Poor
Vitamin deficiencies				
Vitamin A	May be decreased	Often atrophic	May be low	May be suppressed
Thiamin				
Riboflavin		May show atrophy		
Pyridoxine	Oral infections are common	Generally atrophic	May be low	
Pantothenic acid		May show atrophy	Normal	
Cobalamin			Normal	May be depressed
Biotin				
Folic acid			May be low	May be depressed
Ascorbic acid	Decreased	Appear normal	T cell counts low	
Vitamin D	Decreased	Impaired lymphokine production		Impaired lymphocyte replication

Immunoglobulins					
Serum values	Response to new antigens	Delayed dermal hypersensitivity reactions	Monocyte and macrophage abnormalities	Neutrophilic leukocyte abnormalities	Other changes
May be higher than normal	Poor, but not always absent	Diminished or absent		Bactericidal function poor; cytologic and enzyme changes	Achlorohydria Complement depressed Thymulin low
Normal	Depressed	Poor to absent			
Normal	May disappear with prolonged starvation				
Normal	Variable declines	Variable declines		Bactericidal function poor Lactoferrin content low	Microstructural changes in lymphocytes Normal IgA
	T cell-dependent Ig production depressed	Poor, with energy of cell-mediated immunity	Impaired cell production	Impaired chemotaxis	Impaired production of thymic hormones
Low titers of antibodies					Less thymic hormone Low hepatic PG production
	May be poor	May be suppressed	Mobilization may be poor		Serum complement may increase
	May be poor				
Poor primary response					
	Poor	Generally suppressed		Inflammatory response Eosinophilia	Sensitization and anaphylactic mechanisms are intact
	Generally depressed				
				Depressed Megaloblastic bone marrow	
IgA may be low	May be depressed	Depressed			
	May be depressed	May be depressed		Apparently normal, but nuclei are hypersegmented	
	Generally unchanged	Depressed, but with intact sensitization mechanism	Impaired mobilization Cells small and fragile	Poor motility Bactericidal activity may be impaired	Anaphylactic response is normal Thymulin may be low
	Impaired		Impaired monokine production		Impaired genomic expression

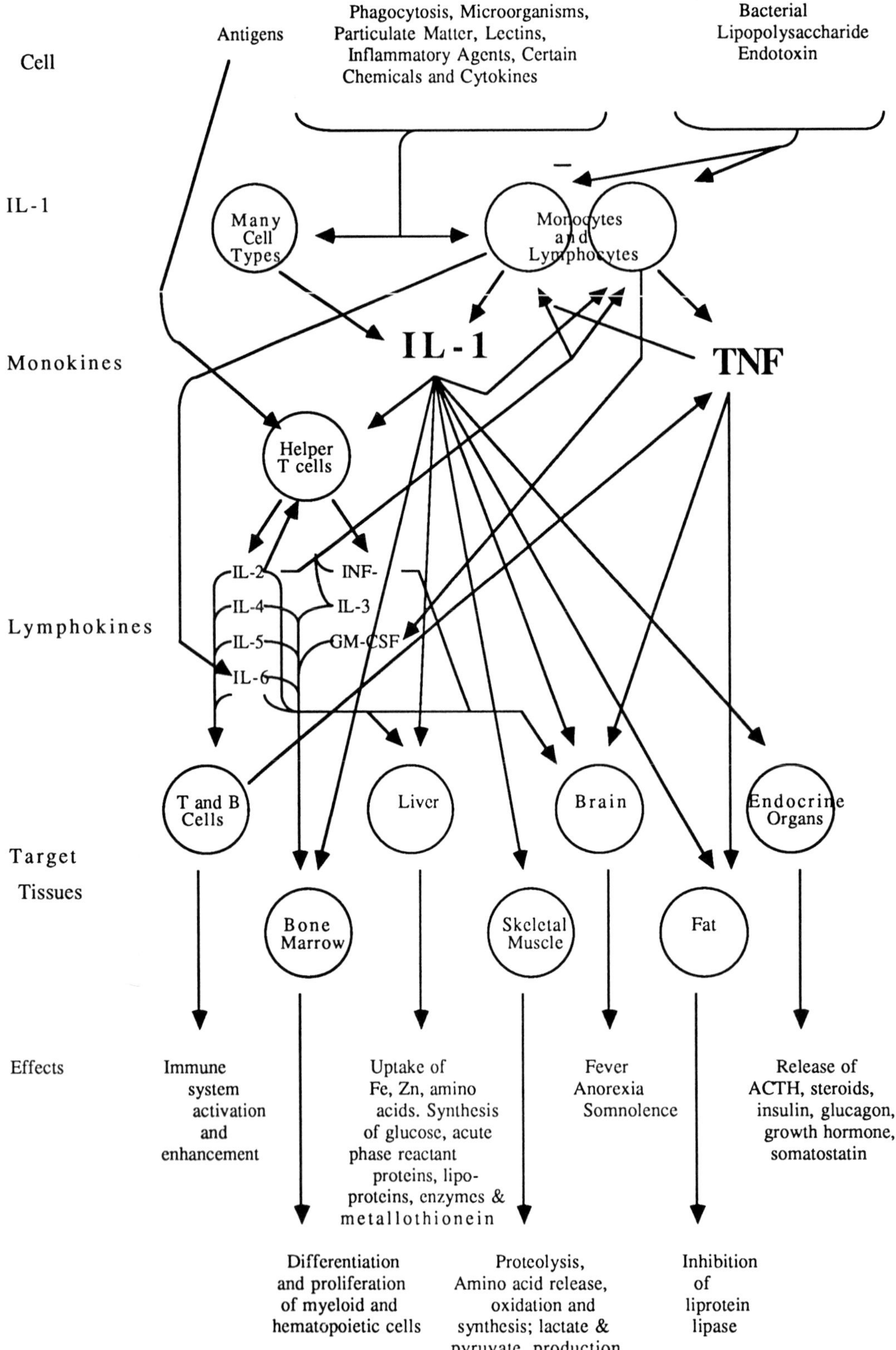

Figure 17.4. Role of cytokines in initiating and modulating the acute phase reaction. A flow diagram is shown depicting the hormonal role of monokines and lymphokines in triggering a wide variety of metabolic and physiologic responses, and the central positions of IL-1 and TNF in coordinating this generalized response to infection.

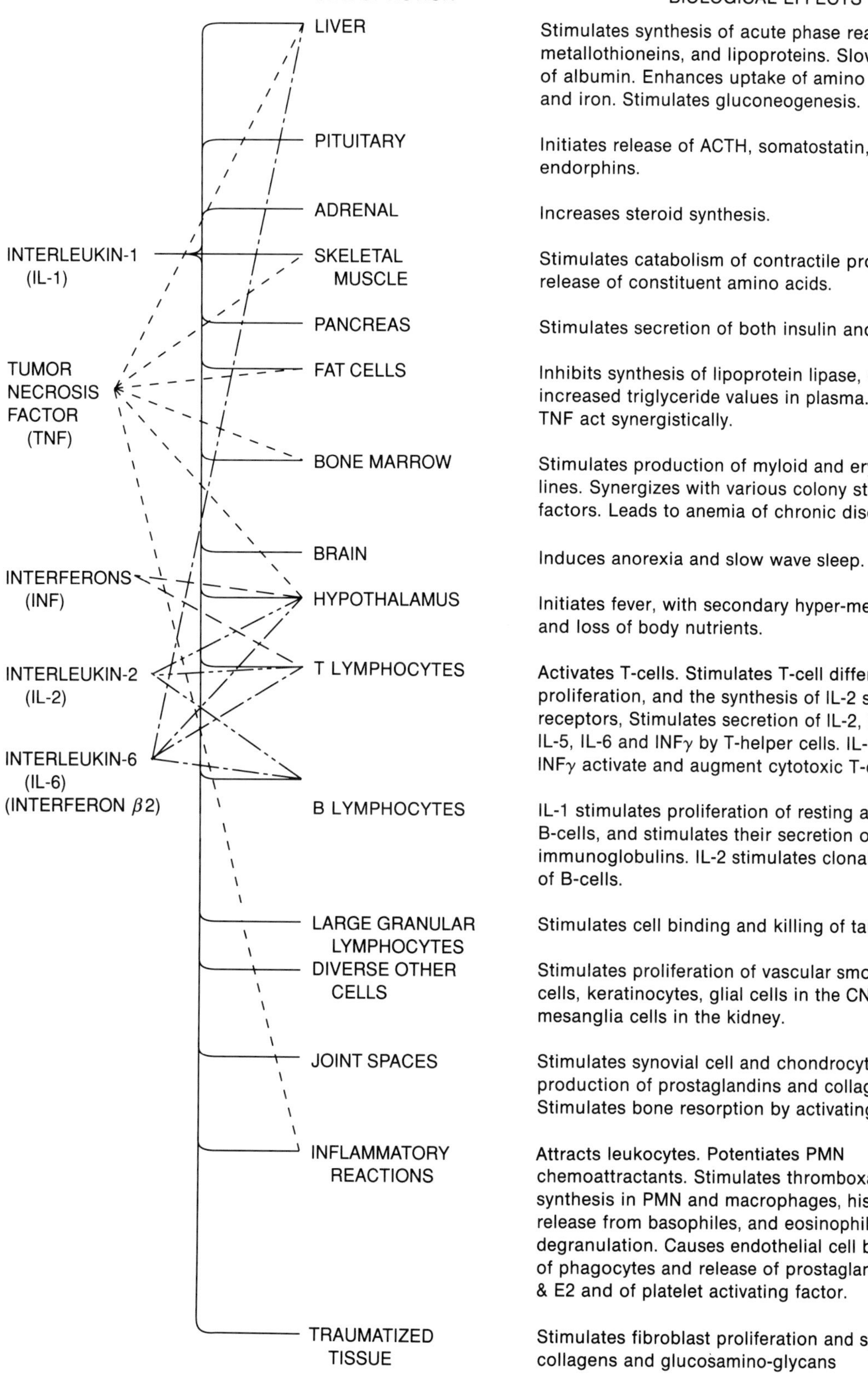

CYTOKINE
SITE OF ACTION
BIOLOGICAL EFFECTS
INTERLEUKIN-1 (IL-1)
TUMOR NECROSIS FACTOR (TNF)
INTERFERONS (INF)
INTERLEUKIN-2 (IL-2)
INTERLEUKIN-6 (IL-6) (INTERFERON β2)
LIVER
Stimulates synthesis of acute phase reactants, metallothioneins, and lipoproteins. Slows synthesis of albumin. Enhances uptake of amino acids, zinc, and iron. Stimulates gluconeogenesis.
PITUITARY
Initiates release of ACTH, somatostatin, and endorphins.
ADRENAL
Increases steroid synthesis.
SKELETAL MUSCLE
Stimulates catabolism of contractile proteins, with release of constituent amino acids.
PANCREAS
Stimulates secretion of both insulin and glucagon.
FAT CELLS
Inhibits synthesis of lipoprotein lipase, causing increased triglyceride values in plasma. IL-1 and TNF act synergistically.
BONE MARROW
Stimulates production of myloid and erythroid cell lines. Synergizes with various colony stimulating factors. Leads to anemia of chronic disease.
BRAIN
Induces anorexia and slow wave sleep.
HYPOTHALAMUS
Initiates fever, with secondary hyper-metabolism and loss of body nutrients.
T LYMPHOCYTES
Activates T-cells. Stimulates T-cell differentiation, proliferation, and the synthesis of IL-2 surface receptors, Stimulates secretion of IL-2, IL-3, IL-4, IL-5, IL-6 and INFγ by T-helper cells. IL-1, IL-2, and INFγ activate and augment cytotoxic T-cell functions.
B LYMPHOCYTES
IL-1 stimulates proliferation of resting and activated B-cells, and stimulates their secretion of immunoglobulins. IL-2 stimulates clonal expansion of B-cells.
LARGE GRANULAR LYMPHOCYTES
Stimulates cell binding and killing of target cells.
DIVERSE OTHER CELLS
Stimulates proliferation of vascular smooth muscle cells, keratinocytes, glial cells in the CNS, and mesanglia cells in the kidney.
JOINT SPACES
Stimulates synovial cell and chondrocyte production of prostaglandins and collagenase. Stimulates bone resorption by activating osteoclasts.
INFLAMMATORY REACTIONS
Attracts leukocytes. Potentiates PMN chemoattractants. Stimulates thromboxane synthesis in PMN and macrophages, histamine release from basophiles, and eosinophil degranulation. Causes endothelial cell binding of phagocytes and release of prostaglandins E1 & E2 and of platelet activating factor.
TRAUMATIZED TISSUE
Stimulates fibroblast proliferation and synthesis of collagens and glucosamino-glycans

Figure 17.5. Cytokines that induce fever and adversely influence host nutrition by their secondary effects.

The immune system, especially its cell-mediated functions, is adversely affected by generalized protein-energy malnutrition as well as by various forms of single-nutrient abnormality (see Table 17.2). Similarly, various forms of malnutrition may have an adverse effect on the function of phagocytic cells. In contrast, the ability of the liver to synthesize acute-phase reactant proteins seems to be sustained even in the presence of the most severe forms of protein and energy deficiencies, in both man and experimental animals (Cockerell, 1973).

Nutritional Responses to Infection

As with many other disease states, acute infections cause metabolic rates and O_2 consumption to increase (Beisel et al., 1980). A concomitant acceleration occurs in both anabolic and catabolic processes despite the seeming incongruity of such a combination. Cells in the liver and lymphoid tissues rapidly increase their rates of synthesis of the proteins needed for host defensive mechanisms, and the proliferation of phagocytic and lymphoid cells is speeded. In order to support these anabolic requirements and to provide the increased fuels needed to maintain high metabolic rates in the presence of anorexia and a diminished food intake, catabolic processes are accelerated also. The stores of labile protein present in muscle fibers and somatic tissues serve to provide the required additional supply of amino acid substrate (Powanda, 1977). These free amino acids are used for glucose production as well as for the synthesis of the new proteins required for host defense. In fueling the increased metabolic activity, the body appears to increase its utilization of glucose. In contrast, utilization of lipid fuels does not appear to be accelerated in acute febrile infections.

Although heightened rates of both anabolism and catabolism occur simultaneously during infection, the catabolic component is far more obvious from a clinical viewpoint. The body loses weight and muscle mass, and its nutrient and fuel stores are consumed in excess of intake. During the acute phase of febrile infections, the body retains water and salt. For a time, fluid retention may mask the extent of weight loss due to catabolism of cellular components. If an infection progresses to a subacute or chronic stage, labile nitrogen stores are expended, fat depots gradually are consumed, and a wasted cachectic state develops.

Protein, Amino Acid, and Nitrogen Metabolism

The importance of protein synthesis in the maintenance of host defense is reflected in the complex readjustments that take place in protein, amino acid, and nitrogen metabolism in the early stages of an acute infection. Labile protein stores in skeletal muscle and other somatic tissues are catabolized at an accelerated rate. Their constituent amino acids are thereby free for reutilization via numerous metabolic pathways in skeletal muscle, the liver, and in many other cells and tissues.

Amino acid metabolism. The amino acid constituents of body proteins, especially the contractile proteins of skeletal muscle, become free as a consequence of protein catabolism. While still within muscle cells, some of the newly released branched-chain free amino acids are deaminated and their carbon skeletons are oxidized as a direct source of cellular energy. The ammonia groups are then reutilized for the de novo synthesis of alanine and glutamine within muscle cells through a combination with two carbon components derived from amino acids, lactate, and/or pyruvate. This synthetic process contributes to the so-called glucose-alanine cycle (see Chapter 4, Figure 4.7) (Felig, 1973). Thus, as free amino acids leave muscle, their relative proportions no longer fully resemble those of the muscle proteins from which they were initially derived.

One of the free amino acids emerging from muscle cells, or more specifically, from the contractile proteins, actin and myosin of skeletal muscle, is 3-methylhistidine. This free amino acid is unique for several reasons: (1) the methyl group is attached only after histidine has first been incorporated into the protein chain of a contractile element of skeletal muscle; (2) once formed, the 3-methylhistidine cannot be reutilized or metabolized further in humans; and (3) after its release during the catabolism of contractile proteins, 3-methylhistidine enters the plasma, is filtered through the renal glomerulus, and is excreted quantitatively in the urine.

Based on these unique phenomena, the urinary excretion of 3-methylhistidine can be used under certain experimental restrictions (i.e., during the avoidance of a meat-containing diet) to estimate the magnitude of catabolism of skeletal muscle protein on a day-to-day basis (Moyer and Powanda, 1981). Such measurements, together with nitrogen balance data, provide indirect evidence for the primary acceleration of muscle protein catabolism during acute febrile infections (Sjolin et al., 1989). As further evidence of skeletal muscle breakdown during severe infection, serum myoglobin and creatinine kinase concentrations may also be increased (Miller et al., 1989).

Although a wide variety of free amino acids reenters the plasma at an accelerated rate during the early stages of an acute febrile infection, plasma concentrations of most of these same free amino acids tend to show a decline, rather than an increase. The minute-to-minute concentration of each free amino acid in plasma represents conceptually the algebraic summation of entry and egress rates into plasma. As both entry and egress rates are accelerated for most free amino acids during early infection, and as a pool size is essentially constant, the falling concentrations of free amino acids must represent an acceleration in egress rates to values greater than those of the entry rates.

Such a postulate has been confirmed in experimental animals. The decline in plasma concentrations of most free amino acids is caused by a marked increase in the movement (or flux) of amino acids from plasma into hepatic cells (Wannemacher, 1977). This phenomenon appears to include the participation of the several different kinds of amino acid transport sites across the outer cell membrane of hepatocytes. This accelerated uptake of amino acids into the liver is believed to be stimulated by the actions of interleukin-1 (IL-1), following its release from activated monocytes, macrophages, and other phagocytic cells. Because an initial interaction of host phagocytic cells with invading microorganisms is one of the earliest host defense responses to infection, it is not surprising that the IL-1-initiated flux of free amino acids from plasma to liver is also one of the earliest of the nonspecific host metabolic responses to an infection (Wannemacher et al., 1973). In fact, declining concentrations of free amino acids were noted early in the incubation period, before the onset of febrile illness, when volunteers were studied longitudinally throughout the course of experimentally induced infections (Moyer and Powanda, 1981).

As pointed out by Wannemacher (1977), the complexities of the infection-induced biochemical and nutritional responses in amino acid metabolism can best be interpreted by determining the responses of individual or closely related small groups of amino acids. The sometimes unique responses of single free amino acids must be considered within the broad framework of the movement of amino acids from catabolized proteins in peripheral somatic tissues, through the plasma pool, to the liver.

The branched-chain amino acids, consisting of leucine, isoleucine, and valine, have emerged as perhaps the most important group of single amino acids contributing to the host responses to infection. In addition to their ability to serve as direct sources of energy within muscle (see Chapter 4), their nitrogen is reutilized for the de novo synthesis of gluconeogenic amino acids (bound for the liver). More importantly, a balanced availability of these branched-chain amino acids is essential to permit an optimal nutritional status within single cells to allow new proteins to be synthesized most efficiently. In support of this concept, Wannemacher et al. (1982) have shown that the intravenous administration of 48% branched-chain amino acid mixtures to infected monkeys receiving only intravenous nutrients could prevent or reverse negative nitrogen balances if given in combination with adequate sources of total energy. No other amino acid combination was as successful in this regard. The greatest decline in plasma concentrations of branched-chain amino acids during human infection has been reported in typhoid fever (Feigin et al., 1968). Experimentally induced nutritional imbalances among the branched-chain amino acids have an adverse impact on immune system competence and function. This adverse impact is greater than that of any other amino acid derangement, with the exception, perhaps, of an absolute deficit in essential amino acids (Beisel, 1982*a*).

Gluconeogenic amino acids are synthesized in muscle and, in addition, come from in vivo protein catabolism or dietary sources. Alanine serves as the major amino acid substrate for glucose production in liver (see Chapter 4, Figure 4.7), and glutamine serves for this purpose primarily in the kidneys. These uses are accelerated during early infection.

The metabolism of tryptophan receives special attention in the liver (see Figure 17.6). An increased activity of tryptophan oxygenase has been shown to occur in rat livers during an infection (Rapoport et al., 1968). This enzyme serves to shunt tryptophan into the vitamin B_6-dependent kynurenine pathway (see Chapter 5, Figure 5.16), where a variety of tryptophan metabolites are formed. These constitute the diazo reactants excreted in the urine. An increased excretion of diazo reactants has been observed in every human infection studied; maximal increases occur in typhoid fever (Rapoport and Beisel, 1971). In-

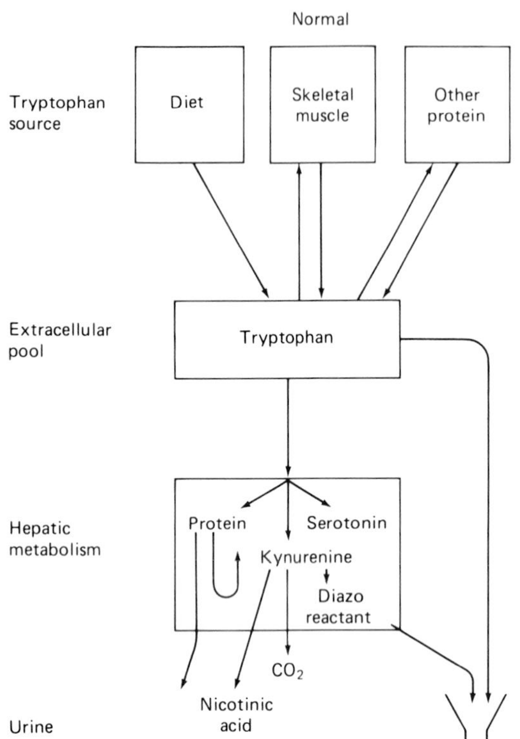

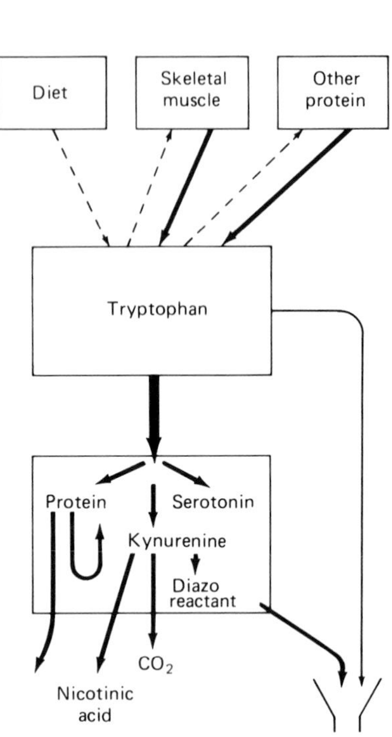

Figure 17.6. Alterations in tryptophan metabolism in infection. A schematic representation of alterations in tryptophan metabolism in infected (right) versus normal (left) animals. Note altered compartment sizes and the decreases (dashed lines) or increases (heavy lines) in pathway usage. [*Source:* Modified from Wannemacher (1977).]

creased activity of the pathways that convert tryptophan into kynurenine metabolites or toward serotonin could help to prevent an excess in plasma of this potentially toxic amino acid.

Phenylalanine is another amino acid that responds uniquely during infections (see Figure 17.7), showing a tendency to increase in concentration, rather than to decrease, as is typical of most other free amino acids. Phenylalanine is linked metabolically to tyrosine to which it can be converted via the action of the hepatic enzyme, phenylalanine hydroxylase (see Chapter 4). Tyrosine itself can be metabolized by tyrosine aminotransferase, an enzyme that also shows increased hepatic activity during acute infection or stress (Shambaugh and Beisel, 1968). Phenylalanine is an amino acid that can be toxic when present in excess. As relatively little phenylalanine is required in the synthesis of new proteins, accelerated metabolism via hepatic pathways would help to prevent a dangerous quantity of phenylalanine from accumulating during infection. Nevertheless, the ratio between phenylalanine and tyrosine concentrations in plasma is consistently increased in infection, due to both the characteristic increase in phenylalanine and the decrease in tyrosine (Wannemacher et al., 1976).

Hepatic synthesis of protein. The accelerated flux of free amino acids into the liver allows them to be used for two primary purposes (i.e., for the synthesis of new proteins or for the production of glucose). Details of hepatic gluconeogenesis are discussed in a subsequent section and in Chapter 4.

For the synthesis of new proteins during infection, the liver cell follows the expected sequence of chromatin template activation within the nucleus, accelerated synthesis of mRNA, mRNA localization to polyribosomes including those on the endoplasmic reticulum, and the formation of nascent protein chains by addition of single amino acids in the proper sequence (Wannemacher, 1975). For hepatic cell production of secreted glycoproteins, the new protein chains are transported through the smooth endoplasmic re-

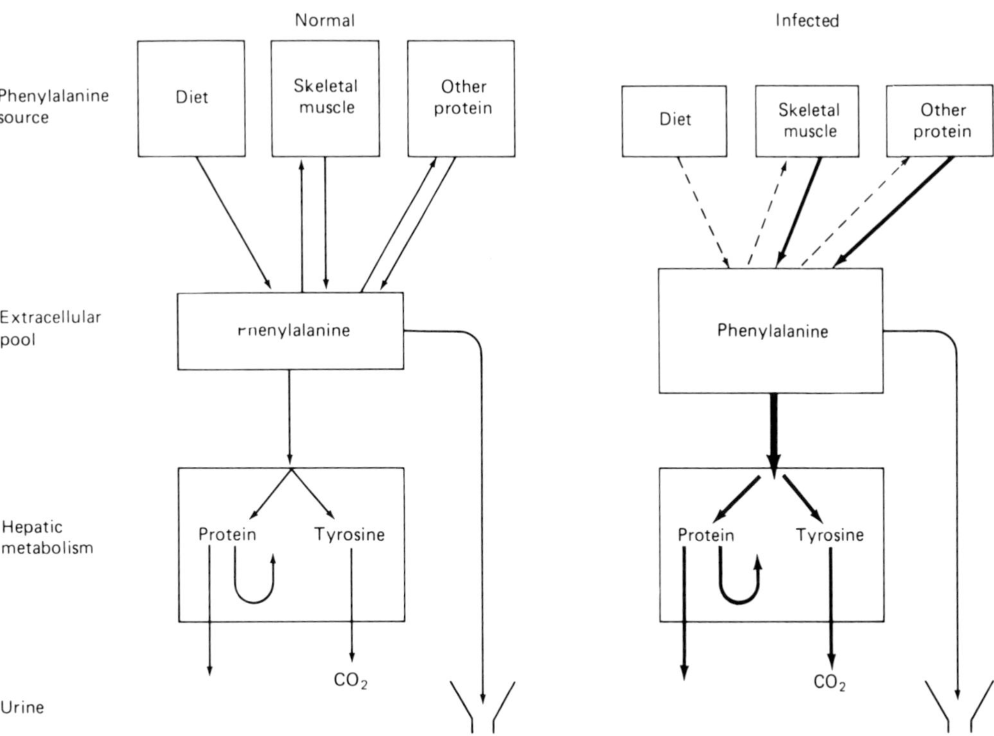

Figure 17.7. Alterations in phenylalanine metabolism in infection. A schematic representation of alterations in phenylalanine metabolism in infected (right) versus normal (left) animals. Note altered compartment sizes and the decreases (dashed lines) or increases (heavy lines) in pathway usage. [*Source:* Modified from Wannemacher (1977).]

ticulum, where carbohydrate molecules are added. The final packaging occurs in the Golgi apparatus prior to release of the glycoproteins into plasma.

Although infection does not alter the molecular mechanisms by which hepatic proteins are produced, it has a profound effect on rates of protein synthesis and the types of proteins being synthesized. The liver accelerates its synthesis of a wide variety of proteins for intracellular use as well as for secretion into plasma (Powanda and Moyer, 1981). Information is not available as to how, or in some instances even why, certain hepatic proteins are selected for accelerated production. These include a number of the enzymes that help regulate the utilization of certain intracellular metabolic pathways within the liver (Rapoport et al., 1968). Increased activities of tryptophan oxygenase, which directs tryptophan into kynurenine metabolites or toward serotonin, and of tyrosine aminotransferase serve as examples. [Both of these can be regulated by glucocorticosteroids, which are released in response to the stress of infection (see below).]

Another example is the rapid synthesis of metallothionein, a unique protein with an extraordinarily high content of cysteine, which serves to bind zinc and sequester it within the liver during active infection (Cousins and Leinart, 1988; Sobocinski et al., 1979). [This again may be controlled by corticosteroids and/or IL-1 (Cousins and Leinart, 1988; Hamer, 1986).]

The majority of newly synthesized hepatic proteins, however, are those classified as acute-phase reactants, a designation that matches their rapid increase in plasma during the acute phase of infectious or inflammatory diseases. These diverse acute-phase reactants are all glycoproteins (see Table 17.3), and include haptoglobin, acid glycoprotein, ceruloplasmin, C-reactive protein, fibrinogen, and—in the rat—macrofetoprotein. It has been postulated (Powanda and Beisel, 1982; Powanda and Moyer, 1981) that each of these proteins has some role to play in the nonspecific aspects of host defense.

Table 17.3. Acute Phase Proteins Found in Increased Concentrations in Plasma in Association with the Acute Phase Response[a]

Haptoglobin
Acid glycoprotein
Ceruloplasmin
α_1 Acid globulin/glycoprotein? (orosomucoid)
C-Reactive protein
Fibrinogen
Complement factor B
Serum amyloid A factor
α_1-Antitrypsin
α_1-Antichymotrypsin
α_1-Macrofetoprotein (in the rat)

[a] These plasma glycoproteins are produced by hepatocytes when stimulated by IL-1, and possibly also by IL-6. The magnitude of the increase in plasma concentrations of these individual glycoproteins provides a rough indication of the severity of the initiating disease process. Although aspects of their individual functions are poorly defined, these acute phase proteins serve in a variety of nonspecific host defense responses.

Although the accelerated influx of free amino acids into the liver could allow for the production of many new protein molecules, Canonico et al. (1977) and Little and Canonico (1981) postulated that increases of some intrahepatic proteins may require decreases of others. This concept is supported by their observations that the activities of some intrahepatic enzymes are diminished during infection. These include catalase, urate oxidase, glucose 6-phosphatase, and 5′-nucleotidase.

A decline in plasma albumin concentrations is perhaps the most consistently observed biochemical change during a wide variety of infectious disease in humans and experimental animals. It has long been assumed that a decreased rate of albumin synthesis was another of the intrahepatic compensatory mechanisms associated with the increase in acute-phase reactant production. However, studies by Wannemacher et al. (1982), performed in Rhesus monkeys with experimentally induced bacterial infections, suggest, instead, that the rates of hepatic synthesis of albumin are neither increased nor decreased during infection. Rather, the rapid fall in plasma albumin concentrations can best be explained by a markedly accelerated catabolism of albumin in peripheral tissues.

In some infections, direct losses of albumin and other plasma proteins may occur through the kidney (febrile proteinuria) or via the intestinal tract (protein-losing enteropathy).

Nitrogen balance. Most infectious illnesses cause the body to lose nitrogen and other nutrient constituents. The amount of loss can be determined by metabolic balance techniques (Beisel et al., 1967). These techniques attempt to achieve an accurate estimation of the difference between body intake and total combined losses over a period of time. Although it is virtually impossible to measure the normally minor losses of nitrogen via hair, sweat, secretions, dermal shedding, expired air, and the like (see Chapter 4, Figure 4.2), reasonably valid estimates can be achieved through careful collection and measurement of consumed foodstuffs and urinary and fecal losses.

Because of the measured losses, the "normal" nitrogen balance of a healthy adult with a stable body weight appears to show a retention of 2–3 g of total nitrogen per day (i.e., an apparent positive balance. Similar values are generally maintained throughout the incubation of the infection, although, in some instances, slightly more positive values may indicate an increase in anabolic activity (see Figure 17.3). Only after fever begins does the nitrogen balance become abruptly negative (Beisel et al., 1967). Daily losses may then range from 2–23 g/day, depending on the presence of anorexia that reduces food intake and the magnitude of hypermetabolism. Febrile hypermetabolism is most important with an average 7% increase in basal metabolic rates per degree Fahrenheit of fever. Losses can be far greater if metabolic rates go even higher, as in patients with severe burns and superimposed infection.

Nitrogen losses from the body occur chiefly via the urine. Virtually every form of urinary nitrogen is increased (i.e., amino nitrogen, creatinine nitrogen, uric acid nitrogen, etc.), but the greatest losses are accounted for by urea nitrogen. As gluconeogenic amino acids are deaminated to provide carbon atoms for glucose production, the nitrogen groups enter into the urea cycle, are converted into urea, and are excreted chiefly in the urine. Unless diarrhea is present, stool nitrogen losses are generally not increased during an infection.

Daily losses of body nitrogen during acute infections reflect the severity and duration of fever. Large initial losses do not resemble those seen at later stages of an infection, for the losses diminish in magnitude if infection persists. Losses can also be influenced by both the age and antecedent nutritional status of a patient. Early losses of nitrogen come chiefly from the so-called labile nitrogen pool, which is represented primarily by the protein in skeletal muscle and other somatic tissues. If an infection enters a subacute or chronic phase, and if the body supplies of labile nitrogen become exhausted, daily losses of nitrogen begin to lessen, and the body enters a new relatively "steady state," but at a wasted cachectic level (Beisel, 1980*a*).

Rapidly growing normal children typically exhibit a strongly positive nitrogen balance. If they become ill with an infection of mild-to-moderate severity, they may not revert to a negative nitrogen balance, but show a less positive balance instead. Daily nitrogen balances may not become appreciably negative in patients who lack adequate stores of labile nitrogen. Such unique findings occur in newborn infants, in the aged, and in previously cachectic patients who have lost large amounts of weight because of starvation, severe injury, or disease processes.

Nitrogen losses can be minimized or even prevented during the infection if the patient consumes, or is given, adequate amounts of amino acids and energy-generating nutrients. Conversely, cumulative losses of nitrogen and other elements can be reversed during the convalescent period. The time required to rebuild lost body stores after an infection may range from weeks to months. This process can be accelerated by providing extra dietary nutrients. Some infants and children experience a period of increased appetite (hyperphagia) when they recover from an infection, and this enables them to achieve "catch-up" growth, if highly nutritious food is available to them.

Carbohydrate Metabolism

The accelerated rates of body metabolism during febrile infections appear to be achieved primarily by oxidation of carbohydrate fuels. This increase in carbohydrate utilization is brought about by a complex variety of metabolic and hormonal responses that coincide in their onset with the beginning of fever.

Some insights into the sequence of carbohydrate-related events was initially gained by studies of laboratory animals given lethal doses of endotoxin. An initial brief period of hyperglycemia was followed by progressive disappearance of glucose from blood, and glycogen from tissue stores. At death, hypoglycemia was severe and the body was virtually devoid of carbohydrate (Berry et al., 1959). During the early period, glucose production was increased, but declined markedly in the hours before death (Wolfe, 1981).

Some aspects of this endotoxin model may be pertinent to infections with living organisms. At the onset of symptomatic illness, fasting blood glucose concentrations may be slightly elevated; if a glucose tolerance test is done, the results resemble those seen in adult diabetic subjects. The initial glucose rise after an intravenous infusion reaches higher than normal concentrations, and the subsequent fall is slower than normal (Shambaugh and Beisel, 1967*a*).

Within hours after the onset of fever in man, fasting plasma insulin values are increased modestly, and the insulin response to infused glucose is greater than normal, resembling in pattern the hyperinsulinemic response of adult-onset diabetic patients. Glucagon concentrations are also high. During a glucose infusion, the response of growth hormone values is paradoxical, showing an abrupt rise rather than the expected decline. A combination of endocrine responses at the onset of acute fever of infectious origin, especially the increased glucagon, has the net result of accelerating hepatic production of new glucose and the release of glucose from stored glycogen (Rayfield et al., 1973; Rocha et al., 1973).

The finding of a slowed rate of glucose disappearance from plasma in the presence of higher than normal insulin values suggests the presence of partial insulin resistance in peripheral tissues (perhaps attributable to a variety of changes in insulin receptor numbers and/or affinities of different target cell populations). This concept is compatible with the time-honored clinical knowledge that insulin-requiring diabetic patients must increase their insulin doses whenever a fever occurs in order to prevent hyperglycemia and glycosuria. The hormonal adjustments to acute febrile illness revert quickly to normal following recovery. The transient nature of the seeming insulin resistance suggests that alterations may have occurred in the number or affinity of insulin receptors on cellular membranes throughout peripheral body tissues.

Although early infectious illnesses are typically accompanied by modest hyperglycemia, there are several clinical situations in which hypoglycemia may be found. In fact, infection-induced hypoglycemia may create a dangerous life-threatening state. Low blood glucose values may be seen clinically in septic gram-negative shock, in newborn or premature infants with generalized infections, or in patients with severe forms of infectious hepatitis (Felig et al., 1970). Each of these situations can be explained by a failure of the liver to sustain an adequate production of glucose. In septic shock or severe hepatitis, the breakdown may occur in the metabolic pathways and in the production of enzymes required for hepatic gluconeogenesis. In infantile hypoglycemia, the breakdown can best be ascribed to an inadequate supply of substrate nutrients. The infant is born with little skeletal muscle protein and too small a pool of labile nitrogen to permit a sizeable diversion of amino acids into gluconeogenic pathways.

There is no evidence to suggest that the usual metabolic pathways for either glycogenolysis or gluconeogenesis (see Chapter 2, Figure 2.4) are altered in any fundamental manner during the infection. Rather, the rates of their utilization are accelerated. The hepatic production and release of glucose are undoubtedly responding to the combined hormonal changes that accompany an infection. Although these hormonal changes will be reviewed in a subsequent section, it should be noted here that, in addition to the already mentioned increases in insulin, glucagon, and growth hormone output, other major glucose-influencing hormones are also involved in the endocrine responses to infection. These include an increased adrenal production of cortisol and other related glucocorticoids, accelerated hepatic metabolism of the thyroid hormones, and, in some infections (especially those that produce hypotensive changes), an increased release of the catecholamines.

In producing the additional glucose, the liver uses all the usual forms of substrate. These include glycerol released from triglycerides during lipolysis in fat depots (see Chapter 4, Figure 4.9) and other tissues, lactic acid and pyruvate created by metabolic activity of cells throughout the body, and, importantly, the gluconeogenic amino acids released from muscle and taken up by the liver at an accelerated rate. The utilization of amino acids as a substrate for glucose production is a costly process for the body in comparison to the use of other substrates (see Chapter 4, Figure 4.8; also Chapter 8). In addition to the diversion of amino acids away from their utilization for protein synthesis, the metabolic costs of deamination and ureagenesis must be subtracted from the energy ultimately derived from the use of amino acids for glucose production. The body seems willing to pay these additional costs in order to overcome and eliminate the invading microorganisms.

An accelerated use of carbohydrate fuels in cellular metabolism has clearly been identified with one important host defensive mechanism—the "respiratory burst," which accompanies the phagocytic activity of neutrophils and macrophages and is fueled by carbohydrate. In rats with *Escherichia coli* sepsis, glucose utilization is increased primarily in macrophage-rich tissues (liver, spleen, ilium) and in several skeletal muscles (Meszaros et al., 1988). On the other hand, it is not clear why an increased use of carbohydrate as a general fuel is of unique value for other aspects of body defense. Glucose appears to be employed to permit the increase in cellular metabolic rates associated with fever (see Chapter 8). Because under normal circumstances, lipid fuels supply the vast majority of body energy needs, it is uncertain why the use of lipid fuels is not appreciably accelerated to provide for the extra energy requirements of fever.

Interrelated metabolic and physiologic aspects of energy metabolism were studied in a group of 14 seriously septic febrile patients who had an increased cardiac output and were not hypotensive (Clowes et al., 1982). These patients showed an increase in blood flow to the legs, with an increase in fasting blood glucose, and an increase in glucose uptake in the legs. Their serum lactate and leg lactate production were increased, but serum free fatty acid values were low. Total free amino acid concentrations were decreased in sepsis, even though leg output of total free amino acids was enhanced. In contrast to most free amino acids, concentrations of plasma phenylalanine and methionine were increased. These findings are in keeping with the preceding discussions of amino acid and carbohydrate metabolism during infection, and the data on lipid metabolism which follow.

Lipid Metabolism

The metabolic responses involving alterations in lipid metabolism during infection are more complex and less well-defined than those involving protein or carbohydrate responses. Altered lipid metabolism, however, can be identified in liver, plasma, and peripheral tissues (see Figure 17.8).

Within liver cells there appears to be an absolute increase in lipogenic activity, with the creation of new fatty acid molecules directly from acetate through the use of conventional lipogenic pathways. Once formed, the fatty acids may be assembled into triglycerides or may be transported as free fatty acids into the mitochondria of the liver cell. Free fatty acids (FFA) taken up by the liver from plasma albumin (which serves as a transport protein) are also transferred into the mitochondria, and both may be used for energy pro-

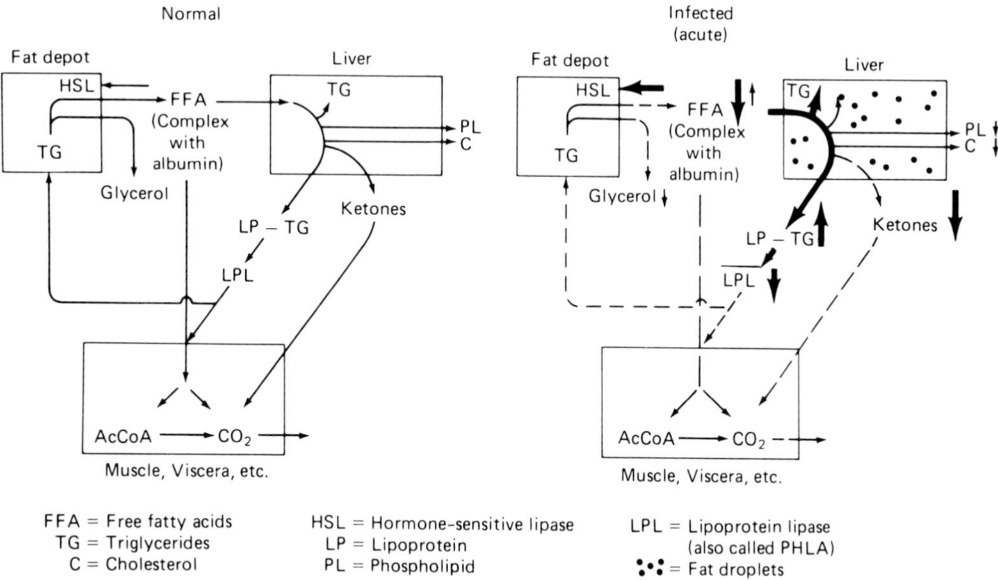

Figure 17.8. Infection and lipid metabolism. A schematic representation of the effects of acute infection (right) on various aspects of host lipid metabolism in rats in comparison to findings in a pair-fed normal control (left) with an equivalent degree of reduced food intake. Pathway or movement (flux) of lipids is shown, with dashed lines indicating decreases and thickened lines indicating increases. Direction and magnitude of change in the concentration of plasma components are shown by short vertical arrows. [*Source:* Reprinted by permission from Beisel et al. (1980).]

duction. The movement of FFA into mitochondria is achieved through carnitine-requiring enzymes (see Chapter 5, Figure 5.37). Detailed studies of hepatic carnitine metabolism during a variety of experimental infections in laboratory animals show that there is no deficiency in the carnitine cofactors required to permit the enzyme-regulated entry of free fatty acids into the mitochondria. The short-chain FFA have no difficulty in being taken up by the mitochondria, but during infection, problems may occur with long-chain FFA (Wannemacher et al., 1981).

The fatty acids assembled into triglycerides may begin to accumulate in hepatocytes during an infection. Sufficient quantities may be generated so as to form lipid droplets within hepatic cells and eventually lead to fatty metamorphosis or lipid degeneration, as seen microscopically. At the same time, the hepatic cell production of lipoproteins is increased. This latter activity is not always sufficient to prevent formation or accumulation of lipid droplets within the cells.

The purposes or potential value of hepatic lipogenesis is uncertain. This activity may be stimulated by the higher than normal baseline concentrations of insulin in plasma.

Very little is known about the hepatic production of phospholipids during infection. Cholesterol production and its hepatic release in complexes with lipoproteins is modestly accelerated (Fiser et al., 1971).

Ketone formation had traditionally been thought to increase during febrile illnesses. However, recent studies show that, when related to the concomitant presence of starvation, ketogenesis is less than expected (Neufeld et al., 1976). This partial inhibition of hepatic ketone production has also been ascribed to the action of insulin, although it may also be related in part to the altered transport of long-chain FFA into liver mitochondria, where ketone body production normally occurs. There is no evidence that ketone body metabolism in peripheral tissues is altered or inhibited by infection.

The plasma concentration and transport of various lipids during infection is influenced by a variety of factors. FFA values typically show a decline that has been ascribed to: (1) a decrease in hormone-stimulated lipolysis in peripheral tissues in part mediated by the presence of higher than normal insulin concentrations; (2) a decrease in plasma albumin levels; (3) an alteration in the rate of flux of FFA from plasma into liver; and (4) changes in rates of FFA uptake as an energy source in peripheral body cells.

The decline in albumin concentrations in plasma is probably the most important factor in terms of actual FFA concentration, whereas the overall movement of FFA from depots to liver and peripheral tissues is more important in terms of lipid utilization for cellular energy production. In any event, plasma FFA concentrations are not a good indicator of rates of either lipolysis or tissue utilization (Wannemacher et al., 1981).

Cholesterol values in plasma do not always follow a clear or consistent pattern during infections. In some instances, they are said to increase, in some to decrease, and in some to remain unchanged. Perhaps the most consistent pattern is a brief decline from normal baseline values in individuals who develop a mild viral illness. It is not certain if the altered concentrations of cholesterol in plasma are due to alterations in rates of cholesterol production, cholesterol uptake by cells or tissues, or to an altered availability of the carrier lipoproteins (Beisel and Fiser, 1970).

Plasma triglycerides show a fairly consistent tendency to increase during most infectious illnesses. This is especially true in gram-negative sepsis, where the rise in triglycerides may cause the plasma to appear milky. The increases in triglyceride values can be accounted for by an increase in hepatic production in combination with a decrease in peripheral uptake and removal rates. The propensity for gram-negative infections to produce an exaggerated hypertriglyceridemia in man was true also in Rhesus monkeys when the triglyceride response was compared in gram-positive (*Streptococcus pneumonia*) and gram-negative (*Salmonella typhimurium*) sepsis (Kaufmann et al., 1976*a*, *b*).

These findings in experimental animals and man can now be explained by the action on fat cells of two monokines, IL-1 and Tumor Necrosis Factor (TNF), both of which reduce the activity of lipoprotein lipase (Tracey et al., 1988), the enzyme in peripheral tissues needed to allow the tissues to take up lipid from the transport lipoproteins (Chapter 3, Figure 3.5). IL-1 is modest in its effects on this enzyme (Dinarello, 1987). In contrast, the effect of TNF, a monokine also called cachectin, is far greater. Since endotoxin is the most potent stimulus for TNF release from monocytes (Urbaschek and Urbaschek, 1987), it is not surprising that the greatest accumulation of triglycerides in plasma occurs during gram-negative sepsis. In addition, TNF stimulates the release of free fatty acids from lipocytes, and thereby contributes to the weight loss and cachexia of chronic or repeated infections.

Mineral and Trace Element Metabolism

The metabolic responses to infection involve virtually all the minerals that can be assayed with accuracy. The principal point in this regard is the observation that the pattern of changes in the balance of intracellular minerals resembles that of nitrogen balance. Patterns of absolute losses of minerals, as determined by balance data, can be estimated using the nitrogen : potassium, nitrogen : phosphorus, and nitrogen : magnesium ratios found in normal skeletal muscle tissue (Beisel et al., 1967).

As applied to body phosphorus losses, this concept has two exceptions. Corrections must be made for the concomitant phosphorus : calcium ratios based on bone mineral and calcium balance, plus the fact that blood and urinary phosphate respond in a unique manner during periods of respiratory hyperventilation. This is due to the accompanying exaggerated loss of CO_2 and the production of respiratory alkalosis. Periods of rapidly rising body temperatures are typically accompanied by tachypnea (rapid breathing), excess respiratory loss of CO_2, and a rising blood pH. Under these circumstances, plasma phosphate concentrations show a dramatic decline, and phosphate virtually disappears from the urine. This is a short-lived phenomenon of early infection; body phosphate losses thereafter follow nitrogen losses, maintaining a phosphorus : nitrogen ratio typical of normal muscle (Beisel et al., 1967).

Most infectious diseases do not have a detectable effect on body balances of calcium, as body losses are chiefly derived from the soft tissues rather than from bone. However, if an infection, such as poliomyelitis, leads to paralysis of skeletal muscles, this complication produces secondary metabolic consequences because of the atrophy of body soft tissues and bone. The period of initial atrophy is accompanied by negative body balances of nitrogen and other intracellular elements from muscle and of calcium, phosphorus, and other minerals from bone.

Although gross changes in calcium balance do not occur in most infections, the recent discovery of calmodulin and its actions suggests that calcium ions participate at the molecular level in many of the host responses to infection and bacterial toxemias. The triggering of a cellular biochemical response to various cytokines is accompanied, in many instances, by an influx of calcium into the target cell (Minghetti and Norman, 1988). (See also Chapter 6.)

Sulfur is a difficult element to quantitate in metabolic balance studies; no balance data are available for any infectious disease. Nevertheless, scattered data from the older literature permit an assumption that sulfur losses follow a pattern similar to those of nitrogen (Beisel et al., 1976).

Zinc is another element that has not been subjected to formal metabolic balance measurements during infectious illnesses. Changes in dietary intake and urinary loss, however, suggest that zinc losses also resemble those of nitrogen. Henkin and Smith (1972) reported a marked reduction in the binding of zinc to plasma macroligands during acute infectious hepatitis. Normally, nearly all of the zinc circulating in plasma is bound to carrier proteins, such as α_2-macroglobulin (see Chapter 7, Figure 7.7). A shift in zinc binding in hepatitis leads to a preponderance of zinc bound to free amino acid microligands, such as histidine. Since zinc–amino acid complexes are small enough to pass through the renal glomerulus, their filtration is followed by sizeable losses of zinc in the urine.

The most notable aspect of altered zinc metabolism during infection, however, is not its loss from the body. Rather, zinc is one of the elements that undergoes a consistent, rapid, and sizeable redistribution within the body. Within hours after the administration of endotoxin or the onset of an infectious process of bacterial or viral origin, plasma concentrations begin to decline. Zinc values typically fall to about half of normal (Kampschmidt, 1981) (see Chapter 7, Figure 7.6). This redistribution has been attributed chiefly to a flux of zinc from plasma to liver and probably results from IL-1-stimulated rapid synthesis of metallothionein, a binding protein that sequesters zinc within the hepatocytes. Both the depression of plasma zinc and its accumulation within the liver during infectious illnesses are components of the acute phase response, which occur as secondary consequences of enhanced hepatic metallothionein synthesis (Cousins and Leinart, 1988). It has been postulated that the hepatic sequestration of zinc may serve a useful purpose in host defense by depressing zinc concentrations in plasma to a range more favorable to effective phagocytic cell function (Pekarek and Englehardt, 1981).

Iron is another mineral that undergoes a dramatic, physiologically controlled redistribution with sequestration in storage forms (Beisel, 1976). Like zinc, the flux of iron from plasma to sequestration sites within the hepatocytes and reticuloendothelial cells is very rapid (see Chapter 7, Figure 7.6), occurring within a matter of hours after experimental administration of bacterial endotoxin to laboratory animals or after the initiation of an infectious illness. Like zinc, the iron stimulates de novo synthesis of, and accumulates in, an intracellular storage protein (ferritin) (Campbell et al., 1989; Hershko and Konijn, 1977; Schiaffonati et al., 1988) (see Chapter 7). Iron differs from zinc in its far greater degree of decline in plasma values, in terms of percent of normal concentrations. While zinc may fall to half of its normal values in plasma, iron can fall to the point where it is virtually nondetectable. The greatest decline in iron values is associated with pyrogenic infections.

IL-1 (Table 17.2) was initially thought to induce this rapid infection-related hypoferremia (Kampschmidt, 1981), but the monokine, TNF, also appears responsible (Moldawer et al., 1989). The decrease in plasma iron may thus be due to an increased uptake by hepatocytes (and by cells of the spleen and other tissues) for sequestration in ferritin. An increase in intracellular ferritin in these cells is brought about by the shift of preexisting ferritin mRNA to the polyribosomes (Campbell et al., 1989). These phenomena provide a molecular mechanism for the redistribution of iron to intracellular sites in the liver and spleen. The synthesis of additional ferritin is thus analogous to the cytokine-induced synthesis of hepatic metallothionein, which provides intracellular binding sites for the sequestration of zinc (Hamer, 1986). The intracellular storage of iron during infection may also be heightened by as yet undetermined mechanisms that inhibit release of intracellular iron (Beisel, 1976).

Removal of iron from the circulation in infection, a phenomenon in which lactoferrin (an iron-binding protein produced by phagocytic cells) also plays a role, is important because it reduces the availability of iron for invading microorganisms (see Chapter 7 and below).

If an infection persists, the cellular sequestration of iron can lead to the so-called "anemia of infection." Rapid hypoferremia induced by TNF is followed, in rats, by a marked decrease in RBC mass. The anemia of infection is characterized by a normal size and hemoglobin content of individual RBCs. If iron is administered therapeutically during an infection, in an attempt to prevent or reverse either the anemia or the low plasma iron values, the administered iron also enters storage sites. Only after the infection is eliminated does the sequestered iron typically become free to serve again its normal physiologic role in hemoglobin production.

Two clinical events have been identified that can lead to release of hepatic iron and hyperferremia (greater than normal concentrations). This may occur during the second or third weeks of acute viral hepatitis. High iron values have also been seen in patients with typhoid fever while they were receiving appropriate antimicrobial therapy (Pekarek and Engelhardt, 1981).

The abrupt decline in plasma iron at the onset of an acute infectious illness appears to serve as a unique mechanism of host defense. Iron is an essential nutrient for the growth and proliferation of bacteria and certain other microorganisms. In fact, many bacteria possess an ability to secrete siderophores, which can bind iron in the surrounding media and thereby increase its availability for the bacteria. On the other hand, the two principal plasma iron-binding proteins of the host have association constants for iron greater than those of the bacterial siderophores. Thus, if host iron-binding proteins, transferrin in plasma and lactoferrin in other places, are in an unsaturated form, they compete quite effectively with bacterial invaders for any available local "free" iron. The movement of iron from plasma to sequestration sites serves to increase the concentration of unsaturated transferrin in the circulating plasma. The direct release of lactoferrin from phagocytic cells in local areas of an inflammatory process also serves to reduce the availability of iron for uptake by bacteria in the inflammatory zone (Pekarek and Engelhardt, 1981).

Copper is a third trace element that undergoes physiologic redistribution during bacterial or viral infection (Beisel, 1976). Copper is an integral component of ceruloplasmin, one of the acute-phase reactant proteins secreted by the liver into the plasma. The increase in plasma copper as a component of ceruloplasmin occurs about 1 day after the more abrupt declines in iron and zinc at the onset of infection. After an infection has been cured, the decline of plasma copper values to normal concentrations is gradual and in accord with the expected half-disappearance time for ceruloplasmin. It is not known if copper is lost from the body during acute infections. Although the purpose of redistribution of copper is not well-defined, it has been postulated that ceruloplasmin may contribute to nonspecific host defenses (Powanda, 1977; Powanda and Beisel, 1982). Ceruloplasmin has at least two different functions, being a source of copper for cells and also a scavenger of superoxide and other oxygen radicals (see Chapter 7). Thus, its roles in inflammation could include copper transport for synthesis of cuproenzymes, modulation of the catecholamine and histamine responses, and/or the inactivation of superoxide and other radicals produced in areas of acute inflammation (Powanda and Moyer, 1981).

Electrolyte and Acid-Base Changes

Changes in electrolyte metabolism characterize the onset and early periods of an acute febrile infection. Initially, there may be a slight increase in the urinary losses of sodium and chloride at the onset of fever. Drenching sweats associated with some patterns of fever can lead to a direct dermal loss of these electrolytes, and vomiting can lead to direct losses of hydrogen and chloride ions.

Within a day or two after the fever has begun, however, renal mechanisms come into play that limit the losses of sodium and chloride in the urine. This renal retention of salt can be ascribed to the actions of aldosterone. Adrenal secretion of this potent mineralocorticoid increases progressively during early fever. Urinary sodium and chloride values decrease concomitantly. Retention of salt is accompanied by retention of water (Beisel, 1981).

An additional hormonal response may emerge in some severe infections to complicate electrolyte changes still further. This involves the secretion of an antidiuretic hormone from the posterior pituitary, which adds an additional stimulus for the retention of body water. In fact, in infections with an intracranial localization, or in Rocky Mountain spotted fever, the production of antidiuretic hormone may become "inappropriate" and contribute to a dangerous water overload and a severe dilutional hyponatremia. In severe disseminated infections, metabolic acidosis and tissue anoxia may impair cellular membrane functions to a degree that allows sodium and hydrogen ions to accumulate in excess within body cells (Beisel, 1981).

Another form of localized infection (i.e., diarrheal disease) has an important effect on water and electrolyte homeostasis. The most severe water and electrolyte losses are seen during Asiatic cholera, and in infants during enterotoxigenic *Escherichia coli* and enterovirus infections. In a matter of hours, the massive fecal losses of an isoosmotic fluid, containing chiefly water and electrolytes, can lead to severe depletion of extracellular fluid, marked hemoconcentration, and hypovolemic hypotension. The pattern of electrolyte loss in diarrheic infections due to the cholera-like enterotoxins that stimulate adenylate cyclase activity is largely controlled by the rate of fluid loss. At the onset of cholera, stool volumes may exceed 500 ml/hr; sodium and bicarbonate content may each exceed 80 meq/L in diarrheic fluids, whereas potassium content is much lower, at 25–30 meq/L (Beisel et al., 1963). As stool production slows over the next several days, the concentrations of sodium and bicarbonate decline and that of potassium increases. Stool losses in milder forms of watery diarrhea are typically high in potassium. In dysenteric infections, direct losses include blood, mucus, cell debris, and protein, which typically are absent from watery stool.

The widely different types of salt and water abnormalities generated by infectious diseases are matched by an equally wide divergence in the kinds of change that can emerge in acid-base relationships. In fact, as illustrated in Figure 17.9, the various aspects or complications of infectious illnesses can induce any one of the four major acid-base derangements.

The onset of fever from any cause is accompanied by an accelerated respiratory rate and an exaggerated loss of CO_2 from the plasma. This leads transiently to typical respiratory alkalosis, with a pronounced increase in plasma pH and a slight decrease in plasma bicarbonate.

Respiratory acidosis is far less common, but can occur if pulmonary gas exchange is compromised by extensive pulmonary consolidation (as in acute pneumonia), lung destruction (as in advanced tuberculosis), or respiratory muscle paralysis (as in poliomyelitis or botulism). In such instances, CO_2 accumulation in plasma causes a decline in pH, together with a modest increase in plasma bicarbonate.

Metabolic acidosis can emerge in severe generalized infections, especially those that are associated with hypotensive shock and tissue anoxia.

Figure 17.9. Acid-base balance in infection. A schematic representation of various types of altered acid-base balance associated with different infectious diseases and their complications. The figure plots plasma HCO_3^- (vertical) versus plasma pH (horizontal). Dashed lines represent isobars for CO_2 pressure.

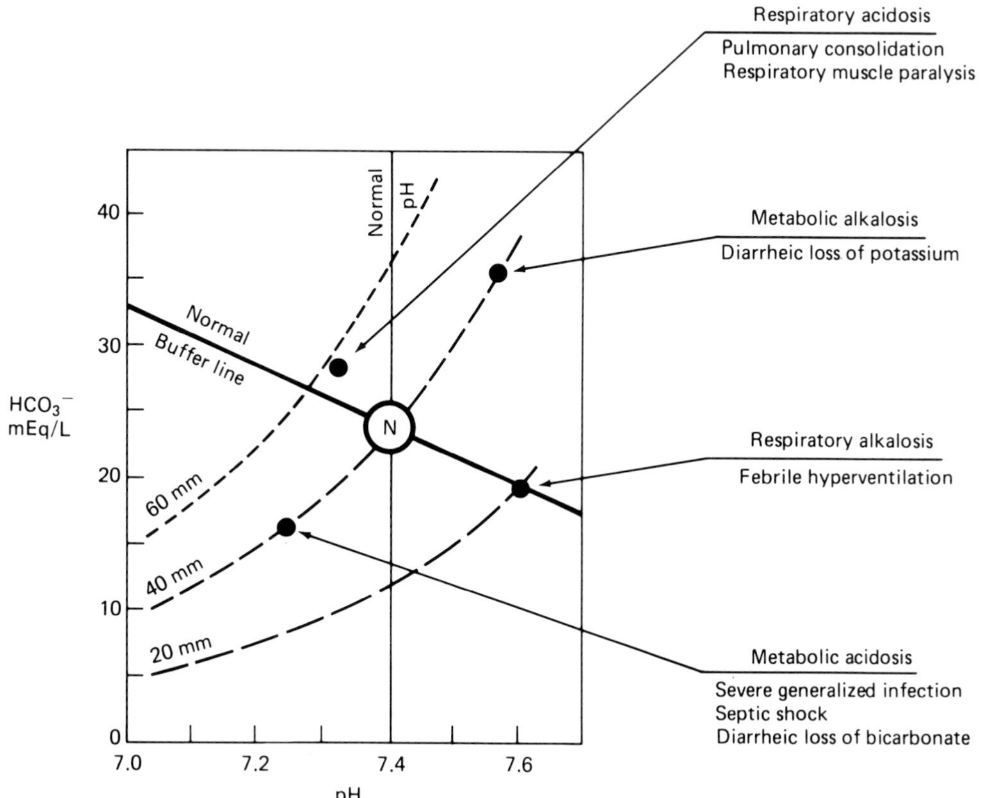

The accumulation of lactic acid and other acidic metabolic products lowers plasma pH and bicarbonate values. This is a relatively common problem, especially when infectious illnesses develop in patients who are already severely ill with other medical or surgical problems, or with a malignancy.

Metabolic alkalosis is relatively uncommon, but does occur as a long-term problem if diarrhea produces a massive depletion of body potassium. In such instances, tissues such as the renal tubules and myocardium develop vascular cellular degenerative changes, and the plasma pH and bicarbonate content are both elevated.

Vitamin Changes

Very little is known about changes in vitamin metabolism during infectious illnesses. It is theorized that body stores of vitamins can be reduced or depleted because of heightened rates of cellular metabolism and/or the altered use of certain metabolic pathways during infectious illnesses. Reduced vitamin intake is common and, possibly, greater direct vitamin losses occur via urine. This concept is in accord with the sparse available data (Beisel et al., 1972). Older clinical observations (Scrimshaw et al., 1968) documented the occasional clinical onset of avitaminoses, such as scurvy, beriberi, or pellagra, during the course of acute infectious illnesses.

The adrenal content of ascorbic acid is reduced during periods of rapid steroidogenesis. Losses of riboflavin via the urine are increased in conjunction with the negative nitrogen balance of acute infection. A large number of vitamins, including pyridoxine, pantothenic acid, and vitamins C, A, and E, contribute to the function of phagocytic cells and/or lymphocytes. Greater activity of these cells undoubtedly accelerates or otherwise influences vitamin metabolism and degradation.

Hormonal Effects

As indicated in the preceding sections, the metabolic responses to infection are modulated and influenced by the interacting effects of many hormones (Beisel, 1981). It is not yet known how this broad complex of endocrine and metabolic responses is orchestrated and interdigitated during the sequential stages of an infectious process. Even without this fundamental understanding of the central regulatory controls, observational data indicate that all major hormones become transiently involved, with the exception of those secreted by the gonads and parathyroid glands.

Adrenocortical Responses

In accord with the concepts of Selye (1948) concerning alarm, stress, and adrenal function, an increased secretion of adrenal glucocorticoids occurs at the onset of acute febrile illnesses, whereas a decreased adrenal output characterizes the cachectic stages of chronic infections, such as tuberculosis. These hormonal events, however, are alone far too limited in magnitude and duration to be a major controlling factor in the numerous host metabolic responses to infection (Beisel and Rapoport, 1969).

In coincidence with, or shortly before, the onset of fever, an increased adrenocortical output of cortisol becomes detectable. Increases in plasma cortisol are not great, however. The initial cortisol response leads to a disappearance of the circadian nadir in plasma values normally seen during afternoon and evening hours. A modest increase above the normal morning time plasma cortisol concentrations may also occur transiently in severe acute infections. However, marked increases are not seen unless there is an agonal failure in hepatic capabilities for converting cortisol to its water-soluble metabolites (Beisel, 1981). None of the changes in plasma cortisol can be attributed to changes in cortisol-binding proteins of plasma. The increased adrenal secretion of cortisol during infection can, however, be ascribed, in part, to an IL-1-stimulated release of ACTH from the anterior pituitary, as well as to possible direct effects of IL-1 on the adrenal cortex itself (Dinarello, 1985; Kluger et al., 1985).

The increase in 24-hr urinary cortisol (and 17-OH corticosteroid) output typically is only two- to threefold above normal during acute infections, but may reach a sixfold increase. This increase is short-lived and returns abruptly to normal when recovery begins, or it falls to subnormal values if an infection becomes chronic. On the other hand, adrenal steroid output is terminated abruptly if a hemorrhagic diathesis leads to adrenal gland infarction (Beisel and Rapoport, 1969).

Typically, the other 17-hydroxy- and 17-ketosteroids of adrenal origin follow the patterns of cortisol secretion, although their increases in output are proportionately smaller.

In contrast, the adrenocortical output of aldosterone follows a different pattern and timing of increase. The onset and rate of increase in plasma values of this mineralocorticoid are more gradual, and the subsequent return to normal is also less abrupt. When the aldosterone effect has ended, the excess of body salt and water retained during the illness is excreted by diuresis in the early convalescent period (Beisel, 1981). It has not yet been determined if the increased adrenal output of aldosterone is an IL-1-stimulated phenomenon.

Adrenomedullary Hormones

Although very few direct measurements of plasma or urinary catecholamines have been reported, relatively small increases (1.2- to 1.6-fold) may occur during mild infections in humans (Mason et al., 1979). Gram-negative sepsis, especially if accompanied by hypotensive shock, leads to greater output of epinephrine and norepinephrine in plasma (Groves et al., 1973).

Thyroid Hormones

The thyroidal hormone responses to infection resemble those that occur during other acute illnesses, trauma, or surgery (Beisel, 1981). Surprisingly, however, the thyroid and its hormones do not appear to participate in or influence the development of fever. Even their contribution to the hypermetabolic state of the febrile patient seems minor.

The changes in thyroid hormone metabolism must be viewed through each of two separate mechanisms: (1) glandular production, storage, and release of the hormones; and (2) peripheral utilization or degradation of these hormones by various tissues. The pattern of longitudinal changes in these mechanisms that occurs during acute infections does not seem to be coordinated. As a result, the hormonal measurements tend to show a biphasic progression.

Early in infection, there is an increase in the rates of thyroid hormone uptake and degradation by the cells of peripheral tissues (Shambaugh and Beisel, 1976*b*; Wartofsky, 1974). The rates of clearance of T_4 and T_3 are generally accelerated, with the liver and peripheral blood neutrophils having important roles in hormonal uptake, deiodination, or conversion to other less active metabolites. A greater percentage of T_4 is converted in the liver to rT_3, rather than to T_3 (Chopra et al., 1975). On the other hand, the clearance rates of T_4 and T_3 may be slowed in patients with malaria (Wartofsky et al., 1972), apparently because of an impairment in hepatic function. The magnitude of the contribution of changes in the thyroid-binding proteins of plasma [i.e., prealbumin and transthyretin (thyroxidine-binding globulin; Harvey, 1971)] to the altered clearance of the hormones or to the decline in protein-bound iodine (Shambaugh and Beisel, 1966, 1967*b*) is not certain.

Both the thyroidal uptake of inorganic iodide and the release of hormonal iodine are slowed during a variety of acute infections in man and the laboratory animal. The apparent slowing-down of thyroid gland function at a time in early infection when thyroid hormones are being utilized at an accelerated rate seems paradoxical. These changes in thyroid gland activities can best be accounted for by sluggish responses of the control mechanism in the hypothalamus, involving thyrotropin-releasing factor (TRF) and thyroid-stimulating hormone (TSH). In convalescence, however, an overshoot of these controls causes a thyroidal rebound with greater than normal hormone values in plasma.

Pituitary Responses

As the master control gland of the endocrine system, the anterior pituitary gland participates importantly in the complex hormonal responses to infection. The posterior pituitary, on the other hand, secretes increased amounts of antidiuretic hormones (ADH) as its principal contribution. ADH secretion may become inappropriately large in some infections, as described earlier.

The release of ACTH from the anterior pituitary during infection, and perhaps the release of several other hormones as well (e.g., somatostatin and growth hormone), are induced by IL-1 (Dinarello, 1985). The increased secretion of anterior pituitary hormones during infection is probably a secondary consequence of IL-1 actions on the hypothalamus which cause the secretion of neurohormonal-releasing factors.

In contrast to the apparent early increase in ACTH, the TSH response is diminished, apparently in response to a diminished output of TRF from the hypothalamus.

Slight increases in morning fasting concentrations of growth hormone in plasma have been noted in a variety of bacterial and viral infections. Growth hormone is one of the hormones secreted in short bursts from the anterior pituitary. Thus, increases are not persistent and do not necessarily correlate in magnitude with the presence or height of fever (Beisel, 1981).

In addition to the slight increases of fasting plasma growth hormone concentrations, Rayfield et al. (1973) found that an intravenous infusion of glucose caused an unexpected further abrupt increase in plasma growth hormone in patients with sandfly fever. A similar phenomenon occurred in monkeys with an experimental gram-negative infection (Rayfield et al., 1974).

Despite this evidence for increased secretion of growth hormone, there is no certainty as to how this increase may influence host defenses or biochemical, metabolic, and nutritional events. The growth hormone response does not prevent the catabolic events or negative nitrogen balances that typify an acute infection. However, the increased concentrations of growth hormone in plasma undoubtedly contribute to the insulin resistance of infection.

Pancreatic Hormones

Among all the infection-induced responses of major hormones, those of insulin and glucagon may be most important metabolically. Infection is unique in that it triggers an increased output of both major pancreatic islet hormones at the same time. The heightened release of insulin during infection, and probably glucagon as well, appears to be due to direct stimulation of pancreatic islet cells by IL-1. In contrast, most aspects of carbohydrate regulation cast insulin and glucagon in opposing or reciprocating roles. As described earlier, the combined responses of insulin and glucagon during early infection have an influence on lipid and amino acid metabolism, as well as on carbohydrate metabolism.

Increased concentrations of immunoreactive glucagon are consistently found in acute infections of man and experimental animals. The hyperglucagonemia of burned patients is further increased in magnitude when superimposed infection develops (Wilmore et al., 1974). In experimental animals, the acute, infection-induced increase in glucagon is accompanied by higher cyclic adenosine monophosphate (cAMP) values in hepatic cells. The increase in plasma glucagon is reversed if high concentrations of glucose are infused intravenously. It is not known if pancreatic alpha cells are the sole source of this infection-induced increase in immunoreactive glucagon.

The magnitude of increase in fasting plasma insulin values is quite modest during acute infections; in some patients, normal fasting values are seen. However, as anorexia is common in infection, the observed insulin values may be much higher than those of noninfected subjects who experience a comparable degree of semistarvation. In any event, the observed insulin concentrations appear sufficient to contribute to the inhibition of hepatic ketogenesis, stimulation of hepatic lipogenesis, inhibition of lipolysis in peripheral tissues and fat depots, and a general anabolic effect on protein synthesis in peripheral tissues accompanied by an increased cellular uptake of glucose and amino acids.

Some of these predicted insulin-stimulated effects are seen in infected patients (i.e., inhibited hepatic ketogenesis, fat depot lipolysis, and stimulated hepatic lipogenesis). The other expected effects of insulin on peripheral glucose metabolism are not fully apparent. The apparent lack of a full display of insulin activity may have two possible explanations. First, the increase in plasma insulin values occurs in the presence of higher-than-normal plasma glucose concentrations; this would indicate some degree of insulin resistance. Second, the increase in plasma insulin values is accompanied by a greater relative increase in plasma glucagon concentrations. This combination causes the molar insulin : glucagon (I : G) ratio to fall. The increase in glucagon alone could trigger the observed hepatic glycogenolysis, whereas insulin resistance alone or in combination with high glucagon values could blunt the expected anabolic effects in peripheral tissues. Further, the declining I : G ratio is a characteristic finding during catabolic illnesses (Unger, 1971).

Other Hormones

There is no evidence that the hormones that participate in pituitary-gonadal interrelationships participate in the host response to infectious illnesses.

Despite evidence for the alterations in phosphate metabolism in soft tissues and the probable role of calcium and calmodulin in molecular events occurring at cell surface membranes, there is little evidence for a direct or indirect parathyroid gland participation in host responses to infection.

Few data are available to document the possible participation during infection of most members of the large family of peptide hormones secreted by cells of the neuroendocrine-gut complex. Such hormones include gastrin, secretin, motilin, bombesin, somatostatin, gastric inhibitory peptide, cholecystokinin, and intestinal glucagon (see Chapter 1). It seems likely, on a theoretical basis, that members of this group should be involved in the transient, infection-induced gastrointestinal dysfunctions that accompany most infections. These include anorexia, nausea and vomiting, altered gastrointestinal mobility, and changes in the digestion and absorption of dietary nutrients. It also seems likely that some of the neuropeptide hormones of this group may be functioning within the central nervous system to influence or modulate the function of the brain centers, such as those that control body temperature, initiate anorexia and the vomiting reflex, or those involved in hormone output by the anterior pituitary gland.

Hormonal cytokines. As shown in Figures 17.4 and 17.5 and Table 17.4, newly identified cytokines play a major role in initiating and regulating the physiologic, metabolic, immunologic, and nonspecific defensive responses of the host to invading microorganisms. Recent advances in biotechnology, which allow individual mammalian genes to be segregated by recombinant methodology and expressed in bacteria or yeasts, are leading to the production and purification of many lymphokines and monokines. Availability of these recombinant polypeptides, such as rIL-1, rIL-2, rTNF, rINF, rGM-CSF, etc., now permit their structure, function, and interactions to be elucidated. In addition to their research value, many of these recombinant cytokines are entering into clinical trials to evaluate their potential therapeutic usefulness, dose range, and possible toxicity.

IL-1 is the most functionally diverse of the cytokines, as might be surmised from its many former aliases. (It was awkwardly termed EP/LEM/LAF in the first edition of this book.) As portrayed in Figure 17.4, IL-1 plays the central role in initiating and orchestrating the acute phase response and in stimulating the release of other cytokines. The prediction that IL-1 would eventually prove to represent a family of closely related molecules (Beisel and Sobocinski, 1980) has been verified (Dinarello, 1985). In man, IL-1 variants α and β are transcribed by different genes, although both are located on chromosome 2. The two rIL-1 polypeptides differ slightly in size, isoelectric point, and considerably in amino acid composition. Although they have only 27% homology in amino acid sequences, almost all of their identified functions are similar.

Both forms of IL-1 are initially transcribed within activated monocytes or macrophages as precursor peptides. At the cell surface they are cleaved by serine proteases, particularly elastase and plasmin, into biologically active circulating peptide hormones (Giri et al., 1984), although significant amounts of biologically active IL-1 remain bound to the cellular membrane. Many other cell types can secrete IL-1 (Table 17.4), but it is not known how important their contribution is to the acute phase reaction.

In stimulating target cells, IL-1 appears to activate cell wall phospholipases, which act on surface membrane phospholipids to release arachidonic acid into the cell interior, a step that can be inhibited, in part, by cortisol. Cells (such as those of the hypothalamus, skeletal muscle, synovia, or fibroblasts), which possess cyclooxygenase enzymes, metabolize the arachidonic acid to prostaglandins, and these serve, in turn, to initiate the cellular effects attributed to IL-1. This pathway can be blocked, in part, by aspirin or ibuprophen. In other cells that possess lipooxygenase enzymes, the arachidonic acid is converted into one of the leukotrines to stimulate alternative cellular responses to IL-1.

When released into the bloodstream, IL-1 can stimulate the wide array of responses shown in Figures 17.4 and 17.5. IL-1 is also known to cause harmful reactions in localized areas, such as the joint spaces, where it can induce an accumulation of inflammatory cells, the endothelial adherence and degranulation of neutrophils, proliferation of fibroblasts, and destruction of bone and cartilage. In other tissues, IL-1 can induce the proliferation of mesanglial and glial cells.

The body also possesses means to counteract IL-1. Corticosteroids can decrease the transcription of IL-1. Substances have been found in plasma or body spaces that can bind to IL-1 or block cell membrane IL-1 receptors. The cytokine can also downregulate its own cellular receptors.

Another recently identified interleukin, IL-6, is also produced by a large variety of body cells and seems to resemble IL-1 in many of its functions. IL-6 concentrations in plasma increase linearly with increasing body temperatures (Nijsten et al., 1987). IL-6 can also induce acute phase protein synthesis in hepatocytes (Sehgal et al., 1989).

Another monokine, tumor necrosis factor (TNF), is released during infectious illnesses, especially those caused by gram-negative bacteria (see Figures 17.4 and 17.5 and Table 17.4). TNF can induce fever, and like IL-1, can inhibit lipoprotein lipase and lead to the hypertriglyceridemia of sepsis. TNF can depolarize skeletal muscle cell membranes, allowing sodium and water to accumulate intracellularly. TNF induces a lactate efflux and glycogen depletion of muscle cells, and

Table 17.4. Cytokines of Importance in Immune Responses, and Host Defenses Against Infection and Trauma

Cytokines	Earlier names	Cells of origin	Inducing stimuli	Primary actions	Other effects
Interleukin-1 (IL-1)	Endogenous pyrogen, leukocytic endogenous mediator, lymphocyte-activating factor, catabolin, osteoclast-activating factor, hemopoietin-1	Macrophages Monocytes Keratinocytes Epithelium Mesangial cells Astrocytes Microglia	Microorganisms Microbial products Antigens Inflammatory agents Plant lectins Lymphokines Certain chemicals	Initiates and orchestrates the acute phase responses (see Figure 17.4) Activates the immune system Stimulates PGE_2 production in many cell types Stimulates growth of fibroblasts, mesanglial, and glial cells	Contributes to the cachexia of severe disease May cause destructive chronic lesions in local areas or closed space In large doses, rIL-1 may inhibit gonadotrophins and cause testicular atrophy in laboratory animals
Interleukin-2 (IL-2)	T cell growth factor	Activated T helper cells expressing IL-2 receptors	T cell activation by IL-1 or antigen T cell mitogens	Stimulates T cell blastic transformation Serves as a growth factor for T subsets and B cells Stimulates transferrin receptors in T and B cells Stimulates formation of INF and TNF Expands populations of lymphokine-activated killer (LAK) cells and tumor-infiltrating lymphocytes	Synergizes with LAK cells in antitumor cytotoxicity Pharmacologic doses of rIL-2 exert toxic effects including fever, weight loss, hypotension, rash, eosinophilia, fluid retention, pulmonary infiltrates, and transient alterations of renal, hepatic, and CNS function
Interleukin-3 (IL-3)	Multi-colony stimulating factor (multi-CSF), mast cell growth factor 1	Activated T helper 1 and 2 cells	T cell activation by IL-1 or antigen	Stimulates differentiation and growth of myloid stem cells and hemopoietic cell lines of many lineages	Stimulates histamine-producing cells and histamine release

Interleukin-4 (IL-4)	B cell growth factor 1, B cell stimulatory factor 1, T cell growth factor 2, mast cell growth factor 2	Activated T helper 2 cells	Direct lymphocyte-to-lymphocyte interaction T cell activation by IL-1, antigen, or endotoxin	Stimulates IgG_1 and IgE synthesis by B cells Stimulates growth and receptor expression in resting B cells Stimulates growth by G_1 phase T cells, thymocytes, and mast cells	Assists IL-3 in causing mast cell division Assists in macrophage development Synergizes with erythropoietin for RBC colony growth
Interleukin-5 (IL-5)	B cell growth factor 2, T cell replacing factor 1, eosinophil colony-stimulating factor (Eo-CSF), eosinophil differentiating factor	Activated T helper 2 cells	T cell activation by IL-1, antigen, or endotoxin	Stimulates growth in B and T cells and in eosinophils Enhances synthesis of IgA and IgM, and IL-4-induced IgE production by B cells Stimulates secretory IgA synthesis and surface immunity	Enhances IL-2-mediated killer cell induction
Interleukin-6 (IL-6)	B cell-stimulating factor 2, hepatocyte-stimulating factor, interferon β_2	Activated helper T cells Macrophages Fibroblasts Endothelial cells	IL-1-stimulated B cells Antigens Mitogens Endotoxin	T cells, macrophages, and hepatocytes Acts on CNS to cause fever	
Interleukin-7 (IL-7)	Pro-B cell growth factor, pre-pre-B cell maturation factor	Marrow stromal cells		Enhances the maturation of pro-B cells to pre-B cells, with rearrangement and expression of Ig heavy-chain genes	
Interleukin-8 (IL-8)	Neutrophil-activating protein-1, neutrophil chemotactic factor, T lymphocyte chemotactic factor	Blood monocytes	Activating stimuli	Dose (concentration)-dependent accumulation of neutrophils and/or lymphocytes in tissues	

(continued)

Table 17.4 *(continued)*

Cytokines	Earlier names	Cells of origin	Inducing stimuli	Primary actions	Other effects
Tumor necrosis factor (TNF)	TNF-α, cachectin, lymphotoxin = TNF-β, endotoxin-induced mediator	Activated macrophages and monocytes Natural killer cells	Bacterial endotoxin Inflammatory agents IL-1 and IFN Amphotericin B Toxic shock toxin 1	Kills tumor cells Stimulates fever Inhibits lipoprotein lipase Accelerates lipolysis Sequesters iron and leads to anemia Alters glucose metabolism in muscle Contributes to inflammatory responses Modulates immune processes Synergizes with IL-1 and IFNs	May contribute to fat depot depletion and cachexia in chronic illness Pharmacologic doses of rTNF may cause fever, chills, anorexia, and neutropenia. High doses may cause CNS toxicity
Interferon-α (IFN-α)	Neutrophil interferon, "classic interferon"	Neutrophils	Viral stimulation of neutrophils Endotoxin	Confers resistance to viral infection on cells Exhibits antitumor cell activity Exerts complex immunomodulatory effects	Pharmacologic doses of rIFN cause dose-dependent fever, myalgia, anorexia, and neutropenia. High doses may cause CNS toxicity
Interferon-β (IFN-β)	Fibrocyte interferon	Fibrocytes	Cytokines	Confers resistance to viral infection in cells	
Interferon-γ (IFN-γ)	Lymphocyte interferon, "immune interferon"	Activated T helper 1 cells	T cell activation by IL-1 or antigen T cell mitogens	Confers resistance to viral infection on cells Exhibits antitumor activity Activates monocytes and natural killer (NK) cells	In pharmacologic doses, rIFN-γ can initiate fever, myalgia, anorexia, and fatigue

Granulocyte–macrophage colony-stimulating factor (GM-CSF)		Activated T helper 1 and 2 cells Fibroblasts Endothelial cells Macrophages	T cell activation by IL-1 or antigen Cytokine stimulation of other cell types	Stimulates colony formation by macrophages, granulocytes, eosinophils, and blast cells Enhances function of cell lines, mature granulocytes and monocytes Stimulates monocyte production of TNF, IL-1, and hydrogen peroxide	Is chemotactic for PMN, macrophages, and eosinophils Stimulates growth in factor hemopoietic cell lines Causes histamine release Pharmacologic doses of rGM-CSF may cause bone pain and slight fever
Granulocyte colony-stimulating factor (G-CSF)		Macrophages Fibroblasts Epithelial cells	Cell activation by IL-1 or mitogen	Stimulates colony formation by neutrophilic granulocytes and their precursors	rG-CSF in pharmacologic doses may cause bone pain, mild fever, and fatigue
Macrophage colony factor	Colony-stimulating factor 1	Monocytes Fibroblasts Endothelial cells	Cell activation by IL-1 or mitogen	Stimulates colony formation by macrophage precursors	

By their physiologic and endocrinologic actions, these cytokines contribute to the biochemical and metabolic components of the multiple host response to infection, and secondarily, to the infection-induced loss of body nutrient stores. Conversely, malnourished cells may not be able to produce normal quantities of these cytokines or their cell surface receptors, or to respond to cytokines in a normal manner. Currently used abbreviations are shown within the table itself. Cytokines produced by recombinant technology are identified by the prefix r (e.g., rIL-1). References for this table include Clark and Kamen (1987), Dinarello (1985), Fletcher and Goldstein (1987), Goodwin et al. (1989), Harriman and Strober (1987), Larsen et al. (1989), Lukasewycz (1990), Moldawer et al. (1989), Nijsten et al. (1987), Ikejima et al. (1988), Miyajima et al. (1988), Paul (1987), Tracey et al. (1988), and Urbaschek and Urbaschek (1987).

stimulates superoxide radical formation in neutrophils (Tracey et al., 1988). The release of a burst of TNF into the bloodstream follows an experimental injection of bacterial endotoxin, with fever, tachycardia, dose-dependent hypotension, and cellular injury (especially to tumor cells). TNF is also believed to contribute importantly to the cachexia of chronic infection.

Unlike IL-1, the lymphokine, IL-2, functions in a far more restricted biological role, serving mainly to heighten immunological responsiveness. IL-2 activates resting T cells. It stimulates them to express high affinity IL-2 receptors and to enter into blastogenic activity. IL-2 also increases the number and activity of cytotoxic T cells. Plasma concentrations of soluble IL-2 receptors rise during infection (Nguyen-Dihn and Greenberg, 1988), as a probable reflection of lymphocyte activation. Conversely, malnutrition inhibits IL-2 production (Kaplan et al., 1988).

In pharmacologic doses, IL-2 can induce fever, nausea, diarrhea, and fatigue. It is not known if the amounts of IL-2 released in vivo during infection contribute to the clinical signs of illness experienced by the patient, or to the nutritional costs of infection.

The lymphokines, IL-4 and IL-5, also have relatively restricted, immunologically focused roles. Operating in concert with IL-2, both IL-4 and IL-5 contribute chiefly to B cell growth and function.

A number of cloned cytokines exert trophic effects on the bone marrow. Of the classical colony-stimulating factors, IL-3 (multi-CSF) stimulates all types of colonies, GM-CSF stimulates myeloid and macrophage colonies, G-CSF stimulates granulocyte colonies, M-CSF stimulates macrophage colonies, and erythropoietin stimulates erythroid colonies. In addition, IL-1, IL-4, and IL-6 have effects in certain stages of marrow development. Body nutrients must be available for the accelerated production of these blood cells which are of major importance in defense against invading microorganisms.

Nutritional Effects on Host Resistance Factors

The preceding sections of this chapter have described the myriad of metabolic, biochemical, and endocrine responses to infection that have a deleterious effect on the nutritional status of the host. Because many infections occur in already malnourished patients, it is important to understand how malnutrition can influence host resistance. In their historic monograph, Scrimshaw et al. (1968) advanced the argument that malnutrition is not always detrimental to the infected host in terms of survival, but that in some instances, the disease process seems less severe than would be expected in a normally nourished host. Hundreds of reported studies of infectious diseases in animals and humans were classified into groups of interactions in which infection seemed more severe (synergistic) or less severe (antagonistic) in the concomitant presence of malnutrition. A third group was recognized in which no evidence could be found for either synergism or antagonism. Most bacterial infections were synergistic, with preexisting malnutrition producing a more severe disease process. Although measles stand as a major example of a synergistic viral infection, a sizeable number of other viral infections in animal studies and many parasitic ones are antagonistic. As the replication of a virus is dependent on metabolic and molecular processes supplied by biochemical functions of the host cell, lack of adequate intracellular nutrients could slow viral growth. Similarly, parasites must obtain nutrients from the host. Bacteria possess their own reproductive mechanisms and have nutritional requirements that, in most instances, are met by the fluids and tissues of a malnourished host. However, iron availability may become a critical rate-limited single nutrient for microorganisms, as previously noted, and severe iron deficiency could cause an antagonistic response in some infections.

It is now widely recognized that various forms of malnutrition can cause derangements in immune system functions, as well as in nonspecific host defense systems (Beisel, 1982*a*; Chandra and Newberne, 1977; Garre et al., 1987; Gershwin et al., 1985; Watson, 1984). Immunological assays can even be used as indirect measurements of nutritional status (Miller, 1978), and a prognostic index can be developed based on the status of nutritional and immunological parameters (Ingenbleek and Carpentier, 1984).

The immunologic dysfunctions associated with malnutrition vary in severity and specificity, depending on the nature of the nutritional derangement and its severity. As outlined in Table 17.2, individual nutrients have special areas of importance in the functioning of lymphocytes, monocytes, macrophages, and other phagocytic cells. Some forms of malnutrition hinder the ability of macrophages to secrete monokines, such as IL-1 (Kaufmann et al., 1986), helper lymphocytes to secrete lymphokines such as IL-2 (Kaufmann et al., 1988), or thymic endothelial cells to secrete thymulin (Jambon et al., 1988).

Every form of immunological dysfunction caused by a nutritional disorder can be classified as an acquired immune deficiency syndrome (AIDS), but fortunately, they are almost always reversible, if the nutritional disorder can be corrected. Palmblad (1987) has suggested that malnutritionally induced AIDS be designated MAIDS, to distinguish it from the far more newsworthy and dangerous form of AIDS caused by the human immunodeficiency viruses, which destroy key subsets of vitally important lymphocytes. Although far more common on a worldwide basis, MAIDS also differs from the relatively rare immune system diseases which are due to genetic defects, and which are generally more severe and usually irreversible.

Malnutrition and Fever

The body's ability to generate a febrile response is dependent on the availability of fuels needed to increase cellular metabolism as well as the mechanisms needed to reduce heat loss. Both factors are impaired by generalized malnutrition. The availability of nitrogen stores and depot fat are reduced in generalized malnutrition. A starvation-induced reduction in body mass occurs without a comparable reduction in body surface area. This makes it more difficult to reduce direct heat loss through the skin. The same heat-loss mechanistic derangements create a problem, even in starving nonfebrile patients. As illustrated during the prolonged siege of the Jewish ghetto in Warsaw by the Nazi invaders, the starving victims continually complained of feeling cold and wore heavy clothing in both summer and winter (Winick, 1979). In the absence of famine and starvation, nutritional inhibition of fever occurs most often in very young infants and premature babies, in the aged, and in patients with severe debilitation due to wasting illnesses.

Fever is a recognized host defensive mechanism, but a relatively weak one. In the preantibiotic era, therapeutically induced fever was used with limited success in an attempt to treat several kinds of infections (i.e., central nervous system syphilis and chronic bacterial arthritis). Kluger (1981) introduced experimental designs that illustrate the value of a modestly increased body temperature in reducing lethality in carefully selected bacterial infections of cold-blooded animals and infant rabbits. Although such demonstrations are of interest, they do not take into account the very real dangers from uncontrolled high fevers in human beings. Many infants are prone to develop severe grand mal seizures with even modest elevations of body temperature. Further, the height and duration of fever are the two most important factors in contributing to nutrient losses during acute infections; such losses can initiate kwashiorkor in children whose nutritional status was previously marginal. The therapeutic aim in modern treatment of infection is to eliminate the invading microorganism as rapidly as possible, to prevent or reduce extreme fevers, and to maintain homeostasis throughout body fluids and physiologic processes to the best extent possible.

Malnutrition and the Inflammatory Reaction

The ability to generate and sustain an inflammatory reaction is of major importance in host defense, for, if successful, it serves to contain invading microorganisms in a localized area and to prevent their widespread dissemination. This is a complex reaction, requiring localized changes in blood vessel flow, caliber, and permeability; the infiltration of leukocytes (with an evolving participation of several different cell types beginning with neutrophils); the accumulation of previously mentioned mediator substances derived from plasma proteins and damaged cells; alterations in localized pH and O_2 content; and an encompassing deposition of fibrin.

Because of this complexity, it is not surprising that malnutrition can have a detrimental effect on the production of inflammatory reactions (see Table 17.2) or on the production of the somewhat analogous reactions that help to localize tubercular lesions. Severely malnourished children often exhibit a wide and unchecked progression of common, easily treated, dermal infections because of the lack of effective localizing mechanisms. It is possible to test for the ability of a malnourished patient to mount an inflammatory response by applying a small drop of a chemical irritant, such as dinitrochlorobenzene (DNCB) to the skin. The skin of a normal subject develops a classical inflamed area with redness, swelling, heat, and even blister formation, while that of a patient with severe protein-energy malnutrition does not. A severe isolated deficiency of vitamin C is also associated with a failure of inflammatory reactions to develop (Axelrod, 1971). These effects of scurvy have been ascribed primarily to impaired chemotactic activity and mobility of neutrophils and macrophages. A deficiency of pyridoxine may also impair the development of an inflammatory response.

If a starving patient is refed, his/her ability to generate local inflammatory and granulomatous reactions and to mount a fever may return with suddenness and potentially dangerous consequences. A starving patient may be harboring infectious microorganisms without manifesting the usual clinical expressions of the disease because of antagonistic effects of malnutrition. A sudden refeeding may then induce the reemergence of host defense mechanisms that convert the clinically latent infections into severely symptomatic ones. The administration of excess parenteral iron to a protein-depleted patient may have similar consequences because of enhanced microorganism proliferation. Emergence of such an apparent therapeutic paradox calls for prompt and specific treatment of the infection while the malnutrition is being reversed.

Malnutrition and Phagocytic Cell Functions

It is possible to test for a variety of phagocytic cell functions by in vitro studies of peripheral blood leukocytes obtained from patients with different kinds of malnutrition (see Table 17.2). These testable functions can include active direct migration toward a chemotactic stimulus, engulfment of test bacteria or inert particulate materials, and the in vitro killing function of ingested test bacteria (Wright, 1981). Related biochemical events can also be measured, such as the respiratory burst that normally accompanies phagocytosis, the generation of superoxide radicals, hexose monophosphate shunt activation, nitroblue tetrazolium dye reduction, or the altered activities of a variety of intracellular enzymes.

Movement of neutrophils toward a chemotactic stimulus is a primary event in the inflammatory reaction. Schopfer and Douglas (1977) found a delayed chemotactic migration in neutrophils obtained from children with kwashiorkor studied in the Ivory Coast. Chemotaxis may also be impaired in isolated vitamin C or zinc deficiency and in polyunsaturated fatty acid (PUFA) excess, whereas an excess of serum iron or vitamin C may each be associated with increased cellular motility (Beisel, 1982*a*).

The ability of neutrophils to engulf bacteria or inert particles is not adversely affected by protein-energy malnutrition (Chandra and Newberne, 1977), but may be depressed by a deficiency in body iron or an excess of PUFA. The ability of neutrophils to kill ingested bacteria is consistently depressed in patients with deficiencies of protein and energy (Chandra and Newberne, 1977; Schopfer and Douglas, 1977) or iron, but is normal in vitamin C deficiency (Beisel, 1982*a*). The depressed bactericidal activity of neutrophils in protein-energy malnutrition may be accompanied by altered biochemical test values in either the resting or postphagocytic state, but reported observations have been too infrequent to demonstrate a consistent overall pattern of responses (Schopfer and Douglas, 1977).

Malnutrition and Humoral Immunity

The development of specific humoral antibodies is dependent initially on the ability of B lymphocytes (with an appropriate preexisting surface receptor configuration), in the presence of macrophages, to match up with a new antigen. Attachment of an antigen to a specific lymphocyte receptor is followed by the activation of the lymphocyte, cellular division, and the replication of cloned daughter cells. These, in turn, differentiate into immunoregulatory lymphocytes or mature immunoglobulin-secreting plasma cells. The memory component of the immune system is provided by the large number of cloned lymphocytes available for matchup if the same antigen is encountered on subsequent occasions. This entire system is delicately balanced under normal circumstances, with helper and suppressor cells serving to regulate the magnitude of immunoglobulin production.

It is possible to evaluate the adequacy of humoral immunity by measuring the titers of specific antibody achieved in response to a newly administered antigen, or to test for the presence and number of antibody-producing cells in peripheral blood or in the spleen of experimental animals.

Nutritional interactions with mechanisms of humoral immunity have been difficult to define and quantitate (Good et al., 1982; Gershwin et al., 1985; Neumann, 1981; Watson et al., 1984). Unfortunately, newly gained information about the workings of the immune system has not been matched by studies to determine how various forms of malnutrition can cause immunological deficits. Table 17.2 summarizes currently available knowledge in this area. Because of the complexity of the immune system and its inherent checks and balances, nutritional inhibition of a blocking function may lead to a greater-than-normal final antibody response. In protein-energy malnutrition, total IgG concentrations in plasma may be normal or increased, as may the concentrations of IgM, IgA, IgD, and IgE. These increases may be due, in part, to the numerous infections and heightened antigenic loads faced by malnourished children in impoverished locales (Beisel, 1979). On the other hand, responses to specific single test antigens may be diminished in generalized malnutrition or in deficiencies of single vitamins, such as pyridoxine, pantothenic acid, riboflavin, biotin, pteroylglutamic acid, folic acid, or vitamin A, or with deficiencies of PUFA or of minerals such as iron, zinc, copper, or selenium (Beisel, 1982*a*; Lukasewycz, 1990).

In situations where an in vivo immunoglobulin response to a test antigen is deficient, in vitro tests of lymphocyte responsiveness to mitogens or to the antigen may also show an impaired function.

Deficiencies have also been demonstrated in secretory antibody production in the saliva, tears, and other mucosal surface fluids of patients with generalized malnutrition.

Observed immunologic responses, however, are not always easy to interpret if secondary infections are present. Studies of humoral responses are also confounded by the molecular configuration of an antigen, its presentation in solution or as a particulate, the presence of adjuvants, or the presence of other antigens. Nutritionally altered primary immune responses to a new antigen may differ from alterations in the secondary responses caused by giving the same antigen on more than one occasion.

Malnutrition and Cell-Mediated Immunity

In contrast to the sometimes ambiguous interpretation of humoral immune responses during states of malnutrition, the responses of cell-mediated immune functions are almost always impaired (see Table 17.2). Cell-mediated immunity is the major host defense mechanism for certain viral diseases, including measles, rubella, and varicella; some bacterial diseases, including tuberculosis, brucellosis, and leprosy; spirochaetal diseases, such as syphilis; some fungal diseases, including histoplasmosis and coccidioidomycosis; and certain parasitic diseases, such as toxoplasmosis and malaria. Cell-mediated immunity is dependent on T lymphocyte function and can be assessed by testing delayed dermal hypersensitivity reactions, graft-versus-host reactions, mixed lymphocyte culture reactions, the responsiveness of lymphocytes to T cell mitogens, and lymphokine production (Neumann, 1981).

Depressed cell-mediated immunity is a characteristic finding in most patients with generalized protein-energy malnutrition (Edelman, 1977). This has been evaluated most commonly in man by using skin tests to common or ubiquitous antigens or by in vitro testing of the responsiveness of peripheral blood lymphocytes to T cell mitogens added to the lymphocyte cultures. Similar tests can be done in laboratory animals, but splenic or thoracic duct lymphocytes are usually used instead of blood lymphocytes. Another useful, but slower, method for testing cell-mediated immunity immunocompetence is to determine if allografts of skin or other tissues will survive. Experimentally induced allergic encephalitis is used as still another test system in animals, which occurs only in the presence of a functionally intact cell-mediated immune system.

A functional loss of cell-mediated immunity is present in most patients with severe generalized malnutrition. This loss occurs whether the malnutrition is initiated by starvation or by a severe medical, surgical, or malignant disease. The functional defect is often corrected with surprising speed if the malnutrition can be corrected. In fact, Bistrain et al. (1975) have judged the return of cell-mediated immunity (as assessed by skin test responsiveness) to be an excellent indicator of a favorable prognosis in individual patients. In contrast, continued skin test anergy is indicative of a poor prognosis.

A number of single nutrients have also been found to influence cell-mediated immunity (Beisel, 1982*a*). Of the vitamins, pyridoxine deficiency is the most consistent cause of defective cell-mediated immune responses in laboratory animals. This has been shown by deficiencies in in vitro lymphocyte responsiveness to mitogens and allogeneic lymphocytes, by delays in allograft rejection, and by loss of delayed dermal hypersensitivity reactions (Axelrod, 1971). Folic acid deficiency will also cause a reduction of T lymphocyte numbers, and mitogenic unresponsiveness and impaired dermal sensitization reactions to DNCB. The derangements in cell-mediated immunity caused by deficiencies of either pyridoxine or folic acid have been ascribed to the importance of these two B vitamins in nuclear DNA metabolism (Beisel, 1982*a*).

A deficiency of vitamin A may also impair cell-mediated immunity. In contrast, an excess of PUFA may prolong allograft survival and prevent the development of allergic encephalitis. The biologically important daughter metabolite of vitamin D, 1,25-diOH-D_3, functions in the manner of a steroid hormone (Minghetti and Norman, 1988). Vitamin D_3 regulates gene expression in many systems, including those that govern the production of lymphokines, and thus may indirectly also affect immune function (Minghetti and Norman, 1988).

Of the mineral effects, zinc deficiency is by far the most consistent and easily produced cause of a severe functional defect in all aspects of cell-mediated immunity studied to date. Zinc deficiency also reduces production of the thymus gland hormone, thymulin (Jambon et al., 1988). The profound derangements in the immune system caused by severe zinc deficiency are accompanied by a markedly increased susceptibility to infection (Fraker et al., 1982). This nutritionally induced impairment is also a very easy one to reverse by the restoration of the zinc stores to normal values (Beisel, 1982*a*). On the other hand, some evidence exists that excessive quantities of zinc may have an adverse effect upon the immune system (Beisel, 1982*a*; Chandra, 1984).

Copper deficiency in experimental animals causes alterations in lymphoid cells, including decreases in thymic weight and splenic T cell populations (Lukasewycz, 1990). Lymphocytes show changes in lipid concentrations of plasma membranes, decreased lymphokine output, decreased natural killer cell activity, decreased antibody production, and hyporesponsiveness when exposed to antigens, mitogens, and mixed lymphocyte tests. In addition, copper-deficient animals are more susceptible to infection, and their hepatic production of prostaglandins may be decreased (Lukasewycz, 1990).

Magnesium deficiency inhibits the induction of experimental allergic encephalitis; this deficiency has not been studied for other possible cell-mediated immune system defects. Cadmium toxicity has been shown in laboratory animals to inhibit delayed dermal hypersensitivity responses and in vitro lymphocyte mitogenic responses.

Summary

This chapter has attempted to define the magnitude and importance of the complex nutritional effects of infectious disease, as well as the effects of altered nutritional states on the ability of the host to defend itself against infectious microorganisms.

Despite the very broad metabolic, biochemical, and endocrine responses that contribute to the generalized host defensive stance during acute states of infection, a reasonably detailed and consistent pattern of changes can now be defined and anticipated. Sufficient numbers of studies with a variety of infections have been reported in humans and experimental animals to allow reasonable confidence that the major patterns of responses have been recognized for the most important major metabolic processes. In some areas, detailed information is also available at the molecular level. Although much work needs to be done, much has already been learned and can be put to practical use in terms of patient management.

The same relatively favorable assessment cannot be made for the state of knowledge concerning nutritional effects on host resistance or on the ability of invading microorganisms to proliferate. The immunological functions are of great importance in this regard, but studies of immunity have not been systematic or comprehensive. None of the major nutrients or single trace nutrients have been studied in sufficient depth to allow a full assessment of their effects on all currently testable aspects of immune system function. Much work needs to be done in this area.

References

Axelrod AE (1971): Am J Clin Nutr 24:265.

Bailey PT, Abeles FB, Hauer EC, Mapes CA (1976): Proc Soc Exp Biol Med 153:419.

Beisel WR (1976): Med Clin North Am 60:831.

Beisel WR (1977): Am J Clin Nutr 30:1236.

Beisel WR (1979): *In* Neuberger A, Jukes TH, eds: Biochemistry of nutrition, Vol 27. Baltimore: University Park Press.

Beisel WR (1980*a*): Fed Proc 39:3105.

Beisel WR (1980*b*): Physiologist 23:38.

Beisel WR (1981): *In* Powanda MC, Canonico PG, eds: Infection. The physiologic and metabolic responses of the host. Amsterdam: Elsevier Biomedical, p 1.

Beisel WR (1982*a*): Am J Clin Nutr 35:415.

Beisel WR (1982*b*): Rev Infect Dis 4:746.

Beisel WR, Fiser RH Jr (1970): Am J Clin Nutr 23:1069.

Beisel WR, Rapoport MI (1969): N Engl J Med 280:541.

Beisel WR, Sobocinski PZ (1980): *In* Lipton JM, ed: Fever. New York: Raven, p 39.

Beisel WR, Herman YF, Sauberlich HE, Herman RH, Bartelloni PJ, Canham JE (1972): Am J Clin Nutr 25:1165.

Beisel WR, Sawyer WD, Ryll ED, Crozier D (1967): Ann Intern Med 67:744.

Beisel WR, Wannemacher RW Jr, Neufeld HA (1980): *In* Kenney JM, ed: Assessment of energy metabolism in health and disease. Columbus, Ohio: Ross Laboratories, p 144.

Beisel WR, Watten RH, Blackwell RQ, Benyajati C, Philips RA (1963): Am J Med 35:58.

Berry LJ, Smythe DS, Young LG (1959): J Exp Med 110:389.

Bistrain BR, Blackburn GL, Scrimshaw NS, Flatt J-P (1975): Am J Clin Nutr 28:1148.

Brown KH, Gilman RH, Gaffar A, Alamgir SM, Strife JL, Kappikian AZ, Sack RB (1981): Nutr Res 1:33.

Campbell CH, Solgonick RM, Linder MC (1989): Biochem Biophys Res Commun 160:453.

Canonico PGH, Ayala E, Rill WL, Little JS (1977): Am J Clin Nutr 30:1359.

Chandra RK (1984): JAMA 252:1443.

Chandra RK, Newberne PM (1977): Nutrition, immunity, and infection. Mechanisms of interactions. New York: Plenum, p 1.

Chopra LJ, Chopra U, Smith SR, Reza M, Solomo DH (1975): J Clin Endocrinol Metab 41:1043.

Clark SC, Kamen R (1987): Science 236:1229.

Clowes GHA Jr, Randall HT, Cha C-J (1982): J Parenter Enter Nutr 4:195.

Cockerell GL (1973): Proc Soc Exp Biol Med 142:1072.

Cousins RJ, Leinart AS (1988): FASEB J 2:2884.

Dinarello CA (1985): J Clin Immunol 5:287.

Dinarello CA (1987): Immunobiology 172:301.

Dinarello CA, Cannon JG, Wolfe SM, Bernheim HA, Beutler B, Cerami A, Figari IS, Palladino MA Jr, O'Connor JV (1986): J Exp Med 163:1433.

Edelman R (1977): *In* Suskind RM, ed: Malnutrition and the immune response. New York: Raven, p 47.

Feigin RD, Klainer AS, Beisel WR, Hornick RB (1968): N Engl J Med 278:293.

Felig P (1973): Metabolism 22:179.

Felig P, Brown WV, Levine RA, Klatskin G (1970): N Engl J Med 283:1436.

Fiser RH, Denniston JC, Rindsig RB, Beisel WR (1971): Proc Soc Exp Biol Med 138:605.

Fletcher M, Goldstein AL (1987): Lymph Res 6:45.

Fraker PJ, Caruso R, Kierszenbaum F (1982): J Nutr 112:1224.

Garre MA, Boles JM, Youinou PY (1987): J Parenter Enter Nutr 11:309.

George DT, Abeles FB, Mapes CA, Sobocinski PZ, Zenser TV, Powanda MC (1977): Am J Physiol 233:E240.

Gershwin ME, Beach RS, Hurley LS, eds (1985): Nutrition and immunity. Orlando: Academic, p 1.

Good RA, Hanson LA, Edelman R (1982): Nutr Rev 40:119.

Goodwin RG, Lupton S, Schmierer A, Hjerrild KJ, Jerzy R, Clevenger W, Gillis S, Cosman D, Namen AE (1989): Immunology 86:302.

Groves AC, Griffiths J, Leung F, Meek RN (1973): Ann Surg 178:102.

Hamer DH (1986): Annu Rev Biochem 55:913.

Harriman GR, Strober W (1987): J Immunol 139:3553.

Harvey RF (1971): Lancet 1:208.

Henkin RI, Smith FR (1972): Am J Med Sci 264:401.

Hershko C, Konijn AM (1977): *In* Brown EB, Aisen P, Fielding J, Crichton RR, eds: Proteins of iron metabolism. New York: Grune & Stratton.

Howard JE, Bigham RS Jr, Mason RE (1946): Trans Assoc Am Physicians 59:242.

Ikejima T, Okusawa S, van der Meer JWM, Dinarello CA (1988): 158:1017.

Ingenbleek Y, Carpentier YA (1984): Int J Vit Nutr Res 55:91.

Jambon B, Ziegler O, Maire B, Hutin M-F, Parent G, Fall M, Burnel D, Duheille J (1988): Am J Clin Nutr 48:335.

Kampschmidt RF (1981): *In* Powanda MC, Canonico PG, eds: Infection. The physiologic and metabolic responses of the host. Amsterdam: Elsevier Biomedical, p 55.

Kaplan J, Hess JW, Prasad AS (1988): J Trace Elem Exp Med 1:3.

Kauffman CA, Jones PG, Kluger MJ (1986): Am J Clin Nutr 44:449.

Kaufmann RL, Matson CF, Beisel WR (1976*a*): J Infect Dis 133:548.

Kaufmann RL, Matson CF, Rowberg AH, Beisel WR (1976*b*): Metabolism 25:615.

Keusch GT, Scrimshaw NS (1986): Rev Infect Dis 8:273.

Kluger MJ (1981): *In* Powanda MC, Canonico PG, eds: Infection. The physiologic and metabolic responses of the host. Amsterdam: Elsevier Biomedical, p 75.

Kluger MJ, Oppenheim JJ, Powanda MC, eds (1985): The physiologic, metabolic, and immunologic actions of interleukin-1. New York: Alan R Liss, p 1.

Larsen CG, Anderson AO, Appella E, Oppenheim JJ, Matsushima K (1989): Science 243:1464.

Lees RS, Fiser RH Jr, Beisel WR, Bartelloni PJ (1972): Metabolism 21:825.

Little JS, Canonico PG (1981): *In* Powanda MC, Canonico PG, eds: Infection. The physiologic and metabolic responses of the host. Amsterdam: Elsevier Biomedical, p 97.

Lukasewycz OD (1990): Ann NY Acad Sci, in press.

Mason JW, Buescher EL, Belfer ML, Artenstein MS, Mougey EH (1979): J Human Stress 5:18.

Mata LJ, Kromal RA, Urrutia JJ, Garcia B (1977): Am J Clin Nutr 30:1215.

Meszaros K, Lang CH, Bagly GJ, Spitzer JJ (1988): FASEB J 2:3083.

Miller CL (1978): J Parenter Enter Nutr 2:554.

Miller KD, White NJ, Lott JA, Roberts JM, Greenwood BM (1989): J Infect Dis 159:139.

Minghetti PP, Norman AW (1988): FASEB J 2:3043.

Miyajima A, Miyatake S, Schreurs J, De Vries J, Arai N, Yokota T, Arai K-I (1988): FASEB J 2:24.

Moldawer LL, Marano MA, Wei H, Fong Y, Silen ML, Kuo G, Manogue KR, Vlassara H, Cohen H, Cerami A, Lowry SF (1989): FASEB J 3:1637.

Moyer ED, Powanda MC (1981): *In* Powanda MC, Canonico PG, eds: Infection. The physiologic and metabolic responses of the host. Amsterdam: Elsevier Biomedical, p 173.

Neufeld HA, Pace JA, White FE (1976): Metabolism 25:877.

Neumann CG (1981): *In* Powanda MC, Canonico PG, eds: Infection. The physiologic and metabolic responses of the host. Amsterdam: Elsevier Biomedical, p 319.

Nguyen-Dinh P, Greenberg AE (1988): J Infect Dis 158:1403.

Nijsten MWN, de Groot ER, ten Duis HJ, Klasen HJ, Hack CE, Aarden LA (1987): Lancet 2:921.

Palmblad J (1987): Acta Med Scand 222:1.

Paul WE (1987): FASEB J 1:456.

Pekarek RS, Engelhardt JA (1981): *In* Powanda MC, Canonico PG, eds: Infection. The physiologic and metabolic responses of the host. Amsterdam: Elsevier Biomedical, p 131.

Powanda MC (1977): Am J Clin Nutr 30:1254.

Powanda MC, Beisel WR (1982): Am J Clin Nutr 35:762.

Powanda MC, Moyer ED (1981): *In* Powanda MC, Canonico PG, eds: Infection. The physiologic and metabolic responses of the host. Amsterdam: Elsevier Biomedical, p 271.

Rapoport ML, Beisel WR (1971): Am J Clin Nutr 24:807.

Rapoport ML, Lust G, Beisel WR (1968): Arch Intern Med 121:11.

Rayfield EJ, George DT, Beisel WR (1973): N Engl J Med 289:618.

Rayfield EJ, George DT, Beisel WR (1974): J Clin Endocrinol Metab 38:746.

Rocha DM, Santeusanio F, Faloona GR, Unger RH (1973): N Engl J Med 288:700.

Schiaffonati L, Rappocciolo E, Tacchini X, et al. (1988): Exp Mol Pathol 48:174.

Schopfer K, Douglas SD (1977): *In* Suskind RM, ed: Malnutrition and the immune response. New York: Raven, p 123.

Scrimshaw NG, Taylor CE, Gordon JE (1968): Interactions of nutrition and infection. Geneva: World Health Organization, p 1.

Sehgal PB, Grieninger G, Tosato G, eds (1989): Ann NY Acad Sci 557.

Selye H (1948): Ann Intern Med 29:403.

Shambaugh GE III, Beisel WR (1966): Endocrinology 79:511.

Shambaugh GE III, Beisel WR (1967*a*): Diabetes 16:369.

Shambaugh GE III, Beisel WR (1967*b*): J Clin Endocrinol Metab 27:1667.

Shambaugh GE III, Beisel WR (1968): Endocrinology 83:965.

Sjolin J, Stjernstrom H, Henneberg S, Hambraeus L, Friman G (1989): Am J Clin Nutr 49:62.

Sobocinski PZ, Canterbury WJ Jr, Hauer EC, Beall FA (1979): Proc Soc Exp Biol Med 160:175.

Tracey KJ, Lowry SF, Cerami A (1988): J Infect Dis 157:413.

Unger RH (1971): Diabetes 20:834.

Urbaschek R, Urbaschek B (1987): Rev Infect Dis 9: S607.

Wannemacher RW Jr (1975): *In* Ghadimi H, ed: Total parenteral nutrition premises and promises. New York: Wiley, p 85.

Wannemacher RW Jr (1977): Am J Clin Nutr 30:1269.

Wannemacher RW Jr, Kaminski MV Jr, Dinterman RE, McCabe TR (1982): J Parenter Enter Nutr 6:100.

Wannemacher RW Jr, Klainer AS, Dinterman RE, Beisel WR (1976): Am J Clin Nutr 29:997.

Wannemacher RW Jr, Pace JG, Neufeld HA (1981): *In* Powanda MC, Canonico PG, eds: Infection. The physiologic and metabolic responses of the host. Amsterdam: Elsevier Biomedical, p 245.

Wannemacher RW Jr, Pekarek RS, Beisel WSR (1973): Am J Clin Nutr 26:460.

Wartofsky L, Martin D, Earll JM (1972): J Clin Invest 51:2215.

Watson RR, ed (1984): Nutrition, disease resistance, and immune function. New York: Marcel Dekker, p 1.

Wilmore DW, Lindsey CA, Moylan JA, Faloona GR, Pruitt BA, Unger RH (1974): Lancet 1:73.

Winick M, ed (1979): Hunger disease (studies by the Jewish physicians in the Warsaw ghetto). New York: Wiley, p 1.

Wolfe RR (1981): *In* Powanda MC, Canonico PG, eds: Infection. The physiologic and metabolic responses of the host. Amsterdam: Elsevier Biomedical, p 213.

Wright DG (1981): *In* Powanda MC, Canonico PG, eds: Infection. The physiologic and metabolic responses of the host. Elsevier Biomedical, p 1.

John B. Stanbury, M.D.*

18

Dietary Treatment of the Inborn Errors of Metabolism

Introduction and Overview

The inborn errors of metabolism are a large group of relatively rare disorders that arise because of inherited deficiency or absence of proteins that have enzymatic, carrier, receptor, structural, or other functional roles. For many of these, the molecular nature of the defect is now quite precisely known, and for some, the chromosomal locus of the defective gene has been mapped. While it is not yet possible to effect a cure of any of these disorders by such techniques as gene replacement or repair, knowledge of the pathophysiology involved often suggests a plan of management that may be palliative or may even permit normal development, activity, and lifespan.

The most frequently identified of the inborn errors are those arising from abnormal or absent proteins that serve an enzymatic function (Stanbury et al., 1983; Tada et al., 1987). A variety of consequences may flow from such defects. An important metabolite may be formed in insufficient quantity, such as in familial goiter or the adrenogenital syndrome. Certain hormonal deficiency states may arise through this mechanism (e.g., diabetes mellitus). Alternatively, reduced enzymatic activity may result in precursor accumulation. Examples are the mucopolysaccharidoses, the lipid storage disorders, and the glycogen storage family of diseases. In some instances, accumulation of precursors may lead to production of toxic products, such as in phenylketonuria and galactosemia. In some disorders, the enzymatic deficiency may result in abnormality of metabolic control. Some types of gout fall into this category, as do the porphyrias and hyperlipidemia type II, in which there is overproduction of these metabolites.

Important carrier proteins may be abnormal on a genetic basis. The best examples are the hemoglobinopathies and the thalassemia syndromes. The abnormal or reduced quantity of hemoglobin, which may have reduced oxygen carrying capacity, may also cause disruption or abnormal adherence of red cells in some instances.

Appreciation of the role of receptors has led to the identification of abnormalities in the cascade of the events that follow from impingement of hormone on cell and the events that normally follow from that encounter. Pseudohypoparathyroidism is a case in point, and another is one form of familial hypothyroidism, in which the hormone fails to act because its specific receptor is absent. It is possible that several puzzling neuropsychiatric disorders may fall into this category. Similarly, defects in receptors for insulin and lipoproteins (like LDL) are emerging as the basis for some forms of diabetes and hyperlipidemias (see earlier chapters).

Certain proteins have a structural role. The Ehlers-Danlos group of inherited disorders in-

* Massachusetts Institute of Technology, Cambridge, MA.

cludes certain patients with hyperextensible skin and joints, easy bruisability, and poor wound healing. These appear to be disorders of the collagen molecule, relating to point mutations in the collagen gene (type IV) or in the lysyl oxidase (a copper protein necessary for its normal cross-linking; see Chapter 7) (types VI and IX) (Scriver et al., 1989). Other proteins have essential roles in the complement system and the blood clotting cascade; errors in the structure of involved proteins may have serious consequences for hemostasis in the one instance and resistance to infection in the other.

Helpful treatment is available for many patients with inborn errors of metabolism. For some, the benefit is marginal, but for many, genuine palliation is possible, and for a number of patients, proper management may permit normal or nearly normal life. Often, the important adjunct is dietary. Table 18.1 lists recognized metabolic errors for which dietary intervention has had some success. It also lists the principal manifestations of the disorders, the strategy for dietary treatment, and an assessment of the value of dietary intervention.

Clearly, it is not possible within the confines of this chapter to review the theory, supporting data, advised treatment, and results of dietary changes for all the described errors. These are described fully in the volume, *The Metabolic Basis of Inherited Disease* (Stanbury et al., 1983), and in the most recent edition by Scriver et al. (1988). Instead, three disorders are selected as examples. These three are chosen because they are representative of the problem, effective therapy is accessible, and because neglect may be disastrous. Many other examples might have been chosen as well.

Glycogen Storage Disease

Glycogen is the most important reservoir for glucose residues used to maintain the constancy of the blood sugar concentration in the daily ebb and flow of energy requirements (see Chapter 2). It is a huge molecule that must be built, continuously restructured, and degraded (in liver and muscle) according to the hexose supply and glucose demand. A number of disorders have been attributed to abnormalities in the various enzymes involved in synthesis and internal restructuring of glycogen and in mobilizing its glucose residues, especially in the liver (Table 18.1).

The first of these disorders to be well understood was *glucose-6-phosphatase* deficiency glycogenosis (glucose-6-phosphatase deficiency). These patients can degrade liver, kidney, and muscle glycogen to glucose-6-phosphate (see Figure 18.1), but the phosphatase in liver and kidney, which releases free glucose for transport across the cell membrane into the blood is missing. The result is accumulation of glycogen in the liver and kidney cells and a hypoglycemia. Episodes of hypoglycemia (excessively low glucose in the plasma) may be frequent, severe, and ultimately fatal. Excessive glycogen accumulation accompanied by acute and chronic hypoglycemia also causes liver and kidney damage and growth retardation. Treatment is not entirely satisfactory, but can do much to restore growth and diminish or eliminate hypoglycemic crises. Treatment strategy is to prevent glycogen accumulation and yet provide some carbohydrate by giving small amounts at a time, frequently or even continuously. Frequent carbohydrate feedings, often including sleep interruption for feedings, may be sufficient, but at times (in the young) nasogastric drip of carbohydrate or even intravenous administration of carbohydrate may be necessary. Absorption of glucose can be slowed and the blood sugar level flattened by giving the glucose with milk curd or in the form of starch. Indeed, a 50% suspension of uncooked starch in tap water (in doses of 2 g/kg body weight) is able to maintain blood glucose levels for up to 6 hr without the trauma of intravenous infusions (Hers et al., 1989). This is because the intestinal α-amylase only digests such starch very slowly, releasing glucose for absorption over a relatively long period. Other patients have been treated with success for several months with glucose delivered intravenously by peristaltic pump through an indwelling catheter (Stacey et al., 1980), although this is much less convenient.

A more recently discovered variant of apparent glucose-6-phosphatase deficiency appears to be a defect in the *translocase* that delivers glucose-6-phosphate to the phosphatase in the lumen of the endoplasmic reticulum (Narisawa et al., 1987). This defect has the same overall effect on hepatic glucose metabolism.

Patients with *amylo-1-6-glucosidase deficiency* (debranching enzyme; Figure 18.1) are limited in their capacity to rupture α1-6 linkages in the arborized glycogen molecule, and accordingly, are thus limited in the mobilization of glucose. Some glucose is available by phosphorolysis of the outer tiers of the molecule, where α1,4 linkages prevail. Because an abnormal glycogen (high in 1,6 linkages) results from this deficiency, car-

Table 18.1. Diet Therapy of the Principal Inborn Errors of Metabolism[a]

Condition	Principal clinical findings	Therapy	Results
	DISORDERS OF CARBOHYDRATE METABOLISM		
Diabetes mellitus			
(A) Insulin-dependent	Hyperglycemia; acidosis	Restricted calories and carbohydrate	Helpful
(B) Noninsulin-dependent	Hyperglycemia	Restricted calories and carbohydrate	Helpful
Glycogen storage disease			
Glucose-6-phosphatase deficiency	Glycogen storage; FTT; hepatic enlargement	Frequent feeding; nasodrip; high carbohydrate intake	Helpful
Amylo-1,6-glucosidase	Glycogen storage	Same	Helpful
Muscle phosphorylase deficiency	Easy muscle fatigue	Oral glucose and fructose	Variable benefit
Galactosemia			
Gal-1-PO_4 transferase deficiency galactosemia	FTT; liver failure; cataracts; mental retardation	Galactose-free diet	Good
Galactokinase galactosemia	Cataracts	Galactose-free diet	Good
Uridine diphosphate gal-4-epimerase deficiency	None	Galactose-free diet	Good
Disorders of fructose metabolism			
Fructokinase deficiency	Fructosuria and fructosemia	Unnecessary	
Fructose-1,6-diphosphatase deficiency	Keto and lactic acidosis; hypotonia; hypoglycemia; seizures	Fructose-free diet; frequent feeding	Good
Fructose-1-phosphate aldolase deficiency	FTT; poor feeding; fructose intolerance; hypoglycemia; hepatic failure	Fructose-free diet; sorbitol	Good
Disorders of pyruvate metabolism			
Pyruvate dehydrogenase deficiency	Psychomotor retardation; lactic acidosis	Ketogenic diet; supplements of thiamine, aspartate, glutamate	Possibly helpful
Pyruvate carboxylase deficiency	Psychomotor retardation; lactic acidosis	Same	Possibly helpful
Primary hyperoxaluria			
Soluble α-ketoglutarate : glyoxalate carboligase deficiency	Oxalate stones; nephrolithiasis (kidney stones)	High pyridoxine diet (supplements needed); high phosphate diet (with supplements)	Good
D-glycerate dehydrogenase deficiency	Same	Same	Good

(continued)

Table 18.1 (*continued*)

Condition	Principal clinical findings	Therapy	Results
DISORDERS OF AMINO ACID METABOLISM			
Phenylketonuria			
Phenylalanine hydroxylase	Mental retardation	Phenylalanine-restricted diet	Fair to good
Dehydropteridine reductase deficiency	Neurologic deficits	Same	? Helpful
Dihydrobiopterine synthetase deficiency	Neurologic deficits	Phenylalanine-restricted diet	Helpful
Tyrosinemia			
Tyrosine aminotransferase deficiency	Mental retardation; skin and corneal changes	Diet low in tyrosine and phenylalanine	Helpful
Fumaryl-acetoacetate hydrolase and maleylacetoacetate hydrolase deficiency	Liver failure; anemia	Diet low in protein, phenylalanine, and tyrosine; vitamin A	Helpful
Neonatal tyrosinemia of multiple causes	Asymptomatic or mild mental retardation	Diet low in protein and tyrosine	Helpful
Alkaptonuria			
Homogentisic acid oxidase deficiency	Pigment deposits; arthritis	—	—
Familial goiter			
Dehalogenase deficiency	Hypothyroidism; goiter	High iodine intake	Helpful
Iodide transport defect	Hypothyroidism; goiter	High iodine intake	Helpful
Hyperornithinemia			
Ornithine-aminotransferase deficiency	Chorioretinal degeneration	Protein restriction; creatine, lysine, and pyrodoxine supplements	Helpful
Hyperornithinemia-hyperammonemia-homocitrullinuria syndrome	Hyperammonemia	Ornithine supplements; protein restriction	Helpful
Disorders of the glutamyl cycle			
Glutathionine synthetase deficiency	Acidosis; hemolysis; CNS dysfunction	Vitamin E	? Effective
Histidinemia			
Histidase deficiency	? Mental deficiency; speech defects	Low histidine diet	? Useful
Chediak-Higashi syndrome	Partial albinism; frequent infections; neuropathy	Vitamin C supplements	Possibly helpful
Disorders of lysine metabolism			
L-lysine NAD; oxidoreductase (periodic hyperlysinemia)	FTT, dehydration; hyperammonemia	Restricted protein diet	Helpful
Persistent hyperlysinemia	Hyperlysinemia and hyperlysinuria; retardation	Low protein diet	Possibly helpful
Disorders of propionate and methylmalonate metabolism			
Propionyl-CoA carboxylase deficiency	Ketoacidosis	Protein restriction; biotin supplements	Helpful

Biotin-dependent multiple carboxylase deficiency	Ketoacidosis; skin disorder; retardation; alopecia	Biotin	Good
Methylmalonyl-CoA mutase deficiency	Methylmalonic acidemia and aciduria	Protein restriction; cobalamin	Helpful
Methylmalonyl-CoA mutase and homocysteine; N^5-methyltetrahydrofolate methyltransferase deficiency	FTT; anemia	Hydroxycobalamin (B_{12})	Helpful
Disorders of transsulfation			
Cystathionine-b-synthase deficiency	Mental retardation; bony changes; dislocated lenses; thromboembolism	Low methionine, cystine-supplemented diet; pyridoxine	Helpful
Disorders of the urea cycle			
N-acetylglutamate synthetase deficiency	Hyperammonemia syndrome	Low protein diet; arginine supplements	Helpful
Carbamoyl-phosphate synthetase deficiency	Same	Same	Helpful
Ornithine carbamoyl transferase deficiency	Same plus orotic aciduria	Low protein diet plus supplements of ketoacid analogues of amino acids	Helpful
Argininosuccinate synthetase deficiency	Hyperammonemia; orotic aciduria; neurologic changes	Protein restriction; arginine supplements	Helpful
Argininosuccinate lyase deficiency	Hyperammonemia; neurologic changes; brittle hair	Same	Helpful
Arginase deficiency	Retardation; neurologic changes; argininuria	Protein-free diet containing essential amino acids, except arginine	Helpful
Multiple urea cycle enzyme defects	Hyperammonemia	Protein restriction; amino acid supplements	Helpful
Hyperdibasic aminoaciduria	Protein intolerance; FTT; retardation; hyperammonemia	Citrulline supplements plus low protein diet	Helpful
Branched chain amino acid and organic acid disorders			
Branched chain transaminase deficiency (hypervalinemia)	Severe retardation	Protein restriction	? Value
Branched chain ketoacid dehydrogenase complex deficiency (maple syrup urine disease)	Retardation; ketoacidosis	Low branched chain amino acid diet; thiamine	Helpful
Isovaleryl-CoA dehydrogenase deficiency (isovaleric acidemia)	FTT; ketoacidosis	Protein restriction; leucine restriction; glycine supplements	Helpful

(continued)

Table 18.1 (*continued*)

Condition	Principal clinical findings	Therapy	Results
Ethyl malonic-adipic aciduria	Hypoglycemia; acidosis	Low fat, high carbohydrate diet	? Helpful
3-Methylcrotonyl-CoA carboxylase deficiency	Hypotonia; muscle atrophy	Low leucine diet	Helpful
3-Hydroxy-3-methyl glutaryl-CoA lyase deficiency	Hypoglycemia; acidosis	Low protein diet; carbohydrate	Helpful
3-Ketothiolase deficiency	Ketoacidosis; psychomotor retardation	Moderate protein restriction	Helpful
Disorders of folate metabolism			
Folate absorption defect	FTT; central nervous system damage; anemia	Parenteral folate	Helpful
Dihydrofolate reductase deficiency	FTT; anemia	Folinic acid supplements	Helpful
Formimino transferase deficiency	FTT; central nervous system damage; anemia	Folate	? Helpful
Tetrahydrofolate methyltransferase deficiency	Anemia; delayed neural development	Folate	Probably not helpful
DISORDERS OF LIPOPROTEIN AND LIPID METABOLISM			
Lipoprotein deficiency			
A-betalipoproteinemia	Ataxia; retinitis pigmentosa; acanthocytosis; fat malabsorption	Restricted long chain triglyceride diet; supplements of vitamins A, K, and E	Helpful
Hypobetalipoproteinemia	Same as above but milder	Same as above if needed	Possibly helpful
Tangier disease	Large orange tonsils; neuromuscular dysfunction	Reduced fat diet	? Useful
Disorders of chylomicron metabolism			
Lipoprotein lipase deficiency	Chylomicronemia; abdominal pain; recurrent pancreatitis; xanthomas	Low fat diet	Helpful
Apolipoprotein C-II deficiency	Hypertriglyceridemia; recurrent pancreatitis	Moderate dietary fat restriction	Helpful
Type V hyperlipoproteinemia	Xanthomas; abdominal pain; recurrent pancreatitis; polyneuropathy	Low calorie, low fat diet; nicotinic acid	Helpful
Lecithin : cholesterol acyl transferase deficiency	Anemia; corneal opacities; renal failure	Restricted fat diet	Helpful
Hypercholesterolemia (familial)	Xanthomas; atherosclerosis	Low cholesterol; low saturated, high unsaturated fat diet with nicotinic acid supplements	Helpful
Sitosterolemia with xanthomatosis	Xanthomas; atherosclerosis	Diet low in plant sterol	Helpful

Phytanic acid storage disease; defective phytanic acid oxidation	Retinitis pigmentosa; peripheral neuropathy; ataxia	Diet low in phytate	Helpful
Glucocerebrosidase deficiency (glucosylceramide lipidosis)	Enlarged viscera; anemia	Vitamins, Fe	Supportive
DISORDERS OF PURINE AND PYRIMIDINE METABOLISM			
Gout (unknown cause; glucose-6-phosphatase deficiency; hypoxanthine-guanine phosphoribosyl-transferase deficiency; phosphoribosyl pyrophosphate synthetase excess activity)	Gouty arthritis; tophi; hyperurecemia	Weight reduction; restricted protein diet; low purine diet; alcohol restriction; high fiber diet	Helpful
Adenine phosphoribosyltransferase deficiency	Renal stones; renal colic	Dietary purine restriction; fluids	Helpful
Myoadenylate deaminase deficiency	Muscle fatigue	High ribose diet and ribose supplements	? Helpful
Xanthine oxidase deficiency	Xanthine urolithiasis (urinary tract stones); sometimes myopathy or polyarthritis	Low purine diet	Helpful
Orotic aciduria			
Orotate phosphoribosyltransferase and orotidine-5-phosphate decarboxylase deficiency	FTT; anemia	Uridine supplements	Helpful
Orotidine-5-phosphate decarboxylase deficiency	Same	Same	Probably not helpful
DISORDERS OF PORPHYRIN AND HEME METABOLISM			
Ferrochelatase deficiency (erythropoietic protoporphyria)	Skin photosensitivity; hepatic damage; anemia	β-carotene supplements; caloric restriction	Helpful
Porphobilinogen deaminase deficiency (acute intermittent porphyria)	Nerve damage; abdominal pain	High carbohydrate diet	? Helpful
Coproporphyrinogen III oxidase deficiency (hereditary coproporphyria)	Abdominal pain; photosensitivity	High carbohydrate diet	? Helpful
Protoporphyrinogen oxidase or ferrochelatase deficiency (variegate porphyria)	Photosensitivity; abdominal pain; neuropathy	High carbohydrate diet	? Helpful
Hepatic uroporphyrinogen decarboxylase deficiency (porphyria cutanea tarda)	Photosensitivity, with skin lesions	Low alcohol; vitamin E supplements; pyridoxal phosphate	Helpful
Uroporphyrinogen III cosynthetase deficiency (congenital erythropoietic porphyria)	Hemolysis; photosensitivity; skin scarring	β-carotene (supplements)	Helpful
DISORDERS INVOLVING CONNECTIVE TISSUE, MUSCLE, AND BONE			
Hypophosphatasia	Rickets; growth retardation	High phosphate	Helpful
Pseudohypoparathyroidism			
Reduced renal cell adenylate cyclase activity	Typical features and habitus; bone changes	Vitamin D (ergocalciferol)	Helpful
Reduced renal cell cyclic AMP effectiveness	Same	Same	

(continued)

Table 18.1 (*continued*)

Condition	Principal clinical findings	Therapy	Results
DISORDERS OF BLOOD AND BLOOD-FORMING TISSUES			
Glucose-6-phosphate dehydrogenase deficiency	Episodic hemolysis	Avoid fava beans (or other inciting substances)	Preventative
NADH cytochrome-b_5-reductase deficiency (methemoglobinemia)	Methemoglobinemia; mental retardation	Diets free of nitrate and nitrite	Preventative
DISORDERS OF TRANSPORT			
Intestinal lactase deficiency	Lactose intolerance; abdominal symptoms	Low lactose diets	Helpful
Sucrase-α-dextrinase deficiency	Sucrose intolerance	Sucrose-free diet	Helpful
Glucose-galactose transport deficiency	Abdominal symptoms; dehydration; diarrhea	Diet substituting fructose for other sugar	Helpful
Hypophosphatemic rickets	Rickets; hypophosphatemia	Oral phosphate (plus 1,25-diOHvitD_3)	Helpful
Vitamin-D-dependent rickets type I	Rickets; FTT; tetany	Vitamin D (large doses)	Helpful
Cystinuria	Cystinuria; cystine stones	Low methionine diet	Variable benefit
Hartnut disease	Skin rash; ataxia; episodic psychosis	Oral nicotinamide	Helpful
Renal tubular acidosis type I	Acidosis; stunting; bicarbonaturia; nephrocalcinosis	Potassium and bicarbonate supplements	Helpful
Renal tubular acidosis type II	Same but less severe	Potassium restriction	Helpful
Pseudohypoaldosteronism type I (with renal tubular acidosis)	FTT; dehydration; hyponatremia	Sodium supplements	Helpful
Pseudohypoaldosteronism type II (with renal tubular acidosis)	Acidosis; hyperkalemia	Chloride restriction	Helpful
Cystinosis	Cystine deposits; renal damage; retinal depigmentation; rickets	Vitamin D; phosphate supplements	Helpful

[a] Only diet therapy is addressed in this table. For many of these conditions, other forms of treatment are available in addition to those related specifically to dietary manipulation. FTT, failure to thrive.

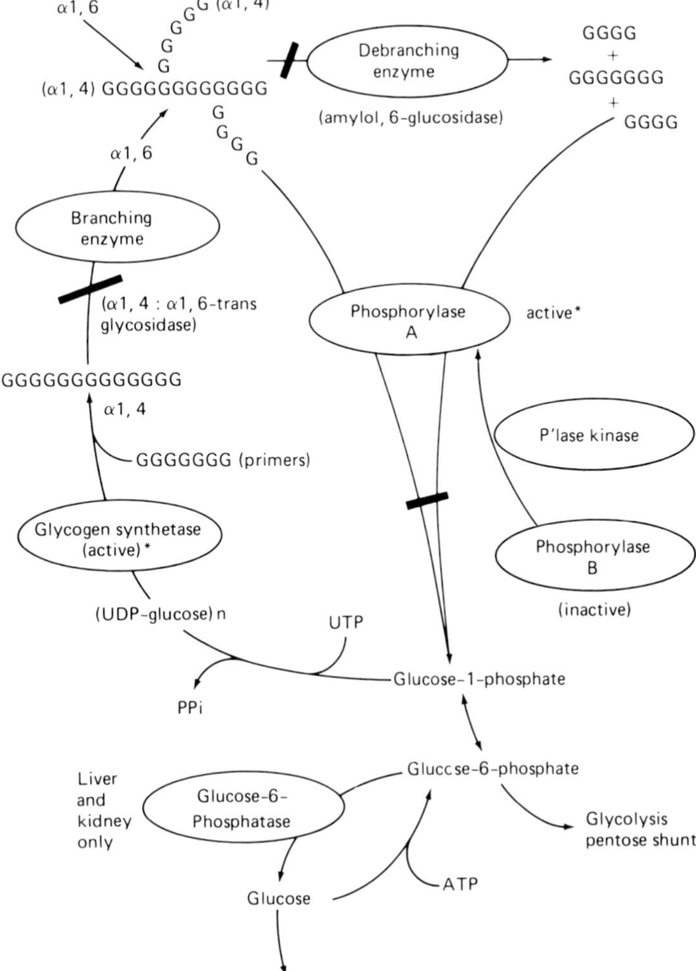

Figure 18.1. Pathways of glycogen synthesis and degradation. Key: G, glucose; ■ inborn enzyme deficiencies that may occur. *See Chapter 2.

diac and skeletal muscle damage may occur. Severe hypoglycemia with seizures may appear, but generally, hypoglycemia is not so severe as in glucose-6-phosphatase deficiency. Treatment is the same, except that, in addition, high protein feedings are helpful because these patients, having glucose-6-phosphatase, can utilize amino acids for liver gluconeogenesis and secrete glucose into the plasma (see Chapters 2 and 4).

Muscle phosphorylase deficiency results in limitation of the phosphorolysis of α1-4 linkages in the glycogen molecule (the majority of linkages present). The result is a limited (but not absent) capacity of the muscle to perform work. While the disorder is inconvenient and limiting, it is not life-threatening. Frequent feeding with small doses of glucose or fructose may be helpful in alleviating symptoms, but the results are not particularly rewarding. Living within one's exercise limitations is usually sufficient.

A related pair of disorders are *hepatic phosphorylase deficiency* (a structurally different protein than muscle phosphorylase), and *deficiency of the activating enzyme phosphorylase B kinase* (see Figure 18.1). Liver enlargement, due to glycogen accumulation, is a feature during the preadolescent years. Symptoms are few, and diet therapy is not necessary unless there is a tendency toward hypoglycemia.

Other forms of glycogen storage disease respond poorly or not at all to diet therapy, possibly because the stored glycogen may have abnormal structure and be damaging to the cells in which it is stored [e.g., α-1,4-glucan : α-1,4-glucan-6-glucosyl transferase (brancher enzyme) deficiency glycogenosis] or because it is inaccessible (acid maltase deficiency). Defects in glycogen synthesis have not yet been established.

Galactosemia

Galactose, which comprises half the lactose molecule, is an exceedingly common hexose. It is metabolized to galactose-1-PO_4 by galactokinase, and further to uridine diphosphate (UDP) galactose by a transferase (Figure 18.2) (see Chapter 2). The sugar nucleotide is further metabolized through a variety of pathways that include formation of complex glycolipids, glycoproteins, glucose, and so on. It is an important constituent of cell membranes.

There are two principal clinical disorders that arise because of impaired galactose metabolism (Table 18.1). *Galactokinase deficiency galactosemia* is a mild disorder, leading to juvenile cataracts. *Transferase deficiency galactosemia* is a much more severe disturbance, which, when untreated, is accompanied by failure to thrive, mental retardation, liver disease, and renal impairment. A group of patients has been identified that also has transferase deficiency but can metabolize galactose to a limited degree through some other undefined pathway and can escape the severe symptoms of the classic form of the disease. Finally, subjects have been identified who lack the epimerase that reversibly catalyzes the conversion of UDP galactose to UDP glucose (Figure 18.2), but in whom the abnormality has no known deleterious effects. As UDP galactose can be made from UDP glucose, galactose deficiency is unknown, and diets low in galactose are not harm-

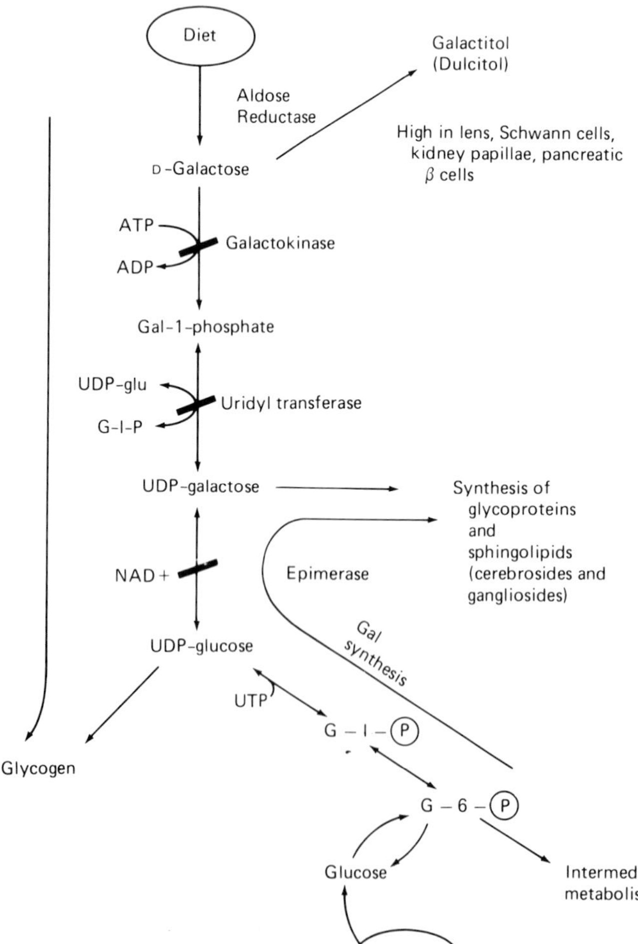

Figure 18.2. Pathways of galactose metabolism. Key: ■ inborn enzyme deficiencies that may occur.

ful, unlike the harmful effects to phenylketonurics of diets that are too low in phenylalanine.

Both galactokinase and the transferase can be measured in erythrocytes, as can the accumulation of galactose-1-phosphate. These tests are widely used for screening neonates and monitoring patients with the disease. In these patients, galactose concentrations are also elevated in the blood, and the sugar may appear in the urine. If a glucose oxidase method is used for determining sugar in the urine, galactose will be missed because of the glucose specificity of this assay.

The cause of cataracts in both forms of galactosemia seems well defined. Galactitol (the sugar alcohol; see Chapter 2), resulting from aldose reductase action on galactose, damages the lens osmotically. These cataracts are rapidly reversed if the patient is placed on a galactose-free diet. The cause of the liver, kidney, and brain damage in transferase deficiency galactosemia is obscure. It may also be due in part to accumulation of galactitol (Figure 18.2) and, in part, to galactonate or to other presently unidentified metabolic products.

Several variant forms of transferase deficiency galactosemia have been identified. These have been less severe than the classic form and are presumably a result of a mutant allelic gene. Among these are Duarte and Indiana variants (Beutler, 1983).

The key element in treatment of galactosemia is a diet as low as possible in galactose. Table 18.2 indicates the galactose content of various foods and many tables have been published (Gardner, 1969; Koch et al., 1963; Robinson and Lawler, 1982), but milk and milk products are the important sources of the sugar. Lactose is also commonly used as a filler (especially in tablets). For the infant, the usual formula is a soy-based product, such as Prosobee (Mead Johnson Co.) or Neomullsoy (Syntax Laboratories), or a preparation based on hydrolyzed and charcoal-treated casein (Mead Johnson Co.). These formulas are supplemented with calcium and vitamins. The soy-based formulas may contain complex carbohydrates, such as stachyose, which contains galactose but is not absorbed. Supplementary feedings may use various foods, except those that contain milk or milk products or have been prepared with lactose. For canned or frozen foods, the labels should be consulted for possible lactose content. There is a consensus that, although some liberalization of the diet is possible with advancing years, there is no significant opening of new and nontoxic pathways of galactose disposal. A lactose-limited diet is the life-long fate of most patients with symptomatic galactosemia.

Table 18.2. Lactose in the Diet

Foods that may contain lactose
- All products that contain or are derived from milk.
  - Bread, crackers, cakes, cookies, french toast, pancakes, waffles, etc., if they are made from milk or milk products (read labels). Butter and margarine may contain lactose. Cheese, cream or cream substitutes whether sweet or sour, ice cream or ice milk, pies and pie crust, sherbets (if milk is used), yogurt
- Cocoa, some soft drinks, instant coffee (read label)
- Other products where lactose content may be inapparent: commercial fruit fillings, custards, cream pies, medications with lactose used as filler, canned or frozen fruits or vegetables (read labels)

Foods low or free of lactose
- Most soft drinks, coffee, tea (consult label)
- Breads and similar products made without milk or milk products (butter, etc.)
- Eggs prepared any style without milk or butter
- All fruits except those prepared with lactose for canning or freezing (consult label)
- Gelatin, puddings, cakes, if prepared without milk or milk products
- Vegetable oils. Some cream substitutes contain no lactose (read label)

Although cataracts regress, constitutional symptoms (such as nausea and vomiting) disappear, and growth begins in the galactosemic child when a galactose-free diet is begun, there is no assurance of normal development. Most, but not all, studies have shown a significant degree of growth and mental retardation in many galactosemic infants (Donnell et al., 1980), and some have even been born with cataracts. This result may derive, in part, from an insufficiently rigorous control of the diet and, in part, from endogenous production of galactose from glucose. Nevertheless, there is full consensus that all galactosemic infants should be vigorously treated with a diet as free of galactose as can be achieved. This results in substantial improvement in symptoms and in development, and in many, it results in a pattern of development well within normal limits. (There is no evidence for abnormality of growth or development of the heterozygote.)

No special treatment is required for the pregnant, homozygous woman with a heterozygous fetus, because the fetus is able to maintain a normal red cell content of galactose-1-phosphate, and this metabolite and galactitol do not accumulate.

What of the homozygous fetus detected by amniocentesis? There are several reports of prenatal detection of transferase-deficient fetuses (Holton and Raymont, 1980). A maternal low galactose diet has been effective in some in preventing manifestations of galactosemia in the neonatal period, but not in others. Whether amniocentesis should be done for detection of a disorder for which reasonably satisfactory treatment exists is a current ethical issue. Some women have elected interruption of pregnancy, while others have proceeded to term; some of the latter group have had normal children and others not. Galactose-1-phosphate is an intracellular compound that does not cross the placenta, and the heterozygous fetus can handle the transplacental galactose that enters its circulation. Nevertheless, it might be prudent to limit sharply the dietary galactose of a pregnant woman with galactosemia. It is especially important that the homozygous infant detected by amniocentesis (done because of a previous sibling with the disorder) should be protected as much as possible from transplacental galactose by rigorous restriction of the maternal diet. Nevertheless, the homozygous fetus is still at risk from maternal endogenous production of galactose. The most sophisticated genetic counseling is in order in such a complex circumstance, where risks are indeterminate and postpartum results not guaranteed even under the best circumstances. Clearly, if one is dealing with transferase deficiency galactosemia, the stakes are much higher than if the disorder is galactokinase deficiency galactosemia.

Disorders of the Urea Cycle, with Hyperammonemia

The urea cycle in humans functions to remove the toxic metabolic product, ammonia, for disposal as urea by renal excretion. A liver mitochondrial enzyme, activated by *N*-acetylglutamate (carbamoyl-phosphate synthetase), catalyzes the formation of carbamoyl-phosphate from NH_4^+, CO_2, and adenosine triphosphate (ATP) (Figure 18.3). This reacts with ornithine, by action of a transferase, to form citrulline. Citrulline in turn combines with aspartate to give arginosuccinate through the action of argininosuccinate synthetase. Argininosuccinate is hydrolyzed to arginine and fumarate, the arginine is hydrolyzed by arginase to urea, and ornithine is regenerated. The enzymes involved in each of these catalytic steps may be deficient in activity, and a set of syndromes may result, all of which may have hyperammonemia as a manifestation (Table 18.1). In certain other respects, the syndromes may differ, and the severity of the disorder varies widely. (See also Tada et al., 1987.)

The overriding principle of therapy for all these diseases is reduction in the concentration of ammonia in the plasma. Frequently, there is urgency in accomplishing this, in that hyperammonemia crises may occur with startling suddenness, especially in the infant, and may be lethal. Several modalities are useful and may be necessary in the event of a crisis. These include peritoneal dialysis, exchange transfusion, charcoal hyperperfusion, administration of sodium benzoate to trap glycine (Figure 18.4), thereby eliminating this major source of ammonia as hippuric acid, or phenylacetate to trap glutamine. These emergency measures must be combined with reduction in the dietary intake of sources of nitrogen (e.g., protein) that might be metabolized to ammonia.

The therapeutic maneuver that concerns us here is dietary manipulation. Reduced production of waste nitrogen can be achieved by limiting protein intake to the minimal levels that will sustain growth. Additional economies can be achieved by substituting essential amino acids for protein intake, reducing intake of nonessential ones, and by use of α-keto or α-hydroxy amino acid analogues. For example, it is possible to substitute the keto analogue of isoleucine, phenylpyruvate for phenylalanine, and the α-keto analogue of methionine. By transamination, these amino acid analogues trap amino nitrogen and reduce the ammonia load (Figure 18.5). (The other analogues are too expensive for chronic use.) However, in severe cases of inborn urea cycle enzyme deficiencies, this dietary approach has failed (Brusilow and Horwich, 1989), probably because turnover of endogenous protein may be enhanced, contributing extra nitrogen and ammonia, when amino acid intake is too much curtailed. These cases are therefore best treated with benzoate and phenylacetate (Figure 18.4).

Variations in the symptom complexes of the related disorders of the urea cycle are attributable to toxic accumulation of intermediates other than ammonia behind enzymatic blocks in the pathway, or to a need for products of blocked reactions other than for urea synthesis. Thus, arginine is a needed metabolite (see Chapter 4) and should be supplemented in patients in this group, except in arginase deficiency.

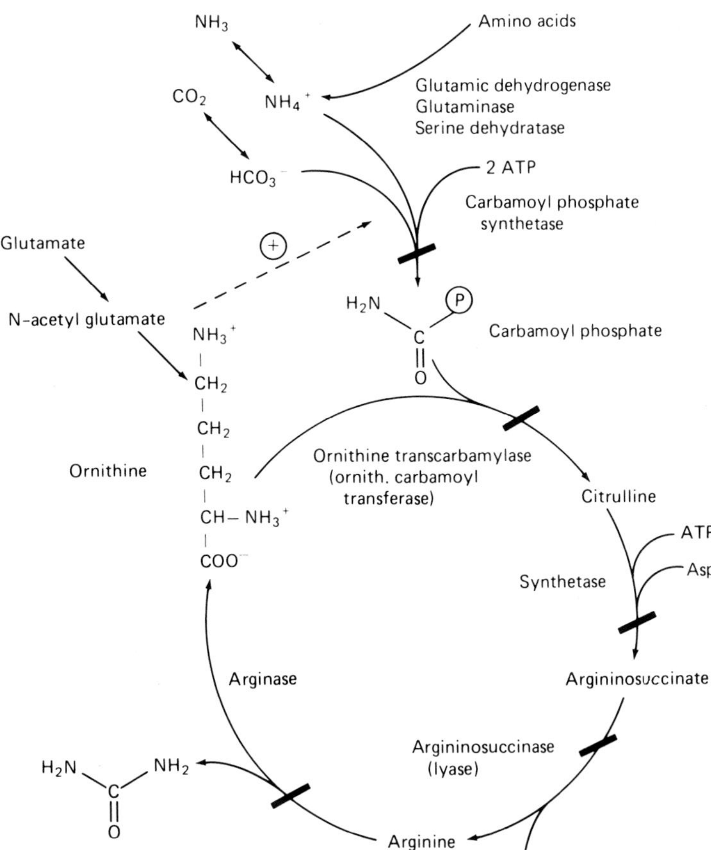

Figure 18.3. Urea cycle enzymes that may be hereditarily deficient. Key: ■ inborn enzyme deficiencies that may occur.

Figure 18.4. Pathways for synthesis of waste nitrogen products (for urinary excretion) upon treatment with benzoate or phenylacetate. [*Source:* modified from Brusilow and Horwich (1989).] **Nitrogen sources.*

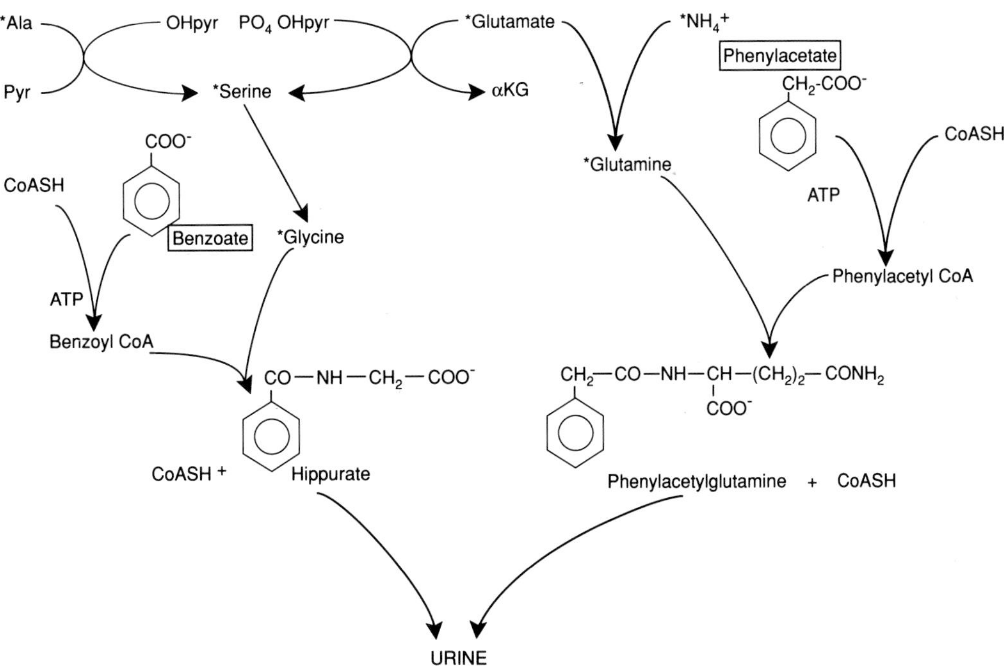

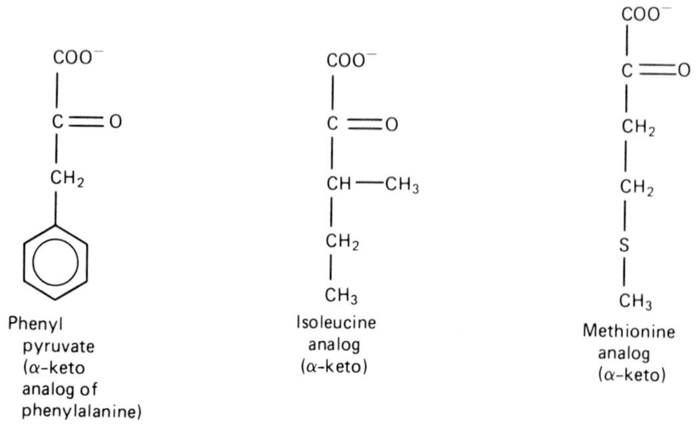

COO^- — C=O — CH_2 — (phenyl)
Phenyl pyruvate (α-keto analog of phenylalanine)

COO^- — C=O — CH—CH_3 — CH_2 — CH_3
Isoleucine analog (α-keto)

COO^- — C=O — CH_2 — CH_2 — S — CH_3
Methionine analog (α-keto)

Figure 18.5. Amino acid analogue used in treating inborn hyperammonemia.

In spite of intensive treatment, *carbamoylphosphate synthetase deficiency* (Figure 18.3) is a dangerous and often (but not always) lethal disorder in the neonatal period. Hyperammonemia and compensatory respiratory acidosis (with lowered respiratory rates) are the obvious findings. A few neonates with *ornithine carbamoyltransferase deficiency* have survived following vigorous therapy. The same may be said for neonatal *argininosuccinate synthetase deficiency*, but a subacute and late onset type are milder and accompanied by episodic hyperammonemia. Argininosuccinic aciduria (*lyase deficiency*) also has neonatal, subacute, and delayed types and is generally a milder disorder. *Arginase deficiency* is usually accompanied by neurologic symptoms, appearing after the neonatal period. Treatment has not been satisfactory, except with highly synthetic structured diets. For example, one patient has been successfully treated from birth with a mixture of nine essential and semiessential amino acids, but omitting arginine as a source of nitrogen for the first several months (Snyderman et al., 1977). The differences in severity of the hyperammonemia in these syndromes may be related to the differences in completeness of the enzyme defect. Residual enzyme activity is demonstrable in some; these patients probably have allelic abnormal genes for the enzyme in question.

From the foregoing, it may be seen that diet therapy is at the center of the clinical management of this group of related disorders. Logically and carefully applied, diet therapy may be the arbiter of survival. However, those more severely affected may resist the more rigorous dietary programs or may require the painstaking care, which could prove very expensive. Early diagnosis is essential for success.

Further Comments: Summary Tables

The three groups of disorders described above illustrate the therapeutic possibilities of dietary manipulation in clinical management. Lifelong galactose restriction is essential in both forms of galactosemia and can permit normal or nearly normal development and activity. Most of the disorders of the urea cycle respond to restriction of protein in the diet. Hypoglycemia and the attendant developmental retardation, and occasional seizures and coma, are features of some of the glycogen storage disorders and can usually be managed successfully with dietary measures designed to maintain normal plasma levels of glucose.

At least two important genetic principles are illustrated by these three groups of inherited diseases. All are noteworthy in that a central laboratory finding, galactosemia (hyperammonemia or glycogen storage with hypoglycemia) may arise from different enzymatic defects in the apparatus related to a coherent metabolic process. All are also noteworthy in that each may appear in multiple degrees of severity, presumably related to the capacity of different allelic forms of the enzyme to function. Thus, what at first appears to have an incomprehensible complexity, becomes relatively accessible through the understanding of a few fundamental and simple principles.

The three groups of disorders cited in the text serve only as examples of the therapeutic resources that are available for the treatment of inborn errors of metabolism. Other examples might equally as well have been chosen, but the principles for all are much the same. These include the addition of a metabolite, such as glucose, which is in short supply because of a metabolic block; detoxification through use of a dietary item that reduces the load of the toxic metabolite, as in the use of ketoacids (or benzoate and phenylacetate) to reduce the ammonia load in the hyperammonemia syndromes; or the use of a diet that is free of a metabolite or precursor that cannot be handled, as in galactosemia. In others, addition of a vitamin that acts as a cofactor may boost the activity of an enzyme that is sluggish because of an inborn error in its structure. Most of the disorders listed in Table 18.1 can be categorized under one or more of these principles. Of course, there are others for which no therapy has yet been devised, and for those for which dietary therapy is useful, there are (in many instances) other therapeutic possibilities for the benefit of the patient. Original sources, or standard texts such as Stanbury et al. (1983) and Scriver et al. (1989), may be consulted when one is faced with the practical necessity of managing one of these patients.

References

Beutler E (1983): *In* Stanbury JB, Wyngaarden JB, Fredrickson DS, Goldstein J, Brown M, eds: The metabolic basis of inherited disease. New York: McGraw-Hill, p 1629.

Brusilow SW, Horwich AL (1989): *In* Scriver CR, Beaudet AL, Sly WS, Valle D, eds: The metabolic basis of inherited disease. New York: McGraw-Hill, p 629.

Donnell GN, Koch R, Fishler K, Ng WG (1980): *In* Burman D, Holton JB, Pennock CA, eds: Inherited disorders of carbohydrate metabolism. Baltimore: University Park Press, p 103.

Gardner LI, ed (1969): Endocrine and genetic disease of childhood. Philadelphia: WB Saunders, p 1036.

Hers H-G, von Hoof F, de Barsy T (1989): *In* Scriver CR, Beaudet AL, Sly WS, Valle D, eds: The metabolic basis of inherited disease. New York: McGraw-Hill, p 425.

Holton JB, Raymont CM (1980): *In* Burman D, Holton JB, Pennock CA, eds: Inherited disorders of carbohydrate metabolism. Baltimore: University Park Press, p 141.

Narisawa K, Igarashi Y, Tada K (1987): Enzyme 38:177.

Koch R, Acosta P, Ragsdale N, Donnell GN (1963): J Am Dietet Assoc 43:216.

Robinson CH, Lawler MR (1982): Normal and therapeutic nutrition (16th ed). New York: Macmillan.

Scriver CR, Beandet AL, Sly WS, Valle D, eds (1989): The metabolic basis of inherited disease (6th ed.). New York: McGraw-Hill.

Snyderman SE, Sansaricq C, Chen WJ, Norton PM, Phansalkar SV (1977): J Pediatr 90:563.

Stacey TE, MacNab A, Strang LB (1980): *In* Burman D, Holton JB, Pennock CA, eds: Inherited disorders of carbohydrate metabolism. Baltimore: University Park Press, p 315.

Stanbury JB, Wyngaarden JB, Fredrickson DS, Goldstein J, Brown M, eds (1983): The metabolic basis of inherited disease. New York: McGraw-Hill.

Tada K, Colombo JP, Desnick RJ, eds (1987): Recent advances in inborn errors in metabolism. Enzyme 38:1.

Daphne A. Roe, M.D.*

19

Interactions of Drugs with Food and Nutrients

Introduction

The drug–nutrient interactions that will be considered are those having direct and/or immediate effects on drug efficacy or safety and those having acute positive or negative effects on nutritional status. All interactions and outcomes of the interactions considered are the results of concurrent drug and nutrient intake or intake in close temporal sequence. Several listings of drug–nutrient interactions have been proposed. Most of these are unsatisfactory, either because the list is incomplete or because the reader is left without means to classify these interactions in an acceptable taxonomic system.

Drug–nutrient interactions can be classified by location (Table 19.1), mechanism (Table 19.2), pharmacologic or nutritional outcomes (Table 19.3), drug group (Table 19.4), nutrient(s) involved (Table 19.5), temporal relationship to food or nutrient ingestion (Table 19.6), patient groups commonly affected (Table 19.7), and risk factors related to regimen (Table 19.8). For each of these classification systems, examples have been given of the type of interaction that occurs. Multiple classification of drug–nutrient interactions is useful in the production of a computerized database; it may be used both as a teaching and research tool and also as a diagnostic tool (Table 19.9).

Biologic scientists and health professionals using drug–nutrient interaction classifications must be reminded that the older definitions separating drugs and nutrients need revision. Nutrients have been defined as chemical agents which, at physiological levels of intake, are necessary to the growth, maintenance, and repair of the body. Recommended intakes of nutrients are those amounts required for optimal health in most people (Passmore et al., 1974). However, intake of certain nutrients at greater than physiologic amounts has been shown to produce pharmacologic effects. For example, the flush reaction, due to niacin, has been known for more than 40 years (Bean and Spies, 1940), and for more than 20 years the hypolipidemic effects of niacin have been utilized in the treatment of familial hyperlipoproteinemia (Yeshurun and Gono, 1976).

The pharmacologic effects of niacin, in turn, are influenced by drug intake. The flush reaction of niacin is abolished by aspirin (Wilkin et al., 1982). However, concurrent intake of niacin with a β-adrenergic blocking agent can cause life-threatening acute hypotension and loss of consciousness due to the peripheral vasodilator effects of the niacin (Roe, 1989).

The hypolipidemic effects of niacin are potentiated by intake of the bile acid sequestrant, colestipol (Illingworth et al., 1981). Therefore, it is apparent that nutrients have druglike properties and that we may be justified at this time in defining overlaps of drug–nutrient, drug–drug, and nutrient–nutrient interactions.

* Division of Nutrition, Cornell University

Table 19.1. Drug–Nutrient Interactions Classified by Site of Occurrence

Interaction site	Interaction/effect	Example
Stomach	(A) Food enhancement of drug dissolution	Fatty food–chlorothiazide
	(B) Drug related reduction of protein digestion	Cimetidine–vitamin B_{12}
Duodenum and jejunum	(A) Food/nutrient enhancement or impairment of drug absorption	Fat–griseofulvin ↑ Food–INH ↓[a]
	(B) Drug impairment of nutrient absorption	Sulfasalazine–folate ↓
Ileum	(A) Selective reduction in nutrient absorption	Biguanides–vitamin B_{12} ↓
Hepatocyte	(A) Food/nutrient enhancement of drug metabolism	Protein–theophylline
	(B) Drug-related enhancement or impairment of nutrient metabolism	Coumarin anticoagulant–vitamin K

[a] INH, isoniazid.

Table 19.2. Classification of Interactions by Mechanisms

Mechanism/ interaction	Example	Effect
Chelation	Calcium–tetracycline	↓ Absorption of both
Adsorption (ionic binding)	Folate–cholestyramine	↓ Folate absorption
Precipitation	Phosphate–aluminum hydroxide	↓ Phosphate absorption
Solubilization	β-carotene–mineral oil	↓ Vitamin absorption
Increased pH	Folate–sodium bicarbonate	↓ Vitamin absorption

Food Effects on Drug Disposition

Until quite recently, we were confident that we could clearly differentiate food effects on drug absorption from food effects on drug metabolism and from food effects on drug excretion. However, increasing knowledge of drug and nutrient disposition and of gastrointestinal physiology has served to blur these distinctions.

Effects of Food and Nutrients in the Diet on Drug Bioavailability

Food, or food components, can influence drug absorption because of physical or chemical interac-

Table 19.3. Grouping of Determinants of Drug–Nutrient Interaction Outcomes by Drug, Diet, and Patient Variables

Drug variables	Diet variables	Patient variables
Chemistry	Macronutrient content/ratio	Age, sex
Physicochemical properties	Micronutrient content	Genetic characteristics
Pharmacologic properties	Nonnutrients present	Physiological status
Formulation	Form	Diet and feeding route
Effect on GI function	Effect on GI function	GI, hepatic, and renal function
Indication	Volume	Diet prescribed
Drug–drug interactions	Cooking method	Social drug use
Dose of each	Mode of administration	Nutrient supplement use
Duration		Nutritional status
Time of administration	Acutal intake	Primary disease
Toxicity	Periods of fasting	Co-morbidity
Plasma level	Change in diet	Pathology
Tissue level	Percent fat	Compliance with regimen
Documentation of Rx changes	Documentation of diet change	Documentation of change in status

Table 19.4. Classification of Drug–Nutrient Interactions by Drug Group and Drug

Drug group	Drug	Nutrient interactions	Effects of reactants: Drugs	Effects of reactants: Nutrients
Antibiotic	Tetracycline	Calcium, magnesium, iron, zinc	If intake within 2 hr of nutrient, absorption reduced	If intake within 2 hr of drug, absorption reduced
Hypolipidemic agents	Colestipol	Folate		Reduced absorption
	Cholestyramine	Vitamins A, D, and K		Reduced absorption
Antacids	Aluminum hydroxide, sodium bicarbonate	Phosphate		Reduced absorption
Laxatives	Mineral oil	β-carotene, vitamins A, D, and K		Reduced absorption
	Phenolphthalein	Fat, calcium		Reduced absorption

Table 19.5. Classification of Drug–Nutrient Interactions by Nutrient

Nutrient	Drugs interacting	Effect on nutrient
Folate	Sodium bicarbonate	↓ Absorption
	Sulfasalazine	↓ Absorption
	Cholestyramine	↓ Absorption
Vitamin A	Cholestyramine	↓ Absorption[a]
	Colestipol	↓ Absorption[a]
	Mineral oil	↓ Absorption

[a] Via bile acid lack.

tions between food and drug or nutrient and drug, or because of physiological changes in the gastrointestinal tract induced by eating or drinking. The net effect may be that drug absorption is reduced, slowed, or increased by food intake. [For reviews, see Welling (1977), Toothaker and Welling (1980), and Melander (1978).] Tables 19.10 and 19.11 list the drugs commonly used for which absorption is significantly altered by food. These same tables also indicate the mechanism whereby effects of food on drug absorption are initiated. When the effect of food on drug absorption is related to interactions between the food and the drug in the gastrointestinal tract, the practical importance of the effect of food on drug absorption is related to the timing of drug intake in relation to eating times (Table 19.6). When the drug is taken at times other than when there is food or food residue in the gastrointestinal tract, interactions will not be observed. Food in the stomach can decrease the rate of drug dissolution. Food can also increase the viscosity of the gastric medium, thereby decreasing the rate of drug diffusion to the mucosal absorption sites, an effect that may slow absorption of aspirin. Food can also

Table 19.6. Drug–Nutrient Interactions Classified by Temporal Relationship of Outcome to Event

Interaction	Example (see text)	Effect	Time to outcome[a]: Days	Hours	Minutes
Food effect on drug bioavailability	Tetracycline–milk (= calcium)	↓ Drug bioavailability		1–3	
Food effect on drug metabolism	Zoxazolamine–flavone	↑ Drug catabolism			<5
	Theophylline–protein	↑ Drug catabolism	≥5		
Drug effect on nutrient availability	Sodium bicarbonate–folic acid	↓ Folate bioavailability		1–2	
	Cholestyramine–folic acid	↓ Folate bioavailability	≥5		

[a] Time between intake of drug and nutrient during which significant effect is observed.

Table 19.7. Drug–Nutrient Interactions, Classified by Patient Groups Affected

Patient group	Drugs	Interactions and outcomes
Arthritic	Aspirin	Decreased folate levels
	Penicillamine	Zinc depletion → taste loss
	NSAIDs	Ulcerogenic effect → iron deficiency anemia
Asthmatic	Theophylline	High fat intake → rapid uptake → acute toxicity High protein intake → rapid Rx metabolism loss of drug effect
Cardiac	Digoxin + furosemide	Potassium depletion → digoxin toxicity
Diabetic	Chlorpropamide	Alcohol ingestion → flush reaction
Epileptic	Phenytoin	High folate intake → seizure recurrence Impaired vitamin D metabolism → rickets
GI (colitis)	Sulfasalazine	Antifolate effect of Rx → megaloblastic anemia
Hypertensive	Thiazides	Potassium depletion → hyperglycemia
Psychotic (manic)	Lithium	Low sodium intake → drug toxicity High sodium intake → loss of drug effect
Tuberculous	Isoniazid	Vitamin B_6 deficiency → neuropathy

alter gastric pH, which can influence the rate of drug dissolution, which in turn affects drug absorption rate.

Fiber components in the diet can adsorb drugs, therefore reducing the amount available for absorption. Mineral components in the diet, including calcium, magnesium, and iron, can form insoluble chelates of drugs, such as the tetracyclines (Table 19.4) (Gibaldi, 1977).

It has been frequently pointed out, and also frequently ignored, that the absorption of *penicillins* and *tetracyclines* is much more efficient when these drugs are taken in the fasting state (Table 19.8). Optimum drug levels for therapeutic efficacy of conventional penicillins are obtained only when these drugs are administered "on an empty stomach." In the case of tetracyclines, food can be taken at the time of drug intake, provided the food does not include dairy products containing calcium or foods high in magnesium or iron. It is generally recommended that tetracyclines be taken at least 2 hr before or after intake of milk, other dairy products, or protein foods. In order to avoid formation of tetracycline-mineral chelates, it is preferable that the patient abstain from all food (other than rusks or crackers) at the time of drug intake.

In a study of 132 hospitals in New York City, conducted by Petrick and Kleinmann (1975), it was shown that there was a wide variety in drug administration schedules and that these often coincided with meal-serving times. Because drug administration times in hospitals are largely set by the pharmacy or therapeutics committee, and mealtimes are decided by the dietitian, it would seem that greater cooperation between these groups is required.

Drug *formulation* influences the rate and extent of drug absorption (Weinberger et al., 1978). Food may differentially affect the absorption of different formulations of a single drug. In circumstances where food delays dissolution of solid drug products, drug absorption will also be delayed. Toothaker and Welling (1980) suggest that there has been a rather general belief that suspensions and solutions of drugs are usually less af-

Table 19.8. Drug–Nutrient Interactions Classified by Risk Factors

Risk factor	Interaction	Example
Food-related		
Change of mealtime Drug fasting[a] Drug with food	Promotion or reduction of drug absorption	Tetracycline absorption ↓ (due to milk)
Change of diet from low protein to high protein	Increase in rate of drug metabolism	Theophylline metabolism ↑ (high protein intake)
Formula diet Liquid nutrition formula administered	Inhibition of drug effect	Warfarin anticoagulant effect ↓ (vitamin K in formula)
Drug-related		
Drug excess Laxative abuse	Reduction in nutrient absorption	Reduction in absorption of β-carotene by mineral oil
Intentional nutrient antagonism	Drug inhibition of nutrient metabolism	Methotrexate inhibition of folate metabolism and function

[a] Drug taken in the fasting state.

fected by the action of food than other dosage forms. However, when phenytoin suspension is administered during continuous nasogastric feeding, serum concentrations of the drug are markedly reduced (Bauer, 1982).

Bogentoft et al. (1978) compared the effect of food on the absorption of enteric-coated *aspirin* tablets versus enteric-coated aspirin granules that were encapsulated. Plasma salicylate levels from the two formations were similar under conditions of fasting. However, food differentially affected the absorption of the two formulations. It appeared not to influence absorption from the granules, while absorption from the aspirin tablets was both decreased and delayed by food intake. There are very marked differences in the effects of food on the absorption of the drug, theophylline, which are dependent on the formulation of the drug (Jonkman, 1989). High fat meals, eaten with certain ultra-slow-releasing theophylline formations, can cause "dose dumping," with a rapid increase in plasma levels of the drug and signs of acute drug toxicity (Hendeles et al., 1985).

Several food-related changes in *gastrointestinal function* that also affect drug absorption include change in stomach-emptying time, change in intestinal motility, change in splanchnic blood flow, change in the bile secretion, as well as in gastric acid secretion, and digestive enzyme secretion. Whereas, in the past, it was accepted that slowing of gastric-emptying time would delay drug absorption, it is now known that the effects of change in stomach-emptying time on drug absorption varies with the drug. Drugs that have very low water solubility are better absorbed when they remain longer in the stomach, as they will after a meal, particularly a large meal, a hot meal, or a high-fat meal. Water-insoluble drugs, such as spironolactone and griseofulvin, are better absorbed when taken directly after a meal. However, absorption of these water-insoluble drugs, and also carbamazepine and nitrofurantoin, is improved when the manufacturer increases the rate of dissolution of tablets by reducing particle size as well as when the product is taken after a meal that allows longer residence of the tablet in the stomach, allowing greater time for dissolution.

Complex Food Effects on Drug Bioavailability

There are a number of drugs for which the effects of food on absorption may be complex. In the case of spironolactone, food promotes disintegration

Table 19.9. Multiple Classification of Drug–Nutrient Interactions by Problem, Drug, or Risk Factor, with Diagnostic Application

Problem	Drug	Nutrient	Risk factor	Drug–nutrient interaction diagnosis
Drug ineffective	Tetracycline	Calcium	High/frequent milk intake	↓ Drug absorption (via chelation)
	Theophylline	Protein	Change to high protein intake	↑ Drug catabolism
Nutrient deficiency		Folate	Antacid abuse	↓ Nutrient absorption
		Folate	Phenytoin	↑ Nutrient metabolism

Table 19.10. Drugs in Common Use for Which Bioavailability Is Reduced or Slowed by Food

Drug	Proposed mechanism of food effect
Penicillin V	Gastric pH ↑
Tetracycline	Mineral chelate formation
Aspirin	Delayed drug diffusion to absorption site
Rifampin	Gastric pH ↑
Isoniazid	Delayed gastric emptying time Nutrient interaction
Methyldopa	Competitive absorption with dietary amino acids

of tablets and improved dissolution of the compound. The possibility has been suggested that the solubility of *spironolactone* also is improved by contact with bile salts released in response to food. Spironolactone undergoes rapid first-pass metabolism in the intestinal mucosa and is converted to canrenone, which is then absorbed into the body. It has been demonstrated that the absorption of canrenone is enhanced when the drug is taken after food (Melander et al., 1977*b*).

Drugs may interact with food components. The food may induce a physiologic change in gastrointestinal function that then facilitates, retards, or impairs drug absorption. These effects may be interactive or additive. For example, it is known that ingestion of food reduces the absorption of *isoniazid*, and this has been explained as being due to a food-related slowing in gastric emptying so that there is a delay in the entry of the drug into the small intestine from which it is optimally absorbed. An alternate explanation of the impairment of isoniazid absorption by food is that the drug interacts with a food substance (Melander et al., 1976). Isoniazid may form Schiff bases with vitamin B_6, although the interaction of the B_6 vitamins with isoniazid is generally considered to occur after absorption (Chin et al., 1978).

In the case of the antihypertensive drug, *methyldopa*, there are also multiple food effects on bioavailability. The drug is a modified neutral amino acid and, as such, is competitively absorbed with dietary amino acids. Stenback et al. (1982) studied the influence of a liquid amino acid mixture and a meal of beef on the rate and extent of the bioavailability of methyldopa in normal volunteers who were given 500 mg of the drug orally. The "absorption" of the unconjugated drug was reduced when the amino acid-containing solution was given and, also, to a great extent, when the subjects ate a beef meal. The pharmacokinetic data obtained showed that the protein-rich meal reduced both the rate and extent of the bioavailability of methyldopa.

Decreased absorption of methyldopa after food may also be explained in part by an increase in "first-pass" metabolism. Methyldopa is extensively sulfoconjugated in the intestinal mucosa (Kwan et al., 1976). It is likely that the formation of sulfoconjugates is dependent on the level of sulfur-containing amino acids in the diet. However, it is not clear at present whether food per se can alter the rate or quantity of sulfoconjugates formed (Myhre et al., 1982).

Multifactorial effects of food on drug absorption have also been considered in relation to the β-blocker drugs, *propranolol* and *metoprolol*. Both of these drugs are better absorbed after food. This has been generally explained as being due to the food-related increase in splanchnic blood flow, together with reduced first-pass metabolism of these drugs either in the intestinal mucosa or in the liver (McLean et al., 1981; Melander et al., 1977*a*).

Table 19.11. Drugs in Common Use for Which Bioavailability Is Enhanced by Food

Drug	Mechanism of food effect
Chlorothiazide Hydrochlorothiazide	Slowed gastric emptying; improved efficiency of intestinal absorption
Hydralazine Propranolol Metoprolol Spironolactone	Increased splanchnic blood flow decreases first-pass metabolism
Griseofulvin Carbamazepine Nitrofurantoin	Food, fat, and bile promote dissolution (and therefore absorption)

Effects of Nutrient Supplements and Substitutes on Drug and Vitamin Absorption

Nutrient supplements can reduce drug absorption. For example, iron supplements such as *ferrous sulfate* tablets, taken with the anti-Parkinson's disease drug, levodopa or levodopa-carbidopa combinations, markedly reduces the absorption of these drugs (Campbell and Hasinoff, 1989). Ferrous sulfate also has been found to reduce the absorption of methyldopa (Campbell et al., 1988).

Mineral supplements can alter the rate or the amount of absorption of therapeutic doses of vitamins. For example, *calcium supplements* taken to retard the progress of osteoporosis can reduce the absorption of therapeutic doses of iron salts (Roe, 1989), and can also reduce the absorption of tetracycline, as when tetracycline is taken with a dairy product that is a rich calcium source. On the other hand, calcium carbonate supplements taken with folic acid supplements do not reduce the absorption of this vitamin as might have been predicted from earlier work with another antacid, sodium bicarbonate (see below).

Folic acid absorption is promoted by glucose (Isak et al., 1972). When folic acid absorption in the human jejunum was measured using tritiated pteroylmonoglutamic acid in a triple lumen perfusion system, it was shown that the addition of glucose to the perfusate caused a marked increase in folic acid absorption, as well as an increase in sodium and water absorption (Gerson et al., 1971). It is suggested by the authors that the effect of glucose is on the passive absorption of folic acid, though they also indicate that their data do not exclude the possibility of an enhancement of active transport. It has also been shown that a glucose polymer (Polycose; Ross Laboratories) enhances the rate of intestinal uptake of folic acid, but does not cause a net increase in folic acid absorption into the blood (Belko et al., 1982).

Caloric diluents (noncaloric macronutrient substitutes) added to the food supply have the potential to alter the absorption of nutrients and drugs. For example, sucrose polyester (Olestra; Procter and Gamble), a fatlike material that has been shown to reduce the absorption of certain fat-soluble vitamins, including vitamin E, does not significantly affect the absorption of a number of lipid-soluble drugs, including propranolol, diazepam, norethindrone, and ethinyl estradiol (Glueck et al., 1983; Roberts and Lef, 1989).

Comparison of Physiological and Pharmacological Factors Affecting Vitamin Absorption

Certain antacids increase intraluminal pH with disturbance of the acid microclimate at the brush border. Decreased absorption of folic acid following administration of sodium bicarbonate was first demonstrated by Benn et al. (1971). By 1976, MacKenzie and Russell, using a triple lumen intestinal infusion technique with tritiated folic acid, found that folic acid absorption was impaired with elevation of the pH of the jejunum. This was later ascribed to decreased hydrolysis of polyglutamates and interference with the transport of pteroylmonoglutamic acid (Halsted, 1980). Impairment of folic acid absorption with change in intrajejunal pH occurred both in normal subjects and in patients with celiac disease (Benn et al., 1971). Evidence has been obtained from these studies that sodium bicarbonate can impair folic acid absorption. Up to the present, however, there has been no clinical proof that folate deficiency with or without an anemia is attributable to antacid usage. To the contrary, calcium carbonate given in amounts of 500 mg or larger doses increases the rate of absorption of folic acid supplements because the dissolution of the folic acid is more rapid when this calcium supplement is in the stomach (Faulkner and Roe, 1989).

Newer semisynthetic carbohydrate sources, such as the oligosaccharide mixture, Polycose (Ross), can affect vitamin absorption. It has long been known that at physiologic levels of intake, food folacins are absorbed by an active transport mechanism, absorption being possible in all segments of the small intestine, but maximal in the jejunum. Gamma glutamylcarboxypeptidase (conjugase), which hydrolyzes the polyglutamate tail from the folacins, has been shown to be present in the small intestinal mucosa and in other tissues (Baugh et al., 1975). Rosenberg et al. (1969) studied the absorption of polyglutamic folacin using everted gut sac preparations and showed that in the process of absorption, intestinal conjugase is necessary to produce smaller folacin peptides which are preferentially absorbed.

When pharmacologic doses of folic acid are administered, folic acid appears in the plasma (Chapman et al., 1978). However, when physiologic levels of folic acid or other folacins are ingested, reduction and methylation occur in the intestinal mucosa, and the major circulating form of folacin is 5-methyltetrahydrofolate (see Chapter 5) (Whitehead et al., 1972).

Riboflavin sources include conventional foods, defined formulae, vitamin or other supplements, and, to a very modest extent, alcoholic beverages, including beers (see Chapter 5). In the U.S. diet, the major sources of riboflavin are milk, cheese, yogurt, and enriched breads and cereals. Other rich sources of riboflavin include liver and yeast. Meat, eggs, and green vegetables contribute to the total daily riboflavin intake. Riboflavin is present in conventional foods, both as protein complexes of the flavin coenzymes, flavin mononucleotide (FMN), and flavin adenine dinucleotide (FAD), and also as free riboflavin or free FMN. Small amounts of flavin peptides are also ingested. In infant formulas and other defined formula diets of monomeric or polymeric types (amino acids/sugars versus proteins, dextrins), riboflavin is present as the free vitamin, except when the formula is prepared for parenteral alimentation, in which case riboflavin is present as FMN (see Chapter 14). In oral vitamin supplements, whether formulated as tablets or liquid preparations, riboflavin is present as free riboflavin; however, in injectable vitamin preparations, FMN is used. Small amounts of riboflavin are present in wines and beers. Riboflavin is absorbed from a saturable site in the proximal small intestine. All riboflavin that is absorbed from the intestine is in the form of the free vitamin. Conversion to FMN and FAD to free riboflavin occurs in the small intestine.

Factors that influence the absorption of pharmacologic doses of riboflavin include the form of the vitamin, the dose, the formulation, the vehicle used, and whether or not the vitamin is taken with food or a phosphate-containing beverage. Stomach-emptying time, gut motility, and gastrointestinal exocrine secretions influence riboflavin absorption, and food- or beverage-related effects on riboflavin uptake are explained by physiologic effects of those GI functions.

When encapsulated forms of riboflavin are administered, efficiency of absorption is dependent on the diluent used for the vitamin. Stewart et al. (1979) showed that riboflavin absorption was greater if the diluent in the capsule was lactose rather than kaolin.

Middleton et al. (1964) demonstrated that tablet disintegration time had a marked effect on the availability of the vitamin. Preparations that have a very slow disintegration time are poorly absorbed.

Factors known to increase the absorption of riboflavin include the form of the vitamin, such that FMN is better absorbed than free riboflavin, which is better absorbed than FAD. Solutions of the vitamin are better absorbed than solid preparations, though this formulation factor mainly affects the rate of absorption, in that solutions are absorbed more rapidly than solid vitamin products (Levy and Jusko, 1966).

Efficient absorption of vitamin B_{12} requires normal gastric functioning, including synthesis and release of hydrochloric acid and pepsin, as well as production of gastric intrinsic factor (GIF), intact pancreatic exocrine function, adequate binding of the B_{12}–GIF complex to the ileal absorption site, and synthesis of transcobalamin II, which is necessary for the initial transport of vitamin B_{12} as it leaves the epithelial cells of the ileum (see Chapter 5) (Toskes and Deren, 1973).

Okuda et al. (1960) investigated the effects of nonionic surfactants on the absorption of vitamin B_{12}. They found that polysorbate 80, polysorbate 85 (polyoxyethylene sorbitan trioleate), and G1096 (polyoxyethylene sorbital hexaoleate) promoted vitamin B_{12} absorption. It was postulated that this was due to the formation of a very viscous mass in the gastric and intestinal lumen that delayed gastric emptying and, therefore, enhanced the absorption of the vitamin. Polyoxyethylene sorbitans are used as food emulsifiers (Taylor, 1980).

Effects of Drugs on Vitamin Absorption

Drugs can promote vitamin absorption. It has also long been known that the chronic administration of particular drugs can result in syndromes of drug-induced malabsorption. The present discussion is concerned with the outcomes of concurrent intakes of drugs and nutrients, and focuses on effects of drugs and food chemicals on the absorption of selected vitamins. Effects of drugs and food chemicals on vitamin absorption can be the outcome of direct interactions or of changes in gastrointestinal function, including motility and secretion, or changes in the transport of the vitamins across the gastrointestinal mucosa. The effects of these factors on absorption of three vitamins are summarized in Table 19.12.

Adverse effects of drugs on vitamin absorption of clinical importance include those induced by drugs that are toxic to enterocytes (e.g., methotrexate, colchicine, and neomycin), as well as those induced by drugs that interact physicochemically with nutrients in the gut. Whether or not an adverse effect is produced by the drug-induced malabsorption relative to impairment of nutritional status depends on the dose of the drug and also, very importantly, on the duration of drug administration. Other factors influencing outcome include the patient's health problems for which the drug is prescribed.

Sulfasalazine, which has been extensively used in the treatment of inflammatory bowel disease, including regional enteritis and ulcerative colitis, has been shown to cause folate malabsorption (Franklin and Rosenberg, 1973). It has further been demonstrated in rats that the inhibitory effect of sulfasalazine on the intestinal transport of

Table 19.12. Factors Influencing the Absorption of Pharmacologic Doses of Vitamins

Vitamin	Factor promoting absorption	Factor reducing absorption
Folic acid	Glucose Glucose polymer (rate only)	Sodium bicarbonate Sulfasalazine Cholestyramine
Riboflavin	Food, fiber, phosphate, glucose polymer, lactose, colas, propantheline bromide	Kaolin
Vitamin B_{12}	Nonionic surfactants, e.g., polyoxyethylene sorbitans	Cimetidine Cholestyramine Biguanides Neomycin, colchicine

folic acid may be explained by inhibition of intestinal folate enzymes (Selhub et al., 1978). Three enzymes required in the interconversion of folacins—namely, dihydrofolate reductase, serine transhydroxymethylase, and methylene tetrahydrofolate reductase (Figure 19.1)—are competitively inhibited by the same concentration of sulfasalazine that inhibits the intestinal transport of folic acid.

Severe folacin deficiency with megaloblastic anemia has rarely been attributed to sulfasalazine. Schneider and Beeley (1977) described a case of megaloblastic anemia associated with sulfasalazine treatment in a patient who had only received the drug for a short period of time (5 months). When the drug was discontinued and he was treated with folic acid, he promptly recovered from the anemia. In a study by Swenson et al. (1981), it was shown that patients with inflammatory bowel disease, who developed anemia or megaloblastosis while receiving sulfasalazine, all had other medical reasons for the development of folate deficiency. These included celiac disease, severe dietary deficiency of folacins, and hemolysis.

As cholestyramine (a nonabsorbable, ion-exchange resin that binds bile acids) can produce a moderate but sustained lowering of serum cholesterol in children and adults with familial type-II hyperlipoproteinemia, without serious side effects, it is recommended in long-term management of this disease. However, cholestyramine does cause moderate folacin depletion over time, apparently because the vitamin is adsorbed onto

Figure 19.1. Metabolic reactions in interconversion of folacins. Numbers and subscripts indicate sites of enzyme inhibition by sulfasalazine. Key: 1, dihydrofolate reductase; 2, 5,10-methylene tetrahydrofolate dehydrogenase; 3, serine hydroxymethylase. [*Source:* Modified from Stockstead and Koch (1967).]

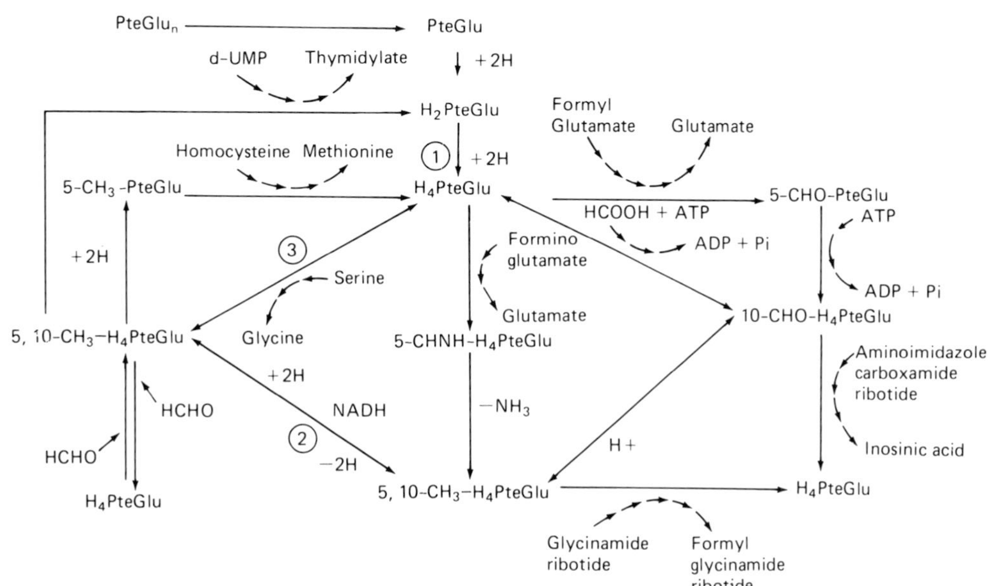

this bile acid sequestrant within the gut lumen (West and Lloyd, 1975).

Riboflavin absorption is promoted by concurrent intake of specific drugs. A cola-type product used for its antiemetic effects, and containing sugar and phosphoric acid, has been shown to enhance the absorption of pharmacologic quantities of riboflavin, as reflected by changes in the urinary excretion of the load dose of this vitamin. In these studies (Brian-Houston and Levy, 1975), riboflavin was administered as FMN (riboflavin 5′-phosphate) in water.

Absorption of riboflavin as FMN is prolonged and increased by the anticholinergic drug, propantheline bromide, which slows gastric emptying (Levy et al., 1972). Absorption of the vitamin is also enhanced by a glucose polymer (Roe, 1981), which retards dissolution of riboflavin and slows gastric emptying.

In theory, vitamin B_{12} malabsorption could be due to interference with any of the functions necessary for efficient absorption of the vitamin. Concurrent drug-induced malabsorption may be due to drug-induced inhibition of gastric secretions or to drug-induced reduction in the binding of the B_{12}-GIF complex to the ileal absorption site.

It has been shown that cimetidine reduces the absorption of food-bound (protein-bound) vitamin B_{12}. It has been proposed that this is due to combined inhibitory effects of this drug on secretion of gastric intrinsic factor and gastric acid (McGuigan, 1980; Okuda et al., 1960).

Cholestyramine (the bile acid-absorbing resin) has been shown to reduce vitamin B_{12} absorption. In vitro studies have indicated that cholestyramine decreases the uptake of vitamin B_{12} by binding sites on the intrinsic factor molecule, which normally bind vitamin B_{12}. Coronato and Jerzy Glass (1973), who carried out this investigation, questioned whether cholestyramine can deplete vitamin B_{12} stores; they suggested that vitamin B_{12} deficiency would only be likely to occur if an individual with depleted vitamin B_{12} stores were to take cholestyramine on a long-term and regular dosage schedule. It should be added that the at-risk individual would ingest cholestyramine concurrently with a single marginal source of vitamin B_{12}.

Biguanides, such as metformin and phenformin, which were once used in the treatment of insulin-independent diabetes, were shown to induce vitamin B_{12} malabsorption (Berchtold et al., 1969; Tomkin et al., 1971). It was proposed that biguanide-induced malabsorption of vitamin B_{12} could be due to competitive inhibition of vitamin absorption in the distal ileum or to drug inactivation of vitamin B_{12}. However, it is perhaps of etiologic significance that, when rats were given biguanide, only those animals also rendered diabetic by administration of alloxan developed chemical evidence of vitamin B_{12} depletion (D.A. Roe, unpublished observations). Alloxan-induced diabetes is associated with impairment of pancreatic exocrine function, which, as previously indicated, adversely affects vitamin B_{12} absorption.

Vitamin B_{12} malabsorption can also be chemically induced by drugs, such as neomycin and colchicine, which cause ileal mucosal damage and may thereby interfere with binding of the GIF–B_{12} complex (Corcino et al., 1970; Race et al., 1970).

Effects of Diet on Drug Metabolism

The liver has been long considered as the main site for metabolism of foreign and endogenous substances. It is now known that there is extensive intestinal drug metabolism, with involvement of mucosal enzymes as well as the intestinal microflora (George, 1981; Hartiala, 1973). The metabolism of environmental chemicals, including therapeutic drugs, and of endogenous chemicals, such as steroids and indoles, is primarily by the microsomal mixed-function oxidase system and also by the conjugating system present within the cell cytosol. The mixed-function oxidase system catalyzes oxidative reactions (phase I reactions) by electron transfer systems in which cytochrome P-450 is the terminal oxidase (Figure 19.2). In conjugating systems, drugs or their oxidized metabolites are converted to glucuronides, ester sulfates, glutathione conjugates, or other conjugates (phase II reactions) (Figure 19.3). Reactions of phase I and II both occur in the liver and in the intestinal mucosa.

Table 19.13. Diet Effects on Drug Metabolism by Mixed Function Oxidase and Conjugation Systems (Liver and Intestine)

Rate increased	Rate decreased
High protein	High carbohydrate
Flavones	
Indoles	
Charcoal broiling	
Sulfur-containing amino acids	

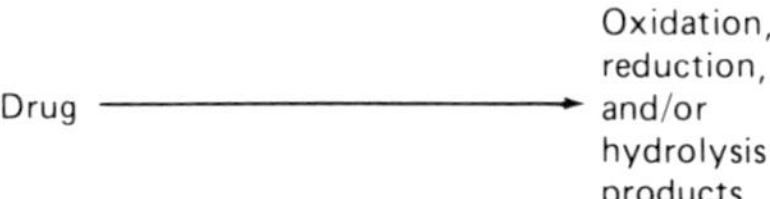

Figure 19.2. Phase 1 metabolism of drugs.

It has already been pointed out that food effects on drug bioavailability may be explained in part by quantitative changes in their availability due to metabolism in the intestinal mucosa or the liver. Dietary factors can influence the rate of drug metabolism, as well as the metabolites produced (Table 19.13). Effects of diet as well as nutritional status on hepatic drug metabolism have been reviewed by Anderson et al. (1982).

Clinical observations have been made of definitive feeding studies carried out to examine the effects of changing macronutrient ratios in the diet on the rate of metabolism of the model drugs *theophylline* and *antipyrine*. A study of hospitalized children with asthma (Feldman et al., 1980) has shown that the rate of theophylline catabolism is increased when a high protein diet is fed, as contrasted to the rate of catabolism of this drug when a high carbohydrate diet is fed. This study was of clinical importance in that it was noted that asthmatic episodes were less frequent when the children were receiving a high carbohydrate, low protein diet (associated with maintenance of therapeutic levels of theophylline in the plasma).

In a study by Anderson et al. (1979), young, healthy, male volunteers were given antipyrine or theophylline during the sequential feeding of high carbohydrate, high fat, or high protein diets. It was shown that rate of drug elimination (as measured by plasma half-life) was slowest when the high carbohydrate diet was fed and fastest during the high protein period. When the high fat diet was fed, there was a small decrease in the rate of antipyrine loss but not with theophylline. However, because of the design of these studies, it is not possible to identify how soon the "protein effect" became manifest after change of diet.

Figure 19.3. Phase 2 metabolism of drugs.

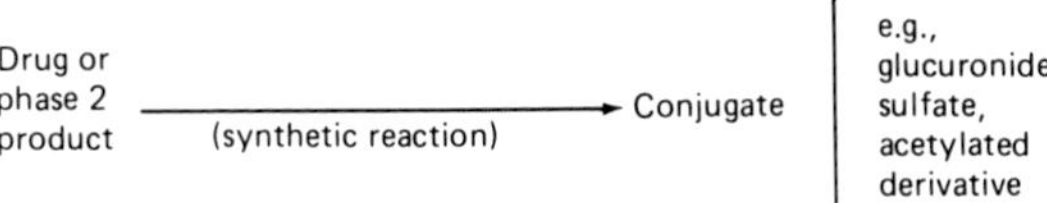

Natural, nonnutrient components of the diet may exert a profound influence on the rate of drug metabolism, and these effects may occur rapidly after food ingestion. Indolic compounds in vegetables of the brassica family, including cabbage and brussels sprouts, stimulate the rate of human drug metabolism (Pantuck et al., 1979).

The effects of these nonnutrient dietary substances on the rate of drug metabolism may be extremely rapid. Lasker et al. (1982) reported that the metabolism of *zoxazolamine* to 6-hydroxyzoxazolamine by liver microsomes from neonatal rats can be stimulated sevenfold by the in vitro addition of a flavone. Flavones (bioflavonoids) are naturally occurring compounds present in citrus and other fruits (see Chapter 5). Laker's group demonstrated clearly that the in vitro metabolism of zoxazolamine is immediately and markedly increased by the concurrent administration of such a substance.

Inhibition of drug metabolism can be brought about by administration of pharmacologic doses of nutrients. Cases have been reported of previously unexplained resistance to coumarin anticoagulants, which were subsequently found to be due to intake of vitamin K in liquid nutritional formulae (Table 19.8) (Lader et al., 1980; Lee et al., 1981). Although some liquid nutrition preparations contain only trace amounts of vitamin K, others contain large amounts, which may interfere with the desired anticoagulant activity of such drugs as warfarin.

However, when megadoses of vitamin E are ingested by patients receiving moderate doses of warfarin to maintain vitamin-K-dependent coagulation factors in a certain range, vitamin E may further depress the levels of these factors, with subsequent hemorrhage (Corrigan and Marcus, 1974). Vitamin E has also been shown to decrease prothrombin levels in mildly vitamin-K-deficient and warfarin-treated rats (Corrigan and Ullers, 1981; Olson and Jones, 1979).

Woolley (1982) showed that DL-α-tocopherolquinone (a metabolite of DL-α-tocopheral) caused hemorrhage and fetal loss in pregnant mice, and Bettger and Olson (1982) found that α-tocopherolquinone inhibits vitamin-K-dependent carboxylase in vitro.

Hence, there is evidence that vitamin E in pharmacologic doses acts as a vitamin K antagonist, although the antagonism of large doses of vitamin E to vitamin K is usually masked by high intake of vitamin K, and is only unmasked when coumarin anticoagulants are administered (Editorial, 1982).

Conclusions

In reviewing drug–nutrient interactions that have direct and immediate effects on drug availability, efficacy, and safety, as well as interactions in which there are adverse outcomes on nutritional status, the theme has been that of predictability. There is now a strong body of evidence which, with knowledge of nutritional physiology and pharmacology, makes it possible to predict and prevent drug–nutrient interactions that adversely affect the intended function of drugs, and vice versa.

Our further investigative responsibility pertains to definition of the precise temporal sequences of drug and food intake that must be avoided when drug–nutrient interactions are unwanted, or must be obtained when drug–nutrient interactions are desirable. Some generalization about concurrent drug–nutrient interactions is permissible. In the situation where a drug's availability is dependent on whether it is taken in the fasting or fed state, the magnitude of the difference must be considered and whether drug efficacy (at the intended dose) is substantially reduced by food. In the interest of safety, efficacy, and patient compliance, it is important that the patient be instructed to take the medication according to a consistent regimen in relation to meals and that favorable food effects on bioavailability be optimized.

As far as possible, the patient's diet should not be changed, especially not from high to low protein or vice versa, when drugs such as theophylline have been prescribed. If the diet is changed, plasma levels of the drug should be monitored. When therapeutic needs dictate prescription of drugs that impair the absorption of vitamins taken concurrently, patient and nurse instruction should be to avoid drug administration at food times. Monitoring of vitamin status (using functional tests) is most desirable, but, above all, it is the physician's responsibility to recognize that avoidance of drug-induced nutritional deficiencies can best be achieved by ensuring that patients receive a daily nutrient intake commensurate with their physiologic and pharmacologic needs.

References

Anderson KE, Conney AH, Kappas A (1982): Nutr Rev 40:161.

Anderson KE, Conney AH, Kappas AA (1979): Clin Pharmacol Ther 26:493.

Bauer LA (1982): Neurol 32:570.

Baugh CM, Krimdieck CL, Baker HJ, Butterworth CE (1975): J Nutr 105:80.

Bean WB, Spies TD (1940): Am Heart J 20:62.

Belko A, Rotter M, Roe DA (1982): J Am Coll Nutr 1:413.

Benn A, Swan CH, Cooke WT, Blair JA, Matte AJ, Smith ME (1971): Br Med J 1:148.

Berchtold P, Bolli P, Arbenz U, Keiser G (1969): Diabetologica 5:405.

Bettger WJ, Olson RE (1982): Fed Proc 41:344.

Bogentoft C, Carlsson J, Ekenved B, Magnusson A (1978): Eur J Clin Pharmacol 14:351.

Brian-Houston J, Levy G (1975): J Pharmacol Sci 64:1504.

Campbell NRC, Hasinoff B (1989): Clin Pharmacol Ther 45:220.

Campbell NRC, Paddock V, Sundaram RS (1988): Clin Pharmacol Ther 43:381.

Chapman SK, Greene BC, Streiff RR (1978): J Chromatogr 145:302.

Chin L, Sievers ML, Laird HE, Herrier RN, Picchioni AL (1978): Toxicol Appl Pharmacol 45:713.

Corcino JJ, Waxman S, Herbert V (1970): Am J Med 48:562.

Coronato A, Jerzy Glass GB (1973): Prog Soc Exp Biol Med 142:1341.

Corrigan J, Marcus FI (1974): JAMA 230:1300.

Corrigan JJ, Ullers LL (1981): Am J Clin Nutr 34:1701.

Editorial (1982): Nutr Rev 40:180.

Faulkner D, Roe DA (1989): FASEB J 3:A727.

Feldman CH, Hutchinson VE, Pippenger CE, Blumenfeld TA, Feldman BR, Davis WJ (1980): Pediatrics 66:956.

Franklin JL, Rosenberg IH (1973): Gastroenterology 64:517.

George CF (1981): Clin Pharmacokinet 6:259.

Gerson CD, Cohen N, Hepner GW, Brown N, Herbert V, Janowitz HD (1971): Gastroenterology 61:224.

Gibaldi M (1977): Biopharmaceutics and clinical pharmacokinetics (2nd ed). Philadelphia: Lea & Febiger, p 15.

Glueck CJ, Jandacek RJ, Hogg E, et al. (1983): Am J Clin Nutr 37:347.

Halsted CH (1980): Annu Rev Med 1:79.

Hartiala K (1973): Physiol Rev 53:496.

Hendeles L, Weinberger M, Milavitz G, Hill M, Vaughan L (1985): Chest 87:758.

Illingworth DRR, Phillipson BE, Rapp JH, Connor WE (1981): Lancet 1:296.

Isak G, Galewski K, Rachmilewitz M, Grossowicz N (1972): Proc Soc Exp Biol Med 140:248.

Jonkman JHG (1989): Clin Pharmacokinet 16:162.

Kwan KC, Foltz EL, Breault GO, Baer JR, Totaro JA (1976): J Pharmacol Exp Ther 198:264.

Lader E, Yang L, Clarke A (1980): Ann Intern Med 93:373.

Lasker JM, Huang M-T, Conney AH (1982): Science 216:1419.

Lee M, Schwartz RN, Sharifi R (1981): Ann Intern Med 94:140.

Levy G, Jusko W (1966): J Pharmacol Sci 55:285.

Levy G, Gibaldi M, Procknal JA (1972): J Pharmacol Sci 61:798.

MacKenzie JF, Russell RL (1976): Clin Sci Mol Med 51:363.

McGuigan JE (1980): Gastroenterology 80:181.

McLean AJ, Isbister C, Bobik A, Dudley FJ (1981): Clin Pharmacol Ther 30:31.

Melander A (1978): Clin Pharmacokinet 3:337.

Melander A, Danielson K, Schersten B, Wahlin E (1977*a*): Clin Pharmacol Ther 22:108.

Melander A, Danielson K, Schersten B, Thulin T, Wahlin E (1977*b*): Clin Pharmacol Ther 22:100.

Melander A, Danielson K, Hanson A, Jansson L, Rerup C, Schersten B, Thulin T, Wahlin E (1976): Acta Med Scand 200:93.

Middleton EJ, Davies JM, Morrison AB (1964): J Pharmacol Sci 53:1378.

Myhre L, Rugstad HE, Hansen T (1982): Clin Pharmacokinet 7:221.

Olson RE, Jones JP (1979): Fed Proc 38:2542.

Okuda K, Duran EW, Chow BF (1960): Proc Soc Exp Biol Med 103:588.

Pantuck EJ, Pantuck CB, Garland WA, Min BH, Wattenberg LW, Anderson KE, Kappas A, Conney AH (1979): Clin Pharmacol Ther 25:88.

Passmore R, Nichol BM, Narayana Rao M (1974): Handbook of nutritional requirements. Monograph series no 61. Geneva: WHO.

Petrick RJ, Kleinmann K (1975): Am J Hosp Pharmacol 32:1008.

Race TF, Paes IC, Faloon WW (1970): Am J Med Sci 259:32.

Roberts RJ, Lef RD (1989): Clin Pharmacol Ther 45:299.

Roe DA (1981): *In* Harper AE, Davis JK, eds: Nutrition in health and disease and international development (Symposium XII international congress on nutrition). New York: Alan R. Liss, p 757.

Roe DA (1989): Diet and drug interactions. New York: Van Nostrand Reinhold, p 90 or 125.

Rosenberg IH, Streiff RR, Godwin HA, Castle WB (1969): N Engl J Med 280:985.

Schneider RE, Beeley L (1977): Br Med J 1:1638.

Selhub J, Dhar GJ, Rosenberg IH (1978): J Clin Invest 61:221.

Stenback O, Myhre L, Rugstad HE, Arnold E, Hansen T (1982): Acta Pharmacol Toxicol 50:225.

Stewart AG, Grant DJW, Newton JM (1979): J Pharm Pharmacol 31:1.

Stockstead ELR, Koch J (1967): Physiol Rev 47:83.

Swenson CM, Perry J, Lumb M, Levi AJ (1981): Gut 22:456.

Taylor RJ (1980): Food additives. New York: Wiley, p 24.

Tomkin GH (1973): Br Med J 3:673.

Tomkin GH, Hadden DR, Weaver JA, Montgomery DAD (1971): Br Med J 2:685.

Toothaker RD, Welling PG (1980): Annu Rev Pharmacol Toxicol 20:173.

Toskes PP, Deren JJ (1973): Gastroenterology 65:662.

Weinberger M, Hendeles L, Bighley L (1978): N Engl J Med 299:852.

Welling PG (1977): J Pharmacokinet Biopharm 5:291.

West RJ, Lloyd JK (1975): Gut 16:93.

Whitehead VM, Pratt R, Viallet A, Cooper BA (1972): Br J Haematol 22:63.

Wilkin JK, Wilken O, Kapp R, Donachie R, Chernosky ME, Buckner J (1982): Clin Pharmacol Ther 31:478.

Woolley DW (1982): Fed Proc 41:344.

Yeshurun D, Gono AM Jr (1976): Am J Med 60:370.

Index

G

H

U